SEVENTH EDITION

DAVIS'S

COMPREHENSIVE HANDBOOK OF Laboratory & Diagnostic Tests

*with **Nursing Implications***

SEVENTH EDITION

DAVIS'S

COMPREHENSIVE HANDBOOK OF

Laboratory & Diagnostic Tests

with Nursing Implications

Anne M. Van Leeuwen

Mickey Lynn Bladh

F.A. Davis Company • Philadelphia

Davis's Comprehensive Handbook of Laboratory and Diagnostic Tests with Nursing Implications

F. A. Davis Company
1915 Arch Street
Philadelphia
PA 19103

www.fadavis.com

Printed in the United States of America

Last digit indicates print number: 10 9 8 7 6 5 4 3 2 1

Publisher: Lisa B. Houck
Art and Design Manager: Carolyn O'Brien
Content Project Manager II: Julia Curcio
Digital Publishing Project Manager: Jacki Albertini

As new scientific information becomes available through basic and clinical research, recommended treatments and drug therapies undergo changes. The authors and publisher have done everything possible to make this book accurate, up to date, and in accord with accepted standards at the time of publication. The authors, editors, and publisher are not responsible for errors or omissions or for consequences from application of the book, and make no warranty, expressed or implied, in regard to the contents of the book. Any practice described in this book should be applied by the reader in accordance with professional standards of care used in regard to the unique circumstances that may apply in each situation. The reader is advised always to check product information (package inserts) for changes and new information regarding dose and contraindications before administering any drug. Caution is especially urged when using new or infrequently ordered drugs.

Library of Congress Cataloging-in-Publication Data

Names: Van Leeuwen, Anne M., author. | Bladh, Mickey Lynn, author.
Title: Davis's comprehensive handbook of laboratory & diagnostic tests with nursing implications / Anne M. Van Leeuwen, Mickey Lynn Bladh.
Other titles: Davis's comprehensive handbook of laboratory and diagnostic tests with nursing implications | Comprehensive handbook of laboratory & diagnostic tests with nursing implications | Comprehensive handbook of laboratory and diagnostic tests with nursing implications
Description: 7th edition. | Philadelphia, PA : F.A. Davis Company, [2017] | Includes index.
Identifiers: LCCN 2016042477 | ISBN 9780803659438 | ISBN 0803659431
Subjects: | MESH: Clinical Laboratory Techniques | Nursing Diagnosis–methods | Handbooks | Nurses' Instruction
Classification: LCC RB38.2 | NLM QY 39 | DDC 616.07/5–dc23 LC record available at https://lccn.loc.gov/2016042477

Dedication

Inspiration springs from Passion. . . . Passion is born from unconstrained love, commitment, and a vision no one else can own.

Lynda—my best friend and an extraordinarily gifted nurse—thank you, I could not have done this without your love, strong support, and belief in me. My gratitude to Mom, Dad, Adele, Gram . . . all my family and friends, for I am truly blessed by your humor and faith. A huge hug for my daughters, Sarah and Margaret—I love you very much. To my puppies, Maggie, Taylor, and Emma, for their endless and unconditional love. Many thanks to my friend and wonderful coauthor Mickey; to all the folks at F.A. Davis, especially Rob and Julia for their guidance, support, and great ideas. And, very special thanks to Lisa Houck, publisher, for her friendship, excellent direction, and unwavering encouragement.

Anne M. Van Leeuwen, MA, BS, MT (ASCP)
Medical Laboratory Scientist & Independent Author
Phoenix, Arizona

An eternity of searching would never have provided me with a man more loving and supportive than my husband, Eric. He is the sunshine in my soul, and I will be forever grateful for the blessing of his presence in my life. I am grateful to my five children, Eric, Anni, Phillip, Mari, and Melissa, for the privilege of being their mom; always remember that you are limited only by your imagination and willingness to try. To Anne, thanks so much for the opportunity to spread my wings, for your patience and guidance, and thanks to Lynda for the miracle of finding me. To all of those at F.A. Davis—Rob, Julia, and Lisa—you are the best. Lastly, to my beloved parents, thanks with hugs and kisses.

Mickey L. Bladh, RN, MSN
Coordinator, Nursing Education
PIH Health Hospital
Whittier, California

We are so grateful to all the people who have helped us make this book possible. We thank our readers for allowing us this important opportunity to touch their lives. We are also thankful for our association with the F.A. Davis Company. We value and appreciate the efforts of all the people associated with F.A. Davis because without their hard work this publication could not succeed. We recognize all the wonderful people in leadership, the editors, freelance consultants, designers, IT gurus, and digital applications developers, as well as those in sales & marketing, distribution, and finance. We have a deep appreciation for the Davis Educational Consultants. They are tasked with being our voice. Their exceptional ability to communicate is what actually

brings our book to the market. We would like to give special acknowledgment to the outstanding publishing professionals who were our core support team throughout the development of this edition:

Lisa Houck, *Publisher*
Robert Allen, *Content Applications Developer*
Julia Curcio, *Content Project Manager II*
Cynthia Naughton, *Production Manager, Digital Solutions*
Jacki Albertini, *Project Manager, Digital Solutions*
Carolyn O'Brien, *Art & Design Manager*
Jaclyn Lux, *Marketing Manager*
Sharon Lee, *Production Manager*

About This Book

This book is a reference for nurses, nursing students, and other health-care professionals. It is useful as a clinical tool as well as a supportive text to supplement clinical courses. It guides the nurse in planning what needs to be assessed, monitored, treated, and taught regarding pretest requirements, intratest procedures, and post-test care. It can be used by nursing students at all levels as a textbook in theory classes, integrating laboratory and diagnostic data as one aspect of nursing care; by practicing nurses to update information; and in clinical settings as a quick reference. Designed for use in academic and clinical settings, *Davis's Comprehensive Handbook of Laboratory and Diagnostic Tests—with Nursing Implications* provides a comprehensive reference that allows easy access to information about laboratory and diagnostic tests and procedures.

WHAT'S NEW IN THE 7TH EDITION?

Four new studies:

- Bioelectric Impedance Analysis
- Antibodies, Fungal
- Prion Disease Testing
- West Nile Virus Testing

New or updated information for more than 50 different tests including further discussion of:

- Genetic and genomic implications for health maintenance
- Molecular testing and companion diagnostics
- Pediatric and older adult considerations
- Specific contraindications and corresponding rationales
- Specific nursing problems, associated patient signs and symptoms, and potential nursing interactions
- Specific complications with corresponding rationales and potential interventions
- Patient education, including references to Web sites for information related to specific health conditions or disease management guidelines
- Expected patient outcomes expressed in terms of understanding, ability, and response. The expected patient outcomes are expressed in statements that reflect the patient's understanding of their medical situation and what it will take to achieve the most positive outcome possible; their demonstrated ability to apply instructions, explanations, and education toward a goal; and their response to various aspects of Safe and Effective Nursing Care used in their situation

Evidence-based practice is reflected throughout in:

- Suggestions for patient teaching that reflect changes in standards of care, particularly with respect to current guidelines for cancer screening
- The most current Centers for Disease Control and Prevention guidelines for communicable diseases such as syphilis, tuberculosis, and HIV

- The most current guidelines for the prevention of cardiovascular disease developed by the American College of Cardiology and the American Heart Association in conjunction with members of the National Heart, Lung, and Blood Institute's ATP IV Expert Panel

Critical Findings sections now include:

- A simple statement that reinforces the role of the nurse in providing timely notification and documentation of critical values
- Conventional and SI units
- Commonly reported adult, pediatric, and neonatal values

Some studies have been combined to consolidate similar tests, and the less frequently used tests have been condensed into a mini-study format that highlights abbreviated test-specific facts, with the full studies for those tests now resident on Fast Find at davispl.us/vanleeuwen7. The mini-study gives each test's full name, synonyms and acronyms, common use, specimen and tube type (laboratory tests) or area of application (diagnostic tests), normal ranges (laboratory tests), contraindications, potential diagnosis (normal and abnormal findings), and critical findings.

The *System Tables* now reside on the Davis*Plus* Web site (http://davispl.us/vanleeuwen7) and indicate the individual studies that contain information regarding genetic testing, so the information, also in the index, can be located quickly.

New: The Intersection of Nursing Care and Lab/Dx Testing

We hear every day from students and instructors that they want a laboratory and diagnostic test reference that will help them "connect-the-dots"—that will show them how to integrate laboratory and diagnostic test results into safe, compassionate, comprehensive, and effective nursing care. So we have revised the 7th edition of the Handbook not only to be the comprehensive reference it was originally designed to be but also to present carefully selected studies that have been enhanced to reflect aspects of Safe and Effective Nursing Care. The enhanced studies allow the reader to drill down further into the nursing implications. More than 92 studies have been expanded and examples include:

- Bilirubin
- Blood Gases
- Blood Groups and Antibodies
- Cerebrospinal Fluid Analysis
- Chlamydia Group Antibody
- Chloride, Sweat
- Complete Blood Count, Hemoglobin; Platelet Count; and WBC Count
- D-Dimer
- Glucose
- Glucose Tolerance Tests
- Newborn Screening
- Prostate-Specific Antigen
- Prothrombin Time and International Normalized Ratio
- Rheumatoid Factor
- Thyroid-Stimulating Hormone
- Tuberculosis Testing

WHAT'S NEW ONLINE?

Davis*Plus*

The following additional information is available at the Davis*Plus* Web site (http://davispl.us/vanleeuwen7):

- A searchable library of studies for all the studies included in the text. Instructors will have access to a searchable, digital version of the print edition. Students will have access to Fast Find: Lab & Dx.
- Eighty-four carefully selected diagnostic studies that have been enhanced to reflect aspects of Safe and Effective Nursing Care. The enhanced studies allow the reader to drill down further into the nursing implications.
- Case studies in both instructor and student versions formatted to help the novice learn how to clinically reason by using the nursing process to problem solve. Cases are purposefully designed to promote discussion of situations that may occur in the clinical setting. Situations may be medical, ethical, family related, patient related, nurse related, or any combination.
- Common potential nursing diagnoses associated with laboratory and diagnostic testing.
- Age-specific nursing care guidelines with suggested approaches to persons at various developmental stages to assist the provider in facilitating cooperation and understanding.
- Transfusion reactions, their signs and symptoms, associated laboratory findings, and potential nursing interventions.
- Introduction to CLIA (Clinical Laboratory Improvement Amendments) with an explanation of the different levels of testing complexity.
- Dietary supplements associated with adverse clinical reactions or drug interactions related to the affected body system.
- Interactive drag-and-drop, quiz-show, flash card, and multiple choice exercises.
- A printable file of critical findings for laboratory and diagnostic tests.
- Alphabetical listings of laboratory and diagnostic tests organized by related body systems. The tables have been revised to quickly identify individual tests in each table that contain information regarding genetic testing.

Instructor Guide and Student Guide

- Organized by nursing curriculum, presentations and case studies with emphasis on laboratory and diagnostic test-related information and nursing implications have been developed for selected conditions and body systems, including sensory, obstetric, and nutrition coverage.
- Open-ended and multiple-choice questions as well as suggested critical-thinking activities are provided.
- Updated with broadened age-related categories designed to enhance clinical communication, each case study includes at least one test that appears in the 7e Handbook as an enhanced study. Information in the enhanced study can be referenced in the Handbook for the material that contains detailed nursing problems, contraindications, complications, patient education, and expected patient outcomes for additional Safe and Effective Nursing Care teaching moments.
- A PowerPoint presentation of laboratory and diagnostic pretest, intratest, and post-test concepts integrated with nursing process is provded.

Alphabetical Order

The tests and procedures are presented in this book in alphabetical order by their complete name, allowing the user to locate information quickly without having to first place tests in a specific category or body system. Wherever possible, information within the Indications, Potential Diagnosis, and Interfering Factors (drug lists) sections also has been organized alphabetically.

Consistent Format

The following information is provided for each laboratory and diagnostic tests:

- Each study is titled by the *test name* and given in its commonly used designation.
- *Synonyms and Acronyms* for each test are listed where appropriate.
- The *Common Use* section includes a brief description of the purpose for the study.
- The *Specimen* section includes the type of specimen usually collected and, where appropriate, the type of collection tube or container commonly recommended. Specimen requirements vary by laboratory, and the testing laboratory should be consulted regarding required specimen volume.
- *Normal Findings* for each laboratory study include age-specific, gender-specific, and ethnicity-specific variations, when indicated. It is important to consider the normal variation of laboratory values over the life span and across cultures; sometimes what might be considered an abnormal value in one circumstance is actually the expected value in another. Normal findings for laboratory tests are given in conventional and standard international (SI) units. The factor used to convert conventional to SI units is also given. Because laboratory values can vary by method, each laboratory reference range is listed along with the associated methodology.
- The *Description* section includes the study's purpose and insight into how and why the test results can affect health. Some test descriptions also provide insight into how test results influence the development of national health guidelines.
- A separate *Contraindications* section has been created to differentiate circumstances that might put the patient at risk if the procedure is performed from interfering factors that may indirectly affect patient care by adversely affecting the results of the study.
- *Indications* are a list of what the test is used for in terms of assessment, evaluation, monitoring, screening, identifying, or assisting in the diagnosis of a clinical condition.
- The *Potential Medical Diagnosis* section presents a list of conditions in which laboratory values may be increased or decreased, in which the findings of diagnostic studies may be abnormal and, in some cases, an explanation of variations that may be encountered.
- *Critical Findings* that may be life threatening or for which particular concern may be indicated are given in conventional and SI units, along with age span considerations where applicable. This section also includes signs and symptoms associated with a critical value as well as possible nursing interventions and the nurse's role in communication of critical findings to the appropriate health-care provider.

- *Interfering Factors* are substances or circumstances that may influence the results of the test, rendering the results invalid or unreliable. Knowledge of interfering factors is an important aspect of quality assurance and includes pharmaceuticals, foods, natural and additive therapies, timing of test in relation to other tests or procedures, collection site, handling of specimen, and underlying patient conditions.
- The *Pretest* section addresses the need to:
  - Positively identify the patient using at least two person-specific identifiers before providing care, treatment, or services.
  - Provide an explanation to the patient, in the simplest terms possible, of the purpose of the study.
  - Obtain pertinent clinical, laboratory, dietary, and therapeutic history of the patient, especially as it pertains to comparison of previous test results, preparation for the test, and identification of potentially interfering factors.
  - Explain the requirements and restrictions related to the procedure as well as what to expect; provide the education necessary for the patient to be properly informed.
  - Anticipate and allay patient and family concerns or anxieties with consideration of social and cultural issues during interactions.
  - Provide for patient safety.

Some studies have an additional section for Potential Nursing Problems at the beginning of the *Pretest* section. The enhanced information presents problems the nurse might encounter relative to the study topic (e.g., glucose), signs and symptoms associated with abnormal study findings, and possible interventions. The additional information provides the reader with the opportunity to drill further down into the nursing implications. It is provided with the thought that incorporating laboratory and diagnostic data, on a day-to-day basis, by using the nursing process can be taught and reinforced using simple examples.

- The *Intratest* section can be used in a quality-control assessment or as a guide for the nurse who may be called on to participate in specimen collection or perform preparatory procedures. It provides:
  - Specific directions for specimen collection and test performance
  - Important information such as patient sensation and expected duration of the procedure
  - Precautions to be taken by the nurse and patient

Some studies have an additional section for study-specific complications and rationales in the *Intratest* section. The additional information is another opportunity to drill further down into the nursing implications. It is provided as a reminder to anticipate the potential for procedural complications and be prepared to identify them across the age continuum.

- The *Post-Test* section provides guidelines regarding:
  - Specific monitoring and therapeutic measures that should be performed after the procedure (e.g., maintaining bedrest, obtaining vital signs to compare with baseline values, signs and symptoms of complications)
  - Specific instructions for the patient and family, such as when to resume usual diet, medications, and activity
  - General nutritional guidelines related to excess or deficit as well as common food sources for dietary replacement

- Indications for interventions from public health representatives or for special counseling related to test outcomes
- Indications for follow-up testing that may be required within specific time frames
- An alphabetical listing of related laboratory and/or diagnostic tests that is intended to provoke a deeper and broader investigation of multiple pieces of information; the tests provide data that, when combined, can form a more complete picture of health or illness
- Reference to the specific body system tables of related laboratory and diagnostic tests that might bear on a patient's situation

Some studies have an additional section for specific patient education and expected patient outcomes in the post-test section. The additional information is another opportunity to drill further down into the nursing implications. It is provided as a reminder of the nurse's role as educator and advocate.

Color and Icons

Design is used to facilitate locating critical information at a glance. On the inside front and back covers is a full-color chart describing tube tops used for various blood tests.

Nursing Process

For each phase of the testing procedure, we describe the nurse's roles and responsibilities as defined by the nursing process.

Index

Completely updated to reflect the addition of new tests, conditions, and other key words.

Assumptions

- The authors recognize that preferences for the use of specific medical terminology may vary by institution. Much of the terminology used in this Handbook is sourced from *Taber's Cyclopedic Medical Dictionary.*
- The definition, implementation, and interpretation of national guidelines for the treatment of various medical conditions changes as new information and new technology emerge. The publication of updated information may at times be contentious among the professional institutions that offer either support or dissent for the proposed changes. This can cause confusion when a patient asks questions about how his or her condition will be identified and managed. The authors believe that the most important discussion about health care occurs between the patient and his or her health-care provider(s). Although the individual studies may point out various screening tests used to identify a disease, the authors often refer the reader to Web sites maintained by nationally recognized authorities on specific topics that reflect the most current information and recommendations for screening, diagnosis, and treatment.
- Most institutions have established policies, protocols, and interdisciplinary teams that provide for efficient and effective patient care within the appropriate scope of practice. It is not our intention that the actual duties a nurse may

perform be misunderstood by way of misinterpreted inferences in writing style, but the information prepared by the authors considers that specific limitations are understood by the licensed professionals and other team members involved in patient care activities and that the desired outcomes are achieved by order of the appropriate health-care provider.

DavisPlus
DavisPlus.fadavis.com

Preface

Laboratory and diagnostic testing. The words themselves often conjure up cold and impersonal images of needles, specimens lined up in collection containers, and high-tech electronic equipment. But they do not stand alone. They are tied to, bound with, and tell of health or disease in the blood and tissue of a person. Laboratory and diagnostic studies augment the health-care provider's assessment of the quality of an individual's physical being. Test results guide the plans and interventions geared toward strengthening life's quality and endurance. Beyond the pounding noise of the MRI, the cold steel of the x-ray table, the sting of the needle, the invasive collection of fluids and tissue, and the probing and inspection is the gathering of evidence that supports the health-care provider's ability to discern the course of a disease and the progression of its treatment. Laboratory and diagnostic data must be viewed with thought and compassion, however, as well as with microscopes and machines. We must remember that behind the specimen and test result is the person from whom it came, a person who is someone's son, daughter, mother, father, husband, wife, or friend.

This book is written to help health-care providers in their understanding and interpretation of laboratory and diagnostic procedures and their outcomes. Just as important, it is dedicated to all health-care professionals who experience the wonders in the science of laboratory and diagnostic testing, performed and interpreted in a caring and efficient manner.

The authors have continued to enhance four areas in this new edition: pathophysiology that affects test results, patient safety, patient education, and integration of related laboratory and diagnostic testing.

First, the Potential Diagnosis section includes an explanation of increased or decreased values, as many of you requested. We have added age-specific reference values for the neonatal, pediatric, and older adult populations at the request of some of our readers. It should be mentioned that standardized information for the complexity of an older adult population is difficult to document. Values may be increased or decreased in older adults due to the sole or combined effects of malnutrition, alcohol use, medications, and the presence of multiple chronic or acute diseases with or without muted symptoms.

Second, the authors appreciate that nurses are the strongest patient advocates with a huge responsibility to protect the safety of their patients, and we have observed student nurses in clinical settings being interviewed by facility accreditation inspectors, so we have updated safety reminders, particularly with respect to positive patient identification, communication of critical information, proper timing of diagnostic procedures, rescheduling of specimen collection for therapeutic drug monitoring, use of evidence-based practices for prevention of surgical site infections, information regarding the move to track or limit exposure to radiation from CT studies for adults, and the Image Gently campaign for pediatric patients who undergo diagnostic studies that utilize radiation. The pretest section reminds the nurse to positively identify the patient before providing care, treatment, or services. The pretest section also addresses hand-off communication of critical information.

The third area of emphasis coaches the student to focus on patient education and prepares the nurse to anticipate and respond to a patient's questions or concerns: describing the purpose of the procedure, addressing concerns about pain, understanding the implications of the test results, and describing postprocedural care. Various related Web sites for patient education are included throughout the book.

And fourth, laboratory and diagnostic tests do not stand on their own—all the pieces fit together to form a picture. The section at the end of each monograph integrates both laboratory and diagnostic tests, providing a more complete picture of the studies that may be encountered in a patient's health-care experience. The authors thought it useful for a nurse to know what other tests might be ordered together—and all the related tests are listed alphabetically for ease of use.

Laboratory and diagnostic studies are essential components of a complete patient assessment. Examined in conjunction with an individual's history and physical examination, laboratory studies and diagnostic data provide clues about health status. Nurses are increasingly expected to integrate an understanding of laboratory and diagnostic procedures and expected outcomes in assessment, planning, implementation, and evaluation of nursing care. The data help develop and support nursing diagnoses, interventions, and outcomes.

Nurses may interface with laboratory and diagnostic testing on several levels, including:

- Interacting with patients and families of patients undergoing diagnostic tests or procedures, and providing pretest, intratest, and post-test information and support
- Maintaining quality control to prevent or eliminate problems that may interfere with the accuracy and reliability of test results
- Providing education and emotional support at the point of care
- Ensuring completion of testing in a timely and accurate manner
- Collaborating with other health-care professionals in interpreting findings as they relate to planning and implementing total patient care
- Communicating significant alterations in test outcomes to appropriate health-care team members
- Coordinating interdisciplinary efforts

Whether the nurse's role at each level is direct or indirect, the underlying responsibility to the patient, family, and community remains the same.

The authors hope that the changes and additions made to the book and its Web-based ancillaries will reward users with an expanded understanding of and appreciation for the place laboratory and diagnostic testing holds in the provision of high-quality nursing care and will make it easy for instructors to integrate this important content in their curricula. The authors would like to thank all the users of the previous editions for helping us identify what they like about this book as well as what might improve its value to them. We want to continue this dialogue. As writers, it is our desire to capture the interest of our readers, to provide essential information, and to continue to improve the presentation of the material in the book and ancillary products. We encourage our readers to provide feedback to the Web site and to the publisher's sales professionals. Your feedback helps us modify the material—to change with your changing needs.

Reviewers

Nell Britton, MSN, RN, CNE
Nursing Faculty
Trident Technical College Nursing Division
Charleston, South Carolina

Cheryl Cassis, MSN, RN
Professor of Nursing
Belmont Technical College
St. Clairsville, Ohio

Pamela Ellis, RN, MSHCA, MSN
Nursing Faculty
Mohave Community College
Bullhead City, Arizona

Stephanie Franks, MSN, RN
Professor of Nursing
St. Louis Community College–Meramec
St. Louis, Missouri

Linda Lott, MSN
AD Nursing Instructor
Itawamba Community College
Fulton, Mississippi

Martha Olson, RN, BSN, MS
Nursing Associate Professor
Iowa Lakes Community College
Emmetsburg, Iowa

Barbara Thompson, RN, BScN, MScN
Professor of Nursing
Sault College
Sault Ste. Marie, Ontario

Edward C. Walton, MS, APN-C, NP-C
Assistant Professor of Nursing
Richard Stockton College of New Jersey
Galloway, New Jersey

Jean Ann Wilson, RN, BSN
Coordinator Norton Annex
Colby Community College
Norton, Kansas

Contents

AVAILABLE ON http://davispl.us/vanleeuwen7:

Acetylcholine Receptor Antibody

SYNONYM/ACRONYM: AChR (AChR-binding antibody, AChR-blocking antibody, and AChR-modulating antibody).

COMMON USE: To assist in confirming the diagnosis of myasthenia gravis (MG).

SPECIMEN: Serum collected in a red-top tube.

NORMAL FINDINGS: (Method: Radioimmunoassay) AChR-binding antibody: Less than 0.4 nmol/L; AChR-blocking antibody: Less than 25% blocking; and AChR-modulating antibody: Less than 30% modulating.

DESCRIPTION: Normally, when impulses travel down a nerve, the nerve ending releases a neurotransmitter called acetylcholine (ACh), which binds to receptor sites in the neuromuscular junction, eventually resulting in muscle contraction. Once the neuromuscular junction is polarized, ACh is rapidly metabolized by the enzyme acetylcholinesterase. When present, AChR-binding antibodies can activate complement and create a complex of ACh, AChR-binding antibodies, and complement. This complex renders ACh unavailable for muscle receptor sites. If AChR-binding antibodies are not detected, and myasthenia gravis (MG) is strongly suspected, AChR-blocking and AChR-modulating antibodies may be ordered. AChR-blocking antibodies impair or prevent ACh from attaching to receptor sites on the muscle membrane, resulting in poor muscle contraction. AChR-modulating antibodies destroy AChR sites, interfering with neuromuscular transmission. The lack of ACh bound to muscle receptor sites results in muscle weakness. Antibodies to AChR sites are present in 90% of patients with generalized MG and in 55% to 70% of patients who either have ocular forms of MG or are in remission. Approximately 10% to 15% of people with confirmed MG do not demonstrate detectable levels of AChR-binding, AChR-blocking, or AChR-modulating antibodies. MG is an acquired autoimmune disorder that can occur at any age. Its exact cause is unknown, and it seems to strike women between ages 20 and 40 yr; men appear to be affected later in life than women. It can affect any voluntary muscle, but muscles that control eye and eyelid movement, facial movement, and swallowing are most frequently affected. Antibodies may not be detected in the first 6 to 12 mo after the first appearance of symptoms. MG is a common complication associated with thymoma. The relationship between the thymus gland and MG is not completely understood. It is believed that miscommunication in the thymus gland directed at developing immune cells may trigger the development of autoantibodies responsible for MG. Remission after thymectomy is associated with a progressive decrease in antibody level. Other markers used in the study of MG include striational muscle antibodies, thyroglobulin, HLA-B8, and HLA-DR3. These antibodies are often undetectable in the early stages of MG.

This procedure is contraindicated for

A

Appropriate timing when scheduling multiple studies should be taken into consideration. Recent radioactive scans or radiation within 1 wk of the test can invalidate test results when radioimmunoassay is the test method.

INDICATIONS

- Confirm the presence but not the severity of MG.
- Detect subclinical MG in the presence of thymoma.
- Monitor the effectiveness of immunosuppressive therapy for MG.
- Monitor the remission stage of MG.

POTENTIAL MEDICAL DIAGNOSIS

Increased in:

- Autoimmune liver disease
- Generalized MG ***(Defective transmission of nerve impulses to muscles evidenced by muscle weakness. It occurs when normal communication between the nerve and muscle is interrupted at the neuromuscular junction. It is believed that miscommunication in the thymus gland directed at developing immune cells may trigger the development of autoantibodies responsible for MG.)***
- Lambert-Eaton myasthenic syndrome
- Primary lung cancer
- Thymoma associated with MG ***(Defective transmission of nerve impulses to muscles evidenced by muscle weakness. It occurs when normal communication between the nerve and muscle is interrupted at the neuromuscular junction. It is believed that miscommunication in the thymus gland directed at developing immune cells may trigger the development of autoantibodies responsible for MG.)***

Decreased in:

- Postthymectomy ***(The thymus gland produces the T lymphocytes responsible for cell-mediated immunity. T cells also help control B-cell development for the production of antibodies. T-cell response is directed at cells in the body that have been infected by bacteria, viruses, parasites, fungi, or protozoans. T cells also provide immune surveillance for cancerous cells. Removal of the thymus gland is strongly associated with a decrease in AChR antibody levels.)***

CRITICAL FINDINGS: N/A

INTERFERING FACTORS

- Drugs and other substances that may increase AChR levels include penicillamine (long-term use may cause a reversible syndrome that produces clinical, serological, and electrophysiological findings indistinguishable from MG).
- Biological false-positive results may be associated with amyotrophic lateral sclerosis, autoimmune hepatitis, Lambert-Eaton myasthenic syndrome, primary biliary cirrhosis, and encephalomyeloneuropathies associated with carcinoma of the lung.
- Immunosuppressive therapy is the recommended treatment for MG; prior immunosuppressive drug administration may result in negative test results.
- Recent radioactive scans or radiation within 1 wk of the test can interfere with test results when radioimmunoassay is the test method.

NURSING IMPLICATIONS AND PROCEDURE

POTENTIAL NURSING PROBLEMS:

Problem	Signs & Symptoms	Interventions
Urination ***(related to neurogenic bladder; spastic bladder; associated with disease process)***	Urinary retention; urinary frequency; urinary urgency; pain and abdominal distention; urinary dribbling	Assess amount of fluid intake, as it may be necessary to limit fluids to control incontinence; assess risk of urinary tract infection with limiting oral intake; begin bladder training program; teach catheterization techniques to family and patient self-catheterization
Self-care ***(related to spasticity; altered level of consciousness; paresis; increasing weakness; paralysis)***	Difficulty fastening clothing; difficulty performing personal hygiene; inability to maintain appropriate appearance; difficulty with independent mobility; declining physical function	Reinforce self-care techniques as taught by occupational therapy; ensure the patient has adequate time to perform self-care; encourage use of assistive devices to maintain independence; assess ability to perform ADLs; provide care assistance appropriate to degree of disability while maintaining as much independence as possible
Mobility ***(related to weakness; tremors; spasticity)***	Unsteady gait; lack of coordination; difficult purposeful movement; inadequate range of motion	Assess gait; assess muscle strength; assess weakness and coordination; assess physical endurance and level of fatigue; assess ability to perform independent ADLs; assess ability for safe, independent movement; identify need for assistive device; encourage safe self-care
Pain ***(related to motor and sensory nerve damage associated with disease process)***	Self-report of pain; emotional symptoms of distress; crying; agitation; facial grimace; moaning; verbalization of pain; rocking motions; irritability; disturbed sleep; diaphoresis; altered blood pressure and heart rate; nausea; vomiting	Keep the immediate environment cool to decrease aggravating MG symptoms; use passive or active range of motion to decrease muscle tightness; administer analgesics, tranquilizers, antispasmodics, and neuropathic pain medication, as ordered

A

PRETEST:

- Positively identify the patient using at least two person-specific identifiers before services, treatments, or procedures are performed.
- ***Patient teaching:*** Inform the patient that the test is used to identify antibodies responsible for decreased neuromuscular transmission and associated muscle weakness.
- Obtain a history of the patient's health concerns, symptoms, surgical procedures, and results of previously performed laboratory and diagnostic studies. Include a list of known allergens, especially allergies or sensitivities to latex, and any prior complications with general anesthesia.
- Note any recent procedures that can interfere with test results.
- Obtain a list of the patient's current medications, including over-the-counter medications and dietary supplements (see Effects of Natural Products on Laboratory Values online at Davis*Plus*).
- Review the procedure with the patient. Inform the patient that specimen collection takes approximately 5 to 10 min. Address concerns about pain, and explain that there may be some discomfort during the venipuncture.
- ***Sensitivity to social and cultural issues,*** as well as concern for modesty, is important in providing psychological support before, during, and after the procedure.
- Note that there are no food, fluid, or medication restrictions unless by medical direction.

INTRATEST:

Potential Complications: N/A

- Avoid the use of equipment containing latex if the patient has a history of allergic reaction to latex.
- Instruct the patient to cooperate fully and to follow directions. Direct the patient to breathe normally and to avoid unnecessary movement.
- Observe standard precautions, and follow the general guidelines in Patient Preparation and Specimen Collection online at Davis*Plus*. Positively identify the patient, and label the appropriate specimen container with the corresponding patient demographics, initials of the person collecting the specimen, date, and time of collection. Perform a venipuncture.
- Remove the needle and apply direct pressure with dry gauze to stop bleeding. Observe/assess venipuncture site for bleeding or hematoma formation and secure gauze with adhesive bandage.
- Promptly transport the specimen to the laboratory for processing and analysis.

POST-TEST:

- Inform the patient that a report of the results will be made available to the requesting health-care provider (HCP),who will discuss the results with the patient.
- Recognize anxiety related to test results, and be supportive of activity challenges related to lack of neuromuscular control, anticipated loss of independence, and fear of death. It is important to note that a diagnosis of MG should be based on abnormal findings from two different diagnostic tests. These tests include AChR antibody assay, anti-MuSK antibody assay (an antibody that is produced in 40% to 70% of the remaining 15% who have MG but test negative for AChR antibody), edrophonium test (which involves injection of edrophonium or Tensilon, a medication that temporarily blocks the degradation of acetylcholine, allowing normal measurable neuromuscular transmission that dissipates as the effects of the injection wear off), repetitive nerve stimulation (small pulses of electricity are repeatedly sent to specific muscles by way of electrodes to measure a decrease in response due to muscle weakening), and single-fiber electromyography (see EMG study for more detailed information). Discuss the implications of positive test results on the patient's lifestyle. Positive test results may lead to testing for other conditions associated with MG.

  Thyrotoxicosis may occur in conjunction with MG; related thyroid testing may be indicated. MG patients may also produce antibodies, such as antinuclear antibody and rheumatoid

factor, not primarily associated with MG that demonstrate measurable reactivity.
- Evaluate test results in relation to future general anesthesia, especially regarding therapeutic management of MG with cholinesterase inhibitors. Succinylcholine-sensitive patients may be unable to metabolize the anesthetic quickly, resulting in prolonged or unrecoverable apnea.
- Provide contact information, if desired, for the Myasthenia Gravis Foundation of America (www.myasthenia.org) and the Muscular Dystrophy Association (www.mdausa.org) 🍁.
- Depending on the results of this procedure, additional testing may be performed to evaluate or monitor progression of the disease process and determine the need for a change in therapy. If a diagnosis of MG is made, a computed tomography (CT) scan of the chest should be performed to rule out thymoma. Evaluate test results in relation to the patient's symptoms and other tests performed.

Patient Education:
- Discuss the implications of positive test results on the patient's lifestyle.
- Provide teaching and information regarding the clinical implications of the test results, as appropriate.
- Educate the patient and family regarding access to counseling services.
- Reinforce information given by the patient's HCP regarding further testing, treatment, or referral to another HCP.
- Answer any questions or address any concerns voiced by the patient or family.
- Teach family to place self-care items within the patients reach to promote as much independence in care as possible.
- Teach the family and patient that assistive devices can improve quality of life and decrease injury risk.

Expected Patient Outcomes:

Understanding
- The patient and family verbalize that spasms can be decreased by adhering to recommended physical therapy.
- The patient and family describe the necessity to promote independent self-care while seeking assistance as necessary to prevent injury.

Ability
- The patient and family demonstrate the ability to perform passive and active range of motion activities.
- The patient and family demonstrate how to apply splints to hands to help control hand spasms.

Response
- The patient and family set personal goals regarding performance of self-care activities that are in realistic proportion to disease progression.
- The patient and family accept the physical limitations related to the disease process.

RELATED STUDIES:
- Related tests include ANA, antithyroglobulin and antithyroid peroxidase antibodies, CT chest, EMG, myoglobin, pseudocholinesterase, RF, TSH, and total T_4.
- Refer to the Musculoskeletal System table online at Davis*Plus* for related tests by body system.

Adrenal Gland Scan

SYNONYM/ACRONYM: Adrenal scintiscan, adrenal scintigraphy, metaiodobenzylguanidine or MIBG scan.

COMMON USE: To assist in the diagnosis of Cushing's syndrome, Conn's syndrome, and adrenal gland tumors (adrenocortical cancer, adenomas, neuroblastomas, and pheochromocytomas).

AREA OF APPLICATION: Adrenal gland.

A

DESCRIPTION: This nuclear medicine study evaluates the function of the adrenal glands. A single adrenal gland is located above each kidney and consists of two parts. The outer cortex is where the adrenal hormones, including cortisol and aldosterone, are produced. The cortex is where the majority of adrenal tumors are identified, most of which are benign. The inner part of the adrenal gland is called the *medulla* and is where the neurohormones epinephrine and norepinephrine are produced. Tumors in the medulla are relatively rare and include neuroblastomas and pheochromocytomas. Most cancers found in the adrenal glands have metastasized from other areas in the body. The secretory function of the adrenal glands is controlled primarily by the anterior pituitary, which produces adrenocorticotropic hormone (ACTH). Adrenal imaging is most useful for adults and children in differentiating hyperplasia from adenoma in primary aldosteronism. Adrenal imaging can be used in combination with other diagnostic tools, such as biopsy, x-ray, CT, MRI, PET, and US. There are a number of radionuclides that may be used in scintiscans such as the MIBG (metaiodobenzylguanidine) scan, I-131 NP-59 (iodomethyl-19-norcholesterol) scan, and octreotide (111-In-labelled pentetreotide) scan. The radionuclides are synthetic analogs of naturally occurring substances in the body known to selectively bind to receptor sites on the tumor cells, visualizing areas of concern. MIBG is an analog of norepinephrine, NP-59 is a cholesterol analog, and octreotide is an analog of somatostatin. The uptake of the radionuclide occurs gradually over time, and imaging is performed within 24 to 48 hours of radionuclide injection and continued daily for 3 to 5 days. The imaging equipment can be a simple gamma camera that produces two-dimensional images; single-photon emission computed tomography (SPECT) imaging taken by a gamma camera that rotates around the body to produce a three-dimensional image; or a combination of technologies such as SPECT-CT, which combines three-dimensional images taken with standard CT imaging equipment followed by imaging provided by a rotating SPECT camera system. Imaging can reveal increased uptake, unilateral or bilateral uptake, or absence of uptake in the detection of pathological processes. Following prescanning treatment with corticosteroids, suppression studies can also be done to differentiate the presence of tumor from hyperplasia of the glands. MBIG is also used therapeutically, at higher doses, to treat adrenal cancer.

This procedure is contraindicated for

- Patients who are pregnant or suspected of being pregnant, unless the potential benefits of a procedure using radiation far outweigh the risk of radiation exposure to the fetus and mother.
- Conditions associated with adverse reactions to contrast medium (e.g., asthma, food allergies, or allergy to contrast medium).

Although patients are asked specifically if they have a known allergy to iodine or shellfish, it has been well established that the reaction is not to iodine; in fact, an actual iodine allergy would be problematic because iodine is required for the production of thyroid hormones. In the case of shellfish, the reaction is to a muscle protein called tropomyosin; in the case of iodinated contrast medium, the reaction is to the noniodinated part of the contrast molecule. Patients with a known hypersensitivity to the medium may benefit from premedication with corticosteroids and diphenhydramine; the use of nonionic contrast or an alternative noncontrast imaging study, if available, may be considered for patients who have severe asthma or who have experienced moderate to severe reactions to ionic contrast medium.

INDICATIONS

- Aid in the diagnosis of Cushing's syndrome and aldosteronism.
- Aid in the diagnosis of gland tissue destruction caused by infection, infarction, neoplasm, or suppression.
- Aid in locating adrenergic tumors.
- Determine adrenal suppressibility with prescan administration of corticosteroid to diagnose and localize adrenal adenoma, aldosteronomas, androgen excess, and low-renin hypertension.
- Differentiate between asymmetric hyperplasia and asymmetry from aldosteronism with dexamethasone suppression test.

POTENTIAL MEDICAL DIAGNOSIS

Normal findings

- No evidence of tumors, infection, infarction, or suppression
- Normal bilateral uptake of radionuclide and secretory function of adrenal cortex
- Normal salivary glands and urinary bladder; vague shape of the liver and spleen sometimes seen

Abnormal findings related to

The radioactive tracer will accumulate in abnormal tissue, and "hot spots" will identify specific areas of concern.

- Adrenal gland suppression
- Adrenal infarction
- Adrenal tumor
- Hyperplasia
- Infection
- Pheochromocytoma

CRITICAL FINDINGS: N/A

INTERFERING FACTORS

Factors that may alter the results of the study

- Retained barium from a previous radiological procedure.
- Inability of the patient to cooperate or remain still during the procedure because of age, significant pain, or mental status.

Other considerations

- Improper injection of the radionuclide may allow the tracer to seep deep into the muscle tissue, producing erroneous hot spots.

NURSING IMPLICATIONS AND PROCEDURE

See Potential Nursing Problems on Fast Find at davispl.us/vanleeuwen7.

PRETEST:

- Positively identify the patient using at least two person-specific identifiers before services, treatments, or procedures are performed.
- ***Patient teaching:*** Inform the patient this procedure can visualize and assess the function of the adrenal gland, which is located near the kidney.
- Obtain a history of the patient's health concerns, symptoms, surgical procedures, and results of previously performed laboratory and diagnostic studies. Include a list of known allergens, especially allergies or sensitivities to latex, anesthetics, contrast medium, or sedatives.

A

- Perform all adrenal blood studies before doing this test.
- Record the date of last menstrual period and determine the possibility of pregnancy in perimenopausal women.
- Obtain a list of the patient's current medications, including over-the-counter medications and dietary supplements (see Effects of Natural Products on Laboratory Values online at Davis*Plus*).
- If iodinated contrast medium is scheduled to be used in patients receiving metformin for type 2 diabetes, the drug should be discontinued on the day of the test and continue to be withheld for 48 hours after the test. Iodinated contrast can temporarily impair kidney function, and failure to withhold metformin may indirectly result in drug-induced lactic acidosis, a dangerous and sometimes fatal adverse effect of metformin ***(related to renal impairment that does not support sufficient excretion of metformin).***
- Review the procedure with the patient. Address concerns about pain and explain that there may be moments of discomfort and some pain experienced during the test. Inform the patient that the procedure is usually performed in a nuclear medicine department by a nuclear medicine technologist with support staff, and it takes approximately 1 to 2 hr each day. Inform the patient the test usually involves a prolonged scanning schedule over a period of days.
- Administer saturated solution of potassium iodide (SSKI or Lugol iodine solution) 24 hr before the study to prevent thyroid uptake of the free radioactive iodine; the solution is usually added to another liquid (e.g., orange juice) and administered orally.
- ***Sensitivity to social and cultural issues,*** as well as concern for modesty, is important in providing psychological support before, during, and after the procedure.
- Explain that an intravenous (IV) line may be inserted to allow infusion of fluids such as saline, anesthetics, sedatives, contrast medium, or emergency medications.
- Note that there are no food, fluid, or medication restrictions unless by medical direction.
- Instruct the patient to remove jewelry and other metallic objects from the area to be examined.
- *Make sure a written and informed consent has been signed prior to the procedure and before administering any medications.*

INTRATEST:

Potential Complications:

Injection of the contrast is an invasive procedure. Complications are rare but do include risk for: allergic reaction ***(related to contrast reaction),*** hematoma ***(related to blood leakage into the tissue following needle insertion),*** bleeding from the puncture site ***(related to a bleeding disorder or the effects of natural products and medications with known anticoagulant, antiplatelet, or thrombolytic properties),*** or infection ***(which might occur if bacteria from the skin surface is introduced at the puncture site).***

- Avoid the use of equipment containing latex if the patient has a history of allergic reaction to latex.
- Observe standard precautions, and follow the general guidelines in Patient Preparation and Specimen Collection online at Davis*Plus*. Positively identify the patient.
- Ensure that the patient has removed external metallic objects from the area to be examined prior to the procedure.
- Have emergency equipment readily available.
- Instruct the patient to void prior to the procedure and to change into the gown, robe, and foot coverings provided.
- Insert an IV line, and inject the radionuclide IV on day 1; images are taken on days 1, 2, and 3. Each image takes 20 min, and total imaging time is 1 to 2 hr per day.

- Instruct the patient to cooperate fully and to follow directions. Instruct the patient to remain still throughout the procedure because movement produces unreliable results.

POST-TEST:

- Inform the patient that a report of the results will be made available to the requesting health-care provider (HCP), who will discuss the results with the patient.
- Advise the patient to drink increased amounts of fluids for 24 to 48 hr to eliminate the radionuclide from the body, unless contraindicated. Inform the patient that radionuclide is eliminated from the body within 24 to 48 hr.
- Do not schedule other radionuclide tests 24 to 48 hr after this procedure.
- Observe/assess the needle site for bleeding, hematoma formation, and inflammation.
- Instruct the patient in the care and assessment of the injection site.
- Instruct the patient to apply cold compresses to the puncture site as needed to reduce discomfort or edema.
- If a woman who is breast-feeding must have a nuclear scan, she should not breast-feed the infant until the radionuclide has been eliminated. This could take as long as 3 days. Instruct her to express the milk and discard it during the 3-day period to prevent cessation of milk production.
- Instruct the patient to immediately flush the toilet and to meticulously wash hands with soap and water after each voiding for 48 hr after the procedure.
- Instruct all caregivers to wear gloves when discarding urine for 48 hr after the procedure. Wash gloved hands with soap and water before removing gloves; then wash ungloved hands.
- Recognize anxiety related to test results. Discuss the implications of abnormal test results on the patient's lifestyle. Provide teaching and information regarding the clinical implications of the test results, as appropriate.
- Reinforce information given by the patient's HCP regarding further testing, treatment, or referral to another HCP. Advise the patient that SSKI (120 mg/day) will be administered for 14 days after the injection of the radionuclide. The iodine solution continues to block uptake of the radioactive iodine by the thyroid gland while the radionuclide is being excreted from the body. Answer any questions or address any concerns voiced by the patient or family. Provide contact information, if desired, for the American Cancer Society (www.cancer.org) 🍁.
- Depending on the results of this procedure, additional testing may be needed to evaluate or monitor progression of the disease process and determine the need for a change in therapy. Evaluate test results in relation to the patient's symptoms and other tests performed.

Patient Education:

- Provide information on the relationship between altered cortisol levels and adrenal disease.
- Ensure the patient understands the injury risks associated with altered cortisol level and adrenal gland disease.

Expected Patient Outcomes:

Understanding

- The patient and family identify foods that are high in calcium and vitamin D.
- The patient and family state the importance of preventing constipation to decrease risk of gastrointestinal bleeding from injury.

Ability

- The patient and family proactively incorporate foods rich in calcium and vitamin D into the diet.
- The patient and family demonstrate how to apply direct pressure to an injury that may be bleeding.

A

Response

- The patient and family continue to participate in social activities.
- The patient and family agree to weigh patient daily and record for HCP review.

RELATED STUDIES:

- Related tests include ACTH and challenge tests, aldosterone, angiography adrenal, catecholamines, CT abdomen, cortisol and challenge tests, HVA, MRI abdomen, metanephrines, potassium, renin, sodium, and VMA.
- Refer to the Endocrine System table online at Davis*Plus* for related tests by body system.

Adrenocorticotropic Hormone (and Challenge Tests)

SYNONYM/ACRONYM: Corticotropin, ACTH.

COMMON USE: To assist in the investigation of adrenocortical dysfunction using ACTH and cortisol levels in diagnosing disorders such as Addison's disease, Cushing's disease, and Cushing's syndrome.

SPECIMEN: Plasma from a lavender-top (EDTA) tube for adrenocorticotropic hormone (ACTH) and serum from a red-top tube for cortisol and 11-deoxycortisol. Collect specimens in a prechilled heparinized plastic syringe, and carefully transfer into collection containers by gentle injection to avoid hemolysis. Alternatively, specimens can be collected in prechilled lavender- and red-top tubes. Gold-tiger- and green-top (heparin) tubes are also acceptable for cortisol, but take care to use the same type of collection container for serial measurements. Immediately transport specimen, tightly capped and in an ice slurry, to the laboratory. The specimens should be immediately processed. Plasma for ACTH analysis should be transferred to a plastic container.

Procedure	Indications	Medication Administered, Adult Dosage	Recommended Collection Times
ACTH stimulation, rapid test	Suspect adrenal insufficiency (Addison's disease) or congenital adrenal hyperplasia	1 mcg (low-dose physiologic protocol) cosyntropin intramuscular (IM) or IV; 250 mcg (standard pharmacologic protocol) cosyntropin IM or intravenous (IV)	Three cortisol levels: baseline immediately before bolus, 30 min after bolus, and 60 min (optional) after bolus. Baseline and 30-min levels are adequate for accurate diagnosis using either dosage; low-dose protocol sensitivity is most accurate for 30-min level only
Corticotropin-releasing hormone (CRH) stimulation	Differential diagnosis between ACTH-dependent conditions such as Cushing's disease (pituitary source) or Cushing's syndrome (ectopic source) and ACTH-independent conditions such as Cushing's syndrome (adrenal source)	IV dose of 1 mcg/kg human CRH	Eight cortisol and eight ACTH levels: baseline collected 15 min before injection, 0 min before injection, and then 5, 15, 30, 60, 120, and 180 min after injection
Dexamethasone suppression (overnight)	Differential diagnosis between ACTH-dependent conditions such as Cushing's disease (pituitary source) or Cushing's syndrome (ectopic source) and ACTH-independent conditions such as Cushing's syndrome (adrenal source)	Oral dose of 1 mg dexamethasone (Decadron) at 2300.	Collect cortisol at 0800 on the morning after the dexamethasone dose
Metyrapone stimulation (overnight)	Suspect hypothalamic/pituitary disease such as adrenal insufficiency, ACTH-dependent conditions such as Cushing's disease (pituitary source) or Cushing's syndrome (ectopic source), and ACTH-independent conditions such as Cushing's syndrome (adrenal source)	Oral dose of 30 mg/kg metyrapone with snack at 2400	Collect cortisol, 11-deoxycortisol, and ACTH at 0800 on the morning after the metyrapone dose

NORMAL FINDINGS: (Method: Immunochemiluminescent assay for ACTH and cortisol; HPLC/MS-MS for 11-deoxycortisol)

A

ACTH

Age	Conventional Units	SI Units (Conventional Units × 0.22)
Cord blood	50–570 pg/mL	11–125 pmol/L
Newborn	10–185 pg/mL	2–41 pmol/L
1 wk–9 yr	5–46 pg/mL	1.1–10.1 pmol/L
10–18 yr	6–55 pg/mL	1.3–12.1 pmol/L
19 yr–Adult		
Male supine (specimen collected in morning)	7–69 pg/mL	1.5–15.2 pmol/L
Female supine (specimen collected in morning)	6–58 pg/mL	1.3–12.8 pmol/L

Values may be unchanged or slightly elevated in healthy older adults. Long-term use of corticosteroids, to treat arthritis and autoimmune diseases, may suppress secretion of ACTH.

ACTH Challenge Tests

ACTH (Cosyntropin) Stimulated, Rapid Test	Conventional Units	SI Units (Conventional Units × 27.6)
Baseline	Cortisol greater than 5 mcg/dL	Greater than 138 nmol/L
30- or 60-min response	Cortisol 18–20 mcg/dL or incremental increase of 7 mcg/dL over baseline value	497–552 nmol/L or incremental increase of 193.2 nmol/L over baseline value

Corticotropin-Releasing Hormone Stimulated	Conventional Units	SI Units (Conventional Units × 27.6)
	Cortisol peaks at greater than 20 mcg/dL within 30–60 min	Greater than 552 nmol/L
		SI Units (Conventional Units × 0.22)
	ACTH increases twofold to fourfold within 30–60 min	Twofold to fourfold increase within 30–60 min

Dexamethasone Suppressed Overnight Test	Conventional Units	SI Units (Conventional Units × 27.6)
	Cortisol less than 1.8 mcg/dL next day	Less than 49.7 nmol/L

Metyrapone Stimulated Overnight Test	Conventional Units	SI Units (Conventional Units × 27.6)
	Cortisol less than 3 mcg/dL next day	Less than 83 nmol/L
		SI Units (Conventional Units × 0.22)
	ACTH greater than 75 pg/mL	Greater than 16.5 pmol/L
		SI Units (Conventional Units × 28.9)
	11-deoxycortisol greater than 7 mcg/dL	Greater than 202 nmol/L

DESCRIPTION: Hypothalamic-releasing factor stimulates the release of ACTH from the anterior pituitary gland. ACTH stimulates adrenal cortex secretion of glucocorticoids, androgens, and, to a lesser degree, mineralocorticoids. Cortisol is the major glucocorticoid secreted by the adrenal cortex. ACTH and cortisol test results are evaluated together because a change in one normally causes a change in the other. ACTH secretion is stimulated by insulin, metyrapone, and vasopressin. It is decreased by dexamethasone. Cortisol excess from any source is termed *Cushing's syndrome*. Cortisol excess resulting from ACTH excess produced by the pituitary is termed *Cushing's disease*. ACTH levels exhibit a diurnal variation, peaking between 0600 and 0800 and reaching the lowest point between 1800 and 2300. Evening levels are generally one-half to two-thirds lower than morning levels. Cortisol levels also vary diurnally, with the peak values occurring during between 0600 and 0800 and reaching the lowest levels between 2000 and 2400. Specimens are typically collected at 0800 and 1600. This pattern may be reversed in individuals who sleep during daytime hours and are active during nighttime hours. Salivary cortisol levels are known to parallel blood levels and can be used to screen for Cushing's disease and Cushing's syndrome.

This procedure is contraindicated for

The metyrapone stimulation test is contraindicated in patients with suspected adrenal insufficiency

A

because it may induce an acute adrenal crisis, a life-threatening condition, in patients whose adrenal function is already compromised. ✤

INDICATIONS

- Determine adequacy of replacement therapy in congenital adrenal hyperplasia.
- Determine adrenocortical dysfunction.
- Differentiate between increased ACTH release with decreased cortisol levels and decreased ACTH release with increased cortisol levels.

POTENTIAL MEDICAL DIAGNOSIS

ACTH Result

Because ACTH and cortisol secretion exhibit diurnal variation with values being highest in the morning, a lack of change in values from morning to evening is clinically significant. Decreased concentrations of hormones secreted by the pituitary gland and its target organs are observed in hypopituitarism. In primary adrenal insufficiency (Addison's disease), because of adrenal gland destruction by tumor, infectious process, or immune reaction, ACTH levels are elevated while cortisol levels are decreased. Both ACTH and cortisol levels are decreased in secondary adrenal insufficiency (i.e., secondary to pituitary insufficiency). Excess ACTH can be produced ectopically by various lung cancers such as oat-cell carcinoma and large-cell carcinoma of the lung and by benign bronchial carcinoid tumor.

Challenge Tests and Results

The* ACTH (cosyntropin) stimulated rapid test *directly evaluates adrenal gland function and indirectly evaluates pituitary gland and hypothalamus function. Cosyntropin is a synthetic form of ACTH. A baseline cortisol level is collected before the injection of cosyntropin. Specimens are subsequently collected at 30- and 60-min intervals. If the adrenal glands function normally, cortisol levels rise significantly after administration of cosyntropin.

The CRH stimulation test works as well as the dexamethasone suppression test (DST) in distinguishing Cushing's disease from conditions in which ACTH is secreted ectopically (e.g., tumors not located in the pituitary gland that secrete ACTH). Patients with pituitary tumors tend to respond to CRH stimulation, whereas those with ectopic tumors do not. Patients with adrenal insufficiency demonstrate one of three patterns depending on the underlying cause:

- ***Primary adrenal insufficiency—high baseline ACTH (in response to IV-administered ACTH) and low cortisol levels pre- and post-IV ACTH.***
- ***Secondary adrenal insufficiency (pituitary)—low baseline ACTH that does not respond to ACTH stimulation. Cortisol levels do not increase after stimulation.***
- ***Tertiary adrenal insufficiency (hypothalamic)—low baseline ACTH with an exaggerated and prolonged response to stimulation. Cortisol levels usually do not reach 20 mcg/dL (SI = 552 nmol/L).***

(The* DST *is useful in differentiating the causes of increased cortisol levels. Dexamethasone is a synthetic glucocorticoid that is significantly more potent than cortisol. It works by negative feedback. It suppresses the release of ACTH in patients with a normal hypothalamus. A cortisol level less than 1.8 mcg/dL (SI = 49.7 nmol/L) usually

excludes Cushing's syndrome. With the DST, a baseline morning cortisol level is collected, and the patient is given a 1-mg dose of dexamethasone at bedtime. A second specimen is collected the following morning. If cortisol levels have not been suppressed, adrenal adenoma is suspected. The DST also produces abnormal results in the presence of certain psychiatric illnesses [e.g., endogenous depression]).

The **metyrapone stimulation test** *is used to distinguish corticotropin-dependent causes (pituitary Cushing's disease and ectopic Cushing's disease) from corticotropin-independent causes (e.g., carcinoma of the lung or thyroid) of increased cortisol levels. Metyrapone inhibits the conversion of 11-deoxycortisol to cortisol. Cortisol levels should decrease to less than 3 mcg/dL if normal pituitary stimulation by ACTH occurs after an oral dose of metyrapone. Specimen collection and administration of the medication are performed as with the overnight dexamethasone test.*

Increased in:
Overproduction of ACTH can occur as a direct result of either disease (e.g., primary or ectopic tumor that secretes ACTH) or stimulation by physical or emotional stress, or it can be an indirect response to abnormalities in the complex feedback mechanisms involving the pituitary gland, hypothalamus, or adrenal glands.

ACTH Increased in
- Addison's disease ***(primary adrenocortical hypofunction)***
- Carcinoid syndrome
- Congenital adrenal hyperplasia
- Cushing's disease ***(pituitary-dependent adrenal hyperplasia)***
- Cushing's syndrome ***(ectopic secretion of ACTH)***
- Depression
- Ectopic ACTH-producing tumors
- Menstruation
- Nelson's syndrome ***(ACTH-producing pituitary tumors)***
- Pregnancy
- Sepsis
- Septic shock
- Type 2 diabetes

Decreased in:
Secondary adrenal insufficiency due to hypopituitarism (inadequate production by the pituitary) can result in decreased levels of ACTH. Conditions that result in overproduction or availability of high levels of cortisol can also result in decreased levels of ACTH.

ACTH Decreased in
- Adrenal adenoma
- Adrenal cancer
- Cushing's syndrome
- Exogenous steroid therapy

Summary of the Relationship Between Cortisol and ACTH Levels in Conditions Affecting the Adrenal and Pituitary Glands

Disease	Cortisol Level	ACTH Level
Addison's disease (adrenal insufficiency)	Decreased	Increased
Cushing's disease (pituitary adenoma)	Increased	Increased
Cushing's syndrome related to ectopic source of ACTH	Increased	Increased
Cushing's syndrome (ACTH independent; adrenal cancer or adenoma)	Increased	Decreased
Congenital adrenal hyperplasia	Decreased	Increased

A

CRITICAL FINDINGS: N/A

INTERFERING FACTORS

- Drugs and other substances that may increase ACTH levels include insulin, metoclopramide, metyrapone, mifepristone (RU 486), spironolactone, and vasopressin.
- Drugs and other substances that may decrease ACTH levels include corticosteroids (e.g., dexamethasone) and pravastatin.
- Test results are affected by the time the test is done because ACTH levels vary diurnally, with the highest values occurring between 0600 and 0800 and the lowest values occurring at night. Samples should be collected at the same time of day, between 0600 and 0800.
- Excessive physical activity can produce elevated levels.
- Metyrapone may cause gastrointestinal distress and/or confusion. Administer oral dose of metyrapone with milk and snack.
- Rapid clearance of metyrapone, resulting in falsely increased cortisol levels, may occur if the patient is taking drugs that enhance steroid metabolism (e.g., phenytoin, rifampin, phenobarbital, mitotane, and corticosteroids). The requesting health-care provider (HCP) should be consulted prior to a metyrapone stimulation test regarding a decision to withhold these medications.

NURSING IMPLICATIONS AND PROCEDURE

POTENTIAL NURSING PROBLEMS:

Problem	Signs & Symptoms	Interventions
Fluid volume (water) ***(related to loss of water secondary to vomiting; diarrhea)***	**Deficient:** Hypotension; decreased cardiac output; decreased urinary output; dry skin/mucous membranes; poor skin turgor; sunken eyeballs; increased urine-specific gravity; hemoconcentration	Monitor intake and output; assess for symptoms of dehydration (dry skin, dry mucous membranes, poor skin turgor, sunken eyeballs); monitor and trend vital signs; monitor for symptoms of poor cardiac output (rapid, weak, thready pulse); monitor and trend daily weight; collaborate with HCP regarding administration of IV fluids to support hydration; monitor laboratory values that reflect alterations in fluid status (potassium, blood urea nitrogen, creatinine, calcium, hemoglobin, and hematocrit, sodium); manage underlying cause of fluid alteration; monitor urine characteristics and respiratory status; establish baseline

Problem	Signs & Symptoms	Interventions
		assessment data; collaborate with HCP to adjust oral and IV fluids to provide optimal hydration status; administer replacement electrolytes, as ordered; adjust diuretics, as appropriate
Infection risk ***(related to impaired immune response secondary to elevated cortisol level)***	Delayed wound healing; inhibited collagen formation; impaired blood flow to edematous tissues; symptoms of infection (temperature; increased heart rate; increased blood pressure; shaking; chills; mottled skin; lethargy; fatigue; swelling; edema; pain; localized pressure; diaphoresis; night sweats; confusion; vomiting; nausea; headache)	Decrease exposure to environment by placing the patient in a private room; monitor and trend vital signs; monitor and trend laboratory values that would indicate an infection (WBC, CRP); promote good hygiene; assist with hygiene, as needed; administer prescribed antibiotics, antipyretics; use cooling measures; administer prescribed IV fluids; monitor vital signs and trend temperatures; encourage oral fluids; adhere to standard or universal precautions; isolate as appropriate; obtain cultures, as ordered; encourage lightweight clothing and bedding
Injury risk ***(related to poor wound healing; decreased bone density; capillary fragility)***	Easy bruising; blood in stool; skin breakdown; fracture; poor wound healing	Assess for bruising; assess stool for occult blood; assess for skin breakdown; assess wound for healing progress; facilitate ordered bone density screening

PRETEST:

- Positively identify the patient using at least two person-specific identifiers before services, treatments, or procedures are performed.
- ***Patient teaching:*** Inform the patient this test can assist in evaluating the amount of hormone produced by the pituitary gland located at the base of the brain.
- Obtain a history of the patient's health concerns, symptoms, surgical procedures, and results of previously performed laboratory and diagnostic studies. Include a list of known allergens, especially allergies or sensitivities to latex.
- Note any recent procedures that can interfere with test results.
- Obtain a list of the patient's current medications, including over-the-counter medications and dietary supplements (see Effects of Natural Products on Laboratory Values online at Davis*Plus*).
- Weigh patient and report weight to pharmacy for dosing of metyrapone

(30 mg/kg body weight to a maximum dose of 3 g).

- Review the procedure with the patient. When ACTH hypersecretion is suspected, a second sample may be requested between 0600 and 0800 to determine if changes are the result of diurnal variation in ACTH levels. Inform the patient that more than one sample may be necessary to ensure accurate results, and samples are obtained at specific times to determine high and low levels of ACTH. Inform the patient that each specimen collection takes approximately 5 to 10 min. Address concerns about pain, and explain that there may be some discomfort during the venipuncture.
- ***Sensitivity to social and cultural issues,*** as well as concern for modesty, is important in providing psychological support before, during, and after the procedure.
- Note that there are no food, fluid, or medication restrictions unless by medical direction.
- Drugs that enhance steroid metabolism may be withheld by medical direction prior to metyrapone stimulation testing.
- Instruct the patient to refrain from strenuous exercise for 12 hr before the test and to remain in bed or at rest for 1 hr immediately before the test. Avoid smoking and alcohol use.
- Prepare an ice slurry in a cup or plastic bag to have on hand for immediate transport of the specimen to the laboratory.

INTRATEST:

Potential Complications:

Adverse reactions to metyrapone include nausea and vomiting (N/V), abdominal pain, headache, dizziness, sedation, allergic rash, decreased white blood cell (WBC) count, and bone marrow depression. Signs and symptoms of overdose or acute adrenocortical insufficiency include cardiac dysrhythmias, hypotension, dehydration, anxiety, confusion, weakness, impairment of consciousness, N/V, epigastric pain, diarrhea, hyponatremia, and hyperkalemia. 🍁

- Ensure that strenuous exercise was avoided for 12 hr before the test and that 1 hr of bed rest was taken immediately before the test. Samples should be collected between 0600 and 0800.
- Have emergency equipment readily available in case of adverse reaction to metyrapone.
- Avoid the use of equipment containing latex if the patient has a history of allergic reaction to latex.
- Instruct the patient to cooperate fully and to follow directions. Direct the patient to breathe normally and to avoid unnecessary movement.
- Observe standard precautions, and follow the general guidelines in Patient Preparation and Specimen Collection online at Davis*Plus*. Positively identify the patient, and label the appropriate tubes with the corresponding patient demographics, date, and time of collection. Perform a venipuncture; collect the specimen in a prechilled plastic heparinized syringe or in prechilled collection containers, as listed under the "Specimen" subheading.
- Remove the needle and apply direct pressure with dry gauze to stop bleeding. Observe/assess venipuncture site for bleeding or hematoma formation, and secure gauze with adhesive bandage.
- Promptly transport the specimen to the laboratory for processing and analysis. The tightly capped sample should be placed in an ice slurry immediately after collection. Information on the specimen label should be protected from water in the ice slurry by first placing the specimen in a protective plastic bag.

POST-TEST:

- Inform the patient that a report of the results will be made available to the requesting HCP, who will discuss the results with the patient.
- Recognize anxiety related to test results, and offer support.
- Observe/assess the patient who has been administered metyrapone for signs and symptoms of an acute adrenal (addisonian) crisis, which

may include abdominal pain, N/V, hypotension, tachycardia, tachypnea, dehydration, excessively increased perspiration of the face and hands, sudden and significant fatigue or weakness, confusion, loss of consciousness, shock, coma. Potential interventions include immediate corticosteroid replacement (IV or IM), airway protection and maintenance, administration of dextrose for hypoglycemia, correction of electrolyte imbalance, and rehydration with IV fluids.

- Depending on the results of this procedure, additional testing may be performed to evaluate or monitor progression of the disease process and determine the need for a change in therapy. If a diagnosis of Cushing's disease is made, pituitary computed tomography (CT) or magnetic resonance imaging (MRI) may be indicated prior to surgery. If a diagnosis of ectopic corticotropin syndrome is made, abdominal CT or MRI may be indicated prior to surgery. Evaluate test results in relation to the patient's symptoms and other tests performed.

Patient Education:

- Instruct the patient to resume normal activity as directed by the HCP.
- Provide contact information, if desired, for the Cushing's Support and Research Foundation (www.csrf.net).
- Reinforce information given by the patient's HCP regarding further testing, treatment, or referral to another HCP.
- Answer any questions or address any concerns voiced by the patient or family.
- Teach the patient and family the effects of the disease process and associated treatments.

Expected Patient Outcomes:

Understanding

- The patient and family state the importance of compliance with the recommended therapeutic regime to health maintenance.
- The patient and family state the necessity of altering the medication regime during times of illness and stress.

Ability

- The patient and family demonstrate proficiency in the administration of prescribed steroids.
- The patient complies with the request to stand slowly to prevent orthostatic hypotension.

Response

- The patient complies with the HCP's request to wear a medic alert bracelet indicating adrenal insufficiency and steroid use.
- The patient and family comply with the HCP's request to increase oral fluid intake with a diet high in sodium and low in potassium (Addison's disease).

RELATED STUDIES:

- Related tests include cortisol and challenge tests, CT abdomen, CT pituitary, MRI abdomen, MRI pituitary, TSH, thyroxine, and US abdomen.
- See the Endocrine System table online at Davis*Plus* for related tests by body system.

Alanine Aminotransferase

SYNONYM/ACRONYM: ALT, SGPT (serum glutamic pyruvic transaminase).

COMMON USE: To assess liver function related to liver disease and/or damage.

SPECIMEN: Serum collected in a gold-, red-, or red/gray-top tube. Plasma collected in a green-top (heparin) tube is also acceptable.

NORMAL FINDINGS: (Method: Spectrophotometry)

Access Canadian content on Fast Find: Lab and Dx at davispl.us/vanleeuwen7

A

Age	Conventional & SI Units
Newborn–12 mo	7–41 units/L
13 mo–60 yr	
Male	19–36 units/L
Female	24–36 units/L
61–90 yr	
Male	13–40 units/L
Female	10–28 units/L
Greater than 90 yr	
Male	6–38 units/L
Female	5–24 units/L

Values may be slightly elevated in older adults due to the effects of medications and the presence of multiple chronic or acute diseases with or without muted symptoms.

DESCRIPTION: Alanine aminotransferase (ALT) is an enzyme produced by the liver. The highest concentration of ALT is found in liver cells; moderate amounts are found in kidney cells; and smaller amounts are found in heart, pancreas, spleen, skeletal muscle, and red blood cells. When liver damage occurs, serum levels of ALT may increase as much as 50 times normal, making this a sensitive test for evaluating liver function. ALT is part of a group of tests known as LFTs, or liver function tests, used to evaluate liver function: ALT; albumin; alkaline phosphatase; aspartate aminotransferase (AST); bilirubin, direct; bilirubin, total; and protein, total.

This procedure is contraindicated for: N/A

INDICATIONS

- Compare serially with AST levels to track the course of liver disease.
- Monitor liver damage resulting from hepatotoxic drugs.
- Monitor response to treatment of liver disease, with tissue repair indicated by gradually declining levels.

POTENTIAL MEDICAL DIAGNOSIS

Increased in:

Related to release of ALT from damaged liver, kidney, heart, pancreas, red blood cells, or skeletal muscle cells.

- Acute pancreatitis
- AIDS ***(related to hepatitis B co-infection)***
- Biliary tract obstruction
- Burns (severe)
- Chronic alcohol misuse
- Cirrhosis
- Fatty liver
- HELLP syndrome of pregnancy (hemolysis, elevated liver enzymes, low platelet count)
- Hepatic carcinoma
- Hepatitis
- Infectious mononucleosis
- Muscle injury from intramuscular injections, trauma, infection, and seizures (recent)
- Muscular dystrophy
- Myocardial infarction
- Myositis
- Pancreatitis
- Pre-eclampsia
- Shock (severe)

Decreased in:

- Pyridoxal phosphate deficiency ***(related to a deficiency of pyridoxal phosphate that results in decreased production of ALT)***

CRITICAL FINDINGS: N/A

INTERFERING FACTORS

- Drugs and other substances that may increase ALT levels by causing cholestasis include anabolic steroids, dapsone, estrogens, ethionamide, oral contraceptives, sulfonylureas, and zidovudine.
- Drugs and other substances that may increase ALT levels by causing

hepatocellular damage include acetaminophen (toxic), acetylsalicylic acid, anticonvulsants, asparaginase, cephalosporins, chloramphenicol, clofibrate, cytarabine, danazol, enflurane, erythromycin, ethambutol, ethionamide, ethotoin, florantyrone, foscarnet, gentamicin, gold salts, halothane, ibufenac, indomethacin, interleukin-2, isoniazid, lincomycin, low-molecular-weight heparin, metahexamide, metaxalone, methoxsalen, methyldopa, naproxen, nitrofurans, oral contraceptives, probenecid, procainamide, and tetracyclines.
- Drugs and other substances that may decrease ALT levels include cyclosporine, interferons, metronidazole (affects enzymatic test methods), and ursodiol.

NURSING IMPLICATIONS AND PROCEDURE

POTENTIAL NURSING PROBLEMS:

Problem	Signs & Symptoms	Interventions
Pain ***(related to organ inflammation and surrounding tissues; excessive alcohol intake; infection)***	Emotional symptoms of distress; crying; agitation; facial grimace; moaning; verbalization of pain; rocking motions; irritability; disturbed sleep; diaphoresis; altered blood pressure and heart rate; nausea; vomiting; self-report of pain; upper abdominal and gastric pain after eating fatty foods or alcohol intake with acute pancreatic disease; pain, which may be decreased or absent in chronic pancreatic disease	Collaborate with the patient and health-care provider (HCP) to identify the best pain management modality to provide relief; refrain from activities that may aggravate pain; use the application of heat or cold to the best effect in managing pain; monitor pain severity
Fluid volume (water) ***(related to vomiting; decreased intake; compromised kidney function; overly aggressive fluid resuscitation; overly aggressive diuresis)***	**Overload:** Edema, shortness of breath, increased weight, ascites, rales, rhonchi, and diluted laboratory values. **Deficient:** Decreased urinary output, fatigue, and sunken eyes, dark urine, decreased blood pressure, increased heart rate, and altered mental status	Complete a daily weight with monitoring of trends; accurate intake and output; collaborate with HCP regarding administration of intravenous (IV) fluids to support hydration; monitor laboratory values that reflect alterations in fluid status (potassium, blood urea nitrogen, creatinine, calcium, hemoglobin, and hematocrit); manage

(table continues on page 22)

A

Problem	Signs & Symptoms	Interventions
		underlying cause of fluid alteration; monitor urine characteristics and respiratory status; establish baseline assessment data; collaborate with HCP to adjust oral and IV fluids to provide optimal hydration status; administer replacement electrolytes, as ordered
Nutrition ***(related to metabolic imbalances)***	Increased liver function tests; hyperglycemia with polyuria, weight loss, weakness, nausea, vomiting; hypocalcemia with confusion, intestinal cramping, diarrhea; hypertriglyceridemia; altered thiamine with weakness, confusion	Administer enteral nutrition; administer parenteral nutrition; monitor laboratory values and collaborate with HCP on replacement strategies; correlate laboratory values with IV fluid infusion and collaborate with the HCP and pharmacist to adjust to patient needs; ensure adequate pain control; monitor vital signs for alterations associated metabolic imbalances
Gastrointestinal (GI) problems ***(related to altered motility; irritation of the GI tract; taste alterations; pancreatic and gastric secretions)***	Nausea; vomiting; abdominal distention; unexplained weight loss; steatorrhea; diarrhea; visible abdominal distention; ascites; diminished or absent bowel sounds	Perform nasogastric intubation (NGT) to remove gastric secretions and decrease pancreatic secretions, which may result in autodigestion; monitor NGT for patency and amount of drainage; assess hydration status; assess bowel sounds frequently; measure abdominal girth to monitor degree of abdominal distention

PRETEST:

- Positively identify the patient using at least two person-specific identifiers before services, treatments, or procedures are performed.
- *Patient teaching:* Inform the patient this test can assist with evaluation of liver function and help identify liver disease.
- Obtain a history of the patient's health concerns, symptoms, surgical procedures, and results of previously performed laboratory and diagnostic studies. Include a list of known allergens, especially allergies or sensitivities to latex.

- Obtain a list of the patient's current medications, including over-the-counter medications and dietary supplements (see Effects of Natural Products on Laboratory Values online at Davis*Plus*).
- Review the procedure with the patient. Inform the patient that specimen collection takes approximately 5 to 10 min. Address concerns about pain, and explain that there may be some discomfort during the venipuncture.
- ***Sensitivity to social and cultural issues,*** as well as concern for modesty, is important in providing psychological support before, during, and after the procedure.
- Note that there are no food, fluid, or medication restrictions unless by medical direction.

INTRATEST:

Potential Complications: N/A

- Avoid the use of equipment containing latex if the patient has a history of allergic reaction to latex.
- Instruct the patient to cooperate fully and to follow directions. Direct the patient to breathe normally and to avoid unnecessary movement.
- Observe standard precautions, and follow the general guidelines in Patient Preparation and Specimen Collection online at Davis*Plus*. Positively identify the patient, and label the appropriate specimen container with the corresponding patient demographics, initials of the person collecting the specimen, date, and time of collection. Perform a venipuncture.
- Remove the needle and apply direct pressure with dry gauze to stop bleeding. Observe/assess venipuncture site for bleeding and hematoma formation and secure gauze with adhesive bandage.
- Promptly transport the specimen to the laboratory for processing and analysis.

POST-TEST:

- Inform the patient that a report of the results will be made available to the requesting HCP, who will discuss the results with the patient.
- ***Nutritional Considerations:*** Increased ALT levels may be associated with liver disease. Dietary recommendations may be indicated and vary depending on the severity of the condition. A low-protein diet may be in order if the patient's liver has lost the ability to process the end products of protein metabolism. A diet of soft foods may be required if esophageal varices have developed. Ammonia levels may be used to determine whether protein should be added to or reduced from the diet. Patients should be encouraged to eat simple carbohydrates and emulsified fats (as in homogenized milk or eggs) rather than complex carbohydrates (e.g., starch, fiber, and glycogen [animal carbohydrates]) and complex fats, which require additional bile to emulsify them so that they can be used. The cirrhotic patient should be carefully observed for the development of ascites, in which case fluid and electrolyte balance requires strict attention.
- Depending on the results of this procedure, additional testing may be performed to evaluate or monitor progression of the disease process and determine the need for a change in therapy. Evaluate test results in relation to the patient's symptoms and other tests performed.

Patient Education:

- Reinforce information given by the patient's HCP regarding further testing, treatment, or referral to another HCP. Recognize anxiety related to test results, and answer any questions or address any concerns voiced by the patient or family.
- Provide teaching and information regarding the clinical implications of the test results, as appropriate.
- Educate the patient regarding access to counseling services. Provide contact information, if desired, for the Centers for Disease Control and Prevention (www.cdc.gov/diseasesconditions) 🍁.
- Provide information regarding disease process and proactive activities that the patient can take in managing health.

A

- Provide samples of dietary selections that can support pancreatic and liver health and that are culturally appropriate.

Expected Patient Outcomes:

Understanding

- The patient and family verbalize causative factors of pancreatitis and liver disease.
- The patient and family verbalize that the disease can reoccur if not adhering to positive actions to change lifestyle.

Ability

- The patient creates a diet plan that supports liver and pancreatic health.
- The patient takes medication as prescribed to limit pancreatic secretions and decrease pain.

Response

- The patient agrees to seek counseling for alcohol abstinence.
- The patient agrees to control potential behaviors that could trigger future disease episodes.

RELATED STUDIES:

- Related tests include acetaminophen, ammonia, AST, bilirubin, biopsy liver, cholangiography percutaneous transhepatic, electrolytes, GGT, hepatitis antigens and antibodies, LDH, liver and spleen scan, US abdomen, and US liver.
- See the Hepatobiliary System table online at Davis*Plus* for related tests by body system.

Albumin and Albumin/Globulin Ratio

SYNONYM/ACRONYM: Alb, A/G ratio.

COMMON USE: To assess liver or kidney function and nutritional status.

SPECIMEN: Serum collected in a gold-, red-, or red/gray-top tube. Plasma collected in a green-top (heparin) tube is also acceptable.

NORMAL FINDINGS: (Method: Spectrophotometry) Normally, the albumin/globulin (A/G) ratio is greater than 1.

Age	Conventional Units	SI Units (Conventional Units × 10)
Cord	2.8–4.3 g/dL	28–43 g/L
Newborn–7 d	2.6–3.6 g/dL	26–36 g/L
8–30 d	2–4.5 g/dL	20–45 g/L
1–3 mo	2–4.8 g/dL	20–48 g/L
4–6 mo	2.1–4.9 g/dL	21–49 g/L
7–12 mo	2.1–4.7 g/dL	21–47 g/L
1–3 yr	3.4–4.2 g/dL	34–42 g/L
4–6 yr	3.5–5.2 g/dL	35–52 g/L
7–19 yr	3.7–5.6 g/dL	37–56 g/L
20–40 yr	3.7–5.1 g/dL	37–51 g/L
41–60 yr	3.4–4.8 g/dL	34–48 g/L
61–90 yr	3.2–4.6 g/dL	32–46 g/L
Greater than 90 yr	2.9–4.5 g/dL	29–45 g/L

A

DESCRIPTION: Most of the body's total protein is a combination of albumin and globulins. Albumin, the protein present in the highest concentrations, is the main transport protein in the body for hormones, therapeutic drugs, calcium, magnesium, heme, and waste products such as bilirubin. Albumin also significantly affects plasma oncotic pressure, which regulates the distribution of body fluid between blood vessels, tissues, and cells. Albumin is synthesized in the liver. Low levels of albumin may be the result of either inadequate intake, inadequate production, or excessive loss. Albumin levels are more useful as an indicator of chronic deficiency than of short-term deficiency. Hypoalbuminemia or low serum albumin, a level less than 3.4 g/dL (SI = 34 g/L), can stem from many causes and may be a useful predictor of mortality. Normally albumin is not excreted in urine. However, in cases of kidney injury or disease, some albumin may be lost due to decreased kidney function, as seen in nephrotic syndrome, and in pregnant women with pre-eclampsia and eclampsia.

Albumin levels are affected by posture. Results from specimens collected in an upright posture are higher than results from specimens collected in a supine position.

The albumin/globulin (A/G) ratio is useful in the evaluation of liver and kidney disease. The ratio is calculated using the following formula:

albumin/(total protein – albumin)

where globulin is the difference between the total protein value and the albumin value. For example, with a total protein of 7 g/dL and albumin of 4 g/dL, the A/G ratio is calculated as 4/(7 – 4) or 4/3 = 1.33. A reversal in the ratio, where globulin exceeds albumin (i.e., ratio less than 1), is clinically significant.

This procedure is contraindicated for: N/A

INDICATIONS
- Assess nutritional status of hospitalized patients, especially older adult patients.
- Evaluate chronic illness.
- Evaluate liver disease.

POTENTIAL MEDICAL DIAGNOSIS

Increased in:

Any condition that results in a decrease of plasma water (e.g., dehydration); look for increase in hemoglobin and hematocrit. Decreases in the volume of intravascular liquid automatically result in concentration of the components present in the remaining liquid, as reflected by an elevated albumin level.
- Hyperinfusion of albumin

Decreased in:
- ***Insufficient intake:***
  - Malabsorption ***(related to lack of amino acids available for protein synthesis)***
  - Malnutrition ***(related to insufficient dietary source of amino acids required for protein synthesis)***
- ***Decreased synthesis by the liver:***
  - Acute and chronic liver disease (e.g., alcoholism, cirrhosis, hepatitis) ***(evidenced by a decrease in normal liver function; the liver is the body's site of protein synthesis)***
  - Genetic analbuminemia ***(related to genetic inability of liver to synthesize albumin)***

A

- ***Inflammation and chronic diseases result in production of acute-phase reactant and other globulin proteins; the increase in globulins causes a corresponding relative decrease in albumin:***
  - Amyloidosis
  - Bacterial infections
  - Monoclonal gammopathies (e.g., multiple myeloma, Waldenström's macroglobulinemia)
  - Neoplasm
  - Parasitic infestations
  - Peptic ulcer
  - Prolonged immobilization
  - Rheumatic diseases
  - Severe skin disease
- ***Increased loss over body surface:***
  - Burns ***(evidenced by loss of interstitial fluid albumin)***
  - Enteropathies (e.g., gluten sensitivity, Crohn's disease, ulcerative colitis, Whipple's disease) ***(evidenced by sensitivity to ingested substances or related to inadequate absorption from intestinal loss)***
  - Fistula (gastrointestinal or lymphatic) ***(related to loss of sequestered albumin from general circulation)***
  - Hemorrhage ***(related to fluid loss)***
  - Kidney disease ***(related to loss from damaged renal tubules)***
  - Pre-eclampsia ***(evidenced by excessive renal loss)***
  - Rapid hydration or overhydration ***(evidenced by dilution effect)***
  - Repeated thoracentesis or paracentesis ***(related to removal of albumin in accumulated third-space fluid)***
- ***Increased catabolism:***
  - Cushing's disease ***(related to excessive cortisol induced protein metabolism)***
  - Heart failure ***(evidenced by dilution effect)***
  - Thyroid dysfunction ***(related to overproduction of albumin binding thyroid hormones)***
- ***Increased blood volume (hypervolemia):***
  - Pre-eclampsia ***(related to fluid retention)***
  - Pregnancy ***(evidenced by increased circulatory volume from placenta and fetus)***

CRITICAL FINDINGS: N/A

INTERFERING FACTORS

- Drugs and other substances that may increase albumin levels include carbamazepine, furosemide, phenobarbital, and prednisolone.
- Drugs and other substances that may decrease albumin levels include acetaminophen (poisoning), amiodarone, asparaginase, dextran, estrogens, ibuprofen, interleukin-2, methotrexate, methyldopa, niacin, nitrofurantoin, oral contraceptives, phenytoin, prednisone, and valproic acid.
- Availability of administered drugs is affected by variations in albumin levels.

NURSING IMPLICATIONS AND PROCEDURE

PRETEST:

- Positively identify the patient using at least two person-specific identifiers before services, treatments, or procedures are performed.
- *Patient teaching:* Inform the patient this test can assist with evaluation of liver and kidney function, as well as chronic disease.
- Obtain a history of the patient's health concerns, symptoms, surgical procedures, and results of previously performed laboratory and

diagnostic studies. Include a list of known allergens, especially allergies or sensitivities to latex. The patient should be assessed for signs of edema or ascites.
- Obtain a list of the patient's current medications, including over-the-counter medications and dietary supplements (see Effects of Natural Products on Laboratory Values online at Davis*Plus*).
- Review the procedure with the patient. Inform the patient that specimen collection takes approximately 5 to 10 min. Address concerns about pain, and explain that there may be some discomfort during the venipuncture.
- ***Sensitivity to social and cultural issues,*** as well as concern for modesty, is important in providing psychological support before, during, and after the procedure.
- Note that there are no food, fluid, or medication restrictions unless by medical direction.

INTRATEST:

Potential Complications: N/A
- Avoid the use of equipment containing latex if the patient has a history of allergic reaction to latex.
- Instruct the patient to cooperate fully and to follow directions. Direct the patient to breathe normally and to avoid unnecessary movement.
- Observe standard precautions, and follow the general guidelines in Patient Preparation and Specimen Collection online at Davis*Plus*. Positively identify the patient, and label the appropriate specimen container with the corresponding patient demographics, initials of the person collecting the specimen, date, and time of collection. Perform a venipuncture.
- Remove the needle and apply direct pressure with dry gauze to stop bleeding. Observe/assess venipuncture site for bleeding or hematoma formation and secure gauze with adhesive bandage.
- Promptly transport the specimen to the laboratory for processing and analysis.

POST-TEST:
- Inform the patient that a report of the results will be made available to the requesting health-care provider (HCP), who will discuss the results with the patient.
- ***Nutritional Considerations:*** Dietary recommendations may be indicated and will vary depending on the severity of the condition. Ammonia levels may be used to determine whether protein should be added to or reduced from the diet.
- Reinforce information given by the patient's HCP regarding further testing, treatment, or referral to another HCP. Recognize anxiety related to test results, and answer any questions or address any concerns voiced by the patient or family.
- Depending on the results of this procedure, additional testing may be performed to evaluate or monitor progression of the disease process and determine the need for a change in therapy. Availability of administered drugs is affected by variations in albumin levels. Patients receiving therapeutic drug treatments should have their drug levels monitored when levels of the transport protein, albumin, are decreased in order to prevent development of toxic drug concentrations. Evaluate test results in relation to the patient's symptoms and other tests performed.

RELATED STUDIES:
- Related tests include ALT, ALP, ammonia, anti–smooth muscle antibodies, AST, bilirubin, biopsy liver, CBC hematocrit, CBC hemoglobin, CT biliary tract and liver, GGT, hepatitis antibodies and antigens, KUB studies, laparoscopy abdominal, liver scan, MRI abdomen, osmolality, potassium, prealbumin, protein total and fractions, radiofrequency ablation liver, sodium, US abdomen, and US liver.
- See the Gastrointestinal, Genitourinary, and Hepatobiliary systems tables online at Davis*Plus* for related tests by body system.

Aldolase

A

SYNONYM/ACRONYM: ALD.

COMMON USE: To assist in the diagnosis of muscle-wasting diseases such as muscular dystrophy or other diseases that cause muscle and cellular damage, such as hepatitis and cirrhosis of the liver.

SPECIMEN: Serum collected in a gold-, red-, or red/gray-top tube.

NORMAL FINDINGS: (Method: Spectrophotometry)

Age	Conventional & SI Units
Newborn–30 d	6–32 units/L
1 mo–2 yr	3.4–11.8 units/L
3–17 yr	1.2–8.8 units/L
Adult	Less than 8.1 units/L

POTENTIAL MEDICAL DIAGNOSIS

Increased in:

ALD is released from any damaged cell in which it is stored, so diseases of skeletal muscle, cardiac muscle, pancreas, RBCs, and liver that cause cellular destruction demonstrate elevated ALD levels.

- Carcinoma (lung, breast, and genitourinary tract and metastasis to liver)
- Dermatomyositis
- Duchenne's muscular dystrophy
- Hepatitis (acute viral or toxic)
- Limb girdle muscular dystrophy
- Myocardial infarction
- Pancreatitis (acute)
- Polymyositis
- Severe crush injuries
- Tetanus
- Trichinosis ***(related to myositis)***

Decreased in:

- Hereditary fructose intolerance ***(evidenced by hereditary deficiency of the aldolase B enzyme)***
- ***Late stages of muscle-wasting diseases in which muscle mass has significantly diminished***

CRITICAL FINDINGS: N/A

Find and print out the full study on Fast Find at davispl.us/vanleeuwen7.

Aldosterone

SYNONYM/ACRONYM: N/A

COMMON USE: To assist in the diagnosis of primary hyperaldosteronism disorders such as Conn's syndrome and Addison's disease. Blood levels fluctuate with dehydration and fluid overload. This test can be used in evaluation of hypertension.

SPECIMEN: Serum collected in a gold-, red-, or red/gray-top tube. Plasma collected in a green-top (heparin) or lavender-top (EDTA) tube is also acceptable.

NORMAL FINDINGS: (Method: Radioimmunoassay)

Age	Conventional Units	SI Units (Conventional Units × 0.0277)
Cord blood	40–200 ng/dL	1.11–5.54 nmol/L
3 d–1 wk	7–184 ng/dL	0.19–5.09 nmol/L
1 mo–1 yr	5–90 ng/dL	0.14–2.49 nmol/L
13–23 mo	7–54 ng/dL	0.19–1.49 nmol/L
2–10 yr		
Supine	3–35 ng/dL	0.08–0.97 nmol/L
Upright (sitting for at least 2 hr)	5–80 ng/dL	0.14–2.22 nmol/L
11–15 yr		
Supine	2–22 ng/dL	0.06–0.61 nmol/L
Upright (sitting for at least 2 hr)	4–48 ng/dL	0.11–1.33 nmol/L
Adult		
Supine	3–16 ng/dL	0.08–0.44 nmol/L
Upright	7–30 ng/dL	0.19–0.83 nmol/L
Older Adult	Levels decline with age	

These values reflect a normal-sodium diet. Values for a low-sodium diet are three to five times higher.

DESCRIPTION: Aldosterone is a mineralocorticoid secreted by the zona glomerulosa of the adrenal cortex and is regulated by the renin-angiotensin system. Changes in renal blood flow trigger or suppress release of renin from the glomeruli. The presence of circulating renin stimulates the liver to produce angiotensin I. Angiotensin I is converted by the lungs and kidneys into angiotensin II, a potent trigger for the release of aldosterone. Aldosterone and the renin-angiotensin system work together to regulate sodium and potassium levels. Aldosterone acts to increase sodium reabsorption in the renal tubules. This results in excretion of potassium, increased water retention, increased blood volume, and increased blood pressure. This test is of little diagnostic value in differentiating primary and secondary aldosteronism unless plasma renin activity is measured simultaneously (see study titled "Renin"). A variety of factors influence serum aldosterone levels, including sodium intake, certain medications, and activity. Secretion of aldosterone is also affected by adrenocorticotropic hormone (ACTH), a pituitary hormone that primarily stimulates secretion of glucocorticoids and minimally affects secretion of mineralocorticosteroids. Patients with serum potassium less than 3.6 mEq/L and 24-hour urine potassium greater than 40 mEq/L fit the general criteria to test for aldosteronism. Renin is low in primary aldosteronism and high in secondary aldosteronism. A ratio of plasma aldosterone to plasma renin activity greater than 50 is significant. Ratios greater than 20 obtained after unchallenged screening may indicate the need for further evaluation with a sodium-loading protocol. A captopril protocol can be substituted for patients who may not tolerate the sodium-loading protocol.

A

This procedure is contraindicated for: N/A

INDICATIONS

- Evaluate hypertension of unknown cause, especially with hypokalemia not induced by diuretics.
- Investigate suspected hyperaldosteronism, as indicated by elevated levels.
- Investigate suspected hypoaldosteronism, as indicated by decreased levels.

POTENTIAL MEDICAL DIAGNOSIS

Increased in:

Increased With Decreased Renin Levels

Primary hyperaldosteronism (evidenced by overproduction related to abnormal adrenal gland function):

- Adenomas (Conn's syndrome)
- Bilateral hyperplasia of the aldosterone-secreting zona glomerulosa cells

Increased With Increased Renin Levels

Secondary hyperaldosteronism (related to conditions that increase renin levels, which then stimulate aldosterone secretion):

- Bartter's syndrome ***(related to excessive loss of potassium by the kidneys, leading to release of renin and subsequent release of aldosterone)***
- Chronic obstructive pulmonary disease
- Cirrhosis with ascites formation ***(related to diluted concentration of sodium by increased blood volume)***
- Diuretic misuse ***(related to direct stimulation of aldosterone secretion)***
- Heart failure ***(related to diluted concentration of sodium by increased blood volume)***
- Hypovolemia ***(secondary to hemorrhage and transudation)***
- Laxative misuse ***(related to direct stimulation of aldosterone secretion)***
- Nephrotic syndrome ***(related to excessive renal protein loss, development of decreased oncotic pressure, fluid retention, and diluted concentration of sodium)***
- Starvation (after 10 days) ***(related to diluted concentration of sodium by development of edema)***
- Thermal stress ***(related to direct stimulation of aldosterone secretion)***
- Toxemia of pregnancy ***(related to diluted concentration of sodium by increased blood volume evidenced by edema; placental corticotropin-releasing hormone stimulates production of maternal adrenal hormones that can also contribute to edema)***

Decreased in:

Without Hypertension

- Addison's disease ***(related to lack of function in the adrenal cortex)***
- Hypoaldosteronism ***(secondary to renin deficiency)***
- Isolated aldosterone deficiency

With Hypertension

- Acute alcohol intoxication ***(related to toxic effects of alcohol on adrenal gland function and therefore secretion of aldosterone)***
- Diabetes ***(related to impaired conversion of prorenin to renin by damaged kidneys, resulting in decreased aldosterone)***
- Excess secretion of deoxycorticosterone ***(related to suppression***

A

of ACTH production by cortisol, which in turn affects aldosterone secretion)

- Turner's syndrome (25% of cases) ***(related to congenital adrenal hyperplasia resulting in underproduction of aldosterone and overproduction of androgens)***

CRITICAL FINDINGS: N/A

INTERFERING FACTORS

- Drugs and other substances that may increase aldosterone levels include amiloride, ammonium chloride, angiotensin, angiotensin II, dobutamine, dopamine, endralazine, fenoldopam, hydralazine, hydrochlorothiazide, laxatives (misuse), metoclopramide, nifedipine, opiates, potassium, spironolactone, and zacopride.
- Drugs and other substances that may decrease aldosterone levels include atenolol, captopril, carvedilol, cilazapril, enalapril, fadrozole, glycyrrhiza (licorice), ibopamine, indomethacin, lisinopril, nicardipine, NSAIDs, perindopril, ranitidine, saline, sinorphan, and verapamil. Prolonged heparin therapy also decreases aldosterone levels.
- Upright body posture, stress, strenuous exercise, and late pregnancy can lead to increased levels.
- Recent radioactive scans or radiation within 1 wk before the test can interfere with test results when radioimmunoassay is the test method.
- Diet can significantly affect results. A low-sodium diet can increase serum aldosterone, whereas a high-sodium diet can decrease levels. Decreased serum sodium and elevated serum potassium increase aldosterone secretion. Elevated serum sodium and decreased serum potassium suppress aldosterone secretion.

NURSING IMPLICATIONS AND PROCEDURE

POTENTIAL NURSING PROBLEMS:

Problem	Signs & Symptoms	Interventions
Fluid volume (water) ***(related to hypovolemia associated with adrenal insufficiency; cortisol insufficiency; hyponatremia, vomiting, diarrhea)***	**Deficient:** Hypotension; decreased cardiac output; decreased urinary output; dry skin/mucous membranes; poor skin turgor; sunken eyeballs; increased urine specific gravity; hemoconcentration; weakness; lethargy; dizziness; tachycardia; low sodium; elevated potassium; hypoglycemia	Monitor intake and output; assess for symptoms of dehydration (dry skin, dry mucous membranes, poor skin turgor, sunken eyeballs), monitor and trend vital signs; monitor for symptoms of poor cardiac output (rapid, weak, thready pulse); monitor daily weight with monitoring of trends; collaborate with health-care provider (HCP) with administration of intravenous (IV) fluids to support hydration; monitor laboratory values

(table continues on page 32)

A

Problem	Signs & Symptoms	Interventions
		that reflect alterations in fluid status (potassium, blood urea nitrogen, creatinine, calcium, hemoglobin, and hematocrit, sodium); manage underlying cause of fluid alteration; monitor urine characteristics and respiratory status; establish baseline assessment data; collaborate with physician to adjust oral and IV fluids to provide optimal hydration status; administer replacement electrolytes, as ordered; adjust diuretics, as appropriate, monitor and trend blood glucose
Tissue perfusion ***(related to inadequate fluid volume; decreased cortisol levels)***	Hypotension; dizziness; cool extremities; pallor; capillary refill greater than 3 sec in fingers and toes; weak pedal pulses; altered level of consciousness; altered sensation; urinary output less than 30 mL/hr	Monitor blood pressure; assess for dizziness; assess extremities for skin temperature, color, warmth; assess capillary refill; assess pedal pulses; monitor for numbness, tingling, hyperesthesia, hypoesthesia; monitor for deep venous thrombosis; carefully use heat and cold on affected areas; use foot cradle to keep pressure off of affected body parts; provide oxygen as required
Self-care ***(related to dizziness, fatigue, weakness, vomiting, diarrhea, anorexia)***	Difficulty fastening clothing; difficulty performing personal hygiene; inability to maintain appropriate appearance; difficulty with independent mobility	Reinforce self-care techniques as taught by occupational therapy; ensure that the patient has adequate time to perform self-care; encourage use of assistive devices to maintain independence; ask if there is any interference with lifestyle activities; assess the ability to engage in activities of daily living

A

Problem	Signs & Symptoms	Interventions
Mobility ***(related to dizziness, fatigue, weakness secondary to adrenal insufficiency and decreased cortisol levels)***	Weakness, muscle wasting, pain in muscles and joints, decreased endurance, activity intolerance, difficult purposeful movement, reluctance to attempt to engage in activity	Provide assistance with mobility with encouraged use of assistive devices; assess emotional response to limited mobility; assess willingness to participate in activity; assess environment of safety concerns; assess the ability to engage in activities of daily living; encourage early mobility to retain as much independent function as possible; allow sufficient time to perform tasks without being rushed; assess nutritional intake

PRETEST:

- Positively identify the patient using at least two person-specific identifiers before services, treatments, or procedures are performed.
- *Patient teaching:* Inform the patient this test evaluates dehydration and can assist in identification of the causes of muscle weakness or high blood pressure.
- Obtain a history of the patient's health concerns, symptoms, surgical procedures, and results of previously performed laboratory and diagnostic studies. Include a list of known allergens, especially allergies or sensitivities to latex.
- Obtain a history of known or suspected fluid or electrolyte imbalance, hypertension, renal function, or stage of pregnancy. Note the amount of sodium ingested in the diet over the past 2 wk.
- Note any recent procedures that can interfere with test results.
- Obtain a list of the patient's current medications, including over-the-counter medications and dietary supplements (see Effects of Natural Products on Laboratory Values online at Davis*Plus*).
- Review the procedure with the patient. Inform the patient that specimen collection takes approximately 5 to 10 min. Inform the patient that multiple specimens may be required. Address concerns about pain, and explain that there may be some discomfort during the venipuncture. Aldosterone levels may also be collected directly from the left and right adrenal veins. This procedure is performed by a radiologist via catheterization and takes approximately 1 hr.
- ***Sensitivity to social and cultural issues,*** as well as concern for modesty, is important in providing psychological support before, during, and after the procedure.
- Inform the patient that the required position, supine/lying down or upright/sitting up, must be maintained for 2 hr before specimen collection.
- Prescribe the patient a normal-sodium diet (1 to 2 g of sodium per day) 🍁 2 to 4 wk before the test. Protocols may vary among facilities.
- Under medical direction, the patient should avoid diuretics, antihypertensive drugs and herbals, and cyclic progestogens and estrogens for 2 to 4 wk before the test. The patient should also be advised to avoid consuming anything that contains licorice for 2 wk before the test. Licorice inhibits short-chain dehydrogenase/

reductase enzymes. These enzymes normally prevent cortisol from binding to aldosterone receptor sites in the kidney. In the absence of these enzymes, cortisol acts on the kidney and triggers the same effects as aldosterone, which include increased potassium excretion, sodium retention, and water retention. Aldosterone levels are not affected by licorice ingestion, but the simultaneous measurements of electrolytes may provide misleading results.

INTRATEST:

Potential Complications: N/A

- Ensure that the patient has complied with dietary, medication, and pretesting preparations regarding activity prior to the study, as instructed.
- Avoid the use of equipment containing latex if the patient has a history of allergic reaction to latex.
- Instruct the patient to cooperate fully and to follow directions. Direct the patient to breathe normally and to avoid unnecessary movement.
- Observe standard precautions, and follow the general guidelines in Patient Preparation and Specimen Collection online at Davis*Plus*. Positively identify the patient, and label the appropriate tubes with the corresponding patient demographics, date, time of collection, patient position (upright or supine), and exact source of specimen (peripheral versus arterial). Perform a venipuncture after the patient has been in the upright (sitting or standing) position for 2 hr. If a supine specimen is requested on an inpatient, the specimen should be collected early in the morning before rising.
- Remove the needle and apply direct pressure with dry gauze to stop bleeding. Observe/assess venipuncture site for bleeding or hematoma formation and secure gauze with adhesive bandage.
- Promptly transport the specimen on ice to the laboratory for processing and analysis.

POST-TEST:

- Inform the patient that a report of the results will be made available to the requesting HCP, who will discuss the results with the patient.
- Instruct the patient to resume usual diet, medication, and activity as directed by the HCP.
- Instruct the patient to notify the HCP of any signs and symptoms of dehydration or fluid overload related to elevated aldosterone levels or compromised sodium regulatory mechanisms.
- ***Nutritional Considerations:*** Aldosterone levels are involved in the regulation of body fluid volume. Educate patients about the importance of proper water balance. Tap water may also contain other nutrients. Water-softening systems replace minerals (e.g., calcium, magnesium, iron) with sodium, so caution should be used if a low-sodium diet is prescribed.
- ***Nutritional Considerations:*** Because aldosterone levels affect sodium levels, some consideration may be given to dietary adjustment if sodium allowances need to be regulated. Educate patients with low sodium levels that the major source of dietary sodium is table salt. Many foods, such as milk and other dairy products, are also good sources of dietary sodium. Most other dietary sodium is available through consumption of processed foods; some examples are baking mixes (pancakes or muffins), sauces (barbecue), butter, canned soups and sauces, dry soup mixes, frozen or microwave meals, ketchup, pickles, and snack foods (potato chips, pretzels). Patients who need to follow low-sodium diets should avoid beverages such as colas, ginger ale, Gatorade, lemon-lime sodas, and root beer. Many over-the-counter medications, including antacids, laxatives, analgesics, sedatives, and antitussives, contain significant amounts of sodium. The best advice

is to emphasize the importance of reading all food, beverage, and medicine labels. Potassium is present in all plant and animal cells, making dietary replacement simple. An HCP or a nutritionist should be consulted before considering the use of salt substitutes. Fruits, vegetables, and meats are rich in potassium (artichokes, avocados, bananas, cantaloupe, dried fruits, kiwi, mango, meats, milk, dried beans, nuts, oranges, peaches, pears, pomegranate, potatoes, prunes, pumpkin, spinach, sunflower seeds, Swiss chard, tomatoes, and winter squash).

- Depending on the results of this procedure, additional testing may be performed to evaluate or monitor progression of the disease process and determine the need for a change in therapy. Evaluate test results in relation to the patient's symptoms and other tests performed.

Patient Education:

- Reinforce information given by the patient's HCP regarding further testing, treatment, or referral to another HCP.
- Answer any questions or address any concerns voiced by the patient and/or family.
- Teach the patient to report any gastric distress or dark stools associated with prescribed medication use.

Expected Patient Outcomes:

Understanding

- The patient and family state the importance of taking prescribed medication regularly.
- The patient and family state that medication will need to be taken continuously for the rest of the patient's life.

Ability

- The patient and family identify diet selections that are lower in potassium and higher in sodium and protein.

Response

- The patient and family comply with medication regime with the understanding that sudden cessation is dangerous.
- The patient and family comply with the request to report infections, or stressors, to HCP for medication adjustments.
- The patient and family agree to weigh patient daily and record for HCP review.

RELATED STUDIES:

- Related tests include adrenal gland scan, biopsy kidney, BUN, catecholamines, cortisol, creatinine, glucose, magnesium, osmolality, potassium, protein urine, renin, sodium, and UA.
- See the Endocrine and Genitourinary systems tables online at Davis*Plus* for related tests by body system.

Alkaline Phosphatase and Isoenzymes

SYNONYM/ACRONYM: Alk Phos, ALP and fractionation, heat-stabile ALP.

COMMON USE: To assist in the diagnosis of liver cancer and cirrhosis, or bone cancer and bone fracture.

SPECIMEN: Serum collected in a gold-, red-, or red/gray-top tube. Plasma collected in a green-top (heparin) tube is also acceptable.

NORMAL FINDINGS: (Method: Spectrophotometry for total alkaline phosphatase, inhibition/electrophoresis for fractionation)

A

Age/Gender	Total ALP Conventional & SI Units	Bone Fraction Conventional & SI Units	Liver Fraction Conventional & SI Units
0–30 d			
Male	75–375 units/L	NA	NA
Female	65–350 units/L	NA	NA
1–11 mo			
Male	70–350 units/L	NA	NA
Female	80–330 units/L	NA	NA
1–5 yr			
Male	56–350 units/L	39–308 units/L	Less than 8–101 units/L
Female	73–378 units/L	56–300 units/L	Less than 8–53 units/L
6–7 yr			
Male	70–364 units/L	50–319 units/L	Less than 8–76 units/L
Female	73–378 units/L	56–300 units/L	Less than 8–53 units/L
8 yr			
Male	70–364 units/L	50–258 units/L	Less than 8–62 units/L
Female	98–448 units/L	78–353 units/L	Less than 8–62 units/L
9–12 yr			
Male	112–476 units/L	78–339 units/L	Less than 8–81 units/L
Female	98–448 units/L	78–353 units/L	Less than 8–62 units/L
13 yr			
Male	112–476 units/L	78–389 units/L	Less than 8–48 units/L
Female	56–350 units/L	28–252 units/L	Less than 8–50 units/L
14 yr			
Male	112–476 units/L	78–389 units/L	Less than 8–48 units/L
Female	56–266 units/L	31–190 units/L	Less than 8–48 units/L
15 yr			
Male	70–378 units/L	48–311 units/L	Less than 8–39 units/L
Female	42–168 units/L	20–115 units/L	Less than 8–53 units/L
16 yr			
Male	70–378 units/L	48–311 units/L	Less than 8–39 units/L
Female	28–126 units/L	14–87 units/L	Less than 8–50 units/L
17 yr			
Male	56–238 units/L	34–190 units/L	Less than 8–39 units/L
Female	28–126 units/L	17–84 units/L	Less than 8–53 units/L
18 yr			
Male	56–182 units/L	34–146 units/L	Less than 8–39 units/L
Female	28–126 units/L	17–84 units/L	Less than 8–53 units/L
19 yr			
Male	42–154 units/L	25–123 units/L	Less than 8–39 units/L
Female	28–126 units/L	17–84 units/L	Less than 8–53 units/L
20 yr			
Male	45–138 units/L	25–73 units/L	Less than 8–48 units/L
Female	33–118 units/L	17–56 units/L	Less than 8–50 units/L
21 yr and older			
Male	35–142 units/L	11–73 units/L	0–93 units/L
Female	25–125 units/L	11–73 units/L	0–93 units/L

Values may be slightly elevated in older adults.

DESCRIPTION: Alkaline phosphatase (ALP) is an enzyme found in the liver; in Kupffer cells lining the biliary tract; and in bones, intestines, and placenta. Additional sources of ALP include the proximal tubules of the kidneys, pulmonary alveolar cells, germ cells, vascular bed, lactating mammary glands, and granulocytes of circulating blood. ALP is referred to as alkaline because it functions optimally at a pH of 9. This test is most useful for determining the presence of liver or bone disease.

Isoelectric focusing methods can identify 12 isoenzymes of ALP. Certain cancers produce small amounts of distinctive Regan and Nagao ALP isoenzymes. Elevations in three main ALP isoenzymes, however, are of clinical significance: ALP_1 of liver origin, ALP_2 of bone origin, and ALP_3 of intestinal origin (normal elevations are present in Lewis antibody–positive individuals with blood types O and B). ALP levels vary by age and gender. Values in children are higher than in adults because of the level of bone growth and development. An immunoassay method is available for measuring bone-specific ALP as an indicator of increased bone turnover and estrogen deficiency in postmenopausal women.

This procedure is contraindicated for: N/A

INDICATIONS

- Evaluate signs and symptoms of various disorders associated with elevated ALP levels, such as biliary obstruction, hepatobiliary disease, and bone disease, including malignant processes.
- Differentiate obstructive hepatobiliary tract disorders from hepatocellular disease; greater elevations of ALP are seen in the former.
- Determine effects of kidney disease on bone metabolism.
- Determine bone growth or destruction in children with abnormal growth patterns.

POTENTIAL MEDICAL DIAGNOSIS

Increased in:

Related to release of alkaline phosphatase from damaged bone, biliary tract, and liver cells.

Liver disease:

- Biliary atresia
- Biliary obstruction (acute cholecystitis, cholelithiasis, intrahepatic cholestasis of pregnancy, primary biliary cirrhosis)
- Cancer
- Chronic active hepatitis
- Cirrhosis
- Diabetes (diabetic hepatic lipidosis)
- Extrahepatic duct obstruction
- Granulomatous or infiltrative liver diseases (sarcoidosis, amyloidosis, tuberculosis)
- Infectious mononucleosis
- Intrahepatic biliary hypoplasia
- Toxic hepatitis
- Viral hepatitis

Bone disease:

- Healing fractures
- Metabolic bone diseases (rickets, osteomalacia)
- Metastatic tumors in bone
- Osteogenic sarcoma
- Osteoporosis
- Paget's disease (osteitis deformans)

Other conditions:

- Advanced pregnancy ***(related to additional sources: placental tissue and new fetal bone growth; marked decline is seen with***

placental insufficiency and imminent fetal demise)
- Cancer of the breast, colon, gallbladder, lung, or pancreas
- Familial hyperphosphatemia
- Heart failure
- HELLP syndrome of pregnancy (hemolysis, elevated liver enzymes, low platelet count)
- Hyperparathyroidism
- Perforated bowel
- Pneumonia
- Pulmonary and myocardial infarctions
- Pulmonary embolism
- Ulcerative colitis

Decreased in:
- Anemia (severe)
- Celiac disease
- Folic acid deficiency
- HIV-1 infection
- Hypervitaminosis D
- Hypophosphatasia ***(related to insufficient phosphorus source for ALP production; congenital and rare)***
- Hypothyroidism (characteristic in infantile and juvenile cases)
- Nutritional deficiency of zinc or magnesium
- Pernicious anemia
- Scurvy ***(related to vitamin C deficiency)***
- Whipple's disease
- Zollinger-Ellison syndrome

CRITICAL FINDINGS: N/A

INTERFERING FACTORS
- Drugs and other substances that may increase ALP levels by causing cholestasis include anabolic steroids, erythromycin, ethionamide, gold salts, imipramine, interleukin-2, isocarboxazid, nitrofurans, oral contraceptives, phenothiazines, sulfonamides, and tolbutamide.
- Drugs and other substances that may increase ALP levels by causing hepatocellular damage include acetaminophen (toxic), amiodarone, anticonvulsants, arsenicals, asparaginase, bromocriptine, captopril, cephalosporins, chloramphenicol, enflurane, ethionamide, foscarnet, gentamicin, indomethacin, lincomycin, methyldopa, naproxen, nitrofurans, probenecid, procainamide, progesterone, ranitidine, tobramycin, tolcapone, and verapamil.
- Drugs and other substances that may cause an overall decrease in ALP levels include alendronate, azathioprine, calcitriol, clofibrate, estrogens with estrogen replacement therapy, and ursodiol.
- Hemolyzed specimens may cause falsely elevated results.
- Elevations of ALP may occur if the patient is nonfasting, usually 2 to 4 hr after a fatty meal, and especially if the patient is a Lewis-positive secretor of blood group B or O.

NURSING IMPLICATIONS AND PROCEDURE

PRETEST:
- Positively identify the patient using at least two person-specific identifiers before services, treatments, or procedures are performed.
- ***Patient teaching:*** Inform the patient this test can assist with determining the presence of liver or bone disease.
- Obtain a history of the patient's health concerns, symptoms, surgical procedures, and results of previously performed laboratory and diagnostic studies. Include a list of known allergens, especially allergies or sensitivities to latex.
- Obtain a list of the patient's current medications, including over-the-counter medications and dietary

supplements (see Effects of Natural Products on Laboratory Values online at Davis*Plus*).

- Review the procedure with the patient. Inform the patient that specimen collection takes approximately 5 to 10 min. Address concerns about pain and explain that there may be some discomfort during the venipuncture.
- ***Sensitivity to social and cultural issues,*** as well as concern for modesty, is important in providing psychological support before, during, and after the procedure.
- Note that there are no food, fluid, or medication restrictions unless by medical direction.

INTRATEST:

Potential Complications: N/A

- Avoid the use of equipment containing latex if the patient has a history of allergic reaction to latex.
- Instruct the patient to cooperate fully and to follow directions. Direct the patient to breathe normally and to avoid unnecessary movement.
- Observe standard precautions, and follow the general guidelines in Patient Preparation and Specimen Collection online at Davis*Plus*. Positively identify the patient, and label the appropriate specimen container with the corresponding patient demographics, initials of the person collecting the specimen, date, and time of collection. Perform a venipuncture.
- Remove the needle and apply direct pressure with dry gauze to stop bleeding. Observe/assess venipuncture site for bleeding and hematoma formation and secure gauze with adhesive bandage.
- Promptly transport the specimen to the laboratory for processing and analysis.

POST-TEST:

- Inform the patient that a report of the results will be made available to the requesting health-care provider (HCP), who will discuss the results with the patient.
- ***Nutritional Considerations:*** Increased ALP levels may be associated with liver disease. Dietary recommendations may be indicated and vary depending on the severity of the condition. A low-protein diet may be in order if the patient's liver has lost the ability to process the end products of protein metabolism. A diet of soft foods may be required if esophageal varices have developed. Ammonia levels may be used to determine whether protein should be added to or reduced from the diet. Patients should be encouraged to eat simple carbohydrates and emulsified fats (as in homogenized milk or eggs) rather than complex carbohydrates (e.g., starch, fiber, and glycogen [animal carbohydrates]) and complex fats, which require additional bile to emulsify them so that they can be used. The cirrhotic patient should be carefully observed for the development of ascites, in which case fluid and electrolyte balance requires strict attention.
- Reinforce information given by the patient's HCP regarding further testing, treatment, or referral to another HCP. Answer any questions or address any concerns voiced by the patient or family.
- Depending on the results of this procedure, additional testing may be performed to evaluate or monitor progression of the disease process and determine the need for a change in therapy. Evaluate test results in relation to the patient's symptoms and other tests performed.

RELATED STUDIES:

- Related tests include acetaminophen, ALT, albumin, ammonia, anti-DNA antibodies, AMA/ASMA, ANA, α_1-antitrypsin, α_1-antitrypsin phenotyping, AST, bilirubin, biopsy

A

bone, biopsy liver, bone scan, BMD, calcium (total and ionized), ceruloplasmin, collagen cross-linked telopeptides, C3 and C4, copper, ERCP, GGT, hepatitis antigens and antibodies, hepatobiliary scan, KUB studies, magnesium, MRI abdomen, MRI venography, osteocalcin, PTH, phosphorus, potassium, protein, protein electrophoresis, PT/INR, salicylate, sodium, US abdomen, US liver, vitamin D, and zinc.

- See the Hepatobiliary and Musculoskeletal systems tables online at Davis*Plus* for related tests by body system.

Allergen-Specific Immunoglobulin E

SYNONYM/ACRONYM: Allergen profile, radioallergosorbent test (RAST), ImmunoCAP Specific immunoglobulin E (IgE).

COMMON USE: To assist in identifying environmental allergens responsible for causing allergic reactions.

SPECIMEN: Serum collected in a gold-, red-, or red/gray-top tube.

NORMAL FINDINGS: (Method: Radioimmunoassay or fluorescence enzyme immunoassay [FEIA])

RAST Scoring Method (Radioimmunoassay) and ImmunoCAP Scoring Guide (FEIA)	Conventional and SI Units Allergen-Specific IgE
Specific IgE Allergen Antibody Level	kU/L
Absent or undetectable allergy	Less than 0.35
Low allergy	0.35–0.7
Moderate allergy	0.71–3.5
High allergy	3.51–17.5
Very high allergy	17.6–50
Very high allergy	51–100
Very high allergy	Greater than 100

DESCRIPTION: Allergen-specific IgE is generally requested for groups of allergens commonly known to incite an allergic response in the affected individual. The test is based on the use of a radiolabelled or non-radiolabelled anti-IgE reagent to detect IgE in the patient's serum, produced in response to specific allergens. The panels include allergens such as animal dander, antibiotics, dust, foods, grasses, insects, trees, mites, molds, venom, and weeds. Allergen testing is useful for evaluating the cause of hay fever, extrinsic asthma, atopic eczema, respiratory allergies, and potentially fatal reactions to insect venom, penicillin, and other drugs or chemicals. RAST and radiolabelled or non-radiolabelled methods are alternatives to skin test anergy and provocation procedures, which can be inconvenient, painful, and potentially hazardous to patients. ImmunoCAP FEIA is a nonradioactive technology with minimal interference from nonspecific binding to total IgE versus allergen-specific IgE.

A nasal smear can be examined for the presence of eosinophils to screen for allergic conditions. Either a single smear or smears of nasal secretions from each side of the nose should be submitted, at room temperature, for Hansel staining and evaluation. Normal findings vary by laboratory but generally, greater than 10% to 15% is considered eosinophilia, or increased presence of eosinophils. Results may be invalid for patients already taking local or systemic corticosteroids.

This procedure is contraindicated for: N/A

INDICATIONS

- Evaluate patients who refuse to submit to skin testing or who have generalized dermatitis or other dermatopathic conditions.
- Monitor response to desensitization procedures.
- Test for allergens when skin testing is inappropriate, such as in infants.
- Test for allergens when there is a known history of allergic reaction to skin testing.
- Test for specific allergic sensitivity before initiating immunotherapy or desensitization shots.
- Test for specific allergic sensitivity when skin testing is unreliable (patients taking long-acting antihistamines may have false-negative skin test).

POTENTIAL MEDICAL DIAGNOSIS

Different scoring systems are used in the interpretation of RAST results.

Increased in:

Related to production of IgE, the antibody that primarily responds to conditions that stimulate an allergic response

- Allergic rhinitis
- Anaphylaxis
- Asthma (exogenous)
- Atopic dermatitis
- *Echinococcus* infection
- Eczema
- Hay fever
- Hookworm infection
- Latex allergy
- Schistosomiasis
- Visceral larva migrans

Decreased in:

- Asthma (endogenous)
- Pregnancy
- Radiation therapy

CRITICAL FINDINGS: N/A

INTERFERING FACTORS

- Recent radioactive scans or radiation within 1 wk of the test can interfere with test results when radioimmunoassay is the test method.

NURSING IMPLICATIONS AND PROCEDURE

PRETEST:

- Positively identify the patient using at least two person-specific identifiers before services, treatments, or procedures are performed.
- ***Patient teaching:*** Inform the patient this test can assist in identification of causal factors related to allergic reaction.
- Obtain a history of the patient's health concerns, symptoms, surgical procedures, and results of previously

performed laboratory and diagnostic studies. Include a list of known allergens, especially allergies or sensitivities to latex.

- Note any recent procedures that can interfere with test results.
- Obtain a list of the patient's current medications, including over-the-counter medications and dietary supplements (see Effects of Natural Products on Laboratory Values online at Davis*Plus*).
- Review the procedure with the patient. Inform the patient that specimen collection takes approximately 5 to 10 min. Address concerns about pain and explain that there may be some discomfort during the venipuncture.
- Note that there are no food, fluid, or medication restrictions unless by medical direction.

INTRATEST:

Potential Complications: N/A

- Avoid the use of equipment containing latex if the patient has a history of allergic reaction to latex.
- Instruct the patient to cooperate fully and to follow directions. Direct the patient to breathe normally and to avoid unnecessary movement.
- Observe standard precautions, and follow the general guidelines in Patient Preparation and Specimen Collection online at Davis*Plus*. Positively identify the patient, and label the appropriate specimen container with the corresponding patient demographics, initials of the person collecting the specimen, date, and time of collection. Inform the laboratory of the specific allergen group to be tested. Perform a venipuncture.
- Remove the needle and apply direct pressure with dry gauze to stop bleeding. Observe/assess venipuncture site for bleeding and hematoma formation and secure gauze with adhesive bandage.
- Promptly transport the specimen to the laboratory for processing and analysis.

POST-TEST:

- Inform the patient that a report of the results will be made available to the requesting health-care provider (HCP), who will discuss the results with the patient.
- ***Nutritional Considerations:*** Should be given to diet if food allergies are present. Lifestyle adjustments may be necessary depending on the specific allergens identified.
- Recognize anxiety related to test results. Administer allergy treatment if ordered. As appropriate, educate the patient in the proper technique for administering his or her own treatments as well as safe handling and maintenance of treatment materials. Treatments may include eye drops, inhalers, nasal sprays, oral medications, or shots. Remind the patient of the importance of avoiding triggers and of complying with the recommended therapy, even if signs and symptoms disappear.
- Reinforce information given by the patient's HCP regarding further testing, treatment, or referral to another HCP. Answer any questions or address any concerns voiced by the patient or family.
- Depending on the results of this procedure, additional testing may be performed to evaluate or monitor progression of the disease process and determine the need for a change in therapy. Evaluate test results in relation to the patient's symptoms and other tests performed.

RELATED STUDIES:

- Related tests include arterial/alveolar oxygen ratio, blood gases, CBC, eosinophil count, fecal analysis, hypersensitivity pneumonitis, IgE, and PFT.
- See the Immune and Respiratory systems tables online at Davis*Plus* for related tests by body system.

Alveolar/Arterial Gradient and Arterial/Alveolar Oxygen Ratio

A

SYNONYM/ACRONYM: Alveolar-arterial difference, A/a gradient, a/A ratio.

COMMON USE: To assist in assessing oxygen delivery and diagnosing causes of hypoxemia such as pulmonary edema, acute respiratory distress syndrome, and pulmonary fibrosis.

SPECIMEN: Arterial blood collected in a heparinized syringe. Specimen should be transported tightly capped and in an ice slurry.

NORMAL FINDINGS: (Method: Selective electrodes that measure Po_2 and Pco_2)

Alveolar/arterial gradient	Less than 10 mm Hg at rest (room air) 20–30 mm Hg at maximum exercise activity (room air)
Arterial/alveolar oxygen ratio	Greater than 0.75 (75%)

POTENTIAL MEDICAL DIAGNOSIS

Increased in:

- Acute respiratory distress syndrome (ARDS) ***(related to thickened edematous alveoli)***
- Atelectasis ***(related to mixing oxygenated and unoxygenated blood)***
- Arterial-venous shunts ***(related to mixing oxygenated and unoxygenated blood)***
- Bronchospasm ***(related to decrease in the diameter of the airway)***
- Chronic obstructive pulmonary disease ***(related to decrease in the elasticity of lung tissue)***
- Congenital cardiac septal defects ***(related to mixing oxygenated and unoxygenated blood)***
- Underventilated alveoli ***(related to mucus plugs)***
- Pneumothorax ***(related to collapsed lung, shunted air, and subsequent decrease in arterial oxygen levels)***
- Pulmonary edema ***(related to thickened edematous alveoli)***
- Pulmonary embolus ***(related to obstruction of blood flow to alveoli)***
- Pulmonary fibrosis ***(related to thickened edematous alveoli)***

CRITICAL FINDINGS: N/A

Find and print out the full study on Fast Find at davispl.us/vanleeuwen7.

Alzheimer's Disease Markers

A

SYNONYM/ACRONYM: CSF tau protein and β-amyloid-42, AD, APP, PS-1, PS-2, Apo E4.

COMMON USE: To assist in diagnosing Alzheimer's disease and monitoring the effectiveness of therapy.

SPECIMEN: Cerebrospinal fluid (CSF) collected in a plain plastic conical tube for tau protein and β-amyloid-42; whole blood from one full lavender-top (EDTA) tube for apolipoprotein E4 (ApoE4) genotyping, β-amyloid precursor protein, presenilin 1, and presenilin 2.

NORMAL FINDINGS: (Method: Enzyme-linked immunosorbent assay) Simultaneous tau protein and β-amyloid-42 measurements in CSF are used in conjunction with detection of apolipoprotein E4 alleles (restriction fragment length polymorphism) and identification of mutations in the β-amyloid precursor protein (APP), presenilin 1 (PS-1) and presenilin 2 (PS-2) genes (polymerase chain reaction and DNA sequencing) as biochemical and genetic markers of Alzheimer's disease (AD). Scientific studies indicate that a combination of elevated tau protein and decreased β-amyloid-42 protein levels are consistent with the presence of AD. The testing laboratory should be consulted for interpretation of results.

POTENTIAL MEDICAL DIAGNOSIS

Increased in:

Tau protein is increased in AD.

Presence of ApoE4 alleles is a genetic risk factor for AD.

Identification of mutations in the APP, PS-1, and PS-2 genes is associated with forms of AD.

Decreased in:

β-Amyloid-42 is decreased in up to 50% of healthy control participants.

- β-Amyloid-42 is decreased in AD ***(related to accumulation in the brain with a corresponding decrease in CSF).***
- β-Amyloid-42 is decreased in Creutzfeldt-Jakob disease.

CRITICAL FINDINGS: N/A

Find and print out the full study on Fast Find at davispl.us/vanleeuwen7.

Amino Acid Screen, Blood

SYNONYM/ACRONYM: N/A

COMMON USE: To assist in diagnosing congenital metabolic disorders in infants, typically homocystinuria, maple syrup urine disease, phenylketonuria (PKU), tyrosinuria, and unexplained mental retardation.

SPECIMEN: Plasma collected in a green-top (heparin) tube.

NORMAL FINDINGS: (Method: Liquid chromatography/mass spectrometry) There are numerous amino acids. Values vary, and the testing laboratory should be consulted for corresponding ranges.

POTENTIAL MEDICAL DIAGNOSIS

Increased in:

Increased amino acid accumulation (total amino acids) occurs when a specific enzyme deficiency prevents its catabolism, with liver disease, or when there is impaired clearance by the kidneys:

- Acute kidney injury ***(related to impaired clearance)***
- Aminoacidopathies ***(usually related to an inherited disorder; specific amino acids are implicated)***
- Burns ***(related to increased protein turnover)***
- Chronic kidney disease ***(related to impaired clearance)***
- Diabetes ***(related to gluconeogenesis, where protein is broken down as a means to generate glucose)***
- Fructose intolerance ***(related to hereditary enzyme deficiency)***
- Malabsorption ***(related to lack of transport and opportunity for catabolism)***
- Reye's syndrome ***(related to liver damage)***
- Severe liver damage ***(related to decreased production of amino acids by the liver)***
- Shock ***(related to increased protein turnover from tissue death and decreased deamination due to impaired liver function)***

Decreased in:

Decreased (total amino acids) in conditions that result in increased renal excretion or insufficient protein intake or synthesis:

- Adrenocortical hyperfunction ***(related to excess cortisol, which assists in conversion of amino acids into glucose)***
- Carcinoid syndrome ***(related to increased consumption of amino acids, especially tryptophan, to form serotonin)***
- Fever ***(related to increased consumption)***
- Glomerulonephritis ***(related to increased renal excretion)***
- Hartnup's disease ***(related to increased renal excretion)***
- Huntington's chorea ***(related to increased consumption due to muscle tremors; possible insufficient intake)***
- Malnutrition ***(related to insufficient intake)***
- Nephrotic syndrome ***(related to increased renal excretion)***
- Pancreatitis (acute) ***(related to increased consumption as part of the inflammatory process and increased ureagenesis)***
- Polycystic kidney disease ***(related to increased renal excretion)***
- Rheumatoid arthritis ***(related to insufficient intake evidenced by lack of appetite)***

CRITICAL FINDINGS: N/A

Find and print out the full study on Fast Find at davispl.us/vanleeuwen7.

Amino Acid Screen, Urine

SYNONYM/ACRONYM: N/A

COMMON USE: To assist in diagnosing congenital metabolic disorders in infants, typically homocystinuria, maple syrup urine disease, phenylketonuria (PKU), tyrosinuria, and unexplained mental retardation.

SPECIMEN: Urine from a random or timed specimen collected in a clean plastic collection container with hydrochloric acid as a preservative.

NORMAL FINDINGS: (Method: Chromatography) There are numerous amino acids. Values vary, and the testing laboratory should be consulted for corresponding ranges.

POTENTIAL MEDICAL DIAGNOSIS

Increased in:

Increased amino acid accumulation (total amino acids) occurs when a specific enzyme deficiency prevents its catabolism or when there is impaired clearance by the kidneys:

- Primary causes ***(inherited):***
  - Aminoaciduria (specific)
  - Cystinosis ***(may be masked because of decreased glomerular filtration rate, so values may be in normal range)***
  - Fanconi's syndrome
  - Fructose intolerance
  - Galactosemia
  - Hartnup's disease
  - Lactose intolerance
  - Lowe's syndrome
  - Maple syrup urine disease
  - Tyrosinemia type I
  - Tyrosinosis
  - Wilson's disease
- Secondary causes ***(noninherited):***
  - Acute leukemia
  - Chronic kidney disease ***(reduced glomerular filtration rate)***
  - Diabetic ketoacidosis
  - Epilepsy ***(transient increase related to disturbed renal function during grand mal seizure)***
  - Folic acid deficiency
  - Hyperparathyroidism
  - Liver necrosis and cirrhosis
  - Multiple myeloma
  - Muscular dystrophy (progressive)
  - Osteomalacia ***(secondary to parathyroid hormone excess)***
  - Pernicious anemia
  - Thalassemia major
  - Vitamin deficiency ***(B, C, and D; vitamin D–deficiency rickets, vitamin D–resistant rickets)***
  - Viral hepatitis ***(related to the degree of hepatic involvement)***

Decreased in: N/A

CRITICAL FINDINGS: N/A

Find and print out the full study on Fast Find at davispl.us/vanleeuwen7.

δ-Aminolevulinic Acid

SYNONYM/ACRONYM: δ-ALA.

COMMON USE: To assist in diagnosing lead poisoning in children, or porphyria, a disorder that disrupts heme synthesis, primarily affecting the liver.

SPECIMEN: Urine from a timed specimen collected in a dark plastic container with glacial acetic acid as a preservative.

NORMAL FINDINGS: (Method: Spectrophotometry)

Conventional Units	SI Units (Conventional Units × 7.626)
1.5–7.5 mg/24 hr	11.4–57.2 micromol/24 hr

POTENTIAL MEDICAL DIAGNOSIS

Increased in:

Related to inhibition of the enzymes involved in porphyrin synthesis; results in accumulation of δ-ALA and is evidenced by exposure to medications, toxins, diet, or infection that can precipitate an attack

- Acute porphyrias
- Aminolevulinic acid dehydrase deficiency ***(related to the inability to convert δ-ALA to porphobilinogen, leading to accumulation of δ-ALA)***
- Hereditary tyrosinemia
- Lead poisoning

Decreased in: N/A

CRITICAL FINDINGS: N/A

Signs and symptoms of an acute porphyria attack include pain (commonly in the abdomen, arms, and legs), nausea, vomiting, muscle weakness, rapid pulse, and high blood pressure. Possible interventions include medication for pain, nausea, and vomiting and, if indicated, respiratory support. Initial treatment following a moderate to severe attack may include identification and cessation of harmful drugs the patient may be taking, intravenous (IV) infusion of carbohydrates, and IV heme therapy (hematin, heme arginate) if indicated by markedly elevated urine δ-ALA and porphyrins.

Find and print out the full study on Fast Find at davispl.us/vanleeuwen7.

Ammonia

SYNONYM/ACRONYM: NH_3.

COMMON USE: To assist in diagnosing liver disease such as hepatitis and cirrhosis and evaluating the effectiveness of treatment modalities. Also used to assist in diagnosing infant Reye's syndrome.

A

SPECIMEN: Plasma collected in completely filled lavender- (EDTA) or green-top (Na or Li heparin) tube. Specimen should be transported tightly capped and in an ice slurry.

NORMAL FINDINGS: (Method: Enzymatic)

Age	Conventional Units	SI Units (Conventional Units × 0.587)
Newborn	170–340 mcg/dL	90–150 micromol/L
10 d–24 mo	70–135 mcg/dL	41–80 micromol/L
25 mo–Adult	15–60 mcg/dL	9–35 micromol/L

DESCRIPTION: Blood ammonia (NH_3) comes from two sources: deamination of amino acids during protein metabolism and degradation of proteins by colon bacteria. The liver converts ammonia in the portal blood to urea, which is excreted by the kidneys. When liver function is severely compromised, especially in situations in which decreased hepatocellular function is combined with impaired portal blood flow, ammonia levels rise. Congenital enzyme defects that prevent the breakdown of ammonia or conditions that affect the ability of the kidneys to excrete ammonia can also result in increased blood levels. Ammonia is potentially toxic to the central nervous system and may result in encephalopathy or coma if toxic levels are reached.

This procedure is contraindicated for: N/A

INDICATIONS

- Evaluate advanced liver disease or other disorders associated with altered serum ammonia levels.
- Identify impending hepatic encephalopathy with known liver disease.
- Monitor the effectiveness of treatment for hepatic encephalopathy, indicated by declining levels.
- Monitor patients receiving hyperalimentation therapy.

POTENTIAL MEDICAL DIAGNOSIS

Increased in:

- Gastrointestinal hemorrhage ***(related to decreased blood volume, which prevents ammonia from reaching the liver to be metabolized)***
- Genitourinary tract infection with distention and stasis ***(related to decreased renal excretion; levels accumulate in the blood)***
- Hepatic coma ***(related to insufficient functioning liver cells to metabolize ammonia; levels accumulate in the blood)***
- Inborn enzyme deficiency ***(evidenced by inability to metabolize ammonia)***
- Liver failure, late cirrhosis ***(related to insufficient functioning liver cells to metabolize ammonia)***
- Reye's syndrome ***(related to insufficient functioning liver cells to metabolize ammonia)***
- Total parenteral nutrition ***(related to ammonia generated from protein metabolism)***

Decreased in: N/A

CRITICAL FINDINGS: N/A

A

INTERFERING FACTORS

- Drugs and other substances that may increase ammonia levels include asparaginase, chlorothiazide, chlorthalidone, fibrin hydrolysate, furosemide, isoniazid, levoglutamide, mercurial diuretics, oral resins, thiazides, and valproic acid.
- Drugs/organisms and other substances that may decrease ammonia levels include diphenhydramine, kanamycin, monoamine oxidase inhibitors, neomycin, tetracycline, and *Lactobacillus acidophilus*.
- Hemolysis falsely increases ammonia levels because intracellular ammonia levels are three times higher than plasma.
- Prompt and proper specimen processing, storage, and analysis are important to achieve accurate results. The specimen should be collected on ice; the collection tube should be filled completely and then kept tightly stoppered. Ammonia increases rapidly in the collected specimen, so analysis should be performed within 20 min of collection.

NURSING IMPLICATIONS AND PROCEDURE

POTENTIAL NURSING PROBLEMS:

Problem	Signs & Symptoms	Interventions
Confusion ***(related to an alteration in fluid and electrolytes, hepatic disease and encephalopathy; acute alcohol consumption; hepatic metabolic insufficiency)***	Disorganized thinking; restlessness; irritability; altered concentration and attention span; changeable mental function over the day; hallucinations; inability to follow directions; disoriented to person, place, time, and purpose; inappropriate affect	Treat the medical condition; correlate confusion with the need to reverse altered electrolytes; evaluate medications; prevent falls and injury through use of postural support, bed alarm, or the appropriate use of restraints; consider pharmacological interventions; track accurate intake and output to assess fluid status; monitor blood ammonia level; determine last alcohol use; assess for symptoms of hepatic encephalopathy such as confusion, sleep disturbances, incoherence; protect the patient from physical harm; administer lactose as prescribed
Nutrition ***(related to excess alcohol intake; insufficient eating habits; altered liver function)***	Known inadequate caloric intake; weight loss; muscle wasting in arms and legs; stool that is pale or gray colored; skin that is flaky with loss of elasticity	Document food intake with possible calorie count; assess barriers to eating; consider using a food diary; monitor continued alcohol use, as it is a barrier to adequate protein nutrition; monitor glucose levels; monitor daily weight; perform dietary consult with assessment of cultural food selections

(table continues on page 50)

A

Problem	Signs & Symptoms	Interventions
Skin ***(related to jaundice and elevated bilirubin levels; excessive scratching)***	Jaundiced skin and sclera; dry skin; itching skin; damage to skin associated with scratching	Apply lotion to keep the skin moisturized; avoid alkaline soaps; discourage scratching; apply mittens if patient is unable to follow direction to avid scratching; administer antihistamines as ordered
Bleeding ***(related to alerted clotting factors; portal hypertension; esophageal bleeding)***	Altered level of consciousness; hypotension; increased heart rate; decreased Hgb and Hct; capillary refill greater than 3 sec; cool extremities	Increase frequency of vital sign assessment with variances in results; monitor for vital sign trends; administer blood or blood products as ordered; administer stool softeners as needed; encourage intake of foods rich in vitamin K; avoid foods that may irritate esophagus

PRETEST:

- Positively identify the patient using at least two person-specific identifiers before services, treatments, or procedures are performed.
- ***Patient teaching:*** Inform the patient this test can assist with the evaluation of liver function related to processing protein waste. May be used to assist in diagnosis of Reye's syndrome in infants.
- Obtain a history of the patient's health concerns, symptoms, surgical procedures, and results of previously performed laboratory and diagnostic studies. Include a list of known allergens, especially allergies or sensitivities to latex.
- Obtain a list of the patient's current medications, including over-the-counter medications and dietary supplements (see Effects of Natural Products on Laboratory Values online at Davis*Plus*).
- Review the procedure with the patient. Inform the patient that specimen collection takes approximately 5 to 10 min. Address concerns about pain and explain that there may be some discomfort during the venipuncture.
- ***Sensitivity to social and cultural issues,*** as well as concern for modesty, is important in providing psychological support before, during, and after the procedure.
- Note that there are no food, fluid, or medication restrictions unless by medical direction.

INTRATEST:

Potential Complications: N/A

- Avoid the use of equipment containing latex if the patient has a history of allergic reaction to latex.
- Instruct the patient to cooperate fully and to follow directions. Direct the patient to breathe normally and to avoid unnecessary movement.
- Observe standard precautions, and follow the general guidelines in Patient Preparation and Specimen Collection online at Davis*Plus*. Positively identify the patient, and label the appropriate specimen container with the corresponding patient demographics, initials of the person collecting the specimen, date, and time of collection. Perform a venipuncture.
- Remove the needle and apply direct pressure with dry gauze to stop bleeding. Observe/assess the venipuncture site for bleeding or hematoma formation and secure the gauze with adhesive bandage.

- Promptly transport the specimen to the laboratory for processing and analysis. The tightly capped sample should be placed in an ice slurry immediately after collection. Information on the specimen label should be protected from water in the ice slurry by first placing the specimen in a protective plastic bag.

POST-TEST:

- Inform the patient that a report of the results will be made available to the requesting health-care provider (HCP), who will discuss the results with the patient.
- *Sensitivity to social and cultural issues,* as well as concern for modesty, is important in providing psychological support before, during, and after the procedure. Recognize anxiety related to test results, and carefully observe the cirrhotic patient for the development of ascites, in which case fluid and electrolyte balance require strict attention. Dietary and fluid restrictions may be required; diuretics may be ordered. The patient should be frequently monitored for weight gain, intake and output, and abdominal girth. Patients who are alcoholics should be encouraged to avoid alcohol and also to seek appropriate counseling.
- *Nutritional Considerations:* Increased ammonia levels may be associated with liver disease. Dietary recommendations may be indicated, depending on the severity of the condition. A low-protein diet may be in order if the patient's liver has lost the ability to process the end products of protein metabolism. A diet of soft foods may be required if esophageal varices have developed. Ammonia levels may be used to determine whether protein should be added to or reduced from the diet. Patients should be encouraged to eat simple carbohydrates and emulsified fats (as in homogenized milk or eggs) rather than complex carbohydrates (e.g., starch, fiber, and glycogen [animal carbohydrates]) and complex fats, which would require additional bile to emulsify them so that they could be used.
- Depending on the results of this procedure, additional testing may be performed to evaluate or monitor progression of the disease process and determine the need for a change in therapy. Evaluate test results in relation to the patient's symptoms and other tests performed.

Patient Education:

- Reinforce information given by the patient's HCP regarding further testing, treatment, or referral to another HCP.
- Answer any questions or address any concerns voiced by the patient or family.
- Teach the patient that small frequent meals throughout the day can increase overall caloric intake and improve nutritional status.
- Teach the patient that scratching can damage the skin and precipitate an infection.

Expected Patient Outcomes:

Understanding

- The patient and family discuss that adherence to eating several small meals can improve caloric intake.
- The patient and family associate compliance with taking lactulose with decreased blood ammonia level to help prevent hepatic encephalopathy.

Ability

- The patient and family modify the diet and select foods that are appropriate for the degree of liver disease (high protein and high carbohydrate can support nutrition until liver disease prohibits these food selections).
- The patient accurately self-administers lactulose as prescribed to reduce absorption of ammonia.

Response

- The patient resolves to participate in counseling for alcohol misuse.
- The patient follows the recommendations of the HCP and family members in supporting positive health decisions.

RELATED STUDIES:

- Related tests include ALT, albumin, analgesic, anti-inflammatory and antipyretic drugs (acetaminophen and acetylsalicylic acid), anion gap, AST, bilirubin, biopsy liver, blood gases, BUN, calcium, CT biliary tract and liver, CT pelvis, cystometry, cystoscopy, EGD, electrolytes, GI blood loss scan, glucose, IVP, MRI pelvis, ketones, lactic acid, Meckel's scan, osmolality, protein, PT/INR, uric acid, and US pelvis.

- See the Gastrointestinal, Genitourinary, and Hepatobiliary systems tables online at Davis*Plus* for related tests by body system.

Amniotic Fluid Analysis and L/S Ratio

SYNONYM/ACRONYM: N/A

COMMON USE: To assist in identification of fetal gender, genetic disorders such as hemophilia and sickle cell anemia, chromosomal disorders such as Down syndrome, anatomical abnormalities such as spina bifida, and hereditary metabolic disorders such as cystic fibrosis. To assess for preterm infant fetal lung maturity to assist in evaluating for potential diagnosis of respiratory distress syndrome (RDS).

SPECIMEN: Amniotic fluid collected in a clean amber glass or plastic container.

NORMAL FINDINGS: (Method: Macroscopic observation of fluid for color and appearance, immunochemiluminometric assay [ICMA] for α_1-fetoprotein, electrophoresis for acetylcholinesterase, spectrophotometry for creatinine and bilirubin, chromatography for lecithin/sphingomyelin [L/S] ratio and phosphatidylglycerol, tissue culture for chromosome analysis, dipstick for leukocyte esterase, and automated cell counter for white blood cell count and lamellar bodies)

Test	Reference Value
Color	Colorless to pale yellow
Appearance	Clear
α_1-Fetoprotein (AFP)	Less than 2 MoM*
Acetylcholinesterase	Absent
Creatinine	1.8–4 mg/dL at term (159.1–353.6 micromol/L) (SI Units = Conventional Units × 88.4)
Bilirubin	Less than 0.075 mg/dL in early pregnancy (Less than 1.28 micromol/L) (SI Units = Conventional Units × 17.1)
	Less than 0.025 mg/dL at term (Less than 0.428 micromol/L)(SI Units = Conventional Units × 17.1)
Bilirubin ΔA_{450}	Less than 0.048 ΔOD in early pregnancy
	Less than 0.02 ΔOD at term
L/S ratio	
Mature (nondiabetic)	Greater than 2:1 in the presence of phosphatidyl glycerol
Borderline	1.5 to 1.9:1

Test	Reference Value
Immature	Less than 1.5:1
Phosphatidylglycerol	Present at term
Chromosome analysis	Normal karyotype
White blood cell count	None seen
Leukocyte esterase	Negative
Lamellar bodies	Findings and interpretive ranges vary depending on the type of instrument used

*MoM = Multiples of the median.

DESCRIPTION: Amniotic fluid is formed in the membranous sac that surrounds the fetus. The total volume of fluid at term is 500 to 2,500 mL. In amniocentesis, fluid is obtained by ultrasound-guided needle aspiration from the amniotic sac. This procedure is generally performed between 14 and 16 weeks' gestation for accurate interpretation of test results, but it also can be done between 26 and 35 weeks' gestation if fetal distress is suspected. Amniotic fluid is tested to identify genetic and neural tube defects, hemolytic diseases of the newborn, fetal infection, fetal renal malfunction, or maturity of the fetal lungs. Examples of genetic defects that are commonly tested for and can be identified from a sample of amniotic fluid include sickle cell anemia, cystic fibrosis, and inborn errors of metabolism. Several rapid tests are also used to differentiate amniotic fluid from other body fluids in a vaginal specimen when premature rupture of membranes (PROM) is suspected. A vaginal swab obtained from the posterior vaginal pool can be used to perform a rapid, waived procedure to aid in the assessment of PROM. Nitrazine paper impregnated with an indicator dye will produce a color change indicative of vaginal pH. Normal vaginal pH is acidic (4.5 to 6), and the color of the paper will not change. Amniotic fluid has an alkaline pH (7.1 to 7.3), and the paper will turn a blue color. False-positive results occur in the presence of semen, blood, alkaline urine, vaginal infection, or if the patient is receiving antibiotics. The amniotic fluid crystallization or Fern test is based on the observation of a fern pattern when amniotic fluid is placed on a glass slide and allowed to air dry. The fern pattern is due to the protein and sodium chloride content of the amniotic fluid. False-positive results occur in the presence of blood, urine, or cervical mucus. Both of these tests can produce false-negative results if only a small amount of fluid is leaked. The reliability of results is also significantly diminished with the passage of time (greater than 24 hr). AmniSure is an immunoassay that can be performed on a vaginal swab sample. It is a rapid test that detects placental alpha microglobulin-1 protein (PAMG-1), which is found in high concentrations in amniotic fluid. AmniSure does not demonstrate the high frequency of false-positive and false-negative results inherent with the pH and fern tests.

RDS is the most common problem encountered in the care of premature infants. RDS, also called *hyaline membrane disease,* results from a deficiency of

A

phospholipid lung surfactants. The phospholipids in surfactant are produced by specialized alveolar cells and stored in granular lamellar bodies in the lung. In normally developed lungs, surfactant coats the surface of the alveoli. Surfactant reduces the surface tension of the alveolar wall during breathing. When there is an insufficient quantity of surfactant, the alveoli are unable to expand normally and gas exchange is inhibited. Amniocentesis, a procedure by which fluid is removed from the amniotic sac, is used to assess fetal lung maturity.

Lecithin is the primary surfactant phospholipid, and it is a stabilizing factor for the alveoli. It is produced at a low but constant rate until the 35th wk of gestation, after which its production sharply increases. Sphingomyelin, another phospholipid component of surfactant, is also produced at a constant rate after the 26th wk of gestation. Before the 35th wk, the L/S ratio is usually less than 1.6:1. The ratio increases to 2 or greater when the rate of lecithin production increases after the 35th wk of gestation. Other phospholipids, such as phosphatidyl glycerol (PG) and phosphatidyl inositol (PI), increase over time in amniotic fluid as well. The presence of PG indicates that the fetus is within 2 to 6 wk of lung maturity (i.e., at full term). Simultaneous measurement of PG with the L/S ratio improves diagnostic accuracy. Production of phospholipid surfactant is delayed in mothers with diabetes. Therefore, caution must be used when interpreting the results obtained from a patient who is diabetic, and a higher ratio is expected to predict maturity.

Testing for common genetically transferred conditions can be performed on either or both prospective parents by blood tests, skin tests, or DNA testing. DNA testing can also be performed on the fetus, in utero, through the collection of fetal cells by amniocentesis or chorionic villus sampling. Genetics is the study and identification of genes, genetic mutations, and inheritance. For example, genetics provides some insight into the likelihood of inheriting a trait such as blue eyes or a medical condition such as cystic fibrosis or errors of amino acid metabolism. Knowledge of genetics assists the nurse in identifying patients and family members who may benefit from additional education, risk assessment, and counseling. Further information regarding inheritance of genes can be found in the study titled "Genetic Testing." Counseling and written, informed consent are recommended and sometimes required before genetic testing.

This procedure is contraindicated for

Women with a history of premature labor, incompetent cervix, or in the presence of placenta previa or abruptio placentae. There is some risk to having an amniocentesis performed, and this should be weighed against the need to obtain the desired diagnostic information. A small percentage (0.5%) of patients have experienced complications including PROM, premature labor, spontaneous abortion, and stillbirth.

INDICATIONS

- Assist in the diagnosis of (in utero) metabolic disorders, such as cystic fibrosis, or errors of

lipid, carbohydrate, or amino acid metabolism.
- Assist in the evaluation of fetal lung maturity when preterm delivery is being considered.
- Detect infection secondary to ruptured membranes.
- Detect fetal ventral wall defects.
- Determine the optimal time for obstetric intervention in cases of threatened fetal survival caused by stresses related to maternal diabetes, toxemia, hemolytic diseases of the newborn, or postmaturity.
- Determine fetal gender when the mother is a known carrier of a sex-linked abnormal gene that could be transmitted to male offspring, such as hemophilia or Duchenne's muscular dystrophy.
- Determine the presence of fetal distress in late-stage pregnancy.
- Evaluate fetus in families with a history of genetic disorders, such as Down syndrome, Tay-Sachs disease, chromosome or enzyme anomalies, or inherited hemoglobinopathies.
- Evaluate fetus in mothers of advanced maternal age (some of the aforementioned tests are routinely requested in mothers age 35 and older).
- Evaluate fetus in mothers with a history of miscarriage or stillbirth.
- Evaluate known or suspected hemolytic disease involving the fetus in an Rh-sensitized pregnancy, indicated by rising bilirubin levels, especially after the 30th wk of gestation.
- Evaluate suspected neural tube defects, such as spina bifida or myelomeningocele, as indicated by elevated α_1-fetoprotein (see study titled "α_1-Fetoprotein" for information related to triple-marker testing).
- Identify fetuses at risk of developing RDS.

POTENTIAL MEDICAL DIAGNOSIS

- Yellow, green, red, or brown fluid ***indicates the presence of bilirubin, blood (fetal or maternal), or meconium, which indicate fetal distress or death, hemolytic disease, or growth retardation.***
- Elevated bilirubin levels ***indicate fetal hemolytic disease or intestinal obstruction. Measurement of bilirubin is not usually performed before 20 to 24 weeks' gestation because no action can be taken before then. The severity of hemolytic disease is graded by optical density (OD) zones: A value of 0.28 to 0.46 OD at 28 to 31 weeks' gestation indicates mild hemolytic disease, which probably will not affect the fetus; 0.47 to 0.9 OD indicates a moderate effect on the fetus; and 0.91 to 1 OD indicates a significant effect on the fetus. A trend of increasing values with serial measurements may indicate the need for intrauterine transfusion or early delivery, depending on the fetal age. After 32 to 33 weeks' gestation, early delivery is preferred over intrauterine transfusion, because early delivery is more effective in providing the required care to the neonate.***
- Creatinine concentration greater than 2 mg/dL (greater than 176.8 micromol/L) (SI Units = Conventional Units × 88.4) ***indicates fetal maturity (at 36 to 37 wk) if maternal creatinine is also within the expected range. This value should be interpreted in conjunction with other parameters evaluated in amniotic fluid and especially with the L/S ratio, because normal lung development depends on normal kidney development.***

A

- An L/S ratio less than 2:1 and absence of phosphatidylglycerol at term ***indicate fetal lung immaturity and possible respiratory distress syndrome. Other conditions that decrease production of surfactants include advanced maternal age, multiple gestation, and polyhydramnios. Conditions that may increase production of surfactant include hypertension, intrauterine growth retardation, malnutrition, maternal diabetes, placenta previa, placental infarction, and premature rupture of the membranes. The expected L/S ratio for the fetus of a mother who is diabetic is higher (3.5:1).***
- ***Lamellar bodies are specialized alveolar cells in which lung surfactant is stored.*** They are approximately the size of platelets. Their presence in sufficient quantities is an indicator of fetal lung maturity. Amniotic fluid lamellar body counts less than 15,000/microL are suggestive of immature lung development and predictive for increased risk of developing RDS; counts greater than 50,000/microL are predictive of mature lung development.
- Elevated AFP levels and presence of acetylcholinesterase may indicate a neural tube defect (see study titled "α_1-Fetoprotein") ***related to leakage from the open spinal cord into the amniotic fluid.*** Elevation of AFP and/or acetylcholinesterase is also indicative of ventral wall defects. The presence of AFP and acetylcholinesterase in amniotic fluid is abnormal; however, the test is not a sensitive marker for neural tube defects; false-positive results can be caused by contamination of the sample with fetal blood, which normally contains measurable levels of AFP and acetylcholinesterase. Abnormal results can be confirmed by testing the amniotic fluid for the presence of fetal hemoglobin (Hgb F). If Hgb F is detected, then the specimen is likely contaminated with fetal blood and the results are unreliable.
- Abnormal karyotype ***indicates genetic abnormality (e.g., Tay-Sachs disease, intellectual disability, chromosome or enzyme anomalies, and inherited hemoglobinopathies).*** (See study titled "Chromosome Analysis, Blood.")
- Elevated white blood cell count and positive leukocyte esterase ***are indicators of infection.***

CRITICAL FINDINGS:

An L/S ratio less than 1.5:1 is predictive of RDS at the time of delivery.

Note and immediately report to the requesting health-care provider (HCP) any critical findings and related symptoms. A listing of these findings varies among facilities. Timely notification of a critical finding for laboratory or diagnostic studies is a role expectation of the professional nurse. The notification processes vary among facilities. Upon receipt of the critical finding, the information should be read back to the caller to verify accuracy.

Infants known to be at risk for RDS can be treated with surfactant by intratracheal administration at birth.

INTERFERING FACTORS

- Bilirubin may be falsely elevated if maternal hemoglobin or meconium is present in the sample; fetal acidosis may also lead to falsely elevated bilirubin levels.
- Bilirubin may be falsely decreased if the sample is exposed to light or if amniotic fluid volume is excessive.
- Maternal serum creatinine should be measured simultaneously for comparison with amniotic fluid creatinine for proper interpretation. Even in circumstances in which

A

the maternal serum value is normal, the results of the amniotic fluid creatinine may be misleading. A high fluid creatinine value in the fetus of a mother who is diabetic may reflect the increased muscle mass of a larger fetus. If the fetus is big, the creatinine may be high, and the fetus may still have immature kidneys.

- Contamination of the sample with blood or meconium or complications in pregnancy may yield inaccurate L/S ratios; fetal blood falsely elevates the L/S ratio.
- α_1-Fetoprotein and acetylcholinesterase may be falsely elevated if the sample is contaminated with fetal blood.
- Karyotyping cannot be performed under the following conditions: (1) failure to promptly deliver samples for chromosomal analysis to the laboratory performing the test or (2) improper incubation of the sample, which causes cell death.

NURSING IMPLICATIONS AND PROCEDURE

POTENTIAL NURSING PROBLEMS:

Problem	Signs & Symptoms	Interventions
Fear ***(related to fetal imperfections secondary to developmental abnormality)***	Verbalization of fear; restlessness; increased tension; continuous questioning; increased blood pressure, heart rate, respiratory rate	Evaluate verbal and nonverbal indicators of fear; assess for the cause of fear; acknowledge the patient's awareness of fear; explain all procedures with simple age and culturally appropriate language; administer proscribed mild tranquilizer; maintain a confident, assured professional manner in all patient interactions; address concerns regarding care of disabled child; recommend support group and provide contact information
Spirituality ***(related to anxiety associated with feral developmental abnormality; unexpected life changes)***	Anger; stated feelings of lack of peace or serenity; stated feelings of alienation from others; stated feelings of hopelessness; request to meet with spiritual leader	Obtain a history of the patient's religious affiliation; identify the patient's willingness to meet with a spiritual leader; encourage verbalization of concerns, feelings of fear and loneliness; acknowledge and support religious practices; accommodate a display of religious objects; facilitate communication between the patient, family, and spiritual leader

(table continues on page 58)

A

Problem	Signs & Symptoms	Interventions
Knowledge ***(related to insufficient information associated with diagnosed developmental abnormality; lack of familiarity or understanding with disease and treatment)***	Lack of interest or questions; multiple questions; anxiety in relation to disease process and management; stating inaccurate information; frustration; confusion	Identify the primary learners and provide specific information that is culturally appropriate and to the correct literacy level; assess for the willingness and ability to learn; identify the patient's priority for learning; identify and dispel any misconceptions associated with the developmental disability; identify the patient's learning style; provide a quiet atmosphere for learning; allow the parents to be self-directed in their learning; provide sufficient time for questions and follow-up; refer to a support group and social services as appropriate

PRETEST:

- Positively identify the patient using at least two person-specific identifiers before services, treatments, or procedures are performed.
- ***Patient teaching:*** Inform the parent this procedure/test can assist in providing a sample of fluid that will allow for evaluation of fetal well-being.
- Obtain a history of the patient's health concerns, symptoms, surgical procedures, and results of previously performed laboratory and diagnostic studies. Include a list of known allergens, especially allergies or sensitivities to latex. Include any family history of genetic disorders such as cystic fibrosis, Duchenne's muscular dystrophy, hemophilia, sickle cell disease, Tay-Sachs disease, thalassemia, and trisomy 21. Obtain maternal Rh type. If Rh-negative, check for prior sensitization. A standard dose of RhIG (Rh immune globulin) or RhoGAM IM or Rhophylac IM or intravenous is indicated after amniocentesis; repeat doses should be considered if repeated amniocentesis is performed.
- Note any recent procedures that can interfere with test results.
- Record the date of the last menstrual period and determine the pregnancy weeks' gestation and expected delivery date.
- Obtain a list of the patient's current medications, including over-the-counter medications and dietary supplements (see Effects of Natural Products on Laboratory Values online at Davis*Plus*).
- Review the procedure with the patient. Warn the patient that normal results do not guarantee a normal fetus. Assure the patient that precautions to avoid injury to the fetus will be taken by localizing the fetus with ultrasound. Address concerns about pain and explain that during the transabdominal procedure, any discomfort associated with a needle biopsy will be minimized with local anesthetics. If the patient is less than 20 weeks' gestation, instruct her to drink extra fluids 1 hr before the test and to refrain from urination. The full bladder assists in raising the uterus up and out of the way to provide better visualization during the ultrasound procedure. Patients who are at 20 weeks' gestation or beyond do not need to drink extra fluids and should void before the test, because an empty bladder is less likely to be accidentally punctured during specimen collection. Encourage relaxation and controlled breathing during the

procedure to aid in reducing any mild discomfort. Inform the patient that specimen collection is performed by an HCP specializing in this procedure and usually takes approximately 20 to 30 min to complete.

- ***Sensitivity to social and cultural issues,*** as well as concern for modesty, is important in providing psychological support before, during, and after the procedure.
- Note that there are no food, fluid, or medication restrictions unless by medical direction.
- *Make sure a written and informed consent has been signed prior to the procedure and before administering any medications.*

INTRATEST:

Potential Complications:
Hemorrhage from highly vascular tissue or infection following amniocentesis. Instruct the patient to look for excessive bleeding, redness of skin, fever, or chills and to notify the HCP if these symptoms occur. An additional risk with amniocentesis is maternal Rh sensitization by fetal red blood cells (RBCs) in the case of an Rh-negative mother carrying an Rh-positive fetus. RhIG or RhoGAM may be administered after amniocentesis to Rh-negative mothers to prevent formation of Rh antibodies.

- Avoid the use of equipment containing latex if the patient has a history of allergic reaction to latex.
- Ensure that the patient has a full bladder before the procedure if gestation is 20 wk or less; have patient void before the procedure if gestation is 21 wk or more.
- Positively identify the patient, and label the appropriate collection containers with the corresponding patient demographics, date, time of collection, and site location.
- Have patient remove clothes below the waist. Assist the patient to a supine position on the examination table with the abdomen exposed. Drape the patient's legs, leaving the abdomen exposed. Raise her head or legs slightly to promote comfort and to relax the abdominal muscles. If the uterus is large, place a pillow or rolled blanket under the patient's right side to prevent hypertension caused by great-vessel compression. Instruct the patient to cooperate fully and to follow directions. Direct the patient to breathe normally and to avoid unnecessary movement during administration of the local anesthetic and the procedure.
- Record maternal and fetal baseline vital signs, and continue to monitor throughout the procedure. Monitor for uterine contractions. Monitor fetal vital signs using ultrasound. Protocols may vary among facilities.
- Have emergency equipment readily available.
- Observe standard precautions, and follow the general guidelines in Patient Preparation and Specimen Collection online at Davis*Plus*. Positively identify the patient, and label the appropriate specimen container with the corresponding patient demographics, initials of the person collecting the specimen, date, and time of collection.
- Assess the position of the amniotic fluid, fetus, and placenta using ultrasound.
- Assemble the necessary equipment, including an amniocentesis tray with solution for skin preparation, local anesthetic, 10- or 20-mL syringe, needles of various sizes (including a 22-gauge, 5-in. spinal needle), sterile drapes, sterile gloves, and foil-covered or amber-colored specimen collection containers.
- Cleanse suprapubic area with an antiseptic solution, and protect with sterile drapes. A local anesthetic is injected. Explain that this may cause a stinging sensation.
- Insert a 22-gauge, 5-in. spinal needle through the abdominal and uterine walls. Explain that a sensation of pressure may be experienced when the needle is inserted. Explain to the patient how to use focused and controlled breathing for relaxation during the procedure.

A

- Apply slight pressure to the site after the fluid is collected and the needle is withdrawn. If there is no evidence of bleeding or other drainage, apply a sterile adhesive bandage to the site.
- Monitor the patient for complications related to the procedure (e.g., premature labor, allergic reaction, anaphylaxis).

POST-TEST:

- Inform the patient that a report of the results will be made available to the requesting HCP, who will discuss the results with the patient.
- Compare fetal heart rate and maternal life signs (i.e., heart rate, blood pressure, pulse, and respiration) with baseline values and closely monitor every 15 min for 30 to 60 min after the amniocentesis procedure. Protocols may vary among facilities.
- Observe/assess for delayed allergic reactions, such as rash, urticaria, tachycardia, hyperpnea, hypertension, palpitations, nausea, or vomiting. Immediately report symptoms to the appropriate HCP.
- Observe/assess the amniocentesis site for bleeding, inflammation, or hematoma formation.
- Instruct the patient in the care and assessment of the amniocentesis site.
- Instruct the patient to report any redness, edema, bleeding, or pain at the amniocentesis site.
- Instruct the patient to expect mild cramping, leakage of small amounts of amniotic fluid, and vaginal spotting for up to 2 days following the procedure. Instruct the patient to report moderate to severe abdominal pain or cramps, change in fetal activity, increased or prolonged leaking of amniotic fluid from abdominal needle site, vaginal bleeding that is heavier than spotting, and either chills or fever.
- Instruct the patient to rest until all symptoms have disappeared before resuming normal levels of activity.
- Administer standard RhIG or RhoGAM dose to maternal Rh-negative patients to prevent maternal Rh sensitization should the fetus be Rh-positive.
- Recognize anxiety related to test results. Discuss the implications of abnormal test results on the patient's lifestyle. Provide teaching and information regarding the clinical implications of the test results, as appropriate. Encourage the family to seek appropriate counseling if concerned with pregnancy termination and to seek genetic counseling if a chromosomal abnormality is determined. Decisions regarding elective abortion should take place in the presence of both parents. Provide a nonjudgmental, nonthreatening atmosphere for discussing the risks and difficulties of delivering and raising a developmentally challenged infant as well as for exploring other options (termination of pregnancy or adoption). It is also important to discuss problems the mother and father may experience (guilt, depression, anger) if fetal abnormalities are detected.
- Depending on the results of this procedure, additional testing may be performed to evaluate or monitor progression of the disease process and determine the need for a change in therapy. Evaluate test results in relation to the patient's symptoms and other tests performed.

Patient Education:

- Reinforce information given by the patient's HCP regarding further testing, treatment, or referral to another HCP.
- Inform the patient that it may be 2 to 4 wk before all results are available.
- Answer any questions or address any concerns voiced by the patient or family.
- Instruct the patient in the use of any ordered medications.

Expected Patient Outcomes:

Understanding

- The patient and family state the importance of adhering to the therapy regimen provided by the HCP.
- The patient and family state the significant adverse effects and

systemic reactions associated with the prescribed medication.

Ability

- The patient and family accurately describe care necessary to support the health of the developmentally disabled infant.
- The patient and family accurately describe the lifestyle changes that will be necessary to provide care for the developmentally disabled infant.

Response

- The patient and family comply with the request to review the literature provided by a pharmacist regarding prescribed medications.
- The patient agrees to meet with support group in relation to diagnosed developmental disability.

RELATED STUDIES:

- Related tests include α_1-fetoprotein, antibodies anticardiolipin, blood groups and antibodies, chromosome analysis, fetal fibronectin, genetic testing, glucose, ketones, Kleihauer-Betke test, lupus anticoagulant antibodies, newborn screening, potassium, US biophysical profile obstetric, and UA.
- Refer to the Reproductive System table online at Davis*Plus* for related tests by body system.

A

Amylase

SYNONYM/ACRONYM: N/A

COMMON USE: To assist in diagnosis and evaluation of the treatment modalities used for pancreatitis.

SPECIMEN: Serum collected in a gold-, red-, or red/gray-top tube. Plasma collected in a green-top (heparin) tube is also acceptable.

NORMAL FINDINGS: (Method: Enzymatic)

Age	Conventional & SI Units
3–90 d	0–30 units/L
3–6 mo	6–40 units/L
7–11 mo	6–70 units/L
1–3 yr	11–80 units/L
4–9 yr	16–91 units/L
10–18 yr	19–106 units/L
Adult–older adult	100–300 units/L

Values may be slightly elevated in pregnancy and in older adults due to the effects of medications and the presence of multiple chronic or acute diseases with or without muted symptoms.

DESCRIPTION: Amylase is a digestive enzyme mainly secreted by the acinar cells of the pancreas and by the parotid glands. Pancreatic amylase is secreted into the pancreatic common bile ducts and then into the duodenum where it assists in the digestion of carbohydrates by splitting starch into disaccharides. Amylase is a sensitive indicator of pancreatic acinar cell damage and pancreatic obstruction. Newborns and children up to age 2 yr have little measurable serum

A

amylase. In the early years of life, most of this enzyme is produced by the salivary glands. Amylase can be separated into pancreatic (P_1, P_2, P_3) and salivary (S_1, S_2, S_3) isoenzymes. Isoenzyme patterns are useful in identifying the organ source. Requests for amylase isoenzymes are rare because of the expense of the procedure and limited clinical utility of the result. Isoenzyme analysis is primarily used to assess decreasing pancreatic function in children 5 yr and older who have been diagnosed with cystic fibrosis and who may be candidates for enzyme replacement. Cyst fluid amylase levels with isoenzyme analysis is useful in differentiating pancreatic neoplasms (low enzyme concentration) and pseudocysts (high enzyme concentration). Lipase is usually ordered in conjunction with amylase because lipase is more sensitive and specific to conditions affecting pancreatic function.

This procedure is contraindicated for: N/A

INDICATIONS

- Assist in the diagnosis of early acute pancreatitis; serum amylase begins to rise within 6 to 24 hr after onset and returns to normal in 2 to 7 days.
- Assist in the diagnosis of macroamylasemia, a disorder seen in alcoholism, malabsorption syndrome, and other digestive problems.
- Assist in the diagnosis of pancreatic duct obstruction, which causes serum amylase levels to remain elevated.
- Detect blunt trauma or inadvertent surgical trauma to the pancreas.
- Differentiate between acute pancreatitis and other causes of abdominal pain that require surgery.

POTENTIAL MEDICAL DIAGNOSIS

Increased in:

Amylase is released from any damaged cell in which it is stored, so conditions that affect the pancreas and parotid glands and cause cellular destruction demonstrate elevated amylase levels.

- Acute appendicitis ***(related to enzyme release from damaged pancreatic tissue)***
- Administration of some drugs (e.g., morphine) is known to increase amylase levels ***(related to increased biliary tract pressure as evidenced by effect of narcotic analgesic drugs)***
- Afferent loop syndrome ***(related to impaired pancreatic duct flow)***
- Aortic aneurysm ***(elevated amylase levels following rupture are associated with a poor prognosis; both S and P subtypes have been identified following rupture. The causes for elevation are mixed and difficult to state as a generalization)***
- Abdominal trauma ***(related to release of enzyme from damaged pancreatic tissue)***
- Alcoholism ***(related to increased secretion; salivary origin most likely)***
- Biliary tract disease ***(related to impaired pancreatic duct flow)***
- Burns and traumatic shock
- Carcinoma of the head of the pancreas (advanced) ***(related to enzyme release from damaged pancreatic tissue)***
- Chronic kidney disease ***(related to decreased renal excretion as evidenced by accumulation in blood)***

- Common bile duct obstruction, common bile duct stones ***(related to impaired pancreatic duct flow)***
- Diabetic ketoacidosis ***(related to increased secretion; salivary origin most likely)***
- Duodenal obstruction ***(accumulation in the blood as evidenced by leakage from the gut)***
- Ectopic pregnancy ***(related to ectopic enzyme production by the fallopian tubes)***
- Extrapancreatic tumors (especially esophagus, lung, ovary)
- Gastric resection ***(accumulation in the blood as evidenced by leakage from the gut)***
- Hyperlipidemias (etiology is unclear, but there is a distinct association with amylasemia)
- Hyperparathyroidism (etiology is unclear, but there is a distinct association with amylasemia)
- Intestinal infarction ***(related to impaired pancreatic duct flow)***
- Intestinal obstruction ***(related to impaired pancreatic duct flow)***
- Macroamylasemia ***(related to decreased ability of renal glomeruli to filter large molecules as evidenced by accumulation in the blood)***
- Mumps ***(related to increased secretion from inflamed tissue; salivary origin most likely)***
- Pancreatic ascites ***(related to release of pancreatic fluid into the abdomen and subsequent absorption into the circulation)***
- Pancreatic cyst and pseudocyst ***(related to release of pancreatic fluid into the abdomen and subsequent absorption into the circulation)***
- Pancreatitis ***(related to enzyme release from damaged pancreatic tissue)***
- Parotitis ***(related to increased secretion from inflamed tissue; salivary origin most likely)***
- Perforated peptic ulcer whether the pancreas is involved or not ***(related to enzyme release from damaged pancreatic tissue; involvement of the pancreas may be unnoticed upon gross examination yet be present as indicated by elevated enzyme levels)***
- Peritonitis ***(accumulation in the blood as evidenced by leakage from the gut)***
- Postoperative period ***(related to complications of the surgical procedure)***
- Pregnancy ***(related to increased secretion; salivary origin most likely related to hyperemesis or hyperlipidemia induced pancreatitis related to increased estrogen levels)***
- Some tumors of the lung and ovaries ***(related to ectopic enzyme production)***
- Tumor of the pancreas or adjacent area ***(related to release of enzyme from damaged pancreatic tissue)***

Decreased in:

- Hepatic disease (severe) ***(may be due to lack of amino acid production necessary for enzyme manufacture)***
- Pancreatectomy
- Pancreatic insufficiency
- Toxemia of pregnancy

CRITICAL FINDINGS: N/A

INTERFERING FACTORS

- Drugs and other substances that may increase amylase levels include acetaminophen, aminosalicylic acid, amoxapine, asparaginase, aspirin, azathioprine, bethanechol, calcitriol, chlorthalidone, cholinergics, clozapine, codeine, corticosteroids, corticotropin, desipramine, dexamethasone, diazoxide, ethyl alcohol, felbamate, fentanyl, fluvastatin, glucocorticoids, hydantoin derivatives, hydrochlorothiazide, hydroflumethiazide, meperidine, mercaptopurine, methacholine, methyclothiazide, methyldopa, metolazone, minocycline, morphine, nitrofurantoin, opium alkaloids, pegaspargase, pentazocine, potassium iodide, prednisone, procyclidine, tetracycline, thiazide diuretics, valproic acid, zalcitabine, and zidovudine.

- Drugs and other substances that may decrease amylase levels include anabolic steroids, citrates, fluorides, and glucose.
- Elevated amylase levels frequently occur (75% of the time) after endoscopic retrograde cholangiopancreatography.

NURSING IMPLICATIONS AND PROCEDURE

POTENTIAL NURSING PROBLEMS:

Problem	Signs & Symptoms	Interventions
Fluid volume (water)***(related to vomiting; decreased oral intake; diaphoresis; NPO with NGT; overly aggressive fluid resuscitation; compromised kidney function; overly aggressive diuresis)***	**Deficient:** Decreased urinary output, fatigue, and sunken eyes, dark urine, decreased blood pressure, increased heart rate, and altered mental status **Overload:** Edema, shortness of breath, increased weight, ascites, rales, rhonchi, and decreased laboratory values ***related to dilutional effect of excess fluid***	Daily weight with monitoring of trends; accurate intake and output; collaboration with health-care provider (HCP) with administration of intravenous (IV) fluids to support hydration; monitor laboratory values that reflect alterations in fluid status (potassium, blood urea nitrogen, creatinine, calcium, hemoglobin, and hematocrit); manage underlying cause of fluid alteration; monitor urine characteristics and respiratory status; establish baseline assessment data; collaborate with HCP to adjust oral and IV fluids to provide optimal hydration status; administer replacement electrolytes as ordered
Nutrition ***(related to altered pancreatic function excess alcohol intake; insufficient eating habits; altered pancreatic function liver function)***	Known inadequate caloric intake; weight loss; muscle wasting in arms and legs; stool that is pale or gray colored; skin that is flaky with loss of elasticity	Document food intake with possible calorie count; assess barriers to eating; consider using a food diary; monitor continued alcohol use as it is a barrier to adequate protein nutrition; monitor glucose levels; check daily weight; arrange dietary consult with assessment of cultural food selections

A

Problem	Signs & Symptoms	Interventions
Gas exchange ***(related to accumulation of pleural fluid, atelectasis, ventilation perfusion mismatch; altered oxygen supply)***	Irregular breathing pattern, use of accessory muscles; altered chest excursion; adventitious breath sounds (crackles, rhonchi, wheezes, diminished breath sounds); copious secretions; signs of hypoxia	Monitor respiratory rate and effort based on assessment of patient condition; assess lung sounds frequently; monitor for secretions; suction as necessary; use pulse oximetry to monitor oxygen saturation; collaborate with HCP to administer oxygen as needed; elevate the head of the bed 30 degrees; monitor IV fluids and avoid aggressive fluid resuscitation
Pain ***(related to pancreatic inflammation and surrounding tissues; excessive alcohol intake; infection)***	Emotional symptoms of distress; crying; agitation; facial grimace; moaning; verbalization of pain; rocking motions; irritability; disturbed sleep; diaphoresis; altered blood pressure and heart rate; nausea; vomiting; self-report of pain; upper abdominal and gastric pain after eating fatty foods or alcohol intake with acute pancreatic disease; pain may be decreased or absent in chronic pancreatic disease	Collaborate with the patient and HCP to identify the best pain management modality to provide relief; refrain from activities that may aggravate pain; use the application of heat or cold to the best effect in managing the pain; monitor pain severity

PRETEST:

- Positively identify the patient using at least two person-specific identifiers before services, treatments, or procedures are performed.
- ***Patient teaching:*** Inform the patient this test can assist in evaluating pancreatic health and/or the effectiveness of medical treatment for pancreatitis.
- Obtain a history of the patient's health concerns, symptoms, surgical procedures, and results of previously performed laboratory and diagnostic studies. Include a list of known allergens, especially allergies or sensitivities to latex.
- Obtain a list of the patient's current medications, including over-the-counter medications and dietary supplements (see Effects of Natural Products on Laboratory Values online at Davis*Plus*).

A

- Review the procedure with the patient. Inform the patient that specimen collection takes approximately 5 to 10 min. Address concerns about pain and explain that there may be some discomfort during the venipuncture.
- *Sensitivity to social and cultural issues,* as well as concern for modesty, is important in providing psychological support before, during, and after the procedure.
- Note that there are no food, fluid, or medication restrictions unless by medical direction.

INTRATEST:

Potential Complications:

- Avoid the use of equipment containing latex if the patient has a history of allergic reaction to latex.
- Instruct the patient to cooperate fully and to follow directions. Direct the patient to breathe normally and to avoid unnecessary movement.
- Observe standard precautions, and follow the general guidelines in Patient Preparation and Specimen Collection online at Davis*Plus*. Positively identify the patient, and label the appropriate specimen container with the corresponding patient demographics, initials of the person collecting the specimen, date, and time of collection. Perform a venipuncture.
- Remove the needle and apply direct pressure with dry gauze to stop bleeding. Observe/assess venipuncture site for bleeding or hematoma formation and secure gauze with adhesive bandage.
- Promptly transport the specimen to the laboratory for processing and analysis.

POST-TEST:

- Inform the patient that a report of the results will be made available to the requesting HCP, who will discuss the results with the patient.
- *Nutritional Considerations:* Increased amylase levels may be associated with gastrointestinal disease or alcoholism. Small, frequent meals work best for patients with gastrointestinal disorders. Consideration should be given to dietary alterations in the case of gastrointestinal disorders. Usually after acute symptoms subside and bowel sounds return, patients are given a clear liquid diet, progressing to a low-fat, high-carbohydrate diet. Vitamin B_{12} may be ordered for parenteral administration to patients with decreased levels, especially if their disease prevents adequate absorption of the vitamin. Patients who are alcoholics should be encouraged to avoid alcohol and to seek appropriate counseling.
- Depending on the results of this procedure, additional testing may be performed to evaluate or monitor progression of the disease process and determine the need for a change in therapy. Evaluate test results in relation to the patient's symptoms and other tests performed.

Patient Education:

- Teach the patient to use the incentive spirometer with deep cough to help maintain open airways and move secretions that interfere with adequate oxygenation
- Teach the patient the symptoms of fluid overload and deficit with an explanation of proper hydration.
- Reinforce information given by the patient's HCP regarding further testing, treatment, or referral to another HCP.
- Recognize anxiety related to test results, and answer any questions or address any concerns voiced by the patient or family.

Expected Patient Outcomes:

Understanding

- The patient and family state the link between alcohol use and disease process.
- The patient and family describe symptoms that indicate being respiratory compromised and should be reported to the HCP.

Ability

- The patient accurately self-administers oxygen.
- The patient proficiently monitors intake and output and records results accurately.

Response

- The patient complies with the therapeutic goals established by the HCP.
- The patient and family verify the necessity in refraining from activities that could cause a disease reoccurrence.

RELATED STUDIES:

- Related tests include ALT, ALP, AST, bilirubin, cancer antigens, calcium, C-peptide, CBC WBC count and differential, CT pancreas, ERCP, fecal fat, GGT, lipase, magnesium, MRI pancreas, mumps serology, peritoneal fluid analysis, triglycerides, US abdomen, and US pancreas.
- See the Gastrointestinal and Hepatobiliary systems tables online at Davis*Plus* for related tests by body system.

Analgesic, Anti-inflammatory, and Antipyretic Drugs: Acetaminophen, Acetylsalicylic Acid

SYNONYM/ACRONYM: *Acetaminophen* (Acephen, Aceta, Apacet, APAP 500, Aspirin Free Anacin, Banesin, Cetaphen, Dapa, Datril, Dorcol, Exocrine, FeverAll, Genapap, Genebs, Halenol, Little Fevers, Liquiprin, Mapap, Myapap, Nortemp, Pain-Eze, Panadol, Paracetamol, Redutemp, Ridenol, Silapap, Tempra, Tylenol, Ty-Pap, Uni-Ace, Valorin) 🍁; *Acetylsalicylic acid* (Anacin, ASA, Aspergum, aspirin, Bufferin, Easprin, Ecotrin, Empirin, Measurin, salicylate, Synalgos, ZORprin) 🍁.

COMMON USE: To assist in monitoring therapeutic drug levels and detect toxic levels of acetaminophen and salicylate in suspected overdose. It should be noted that acetaminophen and acetylsalicylic acid are contained in many other medications, such as cold and cough medicines.

SPECIMEN: Serum collected in a red-top tube.

NORMAL FINDINGS: (Method: Immunoassay)

Drug	Therapeutic Range Conventional Units	Conversion to SI Units	SI Units	Half-Life	Volume of Distribution	Protein Binding	Excretion
Acetaminophen	5–20 mcg/mL	SI units = Conventional units × 6.62	33–132 micromol/L	1–3 hr	0.95 L/kg	10%–25% (dose dependent)	85%–95% hepatic; metabolites, renal
Salicylate	10–30 mg/dL (anti-inflammatory); 2–10 mg/dL (antipyretic/analgesic)	SI units = Conventional units × 0.073	0.7–2.2 mmol/L (anti-inflammatory); 0.2–0.7 mmol/L (antipyretic/analgesic)	2–3 hr	0.1–0.3 L/kg	90%–95%	1° hepatic; metabolites, renal

POTENTIAL MEDICAL DIAGNOSIS

Increased in:

- Acetaminophen
  - Alcoholic cirrhosis ***(related to inability of damaged liver to metabolize the drug)***
  - Liver disease ***(related to inability of damaged liver to metabolize the drug)***
  - Toxicity
- ASA
  - Toxicity

Decreased in:

- Noncompliance with therapeutic regimen

CRITICAL FINDINGS:

Note: The adverse effects of subtherapeutic levels are also important. Care should be taken to investigate signs and symptoms of too little and too much medication.

Note and immediately report to the requesting HCP any critical findings and related symptoms. A listing of these findings varies among facilities. Timely notification of a critical finding for laboratory or diagnostic studies is a role expectation of the professional nurse. The notification processes vary among facilities. Upon receipt of the critical finding, the information should be read back to the caller to verify accuracy.

Acetaminophen:

Greater than 200 mcg/mL (4 hr postingestion): (SI greater than 1,324 micromol/L [4 hr postingestion]) Signs and symptoms of acetaminophen intoxication occur in stages over a period of time. In stage I (0 to 24 hr after ingestion), symptoms may include gastrointestinal irritation, pallor, lethargy, diaphoresis, metabolic acidosis, and possibly coma. In stage II (24 to 48 hr after ingestion), signs and symptoms may include right upper quadrant abdominal pain; elevated liver enzymes, aspartate aminotransferase (AST), and alanine aminotransferase (ALT); and possible decreased kidney function. In stage III (72 to 96 hr after ingestion), signs and symptoms may include nausea, vomiting, jaundice, confusion, coagulation disorders, continued elevation of AST and ALT, decreased kidney function, and coma. Intervention may include gastrointestinal decontamination (stomach pumping) if the patient presents within 6 hr of ingestion or administration of *N*-acetylcysteine (Mucomyst) in the case of an acute intoxication in which the patient presents more than 6 hr after ingestion.

ASA: Greater Than 40 mg/dL: (SI Greater Than 2.9 mmol/L)

Signs and symptoms of salicylate intoxication include ketosis, convulsions, dizziness, nausea, vomiting, hyperactivity, hyperglycemia, hyperpnea, hyperthermia, respiratory arrest, and tinnitus. Possible interventions include administration of activated charcoal as vomiting ceases, alkalinization of the urine with bicarbonate, and a single dose of vitamin K (for rare instances of hypoprothrombinemia).

Find and print out the full study on Fast Find at davispl.us/vanleeuwen7.

Angiography, Abdomen

SYNONYM/ACRONYM: Abdominal angiogram, abdominal arteriography.

COMMON USE: To visualize and assess abdominal organs/structure for tumor, infection, or aneurysm.

AREA OF APPLICATION: Abdomen.

DESCRIPTION: Abdominal angiography allows x-ray visualization of the large and small arteries, veins, and associated branches of the abdominal vasculature and organ parenchyma after contrast medium injection. This visualization is accomplished by the injection of contrast medium through a catheter, which most commonly has been inserted into the femoral artery and advanced through the iliac artery and aorta into the organ-specific artery. Fluoroscopy is used to guide catheter placement, and angiograms (high-speed x-ray images) provide images of the organ of interest and associated vessels that are displayed on a monitor and are recorded for future viewing and evaluation. Digital subtraction angiography (DSA) is a computerized method of removing undesired structures, like bone, from the surrounding area of interest. A digital image is taken prior to injection of the contrast and then again after the contrast has been injected. By subtracting the preinjection image from the postinjection image, a higher-quality, unobstructed image can be created. Patterns of circulation, organ function, and changes in vessel wall appearance can be viewed to help diagnose the presence of vascular abnormalities, aneurysm, tumor, trauma, or lesions. The catheter used to administer the contrast medium to confirm the diagnosis of organ lesions may be used to deliver chemotherapeutic drugs or different types of materials administered to stop bleeding. Catheters with attached inflatable balloons for angioplasty and wire mesh stents are used to widen areas of stenosis and to keep vessels open, frequently replacing surgery. Embolotherapy can also be accomplished through the same catheter when the site of bleeding or extravasation is located. Angiography is one of the definitive tests for organ disease and may be used to evaluate chronic disease and organ failure, treat arterial stenosis, differentiate a vascular cyst from hypervascular cancers, and evaluate the effectiveness of medical or surgical treatment.

This procedure is contraindicated for

- Patients who are pregnant or suspected of being pregnant, unless the potential benefits of a procedure using radiation far outweigh the risk of radiation exposure to the fetus and mother.
- Conditions associated with adverse reactions to contrast medium (e.g., asthma, food allergies, or allergy to contrast medium).

Although patients are asked specifically if they have a known allergy to iodine or shellfish (shellfish contain high levels of iodine), it has been well established that the reaction is not to iodine; an actual iodine allergy would be problematic because iodine is required for the production of thyroid hormones. In the case of shellfish, the reaction is to a muscle protein called *tropomyosin*; in the case of iodinated contrast medium, the reaction is to the noniodinated part of the contrast molecule. Patients with a known hypersensitivity to the medium may benefit from premedication with corticosteroids and diphenhydramine; the use of nonionic contrast or an alternative noncontrast imaging study, if available, may be considered for patients who have severe asthma or who have experienced moderate to severe reactions to ionic contrast medium.

Conditions associated with preexisting renal insufficiency (e.g., chronic kidney disease, single kidney transplant, nephrectomy, diabetes, multiple myeloma, treatment with aminoglycosides and NSAIDs) ***because iodinated contrast is nephrotoxic.***

Patients who are chronically dehydrated before the test, especially older adults and patients whose health is already compromised, ***because of their risk of contrast-induced acute kidney injury.***

Patients with pheochromocytoma, ***because iodinated contrast may cause a hypertensive crisis.***

Patients with bleeding disorders or receiving anticoagulant therapy ***because the puncture site may not stop bleeding.***

INDICATIONS

- Aid in angioplasty, atherectomy, or stent placement.
- Allow infusion of thrombolytic drugs into an occluded artery.
- Detect arterial occlusion, which may be evidenced by a transection of the artery caused by trauma or penetrating injury.
- Detect artery stenosis, evidenced by vessel dilation, collateral vessels, or increased vascular pressure.
- Detect nonmalignant tumors before surgical resection.
- Detect thrombosis, arteriovenous fistula, aneurysms, or emboli in abdominal vessels.
- Detect tumors and arterial supply, extent of venous invasion, and tumor vascularity.
- Detect peripheral arterial disease (PAD).
- Differentiate between tumors and cysts.
- Evaluate organ transplantation for function or organ rejection.
- Evaluate placement of a shunt or stent.
- Evaluate tumor vascularity before surgery or embolization.
- Evaluate the vascular system of prospective organ donors before surgery.

POTENTIAL MEDICAL DIAGNOSIS

Normal findings

- Normal structure, function, and patency of abdominal organ vessels
- Contrast medium normally circulates throughout abdomen symmetrically and without interruption
- No evidence of obstruction, variations in number and size of vessels, malformations, cysts, or tumors

Abnormal findings related to

- Abscess or inflammation ***as seen by edema in the area of the vessel***
- Arterial aneurysm ***visualized by a bulging in a vessel***
- Arterial stenosis, dysplasia, or organ infarction ***indicated by a narrowing or blocked artery***
- Arteriovenous fistula or other abnormalities
- Congenital anomalies
- Cysts visualized by areas with a halo of contrast surrounding them or tumors ***indicated by areas of increased density due to the vascularity which collects the contrast***
- PAD
- Trauma causing tears or other disruption ***indicated by blood outside the vessel***

CRITICAL FINDINGS:

- Abscess
- Aneurysm

Note and immediately report to the requesting health-care provider (HCP) any critical findings and related symptoms. A listing of these findings varies among facilities. Timely notification of

A

a critical finding for laboratory or diagnostic studies is a role expectation of the professional nurse. The notification processes vary among facilities. Upon receipt of the critical finding, the information should be read back to the caller to verify accuracy.

INTERFERING FACTORS

Factors that may alter the results of the study

- Gas or feces in the gastrointestinal tract resulting from inadequate cleansing or failure to restrict food intake before the study.
- Retained barium from a previous radiological procedure.
- Metallic objects within the examination field (e.g., jewelry, body rings), which may inhibit organ visualization and can produce unclear images.
- Inability of the patient to cooperate or remain still during the procedure because of age, significant pain, or mental status.

Other considerations

- This procedure may be terminated if chest pain, severe cardiac dysrhythmias, or signs of a cerebrovascular accident occur.
- Failure to follow dietary restrictions and other pretesting preparations may cause the procedure to be canceled or repeated.

NURSING IMPLICATIONS AND PROCEDURE

See Potential Nursing Problems on Fast Find at davispl.us/vanleeuwen7.

PRETEST:

- Positively identify the patient using at least two person-specific identifiers before services, treatments, or procedures are performed.
- *Patient teaching:* Inform the patient this procedure can assist with the evaluation of abdominal organs.
- Obtain a history of the patient's health concerns, symptoms, surgical procedures, and results of previously performed laboratory and diagnostic studies. Include a list of known allergens, especially allergies or sensitivities to latex, anesthetics, contrast medium, or sedatives. Ensure results of coagulation testing are obtained and recorded prior to the procedure; a creatinine level is also needed before contrast medium is to be used.
- Note any recent procedures that can interfere with test results, including examinations using iodine-based contrast medium or barium. Ensure that barium studies were performed more than 4 days before angiography.
- Record the date of the last menstrual period and determine the possibility of pregnancy in perimenopausal women.
- Obtain a list of the patient's current medications, including over-the-counter medications, dietary supplements, anticoagulants, aspirin and other salicylates (see Effects of Natural Products on Laboratory Values online at Davis*Plus*). Such products should be discontinued by medical direction for the appropriate number of days prior to a surgical procedure. Note the last time and dose of medication taken.
- If iodinated contrast medium is scheduled to be used in patients receiving metformin for type 2 diabetes, the drug should be discontinued on the day of the test and continue to be withheld for 48 hr after the test. Iodinated contrast can temporarily impair kidney function, and failure to withhold metformin may indirectly result in drug-induced lactic acidosis, a dangerous and sometimes fatal adverse effect of metformin ***(related to renal impairment that does not support sufficient excretion of metformin).***
- Review the procedure with the patient. Address concerns about pain and explain that there may be moments of discomfort and some pain experienced during the test. Inform the patient that the procedure

is usually performed in a radiology or vascular suite by an HCP and takes approximately 30 to 60 min.

- *Sensitivity to social and cultural issues,* as well as concern for modesty, is important in providing psychological support before, during, and after the procedure.
- Explain that an intravenous (IV) line may be inserted to allow infusion of fluids such as saline, anesthetics, sedatives, or emergency medications. Explain that the contrast medium will be injected, by catheter, at a separate site from the IV line.
- Inform the patient that a burning and flushing sensation may be felt throughout the body during injection of the contrast medium. After injection of the contrast medium, the patient may experience an urge to cough, flushing, nausea, or a salty or metallic taste.
- Instruct the patient to remove jewelry and other metallic objects from the area to be examined.
- Instruct the patient to fast and restrict fluids, as ordered, for 2 to 4 hr prior to the procedure. Fasting may be ordered as a precaution against aspiration related to possible nausea and vomiting during the administration of contrast. Protocols may vary among facilities.
- *Make sure a written and informed consent has been signed prior to the procedure and before administering any medications.*

INTRATEST:

Potential Complications:

Establishing an IV site and injection of contrast medium by catheter are invasive procedures. Complications are rare but do include risk for allergic reaction ***(related to contrast reaction);*** bleeding from the puncture site ***(related to a bleeding disorder, or the effects of natural products and medications with known anticoagulant, antiplatelet, or thrombolytic properties; postprocedural bleeding from the site is rare because at the conclusion of the procedure a resorbable device, composed of non-latex-containing arterial anchor, collagen plug, and suture, is deployed to seal the puncture site);*** blood clot formation ***(related to thrombus formation on the tip of the catheter sheath surface or in the lumen of the catheter; the use of a heparinized saline flush during the procedure decreases the risk of emboli);*** hematoma ***(related to blood leakage into the tissue following needle insertion);*** infection ***(which might occur if bacteria from the skin surface is introduced at the puncture site);*** tissue damage ***(related to extravasation of the contrast during injection);*** or nerve injury or damage to a nearby organ ***(which might occur if the catheter strikes a nerve or perforates an organ).***

- Observe standard precautions, and follow the general guidelines in Patient Preparation and Specimen Collection online at Davis*Plus.* Positively identify the patient.
- Ensure the patient has complied with dietary and fluid restrictions prior to the study, as instructed. Glucagon or an anticholinergic drug may be given to stabilize movement of the stomach muscles; peristaltic contractions (motion) may alter study findings.
- Ensure the patient has removed all external metallic objects from the area to be examined.
- Administer ordered prophylactic steroids or antihistamines before the procedure if the patient has a history of allergic reaction to any substance or drug.
- Avoid the use of equipment containing latex if the patient has a history of allergic reaction to latex.
- Have emergency equipment readily available.
- Instruct the patient to void prior to the procedure and to change into the gown, robe, and foot coverings provided.
- Instruct the patient to cooperate fully and to follow directions. Instruct the patient to remain still throughout the procedure because movement produces unreliable results.
- Record baseline vital signs, and assess neurological status. Protocols may vary among facilities.

- Establish an IV fluid line for the injection of saline, sedatives, or emergency medications.
- Administer an antianxiety drug, as ordered, if the patient has claustrophobia. Administer a sedative to a child or to an uncooperative adult, as ordered.
- Place electrocardiographic electrodes on the patient for cardiac monitoring. Establish a baseline rhythm; determine if the patient has ventricular dysrhythmias.
- Using a pen, mark the site of the patient's peripheral pulses before angiography; this allows for quicker and more consistent assessment of the pulses after the procedure.
- Place the patient in the supine position on an examination table. Cleanse the selected area, and cover with a sterile drape.
- A local anesthetic is injected at the site, and a small incision is made or a needle inserted under fluoroscopy.
- The contrast medium is injected, and a rapid series of images is taken during and after the filling of the vessels to be examined. Delayed images may be taken to examine the vessels after a time and to monitor the venous phase of the procedure.
- Instruct the patient to inhale deeply and hold his or her breath while the images are taken, and then to exhale after the images are taken.
- Instruct the patient to take slow, deep breaths if nausea occurs during the procedure.
- Monitor the patient for complications related to the procedure (e.g., allergic reaction, anaphylaxis, bronchospasm).
- The needle or catheter is removed, and a pressure dressing is applied over the puncture site.
- Observe/assess the needle/catheter insertion site for bleeding, inflammation, or hematoma formation.

POST-TEST:

- Inform the patient that a report of the results will be made available to the requesting HCP, who will discuss the results with the patient.
- Instruct the patient to resume usual diet, fluids, medications, or activity, as directed by the HCP. Kidney function should be assessed before metformin is resumed.
- Monitor vital signs and neurological status every 15 min for 1 hr, then every 2 hr for 4 hr, and as ordered. Take temperature every 4 hr for 24 hr. Monitor intake and output at least every 8 hr. Compare with baseline values. Protocols may vary among facilities.
- Observe for delayed allergic reactions, such as rash, urticaria, tachycardia, hyperpnea, hypertension, palpitations, nausea, or vomiting.
- Instruct the patient to immediately report symptoms such as fast heart rate, difficulty breathing, skin rash, itching, chest pain, persistent right shoulder pain, or abdominal pain. Immediately report symptoms to the appropriate HCP.
- Assess extremities for signs of ischemia or absence of distal pulse caused by a catheter-induced thrombus.
- Observe/assess the needle/catheter insertion site for bleeding, inflammation, or hematoma formation.
- Instruct the patient in the care and assessment of the site.
- Instruct the patient to apply cold compresses to the puncture site as needed, to reduce discomfort or edema.
- Instruct the patient to maintain bedrest for 4 to 6 hr after the procedure or as ordered.
- Recognize anxiety related to test results, and be supportive of perceived loss of independent function. Discuss the implications of abnormal test results on the patient's lifestyle. Provide teaching and information regarding the clinical implications of the test results, as appropriate.
- Reinforce information given by the patient's HCP regarding further testing, treatment, or referral to another HCP. Answer any questions or address any concerns voiced by the patient or family. Provide contact

A

information, if desired, for the Legs for Life (www.legsforlife.org) 🍁.

- Depending on the results of this procedure, additional testing may be performed to evaluate or monitor progression of the disease process and determine the need for a change in therapy. Evaluate test results in relation to the patient's symptoms and other tests performed.

Patient Education:

- Teach the patient the importance of managing hypertension to decrease bleeding risk.
- Teach the signs and symptoms of transfusion reaction.

Expected Patient Outcomes:

Understanding

- The patient and family discuss the medical versus surgical options for disease management.
- The patient and family discuss the risks and benefits of blood transfusion and the types of transfusion available.

Ability

- The patient and family successfully create a quiet environment.
- The patient successfully demonstrates how to take own blood pressure using an approved medical device.

Response

- The patient and family agree to vigilant follow-up care.
- The patient and family agree to blood replacement therapy.

RELATED STUDIES:

- Related tests include angiography kidneys, BUN, CT abdomen, CT angiography, CT brain and head, CT spleen, CT thoracic, creatinine, KUB, MRA, MRI abdomen, MRI brain, MRI chest, MRI pelvis, aPTT, PT/INR, renogram, US abdomen, and US lower extremity.
- See the Cardiovascular System table online at Davis*Plus* for related tests by body system.

Angiography, Adrenal

SYNONYM/ACRONYM: Adrenal angiogram, adrenal arteriography.

COMMON USE: To visualize and assess the adrenal gland for cancer or other tumors or masses.

AREA OF APPLICATION: Adrenal gland.

DESCRIPTION: Adrenal angiography evaluates adrenal dysfunction by allowing x-ray visualization of the large and small arteries of the adrenal gland vasculature and parenchyma. This visualization is accomplished by the injection of contrast medium through a catheter that has been inserted into the femoral artery for viewing the artery (arteriography) or into the femoral vein for viewing the veins (venography). Fluoroscopy is used to guide catheter placement, and angiograms (high-speed x-ray images) provide images of the adrenal glands and associated vessels surrounding the adrenal tissue which are displayed on a monitor and are recorded for future viewing and evaluation. Digital subtraction angiography (DSA) is a computerized method of removing undesired structures, like bone, from the surrounding area of interest. A digital image is taken prior to injection of the contrast and then again after the

A

contrast has been injected. By subtracting the preinjection image from the postinjection image a higher-quality, unobstructed image can be created. Patterns of circulation, adrenal function, and changes in vessel wall appearance can be viewed to help diagnose the presence of vascular abnormalities, trauma, or lesions. This definitive test for adrenal disease may be used to evaluate chronic adrenal disease, evaluate arterial or venous stenosis, differentiate an adrenal cyst from adrenal tumors, identify pheochromocytoma, and evaluate medical therapy or surgery of the adrenal glands.

Imaging studies cannot always visualize a tumor, especially if it is small. Adrenal venous sampling can be very challenging beginning with proper placement of the catheter; after the catheter is in place, blood samples may be taken from the vein of each gland and the distal portion of the vena cava to assess cortisol and adrenocorticotropic hormone (ACTH) levels. The information is used to assist in determining a diagnosis of ACTH-independent Cushing's syndrome (benign or malignant adrenal growth that secretes cortisol) or primary hyperaldosteronism (excessive adrenal gland production of aldosterone). The gold standard for distinguishing between a cortisol-secreting tumor and unilateral or bilateral adrenal hyperplasia is considered to be measurement of aldosterone/cortisol ratios taken from a series of samples during adrenal angiography. Cortisol levels will be elevated if related to Cushing's syndrome. A ratio of greater than 4:1 is indicative of unilateral hyperplasia. Ratios between each gland are similar and usually less than 3:1 in the presence of bilateral hyperplasia. Obtaining the correct diagnosis from the angiogram is important because treatment for adrenal adenoma and unilateral adrenal hyperplasia is surgical removal of the affected adrenal gland, while bilateral adrenal hypertrophy is treated medically.

This procedure is contraindicated for

- Patients who are pregnant or suspected of being pregnant, unless the potential benefits of a procedure using radiation far outweigh the risk of radiation exposure to the fetus and mother.
- Conditions associated with adverse reactions to contrast medium (e.g., asthma, food allergies, or allergy to contrast medium).

Although patients are asked specifically if they have a known allergy to iodine or shellfish (shellfish contain high levels of iodine), it has been well established that the reaction is not to iodine; an actual iodine allergy would be problematic because iodine is required for the production of thyroid hormones. In the case of shellfish, the reaction is to a muscle protein called *tropomyosin*; in the case of iodinated contrast medium, the reaction is to the noniodinated part of the contrast molecule. Patients with a known hypersensitivity to the medium may benefit from premedication with corticosteroids and diphenhydramine; the use of nonionic contrast or an alternative noncontrast imaging study, if available, may be considered for patients who have severe asthma or who have experienced moderate to severe reactions to ionic contrast medium.

Conditions associated with preexisting renal insufficiency (e.g., chronic kidney disease, single kidney transplant, nephrectomy, diabetes, multiple myeloma, treatment with aminoglycosides and NSAIDs) ***because iodinated contrast is nephrotoxic.***

Patients who are chronically dehydrated before the test, especially older adults and patients whose health is already compromised, ***because of their risk of contrast-induced acute kidney injury.***

Patients with pheochromocytoma ***because iodinated contrast may cause a hypertensive crisis.***

Patients with bleeding disorders or receiving anticoagulant therapy ***because the puncture site may not stop bleeding.***

INDICATIONS

- Assist in the infusion of thrombolytic drugs into an occluded artery.
- Assist with the collection of blood samples from the vein for laboratory analysis.
- Detect adrenal hyperplasia.
- Detect and determine the location of adrenal tumors ***evidenced by arterial supply, extent of venous invasion, and tumor vascularity.***
- Detect arterial occlusion, ***evidenced by a transection of the artery caused by trauma or a penetrating injury.***
- Detect arterial stenosis, ***evidenced by vessel dilation, collateral vessels, or increased vascular pressure.***
- Detect nonmalignant tumors before surgical resection.
- Detect thrombosis, arteriovenous fistula, aneurysms, or emboli in vessels.
- Differentiate between adrenal tumors and adrenal cysts.
- Evaluate tumor vascularity before surgery or embolization.
- Perform angioplasty, perform atherectomy, or place a stent.

POTENTIAL MEDICAL DIAGNOSIS

Normal findings

- Normal structure, function, and patency of adrenal vessels
- Contrast medium circulating throughout the adrenal gland symmetrically and without interruption
- No evidence of obstruction, variations in number and size of vessels and organs, malformations, cysts, or tumors

Abnormal findings related to

- Adrenal adenoma
- Adrenal carcinoma
- Bilateral adrenal hyperplasia
- Pheochromocytoma

CRITICAL FINDINGS: N/A

INTERFERING FACTORS

Factors that may alter the results of the study

- Gas or feces in the gastrointestinal tract resulting from inadequate cleansing or failure to restrict food intake before the study.
- Retained barium from a previous radiological procedure.
- Metallic objects within the examination field (e.g., jewelry, body rings), which may inhibit organ visualization and canproduce unclear images.
- Inability of the patient to cooperate or remain still during the procedure because of age, significant pain, or mental status.

Other considerations

- This procedure may be terminated if chest pain, severe cardiac dysrhythmias, or signs of a cerebrovascular accident occur.
- Failure to follow dietary restrictions and other pretesting preparations may cause the procedure to be canceled or repeated.

A

NURSING IMPLICATIONS AND PROCEDURE

See Potential Nursing Problems on Fast Find at davispl.us/vanleeuwen7.

PRETEST:

- Positively identify the patient using at least two person-specific identifiers before services, treatments, or procedures are performed.
- ***Patient teaching:*** Inform the patient this procedure can assist with evaluation of the adrenal gland (located near the kidney).
- Obtain a history of the patient's health concerns, symptoms, surgical procedures, and results of previously performed laboratory and diagnostic studies. Include a list of known allergens, especially allergies or sensitivities to latex, anesthetics, contrast medium, or sedatives. Ensure results of coagulation testing are obtained and recorded prior to the procedure; a creatinine level is also needed before contrast medium is to be used.
- Note any recent procedures that can interfere with test results, including examinations using iodine-based contrast medium or barium. Ensure that barium studies were performed more than 4 days before angiography.
- Record the date of the last menstrual period and determine the possibility of pregnancy in perimenopausal women.
- Obtain a list of the patient's current medications, including over-the-counter medications, dietary supplements, anticoagulants, aspirin and other salicylates (see Effects of Natural Products on Laboratory Values online at Davis*Plus*). Such products should be discontinued by medical direction for the appropriate number of days prior to a surgical procedure. Note the last time and dose of medication taken.
- If iodinated contrast medium is scheduled to be used in patients receiving metformin for type 2 diabetes, the drug should be discontinued on the day of the test and continue to be withheld for 48 hr after the test. Iodinated contrast can temporarily impair kidney function, and failure to withhold metformin may indirectly result in drug-induced lactic acidosis, a dangerous and sometimes fatal adverse effect of metformin ***(related to renal impairment that does not support sufficient excretion of metformin).***
- Review the procedure with the patient. Address concerns about pain and explain that there may be moments of discomfort and some pain experienced during the test. Inform the patient that the procedure is usually performed in a radiology or vascular suite by a health-care provider (HCP) and takes approximately 30 to 60 min.
- ***Sensitivity to social and cultural issues,*** as well as concern for modesty, is important in providing psychological support before, during, and after the procedure.
- Explain that an intravenous (IV) line may be inserted to allow infusion of fluids such as saline, anesthetics, sedatives, or emergency medications. Explain that the contrast medium will be injected, by catheter, at a separate site from the IV line.
- Inform the patient that a burning and flushing sensation may be felt throughout the body during injection of the contrast medium. After injection of the contrast medium, the patient may experience an urge to cough, flushing, nausea, or a salty or metallic taste.
- Instruct the patient to remove jewelry and other metallic objects from the area to be examined.
- Instruct the patient to fast and restrict fluids, as ordered, for 2 to 4 hr prior to the procedure. Fasting may be ordered as a precaution against aspiration related to nausea and vomiting during the administration of contrast. Protocols may vary among facilities.
- *Make sure a written and informed consent has been signed prior to the procedure and before administering any medications.*

A

INTRATEST:

Potential Complications:

Establishing an IV site and injection of contrast medium by catheter are invasive procedures. Complications are rare but do include risk for allergic reaction ***(related to contrast reaction);*** bleeding from the puncture site ***(related to a bleeding disorder, or the effects of natural products and medications with known anticoagulant, antiplatelet, or thrombolytic properties; postprocedural bleeding from the site is rare because at the conclusion of the procedure a resorbable device, composed of non-latex-containing arterial anchor, collagen plug, and suture, is deployed to seal the puncture site);*** blood clot formation ***(related to thrombus formation on the tip of the catheter sheath surface or in the lumen of the catheter, but the use of a heparinized saline flush during the procedure decreases the risk of emboli);*** hematoma ***(related to blood leakage into the tissue following needle insertion);*** infection ***(which might occur if bacteria from the skin surface is introduced at the puncture site);*** tissue damage ***(related to extravasation of the contrast during injection);*** or nerve injury or damage to a nearby organ ***(which might occur if the catheter strikes a nerve or perforates an organ).***

- Avoid the use of equipment containing latex if the patient has a history of allergic reaction to latex.
- Observe standard precautions, and follow the general guidelines in Patient Preparation and Specimen Collection online at Davis*Plus*. Positively identify the patient.
- Ensure the patient has complied with dietary, fluid, and medication restrictions and pretesting preparations prior to the study, as instructed. Glucagon or an anticholinergic drug may be given to stabilize movement of the stomach muscles; peristaltic contractions (motion) may alter study findings.
- Ensure the patient has removed all external metallic objects from the area to be examined.
- Administer ordered prophylactic steroids or antihistamines before the procedure.
- Have emergency equipment readily available.
- Instruct the patient to void prior to the procedure and to change into the gown, robe, and foot coverings provided.
- Instruct the patient to cooperate fully and to follow directions. Instruct the patient to remain still throughout the procedure because movement produces unreliable results.
- Record baseline vital signs, and continue to monitor throughout the procedure. Protocols may vary among facilities.
- Establish an IV fluid line for the injection of saline, sedatives, or emergency medications.
- Administer an antianxiety drug, as ordered, if the patient has claustrophobia. Administer a sedative to a child or to an uncooperative adult, as ordered.
- Place electrocardiographic electrodes on the patient for cardiac monitoring. Establish a baseline rhythm; determine if the patient has ventricular dysrhythmias.
- Using a pen, mark the site of the patient's peripheral pulses before angiography; this allows for quicker and more consistent assessment of the pulses after the procedure.
- Place the patient in the supine position on an examination table. Cleanse the selected area, and cover with a sterile drape.
- A local anesthetic is injected at the site, and a small incision is made or a needle inserted under fluoroscopy.
- The contrast medium is injected, and a rapid series of images is taken during and after the filling of the vessels to be examined. Delayed images may be taken to examine the vessels after a time and to monitor the venous phase of the procedure.
- Instruct the patient to inhale deeply and hold his or her breath while the x-ray images are taken, and then to exhale after the images are taken.

A

- Instruct the patient to take slow, deep breaths if nausea occurs during the procedure.
- Monitor the patient for complications related to the procedure (e.g., allergic reaction, anaphylaxis, bronchospasm).
- The needle or catheter is removed, and a pressure dressing is applied over the puncture site.
- Observe/assess the needle/catheter insertion site for bleeding, inflammation, or hematoma formation.

POST-TEST:

- Inform the patient that a report of the results will be made available to the requesting HCP, who will discuss the results with the patient.
- Instruct the patient to resume usual diet, fluids, medications, or activity, as directed by the HCP. Kidney function should be assessed before metformin is resumed.
- Monitor vital signs and neurological status every 15 min for 1 hr, then every 2 hr for 4 hr, and as ordered. Take temperature every 4 hr for 24 hr. Monitor intake and output at least every 8 hr. Compare with baseline values. Protocols may vary among facilities.
- Observe for delayed allergic reactions, such as rash, urticaria, tachycardia, hyperpnea, hypertension, palpitations, nausea, or vomiting.
- Instruct the patient to immediately report symptoms such as fast heart rate, difficulty breathing, skin rash, itching, chest pain, persistent right shoulder pain, or abdominal pain. Immediately report symptoms to the appropriate HCP.
- Assess extremities for signs of ischemia or absence of distal pulse caused by a catheter-induced thrombus.
- Observe/assess the needle/catheter insertion site for bleeding, inflammation, or hematoma formation.
- Instruct the patient in the care and assessment of the site.
- Instruct the patient to apply cold compresses to the puncture site as needed, to reduce discomfort or edema.
- Instruct the patient to maintain bed rest for 4 to 6 hr after the procedure or as ordered.
- Recognize anxiety related to test results, and be supportive of perceived loss of independent function. Discuss the implications of abnormal test results on the patient's lifestyle. Provide teaching and information regarding the clinical implications of the test results, as appropriate.
- Reinforce information given by the patient's HCP regarding further testing, treatment, or referral to another HCP. Answer any questions or address any concerns voiced by the patient or family.
- Depending on the results of this procedure, additional testing may be performed to evaluate or monitor progression of the disease process and determine the need for a change in therapy. Evaluate test results in relation to the patient's symptoms and other tests performed.

Patient Education:

- Teach the patient and family the importance of adequate rest in relation to the patient's overall health.
- Teach the patient about the disease process and the available options to treat the disease. Make sure the language used is clear and easily understandable.

Expected Patient Outcomes:

Understanding

- The patient and family verbalize the importance of compliance with the recommended therapeutic regime to health maintenance.
- The patient and family state end-of life options as appropriate to the prognosis.

Ability

- The patient and family demonstrate the use of coping strategies to decrease and manage fear.

- The patient and family collaborate with the HCP to develop a treatment plan that fits with the patient's personal health care goals.

Response

- The patient and family agree to attend a support group that provides emotional support regarding prognosis.
- The patient and family comply with the HCP's recommended therapeutic regime.

RELATED STUDIES:

- Related tests include ACTH and challenge tests, adrenal gland scan, BUN, catecholamines, cortisol and challenge tests, creatinine, CT abdomen, HVA, KUB study, metanephrines, MRI abdomen, aPTT, PT/INR, renin, and VMA.
- Refer to the Endocrine System table online at Davis*Plus* for related tests by body system.

Angiography, Carotid

SYNONYM/ACRONYM: Carotid angiogram, carotid arteriography.

COMMON USE: To visualize and assess the carotid arteries and surrounding tissues for abscess, tumors, aneurysm, and evaluate for atherosclerotic disease related to stroke risk.

AREA OF APPLICATION: Neck/cervical area.

DESCRIPTION: This test evaluates blood vessels in the neck carrying arterial blood to the brain and is accomplished by the injection of contrast material through a catheter that has been inserted into the femoral artery. Fluoroscopy is used to guide catheter placement and angiograms (high-speed x-ray images) provide images of the carotid artery and associated vessels in surrounding tissue which are displayed on a monitor and are recorded for future viewing and evaluation. Digital subtraction angiography (DSA) is a computerized method of removing undesired structures, like bone, from the surrounding area of interest. A digital image is taken prior to injection of the contrast and then again after the contrast has been injected. By subtracting the preinjection image from the postinjection image a higher-quality, unobstructed image can be created. The x-ray equipment is mounted on a C-shaped arm with the x-ray device beneath the table on which the patient lies. Over the patient is an image intensifier that receives the x-rays after they pass through the patient. Patterns of circulation or changes in vessel wall appearance can be viewed to help diagnose the presence of vascular abnormalities, disease, narrowing, enlargement, blockage, trauma, or lesions. This definitive test for arterial disease may be used to evaluate chronic vascular disease, arterial or venous stenosis, and medical therapy or surgery of the vasculature. Catheter angiography still is used in patients who may undergo surgery, angioplasty, or stent placement.

This procedure is contraindicated for

- Patients who are pregnant or suspected of being pregnant, unless the potential benefits of a procedure using radiation far outweigh the risk of radiation exposure to the fetus and mother.
- Conditions associated with adverse reactions to contrast medium (e.g., asthma, food allergies, or allergy to contrast medium).

Although patients are asked specifically if they have a known allergy to iodine or shellfish (shellfish contain high levels of iodine), it has been well established that the reaction is not to iodine; an actual iodine allergy would be problematic because iodine is required for the production of thyroid hormones. In the case of shellfish, the reaction is to a muscle protein called *tropomyosin*; in the case of iodinated contrast medium, the reaction is to the nonionated part of the contrast molecule. Patients with a known hypersensitivity to the medium may benefit from premedication with corticosteroids and diphenhydramine; the use of nonionic contrast or an alternative noncontrast imaging study, if available, may be considered for patients who have severe asthma or who have experienced moderate to severe reactions to ionic contrast medium.

- Conditions associated with preexisting renal insufficiency (e.g., chronic kidney disease, single kidney transplant, nephrectomy, diabetes, multiple myeloma, treatment with aminoglycosides and NSAIDs) ***because iodinated contrast is nephrotoxic.***
- Patients who are chronically dehydrated before the test, especially older adults and patients whose health is already compromised, ***because of their risk of contrast-induced acute kidney injury.***
- Patients with pheochromocytoma ***because iodinated contrast may cause a hypertensive crisis.***
- Patients with bleeding disorders or receiving anticoagulant therapy ***because the puncture site may not stop bleeding.***

INDICATIONS

- Aid in angioplasty, atherectomy, or stent placement.
- Allow infusion of thrombolytic drugs into an occluded artery.
- Detect arterial occlusion, which may be evidenced by a transection of the artery caused by trauma or penetrating injury.
- Detect artery stenosis, evidenced by vessel dilation, collateral vessels, or increased vascular pressure.
- Detect nonmalignant tumors before surgical resection.
- Detect tumors and arterial supply, extent of venous invasion, and tumor vascularity.
- Detect thrombosis, arteriovenous fistula, aneurysms, or emboli in vessels.
- Evaluate placement of a stent.
- Differentiate between tumors and cysts.
- Evaluate tumor vascularity before surgery or embolization.
- Evaluate the vascular system of prospective organ donors before surgery.

POTENTIAL MEDICAL DIAGNOSIS

Normal findings

- Normal structure, function, and patency of carotid arteries
- Contrast medium normally circulates throughout neck symmetrically and without interruption
- No evidence of obstruction, variations in number and size of vessels, malformations, cysts, or tumors

Abnormal findings related to

- Abscess or inflammation
- Arterial stenosis or dysplasia
- Aneurysms

- Arteriovenous fistula or other abnormalities
- Congenital anomalies
- Cysts or tumors
- Trauma causing tears or other disruption
- Vascular blockage or other disruption

CRITICAL FINDINGS: N/A

INTERFERING FACTORS

Factors that may alter the results of the study

- Gas or feces in the gastrointestinal tract resulting from inadequate cleansing or failure to restrict food intake before the study.
- Retained barium from a previous radiological procedure.
- Metallic objects within the examination field (e.g., jewelry, body rings), which may inhibit organ visualization and can produce unclear images.
- Inability of the patient to cooperate or remain still during the procedure because of age, significant pain, or mental status.

Other considerations

- This procedure may be terminated if chest pain, severe cardiac dysrhythmias, or signs of a cerebrovascular accident occur.
- Failure to follow dietary restrictions and other pretesting preparations may cause the procedure to be canceled or repeated.

NURSING IMPLICATIONS AND PROCEDURE

See Potential Nursing Problems on Fast Find at davispl.us/vanleeuwen7.

PRETEST:

- Positively identify the patient using at least two person-specific identifiers before services, treatments, or procedures are performed.
- *Patient teaching:* Inform the patient this procedure can assist with evaluation of the cardiovascular system.
- Obtain a history of the patient's health concerns, symptoms, surgical procedures, and results of previously performed laboratory and diagnostic studies. Include a list of known allergens, especially allergies or sensitivities to latex, anesthetics, contrast medium, or sedatives. Ensure results of coagulation testing are obtained and recorded prior to the procedure; a creatinine level is also needed before contrast medium is to be used.
- Note any recent procedures that can interfere with test results, including examinations using iodine-based contrast medium or barium. Ensure that barium studies were performed more than 4 days before angiography.
- Record the date of the last menstrual period and determine the possibility of pregnancy in perimenopausal women.
- Obtain a list of the patient's current medications, including over-the-counter medications, dietary supplements, anticoagulants, aspirin and other salicylates (see Effects of Natural Products on Laboratory Values online at Davis*Plus*). Such products should be discontinued by medical direction for the appropriate number of days prior to a surgical procedure. Note the last time and dose of medication taken.
- If iodinated contrast medium is scheduled to be used in patients receiving metformin for type 2 diabetes, the drug should be discontinued on the day of the test and continue to be withheld for 48 hr after the test. Iodinated contrast can temporarily impair kidney function, and failure to withhold metformin may indirectly result in drug-induced lactic acidosis, a dangerous and sometimes fatal adverse effect of metformin ***(related to renal impairment that does not support sufficient excretion of metformin).***
- Review the procedure with the patient. Address concerns about pain and explain that there may be moments of discomfort and some pain experienced during the test. Inform the patient that the procedure

A

is usually performed in a radiology or vascular suite by a health-care provider (HCP) and takes approximately 30 to 60 min.

- *Sensitivity to social and cultural issues,* as well as concern for modesty, is important in providing psychological support before, during, and after the procedure.
- Explain that an intravenous (IV) line may be inserted to allow infusion of fluids such as saline, anesthetics, sedatives, or emergency medications. Explain that the contrast medium will be injected, by catheter, at a separate site from the IV line.
- Inform the patient that a burning and flushing sensation may be felt throughout the body during injection of the contrast medium. After injection of the contrast medium, the patient may experience an urge to cough, flushing, nausea, or a salty or metallic taste.
- Instruct the patient to remove jewelry and other metallic objects from the area to be examined.
- Instruct the patient to fast and restrict fluids, as ordered, for 2 to 4 hr prior to the procedure. Fasting may be ordered as a precaution against aspiration related to nausea and vomiting during the administration of contrast. Protocols may vary among facilities.
- *Make sure a written and informed consent has been signed prior to the procedure and before administering any medications.*

INTRATEST:

Potential Complications:

Establishing an IV site and injection of contrast medium by catheter are invasive procedures. Complications are rare but do include risk for: allergic reaction ***(related to contrast reaction);*** bleeding from the puncture site ***(related to a bleeding disorder, or the effects of natural products and medications with known anticoagulant, antiplatelet, or thrombolytic properties—postprocedural bleeding from the site is rare because at the conclusion of the procedure a resorbable device, composed of non-latex-containing arterial anchor, collagen plug, and suture, is deployed to seal the puncture site);*** blood clot formation ***(related to thrombus formation on the tip of the catheter sheath surface or in the lumen of the catheter—the use of a heparinized saline flush during the procedure decreases the risk of emboli);*** hematoma ***(related to blood leakage into the tissue following needle insertion);*** infection ***(that might occur if bacteria from the skin surface is introduced at the puncture site);*** tissue damage ***(related to extravasation of the contrast during injection);*** or nerve injury or damage to a nearby organ ***(which might occur if the catheter strikes a nerve or perforates an organ).***

- Avoid the use of equipment containing latex if the patient has a history of allergic reaction to latex.
- Observe standard precautions, and follow the general guidelines in Patient Preparation and Specimen Collection online at Davis*Plus*. Positively identify the patient.
- Ensure the patient has complied with dietary, fluid, and medication restrictions and pretesting preparations prior to the study, as instructed. Glucagon or an anticholinergic drug may be given to stabilize movement of the stomach muscles; peristaltic contractions (motion) may alter study findings.
- Ensure the patient has removed all external metallic objects from the area to be examined.
- Administer ordered prophylactic steroids or antihistamines before the procedure.
- Have emergency equipment readily available.
- Instruct the patient to void prior to the procedure and to change into the gown, robe, and foot coverings provided.
- Instruct the patient to cooperate fully and to follow directions. Instruct the patient to remain still throughout the procedure because movement produces unreliable results.
- Record baseline vital signs, and assess neurological status. Protocols may vary among facilities.

- Establish an IV fluid line for the injection of saline, sedatives, or emergency medications.
- Administer an antianxiety drug, as ordered, if the patient has claustrophobia. Administer a sedative to a child or to an uncooperative adult, as ordered.
- Place electrocardiographic electrodes on the patient for cardiac monitoring. Establish a baseline rhythm; determine if the patient has ventricular dysrhythmias.
- Using a pen, mark the site of the patient's peripheral pulses before angiography; this allows for quicker and more consistent assessment of the pulses after the procedure.
- Place the patient in the supine position on an examination table. Cleanse the selected area, and cover with a sterile drape.
- A local anesthetic is injected at the site, and a small incision is made or a needle is inserted under fluoroscopy.
- The contrast medium is injected, and a rapid series of images is taken during and after the filling of the vessels to be examined. Delayed images may be taken to examine the vessels after a time and to monitor the venous phase of the procedure.
- Instruct the patient to inhale deeply and hold his or her breath while the images are taken, and then to exhale after the images are taken.
- Instruct the patient to take slow, deep breaths if nausea occurs during the procedure.
- Monitor the patient for complications related to the procedure (e.g., allergic reaction, anaphylaxis, bronchospasm).
- The needle or catheter is removed, and a pressure dressing is applied over the puncture site.
- Observe/assess the needle/catheter insertion site for bleeding, inflammation, or hematoma formation.

POST-TEST:

- Inform the patient that a report of the results will be made available to the requesting HCP, who will discuss the results with the patient.
- Instruct the patient to resume usual diet, fluids, medications, or activity, as directed by the HCP. Kidney function should be assessed before metformin is resumed.
- Monitor vital signs and neurological status every 15 min for 1 hr, then every 2 hr for 4 hr, and as ordered. Take temperature every 4 hr for 24 hr. Monitor intake and output at least every 8 hr. Compare with baseline values. Protocols may vary among facilities.
- Observe for delayed allergic reactions, such as rash, urticaria, tachycardia, hyperpnea, hypertension, palpitations, nausea, or vomiting.
- Instruct the patient to immediately report symptoms such as fast heart rate, difficulty breathing, skin rash, itching, chest pain, persistent right shoulder pain, or abdominal pain. Immediately report symptoms to the appropriate HCP.
- Assess extremities for signs of ischemia or absence of distal pulse caused by a catheter-induced thrombus.
- Observe/assess the needle/catheter insertion site for bleeding, inflammation, or hematoma formation.
- Instruct the patient in the care and assessment of the site.
- Instruct the patient to apply cold compresses to the puncture site as needed, to reduce discomfort or edema.
- Instruct the patient to maintain bedrest for 4 to 6 hr after the procedure or as ordered.
- Recognize anxiety related to test results, and be supportive of perceived loss of independent function. Discuss the implications of abnormal test results on the patient's lifestyle. Provide teaching and information regarding the clinical implications of the test results, as appropriate.
- Reinforce information given by the patient's HCP regarding further testing, treatment, or referral to another HCP. Answer any questions or address any concerns voiced by the patient or family.

A

- Instruct the patient in the use of any ordered medications. Explain the importance of adhering to the therapy regimen. As appropriate, instruct the patient in significant adverse effects associated with the prescribed medication. Encourage him or her to review corresponding literature provided by a pharmacist.
- Depending on the results of this procedure, additional testing may be performed to evaluate or monitor progression of the disease process and determine the need for a change in therapy. Evaluate test results in relation to the patient's symptoms and other tests performed.

Patient Education:

- Teach the pathophysiology of the disease process.
- Teach the patient the importance of requesting pain medication as soon as it is needed for effective pain management.

Expected Patient Outcomes:

Understanding

- The patient and family correctly describe treatment options related to disease process.
- The patient and family acknowledge the importance of family or group counseling related to end-of-life issues.

Ability

- The patient and family demonstrate the ability to maintain a quiet environment for emotional and physical rest.
- The patient and family demonstrate successful coping strategies.

Response

- The patient and family agree to family, individual, and/or group counseling related to prognosis and end of life.
- The patient and family agree to all follow-up diagnostic and laboratory studies needed to monitor health status and the effectiveness of treatment modalities.

RELATED STUDIES:

- Related tests include angiography abdomen, BUN, CT angiography, CT brain and head, creatinine, ECG, exercise stress test, MRA, MRI brain, PT/INR, plethysmography, US arterial Doppler lower extremities, and US peripheral Doppler.
- See the Cardiovascular System table online at Davis*Plus* for related tests by body system.

Angiography, Coronary

SYNONYM/ACRONYM: Angiography of heart, angiocardiography, cardiac angiography, cardiac catheterization, cineangiocardiography, coronary angiography, coronary arteriography.

COMMON USE: To visualize and assess the heart and surrounding structure for abnormalities, defects, aneurysm, atherosclerosis, and tumors.

AREA OF APPLICATION: Heart.

DESCRIPTION: Angiography allows x-ray visualization of the heart, aorta, inferior vena cava, pulmonary artery and vein, and coronary arteries after injection of contrast medium. Contrast medium is injected through a catheter, which has been inserted into a peripheral vein, usually the femoral or brachial vein, for a right heart catheterization or into an artery, usually the femoral or brachial artery, for a left heart catheterization; through the same catheter, cardiac pressures and volumes are recorded. Fluoroscopy is used to guide catheter placement, and angiograms (high-speed x-ray images) provide images of the heart and associated vessels which are displayed on a monitor and are recorded for future viewing and evaluation. Digital subtraction angiography (DSA) is a computerized method of removing undesired structures, like bone, from the surrounding area of interest. A digital image is taken prior to injection of the contrast and then again after the contrast has been injected. By subtracting the preinjection image from the postinjection image, a higher-quality, unobstructed image can be created. Patterns of circulation, cardiac output, cardiac functions, and changes in vessel wall appearance can be viewed to help diagnose the presence of vascular abnormalities or lesions. Pulmonary artery abnormalities are seen with right heart views, and coronary artery and thoracic aorta abnormalities are seen with left heart views. Coronary angiography is useful for evaluating cardiovascular disease and various types of cardiac abnormalities.

Coronary angiography, more commonly called *cardiac catheterization*, is a definitive test for coronary artery disease (CAD). CAD is a condition in which the blood vessels to the heart lose their elasticity and become narrowed by atherosclerotic deposits of plaque. Significant blockage is treatable using coronary artery bypass grafting (CABG) surgery. Cardiac catheterization can also be used in conjunction with less invasive interventional alternatives to CABG surgery, such as percutaneous transluminal coronary angioplasty (PTCA), with or without placement of stents. PTCA is also known as *balloon angioplasty* because once the blockage is identified and determined to be treatable, a balloon catheter is used to help correct the problem. The balloon in the catheter is inflated to compress the plaque against the sides of the affected vessel. The balloon may be inflated multiple times and with increasing size to increase the diameter of the vessel's lumen, which restores more normal blood flow. A stent, which is a small mesh tube, may be placed in the affected vessel to keep it open after the angioplasty is completed.

Carotid endarterectomy (CEA) is another procedure that can be combined with coronary angiography and may also be part of the PTCA procedure. CEA is performed to reduce stroke risk. Stroke results from severe stenosis of the carotid arteries and release of plaque emboli that travel to the brain, block circulation, and cause brain tissue death. The CEA procedure involves insertion of an additional, separate catheter to insert a device that removes plaque from the walls of the carotid arteries. The devices commonly used to perform CEA employ very small drills or rotating blades to remove the plaque. Balloon angioplasty, with or without stent placement, usually follows CEA.

Applications of Cardiac Catheterization for Infants and Pediatric Patients: Cardiac catheterization is very useful in identification of the type of heart defect, determination of the exact location of the defect, and indications regarding the severity of the defect. Some of the common operable heart defects in infants

A

and children include repairs for ventricular septal defects, atrial septic defects, tetralogy of Fallot, valve defects, and arterial switches. Cardiac catheterization can also be used as a palliative procedure prior to arterial switch repair. The catheterization, called a *balloon atrial septostomy*, is used to create a small hole in the inner wall of the heart between the atria that allows a greater volume of oxygenated blood to enter the circulatory system. The improved quality of circulating blood provides some time for very young patients to gain strength prior to the surgical repair. The hole is closed when the corrective surgery is completed.

This procedure is contraindicated for

Patients who are pregnant or suspected of being pregnant, unless the potential benefits of a procedure using radiation far outweigh the risk of radiation exposure to the fetus and mother.

Conditions associated with adverse reactions to contrast medium (e.g., asthma, food allergies, or allergy to contrast medium).

Although patients are asked specifically if they have a known allergy to iodine or shellfish (shellfish contain high levels of iodine), it has been well established that the reaction is not to iodine; an actual iodine allergy would be problematic because iodine is required for the production of thyroid hormones. In the case of shellfish, the reaction is to a muscle protein called *tropomyosin*; in the case of iodinated contrast medium, the reaction is to the noniodinated part of the contrast molecule. Patients with a known hypersensitivity to the medium may benefit from premedication with corticosteroids and diphenhydramine; the use of nonionic contrast or an alternative noncontrast imaging study, if available, may be considered for patients who have severe asthma or who have experienced moderate to severe reactions to ionic contrast medium.

Conditions associated with preexisting renal insufficiency (e.g., chronic kidney disease, single kidney transplant, nephrectomy, diabetes, multiple myeloma, treatment with aminoglycosides and NSAIDs) ***because iodinated contrast is nephrotoxic.***

Patients who are chronically dehydrated before the test, especially older adults and patients whose health is already compromised, ***because of their risk of contrast-induced acute kidney injury.***

Patients with pheochromocytoma ***because iodinated contrast may cause a hypertensive crisis.***

Patients with bleeding disorders or receiving anticoagulant therapy ***because the puncture site may not stop bleeding.***

INDICATIONS

- Allow infusion of thrombolytic drugs into an occluded coronary.
- Detect narrowing of coronary vessels or abnormalities of the great vessels in patients with angina, syncope, abnormal electrocardiogram, hypercholesteremia with chest pain, and persistent chest pain after revascularization.
- Evaluate cardiac muscle function.
- Evaluate cardiac valvular and septal defects.
- Evaluate disease associated with the aortic arch.
- Evaluate previous cardiac surgery or other interventional procedures.
- Evaluate peripheral arterial disease (PAD).

- Evaluate peripheral vascular disease (PVD).
- Evaluate ventricular aneurysms.
- Monitor pulmonary pressures and cardiac output.
- Perform angioplasty, perform atherectomy, or place a stent.
- Quantify the severity of atherosclerotic, occlusive coronary artery disease.

POTENTIAL MEDICAL DIAGNOSIS

Normal findings

- Normal great vessels and coronary arteries

Normal Adult Hemodynamic Pressures and Volumes Monitored During Coronary Angiography (Cardiac Catheterization)

Pressures	Description of What Measured Parameter Represents	Normal Value
Arterial blood pressure (also known as *routine blood pressure*)	The pressure in the brachial artery; one of the significant vital signs, it reflects the pressure the heart exerts to pump blood through the circulatory system	Systolic (100–140) mm Hg/diastolic (60–90) mm Hg
Mean arterial pressure	The average arterial pressure of one cardiac cycle; considered a better indicator of perfusion than routine blood pressure but only obtainable by direct measurement during cardiac catheterization	70–105 mm Hg
Left ventricular pressures	Peak pressure in the left ventricle during systole/peak pressure in the left ventricle at the end of diastole; indication of contractility of the heart muscle	Systolic (90–140) mm Hg/ diastolic (4–12) mm Hg
Central venous pressure (right atrial pressure)	The right-sided ventricular pressures exerted by the central veins closest to the heart (jugular, subclavian, or femoral); used to estimate blood volume and venous return	2–6 mm Hg
Pulmonary artery pressure	The pressures in the pulmonary artery	Systolic (15–30) mm Hg/ diastolic (4–12) mm Hg
Pulmonary artery wedge pressure	The pressure in the pulmonary vessels; used to provide an estimate of left atrial filling pressure, to provide an estimate of left ventricle pressure during end diastole, and as a way to measure ventricular preload	4–12 mm Hg

(table continues on page 90)

A

Pressures	Description of What Measured Parameter Represents	Normal Value
Volumes cardiac output	The amount of blood pumped out by the ventricle of the heart in 1 min	4–8 L/min
Cardiac index	The cardiac output adjusted for body surface to provide the index, which is a more precise measurement; used to assess the function of the ventricle	2.5–4 L/min/m^2
Arterial oxygen saturation	The concentration of oxygen in the blood	95%–100%
Stroke volume	The amount of blood pumped by each ventricle with each contraction in a heartbeat	60–100 mL/beat
Stroke volume index	The stroke volume adjusted for body surface to provide the index, which is a more precise measurement	33–57 mL/m^2
End diastolic volume (EDV)	The amount of blood in the left ventricle at the end of diastole	100–160 mL
EDV index	EDV adjusted for body surface to provide the index, which is a more precise measurement	50–80 mL/m^2
End systolic volume (ESV)	The amount of blood in the left ventricle at the end of systole	50–100 mL
ESV index	ESV adjusted for body surface to provide the index, which is a more precise measurement	25–50 mL/m^2
Ejection fraction	Stroke volume expressed as a percentage of end diastolic volume	55%–70%

Abnormal findings related to

Areas where the contrast medium was not able to circulate will appear dark against the normally white blood vessels and vascular areas of cardiac tissue.

- Aortic atherosclerosis
- Aortic dissection
- Aortitis
- Aneurysms
- Cardiomyopathy
- Congenital anomalies
- Coronary artery atherosclerosis and degree of obstruction
- Graft occlusion
- Heart failure
- PAD
- PVD
- Pulmonary artery abnormalities
- Septal defects
- Trauma causing tears or other disruption
- Tumors
- Valvular disease

CRITICAL FINDINGS:

- Aneurysm
- Aortic dissection

Note and immediately report to the requesting health-care provider (HCP) any critical findings and related symptoms. A listing of these findings varies among facilities.

Timely notification of a critical finding for laboratory or diagnostic studies is a role expectation of the professional nurse. The notification processes vary among facilities. Upon receipt of the critical finding, the information should be read back to the caller to verify accuracy.

INTERFERING FACTORS

Factors that may alter the results of the study

- Gas or feces in the gastrointestinal tract resulting from inadequate cleansing or failure to restrict food intake before the study.
- Retained barium from a previous radiological procedure.
- Metallic objects within the examination field (e.g., jewelry, body rings), which may inhibit organ visualization and can produce unclear images.
- Inability of the patient to cooperate or remain still during the procedure because of age, significant pain, or mental status.

Other considerations

- This procedure may be terminated if chest pain, severe cardiac dysrhythmias, or signs of a cerebrovascular accident occur.
- Failure to follow dietary restrictions and other pretesting preparations may cause the procedure to be canceled or repeated.

NURSING IMPLICATIONS AND PROCEDURE

See Potential Nursing Problems on Fast Find at davispl.us/vanleeuwen7.

PRETEST:

- Positively identify the patient using at least two person-specific identifiers before services, treatments, or procedures are performed.
- ***Patient teaching:*** Inform the patient this procedure can assist with assessment of cardiac function and check for heart disease.
- Obtain a history of the patient's health concerns, symptoms, surgical procedures, and results of previously performed laboratory and diagnostic studies. Include a list of known allergens, especially allergies or sensitivities to latex, anesthetics, contrast medium, or sedatives. The presence of other risk factors, such as family history of heart disease, smoking, obesity, diet, lack of physical activity, hypertension, diabetes, previous myocardial infarction, and previous vascular disease, should be investigated. Knowledge of genetics assists the nurse in identifying patients and family members who may benefit from additional education, risk assessment, and counseling. Genetics is the study and identification of genes, genetic mutations, and inheritance. For example, genetics provides some insight into the likelihood of inheriting a trait such as blue eyes or a medical condition such as CAD. Genomic studies evaluate the interaction of groups of genes. The combined activity or combined expression of groups of genes allows assumptions or predictions to be made. As an example, genomic studies measure the levels of activity in multiple genes to predict how they, along with environmental and lifestyle decisions, influence the development of type 2 diabetes, CAD, myocardial infarction, or ischemic stroke. Further information regarding inheritance of genes can be found in the study titled "Genetic Testing." Ensure results of coagulation testing are obtained and recorded prior to the procedure; a creatinine level is also needed before contrast medium is to be used.
- Note any recent procedures that can interfere with test results, including examinations using iodine-based contrast medium or barium. Ensure that barium studies were

A

performed more than 4 days before angiography.

- Record the date of last menstrual period and determine the possibility of pregnancy in perimenopausal women.
- Obtain a list of the patient's current medications, including over-the-counter medications, dietary supplements, anticoagulants, aspirin and other salicylates (see Effects of Natural Products on Laboratory Values online at Davis*Plus*). Such products should be discontinued by medical direction for the appropriate number of days prior to a surgical procedure. Note the last time and dose of medication taken.
- If iodinated contrast medium is scheduled to be used in patients receiving metformin for type 2 diabetes, the drug should be discontinued on the day of the test and continue to be withheld for 48 hr after the test. Iodinated contrast can temporarily impair kidney function, and failure to withhold metformin may indirectly result in drug-induced lactic acidosis, a dangerous and sometimes fatal adverse effect of metformin ***(related to renal impairment that does not support sufficient excretion of metformin).***
- Review the procedure with the patient. Explain that prior to the procedure, hair in the area near the catheter insertion site (usually groin) will be removed with clippers and the patient will be asked to shower using a special antiseptic soap to cleanse bacteria from the skin in order to reduce the risk for infection. Address concerns about pain and explain that there may be moments of discomfort and some pain experienced during the test. Inform the patient that the procedure is usually performed in a radiology or vascular suite by an HCP and takes approximately 30 to 60 min.
- ***Sensitivity to social and cultural issues,*** as well as concern for modesty, is important in providing psychological support before, during, and after the procedure.
- Explain that an intravenous (IV) line may be inserted to allow infusion of fluids such as saline, anesthetics, sedatives, or emergency medications. Explain that the contrast medium will be injected, by catheter, at a separate site from the IV line.
- Inform the patient that a burning and flushing sensation may be felt throughout the body during injection of the contrast medium. After injection of the contrast medium, the patient may experience an urge to cough, flushing, nausea, or a salty or metallic taste.
- Instruct the patient to remove jewelry and other metallic objects from the area to be examined.
- Instruct the patient to fast and restrict fluids, as ordered, for 2 to 4 hr prior to the procedure. Fasting may be ordered as a precaution against aspiration related to possible nausea and vomiting during the administration of contrast. Protocols may vary among facilities.
- *Make sure a written and informed consent has been signed prior to the procedure and before administering any medications.*

INTRATEST:

Potential Complications:

Establishing an IV site and injection of contrast medium by catheter are invasive procedures. Complications are rare but do include risk for: allergic reaction ***(related to contrast reaction);*** bleeding from the puncture site ***(related to a bleeding disorder, or the effects of natural products and medications with known anticoagulant, antiplatelet, or thrombolytic properties—postprocedural bleeding from the site is rare because at the conclusion of the procedure a resorbable device, composed of non-latex-containing arterial anchor, collagen plug, and suture, is deployed to seal the puncture site);*** blood clot formation ***(related to thrombus formation on the tip of the catheter sheath surface or in the lumen of the catheter—the use of a heparinized***

saline flush during the procedure decreases the risk of emboli); hematoma ***(related to blood leakage into the tissue following needle insertion);*** infection ***(which might occur if bacteria from the skin surface is introduced at the puncture site);*** tissue damage ***(related to extravasation of the contrast during injection);*** or nerve injury or damage to a nearby organ ***(which might occur if the catheter strikes a nerve or perforates an organ).***

- Observe standard precautions, and follow the general guidelines in Patient Preparation and Specimen Collection online at Davis*Plus*. Positively identify the patient.
- Ensure the patient has complied with dietary and fluid restrictions prior to the study, as instructed. Glucagon or an anticholinergic drug may be given to stabilize movement of the stomach muscles; peristaltic contractions (motion) may alter study findings.
- Ensure that the patient has removed external metallic objects from the area to be examined prior to the procedure.
- Administer ordered prophylactic steroids or antihistamines before the procedure.
- Avoid the use of equipment containing latex if the patient has a history of allergic reaction to latex.
- Have emergency equipment readily available.
- Instruct the patient to void prior to the procedure and to change into the gown, robe, and foot coverings provided.
- Instruct the patient to cooperate fully and to follow directions. Instruct the patient to remain still throughout the procedure because movement produces unreliable results.
- Record baseline vital signs, and continue to monitor throughout the procedure. Protocols may vary among facilities.
- Establish an IV fluid line for the injection of saline, sedatives, or emergency medications.
- Administer an antianxiety drug, as ordered, if the patient has claustrophobia. Administer a sedative to a child or to an uncooperative adult, as ordered.
- Place electrocardiographic electrodes on the patient for cardiac monitoring. Establish a baseline rhythm; determine if the patient has ventricular dysrhythmias.
- Using a pen, mark the site of the patient's peripheral pulses before angiography; this allows for quicker and more consistent assessment of the pulses after the procedure.
- Place the patient in the supine position on an examination table. Cleanse the selected area, and cover with a sterile drape.
- A local anesthetic is injected at the site, and a small incision is made or a needle is inserted under fluoroscopy.
- The contrast medium is injected, and a rapid series of images is taken during and after the filling of the vessels to be examined. Delayed images may be taken to examine the vessels after a time and to monitor the venous phase of the procedure.
- Instruct the patient to inhale deeply and hold his or her breath while the x-ray images are taken, and then to exhale after the images are taken.
- Instruct the patient to take slow, deep breaths if nausea occurs during the procedure.
- Monitor the patient for complications related to the procedure (e.g., allergic reaction, anaphylaxis, bronchospasm).
- The needle or catheter is removed, and a pressure dressing is applied over the puncture site.
- Observe/assess the needle/catheter insertion site for bleeding, inflammation, or hematoma formation.

POST-TEST:

- Inform the patient that a report of the results will be made available to the requesting HCP, who will discuss the results with the patient.
- Instruct the patient to resume usual diet, fluids, medications, or activity as

A

directed by the HCP. Kidney function should be assessed before metformin is resumed.

- Monitor vital signs and neurological status every 15 min for 1 hr, then every 2 hr for 4 hr, and then as ordered by the HCP. Take temperature every 4 hr for 24 hr. Monitor intake and output at least every 8 hr. Compare with baseline values. Protocols may vary among facilities.
- Observe for delayed allergic reactions, such as rash, urticaria, tachycardia, hyperpnea, hypertension, palpitations, nausea, or vomiting.
- Instruct the patient to immediately report symptoms such as fast heart rate, difficulty breathing, skin rash, itching, chest pain, persistent right shoulder pain, or abdominal pain. Immediately report symptoms to the appropriate HCP.
- Assess extremities for signs of ischemia or absence of distal pulse caused by a catheter-induced thrombus.
- Observe/assess the needle/catheter insertion site for bleeding, inflammation, or hematoma formation.
- Instruct the patient in the care and assessment of the site and to observe for bleeding, hematoma formation, bile leakage, and inflammation. Any pleuritic pain, persistent right shoulder pain, or abdominal pain should be reported to the appropriate HCP.
- Instruct the patient to apply cold compresses to the puncture site as needed, to reduce discomfort or edema.
- Instruct the patient to maintain bedrest for 4 to 6 hr after the procedure or as ordered.
- ***Nutritional Considerations:*** Nutritional therapy is recommended for the patient identified to be at risk for developing CAD or for individuals who have specific risk factors and/or existing medical conditions (e.g., elevated low-density lipoprotein [LDL] cholesterol levels, other lipid disorders, type 1 diabetes, type 2 diabetes, insulin resistance, or metabolic syndrome). Other changeable risk factors warranting patient education include strategies to encourage patients, especially those who are overweight and with high blood pressure, to safely decrease sodium intake, achieve a normal weight, ensure regular participation of moderate aerobic physical activity three to four times per week, eliminate tobacco use, and adhere to a heart-healthy diet. If triglycerides also are elevated, the patient should be advised to eliminate or reduce alcohol. A variety of dietary patterns are beneficial for people with CAD, and there are many meal-planning approaches with nutritional goals endorsed by the American Diabetes Association (ADA). The Guideline on Lifestyle Management to Reduce Cardiovascular Risk, published by the American College of Cardiology (ACC) and the American Heart Association (AHA) in conjunction with the National Heart, Lung, and Blood Institute (NHLBI), recommends a "Mediterranean"-style diet rather than a low-fat diet. The guideline emphasizes inclusion of vegetables, whole grains, fruits, low-fat dairy, nuts, legumes, and nontropical vegetable oils (e.g., olive, canola, peanut, sunflower, flaxseed) along with fish and lean poultry. 🍁 A similar dietary pattern known as the Dietary Approaches to Stop Hypertension (DASH) diet makes additional recommendations for the reduction of dietary sodium. Both dietary styles emphasize a reduction in consumption of red meats, which are high in saturated fats and cholesterol, and other foods containing sugar, saturated fats, trans fats, and sodium. The ADA also includes a vegetarian diet as well as other potential weight loss diets such as Weight Watchers. 🍁 The nutritional needs of each patient need to be determined individually (especially during

pregnancy) with the appropriate HCPs, particularly professionals educated in nutrition.

- *Sensitivity to social and cultural issues:* Numerous studies point to the prevalence of excess body weight in American children and adolescents. Experts estimate that obesity is present in 25% of the population aged 6 to 11 yr. The medical, social, and emotional consequences of excess body weight are significant. Special attention should be given to instructing the child and caregiver regarding health risks and weight control education. 🍁
- Recognize anxiety related to test results. Discuss the implications of abnormal test results on the patient's lifestyle. Provide teaching and information regarding the clinical implications of the test results, as appropriate. Provide contact information, if desired, for the American Heart Association (www.americanheart.org), National Heart, Lung, and Blood Institute (www.nhlbi.nih.gov), Institute of Medicine of the National Academies (www.iom.edu), the USDA's resource for nutrition (www.choosemyplate.gov), and Legs for Life (www.legsforlife.org) 🍁.
- Reinforce information given by the patient's HCP regarding further testing, treatment, or referral to another HCP. Answer any questions or address any concerns voiced by the patient or family.
- Instruct the patient in the use of any ordered medications. Explain the importance of adhering to the therapy regimen. As appropriate, instruct the patient in significant adverse effects associated with the prescribed medication. Encourage him or her to review corresponding literature provided by a pharmacist.
- Depending on the results of this procedure, additional testing may be needed to evaluate or monitor progression of the disease process and determine the need for a change in therapy. Evaluate test results in relation to the patient's symptoms and other tests performed.

Patient Education:

- Teach the patient the pathophysiology associated with the disease process.
- Teach the patient how personal choices effect successful pain management.

Expected Patient Outcomes:

Understanding

- The patient and family discuss the medical versus surgical options for disease management.

Ability

- The patient and family identify pain management strategies that provide the best relief and communicate those strategies to the HCP.
- The patient and family successfully create a quiet environment.

Response

- The patient and family are willing to make lifestyle changes that will support positive health.
- The patient and family agree to attend a support group to provide emotional support related to diagnosis and prognosis.

RELATED STUDIES:

- Related tests include angiography carotid, blood pool imaging, BNP, BUN, chest x-ray, cholesterol HDL and LDL, cholesterol total, CT abdomen, CT angiography, CT biliary tract and liver, CT cardiac scoring, CT spleen, CT thoracic, CK, creatinine, CRP, electrocardiography, electrocardiography transesophageal, genetic testing, Holter monitor, homocysteine, lipoprotein electrophoresis, MR angiography, MRI abdomen, MRI chest, myocardial perfusion heart scan, plethysmography, aPTT, PT/INR, triglycerides, troponin, and US arterial Doppler carotid.
- Refer to the Cardiovascular System table online at Davis*Plus* for related tests by body system.

Angiography, Kidneys

A

SYNONYM/ACRONYM: Renal angiogram, renal arteriography.

COMMON USE: To visualize and assess the kidneys and surrounding structure for tumor, cancer, absent kidney, and level of renal disease.

AREA OF APPLICATION: Kidney.

DESCRIPTION: Renal angiography allows x-ray visualization of the large and small arteries of the renal vasculature and parenchyma or the renal veins and their branches. Contrast medium is injected through a catheter that has been inserted into the femoral artery or vein and advanced through the iliac artery and aorta into the renal artery or the inferior vena cava into the renal vein. Fluoroscopy is used to guide catheter placement, and angiograms (high-speed x-ray images) provide images of the kidneys and associated vessels which are displayed on a monitor and are recorded for future viewing and evaluation. Digital subtraction angiography (DSA) is a computerized method of removing undesired structures, like bone, from the surrounding area of interest. A digital image is taken prior to injection of the contrast and then again after the contrast has been injected. By subtracting the preinjection image from the postinjection image a higher-quality, unobstructed image can be created. Patterns of circulation, renal function, or changes in vessel wall appearance can be viewed to help diagnose the presence of vascular abnormalities, trauma, or lesions. This definitive test for renal disease may be used to evaluate chronic kidney disease and renal artery stenosis; differentiate a vascular renal cyst from hypervascular renal cancers; and evaluate renal transplant donors, recipients, and the kidney after transplantation.

This procedure is contraindicated for

- Patients who are pregnant or suspected of being pregnant, unless the potential benefits of a procedure using radiation far outweigh the risk of radiation exposure to the fetus and mother.
- Conditions associated with adverse reactions to contrast medium (e.g., asthma, food allergies, or allergy to contrast medium).

Although patients are asked specifically if they have a known allergy to iodine or shellfish (shellfish contain high levels of iodine), it has been well established that the reaction is not to iodine; an actual iodine allergy would be problematic because iodine is required for the production of thyroid hormones. In the case of shellfish, the reaction is to a muscle protein called *tropomyosin*; in the case of iodinated contrast medium, the reaction is to the noniodinated part of the contrast molecule. Patients with a known hypersensitivity to the medium may benefit from premedication with corticosteroids and diphenhydramine; the use of nonionic contrast or an alternative noncontrast imaging study, if available, may be considered for patients who have severe asthma or who have experienced moderate to severe reactions to ionic contrast medium.

- Conditions associated with preexisting renal insufficiency (e.g., chronic kidney disease, single kidney transplant, nephrectomy, diabetes, multiple myeloma, treatment with aminoglycosides and NSAIDs) ***because iodinated contrast is nephrotoxic.***
- Patients who are chronically dehydrated before the test, especially older adults and patients whose health is already compromised, ***because of their risk of contrast-induced acute kidney injury.***
- Patients with pheochromocytoma ***because iodinated contrast may cause a hypertensive crisis.***
- Patients with bleeding disorders receiving an arterial or venous puncture ***because the site may not stop bleeding.***

INDICATIONS

- Aid in angioplasty, atherectomy, or stent placement.
- Allow infusion of thrombolytic drugs into an occluded artery.
- Assist with the collection of blood samples from renal vein for renin analysis.
- Detect arterial occlusion as ***evidenced by a transection of the renal artery caused by trauma or a penetrating injury.***
- Detect nonmalignant tumors before surgical resection.
- Detect renal artery stenosis as ***evidenced by vessel dilation, collateral vessels, or increased renovascular pressure.***
- Detect renal tumors ***as evidenced by arterial supply, extent of venous invasion, and tumor vascularity.***
- Detect small kidney or absence of a kidney.
- Detect thrombosis, arteriovenous fistulae, aneurysms, or emboli in renal vessels.
- Differentiate between renal tumors and renal cysts.
- Evaluate placement of a stent.
- Evaluate postoperative renal transplantation for function or organ rejection.
- Evaluate renal function in chronic kidney disease or hydronephrosis.
- Evaluate the renal vascular system of prospective kidney donors before surgery.
- Evaluate tumor vascularity before surgery or embolization.

POTENTIAL MEDICAL DIAGNOSIS

Normal findings

- Normal structure, function, and patency of renal vessels
- Contrast medium circulating throughout the kidneys symmetrically and without interruption
- No evidence of obstruction, variations in number and size of vessels and organs, malformations, cysts, or tumors

Abnormal findings related to

- Abscess or inflammation
- Arterial stenosis, dysplasia, or infarction
- Arteriovenous fistula or other abnormalities
- Congenital anomalies
- Intrarenal hematoma
- Renal artery aneurysm
- Renal cysts or tumors
- Trauma causing tears or other disruption

CRITICAL FINDINGS: N/A

INTERFERING FACTORS

Factors that may alter the results of the study

- Gas or feces in the gastrointestinal tract resulting from inadequate cleansing or failure to restrict food intake before the study.

A

- Retained barium from a previous radiological procedure.
- Metallic objects within the examination field (e.g., jewelry, body rings), which may inhibit organ visualization and can produce unclear images.
- Inability of the patient to cooperate or remain still during the procedure because of age, significant pain, or mental status.

Other considerations

- This procedure may be terminated if chest pain, severe cardiac dysrhythmias, or signs of a cerebrovascular accident occur.
- Failure to follow dietary restrictions and other pretesting preparations may cause the procedure to be canceled or repeated.

NURSING IMPLICATIONS AND PROCEDURE

See Potential Nursing Problems on Fast Find at davispl.us/vanleeuwen7.

PRETEST:

- Positively identify the patient using at least two person-specific identifiers before services, treatments, or procedures are performed.
- *Patient teaching:* Inform the patient this procedure can assist in assessment of kidney function and check for disease.
- Obtain a history of the patient's health concerns, symptoms, surgical procedures, and results of previously performed laboratory and diagnostic studies. Include a list of known allergens, especially allergies or sensitivities to latex, anesthetics, contrast medium, or sedatives. Ensure results of coagulation testing are obtained and recorded prior to the procedure; a creatinine level is also needed before contrast medium is to be used.
- Note any recent procedures that can interfere with test results, including examinations using iodine-based contrast medium or barium. Ensure that barium studies were performed more than 4 days before angiography.
- Record the date of the last menstrual period and determine the possibility of pregnancy in perimenopausal women.
- Obtain a list of the patient's current medications, including over-the-counter medications, dietary supplements, anticoagulants, aspirin and other salicylates (see Effects of Natural Products on Laboratory Values online at Davis*Plus*). Such products should be discontinued by medical direction for the appropriate number of days prior to a surgical procedure. Note the last time and dose of medication taken.
- If iodinated contrast medium is scheduled to be used in patients receiving metformin for type 2 diabetes, the drug should be discontinued on the day of the test and continue to be withheld for 48 hr after the test. Iodinated contrast can temporarily impair kidney function, and failure to withhold metformin may indirectly result in drug-induced lactic acidosis, a dangerous and sometimes fatal adverse effect of metformin ***(related to renal impairment that does not support sufficient excretion of metformin).***
- Review the procedure with the patient. Address concerns about pain and explain that there may be moments of discomfort and some pain experienced during the test. Inform the patient that the procedure is usually performed in a radiology or vascular suite by a health-care provider (HCP) and takes approximately 30 to 60 min.
- ***Sensitivity to social and cultural issues,*** as well as concern for modesty, is important in providing psychological support before, during, and after the procedure.
- Explain that an intravenous (IV) line may be inserted to allow infusion of fluids such as saline, anesthetics, sedatives, or emergency medications. Explain that the contrast medium will be injected, by catheter, at a separate site from the IV line.

- Inform the patient that a burning and flushing sensation may be felt throughout the body during injection of the contrast medium. After injection of the contrast medium, the patient may experience an urge to cough, flushing, nausea, or a salty or metallic taste.
- Instruct the patient to remove jewelry, and other metallic objects from the area to be examined.
- Instruct the patient to fast and restrict fluids, as ordered, for 2 to 4 hr prior to the procedure. Fasting may be ordered as a precaution against aspiration related to nausea and vomiting during the administration of contrast. Protocols may vary among facilities.
- *Make sure a written and informed consent has been signed prior to the procedure and before administering any medications.*

INTRATEST:

Potential Complications:

Establishing an IV site and injection of contrast medium by catheter are invasive procedures. Complications are rare but do include risk for allergic reaction ***(related to contrast reaction);*** bleeding from the puncture site ***(related to a bleeding disorder, or the effects of natural products and medications with known anticoagulant, antiplatelet, or thrombolytic properties—postprocedural bleeding from the site is rare because at the conclusion of the procedure a resorbable device, composed of non-latex-containing arterial anchor, collagen plug, and suture, is deployed to seal the puncture site);*** blood clot formation ***(related to thrombus formation on the tip of the catheter sheath surface or in the lumen of the catheter—the use of a heparinized saline flush during the procedure decreases the risk of emboli);*** hematoma ***(related to blood leakage into the tissue following needle insertion);*** infection ***(which might occur if bacteria from the skin surface is introduced at the puncture site);*** tissue damage ***(related to extravasation of the contrast during injection)***; or nerve injury or damage to a nearby organ ***(which might occur if the catheter strikes a nerve or perforates an organ).***

- Observe standard precautions, and follow the general guidelines in Patient Preparation and Specimen Collection online at Davis*Plus*. Positively identify the patient.
- Ensure the patient has complied with dietary, fluid, and medication restrictions prior to the study, as instructed. Glucagon or an anticholinergic drug may be given to stabilize movement of the stomach muscles; peristaltic contractions (motion) may alter study findings.
- Ensure the patient has removed all external metallic objects from the area to be examined.
- Administer ordered prophylactic steroids or antihistamines before the procedure.
- Avoid the use of equipment containing latex if the patient has a history of allergic reaction to latex.
- Have emergency equipment readily available.
- Instruct the patient to void prior to the procedure and to change into the gown, robe, and foot coverings provided.
- Instruct the patient to cooperate fully and to follow directions. Instruct the patient to remain still throughout the procedure because movement produces unreliable results.
- Record baseline vital signs, and continue to monitor throughout the procedure. Protocols may vary among facilities.
- Establish an IV fluid line for the injection of saline, sedatives, or emergency medications.
- Administer an antianxiety drug, as ordered, if the patient has claustrophobia. Administer a sedative to a child or to an uncooperative adult, as ordered.
- Place electrocardiographic electrodes on the patient for cardiac monitoring. Establish a baseline rhythm; determine if the patient has ventricular dysrhythmias.
- Using a pen, mark the site of the patient's peripheral pulses before

A

angiography; this allows for quicker and more consistent assessment of the pulses after the procedure.
- Place the patient in the supine position on an examination table. Cleanse the selected area, and cover with a sterile drape.
- A local anesthetic is injected at the site, and a small incision is made or a needle is inserted under fluoroscopy.
- The contrast medium is injected, and a rapid series of images is taken during and after the filling of the vessels to be examined. Delayed images may be taken to examine the vessels after a time and to monitor the venous phase of the procedure.
- Instruct the patient to inhale deeply and hold his or her breath while the images are taken, and then to exhale after the images are taken.
- Instruct the patient to take slow, deep breaths if nausea occurs during the procedure.
- Monitor the patient for complications related to the procedure (e.g., allergic reaction, anaphylaxis, bronchospasm).
- The needle or catheter is removed, and a pressure dressing is applied over the puncture site.
- Observe/assess the needle/catheter insertion site for bleeding, inflammation, or hematoma formation.

POST-TEST:
- Inform the patient that a report of the results will be made available to the requesting HCP, who will discuss the results with the patient.
- Instruct the patient to resume usual diet, fluids, medications, or activity, as directed by the HCP. Kidney function should be assessed before metformin is resumed.
- Monitor vital signs and neurological status every 15 min for 1 hr, then every 2 hr for 4 hr, and as ordered. Take temperature every 4 hr for 24 hr. Monitor intake and output at least every 8 hr. Compare with baseline values. Protocols may vary among facilities.
- Observe for delayed allergic reactions, such as rash, urticaria, tachycardia, hyperpnea, hypertension, palpitations, nausea, or vomiting.
- Instruct the patient to immediately report symptoms such as fast heart rate, difficulty breathing, skin rash, itching, chest pain, persistent right shoulder pain, or abdominal pain. Immediately report symptoms to the appropriate HCP.
- Assess extremities for signs of ischemia or absence of distal pulse caused by a catheter-induced thrombus.
- Observe/assess the needle/catheter insertion site for bleeding, inflammation, or hematoma formation.
- Instruct the patient in the care and assessment of the site.
- Instruct the patient to apply cold compresses to the puncture site as needed, to reduce discomfort or edema.
- Instruct the patient to maintain bedrest for 4 to 6 hr after the procedure or as ordered.
- Recognize anxiety related to test results, and be supportive of perceived loss of independent function. Discuss the implications of abnormal test results on the patient's lifestyle. Provide teaching and information regarding the clinical implications of the test results, as appropriate.
- Reinforce information given by the patient's HCP regarding further testing, treatment, or referral to another HCP. Answer any questions or address any concerns voiced by the patient or family.
- Depending on the results of this procedure, additional testing may be needed to evaluate or monitor progression of the disease process and determine the need for a change in therapy. Evaluate test results in relation to the patient's symptoms and other tests performed.

Patient Education:
- Teach the patient the pathophysiology associated with the disease process.
- Teach the patient the importance of effective pain management.

Expected Patient Outcomes:

Understanding

- The patient and family acknowledge the importance of completing the prescribed antibiotic regime.
- The patient and family acknowledge the therapeutic options provided by the HCP.

Ability

- The patient and family demonstrate how to measure and record intake and output.

Response

- The patient and family agree to diet and lifestyle changes that will facilitate renal health.
- The patient and family agree to HCP-recommended follow-up evaluations.

RELATED STUDIES:

- Related tests include biopsy kidney, BUN, creatinine, CT abdomen, CT angiography, culture urine, cytology urine, KUB study, IVP, MRA, MRI abdomen, aPTT, PT/INR, renin, renogram, US kidney, and UA.
- Refer to the Genitourinary System table online at Davis*Plus* for related tests by body system.

Angiography, Pulmonary

SYNONYM/ACRONYM: Pulmonary angiography, pulmonary arteriography.

COMMON USE: To visualize and assess the lungs and surrounding structure for abscess, tumor, cancer, defects, tuberculosis, and pulmonary embolism.

AREA OF APPLICATION: Pulmonary vasculature.

DESCRIPTION: Pulmonary angiography allows x-ray visualization of the pulmonary vasculature after injection of an iodinated contrast medium into the pulmonary artery or a branch of this great vessel. Contrast medium is injected through a catheter that has been inserted into the vascular system, usually through the femoral or brachial vein. Fluoroscopy is used to guide catheter placement, and angiograms (high-speed x-ray images) provide images of the pulmonary vessels which are displayed on a monitor and are recorded for future viewing and evaluation. Digital subtraction angiography (DSA) is a computerized method of removing undesired structures, like bone, from the surrounding area of interest. A digital image is taken prior to injection of the contrast and then again after the contrast has been injected. By subtracting the preinjection image from the postinjection image a higher-quality, unobstructed image can be created. It is one of the definitive tests for pulmonary embolism, but it is also useful for evaluating other types of pulmonary vascular abnormalities. It is definitive for peripheral pulmonary artery stenosis, anomalous pulmonary venous drainage, and pulmonary fistulae. Hemodynamic measurements during pulmonary angiography can assist in the diagnosis of pulmonary hypertension and cor pulmonale. Pulmonary angiograms are requested less frequently in favor of CT pulmonary angiograms which are less invasive, faster, have fewer complications, and are of similar quality.

This procedure is contraindicated for

- Patients who are pregnant or suspected of being pregnant, unless the potential benefits of a procedure using radiation far outweigh the risk of radiation exposure to the fetus and mother.
- Conditions associated with adverse reactions to contrast medium (e.g., asthma, food allergies, or allergy to contrast medium).

Although patients are asked specifically if they have a known allergy to iodine or shellfish (shellfish contain high levels of iodine), it has been well established that the reaction is not to iodine; an actual iodine allergy would be problematic because iodine is required for the production of thyroid hormones. In the case of shellfish, the reaction is to a muscle protein called tropomyosin; in the case of iodinated contrast medium, the reaction is to the noniodinated part of the contrast molecule. Patients with a known hypersensitivity to the medium may benefit from premedication with corticosteroids and diphenhydramine; the use of nonionic contrast or an alternative noncontrast imaging study, if available, may be considered for patients who have severe asthma or who have experienced moderate to severe reactions to ionic contrast medium.

- Conditions associated with preexisting renal insufficiency (e.g., chronic kidney disease, single kidney transplant, nephrectomy, diabetes, multiple myeloma, treatment with aminoglycosides and NSAIDs) ***because iodinated contrast is nephrotoxic.***
- Patients who are chronically dehydrated before the test, especially older adults and patients whose health is already compromised, ***because of their risk of contrast-induced acute kidney injury.***
- Patients with pheochromocytoma ***because iodinated contrast may cause a hypertensive crisis.***
- Patients with bleeding disorders or receiving anticoagulant therapy ***because the puncture site may not stop bleeding.***

INDICATIONS

- Detect acute pulmonary embolism.
- Detect arteriovenous malformations or aneurysms.
- Detect tumors; aneurysms; congenital defects; vascular changes associated with chronic obstructive pulmonary disease, blebs, and bullae; and heart abnormalities.
- Determine the cause of recurrent or severe hemoptysis.
- Evaluate pulmonary circulation.

POTENTIAL MEDICAL DIAGNOSIS

Normal findings

- Normal pulmonary vasculature; radiopaque iodine contrast medium should circulate symmetrically and without interruption through the pulmonary circulatory system.

Abnormal findings related to

- Aneurysms
- Arterial hypoplasia or stenosis
- Arteriovenous malformations
- Bleeding caused by tuberculosis, bronchiectasis, sarcoidosis, or aspergilloma
- Inflammatory diseases
- Pulmonary embolism (PE) acute or chronic ***(visualized as an area of interrupted opacity in the pulmonary artery)***
- Pulmonary sequestration
- Tumors

CRITICAL FINDINGS:

- PE

Note and immediately report to the requesting health-care provider (HCP) any critical findings and related symptoms. A listing of these findings varies among facilities. Timely notification of a critical finding for laboratory or diagnostic studies is a role expectation of the professional nurse. The notification processes vary among facilities. Upon receipt of the critical finding, the information should be read back to the caller to verify accuracy.

INTERFERING FACTORS

Factors that may alter the results of the study

- Retained barium from a previous radiological procedure.
- Metallic objects within the examination field (e.g., jewelry, body rings), which may inhibit organ visualization and can produce unclear images.
- Inability of the patient to cooperate or remain still during the procedure because of age, significant pain, or mental status.

Other considerations

- This procedure may be terminated if chest pain, severe cardiac dysrhythmias, or signs of a cerebrovascular accident occur.
- Failure to follow dietary restrictions and other pretesting preparations may cause the procedure to be canceled or repeated.

NURSING IMPLICATIONS AND PROCEDURE

See Potential Nursing Problems on Fast Find at davispl.us/vanleeuwen7.

PRETEST:

- Positively identify the patient using at least two person-specific identifiers before services, treatments, or procedures are performed.
- ***Patient teaching:*** Inform the patient this procedure can assist with assessment of lung function and check for disease.
- Obtain a history of the patient's health concerns, symptoms, surgical procedures, and results of previously performed laboratory and diagnostic studies. Include a list of known allergens, especially allergies or sensitivities to latex, anesthetics, contrast medium, or sedatives. Ensure results of coagulation testing are obtained and recorded prior to the procedure; a creatinine level is also needed before contrast medium is to be used.
- Note any recent procedures that can interfere with test results, including examinations using iodine-based contrast medium or barium. Ensure that barium studies were performed more than 4 days before angiography.
- Record the date of the last menstrual period and determine the possibility of pregnancy in perimenopausal women.
- Obtain a list of the patient's current medications, including over-the-counter medications, dietary supplements, anticoagulants, aspirin and other salicylates (see Effects of Natural Products on Laboratory Values online at Davis*Plus*). Such products should be discontinued by medical direction for the appropriate number of days prior to a surgical procedure. Note the last time and dose of medication taken.
- If iodinated contrast medium is scheduled to be used in patients receiving metformin for type 2 diabetes, the drug should be discontinued on the day of the test and continue to be withheld for 48 hr after the test. Iodinated contrast can temporarily impair kidney function, and failure to withhold metformin may indirectly result in drug-induced lactic acidosis, a dangerous and sometimes fatal adverse effect of metformin ***(related to renal impairment that does not support sufficient excretion of metformin).***

A

- Review the procedure with the patient. Address concerns about pain and explain that there may be moments of discomfort and some pain experienced during the test. Inform the patient that the procedure is usually performed in a radiology or vascular suite by an HCP and takes approximately 30 to 60 min.
- *Sensitivity to social and cultural issues,* as well as concern for modesty, is important in providing psychological support before, during, and after the procedure.
- Explain that an intravenous (IV) line may be inserted to allow infusion of fluids such as saline, anesthetics, sedatives, or emergency medications. Explain that the contrast medium will be injected, by catheter, at a separate site from the IV line.
- Inform the patient that a burning and flushing sensation may be felt throughout the body during injection of the contrast medium. After injection of the contrast medium, the patient may experience an urge to cough, flushing, nausea, or a salty or metallic taste.
- Instruct the patient to remove jewelry and other metallic objects from the area to be examined.
- Instruct the patient to fast and restrict fluids, as ordered, for 2 to 4 hr prior to the procedure. Fasting may be ordered as a precaution against aspiration related to nausea and vomiting during the administration of contrast. Protocols may vary among facilities.
- *Make sure a written and informed consent has been signed prior to the procedure and before administering any medications.*

INTRATEST:

Potential Complications:

Injection of the contrast by inserting a catheter into a blood vessel is an invasive procedure. Complications are rare but do include risk for: allergic reaction ***(related to contrast reaction);*** bleeding from the puncture site ***(related to perforation of the blood vessel, a bleeding disorder, or the effects of natural products and medications with known anticoagulant, antiplatelet, or thrombolytic properties—postprocedural bleeding from the site is rare because at the conclusion of the procedure a resorbable device, composed of non-latex-containing arterial anchor, collagen plug, and suture, is deployed to seal the puncture site);*** blood clot formation ***(related to thrombus formation on the tip of the catheter sheath surface or in the lumen of the catheter—the use of a heparinized saline flush during the procedure decreases the risk of emboli);*** hematoma ***(related to blood leakage into the tissue following insertion of the catheter);*** infection ***(which might occur if bacteria from the skin surface is introduced during catheter insertion);*** tissue damage ***(related to extravasation of the contrast during injection);*** or nerve injury or damage to a nearby organ ***(which might occur if the catheter strikes a nerve or perforates an organ).***

- Observe standard precautions, and follow the general guidelines in Patient Preparation and Specimen Collection online at Davis*Plus*. Positively identify the patient.
- Ensure the patient has complied with dietary, fluid, and medication restrictions and pretesting preparations for 2 to 4 hr prior to the procedure. Glucagon or an anticholinergic drug may be given to stabilize movement of the stomach muscles; peristaltic contractions (motion) may alter study findings.
- Ensure the patient has removed all external metallic objects from the area to be examined.
- Administer ordered prophylactic steroids or antihistamines before the procedure.
- Avoid the use of equipment containing latex if the patient has a history of allergic reaction to latex.
- Have emergency equipment readily available.
- Instruct the patient to void prior to the procedure and to change into the gown, robe, and foot coverings provided.

- Instruct the patient to cooperate fully and to follow directions. Instruct the patient to remain still throughout the procedure because movement produces unreliable results.
- Record baseline vital signs, and continue to monitor throughout the procedure. Protocols may vary among facilities.
- Establish an IV fluid line for the injection of saline, sedatives, or emergency medications.
- Administer an antianxiety drug, as ordered, if the patient has claustrophobia. Administer a sedative to a child or to an uncooperative adult, as ordered.
- Place electrocardiographic electrodes on the patient for cardiac monitoring. Establish a baseline rhythm; determine if the patient has ventricular dysrhythmias.
- Using a pen, mark the site of the patient's peripheral pulses before angiography; this allows for quicker and more consistent assessment of the pulses after the procedure.
- Place the patient in the supine position on an examination table. Cleanse the selected area, and cover with a sterile drape.
- A local anesthetic is injected at the site, and a small incision is made or a needle is inserted under fluoroscopy.
- The contrast medium is injected, and a rapid series of images is taken during and after the filling of the vessels to be examined.
- Instruct the patient to inhale deeply and hold his or her breath while the images are taken, and then to exhale after the images are taken.
- Instruct the patient to take slow, deep breaths if nausea occurs during the procedure.
- Monitor the patient for complications related to the procedure (e.g., allergic reaction, anaphylaxis, bronchospasm).
- The needle or catheter is removed, and a pressure dressing is applied over the puncture site.
- Observe/assess the needle/catheter insertion site for bleeding, inflammation, or hematoma formation.

POST-TEST:

- Inform the patient that a report of the results will be made available to the requesting HCP, who will discuss the results with the patient.
- Instruct the patient to resume usual diet, fluids, medications, or activity, as directed by the HCP. Kidney function should be assessed before metformin is resumed.
- Monitor vital signs and neurological status every 15 min for 1 hr, then every 2 hr for 4 hr, and as ordered. Take the temperature every 4 hr for 24 hr. Monitor intake and output at least every 8 hr. Compare with baseline values. Protocols may vary from facility to facility.
- Observe for delayed allergic reactions, such as rash, urticaria, tachycardia, hyperpnea, hypertension, palpitations, nausea, or vomiting.
- Instruct the patient to immediately report symptoms such as fast heart rate, difficulty breathing, skin rash, itching, chest pain, persistent right shoulder pain, or abdominal pain. Immediately report symptoms to the appropriate HCP.
- Assess extremities for signs of ischemia or absence of distal pulse caused by a catheter-induced thrombus.
- Observe/assess the needle/catheter insertion site for bleeding, inflammation, or hematoma formation.
- Instruct the patient in the care and assessment of the site.
- Instruct the patient to apply cold compresses to the puncture site as needed, to reduce discomfort or edema.
- Instruct the patient to maintain bedrest for 4 to 6 hr after the procedure or as ordered.
- Recognize anxiety related to test results, and be supportive of perceived loss of independent function. Discuss the implications of abnormal test results on the patient's lifestyle. Provide teaching and information regarding the clinical implications of the test results, as appropriate.

A

- Reinforce information given by the patient's HCP regarding further testing, treatment, or referral to another HCP. Answer any questions or address any concerns voiced by the patient or family.
- Depending on the results of this procedure, additional testing may be performed to evaluate or monitor progression of the disease process and determine the need for a change in therapy. Evaluate test results in relation to the patient's symptoms and other tests performed.

Patient Education:

- Teach the patient to report signs of bleeding (bleeding gums, black tarry stools, blood in urine, hematoma) if started on thrombolytics.
- Teach the patient the symptoms of pulmonary disease and the importance of timely reporting.

Expected Patient Outcomes:

Understanding

- The patient and family state the importance of remaining on bedrest to prevent oxygen desaturation with activity.
- The patient and family state the importance of keeping oxygen on at all times.

Ability

- The patient demonstrates effective coping mechanisms to decrease anxiety.
- The patient demonstrates how to use controlled breathing to improve breathing patterns.

Response

- The patient and family agree to visit the HCP's office for follow-up studies and review of therapeutic plan.
- The patient agrees to take pain medication to decrease breathing discomfort and improve oxygenation.

RELATED STUDIES:

- Related tests include alveolar/arterial gradient, blood gases, BNP, BUN, chest x-ray, creatinine, CT angiography, CT thoracic, ECG, FDP, lactic acid, lung perfusion scan, lung ventilation scan, MRA, MRI chest, MRI venography, aPTT, and PT/INR.
- Refer to the Cardiovascular and Respiratory systems tables online at Davis*Plus* for related tests by body system.

Angiotensin-Converting Enzyme

SYNONYM/ACRONYM: Angiotensin I-converting enzyme (ACE).

COMMON USE: To assist in diagnosing, evaluating treatment, and monitoring the progression of sarcoidosis, a granulomatous disease that primarily affects the lungs.

SPECIMEN: Serum collected in a gold-, red-, or red/gray-top tube.

NORMAL FINDINGS: (Method: Spectrophotometry)

Age	Conventional Units	SI Units (Conventional Units × 16.667)
0–2 yr	5–83 units/L	83–1,383 nKat/L
3–7 yr	8–76 units/L	133–1,267 nKat/L
8–14 yr	6–89 units/L	100–1,483 nKat/L
Greater than 14 yr	12–68 units/L	200–1,133 nKat/L

POTENTIAL MEDICAL DIAGNOSIS

Increased in:

- Bronchitis (acute and chronic) ***(related to release of ACE from damaged pulmonary tissue)***
- Connective tissue disease ***(related to release of ACE from scarred and damaged pulmonary tissue)***
- Gaucher's disease ***(related to release of ACE from damaged pulmonary tissue; Gaucher's disease is due to the hereditary deficiency of an enzyme that results in accumulation of a fatty substance that damages pulmonary tissue)***
- Hansen's disease (leprosy)
- Histoplasmosis and other fungal diseases
- Hyperthyroidism (untreated) ***(related to possible involvement of thyroid hormones in regulation of ACE)***
- Pulmonary fibrosis ***(related to release of ACE from damaged pulmonary tissue)***
- Rheumatoid arthritis ***(related to development of interstitial lung disease, pulmonary fibrosis, and release of ACE from damaged pulmonary tissue)***
- Sarcoidosis ***(related to release of ACE from damaged pulmonary tissue)***

Decreased in:

- Advanced pulmonary carcinoma ***(related to lack of functional cells to produce ACE)***
- The period following corticosteroid therapy for sarcoidosis ***(evidenced by cessation of effective therapy)***

CRITICAL FINDINGS: N/A

Find and print out the full study on Fast Find at davispl.us/vanleeuwen7.

Anion Gap

SYNONYM/ACRONYM: Agap.

COMMON USE: To assist in diagnosing metabolic disorders that result in metabolic acidosis and electrolyte imbalance such as severe dehydration.

SPECIMEN: Serum for electrolytes (sodium, potassium, chloride, and carbon dioxide) collected in a gold-, red-, or red/gray-top tube. Plasma collected in a green-top (heparin) tube is also acceptable.

NORMAL FINDINGS: (Method: Anion gap is derived mathematically from the direct measurement of sodium, chloride, and total carbon dioxide.) There are differences between serum and plasma values for some electrolytes. The reference ranges listed are based on serum values.

Age	Conventional and SI Units
Child or adult	8–16 mmol/L

A

POTENTIAL MEDICAL DIAGNOSIS

Increased in:

Metabolic acidosis that results from the accumulation of unmeasured anionic substances like proteins, phosphorus, sulfates, ketoacids, or other organic acid waste products of metabolism

- Acute kidney injury
- Chronic kidney disease
- Dehydration (severe)
- End stage renal disease
- Ketoacidosis ***caused by starvation, high-protein/low-carbohydrate diet, diabetes, and alcoholism***
- Lactic acidosis ***(shock, excessive exercise, some malignancies)***
- Poisoning (salicylate, methanol, ethylene glycol, or paraldehyde)
- Uremia

Decreased in:

Conditions that result in metabolic alkalosis

- Chronic vomiting or gastric suction ***(related to alkalosis due to net loss of acid)***
- Excess alkali ingestion
- Hypergammaglobulinemia ***(related to an increase in measurable anions relative to the excessive production of unmeasured cationic M proteins)***
- Hypoalbuminemia ***(related to decreased levels of unmeasured anionic proteins relative to stable and measurable cation concentrations)***
- Hyponatremia ***(related to net loss of cations)***

Significant acidosis or alkalosis can result from increased levels of unmeasured cations like ionized calcium and magnesium or unmeasured anions like proteins, phosphorus, sulfates, or other organic acids, the effects of which may not be accurately reflected by the calculated anion gap.

CRITICAL FINDINGS: N/A

Find and print out the full study on Fast Find at davispl.us/vanleeuwen7.

Antibodies, Actin (Smooth Muscle) and Mitochondrial M2

SYNONYM/ACRONYM: Antiactin antibody, ASMA; mitochondrial M2 antibody, M2 antibody, AMA.

COMMON USE: To assist in the differential diagnosis of chronic liver disease, typically biliary cirrhosis.

SPECIMEN: Serum collected in a red-top tube.

NORMAL FINDINGS: (Method: Immunoassay, enzyme-linked immunosorbent [ELISA])

Actin smooth muscle antibody, IgG

Negative	Less than 20 units
Weak positive	20–30 units
Positive	Greater than 30 units

Mitochondrial M2 antibody, IgG

Negative	Less than 20 units
Weak positive	20.1–24.9 units
Positive	Greater than 25 units

A

POTENTIAL MEDICAL DIAGNOSIS

Increased in:

The exact cause of PBC is unknown. There is a high degree of correlation between the presence of actin smooth muscle antibodies (ASMA) and mitochondrial M2 antibodies (AMA) with PBC, and PBC therefore is thought to be an autoimmune disease. The antibodies have been identified in the sera of patients with other autoimmune diseases.

Actin antibodies (ASMA)
- Autoimmune hepatitis
- Chronic active viral hepatitis
- Infectious mononucleosis
- PBC
- Primary sclerosing cholangitis

Mitochondrial M2 antibodies (AMA)
- Hepatitis (alcoholic, viral)
- PBC
- Rheumatoid arthritis (occasionally)
- Systemic lupus erythematosus (occasionally)
- Thyroid disease (occasionally)

Decreased in: N/A

CRITICAL FINDINGS: N/A

Find and print out the full study on Fast Find at davispl.us/vanleeuwen7.

Antibodies, Anti-Cyclic Citrullinated Peptide

SYNONYM/ACRONYM: Anti-CCP antibodies, ACPA.

COMMON USE: To assist in diagnosing and monitoring rheumatoid arthritis.

SPECIMEN: Serum collected in a gold-, red-, or red/gray-top tube.

NORMAL FINDINGS: IgG Ab (Method: Immunoassay, enzyme-linked immunosorbent assay [ELISA])

Negative	Less than 20 units
Weak positive	20–39 units
Moderate positive	40–59 units
Strong positive	60 units or greater

A

DESCRIPTION: Rheumatoid arthritis (RA) is a chronic, systemic autoimmune disease that damages the joints. Inflammation caused by autoimmune responses can affect other organs and body systems. 🍁 The American Academy of Rheumatology's current criteria focuses on earlier diagnosis of newly presenting patients who have at least one swollen joint unrelated to another condition. The criteria includes four determinants: joint involvement (number and size of joints involved), serological test results (rheumatoid factor [RF] and/or anticitrullinated protein antibody [ACPA]), indications of acute inflammation (C-reactive protein [CRP] and/or erythrocyte sedimentation rate [ESR]), and duration of symptoms. A score of 6 or greater defines the presence of RA. Patients with longstanding RA, whose condition is inactive, or whose prior history would have satisfied the previous classification criteria by having four of seven findings—morning stiffness, arthritis of three or more joint areas, arthritis of hand joints, symmetric arthritis, rheumatoid nodules, abnormal amounts of rheumatoid factor, and radiographic changes—should remain classified as having RA. The study of RA is complex, and it is believed that multiple genes may be involved in the manifestation of RA. Scientific research has revealed an unusual peptide conversion from arginine to citrulline that results in formation of antibodies whose presence provides the basis for this test. Studies show that detection of antibodies formed against citrullinated peptides is specific and sensitive in detecting RA in both early and established disease. Anti-CCP assays have 96% specificity and 78% sensitivity for RA, compared to the traditional IgM RF marker with a specificity of 60% to 80% and sensitivity of 75% to 80% for RA. Anti-CCP antibodies are being used as a marker for erosive disease in RA, and the antibodies have been detected in healthy patients years before the onset of RA symptoms and diagnosed disease. Some studies have shown that as many as 40% of patients seronegative for RF are anti-CCP positive. The combined presence of RF and anti-CCP has a 99.5% specificity for RA. Women are two to three times more likely than men to develop RA. Although RA is most likely to affect people aged 35 to 50, it can affect all ages.

This procedure is contraindicated for: N/A

INDICATIONS

- Assist in the diagnosis of RA in both symptomatic and asymptomatic individuals.
- Assist in the identification of erosive disease in RA.
- Assist in the diagnostic prediction of RA development in undifferentiated arthritis.

POTENTIAL MEDICAL DIAGNOSIS

Increased in:

- RA ***(The immune system produces antibodies that attack the joint tissues. Inflammation of the synovium, membrane that lines the joint, begins a process called synovitis. If untreated, the synovitis can expand beyond the joint tissue to surrounding ligaments, tissues, nerves, and blood vessels.)***

Decreased in: N/A

CRITICAL FINDINGS: N/A

INTERFERING FACTORS: N/A

NURSING IMPLICATIONS AND PROCEDURE

PRETEST:

- Positively identify the patient using at least two person-specific identifiers before services, treatments, or procedures are performed. ***Patient teaching:*** Inform the patient this test can assist in identifying the cause of joint inflammation.
- Obtain a history of the patient's health concerns, symptoms, surgical procedures, and results of previously performed laboratory and diagnostic studies. Include a list of known allergens, especially allergies or sensitivities to latex.
- Obtain a list of the patient's current medications, including over-the-counter medications and dietary supplements (see Effects of Natural Products on Laboratory Values online at Davis*Plus*).
- Review the procedure with the patient. Inform the patient that specimen collection takes approximately 5 to 10 min. Address concerns about pain and explain that there may be some discomfort during the venipuncture.
- ***Sensitivity to social and cultural issues,*** as well as concern for modesty, is important in providing psychological support before, during, and after the procedure.
- Note that there are no food, fluid, or medication restrictions unless by medical direction.

INTRATEST:

Potential Complications: N/A

- Avoid the use of equipment containing latex if the patient has a history of allergic reaction to latex.
- Instruct the patient to cooperate fully and to follow directions. Direct the patient to breathe normally and to avoid unnecessary movement.
- Observe standard precautions, and follow the general guidelines in Patient Preparation and Specimen Collection online at Davis*Plus*. Positively identify the patient, and label the appropriate specimen container with the corresponding patient demographics, initials of the person collecting the specimen, date, and time of collection. Perform a venipuncture.
- Remove the needle and apply direct pressure with dry gauze to stop bleeding. Observe/assess venipuncture site for bleeding or hematoma formation and secure gauze with adhesive bandage.
- Promptly transport the specimen to the laboratory for processing and analysis.

POST-TEST:

- Inform the patient that a report of the results will be made available to the requesting health-care provider (HCP), who will discuss the results with the patient.
- Recognize anxiety related to test results, and be supportive of impaired activity related to anticipated chronic pain resulting from joint inflammation, impairment in mobility, muscular deformity, and perceived loss of independence. Discuss the implications of abnormal test results on the patient's lifestyle. Provide teaching and information regarding the clinical implications of the test results as appropriate. Explain the importance of physical activity in the treatment plan. Educate the patient regarding access to physical therapy, occupational therapy, and counseling services. Provide contact information, if desired, for the American College of Rheumatology (www.rheumatology.org), or the Arthritis Foundation (www.arthritis.org) 🍁. Encourage the patient to take medications as ordered. Treatment with disease-modifying antirheumatic drugs and biologic response modifiers may take as long as 2 to 3 mo to demonstrate their effects.

A

- Reinforce information given by the patient's HCP regarding further testing, treatment, or referral to another HCP. Answer any questions or address any concerns voiced by the patient or family.
- Depending on the results of this procedure, additional testing may be performed to evaluate or monitor progression of the disease process and determine the need for a change in therapy.

RELATED STUDIES:

- Related tests include ANA, arthroscopy, BMD, bone scan, CBC, CRP, ESR, MRI musculoskeletal, radiography bone, RF, synovial fluid analysis, and uric acid.
- Refer to the Immune and Musculoskeletal systems tables online at Davis*Plus* for related tests by body system.

Antibodies, Anti-Glomerular Basement Membrane

SYNONYM/ACRONYM: Goodpasture's antibody, anti-GBM.

COMMON USE: To assist in differentiating Goodpasture's syndrome (an autoimmune disease) from renal dysfunction.

SPECIMEN: Serum collected in a gold-, red-, or red/gray-top tube. Lung or kidney tissue also may be submitted for testing. Refer to related biopsy studies for specimen-collection instructions.

NORMAL FINDINGS: (Method: Enzyme immunoassay) Less than 20 units/mL = negative.

POTENTIAL MEDICAL DIAGNOSIS

Increased in:

- Glomerulonephritis ***(of autoimmune origin as evidenced by the presence of anti-GBM antibodies)***
- Goodpasture's syndrome ***(related to nephritis of autoimmune origin)***
- Idiopathic pulmonary hemosiderosis

Decreased in: N/A

CRITICAL FINDINGS: N/A

Find and print out the full study on Fast Find at davispl.us/vanleeuwen7.

Antibodies, Antineutrophilic Cytoplasmic

SYNONYM/ACRONYM: Cytoplasmic antineutrophil cytoplasmic antibody (c-ANCA), perinuclear antineutrophil cytoplasmic antibody (p-ANCA).

COMMON USE: To assist in diagnosing and monitoring the effectiveness of therapeutic interventions for Wegener's syndrome.

SPECIMEN: Serum collected in a red-top tube.

NORMAL FINDINGS: (Method: Indirect immunofluorescence) Negative.

POTENTIAL MEDICAL DIAGNOSIS

Increased in:

The exact mechanism by which ANCA are developed is unknown. One theory suggests colonization with bacteria capable of expressing microbial superantigens. It is thought that the superantigens may stimulate a strong cellular autoimmune response in genetically susceptible individuals. Another theory suggests the immune system may be stimulated by an accumulation of the antigenic targets of ANCA due to ineffective destruction of old neutrophils or ineffective removal of neutrophil cell fragments containing proteinase, myeloperoxidase, elastase, lactoferrin, or other proteins.

- c-ANCA
  WG and its variants
- p-ANCA
  Alveolar hemorrhage
  Angiitis and polyangiitis
  Autoimmune liver disease
  Capillaritis
  Churg-Strauss syndrome
  Crescentic glomerulonephritis
  Felty's syndrome
  Glomerulonephritis
  Inflammatory bowel disease
  Kawasaki's disease
  Leukocytoclastic skin vasculitis
  Microscopic polyarteritis
  Rheumatoid arthritis
  Vasculitis

Decreased in: N/A

CRITICAL FINDINGS: N/A

Find and print out the full study on Fast Find at davispl.us/vanleeuwen7.

Antibodies, Antinuclear, Anti-DNA, Anticentromere, Antiextractable Nuclear Antigen, Anti-Jo, and Antiscleroderma

SYNONYM/ACRONYM: Antinuclear antibodies (ANA), anti-DNA (anti-ds DNA), antiextractable nuclear antigens (anti-ENA, ribonucleoprotein [RNP], Smith [Sm], SS-A/Ro, SS-B/La), anti-Jo (antihistidyl transfer RNA [tRNA] synthase), and antiscleroderma (progressive systemic sclerosis [PSS] antibody, Scl-70 antibody, topoisomerase I antibody).

COMMON USE: To diagnose multiple systemic autoimmune disorders; primarily used for diagnosing systemic lupus erythematosus (SLE).

SPECIMEN: Serum collected in a red-top tube.

NORMAL FINDINGS: (Method: Indirect fluorescent antibody for ANA and anticentromere; Immunoassay multiplex flow for anti-DNA, ENA, Scl-70, and Jo-1)

ANA and anticentromere: Titer of 1:40 or less. Anti-ENA, Jo-1, and anti-Scl-70: Negative. Reference ranges for anti-DNA, anti-ENA, anti-Scl-70, and anti-Jo-1 vary widely due to differences in methods and the testing laboratory should be consulted directly.

Anti-DNA

A

Negative	Less than 5 international units
Indeterminate	5–9 international units
Positive	Greater than 9 international units

DESCRIPTION: Antinuclear antibodies (ANA) are autoantibodies mainly located in the nucleus of affected cells. The presence of ANA indicates SLE, related collagen vascular diseases, and immune complex diseases. Antibodies against cellular DNA are strongly associated with SLE. Anticentromere antibodies are a subset of ANA. Their presence is strongly associated with CREST syndrome (*c*alcinosis, *R*aynaud's phenomenon, *e*sophageal dysfunction, *s*clerodactyly, and *t*elangiectasia). Women are much more likely than men to be diagnosed with SLE. Jo-1 is an autoantibody found in the sera of some ANA-positive patients. Compared to the presence of other autoantibodies, the presence of Jo-1 suggests a more aggressive course and a higher risk of mortality. The clinical effects of this autoantibody include acute onset fever, dry and crackled skin on the hands, Raynaud's phenomenon, and arthritis. The extractable nuclear antigens (ENAs) include ribonucleoprotein (RNP), Smith (Sm), SS-A/Ro, and SS-B/La antigens. ENAs and antibodies to them are found in various combinations in individuals with combinations of overlapping rheumatologic symptoms. The American College of Rheumatology's current criteria includes a list of 11 signs and/or symptoms to assist in differentiating lupus from similar diseases. The patient should have four or more of these to establish suspicion of lupus; the symptoms do not have to manifest at the same time: malar rash (rash over the cheeks, sometimes described as a butterfly rash), discoid rash (red raised patches), photosensitivity (exposure resulting in development of or increase in skin rash), oral ulcers, nonerosive arthritis involving two or more peripheral joints, pleuritis or pericarditis, renal disorder (as evidenced by excessive protein in urine or the presence of casts in the urine), neurological disorder (seizures or psychosis in the absence of drugs known to cause these effects), hematological disorder (hemolytic anemia, leukopenia, lymphopenia, thrombocytopenia where the leukopenia or lymphopenia occurs on more than two occasions and the thrombocytopenia occurs in the absence of drugs known to cause it), positive ANA in the absence of a drug known to induce lupus, or immunological disorder (evidenced by positive anti-ds DNA, positive anti-Sm, positive antiphospholipid such as anticardiolipin antibody, positive lupus anticoagulant test, or a false-positive serological syphilis test, known to be positive for at least 6 mo and confirmed to be falsely positive by a negative *Treponema pallidum* immobilization or FTA-ABS).

This procedure is contraindicated for: N/A

INDICATIONS

- Assist in the diagnosis and evaluation of SLE.
- Assist in the diagnosis and evaluation of suspected immune disorders, such as rheumatoid arthritis, systemic sclerosis, polymyositis, Raynaud's syndrome, scleroderma, Sjögren's syndrome, and mixed connective tissue disease.
- Assist in the diagnosis and evaluation of idiopathic inflammatory myopathies.

POTENTIAL MEDICAL DIAGNOSIS

ANA Pattern*	Associated Antibody	Associated Condition
Rim and/or homogeneous	Double-stranded DNA	SLE
	Single- or double-stranded DNA	
Homogeneous	Histones	SLE
Speckled	Sm (Smith) antibody	SLE, mixed connective tissue disease, Raynaud's scleroderma, Sjögren's syndrome
	RNP*	Mixed connective tissue disease, various rheumatoid conditions
	SS-B/La, SS-A/Ro	Various rheumatoid conditions
Diffuse speckled with positive mitotic figures	Centromere	PSS with CREST, Raynaud's syndrome
Nucleolar	Nucleolar, RNP	Scleroderma, CREST

*ANA patterns are helpful in that certain conditions are frequently associated with specific patterns. RNP = ribonucleoprotein.

Increased in:

- Anti-Jo-1 ***is associated with dermatomyositis, idiopathic inflammatory myopathies, and polymyositis***
- ANA ***is associated with drug-induced lupus erythematosus***
- ANA ***is associated with lupoid hepatitis***
- ANA ***is associated with mixed connective tissue disease***
- ANA ***is associated with polymyositis***
- ANA ***is associated with progressive systemic sclerosis***
- ANA ***is associated with Raynaud's syndrome***
- ANA ***is associated with rheumatoid arthritis***
- ANA ***is associated with Sjögren's syndrome***
- ANA ***and anti-DNA are associated with SLE***
- Anti-RNP ***is associated with mixed connective tissue disease***
- Anti-Scl 70 ***is associated with progressive systemic sclerosis and scleroderma***
- Anti-SS-A and anti-SS-B ***are helpful in antinuclear antibody (ANA)–negative cases of SLE***
- Anti-SS-A/ANA–positive, anti-SS-B–negative patients ***are likely to have nephritis***
- Anti-SS-A/anti-SS-B–positive sera ***are found in patients with neonatal lupus***

- Anti-SS-A–positive patients ***may also have antibodies associated with antiphospholipid syndrome***
- Anti-SS-A/La ***is associated with primary Sjögren's syndrome***
- Anti-SS-A/Ro ***is a predictor of congenital heart block in neonates born to mothers with SLE***
- Anti-SS-A/Ro–positive patients ***have photosensitivity***

Decreased in: N/A

CRITICAL FINDINGS: N/A

INTERFERING FACTORS

- Drugs and other substances that may cause positive ANA results include acebutolol (diabetics), acetazolamide, anticonvulsants (increases with concomitant administration of multiple antiepileptic drugs), carbamazepine, chlorpromazine, ethosuximide, gemfibrozil, hydralazine, isoniazid, methyldopa, nitrofurantoin, penicillins, phenytoin, primidone, procainamide, quinidine, and trimethadione.
- A patient can have lupus and test ANA-negative.

NURSING IMPLICATIONS AND PROCEDURE

POTENTIAL NURSING PROBLEMS:

Problem	Signs & Symptoms	Interventions
Noncompliance, risk ***(related to failure to comply with recommended therapeutic interventions; failure to accept diagnosis)***	Triggering an acute episode of lupus due to excessive sun exposure during peak periods	Ensure the patient understands the diagnosis and disease process; discuss the risks of noncompliance on overall health
Skin ***(related to rash and lesions associated with the disease process)***	Butterfly rash across bridge of nose; lesions on exposed areas of the skin; nose and mouth ulcers	Encourage patient to avoid sun exposure during high-UV times, use a sunscreen with a UV protection greater than SPF 15 with sun exposure, reapply sunscreen frequently as needed, apply therapeutic creams or ointments to skin as prescribed by the health-care provider (HCP)
Protection ***(related to open sores; decreased immune response; steroid use)***	Fever; tenderness, redness, warmth, drainage, and swelling of open sores	Vigilant hand hygiene to protect from infection; monitor temperature and report any fever; monitor open sores for signs of infection; monitor white blood count; reverse isolation

Problem	Signs & Symptoms	Interventions
		if immune system is compromised; adequate nutrition to promote healing
Body image ***(related to physical changes associated with the disease process)***	Chronic erythematous coin-shaped raised patches (plaque) with scarring from older lesions; fixed erythema, flat or raised rash over the bridge of the nose and the cheekbones; expressions of feelings or concerns over visual physical changes; fear of rejection by others due to appearance	Emphasize strengths; determine the patient's expectations regarding appearance; identify the influence of the patient's culture, religion, ethnicity, and gender on body image perceptions; monitor verbalization of self-criticism

A

PRETEST:

- Positively identify the patient using at least two person-specific identifiers before services, treatments, or procedures are performed.
- ***Patient teaching:*** Inform the patient this test can assist in evaluating immune system function.
- Obtain a history of the patient's health concerns, symptoms, surgical procedures, and results of previously performed laboratory and diagnostic studies. Include a list of known allergens, especially allergies or sensitivities to latex.
- Obtain a list of the patient's current medications, including over-the-counter medications and dietary supplements (see Effects of Natural Products on Laboratory Values online at Davis*Plus*).
- Review the procedure with the patient. Inform the patient that specimen collection takes approximately 5 to 10 min. Address concerns about pain and explain that there may be some discomfort during the venipuncture.
- ***Sensitivity to social and cultural issues,*** as well as concern for modesty, is important in providing psychological support before, during, and after the procedure.
- Note that there are no food, fluid, or medication restrictions unless by medical direction.

INTRATEST:

Potential Complications: N/A

- Avoid the use of equipment containing latex if the patient has a history of allergic reaction to latex.
- Instruct the patient to cooperate fully and to follow directions. Direct the patient to breathe normally and to avoid unnecessary movement.
- Observe standard precautions, and follow the general guidelines in Patient Preparation and Specimen Collection online at Davis*Plus*. Positively identify the patient, and label the appropriate specimen container with the corresponding patient demographics, initials of the person collecting the specimen, date, and time of collection. Perform a venipuncture.

A

- Remove the needle and apply direct pressure with dry gauze to stop bleeding. Observe/assess venipuncture site for bleeding or hematoma formation and secure gauze with adhesive bandage.
- Promptly transport the specimen to the laboratory for processing and analysis.

POST-TEST:

- Inform the patient that a report of the results will be made available to the requesting HCP, who will discuss the results with the patient.
- Recognize anxiety related to test results, and be supportive of perceived loss of independence and fear of shortened life expectancy. Collagen and connective tissue diseases are chronic and, as such, they must be addressed on a continuous basis. Discuss the implications of abnormal test results on the patient's lifestyle. Stress the importance of compliance to the treatment regimen. Instruct patients with SLE to contact the HCP immediately if new symptoms present, including vague or common symptoms such as fever. Educate patients regarding lifestyle changes that must be implemented to protect them from increased risk of infection and development of cardiovascular disease. Patients with lupus should be advised to avoid direct exposure to sunlight or other sources of UV light, such as tanning beds ***(related to hypersensitivity of skin cells in people with lupus to UV light. The exact mechanism for this is not clearly understood, but it is believed that in people with lupus, damaged or dead skin cells are not sloughed as efficiently as occurs in normal individuals. It is also believed that cell contents released from damaged or dead skin cells may instigate an immune response leading to development of a skin rash. Sun exposure is known to damage skin; therefore, avoiding direct exposure reduces the amount of damage incurred).***
- Patients wishing to become pregnant should discuss the possibility with their HCP. The stress of pregnancy and medication regimen may present significant risks to both mother and child; pregnancies should be carefully planned.
- Patients with lupus are at increased risk for infection and should discuss the need for vaccinations with their HCP. Recommendations may include receiving vaccines during periods of remission.
- Depending on the results of this procedure, additional testing may be performed to evaluate or monitor progression of the disease process and determine the need for a change in therapy. Evaluate test results in relation to the patient's symptoms and other tests performed.

Patient Education:

- Educate the patient regarding access to counseling services.
- Educate the patient, as appropriate, regarding the importance of preventing infection, which is a significant cause of death in immunosuppressed individuals.
- Reinforce information given by the patient's HCP regarding further testing, treatment, or referral to another HCP.
- Answer any questions or address any concerns voiced by the patient or family.
- Provide teaching and information regarding the clinical implications of the test results, as appropriate.
- Provide contact information, if desired, for the American College of Rheumatology (www.rheumatology.org), the Lupus Foundation of America (www.lupus.org), or the Arthritis Foundation (www.arthritis.org) 🍁.
- Provide education on caring for open sores to prevent infection.
- Discuss the importance of adequate nutrients in supporting the immune system and preventing infection.

Expected Patient Outcomes:

Understanding

- The patient and family describe the relationship between sun exposure and triggering an acute lupus episode.

- The patient and family explain that wearing loose, long-legged and long-sleeved clothing can enhance sun protection.

Ability

- The patient and family routinely demonstrate good hand hygiene skills.
- The patient and family demonstrate proficiency in the correct application of sunscreen.

Response

- The patient identifies personal strengths to enhance self-esteem.
- The patient discusses change in appearance in a positive manner.

RELATED STUDIES:

- Related tests include antibodies anticyclic citrullinated peptide, arthroscopy, biopsy kidney, biopsy skin, BMD, bone scan, chest x-ray, complement C3 and C4, complement total, CRP, creatinine, ESR, EMG, MRI musculoskeletal, procainamide (antidysrhythmic drugs), radiography bone, RF, synovial fluid analysis, and UA.
- See the Immune and Musculoskeletal systems tables online at Davis*Plus* for related tests by body system.

Antibodies, Antisperm

SYNONYM/ACRONYM: Antispermatozoal antibody, infertility screen.

COMMON USE: To evaluate testicular fertility and identify causes of infertility such as congenital defects, cancer, and torsion.

SPECIMEN: Serum collected in a red-top tube.

NORMAL FINDINGS: (Method: Immunoassay)

Result	Sperm Bound by Immunobead (%)
Negative	0–15
Weak positive	16–30
Moderate positive	31–50
Strong positive	51–100

DESCRIPTION: Normally sperm develop in the seminiferous tubules of the testes separated from circulating blood by the blood-testes barrier. Any situation that disrupts this barrier can expose sperm to detection by immune response cells in the blood and subsequent antibody formation against the sperm. Antisperm antibodies attach to the head, midpiece, or tail of the sperm, impairing motility and ability to penetrate the cervical mucosa. The antibodies can also cause clumping of sperm, which may be noted on a semen analysis. A major cause of infertility in men is blocked efferent testicular ducts. Reabsorption of sperm from the blocked ducts may also result in development of sperm antibodies. Another more specific and sophisticated method than measurement of circulating antibodies is the immunobead sperm

A

antibody test used to identify antibodies directly attached to the sperm. Semen and cervical mucus can also be tested for antisperm antibodies.

This procedure is contraindicated for: N/A

INDICATIONS

- Evaluation of infertility.

POTENTIAL MEDICAL DIAGNOSIS

Increased in:

Conditions that affect the integrity of the blood-testes barrier can result in antibody formation.

- Blocked testicular efferent duct ***(related to absorption of sperm by blocked vas deferens)***
- Congenital absence of the vas deferens ***(related to absorption of sperm by blocked vas deferens)***
- Cryptorchidism ***(related to disruption in the integrity of the blood-testes barrier)***
- Infection (orchitis, prostatitis) ***(related to disruption in the integrity of the blood-testes barrier)***
- Inguinal hernia repair prior to puberty ***(related to disruption in the integrity of the blood-testes barrier)***
- Testicular biopsy ***(related to disruption in the integrity of the blood-testes barrier)***
- Testicular cancer ***(related to disruption in the integrity of the blood-testes barrier)***
- Testicular torsion ***(related to disruption in the integrity of the blood-testes barrier)***
- Varicocele ***(related to disruption in the integrity of the blood-testes barrier)***
- Vasectomy ***(related to absorption of sperm by blocked vas deferens)***
- Vasectomy reversal ***(related to interaction between sperm and autoantibodies developed after vasectomy)***

Decreased in: N/A

CRITICAL FINDINGS: N/A

INTERFERING FACTORS

- The patient should not ejaculate for 3 to 4 days before specimen collection if semen will be evaluated; results may be affected if specimens are collected within 48 hr of ejaculating or after no ejaculation for longer than 5 days.
- Sperm antibodies have been detected in pregnant women and in women with primary infertility.

NURSING IMPLICATIONS AND PROCEDURE

POTENTIAL NURSING PROBLEMS:

Problem	Signs & Symptoms	Interventions
Sexuality ***(related to altered sexual activity; diminished intimacy; testicular disease)***	Decreased sexual satisfaction; diminished sexual function; ongoing infertility	Discuss the possibility of sperm banking for future fertility needs; suggest counseling for patient and family and provide contact information; facilitate a

Problem	Signs & Symptoms	Interventions
		discussion of realistic changes to sexual intimacy associated with testicular disease; provide a relaxed atmosphere to discuss sexuality concerns; provide contact information for a support group
Self-esteem ***(related to altered view of self secondary to altered ability to participate in sexual intimacy; infertility; altered body image)***	Verbalizes feelings that express being a failure as a man; dissatisfaction with present state of intimacy with significant other	Monitor for negative self-statements; assess for withdrawal; monitor for real or perceived rejection of others; encourage verbalization of self-worth; encourage a discussion of perceived changes in family role; monitor for anxiety; recommend personal and family counseling; facilitate support group participation
Fear ***(related to prognosis secondary to diagnosis [cancer]; infertility; permanently altered sexual function; risk of death; loss of control; ineffective coping; unfamiliar therapeutic regime; unknown)***	Expression of fear; preoccupation with fear; increased tension; increased blood pressure; increased heart rate; vomiting; diarrhea; nausea; fatigue; weakness; insomnia; shortness of breath; increased respiratory rate; withdrawal; panic attacks	Discuss the concepts of watchful waiting, surgical intervention, radiation therapy, chemotherapy, in relation to diagnosis; access social services; provide specific and culturally appropriate education; assist the patient and family to recognize effective coping strategies; assist the patient to acknowledge fear; provide a safe environment to decrease fear; explore cultural influences that may enhance fear; use therapeutic touch as appropriate to decrease fear; collaborate with social services to address specific medical problems associated with fear

(table continues on page 122)

A

Problem	Signs & Symptoms	Interventions
Pain ***(related to spermatic cord twisting; disease process [cancer]; infection)***	Sudden testicular pain; swollen, tender testicle; nausea; bloody semen; visually one testicle is higher than the other; testicular lumps; achy discomfort in the lower abdomen; self-report of pain; crying; moaning; sleeplessness; restlessness; emotional symptoms of distress; agitation; facial grimace; irritability; diaphoresis; altered blood pressure and heart rate; nausea; vomiting	Assess pain characteristics, testicular, low abdomen; identify pain modalities that have relieved pain in the past; administer prescribed pain medication; monitor and trend vital signs; recommend use of nonpharmacologic pain management modalities, imagery, distraction, music, relaxation; provide education on postoperative pain management

PRETEST:

- Positively identify the patient using at least two person-specific identifiers before services, treatments, or procedures are performed.
- ***Patient teaching:*** Inform the patient this test can assist in the evaluation of infertility and provide guidance through assistive reproductive techniques.
- Obtain a history of the patient's health concerns, symptoms, surgical procedures, and results of previously performed laboratory and diagnostic studies. Include a list of known allergens, especially allergies or sensitivities to latex.
- Obtain a list of the patient's current medications, including over-the-counter medications and dietary supplements (see Effects of Natural Products on Laboratory Values online at Davis*Plus*).
- Review the procedure with the patient. Inform the patient that blood specimen collection takes approximately 5 to 10 min and that additional specimens may be required. Address concerns about pain and explain that there may be some discomfort during the venipuncture.
- ***Sensitivity to social and cultural issues,*** as well as concern for modesty, is important in providing psychological support before, during, and after the procedure.
- Note that there are no food, fluid, or medication restrictions unless by medical direction.

INTRATEST:

Potential Complications: N/A

- Avoid the use of equipment containing latex if the patient has a history of allergic reaction to latex.
- Instruct the patient to cooperate fully and to follow directions. Direct the patient to breathe normally and to avoid unnecessary movement.
- Observe standard precautions, and follow the general guidelines in Patient Preparation and Specimen Collection online at Davis*Plus*. Positively identify the patient, and label the appropriate specimen container with the corresponding patient demographics, initials of the person collecting the specimen, date, and time of collection. Perform a venipuncture.
- Remove the needle and apply direct pressure with dry gauze to stop bleeding. Observe/assess venipuncture site for bleeding or hematoma formation and secure gauze with adhesive bandage.
- Timing of specimen collection is an important instruction to follow in order to obtain accurate results if semen will be evaluated. The testing facility should be contacted for specific instructions that the patient will need to follow for specimen collection and direct, timely submission to the testing facility.
- Promptly transport the specimen to the laboratory for processing and analysis.

POST-TEST:

- Inform the patient that a report of the results will be made available to the requesting health-care provider (HCP), who will discuss the results with the patient.
- Recognize anxiety related to test results. Discuss the implications of abnormal test results on the patient's lifestyle. Educate the patient regarding access to counseling services. Provide a supportive, nonjudgmental environment when assisting a patient through the process of fertility testing.
- Depending on the results of this procedure, additional testing may be performed to evaluate or monitor progression of the disease process and determine the need for a change in therapy. Evaluate test results in relation to the patient's symptoms and other tests performed.

Patient Education:

- Reinforce information given by the patient's HCP regarding further testing, treatment, or referral to another HCP.
- Answer any questions or address any concerns voiced by the patient or family.
- Educate the patient regarding access to counseling services, as appropriate.

Expected Patient Outcomes:

Understanding

- Patient and family state therapeutic options, as described by HCP.
- Patient and family state that infertility may be permanent.

Skill

- Patient and family actively participate in a support group to address fertility concerns.
- Patient and family describe postoperative symptoms of infection that should be reported to the HCP.

Response

- Patient and family comply with recommendation to attend support group.
- Patient and family comply with the recommendation to attend personal and family counseling in relation to changes in intimacy and fertility.

RELATED STUDIES:

- Related tests include HCG, LH, progesterone, semen analysis, testosterone, and US scrotal.
- See the Reproductive System tables online at Davis*Plus* for related tests by body system.

Antibodies, Antistreptolysin *O*

A

SYNONYM/ACRONYM: Streptozyme, ASO.

COMMON USE: To assist in the diagnosis of streptococcal infection.

SPECIMEN: Serum collected in a red-top tube.

NORMAL FINDINGS: (Method: Immunoturbidimetric) Adult/older adult: Less than 200 international units/mL; 17 yr and younger: Less than 150 international units/mL.

POTENTIAL MEDICAL DIAGNOSIS

Increased in:

Presence of antibodies, especially a rise in titer, is indicative of exposure.

- Endocarditis
- Glomerulonephritis
- Rheumatic fever
- Scarlet fever

Decreased in: N/A

CRITICAL FINDINGS: N/A

Find and print out the full study on Fast Find at davispl.us/vanleeuwen7.

Antibodies, Antithyroglobulin, and Antithyroid Peroxidase

SYNONYM/ACRONYM: Thyroid antibodies, antithyroid peroxidase antibodies (thyroid peroxidase [TPO] antibodies were previously called thyroid antimicrosomal antibodies).

COMMON USE: To assist in diagnosing hypothyroid and hyperthyroid disease.

SPECIMEN: Serum collected in a red-top tube.

NORMAL FINDINGS: (Method: Immunoassay)

Antibody	Conventional Units
Antithyroglobulin antibody	Less than 20 international units/mL
Antiperoxidase antibody	
Newborn–3 d	0–9 international units/mL
4–30 d	0–26 international units/mL
1–12 mo	0–13 international units/mL
13 mo–19 yr	0–20 international units/mL
20 yr–older adult	0–34 international units/mL

POTENTIAL MEDICAL DIAGNOSIS

Increased in:

The presence of these antibodies differentiates the autoimmune origin of these disorders from nonautoimmune causes, which may influence treatment decisions.

- Autoimmune disorders
- Graves' disease
- Goiter
- Hashimoto's thyroiditis
- Idiopathic myxedema
- Pernicious anemia
- Thyroid carcinoma

Decreased in: N/A

CRITICAL FINDINGS: N/A

Find and print out the full study on Fast Find at davispl.us/vanleeuwen7.

A

Antibodies, Cardiolipin, Immunoglobulin A, Immunoglobulin G, and Immunoglobulin M

SYNONYM/ACRONYM: Antiphospholipid antibody, lupus anticoagulant, LA, ACA.

COMMON USE: To detect the presence of antiphospholipid antibodies, which can lead to the development of blood vessel problems and complications including stroke, heart attack, and miscarriage.

SPECIMEN: Serum collected in a red-top tube.

NORMAL FINDINGS: (Method: Immunoassay, enzyme-linked immunosorbent assay [ELISA])

IgA (APL = 1 unit IgA phospholipid)	IgG (GPL = 1 unit IgG phospholipid)	IgM (MPL = 1 unit IgM phospholipid)
Negative: 0–11 APL	Negative: 0–14 GPL	Negative: 0–12 MPL
Indeterminate: 12–19 APL	Indeterminate: 15–19 GPL	Indeterminate: 13–19 MPL
Low-medium positive: 20–80 APL	Low-medium positive: 20–80 GPL	Low-medium positive: 20–80 MPL
Positive: Greater than 80 APL	Positive: Greater than 80 GPL	Greater than 80 MPL

DESCRIPTION: Anticardiolipin (ACA) is one of several identified antiphospholipid antibodies. ACAs are of IgG, IgM, and IgA subtypes, which react with proteins in the blood that are bound to phospholipid and interfere with normal blood vessel function. The two primary types of problems they cause are narrowing and irregularity of the blood vessels and blood clots in the blood vessels. ACAs are found in individuals with lupus erythematosus, lupus-related conditions, infectious diseases, drug reactions, and sometimes fetal loss. ACAs are often found in association with lupus anticoagulant.

A

Increased antiphospholipid antibody levels have been found in pregnant women with lupus who have had miscarriages. β_2 Glycoprotein 1, or apolipoprotein H, is an important facilitator in the binding of antiphospholipid antibodies like ACA. A normal level of β_2 glycoprotein 1 is 19 units or less when measured by ELISA assays. β_2 Glycoprotein 1 measurements are considered to be more specific than ACA because they do not demonstrate nonspecific reactivity as do ACA in sera of patients with syphilis or other infectious diseases. The combination of noninflammatory thrombosis of blood vessels, low platelet count, and history of miscarriage is termed *antiphospholipid antibody syndrome*. It is documented as present if at least one of the clinical and one of the laboratory criteria are met.

Clinical criteria

- Vascular thrombosis: One or more events of arterial, venous, or small vessel thrombosis confirmed by histopathology or imaging studies.
- Pregnancy morbidity defined as either one or more unexplained deaths of a morphologically normal fetus at or beyond the 10th wk of gestation; one or more premature births of a morphologically normal neonate before the 34th wk of gestation due to eclampsia or severe pre-eclampsia; or three or more unexplained consecutive spontaneous abortions before the 10th wk of gestation, where maternal and paternal abnormalities have been excluded.
- Laboratory criteria (all measured by a standardized ELISA, according to recommended procedures).
- ACA IgG, or IgM, detectable at greater than 40 units on two or more occasions at least 12 wk apart.
- Lupus anticoagulant (LA) detectable on two or more occasions at least 12 wk apart.
- Anti-β_2 glycoprotein 1 antibody, IgG, or IgM detectable on two or more occasions at least 12 wk apart.

This procedure is contraindicated for: N/A

INDICATIONS

- Assist in the diagnosis of antiphospholipid antibody syndrome.

POTENTIAL MEDICAL DIAGNOSIS

Increased in:

Although ACAs are observed in specific diseases, the exact mechanism of these antibodies in disease is unclear. In fact, the production of ACA can be induced by bacterial, treponemal, and viral infections. Development of ACA under this circumstance is transient and not associated with an increased risk of antiphospholipid antibody syndrome. Patients who initially demonstrate positive ACA levels should be retested after 6 to 8 wk to rule out transient antibodies that are usually of no clinical significance.

- Antiphospholipid antibody syndrome
- Chorea
- Drug reactions
- Epilepsy
- Infectious diseases
- Mitral valve endocarditis
- Patients with lupus-like symptoms (often antinuclear antibody–negative)
- Placental infarction
- Recurrent fetal loss (strong association with two or more occurrences)
- Recurrent venous and arterial thromboses
- Stroke (in adults under the age of 50 years)
- Systemic lupus erythematosus (SLE)

Decreased in: N/A

CRITICAL FINDINGS: N/A

INTERFERING FACTORS

- Drugs and other substances that may increase anticardiolipin antibody levels include chlorpromazine, hydralazine, penicillin, procainamide, phenytoin, and quinidine.
- Cardiolipin antibody is partially cross-reactive with syphilis reagin antibody and lupus anticoagulant. False-positive rapid plasma reagin results may occur.

A

NURSING IMPLICATIONS AND PROCEDURE

POTENTIAL NURSING PROBLEMS:

Problem	Signs & Symptoms	Interventions
Fear ***(related to possible loss of potential child; disability; death)***	Verbalization of fear; restlessness; increased tension; continuous questioning; increased blood pressure, heart rate, respiratory rate	Provide specific and culturally appropriate education; assist the patient and family to recognize effective coping strategies; assist the patient to acknowledge fear; provide a safe environment to decrease fear; explore cultural influences that may enhance fear; utilize therapeutic touch as appropriate to decrease fear; collaborate with social services to address specific medical problems associated with fear
Grief ***(related to placental infarction associated with placental cell death resulting in loss of potential child)***	Apparent psychological and emotional distress; withdrawal; detachment; loss of appetite; refusal to participate in activities of daily living; anger; blame	Assess decision-making ability; encourage expression of grief; provide contact information for grief support group; assist to identify current support group; provide social services referral as appropriate; allow the patient to recall the loss and express feelings
Spirituality ***(related to significant loss; fear of death; debilitation disease process)***	Forgiveness; acceptance; anger at spiritual leaders; expressed feelings of hopeless, powerlessness; abandonment; refusal or inability to participate in spiritual activities (prayer); expresses	Encourage the verbalization of feelings in a safe, nonjudgmental environment; assess the desire for contact from associated spiritual leader; foster a supportive relationship with the patient and family; encourage a display of objects (spiritual, religious) that provide emotional relief; assess for expressions of hope

(table continues on page 128)

A

Problem	Signs & Symptoms	Interventions
	feelings a lack of meaning in life or lack of serenity	
Family process ***(related to altered role performance secondary to disease progression)***	Inability to perform in supportive family role; alteration in family finances; change in communication patterns; change in the assignment of family tasks and the performance of those tasks; alterations in intimacy	Family counseling; facilitate opportunities for the patient and family to express their feelings; assess the patient and family perception of the problems; evaluate patient and family weaknesses, strengths, and coping strategies; help the family and patient break down concerns into manageable parts

PRETEST:

- Positively identify the patient using at least two person-specific identifiers before services, treatments, or procedures are performed.
- ***Patient teaching:*** Inform the patient this test can assist in evaluating the amount of potentially harmful circulating antibodies.
- Obtain a history of the patient's health concerns, symptoms, surgical procedures, and results of previously performed laboratory and diagnostic studies. Include a list of known allergens, especially allergies or sensitivities to latex.
- Obtain a list of the patient's current medications, including over-the-counter medications and dietary supplements (see Effects of Natural Products on Laboratory Values online at Davis*Plus*).
- Review the procedure with the patient. Inform the patient that specimen collection takes approximately 5 to 10 min. Address concerns about pain and explain that there may be some discomfort during the venipuncture.
- ***Sensitivity to social and cultural issues,*** as well as concern for modesty, is important in providing psychological support before, during, and after the procedure.
- Note that there are no food, fluid, or medication restrictions unless by medical direction.

INTRATEST:

Potential Complications: N/A

- Avoid the use of equipment containing latex if the patient has a history of allergic reaction to latex.
- Instruct the patient to cooperate fully and to follow directions. Direct the patient to breathe normally and to avoid unnecessary movement.
- Observe standard precautions, and follow the general guidelines in Patient Preparation and Specimen Collection online at Davis*Plus*. Positively identify the patient, and label the appropriate specimen container with the corresponding patient demographics, initials of the person collecting the specimen, date, and time of collection. Perform a venipuncture.
- Remove the needle and apply direct pressure with dry gauze to stop bleeding. Observe/assess venipuncture site for bleeding or hematoma formation and secure gauze with adhesive bandage.
- Promptly transport the specimen to the laboratory for processing and analysis.

POST-TEST:

- Inform the patient that a report of the results will be made available to the requesting health-care provider (HCP), who will discuss the results with the patient.

- Recognize anxiety related to test results, and be supportive of fear of shortened life expectancy. Discuss the implications of abnormal test results on the patient's lifestyle. Provide teaching and information regarding the clinical implications of the test results, as appropriate. Educate the patient regarding access to counseling services. Provide contact information, if desired, for the Lupus Foundation of America (www.lupus.org). 🍁
- Depending on the results of this procedure, additional testing may be performed to evaluate or monitor progression of the disease process and determine the need for a change in therapy. Evaluate test results in relation to the patient's symptoms and other tests performed.

Patient Education:

- Reinforce information given by the patient's HCP regarding further testing, treatment, or referral to another HCP.
- Answer any questions or address any concerns voiced by the patient or family.

Expected Patient Outcomes:

Understanding

- The patient and family state fetal loss may be associated with placental infarct.
- The patient and family state the importance in identifying a support system that can assist with coping with the spiritual distress of grief and loss.

Ability

- The patient and family attend recommended grief counseling for emotional and psychological support related to fetal loss.
- The patient actively participates in the provision of self-care associated with the activities of daily living.

Response

- The patient and family seek assistance from spiritual leader to relieve emotional distress associated with loss of potential child or loss of function secondary to disease process.
- The patient and family agree to listen to the designated spiritual leader to assist in decreasing grief, loss.

RELATED STUDIES:

- Related tests include ANA, CBC, CBC platelet count, fibrinogen, lupus anticoagulant antibodies, protein C, protein S, and syphilis serology.
- See the Hematopoietic, Immune, and Reproductive systems tables online at Davis*Plus* for related tests by body system.

Antibodies, Fungal

SYNONYM/ACRONYM: Antifungal antibodies.

COMMON USE: To assist in the diagnosis of fungal infections.

SPECIMEN: Serum collected in a red-top tube.

NORMAL FINDINGS: (Method: Complement fixation, immunodiffusion, serologic testing) Negative or no antibody detected.

DESCRIPTION: Fungi, organisms that normally live in soil, can be introduced into humans through the accidental inhalation of spores or inoculation of spores into tissue through trauma. Yeast are classified as a single-celled fungus. Individuals most susceptible to fungal infections are usually debilitated by chronic disease, are receiving

A

prolonged antibiotic therapy, or have impaired immune systems. Fungal diseases may be classified according to the involved tissue type. Dermatophytoses involve superficial and cutaneous tissue. There are also subcutaneous and systemic mycoses. Systemic fungal infections, especially those caused by fluconazole-resistant fungi, can be life threatening. Identification of the infectious agent and effective therapeutic treatment can be more time sensitive than what is required for the natural course of growth by culture. Fungal antibody testing is used to assist in the diagnosis of fungal infections. Fungal cultures are noted to be slow growing, which causes delays in identification and selection of treatment modalities. Rapid, direct testing platforms are not yet widely available, but molecular-based blood assays are being developed and approved for use in clinical situations. For example, the T2Candida panel employs a combination of molecular technology (DNA amplification) with magnetic resonance technology to identify five common yeast species from a single blood sample in 3 to 5 hr. DNA sequencing of the internal transcribed spacer region of fungal ribosomal ribonucleic acid is another method used to provide relatively rapid identification of many fungi at the genus and species level.

This procedure is contraindicated for: N/A

INDICATIONS

- Identify organisms responsible for nail infections or abnormalities.
- Identify organisms responsible for skin eruptions, drainage, or other evidence of infection.
- Identify organisms responsible for systemic infection and sepsis.

POTENTIAL MEDICAL DIAGNOSIS

Positive Findings in

- *Aspergillus spp.*
- *Blastomyces dermatitidis*
- *Candida albicans*
- *Coccidioides immitis*
- *Cryptococcus neoformans*
- *Histoplasma capsulatum*

CRITICAL FINDINGS:

Lists of specific organisms may vary among facilities; specific organisms are required to be reported to local, state, and national departments of health. 🍁

Note and immediately report to the requesting HCP any critical findings and related symptoms. A listing of these findings varies among facilities. Timely notification of a critical finding for laboratory or diagnostic studies is a role expectation of the professional nurse. The notification processes vary among facilities. Upon receipt of the critical finding, the information should be read back to the caller to verify accuracy.

INTERFERING FACTORS

- Prompt and proper specimen processing, storage, and analysis are important to achieve accurate results.

NURSING IMPLICATIONS AND PROCEDURE

PRETEST:

- Positively identify the patient using at least two person-specific identifiers before services, treatments, or procedures are performed.
- *Patient teaching:* Inform the patient that positive results can indicate fungal

infection; negative results do not rule out a fungal infection, as some antibody titers diminish or disappear altogether 1 to 4 wk after infection has occurred.

- Obtain a history of the patient's health concerns, symptoms, surgical procedures, and results of previously performed laboratory and diagnostic studies. Include a list of known allergens, especially allergies or sensitivities to latex.
- Obtain a list of the patient's current medications, including over-the-counter medications and dietary supplements (see Effects of Natural Products on Laboratory Values online at Davis*Plus*).
- Review the procedure with the patient. Inform the patient that several tests may be necessary to confirm diagnosis. Inform the patient that specimen collection takes approximately 5 to 10 min. Address concerns about pain and explain that there may be some discomfort during the venipuncture.
- ***Sensitivity to social and cultural issues,*** as well as concern for modesty, is important in providing psychological support before, during, and after the procedure.
- Note that there are no food, fluid, or medication restrictions unless by medical direction.

INTRATEST:

Potential Complications: N/A

- Avoid the use of equipment containing latex if the patient has a history of allergic reaction to latex.
- Instruct the patient to cooperate fully and to follow directions. Direct the patient to breathe normally and to avoid unnecessary movement.
- Observe standard precautions, and follow the general guidelines in Patient Preparation and Specimen Collection online at Davis*Plus*. Positively identify the patient, and label the appropriate specimen container with the corresponding patient demographics, initials of the person collecting the specimen, date, and time of collection. Perform a venipuncture.
- Remove the needle, and apply direct pressure with dry gauze to stop bleeding. Observe/assess venipuncture site for bleeding or hematoma formation, and secure gauze with adhesive bandage.
- Promptly transport the specimen to the laboratory for processing and analysis.

POST-TEST:

- Inform the patient that a report of the results will be made available to the requesting HCP, who will discuss the results with the patient.
- Recognize anxiety related to test results. Discuss the implications of abnormal test results on the patient's lifestyle. Provide teaching and information regarding the clinical implications of the test results, as appropriate.
- Reinforce information given by the patient's HCP regarding further testing, treatment, or referral to another HCP. Answer any questions or address any concerns voiced by the patient or family.
- Depending on the results of this procedure, additional testing may be performed to evaluate or monitor progression of the disease process and determine the need for a change in therapy. Evaluate test results in relation to the patient's symptoms and other tests performed.

RELATED STUDIES:

- Related tests include relevant biopsies (lung, lymph node, skin), bronchoscopy, cultures (blood, sputum, skin), CSF analysis, gallium scan, HIV-1/2 antibodies, and pulmonary function tests.
- Refer to the Immune and Reproductive systems tables online at Davis*Plus* for related tests by body system.

A

Antibodies, Gliadin (Immunoglobulin G and Immunoglobulin A), Endomysial (Immunoglobulin A), Tissue Transglutaminase (Immunoglobulin A)

SYNONYM/ACRONYM: Endomysial antibodies (EMA), gliadin deamidated peptide (IgG and IgA) antibodies, tTG.

COMMON USE: To assist in the diagnosis and monitoring of gluten-sensitive enteropathies that may damage intestinal mucosa.

SPECIMEN: Serum collected in a red-top tube. Some genetic test methods utilize samples of saliva or buccal swabs (cells collected from the inside lining of the cheek).

NORMAL FINDINGS: (Method: Enzyme linked immunosorbent assay [ELISA] for gliadin antibody and tissue transglutaminase antibody; indirect immunofluorescence for endomysial antibodies)

	Conventional Units
IgA and IgG gliadin antibody	Less than 20 units
Tissue transglutaminase antibody	Less than 20 units
Endomysial antibodies	Negative

DESCRIPTION: Gliadin is a water-soluble protein found in the gluten of wheat, rye, oats, and barley. The intestinal mucosa of certain individuals does not digest gluten, allowing a toxic buildup of gliadin and intestinal inflammation. The inflammatory response interferes with intestinal absorption of nutrients and damages the intestinal mucosa. In severe cases, intestinal mucosa can be lost. Immunoglobulin G (IgG) and immunoglobulin A (IgA) gliadin antibodies are detectable in the serum of patients with gluten-sensitive enteropathy. Endomysial antibodies and tissue transglutaminase (tTG) antibody are two other serological tests commonly used to investigate gluten-sensitive enteropathies. Gliadin IgA tests are the most sensitive for celiac disease (CD). However, it is also recognized that a significant percentage of patients with CD are also IgA deficient, meaning false-negative IgA results may be misleading in some cases. Estimates of up to 98% of individuals susceptible to CD carry either the DQ2 or DQ8 HLA cell surface receptors, which initiate formation of antibodies to gliadin. While it appears there is a strong association between CD and these gene markers, up to 40% of individuals without CD also carry the DQ2 or DQ8 markers. Molecular testing is available to establish the absence or presence of these susceptibility markers.

CD is an inherited condition with significant impact on quality of life for the affected individual. Genetics is the study and identification of genes, genetic mutations, and inheritance. For example, genetics provides some insight into the likelihood of inheriting a trait such as blue eyes or a medical condition such as CD. Knowledge of genetics assists the nurse in identifying patients and family members who may benefit from additional education, risk assessment, and counseling. Further information regarding inheritance of genes can be found in the study titled "Genetic Testing." Counseling and written, informed consent are recommended and sometimes required before genetic testing. The use of serological markers is useful in disease monitoring because research has established a relationship between amount of gluten in the diet and degree of intestinal damage as reflected by the level of detectable antibodies. CD shares an association with a number of other conditions such as type 1 diabetes, Down's syndrome, and Turner's syndrome.

This procedure is contraindicated for: N/A

INDICATIONS

- Assist in the diagnosis of asymptomatic gluten-sensitive enteropathy in some patients with dermatitis herpetiformis.
- Assist in the diagnosis of gluten-sensitive enteropathies.
- Assist in the diagnosis of nontropical sprue.
- Monitor dietary compliance of patients with gluten-sensitive enteropathies.

POTENTIAL MEDICAL DIAGNOSIS

Increased in:

Evidenced by the combination of detectable gliadin or endomysial antibodies and improvement with a gluten-free diet.

- Asymptomatic gluten-sensitive enteropathy
- Celiac disease
- Dermatitis herpetiformis ***(etiology of this skin manifestation is unknown, but there is an association related to gluten-sensitive enteropathy)***
- Nontropical sprue

Decreased in:

- IgA deficiency ***(related to an inability to produce IgA and evidenced by decreased IgA levels and false-negative IgA gliadin tests)***
- Children under the age of 18 mo ***(related to immature immune system and low production of IgA)***

CRITICAL FINDINGS: N/A

INTERFERING FACTORS

- Conditions other than gluten-sensitive enteropathy can result in elevated antibody levels without corresponding histological evidence. These conditions include Crohn's disease, postinfection malabsorption, and food protein intolerance.
- A negative IgA gliadin result, especially with a positive IgG gliadin result in an untreated patient, does not rule out active gluten-sensitive enteropathy.

NURSING IMPLICATIONS AND PROCEDURE

PRETEST:

- Positively identify the patient using at least two person-specific identifiers before services, treatments, or procedures are performed.

A

- ***Patient teaching:*** Inform the patient this test can assist with evaluating the ability to digest gluten foods such as wheat, rye, and oats.
- Obtain a history of the patient's health concerns, symptoms, surgical procedures, and results of previously performed laboratory and diagnostic studies. Include a list of known allergens, especially allergies or sensitivities to latex.
- Obtain a list of the patient's current medications, including over-the-counter medications and dietary supplements (see Effects of Natural Products on Laboratory Values online at Davis*Plus*).
- Review the procedure with the patient. Inform the patient that specimen collection takes approximately 5 to 10 min. Address concerns about pain and explain that there may be some discomfort during the venipuncture.
- ***Sensitivity to social and cultural issues,*** as well as concern for modesty, is important in providing psychological support before, during, and after the procedure.
- Note that there are no food, fluid, or medication restrictions unless by medical direction.

INTRATEST:

- Avoid the use of equipment containing latex if the patient has a history of allergic reaction to latex.
- Instruct the patient to cooperate fully and to follow directions. Direct the patient to breathe normally and to avoid unnecessary movement.
- Observe standard precautions, and follow the general guidelines in Patient Preparation and Specimen Collection online at Davis*Plus*. Positively identify the patient, and label the appropriate specimen container with the corresponding patient demographics, initials of the person collecting the specimen, date, and time of collection. Perform a venipuncture.
- Remove the needle and apply direct pressure with dry gauze to stop bleeding. Observe/assess venipuncture site for bleeding or hematoma formation and secure gauze with adhesive bandage.
- Promptly transport the specimen to the laboratory for processing and analysis.

POST-TEST:

- Inform the patient that a report of the results will be made available to the requesting health-care provider (HCP), who will discuss the results with the patient.
- ***Nutritional Considerations:*** Encourage the patient with abnormal findings to consult with a qualified nutritionist to plan a gluten-free diet. This dietary planning is complex because patients are often malnourished and have other related nutritional problems.
- Recognize anxiety related to test results, and offer support. Discuss the implications of abnormal test results on the patient's lifestyle. Provide teaching and information regarding the clinical implications of the test results, as appropriate. Educate the patient regarding access to appropriate counseling services. Provide contact information, if desired, for the Celiac Disease Foundation (www.celiac.org) or Children's Digestive Health and Nutrition Foundation (www.cdhnf.org). 🍁
- Reinforce information given by the patient's HCP regarding further testing, treatment, or referral to another HCP. Answer any questions or address any concerns voiced by the patient or family.
- Depending on the results of this procedure, additional testing may be performed to evaluate or monitor progression of the disease process and determine the need for a change in therapy. Evaluate test results in relation to the patient's symptoms and other tests performed.

RELATED STUDIES:

- Related tests include albumin, biopsy intestine, biopsy skin, calcium, capsule endoscopy, colonoscopy, D-xylose tolerance test, electrolytes, fecal analysis, fecal fat, folic acid, genetic testing, immunoglobulins (IgA), iron, and lactose tolerance test.
- See the Gastrointestinal and Immune systems tables online at Davis*Plus* for related tests by body system.

Anticonvulsant Drugs: Carbamazepine, Ethosuximide, Lamotrigine, Phenobarbital, Phenytoin, Primidone, Valproic Acid

SYNONYM/ACRONYM: *Carbamazepine* (Carbamazepinum, Carbategretal, Carbatrol, Carbazep, CBZ, Epitol, Tegretol, Tegretol XR); *ethosuximide* (Suxinutin, Zarontin, Zartalin); *lamotrigine* (Lamictal) *phenobarbital* (Barbital, Comizial, Fenilcal, Gardenal, Phenemal, Phenemalum, Phenobarb, Phenobarbitone, Phenylethylmalonylurea, Solfoton, Stental Extentabs); *phenytoin* (Antisacer, Dilantin, Dintoina, Diphenylan Sodium, Diphenylhydantoin, Ditan, Epanutin, Epinat, Fenitoina, Fenytoin, Fosphenytoin); *primidone* (Desoxyphenobarbital, Hexamidinum, Majsolin, Mylepsin, Mysoline, Primaclone, Prysolin); *valproic acid* (Depacon, Depakote, Depakote XR, Depamide, Dipropylacetic Acid, Divalproex Sodium, Epilim, Ergenyl, Leptilan, 2-Propylpentanoic Acid, 2-Propylvaleric Acid, Valkote, Valproate Semisodium, Valproate Sodium).

COMMON USE: To monitor specific drugs for subtherapeutic, therapeutic, or toxic levels in evaluation of treatment.

SPECIMEN: Serum collected in a red-top tube.

Drug*	Route of Administration
Carbamazepine	Oral
Ethosuximide	Oral
Lamotrigine	Oral
Phenobarbital	Oral
Phenytoin	Oral
Primidone	Oral
Valproic acid	Oral

*Recommended collection time = trough: immediately before next dose (at steady state) or at a consistent sampling time.

NORMAL FINDINGS: (Method: Immunoassay for all except lamotrigine; liquid chromatography/tandem mass spectrometry for lamotrigine)

Drug	Therapeutic Range Conventional Units	Conversion to SI Units	Therapeutic Range SI Units	Half-Life (hr)	Volume of Distribution (L/kg)	Protein Binding (%)	Excretion
Carbamazepine	4–12 mcg/mL	SI units = Conventional units × 4.23	17–51 micromol/L	15–40	0.8–1.8	60–80	Hepatic
Ethosuximide	40–100 mcg/mL	SI units = Conventional units × 7.08	283–708 micromol/L	25–70	0.7	0–5	Renal
Lamotrigine	1–14 mcg/mL	SI units = Conventional units × 3.9	4–55 micromol/L	25–33	0.9–1.3	50–5	Hepatic
Phenobarbital	*Adult:* 15–40 mcg/mL	SI units = Conventional units × 4.31	*Adult:* 65–172 micromol/L	*Adult:* 50–140	0.5–1	40–50	80% hepatic and 20% renal
	Child: 15–30 mcg/mL	SI units = Conventional units × 4.31	*Child:* 65–129 micromol/L	*Child:* 40–70			80% hepatic and 20% renal
Phenytoin	10–20 mcg/mL	SI units = Conventional units × 3.96	40–79 micromol/L	20–40	0.6–0.7	85–95	Hepatic
Primidone	*Adult:* 5–12 mcg/mL	SI units = Conventional units × 4.58	*Adult:* 23–55 micromol/L	4–12	0.5–1	0–20	Hepatic
	Child: 7–10 mcg/mL	SI units = Conventional units × 4.58	*Child:* 32–46 micromol/L				
Valproic acid	50–125 mcg/mL	SI units = Conventional units × 6.93	347–866 micromol/L	8–15	0.1–0.5	85–95	Hepatic

A

POTENTIAL MEDICAL DIAGNOSIS

Level	Response
Normal levels	Therapeutic effect
Subtherapeutic levels	Adjust dose as indicated
Toxic levels	Adjust dose as indicated
Carbamazepine	Hepatic impairment
Ethosuximide	Renal impairment
Lamotrigine	Hepatic impairment
Phenobarbital	Hepatic or renal impairment
Phenytoin	Hepatic impairment
Primidone	Hepatic impairment
Valproic acid	Hepatic impairment

CRITICAL FINDINGS:

It is important to note the adverse effects of toxic and subtherapeutic levels. Care must be taken to investigate signs and symptoms of not enough medication and too much medication.

Note and immediately report to the requesting HCP any critical findings and related symptoms. A listing of these findings varies among facilities. Timely notification of a critical finding for laboratory or diagnostic studies is a role expectation of the professional nurse. The notification processes vary among facilities. Upon receipt of the critical finding, the information should be read back to the caller to verify accuracy.

Carbamazepine: Greater than 20 mcg/mL (SI: Greater than 85 micromol/L)

Signs and symptoms of carbamazepine toxicity include respiratory depression, seizures, leukopenia, hyponatremia, hypotension, stupor, and possible coma. Possible interventions include gastric lavage (contraindicated if ileus is present); airway protection; administration of fluids and vasopressors for hypotension; treatment of seizures with diazepam, phenobarbital, or phenytoin; cardiac monitoring; monitoring of vital signs; and discontinuing the medication. Emetics are contraindicated.

Ethosuximide: Greater than 200 mcg/mL (SI: Greater than 1,416 micromol/L)

Signs and symptoms of ethosuximide toxicity include nausea, vomiting, and lethargy. Possible interventions include administration of activated charcoal, administration of saline cathartic and gastric lavage (contraindicated if ileus is present), airway protection, hourly assessment of neurologic function, and discontinuing the medication.

Lamotrigine: Greater than 20 mcg/mL (SI: Greater than 78 micromol/L)

Signs and symptoms of lamotrigine toxicity include severe skin rash, nausea, vomiting, ataxia, decreased levels of consciousness, coma, increased seizures, nystagmus. Possible interventions include administration of activated charcoal, administration of saline cathartic and gastric lavage (contraindicated if ileus is present), airway protection, hourly assessment of neurologic function, and discontinuing the medication

A

Phenobarbital: Greater than 60 mcg/mL (SI: Greater than 259 micromol/L)
Signs and symptoms of phenobarbital toxicity include cold, clammy skin; ataxia; central nervous system (CNS) depression; hypothermia; hypotension; cyanosis; Cheyne-Stokes respiration; tachycardia; possible coma; and possible renal impairment. Possible interventions include gastric lavage, administration of activated charcoal with cathartic, airway protection, possible intubation and mechanical ventilation (especially during gastric lavage if there is no gag reflex), monitoring for hypotension, and discontinuing the medication.

Phenytoin (Adults): Greater than 40 mcg/mL (SI: Greater than 158 micromol/L)
Signs and symptoms of phenytoin toxicity include double vision, nystagmus, lethargy, CNS depression, and possible coma. Possible interventions include airway support, electrocardiographic monitoring, administration of activated charcoal, gastric lavage with warm saline or tap water, administration of saline or sorbitol cathartic, and discontinuing the medication.

Primidone: Greater than 15 mcg/mL (SI: Greater than 69 micromol/L)
Signs and symptoms of primidone toxicity include ataxia, anemia, CNS depression, lethargy, somnolence, vertigo, and visual disturbances. Possible interventions include airway protection, treatment of anemia with vitamin B_{12} and folate, and discontinuing the medication.

Valproic Acid: Greater than 200 mcg/mL (SI: Greater than 1,386 micromol/L)
Signs and symptoms of valproic acid toxicity include loss of appetite, mental changes, numbness, tingling, and weakness. Possible interventions include administration of activated charcoal and naloxone and discontinuing the medication.

Find and print out the full study on Fast Find at davispl.us/vanleeuwen7.

Antideoxyribonuclease-B, Streptococcal

SYNONYM/ACRONYM: ADNase-B, AntiDNase-B *titer*, antistreptococcal DNase-B *titer*, streptodornase.

COMMON USE: To assist in assessing the cause of recent infection, such as streptococcal exposure, by identification of antibodies.

SPECIMEN: Serum collected in a red-top tube.

NORMAL FINDINGS: (Method: Nephelometry)

Age	Normal Results
1–6 yr	Less than 250 units
7–17 yr	Less than 375 units
18 yr and older	Less than 300 units

Access Canadian content on Fast Find: Lab and Dx at davispl.us/vanleeuwen7

POTENTIAL MEDICAL DIAGNOSIS

Increased in:

Presence of antibodies, especially a rise in* titer, *is indicative of exposure.

- Post streptococcal glomerulonephritis
- Rheumatic fever
- Streptococcal infections (systemic)

Decreased in: N/A

CRITICAL FINDINGS: N/A

Find and print out the full study on Fast Find at davispl.us/vanleeuwen7.

A

Antidepressant Drugs (Cyclic): Amitriptyline, Nortriptyline, Protriptyline, Doxepin, Imipramine ✦

SYNONYM/ACRONYM: *Cyclic antidepressants: amitriptyline* (Elavil, Endep, Etrafon, Limbitrol, Triavil); *nortriptyline* (Allegron, Aventyl HCL, Nortrilen, Norval, Pamelor); *protriptyline* (Vivactil); *doxepin* (Adapin, Co-Dax, Novoxapin, Sinequan, Triadapin); *imipramine* (Berkomine, Dimipressin, Janimine, Pertofrane, Presamine, SK-Pramine, Tofranil PM). ✦

COMMON USE: To monitor subtherapeutic, therapeutic, or toxic drug levels in evaluation of effective treatment modalities.

SPECIMEN: Serum collected in a red-top tube.

Drug	Route of Administration	Recommended Collection Time
Amitriptyline ✦	Oral	Trough: immediately before next dose (at steady state)
Nortriptyline ✦	Oral	Trough: immediately before next dose (at steady state)
Protriptyline	Oral	Trough: immediately before next dose (at steady state)
Doxepin ✦	Oral	Trough: immediately before next dose (at steady state)
Imipramine ✦	Oral	Trough: immediately before next dose (at steady state)

NORMAL FINDINGS: (Method: Chromatography for amitriptyline, nortriptyline, protriptyline, and doxepin; immunoassay for imipramine)

Drug	Therapeutic Range Conventional Units	Conversion to SI Units	Therapeutic Range SI Units	Half-Life (h)	Volume of Distribution (L/kg)	Protein Binding (%)	Excretion
Amitriptyline ✱	125–250 ng/mL	SI units = Conventional units × 3.6	450–900 nmol/L	20–40	10–36	85–95	Hepatic
Nortriptyline ✱	50–150 ng/mL	SI units = Conventional units × 3.8	190–570 nmol/L	20–60	15–23	90–95	Hepatic
Protriptyline	70–250 ng/mL	SI units = Conventional units × 3.8	266–950 nmol/L	60–90	15–31	91–93	Hepatic
Doxepin ✱	110–250 ng/mL	SI units = Conventional units × 3.58	394–895 nmol/L	10–25	10–30	75–85	Hepatic
Imipramine ✱	180–240 ng/mL	SI units = Conventional units × 3.57	643–857 nmol/L	6–18	9–23	60–95	Hepatic

A

POTENTIAL MEDICAL DIAGNOSIS

Level	Response
Normal levels	Therapeutic effect
Subtherapeutic levels	Adjust dose as indicated
Toxic levels	Adjust dose as indicated
Amitriptyline 🍁	Hepatic impairment
Nortriptyline 🍁	Hepatic impairment
Protriptyline	Hepatic impairment
Doxepin 🍁	Hepatic impairment
Imipramine 🍁	Hepatic impairment

CRITICAL FINDINGS:
It is important to note the adverse effects of toxic and subtherapeutic levels of antidepressants. Care must be taken to investigate signs and symptoms of too little and too much medication.

Note and immediately report to the requesting HCP any critical findings and related symptoms. A listing of these findings varies among facilities. Timely notification of a critical finding for laboratory or diagnostic studies is a role expectation of the professional nurse. The notification processes vary among facilities. Upon receipt of the critical finding, the information should be read back to the caller to verify accuracy.

Cyclic Antidepressants

- Amitriptyline: Greater than 500 ng/mL (SI: Greater than 1,800 nmol/L)
- Nortriptyline: Greater than 500 ng/mL (SI: Greater than 1,900 nmol/L)
- Protriptyline: Greater than 500 ng/mL (SI: Greater than 1,900 nmol/L)
- Doxepin: Greater than 500 ng/mL (SI: Greater than 1,790 nmol/L)
- Imipramine: Greater than 500 ng/mL (SI: Greater than 1,785 nmol/L)

Signs and symptoms of cyclic antidepressant toxicity include agitation, drowsiness, hallucinations, confusion, seizures, dysrhythmias, hyperthermia, flushing, dilation of the pupils, and possible coma. Possible interventions include administration of activated charcoal; emesis; gastric lavage with saline; administration of physostigmine to counteract seizures, hypertension, or respiratory depression; administration of bicarbonate, propranolol, lidocaine, or phenytoin to counteract dysrhythmias; and electrocardiographic monitoring.

Find and print out the full study on Fast Find at davispl.us/vanleeuwen7.

Antidiuretic Hormone

SYNONYM/ACRONYM: Vasopressin, arginine vasopressin hormone, ADH.

COMMON USE: To evaluate disorders that affect urine concentration related to fluctuations of ADH secretion, such as diabetes insipidus.

SPECIMEN: Plasma collected in a lavender-top (EDTA) tube.

NORMAL FINDINGS: (Method: Radioimmunoassay)

A

Age	Antidiuretic Hormone*	SI Units (Conventional Units × 0.923)
Neonates	Less than 1.5 pg/mL	Less than 1.4 pmol/L
1 day–18 yr (normally hydrated)	0.5–1.7 pg/mL	Less than 0.5–1.6 pmol/L
Adult (normally hydrated)	1–5 pg/mL	0.9–4.6 pmol/L

*Conventional units.

Recommendation

This test should be ordered and interpreted with results of a serum osmolality.

Serum Osmolality*	Antidiuretic Hormone	SI Units (Conventional Units × 0.923)
270–280 mOsm/kg	Less than 1.5 pg/mL	Less than 1.4 pmol/L
280–285 mOsm/kg	Less than 2.5 pg/mL	Less than 2.3 pmol/L
285–290 mOsm/kg	1–5 pg/mL	0.9–4.6 pmol/L
290–295 mOsm/kg	2–7 pg/mL	1.8–6.5 pmol/L
295–300 mOsm/kg	4–12 pg/mL	3.7–11.1 pmol/L

*Conventional units.

POTENTIAL MEDICAL DIAGNOSIS

Increased in:

- Acute intermittent porphyria ***(speculated to be related to the release of ADH from damaged cells in the hypothalamus and effect of hypovolemia; the mechanisms are unclear)***
- Brain tumor ***(related to ADH production from the tumor or release from damaged cells in an adjacent affected area)***
- Disorders involving the central nervous system, thyroid gland, and adrenal gland ***(numerous conditions influence the release of ADH)***
- Ectopic production ***(related to ADH production from a systemic neoplasm)***
- Guillain-Barré syndrome ***(relationship to syndrome of inappropriate ADH [SIADH] is unclear)***
- Hypovolemia ***(potent instigator of ADH release)***
- Nephrogenic diabetes insipidus ***(related to lack of renal system response to ADH stimulation; evidenced by increased secretion of ADH)***
- Pain, stress, or exercise ***(all are potent instigators of ADH release)***
- Pneumonia ***(related to SIADH)***
- Pulmonary tuberculosis ***(related to SIADH)***
- SIADH ***(numerous conditions influence the release of ADH)***
- Tuberculous meningitis ***(related to SIADH)***

Decreased in:

Decreased production or secretion of ADH in response to changes in blood volume or pressure.

- Hypervolemia ***(related to increased blood volume, which inhibits secretion of ADH)***
- Nephrotic syndrome ***(related to destruction of pituitary cells that secrete ADH)***
- Pituitary (central) diabetes insipidus ***(related to destruction of pituitary cells that secrete ADH)***
- Pituitary surgery ***(related to destruction or removal of pituitary cells that secrete ADH)***

- Psychogenic polydipsia ***(evidenced by decreased osmolality, which inhibits secretion of ADH)***

CRITICAL FINDINGS:
Effective treatment of SIADH depends on identifying and resolving the cause of increased ADH production. Signs and symptoms of SIADH are the same as those for hyponatremia, including irritability, tremors, muscle spasms, convulsions, and neurologic changes. The patient has enough sodium, but it is diluted in excess retained water.

Find and print out the full study on Fast Find at davispl.us/vanleeuwen7.

Antidysrhythmic Drugs ✱: Amiodarone, Digoxin, Disopyramide, Flecainide, Lidocaine, Procainamide, Quinidine ✱

SYNONYM/ACRONYM: *Amiodarone* (Cordarone); *digoxin* (Digitek, Lanoxicaps, and Lanoxin); *disopyramide* (Norpace, Norpace CR); *flecainide* (Tambocor); *lidocaine* (Xylocaine); *procainamide* (Procanbid, Pronestyl, Pronestyl SR); *quinidine* (Quinidex Extentabs, Quinidine sulfate SR, Quinidine gluconate SR).

COMMON USE: To evaluate specific drugs for subtherapeutic, therapeutic, or toxic levels in treatment of heart failure and cardiac dysrhythmias.

SPECIMEN: Serum collected in a red-top tube.

Drug	Route of Administration	Recommended Collection Time
Amiodarone	Oral	Trough: immediately before next dose
Digoxin	Oral	Trough: 12–24 hr after dose Never draw peak samples
Disopyramide	Oral	Trough: immediately before next dose Peak: 2–5 hr after dose
Flecainide	Oral	Trough: immediately before next dose Peak: 3 hr after dose
Lidocaine	Intravenous (IV)	15 min; 1 hr; then every 24 hr
Procainamide	IV	15 min; 2, 6, 12 hr; then every 24 hr
Procainamide	Oral	Trough: immediately before next dose Peak: 75 min after dose
Quinidine sulfate	Oral	Trough: immediately before next dose Peak: 1 hr after dose
Quinidine gluconate	Oral	Trough: immediately before next dose Peak: 5 hr after dose
Quinidine polygalacturonate	Oral	Trough: immediately before next dose Peak: 2 hr after dose

NORMAL FINDINGS: (Method: Immunoassay)

Drug (Indication)	Therapeutic Range Conventional Units	Conversion to SI Units	SI Units	Half-Life (hr)	Volume of Distribution (L/kg)	Protein Binding (%)	Excretion
Amiodarone	0.5–2.5 mcg/mL	SI units = Conventional units × 1.55	0.8–3.9 micromol/L	250–1200	20–100	95–97	1° hepatic
Digoxin	0.5–2 ng/mL	SI units = Conventional units × 1.28	0.6–2.6 nmol/L	20–60	7	20–30	1° renal
Disopyramide	2.8–7 mcg/mL	SI units = Conventional units × 2.95	8.3–20.6 micromol/L	4–10	0.7–0.9	20–60	1° renal
Flecainide	0.2–1 mcg/mL	SI units = Conventional units × 2.41	0.5–2.4 micromol/L	7–19	5–13	40–50	1° renal
Lidocaine	1.5–5 mcg/mL	SI units = Conventional units × 4.27	6.4–21.4 micromol/L	1.5–2	1–1.5	60–80	1° hepatic
Procainamide	4–10 mcg/mL	SI units = Conventional units × 4.25	17–42 micromol/L	2–6	2–4	10–20	1° renal
N-acetyl procainamide	10–20 mcg/mL	SI units = Conventional units × 4.25	42–85 micromol/L	8			1° renal
Quinidine	2–5 mcg/mL	SI units = Conventional units × 3.08	6–15 micromol/L	6–8	2–3	70–90	Renal and hepatic

POTENTIAL MEDICAL DIAGNOSIS

Level	Response
Normal levels	Therapeutic effect
Subtherapeutic levels	Adjust dose as indicated
Toxic levels	Adjust dose as indicated
Amiodarone	Hepatic impairment, older results
Digoxin	Renal impairment, HF,* **older adults**
Disopyramide	Renal impairment
Flecainide	Renal impairment, HF
Lidocaine	Hepatic impairment, HF
Procainamide	Renal impairment
Quinidine	Renal and hepatic impairment, HF, older adults

*HF = heart failure.

CRITICAL FINDINGS:

Adverse effects of subtherapeutic levels are important. Care should be taken to investigate the signs and symptoms of too little and too much medication.

Note and immediately report to the requesting HCP any critical findings and related symptoms. A listing of these findings varies among facilities. Timely notification of a critical finding for laboratory or diagnostic studies is a role expectation of the professional nurse. The notification processes vary among facilities. Upon receipt of the critical finding, the information should be read back to the caller to verify accuracy.

Amiodarone: Greater than 2.5 mcg/mL (SI: Greater than 3.9 micromol/L)

Signs and symptoms of pulmonary damage related to amiodarone toxicity include bronchospasm, wheezing, fever, dyspnea, cough, hemoptysis, and hypoxia. Possible interventions include discontinuing the medication, monitoring pulmonary function with chest x-ray, monitoring liver function tests to assess for liver damage, monitoring thyroid function tests to assess for thyroid damage (related to the high concentration of iodine contained in the medication), and electrocardiographic (ECG) monitoring for worsening of dysrhythmia.

Digoxin: Greater than 2.5 ng/mL (SI: Greater than 3.2 nmol/L)

Signs and symptoms of digoxin toxicity include dysrhythmias, anorexia, hyperkalemia, nausea, vomiting, diarrhea, changes in mental status, and visual disturbances (objects appear yellow or have halos around them). Possible interventions include discontinuing the medication, continuous ECG monitoring (prolonged P-R interval, widening QRS interval, lengthening Q-Tc interval, and atrioventricular block), transcutaneous pacing, administration of activated charcoal (if the patient has a gag reflex and central nervous system function), support and treatment of electrolyte disturbance, and administration of Digibind or DigiFab (digoxin immune Fab). The amount of Digibind or DigiFab given depends on the level of digoxin to be neutralized. Digoxin levels must be measured before the administration of Digibind or DigiFab. Digoxin levels should not be measured for several days after administration of Digibind or DigiFab in patients with normal

A

kidney function (1 wk or longer in patients with decreased kidney function). Digibind or DigiFab cross-reacts in the digoxin assay and may provide misleading elevations or decreases in values depending on the particular assay in use by the laboratory.

Disopyramide: Greater than 7 mcg/mL (SI: Greater than 20.6 micromol/L)
Signs and symptoms of disopyramide toxicity include prolonged Q-T interval, ventricular tachycardia, hypotension, and heart failure. Possible interventions include discontinuing the medication, airway support, and ECG and blood pressure monitoring.

Flecainide : Greater than 1 mcg/mL (SI: Greater than 2.41 micromol/L)
Signs and symptoms of flecainide toxicity include exaggerated pharmacological effects resulting in dysrhythmia. Possible interventions include discontinuing the medication as well as continuous ECG, respiratory, and blood pressure monitoring.

Lidocaine: Greater than 6 mcg/mL (SI: Greater than 25.6 micromol/L)
Signs and symptoms of lidocaine toxicity include slurred speech, central nervous system depression, cardiovascular depression, convulsions, muscle twitches, and possible coma. Possible interventions include continuous ECG monitoring, airway support, and seizure precautions.

Procainamide: Greater than 10 mcg/mL (SI: Greater than 42.5 micromol/L)

***N*-Acetyl Procainamide: Greater than 40 mcg/mL (SI: Greater than 170 micromol/L);**
The active metabolite of procainamide is *N*-acetyl procainamide (NAPA). Signs and symptoms of procainamide toxicity include torsade de pointes (ventricular tachycardia), nausea, vomiting, agranulocytosis, and hepatic disturbances. Possible interventions include airway protection, emesis, gastric lavage, and administration of sodium lactate.

Quinidine: Greater than 6 mcg/mL (SI: Greater than 18.5 micromol/L)
Signs and symptoms of quinidine toxicity include ataxia, nausea, vomiting, diarrhea, respiratory system depression, hypotension, syncope, anuria, dysrhythmias (heart block, widening of QRS and Q-T intervals), asystole, hallucinations, paresthesia, and irritability. Possible interventions include airway support, emesis, gastric lavage, administration of activated charcoal, administration of sodium lactate, and temporary transcutaneous or transvenous pacemaker.

Find and print out the full study on Fast Find at davispl.us/vanleeuwen7.

Antimicrobial Drugs—Aminoglycosides: Amikacin, Gentamicin, Tobramycin; Tricyclic Glycopeptide: Vancomycin 🍁

SYNONYM/ACRONYM: *Amikacin* (generic only); *gentamicin* (Garamycin, Genoptic, Gentacidin, Gentafair, Gentak, Gentamar, Gentrasul, G-myticin, Oco-Mycin, Spectro-Genta); *tobramycin* (Nebcin, Tobrex); *vancomycin* (Lyphocin, Vancocin, Vancoled).

COMMON USE: To evaluate specific drugs for subtherapeutic, therapeutic, or toxic levels in treatment of infection.

SPECIMEN: Serum collected in a red-top tube.

Drug	Route of Administration	Recommended Collection Time*
Amikacin	IV, IM	Trough: immediately before next dose Peak: 30 min after the end of a 30-min IV infusion
Gentamicin	IV, IM	Trough: immediately before next dose Peak: 30 min after the end of a 30-min IV infusion
Tobramycin	IV, IM	Trough: immediately before next dose Peak: 30 min after the end of a 30-min IV infusion
Tricyclic glycopeptide and vancomycin	IV, PO	Trough: immediately before next dose Peak: 30–60 min after the end of a 60-min IV infusion

*Usually after fifth dose if given every 8 hr or third dose if given every 12 hr.
IM = intramuscular; IV = intravenous; PO = by mouth.

NORMAL FINDINGS: (Method: Immunoassay)

A

Drug	Therapeutic Range Conventional Units	Conversion to SI Units	SI Units	Half-Life (hr)	Distribution (L/kg)	Volume of Binding (%)	Excretion
Amikacin							
Peak	15–30 mcg/mL	SI units = Conventional units × 1.71	26–51 micromol/L	4–8	0.4–1.3	50	1° renal
Trough	4–8 mcg/mL	SI units = Conventional units × 1.71	7–14 micromol/L				1° renal
Gentamicin (Standard dosing)							
Peak	5–10 mcg/mL	SI units = Conventional units × 2.09	10–21 micromol/L	4–8	0.4–1.3	50	1° renal
Trough	Less than 2 mcg/mL	SI units = Conventional units × 2.09	Less than 4 micromol/L				1° renal
Tobramycin (Standard dosing)							
Peak	4–8 mcg/mL	SI units = Conventional units × 2.09	8.4–16 micromol/L	4–8	0.4–1.3	50	1° renal
Trough	Less than 1 mcg/mL	SI units = Conventional units × 2.09	Less than 2.1 micromol/L				1° renal

Tobramycin (Once daily dosing)							
Peak	8–12 mcg/mL	SI units = Conventional units × 2.09	16.7–25 micromol/L	4–8	0.4–1.3	50	1° renal
Trough	Less than 0.5 mcg/mL	SI units = Conventional units × 2.09	Less than 1 micromol/L				1° renal
Vancomycin							
Trough (general) values vary with indication	5–15 mcg/mL	SI units = Conventional units × 0.69	3–10 micromol/L	6–12	0.4–1	10–15	1° renal

POTENTIAL MEDICAL DIAGNOSIS

A

Level	Response
Normal levels	Therapeutic effect
Subtherapeutic levels	Adjust dose as indicated
Toxic levels	Adjust dose as indicated
Amikacin	Renal, hearing impairment
Gentamicin	Renal, hearing impairment
Tobramycin	Renal, hearing impairment
Vancomycin	Renal, hearing impairment

CRITICAL FINDINGS:

The adverse effects of subtherapeutic levels are important. Care should be taken to investigate signs and symptoms of too little and too much medication.

Note and immediately report to the requesting HCP any critical findings and related symptoms. A listing of these findings varies among facilities. Timely notification of a critical finding for laboratory or diagnostic studies is a role expectation of the professional nurse. The notification processes vary among facilities. Upon receipt of the critical finding, the information should be read back to the caller to verify accuracy.

Signs and symptoms of toxic levels of these antibiotics are similar and include loss of hearing and decreased renal function. Suspected hearing loss can be evaluated by audiometry testing. Impaired renal function may be identified by monitoring BUN and creatinine levels as well as intake and output. The most important intervention is accurate therapeutic drug monitoring so the medication can be discontinued before irreversible damage is done.

Amikacin: Greater than 10 mcg/mL (SI: Greater than 17 micromol/L)

Gentamicin: Peak greater than 12 mcg/mL, trough greater than 2 mcg/mL (SI: Peak greater than 25 micromol/L, trough greater than 4 micromol/L)

Tobramycin: Peak greater than 12 mcg/mL, trough greater than 2 mcg/mL (SI: Peak greater than 25 micromol/L, trough greater than 4 micromol/L)

Vancomycin: Trough greater than 30 mcg/mL (SI: Trough greater than 21 micromol/L)

Find and print out the full study on Fast Find at davispl.us/vanleeuwen7.

Antipsychotic Drugs and Antimanic Drugs: Haloperidol, Lithium 🍁

SYNONYM/ACRONYM: *Antipsychotic drugs: haloperidol* (Dozic, Fortunan, Haldol, Haldol Decanoate, Haloneural, Serenace); *antimanic drugs: lithium* (Cibalith-S, Eskalith, Lithane, Lithobid, Lithonate, Lithotabs, PFI-Lith, Phasal).

COMMON USE: To assist in monitoring subtherapuetic, therapeutic, or toxic drug levels related to medical interventions.

SPECIMEN: Serum collected in a red-top tube.

Drug	Route of Administration	Recommended Collection Time
Haloperidol	Oral	Peak: 3–6 hr
Lithium	Oral	Trough: at least 12 hr after last dose; steady state occurs at 90–120 hr

NORMAL FINDINGS: (Method: Chromatography for haloperidol; ion-selective electrode for lithium)

A

Drug	Therapeutic Range Conventional Units	Conversion to SI Units	Therapeutic Range SI Units	Half-Life (hr)	Volume of Distribution (L/kg)	Protein Binding (%)	Excretion
Haloperidol	6–24 ng/mL	SI units = Conventional units x 2.66	16–64 nmol/L	15–40	18–30	90	Hepatic
Lithium (chronic)	0.6–1.2 mEq/L	SI units = Conventional units x 1	0.6–1.2 mmol/L	18–24	0.7–1	0	Renal

A

POTENTIAL MEDICAL DIAGNOSIS

Level	Response
Normal levels	Therapeutic effect
Subtherapeutic levels	Adjust dose as indicated
Toxic levels	Adjust dose as indicated
Haloperidol	Hepatic impairment
Lithium	Renal impairment

CRITICAL FINDINGS:

It is important to note the adverse effects of toxic and subtherapeutic levels. Care must be taken to investigate signs and symptoms of not enough medication and too much medication.

Note and immediately report to the requesting health-care provider (HCP) any critical findings and related symptoms. A listing of these findings varies among facilities. Timely notification of a critical finding for laboratory or diagnostic studies is a role expectation of the professional nurse. The notification processes vary among facilities. Upon receipt of the critical finding, the information should be read back to the caller to verify accuracy.

Haloperidol: Greater than 42 ng/mL (SI: Greater than 112 nmol/L)

Signs and symptoms of haloperidol toxicity include hypotension, myocardial depression, respiratory depression, and extrapyramidal neuromuscular reactions. Possible interventions include emesis (contraindicated in the absence of gag reflex or central nervous system depression or excitation) and gastric lavage followed by administration of activated charcoal.

Lithium: Greater than 2 mEq/L (SI: Greater than 2 mmol/L)

Signs and symptoms of lithium toxicity include ataxia, coarse tremors, muscle rigidity, vomiting, diarrhea, confusion, convulsions, stupor, T-wave flattening, loss of consciousness, and possible coma. Possible interventions include administration of activated charcoal, gastric lavage, and administration of intravenous fluids with diuresis.

Find and print out the full study on Fast Find at davispl.us/vanleeuwen7.

Antithrombin III

SYNONYM/ACRONYM: Heparin cofactor assay, AT-III.

COMMON USE: To assist in diagnosing heparin resistance or disorders resulting from a hypercoagulable state such as thrombus.

SPECIMEN: Plasma collected in a completely filled blue-top (3.2% sodium citrate) tube. If the patient's hematocrit exceeds 55%, the volume of citrate in the collection tube must be adjusted.

NORMAL FINDINGS: (Method: Chromogenic Immunoturbidimetric)

Age	AT-III Activity Conventional Units (% of Normal)
1–4 days	39–87
5–29 days	41–93
1–3 mo	48–108
3–6 mo	73–121
6–12 mo	84–124
1–5 yr	82–139
6–17 yr	90–131
18 yr–older adult	80–120
	AT-III antigen
Newborn	40–60
6 mo–Adult	82–136

POTENTIAL MEDICAL DIAGNOSIS

Increased in:

- Acute hepatitis
- Kidney transplantation ***(Some studies have demonstrated high levels of AT III in proximal tubule epithelial cells at the time of renal transplant. The exact relationship between the kidneys and AT III levels is unknown. It is believed the kidneys may play a role in maintaining plasma levels of AT III as evidenced by the correlation between renal disease and low AT III levels.)***
- Vitamin K deficiency ***(decreased consumption related to impaired coagulation factor function)***

Decreased in:

- Carcinoma ***(related to decreased synthesis)***
- Chronic liver failure ***(related to decreased synthesis)***
- Cirrhosis ***(related to decreased synthesis)***
- Congenital deficiency
- DIC ***(related to increased consumption)***
- Liver transplantation or partial hepatectomy ***(related to decreased synthesis)***
- Nephrotic syndrome ***(related to increased protein loss)***
- Pulmonary embolism ***(related to increased consumption)***
- Septic shock ***(related to increased consumption and decreased synthesis due to hepatic impairment)***
- Venous thrombosis ***(related to increased consumption)***

CRITICAL FINDINGS: N/A

Find and print out the full study on Fast Find at davispl.us/vanleeuwen7.

α_1-Antitrypsin and α_1-Antitrypsin Phenotyping

SYNONYM/ACRONYM: α_1-antitrypsin: A_1AT, α_1-AT, AAT; α_1-antitrypsin phenotyping: A_1AT phenotype, α_1-AT phenotype, AAT phenotype, Pi phenotype.

COMMON USE: To assist in the identification of chronic obstructive pulmonary disease (COPD) and liver disease associated with α_1-antitrypsin (α_1-AT) deficiency.

SPECIMEN: Serum for α_1-AT and α_1-AT phenotyping collected in a gold-, red-, or red/gray-top tube. Whole blood from one full lavender-top (EDTA) is also acceptable.

NORMAL FINDINGS: (Method: Rate nephelometry for α_1-AT, isoelectric focusing/high-resolution electrophoresis for α_1-AT phenotyping)

α_1-Antitrypsin

Age	Conventional Units	SI Units (Conventional Units × 0.01)
0–1 mo	124–348 mg/dL	1.24–3.48 g/L
2–6 mo	111–297 mg/dL	1.11–2.97 g/L
7 mo–2 yr	95–251 mg/dL	0.95–2.51 g/L
3–19 yr	110–279 mg/dL	1.1–2.79 g/L
Adult	126–226 mg/dL	1.26–2.26 g/L

α_1-Antitrypsin Phenotyping

There are three major protease inhibitor phenotypes:

- MM—Normal
- SS—Intermediate; heterozygous
- ZZ—Markedly abnormal; homozygous

The total level of measurable α_1-AT varies with genotype. The effects of α_1-AT deficiency depend on the patient's personal habits but are most severe in patients who smoke tobacco.

POTENTIAL MEDICAL DIAGNOSIS

Increased in:

- Acute and chronic inflammatory conditions ***(related to rapid, nonspecific response to inflammation)***
- Carcinomas ***(related to rapid, nonspecific response to inflammation)***
- Estrogen therapy
- Postoperative recovery ***(related to rapid, nonspecific response to inflammation or stress)***
- Pregnancy ***(related to rapid, nonspecific response to stress)***
- Steroid therapy
- Stress (extreme physical) ***(related to rapid, nonspecific response to stress)***

Decreased in:

- COPD ***(related to malnutrition and evidenced by decreased protein synthesis)***
- Homozygous α_1-AT-deficient patients ***(related to decreased protein synthesis)***
- Liver disease (severe) ***(related to decreased protein synthesis)***
- Liver cirrhosis (infant or child) ***(related to decreased protein synthesis)***
- Malnutrition ***(related to insufficient protein intake)***
- Nephrotic syndrome ***(related to increased protein loss from diminished renal function)***

CRITICAL FINDINGS: N/A

Find and print out the full study on Fast Find at davispl.us/vanleeuwen7.

Apolipoproteins: A, B, and E

A

SYNONYM/ACRONYM: Apo A (Apo A1), Apo B (Apo B100), and Apo E.

COMMON USE: To identify levels of circulating lipoprotein to evaluate the risk of coronary artery disease (CAD).

SPECIMEN: Serum collected in a gold-, red-, or red/gray-top tube or plasma collected in a green- (heparin) or lavender-top (EDTA) tube for Apo A and Apo B; Plasma collected in a lavender-top (EDTA) tube.

NORMAL FINDINGS: (Method: Immunonephelometry for Apo A and Apo B; PCR with restriction length enzyme digestion and polyacrylamide gel electrophoresis for Apo E)

Apolipoprotein A

Age	Conventional Units	SI Units (Conventional Units × 0.01)
Newborn		
Male	41–93 mg/dL	0.41–0.93 g/L
Female	38–106 mg/dL	0.38–1.06 g/L
6 mo–4 yr		
Male	67–163 mg/dL	0.67–1.63 g/L
Female	60–148 mg/dL	0.6–1.48 g/L
Adult		
Male	81–166 mg/dL	0.81–1.66 g/L
Female	80–214 mg/dL	0.80–2.14 g/L

Apolipoprotein B

Age	Conventional Units	SI Units (Conventional Units × 0.01)
Newborn–5 yr	11–31 mg/dL	0.11–0.31 g/L
5–17 yr		
Male	47–139 mg/dL	0.47–1.39 g/L
Female	41–96 mg/dL	0.41–0.96 g/L
Adult		
Male	46–174 mg/dL	0.46–1.74 g/L
Female	46–142 mg/dL	0.46–1.42 g/L

Normal Apo E: Homozygous phenotype for e3/e3.

POTENTIAL MEDICAL DIAGNOSIS

Apolipoproteins are the protein portion of lipoproteins. Their function is to transport and to assist in cell surface receptor recognition and cellular absorption of lipoproteins to be used as energy. While studies of the exact role of apolipoproteins

A

in health and disease continue, there is a very strong association between Apo A and HDL "good" cholesterol and Apo B and LDL "bad" cholesterol.

Apolipoprotein A

Increased in:

- Familial hyper-α-lipoproteinemia
- Pregnancy
- Weight reduction

Decreased in:

- Abetalipoproteinemia
- Cholestasis
- Chronic kidney disease
- Coronary artery disease
- Diabetes (uncontrolled)
- Diet high in carbohydrates or polyunsaturated fats
- Familial deficiencies of related enzymes and lipoproteins (e.g., Tangier's disease)
- Hemodialysis
- Hepatocellular disorders
- Hypertriglyceridemia
- Nephrotic syndrome
- Premature coronary artery disease
- Smoking

Apolipoprotein B

Increased in:

- Anorexia nervosa
- Biliary obstruction
- Chronic kidney disease
- Coronary artery disease
- Cushing's syndrome
- Diabetes
- Dysglobulinemia
- Emotional stress
- End-stage renal disease
- Hemodialysis
- Hepatic disease
- Hepatic obstruction
- Hyperlipoproteinemias
- Hypothyroidism
- Infantile hypercalcemia
- Nephrotic syndrome
- Porphyria
- Pregnancy
- Premature CAD
- Werner's syndrome

Decreased in:

- Acute stress (burns, illness)
- Chronic anemias
- Chronic pulmonary disease
- Familial deficiencies of related enzymes and lipoproteins (e.g., Tangier's disease)
- Hyperthyroidism
- Inflammatory joint disease
- Intestinal malabsorption
- α-Lipoprotein deficiency (Tangier's disease)
- Malnutrition
- Myeloma
- Reye's syndrome
- Weight reduction

CRITICAL FINDINGS: N/A

Find and print out the full study on Fast Find at davispl.us/vanleeuwen7.

Arthrogram

SYNONYM/ACRONYM: Joint study.

COMMON USE: To assess and identify the cause of persistent joint pain and monitor the progression of joint disease.

AREA OF APPLICATION: Shoulder, elbow, wrist, hip, knee, ankle, temporomandibular joint.

A

DESCRIPTION: An arthrogram evaluates the cartilage, ligaments, and bony structures that compose a joint. After a local anesthetic is administered to the area of interest, a fluoroscopically guided small-gauge needle is inserted into the joint space. Fluid in the joint space is aspirated and sent to the laboratory for analysis. A water-based or air-contrast medium is injected into the joint space to outline the soft tissue structures and the contour of the joint. After a brief exercise of the joint, radiographs, computed tomography (CT), or magnetic resonance images (MRIs) are obtained.

Arthrography is instrumental in evaluating ongoing joint pain or dysfunction, damage from recurrent dislocations of a joint, visualizing synovial cysts, and identifying acute or chronic tears in the soft tissue of the joint. Arthrography can also be used therapeutically to remove fluid in the joint space or to inject medications for pain relief.

Pediatrics: Arthrography is usually performed on young athletes with a suspected chronic joint injury or acute joint trauma. Hip arthrography is performed most often in children to evaluate congenital hip dislocation, hip dysplasia, or Perthes' disease, before and after treatment. Young children may need to be sedated in order to remain still during the procedure. Parents should be encouraged to ask about preparation for sedation prior to the procedure including any ordered medications or restrictions regarding medications, diet, and activity.

This procedure is contraindicated for

- Patients who are pregnant or suspected of being pregnant, unless the potential benefits of a procedure using radiation far outweigh the risk of radiation exposure to the fetus.
- Conditions associated with adverse reactions to contrast medium (e.g., asthma, food allergies, or allergy to contrast medium).

Although patients are asked specifically if they have a known allergy to iodine or shellfish, it has been well established that the reaction is not to iodine, in fact an actual iodine allergy would be problematic because iodine is required for the production of thyroid hormones. In the case of shellfish, the reaction is to a muscle protein called tropomyosin; in the case of iodinated contrast medium, the reaction is to the noniodinated part of the contrast molecule. Patients with a known hypersensitivity to the medium may benefit from premedication with corticosteroids and diphenhydramine; the use of nonionic contrast or an alternative noncontrast imaging study, if available, may be considered for patients who have severe asthma or who have experienced moderate to severe reactions to ionic contrast medium.

- Patients with infection in the joint of interest.
- Patients with active arthritis.
- Patients with bleeding disorders receiving an arthrogram, ***because the injection site may not stop bleeding.***
- Patients with metal in their body, such as shrapnel or ferrous metal in the eye, and who will be having associated MRI studies.
- Patients with cardiac pacemakers, and who will be having associated MRI studies ***because the pacemaker can be deactivated by MRI.***

Use of gadolinium-based contrast medium (GBCAs) is contraindicated in patients with acute or chronic severe renal insufficiency (glomerular filtration rate less than 30 mL/min/1.73 m²). Patients should be screened for renal dysfunction prior to administration. The use of GBCAs should be avoided in these patients unless the benefits of the studies outweigh the risks, and if essential diagnostic information is not available using non-contrast-enhanced diagnostic studies.

Patients who are chronically dehydrated before the test, especially older adults and patients whose health is already compromised, ***because of their risk of contrast-induced acute kidney injury.***

INDICATIONS

- Evaluate pain, swelling, or dysfunction of a joint.
- Monitor disease progression.

POTENTIAL MEDICAL DIAGNOSIS

Normal findings

- Normal bursae, menisci, ligaments, and articular cartilage of the joint (note: the cartilaginous surfaces and menisci should be smooth, without evidence of erosion, tears, or disintegration).

Abnormal findings related to

- Arthritis
- Cysts
- Diseases of the cartilage (chondromalacia)
- Injury to the ligaments
- Joint derangement
- Meniscal tears or laceration
- Muscle tears
- Osteochondral fractures
- Osteochondritis dissecans
- Synovial tumor
- Synovitis

CRITICAL FINDINGS: N/A

INTERFERING FACTORS

Factors that may alter the results of the study

- Metallic objects within the examination field which may inhibit organ visualization and can produce unclear images
- Inability of the patient to cooperate or remain still during the procedure because of age, significant pain, or mental status

Other considerations N/A

NURSING IMPLICATIONS AND PROCEDURE

PRETEST:

- Positively identify the patient using at least two person-specific identifiers before services, treatments, or procedures are performed.
- ***Patient teaching:*** Inform the patient this procedure can assist in assessing the joint being examined.
- Obtain a history of the patient's health concerns, symptoms, surgical procedures, and results of previously performed laboratory and diagnostic studies. Include a list of known allergens, especially allergies or sensitivities to latex, anesthetics, contrast medium, or sedatives. Ensure results of coagulation testing are obtained and recorded prior to the procedure; a creatinine level is also needed before contrast medium is to be used. Obtain an eGFR (estimated glomerular filtration rate) and a history of renal dysfunction if the use of iodinated contrast medium (CT) or GBCA (MRI) is anticipated.
- Record the date of the last menstrual period and determine the possibility of pregnancy in perimenopausal women.
- Obtain a list of the patient's current medications, including over-the-counter medications, dietary supplements, anticoagulants, aspirin and other salicylates (see Effects of Natural Products on Laboratory Values online at Davis*Plus*). Such products should be discontinued by

A

medical direction for the appropriate number of days prior to a surgical procedure. Note the last time and dose of medication taken.

- If iodinated contrast medium is scheduled to be used in patients receiving metformin (Glucophage) for type 2 diabetes, the drug should be discontinued on the day of the test and continue to be withheld for 48 hr after the test. Iodinated contrast can temporarily impair kidney function, and failure to withhold metformin may indirectly result in drug-induced lactic acidosis, a dangerous and sometimes fatal adverse effect of metformin ***(related to renal impairment that does not support sufficient excretion of metformin).***
- Review the procedure with the patient. Address concerns about pain and explain that there may be moments of discomfort and some pain experienced during the test. Inform the patient that the procedure is usually performed in the radiology department by a health-care provider (HCP) and takes approximately 30 to 60 min.
- ***Sensitivity to social and cultural issues,*** as well as concern for modesty, is important in providing psychological support before, during, and after the procedure.
- Explain that an intravenous line may be inserted to allow infusion of fluids such as saline, anesthetics, contrast medium, or sedatives.
- Note that there are no food, fluid, or medication restrictions unless by medical direction.
- *Make sure a written and informed consent has been signed prior to the procedure and before administering any medications.*

INTRATEST:

Potential Complications:

Injection of the contrast is an invasive procedure. Complications are rare but do include risk for allergic reaction ***(related to contrast reaction);*** cardiac dysrhythmias; hematoma ***(related to blood leakage into the tissue following needle insertion);*** bleeding from the puncture site ***(related to a bleeding disorder, or the effects of natural products and medications with known anticoagulant, antiplatelet or thrombolytic properties);*** infection ***(which might occur if bacteria from the skin surface is introduced at the puncture site);*** and vascular or nerve injury ***(which might occur if the needle strikes a nerve or nearby blood vessel).***

- Avoid the use of equipment containing latex if the patient has a history of allergic reaction to latex.
- Observe standard precautions, and follow the general guidelines in Patient Preparation and Specimen Collection online at Davis*Plus*. Positively identify the patient.
- Ensure that the patient has removed all external metallic objects prior to the procedure.
- Have emergency equipment readily available.
- Administer ordered prophylactic steroids or antihistamines before the procedure if the patient has a history of allergic reactions to any substance or drug to be used in the procedure.
- Have emergency equipment readily available.
- Instruct the patient to void prior to the procedure and to change into the gown, robe, and foot coverings provided.
- Place the patient on the table in a supine position.
- The skin surrounding the joint is aseptically cleaned and anesthetized.
- A small-gauge needle is inserted into the joint space.
- Any fluid in the space is aspirated and sent to the laboratory for analysis.
- Contrast medium is inserted into the joint space with fluoroscopic guidance.
- The needle is removed, and the joint is exercised to help distribute the contrast medium.
- X-rays or MRIs are taken of the joint.

- Instruct the patient to cooperate fully and to follow directions. Instruct the patient to remain still throughout the procedure because movement produces unreliable results.
- During x-ray imaging, lead protection is placed over the gonads to prevent their irradiation.
- If MRI images are taken, supply earplugs to the patient to block out the loud, banging sounds that occur during the test. Instruct the patient to communicate with the technologist during the examination via a microphone within the scanner.

POST-TEST:

- Inform the patient that a report of the results will be made available to the requesting HCP, who will discuss the results with the patient.
- Observe/assess the joint for swelling after the test. Apply ice as needed.
- Instruct the patient to use a mild analgesic (aspirin, acetaminophen), as ordered, if there is discomfort.
- Advise the patient to avoid strenuous activity until approved by the HCP.
- Instruct the patient to notify the HCP if fever, increased pain, drainage, warmth, edema, or swelling of the joint occurs.
- Inform the patient that noises from the joint after the procedure are common and should disappear 24 to 48 hr after the procedure.
- Recognize anxiety related to test results, and be supportive of impaired activity related to anticipated persistent pain resulting from joint inflammation, impairment in mobility, musculoskeletal deformity, and loss of independence. Discuss the implications of abnormal test results on the patient's lifestyle. Provide teaching and information regarding the clinical implications of the test results, as appropriate. Educate the patient regarding access to counseling services, as appropriate. Provide contact information, if desired, for the American College of Rheumatology (www.rheumatology.org) or the Arthritis Foundation (www.arthritis.org) ✦.
- Reinforce information given by the patient's HCP regarding further testing, treatment, or referral to another HCP. Answer any questions or address any concerns voiced by the patient or family.
- Depending on the results of this procedure, additional testing may be needed to evaluate or monitor progression of the disease process and determine the need for a change in therapy. Evaluate test results in relation to the patient's symptoms and other tests performed.

RELATED STUDIES:

- Related tests include antibodies anticyclic citrullinated peptide, ANA, arthroscopy, BMD, bone scan, BUN, CBC, CRP, creatinine, ESR, MRI musculoskeletal, PT/INR, radiography bone, RF, synovial fluid analysis, and uric acid.
- Refer to the Musculoskeletal System table online at Davis*Plus* for related tests by body system.

Arthroscopy

SYNONYM/ACRONYM: N/A

COMMON USE: To obtain direct visualization of a specific joint to assist in diagnosis of joint injury or disease, and assessment of response to treatment.

AREA OF APPLICATION: Joints.

A

DESCRIPTION: Arthroscopy provides direct visualization of a joint, usually a major joint such as the ankle, knee, hip, or shoulder, through the use of a fiberoptic endoscope. The arthroscope has a light, fiberoptics, and lenses; it connects to a monitor, and the images are recorded for future study and comparison. This procedure is used for inspection of joint structures, performance of a biopsy, and surgical repairs to the joint. Meniscus removal, spur removal, and ligamentous repair are some of the surgical procedures that may be performed.

This procedure is contraindicated for

Patients with bleeding disorders undergoing arthroscopy, ***because the insertion site may not stop bleeding.***

Patients with infection in the joint of interest or on the skin surrounding the area of the insertion site ***because the infection can be introduced into the joint by the contaminated arthroscope.***

Patients who have had an arthrogram within the last 14 days ***related to residual inflammation from the contrast.***

INDICATIONS

- Detect torn ligament or tendon.
- Evaluate joint pain and damaged cartilage.
- Evaluate meniscal, patellar, condylar, extrasynovial, and synovial injuries or diseases of the knee.
- Evaluate the extent of arthritis.
- Evaluate the presence of gout.
- Monitor effectiveness of therapy.
- Remove loose objects.

POTENTIAL MEDICAL DIAGNOSIS

Normal findings

- Normal muscle, ligament, cartilage, synovial, and tendon structures of the joint, which is lined with a smooth, finely vascularized synovial membrane. The normal appearance of the cable-like ligaments and tendons visible in joints is smooth and silvery; the cartilage appears smooth and white.

Abnormal findings related to

- Arthritis (rheumatoid)
- Chondromalacia
- Cysts
- Degenerative joint changes (osteoarthritis)
- Fractures
- Ganglion or Baker's cyst
- Gout or pseudogout
- Hemarthrosis
- Infection
- Joint tumors
- Loose bodies
- Meniscal disease
- Osteochondritis
- Rheumatoid arthritis
- Subluxation, fracture, or dislocation
- Synovial rupture
- Synovitis
- Torn cartilage
- Torn ligament
- Torn rotator cuff
- Trapped synovium

CRITICAL FINDINGS: N/A

INTERFERING FACTORS

Factors that may alter the results of the study

- Inability of the patient to cooperate or remain still during the procedure because of age, significant pain, or mental status.
- Fibrous ankylosis of the joint preventing effective use of the arthroscope.
- Joints with flexion of less than 50°.

A

Other considerations

- Failure to follow dietary restrictions before the procedure may cause the procedure to be canceled or repeated.

NURSING IMPLICATIONS AND PROCEDURE

See Potential Nursing Problems on Fast Find at davispl.us/vanleeuwen7.

PRETEST:

- Positively identify the patient using at least two person-specific identifiers before services, treatments, or procedures are performed.
- *Patient teaching:* Inform the patient this procedure can assist in assessing the joint being examined.
- Obtain a history of the patient's health concerns, symptoms, surgical procedures, and results of previously performed laboratory and diagnostic studies. Include a list of known allergens, especially allergies or sensitivities to latex and anesthetics.
- Record the date of the last menstrual period and determine the possibility of pregnancy in perimenopausal women.
- Obtain a list of the patient's current medications, including over-the-counter medications, dietary supplements, anticoagulants, aspirin and other salicylates (see Effects of Natural Products on Laboratory Values online at Davis*Plus*). Such products should be discontinued by medical direction for the appropriate number of days prior to a surgical procedure. Note the last time and dose of medication taken.
- Review the procedure with the patient. Address concerns about pain, and explain that some discomfort and pain may be experienced during the test. Inform the patient that the procedure is performed by a health-care provider (HCP), usually in the surgery department, and takes approximately 30 to 120 min, depending on the joint studied.
- Explain that a preprocedure sedative may be administered to promote relaxation, as ordered.
- Crutch walking should be taught before the procedure if it is anticipated postoperatively.
- Hair around the joint area and areas 5 to 6 in. above and below the joint are clipped and prepared for the procedure.
- ***Sensitivity to social and cultural issues,*** as well as concern for modesty, is important in providing psychological support before, during, and after the procedure.
- Explain that an intravenous line may be inserted to allow infusion of fluids such as saline, anesthetics, sedatives, or emergency medications.
- Instruct the patient that to reduce the risk of aspiration related to nausea and vomiting, solid food and milk or milk products have been restricted for at least 6 hr, and clear liquids have been restricted for at least 2 hr prior to general anesthesia, regional anesthesia, or sedation/analgesia (monitored anesthesia). The American Society of Anesthesiologists has fasting guidelines for risk levels according to patient status. More information can be located at www.asahq.org. 🍁 Patients on beta blockers before the surgical procedure should be instructed to take their medication as ordered during the perioperative period. Protocols may vary among facilities.
- *Make sure a written and informed consent has been signed prior to the procedure and before administering any medications.*

INTRATEST:

Potential Complications:

Possible complications include infection, phlebitis, hemarthrosis, hematoma, swelling, formation of blood clots, and synovial sac rupture.

- Avoid the use of equipment containing latex if the patient has a history of allergic reaction to latex.

A

- Observe standard precautions, and follow the general guidelines in Patient Preparation and Specimen Collection online at Davis*Plus*. Positively identify the patient.
- Ensure the patient has complied with food and fluid restrictions as instructed, prior to the procedure.
- Resuscitation equipment and patient monitoring equipment must be available.
- Instruct the patient to void prior to the procedure and to change into the gown, robe, and foot coverings provided.
- The extremity is scrubbed, elevated, and wrapped with an elastic bandage from the distal portion of the extremity to the proximal portion to drain as much blood from the limb as possible.
- A pneumatic tourniquet placed around the proximal portion of the limb is inflated, and the elastic bandage is removed.
- As an alternative to a tourniquet, a mixture of lidocaine with epinephrine and sterile normal saline may be instilled into the joint to help reduce bleeding.
- The joint is placed in a 45° angle, and a local anesthetic is administered.
- A small incision is made in the skin in the lateral or medial aspect of the joint.
- The arthroscope is inserted into the joint spaces. The joint is manipulated as it is visualized. Added puncture sites may be needed to provide a full view of the joint.
- Biopsy or treatment can be performed at this time, and photographs should be taken for future reference.
- After inspection, specimens may be obtained for cytological and microbiological study. All specimens are placed in appropriate containers, labelled with the corresponding patient demographics, date and time of collection, site location, and promptly sent to the laboratory.
- The joint is irrigated, and the arthroscope is removed. Manual pressure is applied to the joint to remove remaining irrigation solution.
- The incision sites are sutured, and a pressure dressing is applied.
- Sterile gloves and gowns are worn throughout the procedure.

POST-TEST:

- Inform the patient that a report of the results will be made available to the requesting HCP, who will discuss the results with the patient.
- Advise the patient to avoid strenuous activity involving the joint until approved by the HCP. Driving may be restricted for a period of time, as ordered by the HCP.
- Instruct the patient to resume normal diet and medications, as directed by the HCP. The patient may be given specific activity restrictions and may also need to be taught to use crutches.
- Monitor the patient's circulation and sensations in the joint area.
- Instruct the patient to immediately report symptoms such as fever, excessive bleeding, difficulty breathing, incision site redness, swelling, coldness, numbness, tingling, change in skin color (blue or dusky), and tenderness.
- Instruct the patient to elevate the joint when sitting and to avoid flexion of the joint to reduce swelling and formation of blood clots.
- Instruct the patient to take an analgesic for joint discomfort after the procedure; ice bags may be used to reduce postprocedure swelling.
- Inform the patient to shower after 48 hr but to avoid a tub bath until after his or her appointment with the HCP.
- Recognize anxiety related to test results, and be supportive of impaired activity related to anticipated chronic pain resulting from joint inflammation, impairment in mobility, musculoskeletal deformity, and loss of independence. Discuss

the implications of abnormal test results on the patient's lifestyle. Provide teaching and information regarding the clinical implications of the test results, as appropriate. Educate the patient regarding access to counseling services, as appropriate. Provide contact information, if desired, for the American College of Rheumatology (www.rheumatology.org) or for the Arthritis Foundation (www.arthritis.org) 🍁.

- Reinforce information given by the patient's HCP regarding further testing, treatment, or referral to another HCP. Answer any questions or address any concerns voiced by the patient or family.
- Depending on the results of this procedure, additional testing may be needed to evaluate or monitor progression of the disease process and determine the need for a change in therapy. Evaluate test results in relation to the patient's symptoms and other tests performed.

Patient Education:

- Teach the patient the importance of refraining from activities that will aggravate the pain.
- Teach the patient the importance of heat and cold therapy for decreasing joint pain and improving mobility.

Expected Patient Outcomes:

Understanding

- The patient and family state the necessity of accurately reporting pain characteristics so that an appropriate pain management plan can be developed.
- The patient and family state that pacing activities is important to decrease joint stress and pain.

Ability

- The patient self-administers ordered medication (NSAIDs, corticosteroids, muscle relaxants) correctly.
- The patient demonstrates how to correctly perform range-of-motion exercises.

Response

- The patient verbalizes the importance of accurate and timely self-medication to adequately manage joint pain.
- The patient agrees to take prescribed medications.

RELATED STUDIES:

- Related tests include anticyclic citrullinated peptide, ANA, arthrogram, BMD, bone scan, CBC, CRP, ESR, MRI musculoskeletal, radiography of the bone, RF, synovial fluid analysis, and uric acid.
- Refer to the Musculoskeletal System table online at Davis*Plus* for related tests by body system.

Aspartate Aminotransferase

SYNONYM/ACRONYM: AST, SGOT (serum glutamic-oxaloacetic transaminase).

COMMON USE: Considered an indicator of cellular damage in liver disease, such as hepatitis or cirrhosis.

SPECIMEN: Serum collected in a gold-, red-, or red/gray-top tube.

NORMAL FINDINGS: (Method: Spectrophotometry, enzymatic at 37°C)

A

Age	Conventional & SI Units	SI Units Expressed as microkat/L = (Units/L × 0.017)
Newborn	25–75 units/L	0.43–1.28 microkat/L
10 days–23 mo	15–60 units/L	0.26–1.02 microkat/L
2–3 yr	10–56 units/L	0.17–0.95 microkat/L
4–6 yr	20–39 units/L	0.34–0.66 microkat/L
7–19 yr	12–32 units/L	0.2–0.54 microkat/L
20–49 yr		
Male	20–40 units/L	0.34–0.68 microkat/L
Female	15–30 units/L	0.26–0.51 microkat/L
Greater than 50 yr (older adult)		
Male	10–35 units/L	0.17–0.6 microkat/L
Greater than 45 yr (older adult)		
Female	10–35 units/L	0.17–0.6 microkat/L

Values may be slightly elevated in older adults due to the effects of medications and the presence of multiple chronic or acute diseases with or without muted symptoms.

DESCRIPTION: Aspartate aminotransferase (AST) is an enzyme that catalyzes the reversible transfer of an amino group between aspartate and α-ketoglutaric acid in the citric acid or Krebs cycle, a powerful and essential biochemical pathway for releasing stored energy. AST exists in large amounts in liver and myocardial cells and in smaller but significant amounts in skeletal muscle, kidneys, pancreas, red blood cells, and the brain. Serum AST rises when there is damage to the tissues and cells where the enzyme is found and levels directly reflect the extent of damage. AST values greater than 500 units/L (SI = 8.5 microkat/L) are usually associated with hepatitis and other hepatocellular diseases in an acute phase. AST levels are very elevated at birth, decrease with age to adulthood, and increase slightly in older adults.

This procedure is contraindicated for: N/A

INDICATIONS

- Compare serially with alanine aminotransferase levels to track the course of hepatitis.
- Monitor response to therapy with potentially hepatotoxic or nephrotoxic drugs.
- Monitor response to treatment for various disorders of hepatic function in which AST may be elevated, with tissue repair indicated by declining levels.

POTENTIAL MEDICAL DIAGNOSIS

Increased in:

AST is released from any damaged cell in which it is stored, so conditions that affect the liver, kidneys, heart, pancreas, red blood cells, or skeletal muscle, and cause cellular destruction demonstrate elevated AST levels.

Significantly Increased in: (greater than five times normal levels)

- Acute hepatitis ***(AST is very elevated in acute viral hepatitis)***
- Acute hepatocellular disease ***(especially related to chemical***

toxicity or drug overdose; moderate doses of acetaminophen have initiated severe hepatocellular disease in patients who are alcoholics)
- Acute pancreatitis
- Shock

Moderately Increased in: (three to five times normal levels)
- Alcohol misuse (chronic)
- Biliary tract obstruction
- Cardiac dysrhythmias
- Cardiac catheterization, angioplasty, or surgery
- Cirrhosis
- Chronic hepatitis
- Heart failure
- HELLP (hemolysis , elevated liver enzymes, low platelet count) syndrome of pregnancy
- Infectious mononucleosis
- Liver tumors
- Muscle diseases (e.g., dermatomyositis, dystrophy, gangrene, polymyositis, trichinosis)
- Myocardial infarction
- Reye's syndrome
- Trauma ***(related to injury or surgery of liver, head, and other sites where AST is found)***

Slightly Increased in: (two to three times normal)
- Cerebrovascular accident
- Cirrhosis, fatty liver ***(related to obesity, diabetes, jejunoileal bypass, administration of total parenteral nutrition)***
- Delirium tremens
- Hemolytic anemia
- Pericarditis
- Pulmonary infarction

Decreased in:
- Hemodialysis ***(presumed to be related to a corresponding deficiency of vitamin B_6 observed in hemodialysis patients)***
- Uremia ***(related to a buildup of toxins which modify the activity of coenzymes required for transaminase activity)***
- Vitamin B_6 deficiency ***(related to the lack of vitamin B_6, a required cofactor for the transaminases)***

CRITICAL FINDINGS: N/A

INTERFERING FACTORS
- Drugs and other substances that may increase AST levels by causing cholestasis include amitriptyline, anabolic steroids, androgens, benzodiazepines, chlorothiazide, chlorpropamide, dapsone, erythromycin, estrogens, ethionamide, gold salts, imipramine, mercaptopurine, nitrofurans, oral contraceptives, penicillins, phenothiazines, progesterone, sulfonamides, tamoxifen, and tolbutamide.
- Drugs and other substances that may increase AST levels by causing hepatocellular damage include acetaminophen, acetylsalicylic acid, allopurinol, amiodarone, anabolic steroids, anticonvulsants, asparaginase, azithromycin, bromocriptine, captopril, cephalosporins, chloramphenicol, clindamycin, clofibrate, danazol, enflurane, ethambutol, ethionamide, fenofibrate, fluconazole, fluoroquinolones, foscarnet, gentamicin, indomethacin, interferon, interleukin-2, levamisole, levodopa, lincomycin, low-molecular-weight heparin, methyldopa, monoamine oxidase inhibitors, naproxen, nifedipine, nitrofurans, oral contraceptives, probenecid, procainamide, quinine, ranitidine, retinol, ritodrine, sulfonylureas, tetracyclines, tobramycin, and verapamil .
- Drugs and other substances that may decrease AST levels include allopurinol, cyclosporine, interferon

A

alpha, naltrexone, progesterone, trifluoperazine, and ursodiol.

- **Hemolysis falsely increases AST values.**
- **Hemodialysis falsely decreases AST values.**

NURSING IMPLICATIONS AND PROCEDURE

PRETEST:

- Positively identify the patient using at least two person-specific identifiers before services, treatments, or procedures are performed.
- *Patient teaching:* Inform the patient this test can assist in assessing liver function.
- Obtain a history of the patient's health concerns, symptoms, surgical procedures, and results of previously performed laboratory and diagnostic studies. Include a list of known allergens, especially allergies or sensitivities to latex.
- Obtain a list of the patient's current medications, including over-the-counter medications and dietary supplements (see Effects of Natural Products on Laboratory Values online at Davis*Plus*).
- Review the procedure with the patient. Inform the patient that specimen collection takes approximately 5 to 10 min. Address concerns about pain, and explain to the patient that there may be some discomfort during the venipuncture.
- *Sensitivity to social and cultural issues,* as well as concern for modesty, is important in providing psychological support before, during, and after the procedure.
- Note that there are no food, fluid, or medication restrictions unless by medical direction.

INTRATEST:

Potential Complications: N/A

- Avoid the use of equipment containing latex if the patient has a history of allergic reaction to latex.
- Instruct the patient to cooperate fully and to follow directions. Direct the patient to breathe normally and to avoid unnecessary movement.
- Observe standard precautions, and follow the general guidelines in Patient Preparation and Specimen Collection online at Davis*Plus*. Positively identify the patient, and label the appropriate specimen container with the corresponding patient demographics, initials of the person collecting the specimen, date, and time of collection. Perform a venipuncture.
- Remove the needle and apply direct pressure with dry gauze to stop bleeding. Observe/assess venipuncture site for bleeding or hematoma formation and secure gauze with adhesive bandage.
- Promptly transport the specimen to the laboratory for processing and analysis.

POST-TEST:

- Inform the patient that a report of the results will be made available to the requesting health-care provider (HCP), who will discuss the results with the patient.
- *Nutritional Considerations:* Increased AST levels may be associated with liver disease. Dietary recommendations may be indicated and will vary depending on the condition and its severity. Currently, there are no specific medications that can be given to cure hepatitis, but elimination of alcohol ingestion and a diet optimized for convalescence are commonly included in the treatment plan. A high-calorie, high-protein, moderate-fat diet with a high fluid intake is often recommended for patients with hepatitis. Treatment of cirrhosis is different; a low-protein diet may be in order if the patient's liver can no longer process the end products of protein metabolism. A diet of soft foods may be required if esophageal varices have developed. Ammonia levels may be used to determine

A

whether protein should be added to or reduced from the diet. Patients should be encouraged to eat simple carbohydrates and emulsified fats (as in homogenized milk or eggs) rather than complex carbohydrates (e.g., starch, fiber, and glycogen [animal carbohydrates]) and complex fats, which require additional bile to emulsify them so that they can be used. The patient with cirrhosis should be observed carefully for the development of ascites, in which case fluid and electrolyte balance requires strict attention.

- Recognize anxiety related to test results, and be supportive of fear of shortened life expectancy. Discuss the implications of abnormal test results on the patient's lifestyle. Provide teaching and information regarding the clinical implications of the test results, as appropriate. Educate the patient regarding access to counseling services.
- Instruct the patient to immediately report chest pain and changes in breathing pattern to the HCP.
- Reinforce information given by the patient's HCP regarding further testing, treatment, or referral to another HCP. Answer any questions or address any concerns voiced by the patient or family.
- Depending on the results of this procedure, additional testing may be performed to evaluate or monitor progression of the disease process and determine the need for a change in therapy. Evaluate test results in relation to the patient's symptoms and other tests performed.

RELATED STUDIES:

- Related tests include acetaminophen, ALT, albumin, ALP, ammonia, AMA/ASMA, α_1-antitrypsin/phenotyping, bilirubin and fractions, biopsy liver, cholangiography percutaneous transhepatic, cholangiography post-op, CT biliary tract and liver, ERCP, ethanol, ferritin, GGT, hepatitis antigens and antibodies, hepatobiliary scan, iron/total iron-binding capacity, liver and spleen scan, protein and fractions, PT/INR, US abdomen, and US liver.
- See the Hepatobiliary System table online at Davis*Plus* for related tests by body system.

Atrial Natriuretic Peptide

SYNONYM/ACRONYM: Atrial natriuretic hormone, atrial natriuretic factor, ANF, ANH, ANP.

COMMON USE: To assist in diagnosing and monitoring heart failure (HF) and to differentiate HF from other causes of dyspnea.

SPECIMEN: Plasma collected in a chilled, lavender-top tube. Specimen should be transported tightly capped and in an ice slurry.

NORMAL FINDINGS: (Method: Radioimmunoassay)

Conventional Units	SI Units (Conventional Units × 1)
20–77 pg/mL	20–77 ng/L

A

POTENTIAL MEDICAL DIAGNOSIS

Increased in:

ANP is secreted in response to increased hemodynamic load caused by physiological stimuli as with atrial stretch or endocrine stimuli from the aldosterone/renin system.

- Asymptomatic cardiac volume overload
- Atherosclerosis
- Coronary heart disease (CHD)
- Elevated cardiac filling pressure
- HF
- Paroxysmal atrial tachycardia

Decreased in: N/A

CRITICAL FINDINGS: N/A

Find and print out the full study on Fast Find at davispl.us/vanleeuwen7.

Audiometry, Hearing Loss

SYNONYM/ACRONYM: N/A

COMMON USE: To evaluate hearing loss in newborns and school-age children but can be used for all ages.

AREA OF APPLICATION: Ears.

DESCRIPTION: Tests to estimate hearing ability can be performed on patients of any age (e.g., at birth before discharge from a hospital or birthing center, as part of a school screening program, or as adults if indicated). Hearing loss audiometry includes quantitative testing for a hearing deficit. An audiometer is used to measure and record thresholds of hearing by air conduction and bone conduction tests. The test results determine if hearing loss is conductive, sensorineural, or a combination of both. An elevated air-conduction threshold with a normal bone-conduction threshold indicates a conductive hearing loss. An equally elevated threshold for both air and bone conduction indicates a sensorineural hearing loss. An elevated threshold of air conduction that is greater than an elevated threshold of bone conduction indicates a composite of both types of hearing loss. A conductive hearing loss is caused by an abnormality in the external auditory canal or middle ear, and a sensorineural hearing loss by an abnormality in the inner ear or of the VIII (auditory) nerve. Sensorineural hearing loss can be further differentiated clinically by sensory (cochlear) or neural (VIII nerve) lesions. Sensorineural hearing loss is permanent. Additional information for comparing and differentiating between conductive and sensorineural hearing loss can be obtained from hearing loss tuning fork tests. Every state and territory in the United States has a newborn screening program that includes early hearing loss detection and intervention (EHDI). The goal of EHDI is to assure that permanent hearing loss is identified before 3 mo of age, appropriate and timely intervention services are provided before 6 mo of age, families of infants with hearing loss receive culturally competent support, and tracking and data management systems for newborn hearing screens are linked with other relevant public health information systems. 🍁

This procedure is contraindicated for: N/A

INDICATIONS

- Determine the need for a type of hearing aid and evaluate its effectiveness.
- Determine the type and extent of hearing loss and if further radiological, audiological, or vestibular procedures are needed to identify the cause.
- Evaluate communication disabilities and plan for rehabilitation interventions.
- Evaluate degree and extent of preoperative and postoperative hearing loss following stapedectomy in patients with otosclerosis.
- Screen for hearing loss in infants and children and determine the need for a referral to an audiologist.

POTENTIAL MEDICAL DIAGNOSIS

If findings are normal, the patient should have normal hearing. The test is conducted using earphones and/or a device placed behind the ear to deliver sounds of varying intensities. Results are categorized using ranges of pure tone recorded in decibels.

ASHA Category	Pure Tone Averages
Normal range or no impairment	−10–15 dB
Slight loss	16–25 dB
Mild loss	26–40 dB
Moderate loss	41–55 dB
Moderately severe loss	56–70 dB
Severe loss	71–90 dB
Profound loss	Greater than 91 dB

dB = decibel.

Normal findings

- Normal pure tone average of −10 to 15 dB for infants, children, or adults

Abnormal findings related to

- Causes of conductive hearing loss
  - Impacted cerumen
  - Hole in eardrum
  - Malformed outer ear, ear canal, or middle ear
  - Obstruction of external ear canal ***(related to presence of a foreign body)***
  - Otitis externa ***(related to infection in ear canal)***
  - Otitis media ***(related to poor eustachian tube function or infection)***
  - Otitis media serous ***(related to fluid in middle ear due to allergies or a cold)***
  - Otosclerosis
- Causes of sensorineural hearing loss
  - Congenital damage or malformations of the inner ear
  - Ménière's disease
  - Ototoxic drugs administered orally, topically, as otic drops, by intravenous, or passed to the fetus in utero ***(aminoglycoside antibiotics, e.g., gentamicin or tobramycin, and chemotherapeutic drugs, e.g., cisplatin and carboplatin, are known to cause permanent hearing loss; quinine, loop diuretics, and salicylates, e.g., aspirin, are known to cause temporary hearing loss; other categories***

of drugs known to be ototoxic include anesthetics, cardiac medications, mood altering medications, and glucocorticosteroids, e.g., cortisone, steroids)

Presbycusis ***(gradual hearing loss experienced in advancing age related to degeneration of the cochlea)***

Serious infections ***(meningitis, measles, mumps, other viral, syphilis)***

Trauma to the inner ear ***(related to exposure to noise in excess of 90 dB or as a result of physical trauma)***

Tumor ***(e.g., acoustic neuroma, cerebellopontine angle tumor, meningioma)***

Vascular disorders

CRITICAL FINDINGS: N/A

INTERFERING FACTORS

Factors that may impair the results of the examination

- Effects of ototoxic medications can cause temporary, intermittent, or permanent hearing loss.
- Failure to follow pretesting preparations before the procedure may cause the procedure to be canceled or repeated.
- Improper earphone fit or audiometer calibration can affect results.
- Inability of the patient to cooperate or remain still during the procedure because of age, language barriers, significant pain, or mental status may interfere with the test results.
- Noisy environment or extraneous movements can affect results.
- Tinnitus or other sensations can cause abnormal responses.

NURSING IMPLICATIONS AND PROCEDURE

PRETEST:

- Positively identify the patient using at least two person-specific identifiers before services, treatments, or procedures are performed.
- *Patient teaching:* Inform the patient/caregiver this procedure can assist in detecting hearing loss.
- Obtain a history of the patient's health concerns (especially the patient's known or suspected hearing loss, including type and cause; ear conditions with treatment regimens), symptoms, surgical procedures (especially related to the ears), and results of previously performed laboratory and diagnostic studies. Include a list of known allergens, especially allergies or sensitivities to latex.
- Obtain a list of the patient's current medications, including over-the-counter medications and dietary supplements (see Effects of Natural Products on Laboratory Values online at Davis*Plus*).
- Review the procedure with the patient. Address concerns about pain and explain that no discomfort will be experienced during the test. Inform the patient that an audiologist or health-care provider (HCP) specializing in this procedure performs the test in a quiet, soundproof room and that the test can take up to 20 min to evaluate both ears. Explain that each ear will be tested separately by using earphones and/or a device placed behind the ear to deliver sounds of varying intensities. Address concerns about claustrophobia, as appropriate. Explain and demonstrate to the patient how to communicate with the audiologist and how to exit from the room.
- *Sensitivity to social and cultural issues,* as well as concern for modesty, is important in providing psychological support before, during, and after the procedure.
- Note that there are no food, fluid, or medication restrictions unless by medical direction.
- Ensure that the external auditory canal is clear of impacted cerumen.
- *Make sure a written and informed consent has been signed prior to the procedure and before administering any medications.*

INTRATEST:

Potential Complications: N/A

- Observe standard precautions, and follow the general guidelines in Patient Preparation and Specimen Collection online at Davis*Plus*. Positively identify the patient.
- Instruct the patient to cooperate fully and to follow directions. Instruct the patient to remain still during the procedure because movement produces unreliable results.
- Perform otoscopy examination to ensure that the external ear canal is free from any obstruction (see study titled "Otoscopy").
- Test for closure of the canal from the pressure of the earphones by compressing the tragus. Tendency for the canal to close (often the case in children and older adult patients) can be corrected by the careful insertion of a small stiff plastic tube into the anterior canal.
- Place the patient in a sitting position in comfortable proximity to the audiometer in a soundproof room. The ear not being tested is masked to prevent crossover of test tones, and the earphones are positioned on the head and over the ear canals. Infants and children may be tested using earphones that are inserted into the ear, unless contraindicated. An oscillating probe may be placed over the mastoid process behind the ear or on the forehead if bone conduction testing is to be performed as part of the hearing assessment.
- Start the test by providing a trial tone of 15 to 20 dB above the expected threshold to the ear for 1 to 2 sec to familiarize the patient with the sounds. Instruct the patient to press the button each time a tone is heard, no matter how loudly or faintly it is perceived. If no response is indicated, the level is increased until a response is obtained and then raised in 10-dB increments or until the audiometer's limit is reached for the test frequency. The test results are plotted on a graph called an *audiogram* using symbols that indicate the ear tested and responses using earphones (air conduction) or oscillator (bone conduction).

Air Conduction

- Air conduction is tested first by starting at 1,000 Hz and gradually decreasing the intensity 10 dB at a time until the patient no longer presses the button, indicating that the tone is no longer heard. The intensity is then increased 5 dB at a time until the tone is heard again. The tone is delivered to an infant through insert earphones or ear muffs, and the auditory response is measured through electrodes placed on the infant's scalp. This process is repeated until the same response is achieved at a 50% response rate at the same hertz level. The threshold is derived from the lowest decibel level at which the patient correctly identifies three out of six responses to a tone at that hertz level. The test is continued for each ear, testing the better ear first, with tones delivered at 1,000 Hz, 2,000 Hz, 4,000 Hz, and 8,000 Hz and then again at 1,000 Hz, 500 Hz, and 250 Hz to determine a second threshold. Results are recorded on an audiogram. Averaging the air conduction thresholds at the 500-Hz, 1,000-Hz, and 2,000-Hz levels reveals the degree of hearing loss and is called the pure tone average (PTA).

Bone Conduction

- Bone conduction testing is performed in a similar manner to air conduction testing; a vibrator placed on the skull is used to deliver tones to an infant. The raised and lowered tones are delivered as in air conduction using 250 Hz, 500 Hz, 1,000 Hz, 2,000 Hz, and 4,000 Hz to determine the thresholds. An analysis of thresholds for air and bone conduction tones is done to determine the type of hearing loss (conductive, sensorineural, or mixed).
- In children between 6 mo and 2 yr of age, minimal response levels can be determined by behavioral responses to test tone. In the child 2 yr and

A

older, play audiometry that requires the child to perform a task or raise a hand in response to a specific tone is performed. In children 12 yr and older, the child is asked to follow directions in identifying objects; response to speech of specific intensities can be used to evaluate hearing loss that is affected by speech frequencies.

POST-TEST:

- Inform the patient that a report of the results will be made available to the requesting HCP, who will discuss the results with the patient.
- Instruct the patient to resume usual activity, as directed by the HCP.
- Recognize anxiety related to test results, and be supportive of impaired activity related to hearing loss or perceived loss of independence. As appropriate, instruct the patient in the use, cleaning, and storing of a hearing aid. Discuss the implications of abnormal test results on the patient's lifestyle. Provide teaching and information regarding the clinical implications of the test results, as appropriate. Profound hearing loss can have a long-range impact personally, socially, and professionally. Consideration needs to be given to support groups that may guide the patient toward a realistic transition toward life management with an auditory deficit. Educate the patient regarding access to counseling services. Provide contact information, if desired, for the National Center for Hearing Assessment and Management (http://infanthearing.org), American Speech-Language-Hearing Association (www.asha.org) or for assistive technology at ABLEDATA, sponsored by the National Institute on Disability and Rehabilitation Research (www.abledata.com) 🍁. When caring for a patient with altered auditory function, forms of communication should be adapted to meet the patient's needs. The process of communication chosen should be documented on the plan of care to ensure consistency and decrease frustration.
- Reinforce information given by the patient's HCP regarding further testing, treatment, or referral to another HCP. As appropriate, instruct the patient in the use, cleaning, and storing of a hearing aid. Answer any questions or address any concerns voiced by the patient or family.
- Depending on the results of this procedure, additional testing may be performed to evaluate or monitor progression of the disease process and determine the need for a change in therapy. Evaluate test results in relation to the patient's symptoms and other tests performed.

RELATED STUDIES:

- Related tests include analgesic and antipyretic drugs, antimicrobial drugs, cultures bacterial (ear), evoked brain potential studies for hearing loss, Gram stain, newborn screening, otoscopy, spondee speech reception threshold, and tuning fork tests (Webber, Rinne).
- Refer to the table of tests associated with the auditory system online at Davis*Plus*.

β_2-Microglobulin, Blood and Urine

SYNONYM/ACRONYM: β_2-M, BMG.

COMMON USE: To assist in diagnosing malignancy such as lymphoma, leukemia, or multiple myeloma. Also valuable in assessing for chronic severe inflammatory and kidney diseases.

SPECIMEN: Serum collected in a red- or red/gray-top tube or urine from a timed collection in a clean plastic container with 1 N NaOH as a preservative. Urine from an unpreserved random collection may also be requested.

NORMAL FINDINGS: (Method: Immunochemiluminometric assay)

Sample	Conventional & SI Units
Serum	
Newborn–1 mo	1.6–4.8 mg/L
2–6 mo	1–3.8 mg/L
7–11 mo	0.9–3.1 mg/L
1–6 yr	0.6–2.4 mg/L
7–18 yr	0.7–2 mg/L
Adult	0.6–2.4 mg/L
Urine	0–300 mcg/L

DESCRIPTION: β_2-Microglobulin (BMG) is a protein component of human leukocyte antigen (HLA) complexes. BMG is on the surface of most cells and is therefore a useful indicator of cell death or unusually high levels of cell production. BMG is a small protein and is readily reabsorbed by kidneys with normal function. Cerebrospinal fluid (CSF) levels parallel serum levels. BMG increases in inflammatory conditions and when lymphocyte turnover increases, such as in lymphocytic leukemia or when T-lymphocyte helper (OKT4) cells are attacked by HIV. Serum BMG becomes elevated with malfunctioning glomeruli but decreases with malfunctioning tubules because it is metabolized by the renal tubules. Conversely, urine BMG decreases with malfunctioning glomeruli but becomes elevated with malfunctioning tubules.

This procedure is contraindicated for: N/A

INDICATIONS

- Detect aminoglycoside toxicity.
- Detect chronic lymphocytic leukemia, multiple myeloma, lung cancer, hepatoma, or breast cancer.
- Detect HIV infection. (*Note:* Levels do not correlate with stages of infection.)
- Evaluate kidney disease to differentiate glomerular from tubular dysfunction.
- Evaluate kidney transplant viability and predict rejection.
- Monitor antiretroviral therapy.

POTENTIAL MEDICAL DIAGNOSIS

Increased in:

- AIDS ***(related to increased lymphocyte turnover)***
- Aminoglycoside toxicity ***(related to acute kidney injury; urine BMG becomes elevated before creatinine)***
- Amyloidosis ***(related to chronic inflammatory conditions associated with increased BMG and other acute-phase reactant proteins; also related to deposition of amyloid in joints and tissues***

B

of patients receiving long-term hemodialysis)
- Autoimmune disorders ***(related to increased lymphocyte turnover)***
- Breast cancer ***(related to increased lymphocyte turnover; serum BMG indicates tumor growth rate, size, and response to treatment)***
- Crohn's disease ***(related to chronic inflammatory conditions associated with increased BMG and other acute-phase reactant proteins)***
- Felty's syndrome ***(related to chronic inflammatory conditions associated with increased BMG and other acute-phase reactant proteins)***
- Heavy metal poisoning
- Hepatitis ***(related to increased lymphocyte turnover in response to viral infection)***
- Hepatoma ***(related to increased lymphocyte turnover; serum BMG indicates tumor growth rate, size, and response to treatment)***
- Hyperthyroidism ***(related to increased lymphocyte turnover in immune thyroid disease)***
- Kidney disease (glomerular): serum only ***(related to ability of kidney tubule to reabsorb BMG)***
- Kidney disease (tubular): urine only ***(related to ability of kidney tubule to reabsorb BMG)***
- Leukemia (chronic lymphocytic) ***(related to increased lymphocyte turnover; serum BMG indicates tumor growth rate, size, and response to treatment)***
- Lung cancer ***(related to increased lymphocyte turnover; serum BMG indicates tumor growth rate, size, and response to treatment)***
- Lymphoma ***(related to increased lymphocyte turnover; serum BMG indicates tumor growth rate, size, and response to treatment)***
- Multiple myeloma ***(related to increased lymphocyte turnover)***
- Poisoning with heavy metals, such as mercury or cadmium ***(related to kidney damage that decreases BMG absorption)***
- Renal dialysis ***(related to ability of kidney tubule to reabsorb BMG)***
- Sarcoidosis
- Sjögren's disease
- Systemic lupus erythematosus ***(related to chronic inflammatory conditions associated with increased BMG and other acute-phase reactant proteins)***
- Vasculitis ***(related to chronic inflammatory conditions associated with increased BMG and other acute-phase reactant proteins)***
- Viral infections (e.g., cytomegalovirus) ***(related to increased lymphocyte turnover)***

Decreased in:
- Kidney disease (glomerular): urine only
- Kidney disease (tubular): serum only
- Response to zidovudine (AZT) ***(related to decreased viral replication and lymphocyte destruction)***

CRITICAL FINDINGS: N/A

INTERFERING FACTORS
- Drugs and other substances that may increase serum BMG levels include cyclosporin A, gentamicin, interferon alfa, and lithium.
- Drugs and other substances that may decrease serum BMG levels include zidovudine.
- Drugs and other substances that may increase urine BMG levels include azathioprine, cisplatin, cyclosporin A, furosemide, gentamicin, iodixanol, iopentol, mannitol, nifedipine, sisomicin, and tobramycin.
- Urinary BMG is unstable at pH less than 5.5.

NURSING IMPLICATIONS AND PROCEDURE

POTENTIAL NURSING PROBLEMS:

Problem	Signs & Symptoms	Interventions
Fatigue ***(related to metastatic disease; tumor; pain; radiation therapy; chemotherapy; anemia; insufficient nutrition; anxiety)***	Report of tiredness; inability to maintain activities of daily living at current level; inability to restore energy after rest or sleep	Discuss the implementation of energy conservation activities (even pace when working, frequent rest periods, frequent items in easy reach, push items instead of pulling); limit naps to increase nighttime sleeping; set priorities for energy expenditures; order transfusion of ordered blood or blood products to treat anemia; administer ordered psychostimulants as appropriate; encourage participation in ordered psychotherapy
Spirituality ***(related to diagnosis of terminal illness; active dying; ongoing chronic illness; anxiety; fear; hopelessness)***	Disharmony between personal beliefs, value system, and threat to life; anger; lack of courage; no purpose or meaning to life; lack of acceptance of diagnosis, disease process; separation from support system; disinterest in connecting with others	Assess for the presence of religious affiliation; assess cultural factors that influence spirituality; encourage verbalization of feelings; work proactively to develop a positive relationship with the patient; assist decision making working within patient's value system; facilitate interaction with spiritual leaders; support faith-based rituals

(table continues on page 178)

Problem	Signs & Symptoms	Interventions
Infection ***(related to altered immune response associated with chemotherapy and radiation therapy; opportunistic hosts)***	Fever; evidence of local or systemic infection; blood cultures positive for infection; sputum culture positive for infection; increased heart rate and respiratory rate; chills; change in mental status; fatigue; malaise; weakness; anorexia; headache; nausea; elevated blood glucose; hypotension; diminished oxygen saturation; elevated WBC; elevated C-reactive protein	Provide standard precautions in the provision of care; correlate symptoms with laboratory values and disease process; trend vital signs and laboratory values to monitor for improvement; administer prescribed antibiotics and medications for fever reduction; administer cooling measures; be vigilant with hand hygiene; educate patient and family regarding good hand hygiene; infuse ordered intravenous fluids to support adequate hydration; ensure implementation of infection prevention measures with consideration of age and culture such as adequate nutrition; perform aseptic wound care; ensure skin care; ensure oral care; ensure adequate rest; avoid exposure to opportunistic hosts; send cultures to the laboratory as ordered; correlate culture findings with selected antibiotics; avoid mouthwashes with high alcohol content; notify health-care provider (HCP) of temperature spikes or flu-like symptoms; discuss implementation of protective isolation for neutrophil count less than 0.5 to 1 × 10^3/microL
Bleeding ***(related to altered bone marrow function secondary to radiation therapy and chemotherapy)***	Decreased platelet count; altered level of consciousness; hypotension; increased heart rate; decreased Hgb and Hct; capillary refill greater than 3 sec; cool extremities	Administer prescribed platelets or blood as ordered; monitor and trend platelet count; increase frequency of vital sign assessment with variances in results; monitor for vital sign trends; administer stool softeners as needed; monitor stool for blood; encourage intake of foods rich in vitamin K; monitor and trend Hgb/Hct; assess skin for petechiae, purpura, hematoma; monitor for blood in emesis or sputum; institute bleeding precautions (prevent unnecessary venipuncture; avoid intramuscular [IM] injections; prevent trauma; be gentle with oral care, suctioning; avoid use of a sharp razor); coordinate laboratory draws to decrease number of sticks; review transfusion reaction symptoms

PRETEST:

- Positively identify the patient using at least two person-specific identifiers before services, treatments, or procedures are performed.
- *Patient Teaching:* Inform the patient that the test is used to evaluate kidney disease, AIDS, and certain malignancies.
- Obtain a history of the patient's health concerns, symptoms, surgical procedures, and results of previously performed laboratory and diagnostic studies. Include a list of known allergens, especially allergies or sensitivities to latex.
- Note any recent procedures that can interfere with test results.
- Obtain a list of the patient's current medications, including over-the-counter medications and dietary supplements (see Effects of Natural Products on Laboratory Values online at Davis*Plus*).
- *Sensitivity to social and cultural issues,* as well as concern for modesty, are important in providing psychological support before, during, and after the procedure.
- Note that there are no food, fluid, or medication restrictions unless by medical direction.

Blood

- Review the procedure with the patient. Inform the patient that specimen collection takes approximately 5 to 10 min. Address concerns about pain and explain that there may be some discomfort during the venipuncture.

Urine

- Review the procedure with the patient. Provide a nonmetallic urinal, bedpan, or toilet-mounted collection device.
- Usually, a 24-hr urine collection is ordered. Inform the patient that all urine over a 24-hr period must be saved; instruct the patient to avoid defecating in the collection device and to keep toilet tissue out of the collection device to prevent contamination of the specimen. Place a sign in the bathroom as a reminder to save all urine.
- Instruct the patient to void all urine into the collection device and then pour the urine into the laboratory collection container. Alternatively, the specimen can be left in the collection device for a health-care staff member to add to the laboratory collection container.

INTRATEST:

Potential Complications: N/A

- Instruct the patient to cooperate fully and to follow directions. Direct the patient to breathe normally and to avoid unnecessary movement during the venipuncture.
- Observe standard precautions, and follow the general guidelines in Patient Preparation and Specimen Collection online at Davis*Plus*. Positively identify the patient, and label the appropriate specimen container with the corresponding patient demographics, initials of the person collecting the specimen, date, and time of collection. Perform a venipuncture as appropriate.

Blood

- Avoid the use of equipment containing latex if the patient has a history of allergic reaction to latex.
- Perform a venipuncture.
- Remove the needle and apply direct pressure with dry gauze to stop bleeding. Observe/assess venipuncture site for bleeding or hematoma formation, and secure gauze with adhesive bandage.

Urine

- Obtain a clean 3-L urine specimen container, toilet-mounted collection device, and plastic bag (for transport of the specimen container). The specimen must be refrigerated or kept on ice throughout the entire collection period. If an indwelling urinary catheter is in place, the drainage bag must be kept on ice.
- If possible, begin the test between 0600 and 0800. Collect first voiding and discard. Record the time the specimen was discarded as the beginning of the timed collection period. At the same time the next morning, ask the patient to void and

B

add this last voiding to the container. Urinary output should be recorded throughout the collection time.

- If an indwelling catheter is in place, replace the tubing and container system at the start of the collection time. Keep the container system on ice during the collection period, or empty the urine into a larger container periodically during the collection period; monitor to ensure continued drainage, and conclude the test the next morning at the same hour the collection started.
- Compare the quantity of urine with the urinary output record for the collection at the conclusion of the test. If the specimen contains less than what was recorded as output, some urine may have been discarded, thus invalidating the test.

Blood or Urine

- Promptly transport the specimen to the laboratory for processing and analysis. Include on the urine specimen label the amount of urine and ingestion of any medications that can affect test results.

POST-TEST:

- Inform the patient that a report of the results will be made available to the requesting HCP, who will discuss the results with the patient.
- ***Nutritional Considerations:*** Stress the importance of good nutrition, and suggest that the patient meet with a nutritional specialist. Also, stress the importance of following the care plan for medications and follow-up visits.
- ***Social and Cultural Considerations:*** Recognize anxiety related to test results, and be supportive of impaired activity related to weakness, perceived loss of independence, and fear of shortened life expectancy. Discuss the implications of abnormal test results on the patient's lifestyle. Provide teaching and information regarding the clinical implications of the test results, as appropriate. Educate the patient regarding access to counseling services. Provide contact information, if desired, for cancer information provided by the American Cancer Society (www.cancer.org) 🍁. Provide contact information, if desired, for AIDS information provided by the National Institutes of Health (www.aidsinfo.nih.gov), American Congress of Obstetricians and Gynecologists (www.acog.org), or Centers for Disease Control and Prevention (www.cdc.gov) 🍁.
- ***Social and Cultural Considerations:*** Counsel the patient, as appropriate, regarding risk of transmission and proper prophylaxis, and reinforce the importance of strict adherence to the treatment regimen.
- ***Social and Cultural Considerations:*** Offer support, as appropriate, to patients who may be the victims of sexual assault.
- Depending on the results of this procedure, additional testing may be performed to evaluate or monitor progression of the disease process and determine the need for a change in therapy. Evaluate test results in relation to the patient's symptoms and other tests performed.

Patient Education:

- Educate the patient regarding the risk of infection related to immunosuppressed inflammatory response and fatigue related to decreased energy production.
- Educate the patient regarding access to counseling services.
- Provide a nonjudgmental, nonthreatening atmosphere for a discussion during which risks of sexually transmitted infections are explained.
- Discuss emotional problems the patient may experience (e.g., guilt, depression, anger).
- Reinforce information given by the patient's HCP regarding further testing, treatment, or referral to another HCP.
- Inform the patient that retesting may be necessary.
- Answer any questions or address any concerns voiced by the patient or family.

Expected Patient Outcomes:

Understanding

- The patient and family state the normal range of a platelet count.
- The patient and family state the rationale for bleeding precautions to overall health.

Ability

- The patient demonstrates proficient use of nasal spray and lip lubricant to decrease cracking and bleeding.
- The patient demonstrates proficiency in protecting self from injury and trauma with associated bleeding risk.

Response

- The patient and family comply with the request for type and cross match for possible platelet transfusion.
- The patient and family comply with recommendation to attend support groups to assist with managing end-of-life concerns.

RELATED STUDIES:

- Related tests include antimicrobial drugs, ANA, barium enema, biopsy (bone marrow, biopsy breast, biopsy liver, biopsy lung, biopsy lymph node), BUN, capsule endoscopy, CD4/CD8 enumeration, colonoscopy, CRP, cancer antigens, CBC, creatinine, cultures (mycobacteria, sputum, viral), cytology sputum, CMV, ESR, gallium scan, GGT, hepatitis antigens and antibodies (A, B, C), HIV-1/HIV-2 serology, immunofixation electrophoresis, immunoglobulins (A, G, and M), liver and spleen scan, lymphangiogram, MRI breast, mammogram, microalbumin, osmolality, protein total and fractions, renogram, RF, stereotactic breast biopsy, TB tests, US (breast, liver, lymph node), and UA.
- Refer to the Genitourinary and Immune systems tables online at Davis*Plus* for related tests by body system.

Barium Enema

SYNONYM/ACRONYM: Air-contrast barium enema, double-contrast barium enema, lower GI series, BE.

COMMON USE: To assist in diagnosing bowel disease in the colon such as tumors and polyps.

AREA OF APPLICATION: Colon.

DESCRIPTION: This radiological examination of the colon, distal small bowel, and occasionally the appendix follows instillation of barium (single contrast study) using a rectal tube inserted into the rectum or an existing ostomy; the patient retains the contrast while a series of images are obtained. Visualization can be improved by draining the barium and using air contrast (double contrast study). Some of the barium remains on the surface of the colon wall, allowing for greater detail in the images. A combination of x-ray and fluoroscopic techniques are used to complete the study. This test is especially useful in the evaluation of patients experiencing lower abdominal pain, changes in bowel habits, or the passage of stools containing blood or mucus, and for visualizing polyps, diverticula, and tumors. A barium enema may be therapeutic by reducing an obstruction caused by intussusception, or telescoping of the small intestine into the large intestine; this is a condition that most commonly affects children.

B

This procedure is contraindicated for

Patients who are pregnant or suspected of being pregnant, unless the potential benefits of a procedure using radiation far outweigh the risk of radiation exposure to the fetus and mother.

Patients with suspected perforation of the colon should receive a water-soluble iodinated contrast medium, such as Gastrografin, to prevent barium from spilling into the retroperitoneum and causing an inflammatory reaction in the surrounding tissue.

Patients with conditions associated with adverse reactions to contrast medium (e.g., asthma, food allergies, or allergy to contrast medium).

Although patients are asked specifically if they have a known allergy to iodine or shellfish, it has been well established that the reaction is not to iodine, in fact an actual iodine allergy would be problematic because iodine is required for the production of thyroid hormones. In the case of shellfish the reaction is to a muscle protein called tropomyosin; in the case of iodinated contrast medium the reaction is to the noniodinated part of the contrast molecule. Patients with a known hypersensitivity to the medium may benefit from premedication with corticosteroids and diphenhydramine; the use of nonionic contrast or an alternative noncontrast imaging study, if available, may be considered for patients who have severe asthma or who have experienced moderate to severe reactions to ionic contrast medium.

Patients who are uncooperative and who may not be able to retain the barium for imaging.

Patients with conditions such as rapid heart rate, intestinal obstruction, megacolon, acute ulcerative colitis, acute diverticulitis, or suspected rupture of the colon; ***barium or water from the enema may make the condition worse.***

INDICATIONS

- Determine the cause of rectal bleeding, blood, pus, or mucus in feces.
- Evaluate suspected inflammatory process, congenital anomaly, motility disorder, or structural change.
- Evaluate unexplained weight loss, anemia, or a change in bowel pattern.
- Identify and locate benign or malignant polyps or tumors.

POTENTIAL MEDICAL DIAGNOSIS

Normal findings

- Normal size, filling, shape, position, and motility of the colon
- Normal filling of the appendix and terminal ileum

Abnormal findings related to

- Appendicitis
- Colorectal cancer
- Congenital anomalies
- Crohn's disease
- Diverticular disease
- Fistulas
- Gastroenteritis
- Granulomatous colitis
- Hirschsprung's disease
- Intussusception
- Perforation of the colon
- Polyps
- Sarcoma
- Sigmoid torsion
- Sigmoid volvulus
- Stenosis
- Tumors
- Ulcerative colitis

CRITICAL FINDINGS: N/A

INTERFERING FACTORS

Factors that may alter the results of the study

- Gas or feces in the gastrointestinal (GI) tract resulting from inadequate cleansing or failure to restrict food intake before the study.
- Retained barium from a previous radiological procedure.
- Metallic objects within the examination field (e.g., jewelry, body rings).
- Improper adjustment of the radiographic equipment to accommodate patients who are obese or thin.
- Incorrect patient positioning, which may produce poor visualization of the area to be examined.
- Inability of the patient to cooperate or remain still during the procedure because of age, significant pain, or mental status.
- Spasm of the colon, which can mimic the radiographic signs of cancer. (*Note:* The use of intravenous glucagon minimizes spasm.)
- Inability of the patient to tolerate introduction of or retention of barium, air, or both in the bowel.
- Residual stool in the colon, which can obscure visualization of the bowel wall and can mimic a polyp.

Other considerations

- Barium enema should be performed before an upper GI study or barium swallow to avoid retention of residual barium which may obscure details of interest.
- The procedure may be terminated if chest pain or severe cardiac dysrhythmias occur.
- Failure to follow dietary restrictions and other pretesting preparations may cause the procedure to be canceled or repeated.

NURSING IMPLICATIONS AND PROCEDURE

See Potential Nursing Problems on Fast Find at davispl.us/vanleeuwen7.

PRETEST:

- Positively identify the patient using at least two person-specific identifiers before services, treatments, or procedures are performed.
- ***Patient Teaching:*** Inform the patient this procedure can assist in assessing the colon.
- Obtain a history of the patient's health concerns, symptoms, surgical procedures, and results of previously performed laboratory and diagnostic studies. Include a list of known allergens, especially allergies or sensitivities to latex, anesthetics, contrast medium, or sedatives.
- Verify that this procedure is performed before an upper GI study or barium swallow.
- Record the date of the last menstrual period and determine the possibility of pregnancy in perimenopausal women.
- Obtain a list of the patient's current medications, including over-the-counter medications, dietary supplements, anticoagulants, aspirin and other salicylates (see Effects of Natural Products on Laboratory Values online at Davis*Plus*). Such products should be discontinued by medical direction for the appropriate number of days prior to a surgical procedure. Note the last time and dose of medication taken.
- If iodinated contrast medium (e.g., Gastrografin) is scheduled to be used in patients receiving metformin (Glucophage) for type 2 diabetes, the drug should be discontinued on the day of the test and continue to be withheld for 48 hr after the test. Iodinated contrast can temporarily impair kidney function, and failure to withhold metformin may indirectly result in drug-induced lactic acidosis, a dangerous and sometimes fatal adverse effect of metformin ***(related to kidney impairment that does not support sufficient excretion of metformin)***.

B

- Review the procedure with the patient. Address concerns about pain and explain that there may be moments of discomfort and some pain experienced during the test. Inform the patient that the procedure is performed in a radiology department, by a health-care provider (HCP) specializing in this procedure, with support staff, and takes approximately 30 min. **Pediatric Considerations:** Preparing children for a barium enema depends on the age of the child. Encourage parents to be truthful about unpleasant sensations (cramping, pressure, fullness) the child may experience during the procedure and to use words that they know their child will understand. Toddlers and preschool-age children have a short attention span, so the best time to talk about the test is right before the procedure. The child should be assured that he or she will be allowed to bring a favorite comfort item into the examination room, and if appropriate, that a parent will be with them during the procedure. Explain that there will be monitors in the room, and they will be able to watch their procedure along with their health-care team.
- ***Sensitivity to social and cultural issues,*** as well as concern for modesty, is important in providing psychological support before, during, and after the procedure.
- Instruct the patient to eat a low-residue diet for several days before the procedure, consume only clear liquids during the 24 hr before the procedure, including the evening before the test. The patient should fast and restrict fluids for 8 hr prior to the procedure. Protocols may vary among facilities. Inform the patient that a laxative and cleansing enema may be needed the day before the procedure, with cleansing enemas on the morning of the procedure, depending on the institution's policy.

Pediatric Preps

2 years or younger	Clear liquid diet 24 hr prior to the procedure; a pediatric Fleet enema (a half or whole suppository [glycerin or bisacodyl (Dulcolax)] may be ordered instead of the enema) on the evening before and morning of the procedure up to 3 hr prior to the procedure; NPO for 4 hr before procedure
3–16 years	• Low-residue diet for 48 hr prior to procedure • Clear liquid diet for 24 hr prior to procedure; castor oil or Neoloid, a flavored castor oil may be ordered the night before the procedure; dose is based on either weight or age—for castor oil, 26–80 lb, give 1 oz, 81 lb or greater, give 2 oz; for Neoloid, 2–5 yr give 2 teaspoons, 6–8 yr give 1 tablespoon, 8–18 yr give 2 tablespoons—or bisacodyl oral tablet may be substituted based on age (3–8 yr give 1 tablet, 9 yr and older give 2 tablets) • Fleet enemas, until fecal return is clear, up to 3 hr prior to procedure • NPO for 4 hr prior to procedure

- Patients with a colostomy will be ordered special preparations and colostomy irrigation.
- Instruct the patient to remove all metallic objects from the area of the procedure as the metal may impair clear imaging.

INTRATEST:

Potential Complications:

Complications include allergic reaction ***(related to contrast reaction),*** abdominal discomfort and cramping

(related to retention of barium), peritonitis ***(related to leakage of barium into the peritoneal cavity, perforation of the colon or hemorrhage, resulting from changes in hydrostatic pressure during administration of the enema or manipulations of the tip of the enema tubing during barium administration to patients with a weak colon; a rare complication that may occur in children, immunocompromised patients, or patients whose colon is already weakened by disease),*** and constipation, fecal impaction, or bowel obstruction ***(related to dehydration and/or retained barium).***

- Avoid the use of equipment containing latex if the patient has a history of allergic reaction to latex.
- Observe standard precautions, and follow the general guidelines in Patient Preparation and Specimen Collection online at Davis*Plus*. Positively identify the patient.
- Ensure the patient has complied with dietary, fluid, and medication restrictions and pretesting preparations prior to the study, as instructed.
- Ensure the patient has removed all external metallic objects from the area to be examined.
- Assess for completion of bowel preparation according to the institution's procedure.
- Have emergency equipment readily available.
- Instruct the patient to void prior to the procedure and to change into the gown, robe, and foot coverings provided. **Older Adult Considerations:** Older adult patients present with a variety of concerns when undergoing diagnostic procedures. Level of cooperation and fall risk may be complicated by underlying problems such as visual and hearing impairment, joint and muscle stiffness, physical weakness, mental confusion, and the effects of medications. A fall injury can be avoided by providing assistance getting on and off the x-ray table and on and off the toilet at the end of the exam. Older adult patients are often chronically dehydrated; anticipating the effects of hypovolemia and orthostasis can also help prevent falls.
- Instruct the patient to cooperate fully and to follow directions. Instruct the patient to remain still throughout the procedure because movement produces unreliable results.
- Place the patient in the supine position on an examination table and take an initial image.
- Instruct the patient to lie on his or her left side (Sims' position). A rectal tube is inserted into the anus and an attached balloon is inflated after it is situated against the anal sphincter. **Older Adult and Pediatric Considerations:** Reduced muscle tone occurs with advanced age, and fully developed muscle tone may not be present in children. Therefore, older adult patients and children may have difficulty holding the barium in the colon while the images are taken. A balloon tip may be used to assist with retention of the barium; the buttocks may be gently held together with tape if necessary.
- Barium is instilled into the colon by gravity, and its movement through the colon is observed by fluoroscopy.
- For patients with a colostomy, an indwelling urinary catheter is inserted into the stoma and barium is administered.
- Images are taken with the patient in different positions to aid in the diagnosis.
- If a double-contrast barium enema has been ordered, air is then instilled in the intestine and additional images are taken.
- After the procedure, most of the barium is removed using the rectal tube. The patient is helped to the bathroom to expel residual barium or placed on a bedpan if unable to ambulate.
- A postevacuation image is taken of the colon to verify expulsion of the barium.

POST-TEST:

- Inform the patient that a report of the results will be made available to the requesting HCP, who will discuss the results with the patient.

B

- Instruct the patient to resume usual diet, medications, or activity, as directed by the HCP.
- Instruct the patient to take a mild laxative and increase fluid intake (four 8-oz glasses) to aid in elimination of barium, unless contraindicated. **Pediatric Considerations:** Instruct the parents of pediatric patients to hydrate the child with electrolyte fluid post barium enema. **Older Adult Considerations:** Chronic dehydration can also result in frequent bouts of constipation. Therefore, after the procedure, older adult patients should be encouraged to hydrate with fluids containing electrolytes (e.g., Gatorade, Gatorade low calorie for individuals with diabetes, or Pedialyte) and to use a mild laxative daily until the stool is back to normal color.
- Carefully monitor the patient for fatigue and fluid and electrolyte imbalance.
- Instruct the patient that stools will be white or light in color for 2 to 3 days. If the patient is unable to eliminate the barium, or if stools do not return to normal color, the patient should notify the HCP.
- Advise patients with a colostomy that tap water colostomy irrigation may aid in barium removal.
- Recognize anxiety related to test results. Discuss the implications of abnormal test results on the patient's lifestyle. Provide teaching and information regarding the clinical implications of the test results, as appropriate.
- Reinforce information given by the patient's HCP regarding further testing, treatment, or referral to another HCP. Decisions regarding the need for and frequency of occult blood testing, colonoscopy, or other cancer screening procedures should be made after consultation between the patient and HCP. The most current guidelines for colon cancer screening of the general population as well as individuals with increased risk are available from the American Cancer Society (www.cancer.org), U.S. Preventive Services Task Force (www.uspreventiveservicestaskforce.org), and American College of Gastroenterology (www.gi.org) 🍁. Answer any questions or address any concerns voiced by the patient or family.
- Depending on the results of this procedure, additional testing may be performed to evaluate or monitor progression of the disease process and determine the need for a change in therapy. Evaluate test results in relation to the patient's symptoms and other tests performed.

Patient Education:

- Teach the patient and family about the disease process and the available options to treat the disease; make sure the language used is clear and easily understandable.
- Teach the patient and family dietary changes that are necessary to decrease pain and GI irritation.

Expected Patient Outcomes:

Understanding

- The patient and family verbalize the treatment options that are available for the diagnosed GI disorder.
- The patient and family verbalize the importance of adjusting the diet to decrease GI irritation.

Ability

- The patient and family demonstrate how to splint abdomen when moving to decrease incisional pain postoperatively.
- The patient and family collaborate with the HCP to develop a treatment plan that fits with the patient's personal health-care goals.

Response

- The patient and family accept information regarding disease progression and recommended medical treatment.
- The patient and family are willing to attend a support group for grief counseling and end-of-life care.

RELATED STUDIES:

- Related tests include cancer antigens, colonoscopy, colposcopy,

CT abdomen, fecal analysis, MRI abdomen, PET pelvis, and proctosigmoidoscopy.

➧ Refer to the Gastrointestinal System table online at Davis*Plus* for related tests by body system.

Barium Swallow

SYNONYM/ACRONYM: Esophagram, video swallow, esophagus x-ray, swallowing function, esophagography.

COMMON USE: To assist in diagnosing disease of the esophagus such as stricture or tumor.

AREA OF APPLICATION: Esophagus.

DESCRIPTION: This radiological examination of the esophagus evaluates motion and anatomic structures of the esophageal lumen by recording images of the lumen while the patient swallows a barium solution of milkshake consistency and a chalky taste. The procedure is a dynamic study and uses fluoroscopic and cineradiographic techniques. A dynamic study is one in which there is continuous monitoring of the motion being studied as opposed to a static study in which the patient and equipment are held in one position until the image has been taken. The barium swallow is often performed as part of an upper gastrointestinal (GI) series or cardiac series and is indicated for patients with a history of dysphagia and gastric reflux. The standard barium swallow study focuses on the esophageal structures of the GI tract and may identify reflux of the barium from the stomach back into the esophagus. Muscular abnormalities such as achalasia, as well as diffuse esophageal spasm, can be easily detected with this procedure. Gastroesophageal reflux disease (GERD) is a disorder of the gastrointestinal system commonly seen in the older adult. Because of the physiological changes associated with the aging process, numerous factors may negatively impact quality of life and contribute to the development of significant complications in older adult patients as a result of GERD.

The **modified barium swallow** focuses on the oropharyngeal structures and is also used to evaluate dysphagia, or difficulty swallowing. The test may be performed and observed in the presence of a radiologist and radiology technician with or without a feeding specialist or speech pathologist depending on the reason for the examination. Nurses will encounter patients who struggle with swallowing disorders in different settings such as intensive care units, nurseries, rehabilitative units, or skilled nursing care units. Situations that might indicate a modified barium swallow include the evaluation of a patient's ability to swallow food after a stroke or the inability of a child to swallow food of varying consistencies without gagging and choking during feeding.

B

This procedure is contraindicated for

Patients who are pregnant or suspected of being pregnant, unless the potential benefits of a procedure using radiation far outweigh the risk of radiation exposure to the fetus and mother.

Patients who are unable to cooperate by swallowing upon request.

Patients with an obstruction, ulcer, or suspected esophageal rupture, unless water-soluble iodinated contrast medium, such as Gastrografin, is used.

Patients with conditions associated with adverse reactions to contrast medium (e.g., asthma, food allergies, or allergy to contrast medium).

Although patients are asked specifically if they have a known allergy to iodine or shellfish, it has been well established that the reaction is not to iodine, in fact an actual iodine allergy would be problematic because iodine is required for the production of thyroid hormones. In the case of shellfish the reaction is to a muscle protein called tropomyosin; in the case of iodinated contrast medium the reaction is to the noniodinated part of the contrast molecule. Patients with a known hypersensitivity to the medium may benefit from premedication with corticosteroids and diphenhydramine; the use of nonionic contrast or an alternative noncontrast imaging study, if available, may be considered for patients who have severe asthma or who have experienced moderate to severe reactions to ionic contrast medium.

Patients with severe constipation or bowel obstruction, as barium may make the condition worse.

Patients with a severe swallowing disorder ***to the extent that aspiration might occur.***

Patients with suspected tracheoesophageal fistula, unless barium is used.

INDICATIONS

- Confirm the integrity of esophageal anastomoses in the postoperative patient.
- Detect esophageal reflux, tracheoesophageal fistulas, and esophageal varices.
- Determine the cause of dysphagia or heartburn.
- Determine the type and location of foreign bodies within the pharynx and esophagus.
- Evaluate suspected esophageal motility disorders.
- Evaluate suspected polyps, strictures, Zenker's diverticula, tumor, or inflammation.

POTENTIAL MEDICAL DIAGNOSIS

Normal findings

- Normal peristalsis through the esophagus into the stomach with normal size, filling, patency, and shape of the esophagus

Abnormal findings related to

- Achalasia
- Acute or chronic esophagitis
- Benign or malignant tumors
- Chalasia
- Congenital diaphragmatic hernia
- Diverticula
- Dysphagia with or without pain ***related to constrictions, arteria lusoria, paralysis, muscle spasms, etc.)***
- Esophageal motility issues ***related to other conditions such as scleroderma or advancing age***
- Esophageal ulcers
- Esophageal varices
- Gastroesophageal reflux disease

- Hiatal hernia
- Perforation of the esophagus
- Strictures or polyps

CRITICAL FINDINGS: N/A

INTERFERING FACTORS

Factors that may alter the results of the study

- Metallic objects within the examination field.
- Improper adjustment of the radiographic equipment to accommodate obese or thin patients, which can cause overexposure or underexposure.
- Incorrect patient positioning, which may produce poor visualization of the area to be examined.
- Inability of the patient to cooperate or remain still during the procedure because of age, significant pain, or mental status.

Other considerations

- Failure to follow dietary restrictions and other pretesting preparations may cause the procedure to be canceled or repeated.
- Ensure that the procedure is done after cholangiography and barium enema.

NURSING IMPLICATIONS AND PROCEDURE

See Potential Nursing Problems on Fast Find at davispl.us/vanleeuwen7.

PRETEST:

- Positively identify the patient using at least two person-specific identifiers before services, treatments, or procedures are performed.
- *Patient Teaching:* Inform the patient this procedure can assist in assessing the esophagus.
- Obtain a history of the patient's health concerns, symptoms, surgical procedures, and results of previously performed laboratory and diagnostic studies. Include a list of known allergens, especially allergies or sensitivities to latex, anesthetics, contrast medium, or sedatives.
- Ensure that this procedure is performed before an upper GI study or video swallow.
- Record the date of the last menstrual period and determine the possibility of pregnancy in perimenopausal women.
- Obtain a list of the patient's current medications, including over-the-counter medications, dietary supplements, anticoagulants, aspirin and other salicylates (see Effects of Natural Products on Laboratory Values online at Davis*Plus*). Such products should be discontinued by medical direction for the appropriate number of days prior to a surgical procedure. Note the last time and dose of medication taken.
- If iodinated contrast medium (e.g., Gastrografin) is scheduled to be used in patients receiving metformin (Glucophage) for type 2 diabetes, the drug should be discontinued on the day of the test and continue to be withheld for 48 hr after the test. Iodinated contrast can temporarily impair kidney function, and failure to withhold metformin may indirectly result in drug-induced lactic acidosis, a dangerous and sometimes fatal adverse effect of metformin ***(related to renal impairment that does not support sufficient excretion of metformin).***
- Explain to the patient that no pain should be experienced during the test. Review the procedure with the patient and explain the need to swallow a barium contrast medium. Inform the patient that the procedure is performed in a radiology department by a health-care provider (HCP) and takes approximately 15 to 30 min.
- *Sensitivity to social and cultural issues,* as well as concern for modesty, is important in providing psychological

support before, during, and after the procedure.

- Instruct the patient to remove all external metallic objects from the area to be examined.
- Instruct the patient to fast and restrict fluids for 6 hr prior to the procedure. Protocols may vary among facilities. **Pediatric Considerations:** The fasting period prior to the time of the examination depends on the child's age. General guidelines are as follows: birth to 6 mo, 3 hr; 7 months to 2 yr, 4 hr; 3 yr and older, 6 hr.

INTRATEST:

Potential Complications:

Although complications are rare, they may include allergic reaction ***(related to contrast reaction),*** constipation, impaction, or bowel obstruction ***(related to retained barium),*** and aspiration of barium ***(related to extreme swallowing disorders).***

- Avoid the use of equipment containing latex if the patient has a history of allergic reaction to latex.
- Observe standard precautions, and follow the general guidelines in Patient Preparation and Specimen Collection online at Davis*Plus*. Positively identify the patient.
- Ensure the patient has complied with dietary and fluid restrictions prior to the study, as instructed.
- Ensure the patient has removed all external metallic objects from the area to be examined.
- Instruct the patient to void prior to the procedure and to change into the gown, robe, and foot coverings provided.
- Instruct the patient to cooperate and follow directions. Instruct the patient to remain still throughout the procedure because movement produces unreliable results.
- Instruct the patient to stand in front of the x-ray fluoroscopy screen. Place the patient supine on the radiographic table if he or she is unable to stand.
- An initial image is taken, and the patient is asked to swallow a barium solution with or without a straw.
- Multiple images at different angles may be taken.
- The patient may be asked to drink additional barium to complete the study. Swallowing the additional barium evaluates the passage of barium from the esophagus into the stomach.

POST-TEST:

- Inform the patient that a report of the results will be made available to the requesting HCP, who will discuss the results with the patient.
- Instruct the patient to resume usual diet, fluids, medications, and activity, as directed by the HCP.
- Carefully monitor the patient for fatigue and fluid and electrolyte imbalance.
- Instruct the patient to take a mild laxative and increase fluid intake (four 8-oz glasses) to aid in elimination of barium, unless contraindicated. **Pediatric Considerations:** Instruct the parents of pediatric patients to hydrate children with electrolyte fluids post barium swallow. **Considerations for Older Adults:** Chronic dehydration can also result in frequent bouts of constipation. Therefore, after the procedure, older adult patients should be encouraged to use a mild laxative daily until the stool is back to normal color.
- Instruct the patient that stools will be white or light in color for 2 to 3 days. If the patient is unable to eliminate the barium, or if stools do not return to normal color, the patient should notify the requesting HCP.
- Recognize anxiety related to test results. Discuss the implications of abnormal test results on the patient's lifestyle. Provide teaching and information regarding the clinical implications of the test results, as appropriate.

- Reinforce information given by the patient's HCP regarding further testing, treatment, or referral to another HCP. Answer any questions or address any concerns voiced by the patient or family.
- Depending on the results of this procedure, additional testing may be performed to evaluate or monitor progression of the disease process and determine the need for a change in therapy. Evaluate test results in relation to the patient's symptoms and other tests performed.

Patient Education:

- Teach the patient the causes of bleeding and actions that can be taken to decrease bleeding risk.
- Explain why it is important to avoid taking substances that can cause gastric irritation and result in bleeding (NSAIDs, aspirin, steroids, alcohol).

Understanding

- The patient and family recognize the importance of tracking and reporting bloody or coffee ground emesis.
- The patient and family acknowledge the causes of GI bleeding.

Ability

- The patient demonstrates the ability to decrease fall risk by calling for assistance in the presence of hypotension and dizziness.
- The patient and family demonstrate the ability to monitor stools and record and report color, consistency, amount, and odor.

Response

- The patient agrees to abstain from alcohol use.
- The patient proactively collaborates with the HCP and family members in supporting positive health decisions.

RELATED STUDIES:

- Related tests include capsule endoscopy, chest x-ray, CT thoracic, endoscopy, esophageal manometry, gastroesophageal reflux scan, MRI chest, and thyroid scan.
- Refer to the Gastrointestinal System table online at Davis*Plus* for related tests by body system.

Bilirubin and Bilirubin Fractions

SYNONYM/ACRONYM: Conjugated/direct bilirubin, unconjugated/indirect bilirubin, delta bilirubin, TBil.

COMMON USE: A multipurpose laboratory test that acts as an indicator for various diseases of the liver, for disease that affects the liver, or conditions associated with red blood cell (RBC) hemolysis.

SPECIMEN: Serum collected in gold-, red-, or red/gray-top tube. Plasma collected in green-top (heparin) tube or in a heparinized Microtainer is also acceptable. Protect sample from direct light.

NORMAL FINDINGS: (Method: Spectrophotometry) Total bilirubin levels in infants should decrease to adult levels by day 10 as the development of the hepatic circulatory system matures. Values in breastfed infants may take longer to reach normal adult levels. Values in premature infants may initially be higher than in full-term infants and also take longer to decrease to normal levels.

Age	Conventional Units	SI Units (Conventional Units × 17.1)
Total bilirubin		
Newborn–1 d	Less than 5.8 mg/dL	Less than 99 micromol/L
1–2 d	Less than 8.2 mg/dL	Less than 140 micromol/L
3–5 d	Less than 11.7 mg/dL	Less than 200 micromol/L
6–7 d	Less than 8.4 mg/dL	Less than 144 micromol/L
8–9 d	Less than 6.5 mg/dL	Less than 111 micromol/L
10–11 d	Less than 4.6 mg/dL	Less than 79 micromol/L
12–13 d	Less than 2.7 mg/dL	Less than 46 micromol/L
14–30 d	Less than 0.8 mg/dL	Less than 14 micromol/L
1 mo–older adult	Less than 1.2 mg/dL	Less than 21 micromol/L
Unconjugated bilirubin	Less than 1.1 mg/dL	Less than 19 micromol/L
Conjugated bilirubin		
Neonate	Less than 0.6 mg/dL	Less than 10 micromol/L
29 d–older adult	Less than 0.3 mg/dL	Less than 5 micromol/L
Delta bilirubin	Less than 0.2 mg/dL	Less than 3 micromol/L

DESCRIPTION: The spleen removes old or damaged RBCs from circulation. When RBCs are destroyed, the cellular contents are recycled (e.g., iron from hemoglobin) or excreted (e.g., the heme from hemoglobin). Bilirubin is a by-product of heme catabolism from aged RBCs and is primarily produced in the liver and spleen. Unconjugated bilirubin is carried to the liver by albumin, where it is conjugated with glucuronic acid. Conjugated bilirubin is water soluble and more easily excreted. Most of the conjugated bilirubin enters the bile and is transported directly into the small intestine; a small portion of the conjugated bilirubin remains in the bile and is stored in the gallbladder. Bacteria in the small intestine convert the conjugated bilirubin to urobilinogen, which is then converted to stercobilin and urobilin. Stercobilin, a pigmented waste product of bilirubin, is excreted in feces; stercobilin gives feces its normal brown color. Small amounts of urobilin, another pigmented waste product of bilirubin, are excreted in urine; urobilin gives urine its characteristic yellow color. Defects in bilirubin excretion can be identified by the presence of urobilinogen in a routine urinalysis. Increases in levels of bilirubin or its metabolites can result from prehepatic, hepatic, and/or posthepatic conditions, making fractionation useful in determining the cause of the increase in total bilirubin levels. Total bilirubin is the sum of unconjugated or indirect bilirubin, monoglucuronide and diglucuronide (conjugated or direct bilirubin), and albumin-bound delta bilirubin. Delta bilirubin has a longer half-life than the other bilirubin fractions and therefore remains elevated during convalescence after the other fractions have decreased to normal levels. Delta bilirubin can be calculated using this formula:

Delta bilirubin = Total bilirubin – (Indirect bilirubin + Direct bilirubin)

When bilirubin concentration increases, the yellowish pigment deposits in skin and sclera. This increase in yellow pigmentation is termed *jaundice* or *icterus*. Bilirubin levels can also be checked using noninvasive methods. Hyperbilirubinemia in neonates can be reliably evaluated using transcutaneous measurement devices.

This procedure is contraindicated for: N/A

INDICATIONS

- Assist in the differential diagnosis of obstructive jaundice.
- Assist in the evaluation of liver and biliary disease.
- Monitor the effects of drug reactions on liver function.
- Monitor the effects of phototherapy on jaundiced newborns.
- Monitor physiological jaundice in newborn patients.

POTENTIAL MEDICAL DIAGNOSIS

Increased in:

- Prehepatic (hemolytic) jaundice ***(related to excessive amounts of heme released from RBC destruction. Heme is catabolized to bilirubin in concentrations that exceed the liver's conjugation capacity, and indirect bilirubin accumulates)***
  Erythroblastosis fetalis
  Hematoma
  Hemolytic anemia
  Pernicious anemia
  Physiological jaundice of the newborn
  The post blood transfusion period, when a number of units are rapidly infused or in the case of a delayed transfusion reaction
  RBC enzyme abnormalities (i.e., glucose-6-phosphate dehydrogenase, pyruvate kinase, spherocytosis)
- Hepatic jaundice ***(related to bilirubin conjugation failure)***
  Crigler-Najjar syndrome
- Hepatic jaundice ***(related to disturbance in bilirubin transport)***
  Dubin-Johnson syndrome ***(related to preconjugation transport failure)***
  Gilbert's syndrome ***(related to postconjugation transport failure)***
- Hepatic jaundice ***(evidenced by liver damage or necrosis that interferes with excretion into bile ducts either by physical obstruction or drug inhibition and bilirubin accumulates)***
  Alcoholism
  Cholangitis
  Cholecystitis
  Cholestatic drug reactions
  Cirrhosis
  Hepatitis
  Hepatocellular damage
  Infectious mononucleosis
- Posthepatic jaundice ***(evidenced by blockage that interferes with excretion into bile ducts, resulting in accumulated bilirubin)***
  Advanced tumors of the liver
  Biliary obstruction
- Other conditions
  Anorexia or starvation ***(related to liver damage)***
  HELLP syndrome of pregnancy (hemolysis, elevated liver enzymes, low platelet count) ***(related to RBC hemolysis)***
  Hypothyroidism ***(related to effect on the liver whereby hepatic enzyme activity for formation of conjugated or direct bilirubin is enhanced in combination with decreased flow of bile and secretion of bile acids; results in accumulation of direct bilirubin)***
  Premature or breastfed infants ***(evidenced by diminished hepatic***

function of the liver in premature infants; related to inability of neonate to feed in sufficient quantity. Insufficient breast milk intake results in weight loss, decreased stool formation, and decreased elimination of bilirubin)

B

Decreased in: N/A

CRITICAL FINDINGS:

Adults and children
- Greater than 15 mg/dL (SI: Greater than 257 micromol/L)

Newborns
- Greater than 13 mg/dL (SI: Greater than 222 micromol/L)

Note and immediately report to the requesting health-care provider (HCP) any critical findings and related symptoms. A listing of these findings varies among facilities. Timely notification of a critical finding for laboratory or diagnostic studies is a role expectation of the professional nurse. The notification processes vary among facilities. Upon receipt of the critical finding, the information should be read back to the caller to verify accuracy.

Consideration may be given to verification of critical findings before action is taken. Policies vary among facilities and may include requesting recollection and retesting by the laboratory.

Sustained hyperbilirubinemia can result in brain damage. Kernicterus refers to the deposition of bilirubin in the basal ganglia and brainstem nuclei. There is no exact level of bilirubin that puts infants at risk for developing kernicterus. Symptoms of kernicterus in infants include lethargy, poor feeding, upward deviation of the eyes, and seizures. Intervention for infants may include early frequent feedings to stimulate gastrointestinal motility, phototherapy, and exchange transfusion.

INTERFERING FACTORS

- Drugs and other substances that may increase bilirubin levels by causing cholestasis include anabolic steroids, androgens, butaperazine, chlorothiazide, chlorpromazine, chlorpropamide, dapsone, dienoestrol, erythromycin, estrogens, ethionamide, gold salts, imipramine, iproniazid, isocarboxazid, isoniazid, meprobamate, mercaptopurine, meropenem, nitrofurans, nortriptyline, oleandomycin, oral contraceptives, penicillins, phenothiazines, prochlorperazine, progesterone, promethazine, protriptyline, sulfonamides, tacrolimus, thiouracil, tolazamide, tolbutamide, thiacetazone, trifluoperazine, and trimeprazine.
- Drugs and other substances that may increase bilirubin levels by causing hepatocellular damage include acetaminophen (toxic), acetylsalicylic acid, allopurinol, aminothiazole, anabolic steroids, asparaginase, azathioprine, azithromycin, carbamazepine, chloramphenicol, clindamycin, clofibrate, chlorambucil, chloramphenicol, chlordane, chloroform, chlorzoxazone, clonidine, colchicine, coumarin, cyclophosphamide, cyclopropane, cycloserine, cyclosporine, dactinomycin, danazol, desipramine, diazepam, diethylstilbestrol, enflurane, ethambutol, ethionamide, ethoxazene, factor IX complex, felbamate, flavaspidic acid, flucytosine, fusidic acid, gentamicin, glycopyrrolate, guanoxan, haloperidol, halothane, hycanthone, hydroxyacetamide, ibuprofen, interferon, interleukin-2, isoniazid, kanamycin, labetalol, levamisole, lincomycin, melphalan, mesoridazine, metahexamide, metaxalone, methotrexate, methoxsalen, methyldopa, nitrofurans, oral contraceptives, oxamniquine, pemoline, penicillin,

perphenazine, phenazopyridine, phenelzine, pheniprazine, phenothiazines, piroxicam, probenecid, procainamide, pyrazinamide, quinine, sulfonylureas, thiothixene, timolol, tobramycin, tolcapone, tretinoin, trimethadione, urethan, and verapamil.

- Drugs and other substances that may increase bilirubin levels by causing hemolysis include amphotericin B, carbamazepine, cephaloridine, cephalothin, chloroquine, dimercaprol, dipyrone, furazolidone, mefenamic acid, melphalan, methylene blue, nitrofurans, nitrofurazone, pamaquine, penicillins, pentaquine, phenylhydrazine, piperazine, pipobroman, primaquine, procainamide, quinacrine, quinidine, quinine, stibophen, streptomycin, sulfonamides, triethylenemelamine, tyrothricin, and vitamin K.
- Drugs and other substances that may decrease bilirubin levels include anticonvulsants, barbiturates (newborns), chlorophenothane, cyclosporine, flumecinolone (newborns), and salicylates.
- Bilirubin is light sensitive. Therefore, the collection container should be suitably covered to protect the specimen from light between the time of collection and analysis.

B

NURSING IMPLICATIONS AND PROCEDURE

POTENTIAL NURSING PROBLEMS:

Problem	Signs & Symptoms	Interventions
Body image ***(related to jaundice; ascites; dry flaky itchy skin)***	Yellowing of sclera and skin, open sores due to aggressive itching; repeated self-criticism; refusal to discuss altered physical appearance; withdrawal from social situations; conceals physical self with clothing	Assess skin for patches of itching; monitor liver function tests; monitor bilirubin levels; assess for yellowing of the sclera and skin; provide mitts to decrease scratching; assess patient's perception of self related to current medical status; monitor for self-criticism; acknowledge normal response to changed appearance
Nutrition ***(related to poor eating habits; excessive alcohol use; altered liver function; nausea; vomiting)***	Known inadequate caloric intake; weight loss; muscle wasting in arms and legs; stool that is pale or gray colored; skin that is flaky with loss of elasticity	Document food intake with possible calorie count; assess barriers to eating; consider using a food diary; monitor continued alcohol use, as it is a barrier to adequate nutrition; monitor glucose levels; check daily weight; perform dietary

(table continues on page 196)

Problem	Signs & Symptoms	Interventions
		consult with assessment of cultural food selections; consider a high-carbohydrate diet; administer multivitamin as prescribed; administer parenteral and enteral nutrition as needed; assess liver function tests (ALT, AST, ALP, total protein, albumin, bilirubin), folic acid, glucose, thiamine, and electrolytes
Confusion; altered sensory perception ***(related to hepatic encephalopathy; acute alcohol consumption; hepatic metabolic insufficiency)***	Altered attention span; unable to follow directions; disoriented to person, place, time, and purpose; inappropriate affect	Monitor blood ammonia level; determine last alcohol use; assess for symptoms of hepatic encephalopathy such as confusion, sleep disturbances, incoherence; protect the patient from physical harm; administer lactulose as prescribed
Gas exchange ***(related to accumulation of pleural fluid, atelectasis, ventilation perfusion mismatch; altered oxygen supply)***	Irregular breathing pattern, use of accessory muscles; altered chest excursion; adventitious breath sounds (crackles, rhonchi, wheezes, diminished breath sounds); copious secretions; signs of hypoxia	Monitor respiratory rate and effort based on assessment of patient condition; assess lung sounds frequently; monitor for secretions; suction as necessary; perform pulse oximetry to monitor oxygen saturation; collaborate with HCP to administer oxygen as needed; elevate the head of the bed 30 degrees; monitor intravenous (IV) fluids and avoid aggressive fluid resuscitation; monitor degree of abdominal ascites

PRETEST:

- Positively identify the patient using at least two person-specific identifiers before services, treatments, or procedures are performed.
- *Patient Teaching:* Inform the patient this test can assist in assessing liver function and conditions that cause jaundice.
- Obtain a history of the patient's health concerns, symptoms, surgical procedures, and results of previously performed laboratory and diagnostic studies. Include a list of known

allergens, especially allergies or sensitivities to latex.

- Obtain a list of the patient's current medications, including over-the-counter medications and dietary supplements (see Effects of Natural Products on Laboratory Values online at Davis*Plus*).
- Review the procedure with the patient. Inform the patient that specimen collection takes approximately 5 to 10 min. Address concerns about pain and explain that there may be some discomfort during the venipuncture.
- ***Sensitivity to social and cultural issues,*** as well as concern for modesty, is important in providing psychological support before, during, and after the procedure.
- Note that there are no food, fluid, or medication restrictions unless by medical direction.

INTRATEST:

Potential Complications:

There are several types of jaundice that may occur in the neonate, and it is important to quickly determine the cause so effective treatment can be initiated.

- Physiologic jaundice occurs as a normal response to the neonate's limited ability to excrete bilirubin in the first days of life. Intervention may include early frequent feeding to stimulate gastrointestinal motility and phototherapy. This type of jaundice usually lasts 10 to 14 days (premature neonates may take up to a month) and resolves in reverse to the pattern of development with the legs looking normal first and the face remaining yellowish longer.
- Breastfeeding jaundice is seen in breastfed neonates during the first week of life, peaking during the second or third week. It occurs due to dehydration in neonates who do not nurse well or if the mother's milk is slow to come in; the bilirubin levels are elevated relative to the decreased total fluid volume. The goal is to provide adequate fluid and nutrition to the breastfeeding neonate by providing water or formula between feedings and until the mother's milk supply is adequate. Phototherapy may also be ordered in order to accelerate the breakdown of bilirubin and prevent accumulation to dangerous levels. Skin turgor, input and output, vital signs, and number/quality of stools should be frequently monitored. Total bilirubin and fractions should be monitored regularly until levels decrease to normal neonatal values.
- Breast milk jaundice is different than breastfeeding jaundice, occurs in about 2 percent of breastfed neonates after the first week of life, takes up to 12 wk to resolve, and is believed to have a familial relationship; assessment for family history is helpful. Hyperbilirubinemia occurs due to substances in the mother's milk that interfere with development of enzymes required to break down bilirubin. The main goals are to increase fluids by more frequent feeding or additional fluids given orally or by IV and through the use of phototherapy. Fiberoptic blankets and special beds that shine light up from the mattresses are available.
- Severe jaundice may occur as the result of an ABO or Rh incompatibility between the mother and baby. The jaundice occurs as the result of hemolysis or RBC breakdown due to the incompatibility.
- Avoid the use of equipment containing latex if the patient has a history of allergic reaction to latex.
- Instruct the patient to cooperate fully and to follow directions. Direct the patient to breathe normally and to avoid unnecessary movement.
- Observe standard precautions, and follow the general guidelines in Patient Preparation and Specimen Collection online at Davis*Plus*. Positively identify the patient, and label the appropriate specimen container with the corresponding patient demographics, initials of the person collecting the specimen,

date, and time of collection. Perform a venipuncture.
- Remove the needle and apply direct pressure with dry gauze to stop bleeding. Observe/assess venipuncture site for bleeding or hematoma formation and secure gauze with adhesive bandage.
- Protect the specimen from light and promptly transport the specimen to the laboratory for processing and analysis.

POST-TEST:
- Inform the patient that a report of the results will be made available to the requesting HCP, who will discuss the results with the patient.
- ***Nutritional Considerations:*** Increased bilirubin levels may be associated with liver disease. Dietary recommendations may be indicated depending on the condition and severity of the condition. Currently, there are specific drugs being used to treat different types of viral hepatitis. For example, there are a number of drugs used to treat hepatitis B such as peglated interferon (adults only), interferon alpha (adults and children), and lamivudine (adults and children); harvoni and solvaldi are examples of drugs used to treat hepatitis C. There are also drugs that can be given to treat and reverse the symptoms of nonviral hepatitis once the primary cause of hepatic inflammation is identified. Elimination of alcohol consumption and a diet optimized for convalescence are commonly included in the treatment plan. A high-calorie, high-protein, moderate-fat diet with a high fluid intake is often recommended for the patient with hepatitis. Treatment of cirrhosis is different because a low-protein diet may be in order if the patient's liver has lost the ability to process the end products of protein metabolism. A diet of soft foods may also be required if esophageal varices have developed. Ammonia levels may be used to determine whether protein should be added to or reduced from the diet. Patients should be encouraged to eat simple carbohydrates and emulsified fats (as in homogenized milk or eggs) rather than complex carbohydrates (e.g., starch, fiber, and glycogen [animal carbohydrates]) and complex fats, which require additional bile to emulsify them so that they can be used. The cirrhotic patient should be carefully observed for the development of ascites, in which case fluid and electrolyte balance requires strict attention. Patients who are alcoholics should be encouraged to avoid alcohol and also to seek appropriate counseling.
- Depending on the results of this procedure, additional testing may be performed to evaluate or monitor progression of the disease process and determine the need for a change in therapy. Evaluate test results in relation to the patient's symptoms and other tests performed.

Patient Education:
- Educate the patient regarding the cause of the hyperbilirubinemia. Reinforce information given by the patient's HCP regarding further testing, treatment, or referral to another HCP.
- Recognize anxiety related to test results, and answer any questions or address any concerns voiced by the patient or family.
- Assist patient to identify coping strategies that have worked in the past to manage disease-related anxiety.
- Explain the importance of adhering to scheduled laboratory appointments to monitor liver function and disease progress.
- Explain the importance of adequate fluid intake and teach the patient skin care for the neonate.

Expected Patient Outcomes:

Understanding
- The patient and family recognize that jaundice may resolve with treatment of the liver disease.

- The patient and family relate the importance of nutritional supplements to help prevent malnutrition.

Ability
- The patient follows dietary recommendations to gain and maintain adequate weight.
- The patient naturally verbalizes feelings about changed appearance in a positive manner.

Response
- The patient and family resolve to take proactive steps to ensure positive health maintenance.
- The patient and family comply with the recommendation to attend support groups to assist in adapting to changed physical appearance.

RELATED STUDIES:
- Related tests include ALT, albumin, ALP, ammonia, amylase, antibodies actin and mitochondrial M2, α_1-antitrypsin/phenotyping, AST, biopsy liver, cholesterol, coagulation factor assays, CBC, cholangiography percutaneous transhepatic, cholangiography post-op, CT biliary tract and liver, copper, ERCP, GGT, hepatobiliary scan, hepatitis serologies, infectious mononucleosis screen, lipase, liver and spleen scan, protein blood total and fractions, PT/INR, US abdomen, US liver, and UA.
- See the Hepatobiliary System table online at Davis*Plus* for related tests by body system.

B

Bioelectric Impedance Analysis

SYNONYM/ACRONYM: BIA.

COMMON USE: To estimate and assess body composition.

AREA OF APPLICATION: Hands and feet (single frequency or whole body BIA).

DESCRIPTION: Electrical impulses run continuously through the cells, tissues, and organs involved in any type of metabolic process. A few examples include the musculoskeletal, cardiovascular, and nervous systems. The impulses are conducted and sustained through complex chain reactions involving electrolytes such as sodium, potassium, calcium, and magnesium. The ability of tissues to conduct or prevent the passage of electrical energy varies with changes in the concentration of electrolytes in intra- and extracellular fluids, changes in cell membrane permeability, cellular composition, and water content. When an electric current is passed through the body, it is conducted through the intra- and extracellular fluids containing water and electrolytes. Lean tissue contains more water than fatty tissue; therefore, the flow of current occurs easily through muscle but is impeded by fat, which is the basis for bioelectric impedance analysis (BIA). Bioelectric impedance measurements are a reflection of the structure, composition, and function of specific tissues. Measurements of the electrical properties of normal tissue have been expanded to explore tissue profiles along a continuum of cellular change from damaged to expired. These advances may make it possible to diagnose diseases earlier, predict survival, and guide the progress of therapeutic

B

interventions. The technology has appeal because it is simple, portable, noninvasive, relatively inexpensive, and has rapid turnaround to results. In practice, it is usually conducted by contact with electrodes at the site of interest, such as wrist to ankle, hand to hand, or foot to foot. Estimates of body fat percentage are derived from the measurements set against validated formulas that consider factors to include a person's age, height, weight, gender, and ethnicity. The development of medical applications based on BIA include impedance plethysmography; electroencephalography; hydration management for patients with hemodynamic disturbances; nutritional interventions for malnourished, critically ill patients; and assessment of body composition as a risk factor for developing diseases such as heart disease, diabetes, hypertension, and some types of cancer. Nutritionists, athletic club trainers, and members of sports organizations are using BIA to assess health and assist patients in successful weight management. Health assessment has become part of some employee wellness programs. Participation in health assessment is also tied to some employer-sponsored health insurance plans that offer discounts to employees who participate and penalties for those who do not participate. Drawbacks to some of the simpler equipment used to measure body composition in normal subjects are inconsistent readings due to variations in hydration level, skin temperature, and testing environment, as well as the skill level of the person administering the measurements.

This procedure is contraindicated for

- Patients who are pregnant may be excluded from participating in the study; protocols vary among facilities. Fluid volumes change significantly throughout the course of a pregnancy, and interpretation of results may not be accurate or useful.
- Patients with a pacemaker.
- Patients with extremely abnormal body weight (obese or emaciated) or physical deformities that present an irregular distribution in body composition may be excluded from participating in the study; protocols vary among facilities. Interpretation of results may not be accurate or useful.
- Patients with a skin condition that would interfere with placement of electrodes.
- Patients with sudden and significant changes in hydration status (hyper- or hypovolemia).
- Young patients (neonate to adolescent) and older adult patients may be excluded from participating in the study; protocols vary among facilities. Validated formulas for younger and older adult patients may not be available, and interpretation of results may not be accurate or useful.

INDICATIONS

- Assessment of nutritional therapy for the treatment of a chronic disease.
- Assist in evaluating prognosis for patients with chronic conditions such as cancer or liver disease or who are critically ill with an infectious disease.
- Estimation of body composition as part of a biophysical health assessment.

POTENTIAL MEDICAL DIAGNOSIS

Normal findings

- Healthy adults

Abnormal findings related to

- Chronic conditions (e.g., cancer, HIV, liver disease) ***related to diminished electrical conductivity as a result of cachexia***
- Patients receiving nutritional therapy related to weight issues or chronic conditions ***(in order to assess and monitor the efficacy of therapy)***

CRITICAL FINDINGS: N/A

INTERFERING FACTORS

Factors that may alter the results of the study

- Inability of the patient to cooperate or remain still during the procedure because of age, significant pain, or mental status.
- The quality of the BIA study is dependent on the skill of the person performing the study.
- Poor electrode conduction.

NURSING IMPLICATIONS AND PROCEDURE

PRETEST:

- Positively identify the patient using at least two person-specific identifiers before services, treatments, or procedures are performed.
- ***Patient Teaching:*** Inform the patient that this procedure is performed to measure the amount of fat and lean muscle mass in the body.
- Obtain a history of the patient's health concerns, symptoms, surgical procedures, and results of previously performed laboratory and diagnostic studies. Include a list of known allergens, especially allergies or sensitivities to latex.
- Obtain a list of the patient's current medications, including over-the-counter medications and dietary supplements (see Effects of Natural Products on Laboratory Values online at Davis*Plus*).
- Review the procedure with the patient. Address concerns about pain related to the procedure, and inform the patient that there should be no discomfort. Advise the patient that the application of an electrical current is brief, will not be felt, and is not harmful. Inform the patient that the procedure is performed by a health-care provider (HCP) or other person trained to perform the BIA, and it takes approximately 3 to 5 min to complete.
- ***Sensitivity to social and cultural issues,*** as well as concern for modesty, is important in providing psychological support before, during, and after the procedure.
- Note that there are no food, fluid, or medication restrictions unless by specific direction; protocols vary among facilities.
- Instruct the patient to remove jewelry and other metallic objects from the area to be examined.

INTRATEST:

Potential Complications: N/A

- Observe standard precautions, and follow the general guidelines in Patient Preparation and Specimen Collection online at Davis*Plus*. Positively identify the patient.
- Ensure that the patient has removed all external metallic objects from the area to be examined prior to the procedure.
- In some types of studies, the patient may stand and hold a device containing hand-to-hand electrodes to record body composition, and in other types of studies, the patient may stand on a device used to record body composition using foot-to-foot measurements. A third type of measurement is taken with the patient lying down (hand-to-foot study).

Hand-to-foot study:

- Place the patient in a supine position for 5 to 10 min prior to the study in order to achieve a relatively even distribution of body fluids.
- Instruct the patient to void prior to the procedure and to change into the gown, robe, and foot coverings provided.

B

- Avoid the use of equipment containing latex if the patient has a history of allergic reaction to latex.
- Thoroughly cleanse the skin where the electrodes will be placed with alcohol pads to remove any fatty substances such as lotion or other types of residue that may interfere with the study measurements.
- Ask the patient to lie on the examination table facing up with the arms abducted 30 degrees from the sides of the body and legs positioned such that the thighs do not touch. The person performing the study may place a thin piece of acrylic fabric between the arms and trunk or between the thighs if necessary.
- Apply two sets of electrodes: one to the patient's right hand and one to the patient's right foot. Each set of electrodes has one electrode that provides the source of the current and another that serves as a voltage detector.
- When the procedure is complete, remove the electrodes.
- Monitor electrode sites for inflammation.

POST-TEST:

- Inform the patient that a report of the results will be made available to the requesting HCP, who will discuss the results with the patient.
- Instruct the patient to resume usual diet, medication, and activity, as directed by the HCP.
- Recognize anxiety related to test results. Discuss the implications of abnormal test results on the patient's lifestyle. Provide teaching and information regarding the clinical implications of the test results, as appropriate.
- Reinforce information given by the patient's HCP regarding further testing, treatment, or referral to another HCP. Answer any questions or address any concerns voiced by the patient or family.
- Depending on the results of this procedure, additional testing may be performed to evaluate or monitor progression of the disease process and determine the need for a change in therapy. Evaluate test results in relation to the patient's symptoms and other tests performed.

RELATED STUDIES:

- Related tests include albumin, anion gap, chloride, osmolality, potassium, prealbumin, sodium, urea nitrogen (blood), and tests related to the specific health condition for which the patient is being treated (e.g., weight disorder, infectious disease, or cancer).
- Refer to the Immune System and Nutritional Considerations tables online at Davis*Plus* for related tests by body system.

Biopsy, Bladder

SYNONYM/ACRONYM: N/A

COMMON USE: To assist in diagnosing bladder cancer.

SPECIMEN: Bladder tissue or cells.

NORMAL FINDINGS: (Method: Macroscopic and microscopic examination of tissue) No abnormal tissue or cells.

POTENTIAL MEDICAL DIAGNOSIS

- Positive findings in neoplasm of the bladder or ureter

CRITICAL FINDINGS:

- Assessment of clear margins after tissue excision

- Classification or grading of tumor
- Identification of malignancy

Note and immediately report to the requesting health-care provider (HCP) any critical findings and related symptoms. A listing of these findings varies among facilities. Timely notification of a critical finding for laboratory or diagnostic studies is a role expectation of the professional nurse. The notification processes vary among facilities. Upon receipt of the critical finding, the information should be read back to the caller to verify accuracy.

Find and print out the full study on Fast Find at davispl.us/vanleeuwen7.

Biopsy, Bone

SYNONYM/ACRONYM: N/A

COMMON USE: To assist in diagnosing bone cancer.

SPECIMEN: Bone tissue.

NORMAL FINDINGS: (Method: Microscopic study of bone samples) No abnormal tissue or cells.

DESCRIPTION: Biopsy is the excision of a sample of tissue that can be analyzed microscopically to determine cell morphology and the presence of tissue abnormalities. This test is used to assist in confirming the diagnosis of cancer when clinical symptoms or x-rays are suspicious. After surgical biopsy by incision to reveal the affected area, a bone biopsy is obtained. An alternative collection method is needle biopsy. There are two types of needle biopsy: fine-needle biopsy in which fluid and tumor cells are aspirated from the tumor site and core-needle biopsy in which a plug of bone is removed using a special serrated needle. The choice of biopsy method is based on the type of tumor expected, whether the tumor is benign or malignant, and the surgeon's anticipated plan regarding removal of the tumor.

This procedure is contraindicated for

Patients with bleeding disorders ***(related to the potential for prolonged bleeding from the biopsy site)***

INDICATIONS

- Differentiation of a benign from a malignant bone lesion.
- Radiographic evidence of a bone lesion.

POTENTIAL MEDICAL DIAGNOSIS

Abnormal findings related to

- Ewing's sarcoma
- Multiple myeloma
- Osteoma
- Osteosarcoma

CRITICAL FINDINGS:

- Classification or grading of tumor
- Identification of malignancy

Note and immediately report to the requesting health-care provider (HCP) any critical findings and related symptoms. A listing of these findings varies among facilities. Timely notification of a critical finding for laboratory or diagnostic studies is a role expectation of the professional nurse. The notification processes vary among facilities. Upon receipt of the critical finding, the information should be read back to the caller to verify accuracy.

B

INTERFERING FACTORS

- Failure to follow dietary restrictions before the procedure may cause the procedure to be canceled or repeated.

NURSING IMPLICATIONS AND PROCEDURE

PRETEST:

- Positively identify the patient using at least two person-specific identifiers before services, treatments, or procedures are performed.
- *Patient Teaching:* Inform the patient this procedure can assist to establish a diagnosis of bone disease.
- Obtain a history of the patient's health concerns, symptoms, surgical procedures, and results of previously performed laboratory and diagnostic studies. Include a list of known allergens, especially allergies or sensitivities to latex or anesthetics.
- Record the date of the last menstrual period and determine the possibility of pregnancy in perimenopausal women.
- Note any recent procedures that can interfere with test results.
- Obtain a list of the patient's current medications, including over-the-counter medications, dietary supplements, anticoagulants, aspirin and other salicylates (see Effects of Natural Products on Laboratory Values online at Davis*Plus*). Such products should be discontinued by medical direction for the appropriate number of days prior to a surgical procedure. Note the last time and dose of medication taken.
- Review the procedure with the patient. Inform the patient that it may be necessary to remove hair from the site before the procedure. Instruct the patient that prophylactic antibiotics may be administered before the procedure. Address concerns about pain and explain that a sedative and/or analgesia will be administered to promote relaxation and reduce discomfort prior to the percutaneous biopsy; general anesthesia will be administered prior to the open biopsy. Explain to the patient that no pain will be experienced during the test when general anesthesia is used but that any discomfort with a needle biopsy will be minimized with local anesthetics and systemic analgesics. Inform the patient that the biopsy is performed under sterile conditions by an HCP specializing in this procedure. The surgical procedure usually takes about 30 min to complete, and sutures may be necessary to close the site. A needle biopsy usually takes about 20 min to complete.
- ***Sensitivity to social and cultural issues,*** as well as concern for modesty, is important in providing psychological support before, during, and after the procedure.
- Explain that an intravenous (IV) line will be inserted to allow infusion of fluids such as saline, anesthetics, analgesics, or IV sedation.
- Instruct the patient that to reduce the risk of aspiration related to nausea and vomiting, solid food and milk or milk products are restricted for at least 6 hr, and clear liquids are restricted for at least 2 hr prior to general anesthesia, regional anesthesia, or sedation/analgesia (monitored anesthesia). The American Society of Anesthesiologists has fasting guidelines for risk levels according to patient status. More information can be located at www.asahq.org. 🍁 Patients on beta blockers before the surgical procedure should be instructed to take their medication as ordered during the perioperative period. Protocols may vary among facilities.

- *Make sure a written and informed consent has been signed prior to the procedure and before administering any medications.*

INTRATEST:

Potential Complications:

Bleeding ***(related to a bleeding disorder, or the effects of natural products and medications with known anticoagulant, antiplatelet, or thrombolytic properties)*** or seeding of the biopsy tract with tumor cells.

- Ensure that the patient has complied with dietary restrictions prior to the study, as instructed.
- Ensure that anticoagulant therapy has been withheld for the appropriate number of days prior to the procedure. Number of days to withhold medication is dependent on the type of anticoagulant. Notify the HCP if patient anticoagulant therapy has not been withheld. Ensure that patients on beta-blocker therapy have continued their medication regimen as ordered.
- Avoid the use of equipment containing latex if the patient has a history of allergic reaction to latex.
- Have emergency equipment readily available.
- Have the patient void before the procedure.
- Observe standard precautions, and follow the general guidelines in Patient Preparation and Specimen Collection online at Davis*Plus*. Positively identify the patient, and label the appropriate specimen containers with the corresponding patient demographics, initials of the person collecting the specimen, date and time of collection, and site location.
- Assist the patient to the desired position depending on the test site to be used, and direct the patient to breathe normally during the beginning of the general anesthetic. Instruct the patient to cooperate fully and to follow directions. For the patient undergoing local anesthesia, direct him or her to breathe normally and to avoid unnecessary movement during the procedure.
- Record baseline vital signs, and continue to monitor throughout the procedure. Protocols may vary among facilities.
- After the administration of general or local anesthesia, cleanse the site with an antiseptic solution and drape the area with sterile towels.

Open Biopsy

- Adhere to Surgical Care Improvement Project (SCIP) quality measures. Administer ordered prophylactic antibiotics 1 hr before incision, use antibiotics that are consistent with current guidelines specific to the procedure, and use clippers to remove hair from the surgical site if appropriate 🍁.
- After administration of general anesthesia and surgical preparation are completed, an incision is made, suspicious area(s) are located, and tissue samples are collected.

Needle Biopsy

- Instruct the patient to take slow, deep breaths when the local anesthetic is injected. Protect the site with sterile drapes. A small incision is made and the biopsy needle is inserted to remove the specimen. Pressure is applied to the site for 3 to 5 min, then a sterile pressure dressing is applied.

General

- Monitor the patient for complications related to the procedure (e.g., allergic reaction, anaphylaxis).
- Place tissue samples in properly labelled specimen container containing formalin solution, and promptly transport the specimen to the laboratory for processing and analysis.

POST-TEST:

- Inform the patient that a report of the results will be made available to the requesting HCP, who will discuss the results with the patient.
- Instruct the patient to resume preoperative diet, as directed by the HCP. Assess the patient's ability to swallow before allowing the patient to attempt liquids or solid foods.
- Monitor vital signs and neurological status every 15 min for 1 hr, then

every 2 hr for 4 hr, and then as ordered by the HCP. Monitor temperature every 4 hr for 24 hr. Monitor intake and output at least every 8 hr. Compare with baseline values. Notify the HCP if temperature is elevated. Discontinue prophylactic antibiotics within 24 hr after the conclusion of the procedure. Protocols may vary among facilities.

- Observe/assess for delayed allergic reactions, such as rash, urticaria, tachycardia, hyperpnea, hypertension, palpitations, nausea, or vomiting.
- Observe/assess the biopsy site for bleeding, inflammation, or hematoma formation.
- Instruct the patient in the care and assessment of the site.
- Instruct the patient to report any redness, edema, bleeding, or pain at the biopsy site. Instruct the patient to immediately report chills or fever.
- Assess for nausea and pain. Administer antiemetic and analgesic medications as needed and as directed by the HCP.
- Administer antibiotic therapy if ordered. Remind the patient of the importance of completing the entire course of antibiotic therapy, even if signs and symptoms disappear before completion of therapy.
- Recognize anxiety related to test results. Discuss the implications of abnormal test results on the patient's lifestyle. Provide teaching and information regarding the clinical implications of the test results, as appropriate. Educate the patient regarding access to counseling services.
- Reinforce information given by the patient's HCP regarding further testing, treatment, or referral to another HCP. Inform the patient of a follow-up appointment for removal of sutures, if indicated. Answer any questions or address any concerns voiced by the patient or family.
- Instruct the patient in the use of any ordered medications. Explain the importance of adhering to the therapy regimen. As appropriate, instruct the patient in significant adverse effects associated with the prescribed medication. Encourage him or her to review corresponding literature provided by a pharmacist.
- Depending on the results of this procedure, additional testing may be performed to evaluate or monitor progression of the disease process and determine the need for a change in therapy. Evaluate test results in relation to the patient's symptoms and other tests performed.

RELATED STUDIES:

- Related tests include ALP, biopsy bone marrow, bone scan, calcium, CBC, CT spine, immunofixation electrophoresis, immunoglobulins (A, G, and M), β_2-microglobulin, MRI musculoskeletal, PTH, phosphorus, total protein and fractions, radiography bone, UA, and vitamin D.
- See the Immune and Musculoskeletal systems tables online at Davis*Plus* for related tests by body system.

Biopsy, Bone Marrow

SYNONYM/ACRONYM: N/A

COMMON USE: To assist in diagnosing hematological diseases and in identifying and staging myeloproliferative neoplasms and leukemias.

SPECIMEN: Bone marrow aspirate, bone core biopsy, marrow and peripheral smears.

NORMAL FINDINGS: (Method: Microscopic study of bone and bone marrow samples, flow cytometry) Reference ranges are subject to many variables, and therefore the laboratory should be consulted for their specific interpretation. Some generalities may be commented on regarding findings as follows:

- Ratio of marrow fat to cellular elements is related to age, with the amount of fat increasing with increasing age.
- Normal cellularity, cellular distribution, presence of megakaryocytes, and absence of fibrosis or tumor cells.
- The myeloid-to-erythrocyte ratio (M:E) is 2:1 to 4:1 in adults. It may be slightly higher in children.

Differential Parameter	Conventional Units
Erythrocyte precursors	18%–32%
Myeloblasts	0%–2%
Promyelocytes	2%–6%
Myelocytes	9%–17%
Metamyelocytes	7%–25%
Bands	10%–16%
Neutrophils	18%–28%
Eosinophils and precursors	1%–5%
Basophils and precursors	0%–1%
Monocytes and precursors	1%–5%
Lymphocytes	9%–19%
Plasma cells	0%–1%

DESCRIPTION: This test involves the removal of a small sample of bone marrow by aspiration, needle biopsy, or open surgical biopsy for a complete hematological analysis. The marrow is a suspension of blood, fat, and developing blood cells, which is evaluated for morphology and examined for all stages of maturation; iron stores; and myeloid-to-erythrocyte ratio (M:E). Sudan black B and periodic acid–Schiff (PAS) stains can be performed for microscopic examination to differentiate the types of leukemia, although flow cytometry and cytogenetics have become more commonly used techniques for this purpose. Immunophenotyping by flow cytometry uses markers directed at specific antigens on white blood cell membranes to provide rapid enumeration and identification of white blood cell types as well as detection of abnormal increases or decreases in specific cell lines. Cytogenetics is a specialization within the area of genetics that includes chromosome analysis or karyotyping. Bone marrow cells are incubated in culture media to increase the number of cells available for study and to allow for hybridization of the cellular DNA with fluorescent DNA probes in a technique called fluorescence in situ hybridization (FISH). The probes are designed to target areas of the chromosome known to correlate with genetic risk for a particular disease. When a suitable volume of hybridized

B

sample is achieved, cell growth is chemically inhibited during the prophase and metaphase stages of mitosis (cell division) and cellular DNA is examined to detect fluorescence, which represents chromosomal abnormalities, in the targeted areas. Real-time polymerase chain reaction (RT-PCR) and cell-based polymerase chain reaction (PCR) are newer, more sensitive methods for quantitation of genetic material. There are a number of chromosome markers used to diagnose, develop potential treatment regimens, and monitor treatment outcomes. Some chromosome markers commonly evaluated on whole blood and bone marrow include BCR-ABL1 and/or Philadelphia chromosome to diagnose chronic myelogenous leukemia (CML); JAK2 V617F mutation, which is associated with polycythemia vera (PV), essential thrombocytosis (ET), and primary myelofibrosis (PMF); and promyelocytic leukemia/retinoic acid receptor alpha (PML-RARA) which is used to help diagnose acute promyelocytic leukemia.

This procedure is contraindicated for

Patients with bleeding disorders ***(related to the potential for prolonged bleeding from the biopsy site).***

INDICATIONS

- Determine marrow differential (proportion of the various types of cells present in the marrow) and M:E.
- Evaluate abnormal results of complete blood count or white blood cell count with differential showing increased numbers of leukocyte precursors.
- Evaluate hepatomegaly or splenomegaly.
- Identify bone marrow hyperplasia or hypoplasia.
- Identify infectious organisms present in the bone marrow (histoplasmosis, mycobacteria, cytomegalovirus, parvovirus inclusions).
- Monitor effects of exposure to bone marrow depressants.
- Monitor bone marrow response to chemotherapy or radiation therapy.

POTENTIAL MEDICAL DIAGNOSIS

Increased Reticulocytes

- Compensated red blood cell (RBC) loss
- Response to vitamin B_{12} therapy

Decreased Reticulocytes

- Aplastic crisis of sickle cell anemia or hereditary spherocytosis

Increased Leukocytes

- ***General associations include compensation for infectious process, leukemias, or leukemoid drug reactions***

Decreased Leukocytes

- ***General associations include reduction in the marrow space as seen in myelofibrosis, lack of production of cells, lower production of cells as seen in older adults, or following suppressive therapy such as chemotherapy or radiation***

Increased Neutrophils (total)

- Acute myeloid leukemia
- Chronic myeloid leukemia
- Compensation for bone marrow aplasia
- Myelofibrosis
- Polycythemia vera

Decreased Neutrophils (total)

- Aplastic anemia

- Leukemias (monocytic and lymphoblastic)
- Myelodysplastic syndrome

Increased Lymphocytes
- Compensation for bone marrow aplasia
- Infections (chronic infection, viral infections, e.g., Epstein-Barr, hepatitis, HTLV-1, parvovirus B19)
- Lymphoblastic leukemia
- Lymphomas: Hodgkin's disease and all other non-Hodgkin lymphomas; Waldenström's macroglobulinemia is a type of non-Hodgkin lymphoma, also called lymphoplasmacytic lymphoma

Decreased Lymphocytes
- Aplastic anemia

Increased Plasma Cells
- Cirrhosis of the liver
- Connective tissue disorders
- Hypersensitivity reactions
- Infections and conditions of chronic inflammation
- Multiple myeloma
- Ulcerative colitis

Increased Monocytes
- Acute monocytic leukemia
- Acute myelomonocytic leukemia
- Chronic myelomonocytic leukemia
- Compensation for bone marrow aplasia
- Hodgkin and non-Hodgkin lymphomas

Decreased Monocytes
- Compensation for bone marrow aplasia
- Hairy cell leukemia

Increased Eosinophils
- Lymphadenoma
- Myeloid leukemia
- Polycythemia vera

Decreased Eosinophils
- Aplastic anemia

Increased Basophils
- Acute basophilic leukemia
- Myelodysplastic syndrome
- Myeloid leukemia
- Polycythemia vera

Decreased Basophils
- Aplastic anemia

Increased Megakaryocytes
- Hemorrhage ***related to bone marrow response for compensatory replacement***
- Increasing age
- Infections
- Myeloid leukemia
- Polycythemia vera
- Thrombocytopenia ***related to bone marrow response for compensatory replacement***

Decreased Megakaryocytes
- Aplastic anemia
- Cirrhosis of the liver
- Myelodysplastic syndrome
- Radiation or chemotherapy
- Thrombocytopenic purpura

Increased M:E
- Bone marrow failure
- Infections
- Leukemoid reactions
- Myeloid leukemia

Decreased M:E
- Anemias
- Hepatic disease
- Polycythemia vera
- Posthemorrhagic hematopoiesis

Increased Normoblasts
- Anemias
- Chronic blood loss
- Polycythemia vera

Decreased Normoblasts
- Aplastic anemia
- Folic acid or vitamin B_{12} deficiency
- Hemolytic anemia

CRITICAL FINDINGS:

- Classification or grading of tumor
- Identification of malignancy

Note and immediately report to the requesting health-care provider (HCP) any critical findings and related symptoms. A listing of these findings varies among facilities. Timely notification of a critical finding for laboratory or diagnostic studies is a role expectation of the professional nurse. The notification processes vary among facilities. Upon receipt of the critical finding, the information should be read back to the caller to verify accuracy.

INTERFERING FACTORS

- Recent blood transfusions, iron therapy, or administration of cytotoxic drugs may alter test results.
- Failure to follow dietary restrictions before the procedure may cause the procedure to be canceled or repeated.

NURSING IMPLICATIONS AND PROCEDURE

POTENTIAL NURSING PROBLEMS:

Problem	Signs & Symptoms	Interventions
Fear ***(related to lack of understanding of disease process and management; potential death)***	Anxiety; apprehension; stated fear; restlessness; increased tension; continuous questioning; increased blood pressure, heart rate, and respiratory rate	Evaluate both verbal and nonverbal cues of fear; assess for the cause of the fear; acknowledge the patient's awareness of his or her fear; explain all procedures in simple-to-understand, culturally, and age-appropriate terms; administer ordered tranquilizer; maintain a confident, assured, professional manner in all patient interactions
Inadequate coping ***(related to new disease process; fear of prognosis [death])***	Verbal expression of fear; restlessness; anxiety; withdrawal; crying; apparent emotional distress	Assess coping mechanism; support positive coping mechanism; recommend support group; provide clear, concise, appropriate information; administer ordered antianxiety medication; provide contact information for spiritual advisor; provide information related to advance directives; maintain a calm, quiet environment

B

Problem	Signs & Symptoms	Interventions
Knowledge ***(related to medical and postprocedural care and treatment secondary to interventions associated with tumor; cancer; disease [sickle cell, leukemia, lymphoma, mononucleosis, viral infection, anemia, infection, vitamin deficiency])***	Lack of interest or multiple questions; anxiety in relation to disease process and management; verbalization of inaccurate information	Assess the patient's understanding of the need for further treatment (radiation therapy, chemotherapy); discuss postprocedural care (bone marrow retrieval); discuss potential complications; review the signs and symptoms of the disease process as applies to the diagnostic findings

PRETEST:

- Positively identify the patient using at least two person-specific identifiers before services, treatments, or procedures are performed.
- *Patient Teaching:* Inform the patient this procedure can assist in establishing a diagnosis of bone marrow and immune system disease.
- Obtain a history of the patient's health concerns, symptoms, surgical procedures, and results of previously performed laboratory and diagnostic studies. Include a list of known allergens, especially allergies or sensitivities to latex or anesthetics.
- Record the date of the last menstrual period and determine the possibility of pregnancy in perimenopausal women.
- Note any recent procedures that can interfere with test results.
- Obtain a list of the patient's current medications, including over-the-counter medications, dietary supplements, anticoagulants, aspirin and other salicylates (see Effects of Natural Products on Laboratory Values online at Davis*Plus*). Such products should be discontinued by medical direction for the appropriate number of days prior to a surgical procedure. Note the last time and dose of medication taken.
- Review the procedure with the patient. Inform the patient that it may be necessary to remove hair from the site before the procedure. Address concerns about pain and explain that a sedative and/or analgesia will be administered to promote relaxation and reduce discomfort prior to the percutaneous biopsy. Explain to the patient that any discomfort with the needle biopsy will be minimized with local anesthetics and systemic analgesics. Explain that the patient may feel some pain when the lidocaine is injected and some discomfort at the stage in the procedure when the specimen is aspirated. Inform the patient that the biopsy is performed under sterile conditions by an HCP specializing in this procedure. A needle biopsy usually takes about 20 min to complete.
- *Sensitivity to social and cultural issues,* as well as concern for modesty, is important in providing psychological support before, during, and after the procedure.
- Explain that an intravenous line may be inserted to allow infusion of fluids such as saline, anesthetics, or sedatives.
- Instruct the patient that to reduce the risk of aspiration related to nausea and vomiting, solid food and milk or milk products are restricted for at least 6 hr, and clear liquids are restricted for at least 2 hr prior to general anesthesia, regional anesthesia,

B

or sedation/analgesia (monitored anesthesia). The American Society of Anesthesiologists has fasting guidelines for risk levels according to patient status. More information can be located at www.asahq.org. 🍁 Protocols may vary among facilities.

- *Make sure a written and informed consent has been signed prior to the procedure and before administering any medications.*

INTRATEST:

Potential Complications:

Bleeding ***(related to a bleeding disorder, or the effects of natural products and medications with known anticoagulant, antiplatelet, or thrombolytic properties)***

- Ensure that the patient has complied with dietary restrictions prior to the study, as instructed.
- Ensure that anticoagulant therapy has been withheld for the appropriate number of days prior to the procedure. Number of days to withhold medication is dependent on the type of anticoagulant. Notify the HCP if patient anticoagulant therapy has not been withheld.
- Avoid the use of equipment containing latex if the patient has a history of allergic reaction to latex.
- Have emergency equipment readily available.
- Have the patient void before the procedure.
- Observe standard precautions, and follow the general guidelines in Patient Preparation and Specimen Collection online at Davis*Plus*. Positively identify the patient, and label the appropriate specimen containers with the corresponding patient demographics, initials of the person collecting the specimen, date and time of collection, and site location.
- Assist the patient to the desired position depending on the test site to be used. In young children, the most frequently chosen site is the proximal tibia. Vertebral bodies T10 through L4 are preferred in older children. In adults, the sternum or iliac crests are the preferred sites. Place the patient in the prone, sitting, or side-lying position for the vertebral bodies; the side-lying position for iliac crest or tibial sites; or the supine position for the sternum. Instruct the patient to cooperate fully and to follow directions. Direct the patient to breathe normally and to avoid unnecessary movement during administration of the local anesthetic and during the procedure.
- Record baseline vital signs, and continue to monitor throughout the procedure. Protocols may vary among facilities.
- After the administration of local anesthetic, use clippers to remove hair from the biopsy site if appropriate, cleanse the site with an antiseptic solution, and drape the area with sterile towels.

Needle Aspiration

- The HCP will anesthetize the site with lidocaine, and then insert a needle with stylet into the marrow. The stylet is removed, a syringe attached, and a 0.5-mL aliquot of marrow withdrawn. The needle is removed, and pressure is applied to the site. The aspirate is applied to slides, and, when dry, a fixative is applied.

Needle Biopsy

- Instruct the patient to take slow deep breaths when the local anesthetic is injected. Protect the site with sterile drapes.
- Local anesthetic is introduced deeply enough to include periosteum. A cutting biopsy needle is introduced through a small skin incision and bored into the marrow cavity. A core needle is introduced through the cutting needle, and a plug of marrow is removed. The needles are withdrawn, and the specimen is placed in a preservative solution. Pressure is applied to the site for 3 to 5 min, and then a pressure dressing is applied.

General

- Monitor the patient for complications related to the procedure (e.g., allergic reaction, anaphylaxis).

- Place tissue samples in properly labelled specimen container containing formalin solution, and promptly transport the specimen to the laboratory for processing and analysis.

POST-TEST:

- Inform the patient that a report of the results will be made available to the requesting HCP, who will discuss the results with the patient.
- Instruct the patient to resume preoperative diet, as directed by the HCP.
- Monitor vital signs and neurological status every 15 min for 1 hr, then every 2 hr for 4 hr, and then as ordered by the HCP. Monitor temperature every 4 hr for 24 hr. Monitor intake and output at least every 8 hr. Compare with baseline values. Notify the HCP if temperature is elevated. Protocols may vary among facilities.
- Observe for delayed allergic reactions, such as rash, urticaria, tachycardia, hyperpnea, hypertension, palpitations, nausea, or vomiting.
- Observe/assess the biopsy site for bleeding, inflammation, or hematoma formation.
- Instruct the patient in the care and assessment of the site.
- Instruct the patient to report any redness, edema, bleeding, or pain at the biopsy site. Instruct the patient to immediately report chills or fever.
- Assess for nausea and pain. Administer antiemetic and analgesic medications as needed and as directed by the HCP.
- Administer antibiotic therapy if ordered. Remind the patient of the importance of completing the entire course of antibiotic therapy, even if signs and symptoms disappear before completion of therapy.
- Recognize anxiety related to test results. Discuss the implications of abnormal test results on the patient's lifestyle. Provide teaching and information regarding the clinical implications of the test results, as appropriate. Educate the patient and family members regarding access to counseling and other supportive services. Provide contact information, if desired, for the National Marrow Donor Program (www.marrow.org) 🍁.
- Reinforce information given by the patient's HCP regarding further testing, treatment, or referral to another HCP. Inform the patient of a follow-up appointment for removal of sutures, if indicated. Answer any questions or address any concerns voiced by the patient or family.
- Instruct the patient in the use of any ordered medications. Explain the importance of adhering to the therapy regimen. As appropriate, instruct the patient in significant adverse effects associated with the prescribed medication. Encourage him or her to review corresponding literature provided by a pharmacist.
- Depending on the results of this procedure, additional testing may be performed to evaluate or monitor progression of the disease process and determine the need for a change in therapy. Evaluate test results in relation to the patient's symptoms and other tests performed.

Patient Education:

- Teach the pathophysiology associated with cancer, disease, as well as ongoing treatment and screenings.
- Explain that a health-care specialist may need to be consulted to manage the disease and therapeutic interventions.

Expected Patient Outcomes:

Understanding

- The patient and family discuss the medical versus surgical options for disease management.
- The patient and family acknowledge end-of-life treatment options as appropriate.

Ability

- The patient and family demonstrate positive coping strategies.
- The patient and family successfully demonstrate care of surgical site, biopsy site.

Response

- The patient and family agree to attend disease-specific support group meetings.
- The patient and family agree to seek psychological counseling to adjust to lifestyle changes associated with positive therapeutic management strategies.

B

RELATED STUDIES:

- Related tests include biopsy lymph node, CBC, LAP, genetic testing, immunofixation electrophoresis, mediastinoscopy, and vitamin B_{12}.
- Refer to the Hematopoietic and Immune systems tables online at Davis*Plus* for related tests by body system.

Biopsy, Breast

SYNONYM/ACRONYM: N/A

COMMON USE: To assist in establishing a diagnosis of breast disease; in the presence of breast cancer, this test is also used to assist in evaluating prognosis and management of response to therapy.

SPECIMEN: Breast tissue or cells.

NORMAL FINDINGS: (Method: Macroscopic and microscopic examination of tissue for biopsy; cytochemical or immunohistochemical for estrogen and progesterone receptors, Ki67, PCNA, P53; flow cytometry for DNA ploidy and S-phase fraction; immunohistochemical or FISH for Her-2/neu) Fluorescence in situ hybridization (FISH) is a cytogenic technique that uses fluorescent-labelled DNA probes to detect specific chromosome abnormalities. Favorable findings:

- Biopsy: No abnormal cells or tissue.
- DNA ploidy: Majority diploid cell population.
- SPF: Low fraction of replicating cells in total cell population.
- Her-2/neu, Ki67, PCNA, and P53: Negative to low percentage of stained cells.
- Estrogen and progesterone receptors: High percentage of stained cells.

DESCRIPTION: Breast cancer is the most common newly diagnosed cancer in American women. It is the second leading cause of cancer-related death. Biopsy is the excision of a sample of tissue that can be analyzed microscopically to determine cell morphology and the presence of tissue abnormalities. Fine-needle and open biopsies of the breast have become more commonly ordered in recent years as increasing emphasis on early detection of breast cancer has become stronger. Breast biopsies are used to assist in the identification and prognosis of breast cancer. A number of tests can be performed on breast tissue to assist in identification and management of breast cancer. ***Estrogen and progesterone receptor assays (ER and PR)*** are used to identify patients with a type of breast cancer that may be more responsive than other types of tumors to estrogen-deprivation (antiestrogen) therapy or removal of the ovaries. Patients with these types of tumors generally have a better prognosis. ***DNA ploidy*** testing by flow cytometry may also be performed on suspicious tissue. Cancer is the unchecked proliferation of tumor cells that contain abnormal amounts of DNA. The higher the grade of tumor cells, the more likely abnormal DNA will be detected. The ***ploidy*** (number of chromosome sets in the nucleus) is an indication of the speed of cell replication and tumor growth. Cells synthesize DNA in the S phase of mitosis. ***S-phase fraction (SPF)*** is an indicator of the number of cells undergoing replication. Normal tissue has a higher percentage of resting diploid cells, or cells containing two chromosomes. Aneuploid cells contain multiple chromosomes. Genes on the chromosomes are coded to produce specific proteins. ***Ki67 and proliferating cell nuclear antigen (PCNA)*** are examples of proteins that can be measured to indicate the degree of cell proliferation in biopsied tissue. Overexpression of a protein called ***human epidermal growth factor receptor 2*** (HER-2/neu oncoprotein) is helpful in establishing histological evidence of metastatic breast cancer. Metastatic breast cancer patients with high levels of HER-2/neu oncoprotein have a poor prognosis. They have rapid tumor progression, increased rate of recurrence, poor response to standard therapies, and a lower survival rate. Herceptin (trastuzumab) is indicated for treatment of HER-2/neu overexpression. ***P53*** is a suppressor protein that normally prevents cells with abnormal DNA from multiplying. Mutations in the P53 gene cause the loss of P53 functionality; the checkpoint is lost, and cancerous cells are allowed to proliferate.

Knowledge of genetics assists the nurse in identifying patients and family members who may benefit from additional education, risk assessment, and counseling. Genetics is the study and identification of genes, genetic mutations, and inheritance. For example, genetics provides some insight into the likelihood of inheriting a trait such as blue eyes or a condition associated with a type of cancer such as breast cancer. Genomic studies evaluate the interaction of groups of genes. The combined activity or combined expression of groups of genes allows assumptions or predictions to be made. As an example, genomic studies measure the levels of activity in multiple genes to predict how they influence the development and growth of a tumor. Further information regarding inheritance of genes can be found in the study titled "Genetic Testing." Presently, there are four genomic tests for breast cancer: Oncotype DX, MammaPrint, Mammostrat, and Prosigna Breast Cancer Prognostic Gene Signature Assay 🍁.

- Oncotype DX measures the activity of 21 genes that influence the likelihood that breast cancer will develop and, if so, how well it will respond to chemotherapy (early-stage invasive) or radiation treatments (ductal carcinoma in situ [DCIS]). Candidates include patients who have been diagnosed with early-stage breast cancer, recently diagnosed with estrogen receptor–positive breast cancer, recently diagnosed with

DCIS, or scheduled to have a lumpectomy to remove the ductal carcinoma in situ. Test results from this assay have been robustly validated in research studies. The assay is included in the National Comprehensive Cancer Network (NCCN) and the American Society of Clinical Oncology (ASCO) treatment guidelines for early-stage breast cancer. Use of the test for DCIS is growing, but it has not yet been included in the NCCN or ASCO treatment guidelines.

- MammaPrint measures the activity of 70 genes. Candidates include patients who have been diagnosed with state I or state II cancer—whether estrogen receptor positive or negative—that is invasive, smaller than 5 cm, or present in three or fewer lymph nodes.
- Mammostrat measures the activity of five genes. Candidates include patients who have been diagnosed with stage I or stage II cancer. It is not widely used to make treatment decisions.
- Prosigna measures the activity of 58 genes. Candidates are limited to postmenopausal patients who have been diagnosed with:
  A. Stage I or stage II breast cancer that is lymph node negative
  B. Stage II breast cancer with one to three positive nodes
  C. Breast cancer and are hormone receptor positive
  D. Breast cancer that is invasive
  E. Breast cancer and have been treated with surgery and hormone therapy

  It is not widely used to make treatment decisions. ✤

Fluid from breast cysts or nipple discharge may be collected by aspiration and examined microscopically for benign or cancerous findings. Mammography should be performed before aspiration of cyst fluid because of the potential interference to the mammogram from bleeding. Potential complications of aspiration include infection, pneumothorax, and hematoma.

This procedure is contraindicated for

Patients with bleeding disorders ***(related to the potential for prolonged bleeding from the biopsy site).***

INDICATIONS

- Evidence of breast lesion by palpation, mammography, or ultrasound.
- Identify patients with breast or other types of cancer that may respond to hormone or antihormone therapy.
- Monitor responsiveness to hormone or antihormone therapy.
- Observable breast changes such as "peau d'orange" skin, scaly skin of the areola, drainage from the nipple, or ulceration of the skin.

POTENTIAL MEDICAL DIAGNOSIS

Positive Findings in

- Cancer
- Hormonal therapy (ER and PR)
- Receptor-positive tumors (ER and PR)

CRITICAL FINDINGS:

- Assessment of clear margins after tissue excision
- Classification or grading of tumor
- Identification of malignancy

Note and immediately report to the requesting health-care provider (HCP) any critical findings and related symptoms. A listing of these findings varies among facilities. Timely notification of a critical finding for laboratory or diagnostic studies is a role expectation of the professional nurse. The notification processes vary among facilities. Upon receipt of the critical finding, the information should be read back to the caller to verify accuracy.

INTERFERING FACTORS

- Antiestrogen preparations (e.g., tamoxifen) ingested 2 mo before tissue sampling will affect test results [ER and PR]).
- Pretesting preservation of the tissue is method and test dependent. The testing laboratory should be consulted for proper instructions prior to the biopsy procedure.
- Failure to transport specimen to the laboratory immediately can result in degradation of tissue. Prompt and proper specimen processing, storage, and analysis are important to achieve accurate results.
- Massive tumor necrosis or tumors with low cellular composition falsely decrease results.
- Failure to follow dietary restrictions before the procedure may cause the procedure to be canceled or repeated.

NURSING IMPLICATIONS AND PROCEDURE

POTENTIAL NURSING PROBLEMS:

Problem	Signs & Symptoms	Interventions
Inadequate coping ***(related to new disease process; fear of prognosis [death]; loss of breast; perceived loss of desirability)***	Verbal expression of fear; restlessness; anxiety; withdrawal; crying; apparent emotional distress	Assess coping mechanism; support positive coping mechanism; recommend support group; provide clear, concise, appropriate information; administer ordered antianxiety medication; provide contact information for spiritual leader provide information related to advance directives; maintain a calm, quiet environment
Fear ***(related to lack of understanding of disease process and management; potential death)***	Anxiety; apprehension; stated fear; restlessness; increased tension; continuous questioning; increased blood pressure, heart rate, and respiratory rate	Evaluate both verbal and nonverbal cues of fear; assess for the cause of the fear; acknowledge the patient's awareness of her fear; explain all procedures in simple-to-understand, culturally and age-appropriate terms; administer ordered tranquilizer; maintain a confident, assured, professional manner in all patient interactions

(table continues on page 218)

B

Problem	Signs & Symptoms	Interventions
Insufficient knowledge ***(related to postoperative care and treatment secondary to surgical intervention associated with breast cancer)***	Lack of interest or multiple questions; anxiety in relation to disease process and management; verbalization of inaccurate information	Assess the patient's understanding of the need for further treatment (radiation therapy, chemotherapy); discuss postoperative care and potential complications; review the signs and symptoms of infection; discuss the possibility of postoperative self-image dysfunction due to breast removal

PRETEST:

- Positively identify the patient using at least two person-specific identifiers before services, treatments, or procedures are performed.
- ***Patient Teaching:*** Inform the patient this procedure can assist in evaluating breast health.
- Obtain a history of the patient's health concerns, symptoms, surgical procedures, and results of previously performed laboratory and diagnostic studies. Include a list of known allergens, especially allergies or sensitivities to latex or anesthetics.
- Record the date of the last menstrual period and determine the possibility of pregnancy in perimenopausal women.
- Note any recent procedures that can interfere with test results. Ensure that the patient has not received antiestrogen therapy within 2 mo of the test.
- Obtain a list of the patient's current medications, including over-the-counter medications, dietary supplements, anticoagulants, aspirin and other salicylates (see Effects of Natural Products on Laboratory Values online at Davis*Plus*). Such products should be discontinued by medical direction for the appropriate number of days prior to a surgical procedure. Note the last time and dose of medication taken.
- Review the procedure with the patient. Inform the patient that it may be necessary to remove hair from the site before the procedure. Instruct that prophylactic antibiotics may be administered prior to the procedure. Address concerns about pain and explain that a sedative and/or analgesia will be administered to promote relaxation and reduce discomfort prior to the percutaneous biopsy; a general anesthesia will be administered prior to the open biopsy. Explain to the patient that no pain will be experienced during the test when general anesthesia is used but that any discomfort with a needle biopsy will be minimized with local anesthetics and systemic analgesics. Inform the patient that the biopsy is performed under sterile conditions by an HCP specializing in this procedure. The surgical procedure usually takes about 20 to 30 min to complete, and sutures may be necessary to close the site. A needle biopsy usually takes about 15 min to complete.
- ***Sensitivity to social and cultural issues,*** as well as concern for modesty, is important in providing psychological support before, during, and after the procedure.
- Explain that an intravenous line may be inserted to allow infusion of fluids such as saline, anesthetics, analgesics, or sedation.
- Instruct the patient that to reduce the risk of aspiration related to nausea and vomiting, solid food and milk or milk products are restricted for at least 6 hr, and clear liquids are restricted for at least 2 hr prior to general anesthesia, regional anesthesia, or sedation/analgesia (monitored anesthesia).

The American Society of Anesthesiologists has fasting guidelines for risk levels according to patient status. More information can be located at www.asahq.org ♣. Patients on beta blockers before the surgical procedure should be instructed to take their medication as ordered during the perioperative period. Protocols may vary among facilities.

- *Make sure a written and informed consent has been signed prior to the procedure and before administering any medications.*

INTRATEST:

Potential Complications:

Bleeding ***(related to a bleeding disorder, or the effects of natural products and medications with known anticoagulant, antiplatelet, or thrombolytic properties)*** or seeding of the biopsy tract with tumor cells.

- Ensure that the patient has complied with dietary restrictions prior to the study, as instructed. Ensure that the patient has not received antiestrogen therapy within 2 mo of the test.
- Ensure that anticoagulant therapy has been withheld for the appropriate number of days prior to the procedure. Number of days to withhold medication is dependent on the type of anticoagulant. Notify the HCP if patient anticoagulant therapy has not been withheld. Ensure that patients on beta-blocker therapy have continued their medication regimen as ordered.
- Avoid the use of equipment containing latex if the patient has a history of allergic reaction to latex.
- Have emergency equipment readily available.
- Have the patient void before the procedure.
- Observe standard precautions, and follow the general guidelines in Patient Preparation and Specimen Collection online at Davis*Plus*. Positively identify the patient, and label the appropriate specimen containers with the corresponding patient demographics, initials of the person collecting the specimen, date and time of collection, and site location, especially right or left breast.
- Assist the patient to the desired position depending on the test site to be used, and direct the patient to breathe normally during the beginning of the general anesthetic. Instruct the patient to cooperate fully and to follow directions. For the patient undergoing local anesthesia, direct him or her to breathe normally and to avoid unnecessary movement during the procedure.

Open Biopsy

- Adhere to Surgical Care Improvement Project (SCIP) quality measures. Administer ordered prophylactic antibiotics 1 hr before incision, use antibiotics that are consistent with current guidelines specific to the procedure, and use clippers to remove hair from the surgical site if appropriate ♣.
- After administration of general anesthetic and surgical preparation are completed, an incision is made, suspicious area(s) are located, and tissue samples are collected.
- Record baseline vital signs, and continue to monitor throughout the procedure. Protocols may vary among facilities.

Needle Biopsy

- Direct the patient to take slow deep breaths when the local anesthetic is injected. Protect the site with sterile drapes. Instruct the patient to take a deep breath, exhale forcefully, and hold the breath while the biopsy needle is inserted and rotated to obtain a core of breast tissue. Once the needle is removed, the patient may breathe. Pressure is applied to the site for 3 to 5 min, then a sterile pressure dressing is applied.

General

- Monitor the patient for complications related to the procedure (e.g., allergic reaction, anaphylaxis).
- Place tissue samples in formalin solution. Label the specimen, indicating site location, and promptly transport the specimen to the laboratory for processing and analysis.

B

POST-TEST:

- Inform the patient that a report of the results will be made available to the requesting HCP, who will discuss the results with the patient.
- Instruct the patient to resume preoperative diet, as directed by the HCP. Assess the patient's ability to swallow before allowing the patient to attempt liquids or solid foods.
- Monitor vital signs and neurological status every 15 min for 1 hr, then every 2 hr for 4 hr, and then as ordered by the HCP. Monitor temperature every 4 hr for 24 hr. Monitor intake and output at least every 8 hr. Compare with baseline values. Notify the HCP if temperature is elevated. Discontinue prophylactic antibiotics within 24 hr after the conclusion of the procedure. Protocols may vary among facilities.
- Observe/assess for delayed allergic reactions, such as rash, urticaria, tachycardia, hyperpnea, hypertension, palpitations, nausea, or vomiting.
- Observe/assess the biopsy site for bleeding, inflammation, or hematoma formation.
- Instruct the patient in the care and assessment of the site.
- Instruct the patient to report any redness, edema, bleeding, or pain at the biopsy site. Instruct the patient to immediately report chills or fever.
- Assess for nausea and pain. Administer antiemetic and analgesic medications as needed and as directed by the HCP.
- Administer antibiotic therapy if ordered. Remind the patient of the importance of completing the entire course of antibiotic therapy, even if signs and symptoms disappear before completion of therapy.
- Recognize anxiety related to test results. Discuss the implications of abnormal test results on the patient's lifestyle. Provide teaching and information regarding the clinical implications of the test results, as appropriate. Educate the patient regarding access to counseling services. Provide contact information, if desired, for the American Cancer Society (www.cancer.org).
- Reinforce information given by the patient's HCP regarding further testing, treatment, or referral to another HCP. Inform the patient of a follow-up appointment for removal of sutures, if indicated. Decisions regarding the need for and frequency of breast self-examination, mammography, magnetic resonance imaging (MRI) breast, or other cancer screening procedures should be made after consultation between the patient and HCP. The most current guidelines for breast cancer screening of the general population as well as of individuals with increased risk are available from the American Cancer Society (ACS) (www.cancer.org), the American College of Obstetricians and Gynecologists (ACOG) (www.acog.org), and the American College of Radiology (www.acr.org). The ACS recommends breast examinations be performed every 3 yr for women between the ages of 20 and 39 yr and annually for women over 40 yr of age; annual mammograms should be performed on women 40 yr and older as long as they are in good health. The ACS also recommends annual MRI testing, in addition to an annual mammogram, for women at high risk of developing breast cancer. 🍁 Genetic testing for inherited mutations (BRCA1 and BRCA2) associated with increased risk of developing breast cancer may be ordered for women at risk. The test is performed on a blood specimen. Answer any questions or address any concerns voiced by the patient or family.
- Instruct the patient in the use of any ordered medications. Explain the importance of adhering to the therapy regimen. As appropriate, instruct the patient in significant adverse effects associated with the prescribed medication. Encourage the patient to review corresponding literature provided by a pharmacist.
- Depending on the results of this procedure, additional testing may be performed to evaluate or monitor progression of the disease process

and determine the need for a change in therapy. Evaluate test results in relation to the patient's symptoms and other tests performed.

Patient Education:

- Teach the patient the pathophysiology associated with breast cancer as well as ongoing treatment and screenings.
- Explain that a health-care specialist may need to be consulted to manage the disease and therapeutic interventions.

Expected Patient Outcomes:

Understanding

- The patient and family discuss the medical versus surgical options for breast cancer management.
- The patient and family acknowledge end-of-life treatment options as appropriate.

Ability

- The patient and family demonstrate positive coping strategies.
- The patient and family demonstrate care of surgical site.

Response

- The patient and family agree to attend cancer support group meetings.
- The patient and family agree to seek psychological counseling to adjust to body changes and intimacy concerns.

RELATED STUDIES:

- Related tests include cancer antigens, ductography, genetic testing, mammogram, MRI breast, stereotactic biopsy breast, and US breast.
- Refer to the Reproductive System table online at Davis*Plus* for related tests by body system.

B

Biopsy, Cervical

SYNONYM/ACRONYM: Cone biopsy, LEEP.

COMMON USE: To assist in diagnosing and staging cervical cancer.

SPECIMEN: Cervical tissue.

NORMAL FINDINGS: (Method: Microscopic examination of tissue cells) No abnormal cells or tissue.

DESCRIPTION: Biopsy is the excision of a sample of tissue that can be analyzed microscopically to determine cell morphology and the presence of tissue abnormalities. The cervical biopsy is used to assist in confirmation of cancer when screening tests are positive. Cervical biopsy is obtained using an instrument that punches into the tissue and retrieves a tissue sample. Schiller's test entails applying an iodine solution to the cervix. Normal cells pick up the iodine and stain brown. Abnormal cells do not pick up any color. Punch biopsy results may indicate the need for a cone biopsy of the cervix. Cone biopsy involves removing a wedge of tissue from the cervix by using a surgical knife, a carbon dioxide laser, or a loop electrosurgical excision procedure (LEEP). LEEP can be performed by placing the patient under a general anesthetic; by a regional anesthesia, such as a spinal or epidural; or by a cervical block whereby a local anesthetic is injected into the cervix. The patient is given oral or intravenous (IV) pain medicine in conjunction with the local anesthetic when this method is used. Following colposcopy or cervical biopsy, LEEP can be used to treat abnormal tissue identified on biopsy.

B

This procedure is contraindicated for

Patients with bleeding disorders ***(related to the potential for prolonged bleeding from the biopsy site)*** or acute pelvic inflammatory disease.

INDICATIONS

- Follow-up to abnormal Papanicolaou (Pap) smear, Schiller's test, or colposcopy.
- Suspected cervical malignancy.

POTENTIAL MEDICAL DIAGNOSIS

Positive findings in

- Carcinoma in situ
- Cervical dysplasia
- Cervical polyps

CRITICAL FINDINGS:

- Assessment of clear margins after tissue excision
- Classification or grading of tumor
- Identification of malignancy

Note and immediately report to the requesting health-care provider (HCP) any critical findings and related symptoms. A listing of these findings varies among facilities. Timely notification of a critical finding for laboratory or diagnostic studies is a role expectation of the professional nurse. The notification processes vary among facilities. Upon receipt of the critical finding, the information should be read back to the caller to verify accuracy.

INTERFERING FACTORS

- This test should not be performed while the patient is menstruating.
- Failure to follow dietary restrictions before the procedure may cause the procedure to be canceled or repeated.

NURSING IMPLICATIONS AND PROCEDURE

POTENTIAL NURSING PROBLEMS:

Problem	Signs & Symptoms	Interventions
Fear ***(related to lack of understanding of disease process and management; potential death)***	Anxiety; apprehension; stated fear; restlessness; increased tension; continuous questioning; increased blood pressure, heart rate, and respiratory rate	Evaluate both verbal and nonverbal cues of fear; assess for the cause of the fear; acknowledge the patient's awareness of her fear; explain all procedures in simple-to-understand, culturally and age-appropriate terms; administer ordered tranquilizer; maintain a confident, assured, professional manner in all patient interactions

Problem	Signs & Symptoms	Interventions
Inadequate coping ***(related to new disease process; fear of prognosis [death]; loss of childbearing potential)***	Verbal expression of fear; restlessness; anxiety; withdrawal; crying; apparent emotional distress	Assess coping mechanism; support positive coping mechanism; recommend support group; provide clear, concise, appropriate information; administer ordered antianxiety medication; provide contact information for spiritual advisor; provide information related to advance directives; maintain a calm, quiet environment
Insufficient knowledge ***(related to postoperative care and treatment secondary to surgical intervention associated with cancer, tumor, dysplasia, polyps)***	Lack of interest or multiple questions; anxiety in relation to disease process and management; verbalization of inaccurate information	Assess the patient's understanding of the need for further treatment (radiation therapy, chemotherapy); discuss postoperative care and potential complications; review the signs and symptoms of infection; discuss the possibility of postoperative self-image dysfunction due to loss of childbearing potential

PRETEST:

- Positively identify the patient using at least two person-specific identifiers before services, treatments, or procedures are performed.
- *Patient Teaching:* Inform the patient this procedure can assist in establishing a diagnosis of cervical disease.
- Obtain a history of the patient's health concerns (especially any bleeding disorders), symptoms, surgical procedures, and results of previously performed laboratory and diagnostic studies. Include a list of known allergens, especially allergies or sensitivities to latex or anesthetics.
- Record the date of the last menstrual period and determine the possibility of pregnancy in perimenopausal women.
- Obtain a list of the patient's current medications, including over-the-counter medications, dietary supplements, anticoagulants, aspirin and other salicylates (see Effects of Natural Products on Laboratory Values online at Davis*Plus*). Such products should be discontinued by medical direction for the appropriate

B

number of days prior to a surgical procedure. Note the last time and dose of medication taken.

- Review the procedure with the patient. Inform the patient that it may be necessary to remove hair from the site before the procedure. Instruct the patient that prophylactic antibiotics may be administered before the procedure. Address concerns about pain and explain that a sedative and/or analgesia will be administered to promote relaxation and reduce discomfort prior to the percutaneous biopsy; general anesthesia will be administered prior to the open biopsy. Explain that no pain will be experienced during the test when general anesthesia is used but that any discomfort with a needle biopsy will be minimized with local anesthetics and systemic analgesics. Inform the patient the biopsy is performed under sterile conditions by an HCP specializing in this procedure. The biopsy can be performed in the HCP's office and takes approximately 5 to 10 min to complete. The open biopsy is performed in a surgical suite, usually takes about 20 to 30 min to complete, and sutures may be necessary to close the site.
- ***Sensitivity to social and cultural issues,*** as well as concern for modesty, is important in providing psychological support before, during, and after the procedure.
- Explain that an IV line may be inserted to allow infusion of fluids such as saline, anesthetics, analgesics, or IV sedation.
- Instruct the patient that to reduce the risk of aspiration related to nausea and vomiting, solid food and milk or milk products are restricted for at least 6 hr, and clear liquids are restricted for at least 2 hr prior to general anesthesia, regional anesthesia, or sedation/analgesia (monitored anesthesia). The American Society of Anesthesiologists has fasting guidelines for risk levels according to patient status. More information can be located at www.asahq.org ✦. Patients on beta blockers before the surgical procedure should be instructed to take their medication as ordered during the perioperative period. Protocols may vary among facilities.
- *Make sure a written and informed consent has been signed prior to the procedure and before administering any medications.*

INTRATEST:

Potential Complications:

Bleeding ***(related to a bleeding disorder, or the effects of natural products and medications with known anticoagulant, antiplatelet, or thrombolytic properties)***

- Ensure that the patient has complied with dietary restrictions prior to the study, as instructed.
- Ensure that anticoagulant therapy has been withheld for the appropriate number of days prior to the procedure. Number of days to withhold medication is dependent on the type of anticoagulant. Notify HCP if patient anticoagulant therapy has not been withheld. Ensure that patients on beta-blocker therapy have continued their medication regimen as ordered.
- Avoid the use of equipment containing latex if the patient has a history of allergic reaction to latex.
- Have emergency equipment readily available.
- Have the patient void before the procedure.
- Observe standard precautions, and follow the general guidelines in Patient Preparation and Specimen Collection online at Davis*Plus*. Positively identify the patient, and label the appropriate specimen containers with the corresponding patient demographics, initials of the person collecting the specimen, date and time of collection, and site location.
- Have the patient remove clothes below the waist. Assist the patient into a lithotomy position on a gynecological examination table (with feet in stirrups). Drape the patient's legs.

Instruct the patient to cooperate fully and to follow directions. Direct the patient to breathe normally and to avoid unnecessary movement during the local or general anesthetic and the procedure.

Punch Biopsy

- Iodine solution is used to cleanse the cervix and distinguish normal from abnormal tissue. Local anesthetics, analgesics, or both, are administered to minimize discomfort.
- A small, round punch is rotated into the skin to the desired depth. The cylinder of skin is pulled upward with forceps and separated at its base with a scalpel or scissors.

LEEP in the HCP's Office

- A speculum is inserted into the vagina and is opened to gently spread apart the vagina for inspection of the cervix.
- Iodine solution is used to cleanse the cervix and distinguish normal from abnormal tissue. Local anesthetics, analgesics, or both, are administered to minimize discomfort.
- The diseased tissue is removed along with a small amount of healthy tissue along the margins of the biopsy to ensure that no diseased tissue is left in the cervix after the procedure.

Open Biopsy

- Adhere to Surgical Care Improvement Project (SCIP) quality measures. Administer ordered prophylactic antibiotics 1 hr before incision, use antibiotics that are consistent with current guidelines specific to the procedure, and use clippers to remove hair from the surgical site if appropriate 🍁.
- After administration of general anesthetics and surgical preparation are completed, the procedure is carried out as noted above.

General

- Monitor the patient for complications related to the procedure (e.g., allergic reaction, anaphylaxis).
- Place tissue samples in properly labelled specimen container containing formalin solution, and promptly transport the specimen to the laboratory for processing and analysis.

POST-TEST:

- Inform the patient that a report of the results will be made available to the requesting HCP, who will discuss the results with the patient.
- Instruct the patient to resume preoperative diet, as directed by the HCP. Assess the surgical patient's ability to swallow before allowing the patient to attempt liquids or solid foods.
- Monitor vital signs and neurological status every 15 min for 1 hr, then every 2 hr for 4 hr, and then as ordered by the HCP. Monitor temperature every 4 hr for 24 hr. Monitor intake and output at least every 8 hr. Compare with baseline values. Notify the HCP if temperature is elevated. Discontinue prophylactic antibiotics within 24 hr after the conclusion of the procedure. Protocols may vary among facilities.
- Observe/assess for delayed allergic reactions, such as rash, urticaria, tachycardia, hyperpnea, hypertension, palpitations, nausea, or vomiting.
- Advise the patient to expect a gray-green vaginal discharge for several days, that some vaginal bleeding may occur for up to 1 wk but should not be heavier than a normal menses, and that some pelvic pain may occur. Instruct the patient to wear a sanitary pad, and advise the patient that tampons should not be used for 1 to 3 wk. Patients who have undergone a simple cervical punch biopsy can usually resume normal activities immediately following the procedure. Instruct patients who have undergone LEEP or open biopsy to avoid strenuous activity for 8 to 24 hr; to avoid douching or intercourse for 2 to 4 wk or as instructed; and to report excessive bleeding, chills, fever, or any other unusual findings to the HCP.

B

- Assess for nausea and pain. Administer antiemetic and analgesic medications as needed and as directed by the HCP.
- Administer antibiotic therapy if ordered. Remind the patient of the importance of completing the entire course of antibiotic therapy, even if signs and symptoms disappear before completion of therapy.
- Recognize anxiety related to test results, and offer support. Discuss the implications of abnormal test results on the patient's lifestyle. Provide teaching and information regarding the clinical implications of the test results, as appropriate. Educate the patient regarding access to counseling services.
- Reinforce information given by the patient's HCP regarding further testing, treatment, or referral to another HCP. Decisions regarding the need for and frequency of conventional or liquid-based Pap tests or other cancer screening procedures should be made after consultation between the patient and HCP. The American Cancer Society's (ACS) guidelines for preventing cervical cancer recommend cytological screening every 3 yr for women age 21 to 29 yr and co-testing for human papillomavirus (HPV) and cytological screening every 5 yr for women age 30 to 65 yr; no screening is recommended for women who have had a hysterectomy. The most current guidelines for cervical cancer screening of the general population as well as of individuals with increased risk are available from the ACS (www.cancer.org) and the American College of Obstetricians and Gynecologists (ACOG) (www.acog.org). 🍁 Answer any questions or address any concerns voiced by the patient or family.
- Instruct the patient in the use of any ordered medications. Explain the importance of adhering to the therapy regimen. As appropriate, instruct the patient in significant adverse effects associated with the prescribed medication. Encourage her to review corresponding literature provided by a pharmacist.
- Depending on the results of this procedure, additional testing may be performed to evaluate or monitor progression of the disease process and determine the need for a change in therapy. Evaluate test results in relation to the patient's symptoms and other tests performed.

Patient Education:

- Teach the patient the pathophysiology associated with cancer, disease, as well as ongoing treatment and screenings.
- Explain that a health-care specialist may need to be consulted to manage the disease and therapeutic interventions.

Expected Patient Outcomes:

Understanding

- The patient and family discuss the medical versus surgical options for disease management.
- The patient and family acknowledge end-of-life treatment options as appropriate.

Ability

- The patient and family demonstrate positive coping strategies.
- The patient and family successfully demonstrate postoperative care.

Response

- The patient and family agree to attend disease-specific support group meetings.
- The patient and family agree to seek psychological counseling to adjust to lifestyle changes associated with positive therapeutic management strategies.

RELATED STUDIES:

- Related tests include *Chlamydia* group antibodies, colposcopy, culture anal/genital, culture viral, Pap smear, and syphilis serology.
- See the Reproductive System table online at Davis*Plus* for related tests by body system.

Biopsy, Chorionic Villus

SYNONYM/ACRONYM: N/A

COMMON USE: To assist in diagnosing genetic fetal abnormalities such as Down syndrome.

SPECIMEN: Chorionic villus tissue.

NORMAL FINDINGS: (Method: Tissue culture) Normal karyotype.

DESCRIPTION: This test is used to detect fetal abnormalities caused by numerous genetic disorders. Examples of genetic defects that are commonly tested for and can be identified from a chorionic villus sampling include sickle cell anemia and cystic fibrosis. The advantage over amniocentesis is that it can be performed as early as the 8th week of pregnancy, permitting earlier decisions regarding termination of pregnancy. However, unlike amniocentesis, this test will not detect neural tube defects.

Knowledge of genetics assists the nurse in identifying patients and family members who may benefit from additional education, risk assessment, and counseling. Genetics is the study and identification of genes, genetic mutations, and inheritance. For example, genetics provides some insight into the likelihood of inheriting a trait such as blue eyes or a medical condition such as sickle cell anemia. Some conditions are the result of mutations involving a single gene, and other conditions may involve multiple genes and/or multiple chromosomes. Sickle cell anemia and cystic fibrosis are examples of autosomal recessive, single-gene disorders. Down syndrome is an example of a chromosome disorder in which the cells have three copies of chromosome 21 (trisomy) instead of the normal two copies. Hemophilia is an example of a recessive, sex-linked genetic disorder passed on from a mother to male children. Further information regarding inheritance of genes can be found in the study titled "Genetic Testing."

This procedure is contraindicated for

Patients with a history of or in the presence of incompetent cervix, vaginal infection, or Rh sensitization.

INDICATIONS

- Assist in the diagnosis of in utero metabolic disorders such as cystic fibrosis or other errors of lipid, carbohydrate, or amino acid metabolism.
- Detect abnormalities in the fetus of women of advanced maternal age.
- Determine fetal gender when the mother is a known carrier of a sex-linked abnormal gene that could be transmitted to male offspring, such as hemophilia or Duchenne's muscular dystrophy.
- Evaluate fetus in families with a history of genetic disorders, such as Down syndrome, Tay-Sachs disease, chromosome or enzyme anomalies, or inherited hemoglobinopathies.

B

POTENTIAL MEDICAL DIAGNOSIS

Abnormal karyotype: ***Numerous genetic disorders. Generally, the laboratory provides detailed interpretive information regarding the specific chromosome abnormality detected.***

CRITICAL FINDINGS:

- Identification of abnormalities in chorionic villus tissue

Note and immediately report to the requesting health-care provider (HCP) any critical findings and related symptoms. A listing of these findings varies among facilities. Timely notification of a critical finding for laboratory or diagnostic studies is a role expectation of the professional nurse. The notification processes vary among facilities. Upon receipt of the critical finding, the information should be read back to the caller to verify accuracy.

INTERFERING FACTORS

- Failure to follow dietary restrictions before the procedure may cause the procedure to be canceled or repeated.

NURSING IMPLICATIONS AND PROCEDURE

PRETEST:

- Positively identify the patient using at least two person-specific identifiers before services, treatments, or procedures are performed.
- *Patient Teaching:* Inform the patient this procedure can assist in establishing a diagnosis of in utero genetic disorders.
- Obtain a history of the patient's health concerns, symptoms, surgical procedures, and results of previously performed laboratory and diagnostic studies. Include any family history of genetic disorders such as cystic fibrosis, Duchenne's muscular dystrophy, hemophilia, sickle cell anemia, Tay-Sachs disease, thalassemia, and trisomy 21. Obtain maternal Rh type. If Rh-negative, check for prior sensitization. Include a list of known allergens, especially allergies or sensitivities to latex or anesthetics.
- Record the date of the last menstrual period and determine that the pregnancy is in the first trimester between the 10th and 12th weeks.
- Obtain a history of intravenous (IV) drug use, high-risk sexual activity, or occupational exposure.
- Obtain a list of the patient's current medications, including over-the-counter medications and dietary supplements (see Effects of Natural Products on Laboratory Values online at Davis*Plus*).
- Review the procedure with the patient. Warn the patient that normal results do not guarantee a normal fetus. Assure the patient that precautions to avoid injury to the fetus will be taken by locating the fetus with ultrasound. Address concerns about pain related to the procedure. Explain that during the transabdominal procedure, any discomfort with a needle biopsy will be minimized with local anesthetics. Explain that during the transvaginal procedure, some cramping may be experienced as the catheter is guided through the cervix. Encourage relaxation and controlled breathing during the procedure to aid in reducing any mild discomfort. Inform the patient that specimen collection is performed by an HCP specializing in this procedure and usually takes approximately 10 to 15 min to complete.
- ***Sensitivity to social and cultural issues,*** as well as concern for modesty, is important in providing psychological support before, during, and after the procedure.
- Note that there are no food, fluid, or medication restrictions unless by medical direction.
- Instruct the patient to drink 1 to 2 glasses of water about 30 min prior to testing so that the bladder is full. This elevates the uterus higher in the pelvis. The patient should not void before the procedure.

- *Make sure a written and informed consent has been signed prior to the procedure and before administering any medications.*

INTRATEST:

Potential Complications:

Women at risk for or with known cervical abnormalities should be aware of the risks of miscarriage due to incompetent (loose) cervix ***(related to passing a catheter or other instrument through the cervix, weakening the cervix).*** Rh-negative women risk mixing of the maternal and fetal blood supply ***(related to the invasive nature of the procedure and potentially resulting in development of maternal antibodies directed against fetal blood cells; a situation that can develop into hemolytic disease of the newborn).***

- Ensure that the patient has a full bladder before the procedure.
- Avoid the use of equipment containing latex if the patient has a history of allergic reaction to latex.
- Have emergency equipment readily available.
- Observe standard precautions, and follow the general guidelines in Patient Preparation and Specimen Collection online at Davis*Plus*. Positively identify the patient, and label the appropriate specimen containers with the corresponding patient demographics, initials of the person collecting the specimen, date and time of collection, and site location.
- Have the patient remove clothes below the waist. *Transabdominal:* Assist the patient into a supine position on the examination table with abdomen exposed. Drape the patient's legs, leaving abdomen exposed. *Transvaginal:* Assist the patient into a lithotomy position on a gynecologic examination table (with feet in stirrups). Drape the patient's legs. Instruct the patient to cooperate fully and to follow directions. Direct the patient to breathe normally and to avoid unnecessary movement during the local anesthetic and the procedure.
- Record maternal and fetal baseline vital signs, and continue to monitor throughout the procedure. Monitor for uterine contractions. Monitor fetal vital signs using ultrasound. Protocols may vary among facilities.
- After the administration of the local anesthetic, use clippers to remove hair from the surgical site if appropriate, cleanse the site with an antiseptic solution, and drape the area with sterile towels.

Transabdominal Biopsy

- Assess the position of the amniotic fluid, fetus, and placenta using ultrasound.
- A needle is inserted through the abdomen into the uterus, avoiding contact with the fetus. A syringe is connected to the needle, and the specimen of chorionic villus cells is withdrawn from the uteroplacental area. Pressure is applied to the site for 3 to 5 min, and then a sterile pressure dressing is applied.

Transvaginal Biopsy

- Assess the position of the fetus and placenta using ultrasound.
- A speculum is inserted into the vagina and is opened to gently spread apart the vagina for inspection of the cervix. The cervix is cleansed with a swab of antiseptic solution.
- A catheter is inserted through the cervix into the uterus, avoiding contact with the fetus. A syringe is connected to the catheter, and the specimen of chorionic villus cells is withdrawn from the uteroplacental area.

General

- Monitor the patient for complications related to the procedure (e.g., premature labor, allergic reaction, anaphylaxis).
- Place tissue samples in formalin solution. Label the specimen, indicating site location, and promptly transport the specimen to the laboratory for processing and analysis.

POST-TEST:

- Inform the patient that a report of the results will be made available to the

B

requesting HCP, who will discuss the results with the patient.

- After the procedure, the patient is placed in the left side-lying position, and both maternal and fetal vital signs are monitored for at least 30 min. Protocols may vary among facilities.
- Observe/assess for delayed allergic reactions, such as rash, urticaria, tachycardia, hyperpnea, hypertension, palpitations, nausea, or vomiting.
- Observe/assess the biopsy site for bleeding, inflammation, or hematoma formation.
- Instruct the patient in the care and assessment of the site.
- Instruct the patient to report any redness, edema, bleeding, or pain at the biopsy site.
- Advise the patient to expect mild cramping, leakage of small amount of amniotic fluid, and vaginal spotting for up to 2 days following the procedure. Instruct the patient to report moderate to severe abdominal pain or cramps, increased or prolonged leaking of amniotic fluid from vagina or abdominal needle site, vaginal bleeding that is heavier than spotting, and either chills or fever.
- Administer Rh(D) immune globulin RhoGAM IM or Rhophylac IM or IV to maternal Rh-negative patients to prevent maternal Rh sensitization should the fetus be Rh-positive.
- Administer mild analgesic and antibiotic therapy as ordered. Remind the patient of the importance of completing the entire course of antibiotic therapy, even if signs and symptoms disappear before completion of therapy.
- Recognize anxiety related to test results. Discuss the implications of abnormal test results on the patient's lifestyle. Provide teaching and information regarding the clinical implications of the test results, as appropriate. Encourage family to seek counseling if concerned with pregnancy termination or to seek genetic counseling if chromosomal abnormality is determined. Decisions regarding elective abortion should take place in the presence of both parents. Provide a nonjudgmental, nonthreatening atmosphere for a discussion during which risks of delivering a developmentally challenged infant are discussed with options (termination of pregnancy or adoption). It is also important to discuss problems the mother and father may experience (guilt, depression, anger) if fetal abnormalities are detected.
- Reinforce information given by the patient's HCP regarding further testing, treatment, or referral to another HCP. Answer any questions or address any concerns voiced by the patient or family.
- Instruct the patient in the use of any ordered medications. Explain the importance of adhering to the therapy regimen. As appropriate, instruct the patient in significant adverse effects associated with the prescribed medication. Encourage her to review corresponding literature provided by a pharmacist.
- Depending on the results of this procedure, additional testing may be performed to evaluate or monitor progression of the disease process and determine the need for a change in therapy. There are numerous tests for fetal genetic testing associated with inherited diseases and congenital abnormalities. The tests can be performed from chorionic villus sampling or amniotic fluid by methods that include polymerase chain reaction, microarray, and cell culture with karyotyping comparison. Evaluate test results in relation to the patient's symptoms and other tests performed.

RELATED STUDIES:

- Related tests include amniotic fluid analysis and L/S ratio, chromosome analysis, α_1 fetoprotein, genetic testing, HCG, hexosaminidase A and B, newborn screening, US biophysical profile, and US obstetric.
- Refer to the Reproductive System table online at Davis*Plus* for related tests by body system.

Biopsy, Intestinal

SYNONYM/ACRONYM: N/A

COMMON USE: To assist in confirming a diagnosis of intestinal cancer or disease.

SPECIMEN: Intestinal tissue or cells.

NORMAL FINDINGS: (Method: Macroscopic and microscopic examination of tissue) No abnormal tissue or cells.

DESCRIPTION: Intestinal biopsy is the excision of a tissue sample from the small intestine for microscopic analysis to determine cell morphology and the presence of tissue abnormalities. This test assists in confirming the diagnosis of cancer or intestinal disorders. Biopsy specimen is usually obtained during endoscopic examination.

This procedure is contraindicated for

Patients with bleeding disorders ***(related to the potential for prolonged bleeding from the biopsy site)*** or aortic arch aneurysm.

INDICATIONS

- Assist in the diagnosis of various intestinal disorders, such as lactose and other enzyme deficiencies, celiac disease, and parasitic infections.
- Confirm suspected intestinal malignancy.
- Confirm suspicious findings during endoscopic visualization of the intestinal wall.

POTENTIAL MEDICAL DIAGNOSIS

Abnormal findings related to

- Cancer
- Celiac disease
- Lactose deficiency
- Parasitic infestation
- Tropical sprue

CRITICAL FINDINGS:

- Assessment of clear margins after tissue excision
- Classification or grading of tumor
- Identification of malignancy

Note and immediately report to the requesting health-care provider (HCP) any critical findings and related symptoms. A listing of these findings varies among facilities. Timely notification of a critical finding for laboratory or diagnostic studies is a role expectation of the professional nurse. The notification processes vary among facilities. Upon receipt of the critical finding, the information should be read back to the caller to verify accuracy.

INTERFERING FACTORS

- Barium swallow within 48 hr of small intestine biopsy affects results.
- Failure to follow dietary restrictions before the procedure may cause the procedure to be canceled or repeated.

NURSING IMPLICATIONS AND PROCEDURE

PRETEST:

- Positively identify the patient using at least two person-specific identifiers before services, treatments, or procedures are performed.
- *Patient Teaching:* Inform the patient this procedure can assist in establishing a diagnosis of intestinal disease.

B

- Obtain a history of the patient's health concerns, symptoms, surgical procedures, and results of previously performed laboratory and diagnostic studies. Include a list of known allergens, especially allergies or sensitivities to latex or anesthetics.
- Record the date of the last menstrual period and determine the possibility of pregnancy in perimenopausal women.
- Note any recent procedures that can interfere with test results.
- Obtain a list of the patient's current medications, including over-the-counter medications, dietary supplements, anticoagulants, aspirin and other salicylates (see Effects of Natural Products on Laboratory Values online at Davis*Plus*). Such products should be discontinued by medical direction for the appropriate number of days prior to a surgical procedure. Note the last time and dose of medication taken.
- Review the procedure with the patient. Address concerns about pain and explain that a sedative may be administered to promote relaxation during the procedure. Inform the patient that the procedure is performed by an HCP specializing in this procedure and usually takes about 60 min to complete.
- ***Sensitivity to social and cultural issues,*** as well as concern for modesty, is important in providing psychological support before, during, and after the procedure.
- Explain that an intravenous line will be inserted to allow infusion of fluids such as saline, anesthetics, and analgesics.
- Explain that a clear liquid diet is to be consumed 1 day prior to the procedure. Instruct the patient that to reduce the risk of aspiration related to nausea and vomiting, clear liquids are restricted for at least 2 hr prior to general anesthesia, regional anesthesia, or sedation/analgesia (monitored anesthesia). The American Society of Anesthesiologists has fasting guidelines for risk levels according to patient status. More information can be located at www.asahq.org 🍁. Patients on beta blockers before the surgical procedure should be instructed to take their medication as ordered during the perioperative period. Protocols may vary among facilities.
- Provide the patient with a gown, robe, and foot coverings and instruct him or her to void prior to the procedure.
- Instruct the patient to remove dentures. Inform the HCP if the patient has any crowns or caps on the teeth.
- *Make sure a written and informed consent has been signed prior to the procedure and before administering any medications.*

INTRATEST:

Potential Complications:

Bleeding ***(related to a bleeding disorder, or the effects of natural products and medications with known anticoagulant, antiplatelet, or thrombolytic properties)*** or seeding of the biopsy tract with tumor cells.

- Ensure that the patient has complied with dietary restrictions prior to the study, as instructed.
- Ensure that anticoagulant therapy has been withheld for the appropriate number of days prior to the procedure. Number of days to withhold medication is dependent on the type of anticoagulant. Notify the HCP if patient anticoagulant therapy has not been withheld.
- Avoid the use of equipment containing latex if the patient has a history of allergic reaction to latex.
- Have emergency equipment readily available.
- Observe standard precautions, and follow the general guidelines in Patient Preparation and Specimen Collection online at Davis*Plus*. Positively identify the patient, and label the appropriate specimen containers with the corresponding patient demographics, initials of the person collecting the specimen, date and time of collection, and site location.
- Assist the patient into a semireclining position. Instruct the patient to cooperate fully and to follow directions.

Direct the patient to breathe normally and to avoid unnecessary movement.
- Record baseline vital signs, and continue to monitor throughout the procedure. Protocols may vary among facilities.

Esophagogastroduodenoscopy (EGD) Biopsy

- A local anesthetic is sprayed into the throat. A protective tooth guard and a bite block may be placed in the mouth.
- The flexible endoscope is passed into and through the mouth, and the patient is asked to swallow. Once the endoscope passes into the esophagus, assist the patient into the left lateral position. A suction device is used to drain saliva.
- The esophagus, stomach, and duodenum are visually examined as the endoscope passes through each section. A biopsy specimen can be taken from any suspicious sites.
- Tissue samples are obtained by inserting a cytology brush or biopsy forceps through the endoscope.
- When the examination and tissue removal are complete, the endoscope and suction device are withdrawn and the tooth guard and bite block are removed.
- Monitor the patient for complications related to the procedure (e.g., allergic reaction, anaphylaxis).
- Place tissue samples in formalin solution. Label the specimen, indicating site location, and promptly transport the specimen to the laboratory for processing and analysis.

POST-TEST:

- Inform the patient that a report of the results will be made available to the requesting HCP, who will discuss the results with the patient.
- Instruct the patient to resume usual diet, as directed by the HCP. Assess the patient's ability to swallow before allowing the patient to attempt liquids or solid foods.
- Monitor vital signs and neurological status every 15 min for 1 hr, then every 2 hr for 4 hr, and then as ordered by the HCP. Monitor temperature every 4 hr for 24 hr. Monitor intake and output at least every 8 hr. Compare with baseline values. Notify the HCP if temperature is elevated. Protocols may vary among facilities.
- Observe/assess for delayed allergic reactions, such as rash, urticaria, tachycardia, hyperpnea, hypertension, palpitations, nausea, or vomiting.
- Instruct the patient to report any chest pain, upper abdominal pain, pain on swallowing, difficulty breathing, or expectoration of blood. Report these to the HCP immediately.
- Administer mild analgesic and antibiotic therapy as ordered. Remind the patient of the importance of completing the entire course of antibiotic therapy, even if signs and symptoms disappear before completion of therapy.
- Recognize anxiety related to test results. Discuss the implications of abnormal test results on the patient's lifestyle. Provide teaching and information regarding the clinical implications of the test results, as appropriate. Educate the patient regarding access to counseling services.
- Reinforce information given by the patient's HCP regarding further testing, treatment, or referral to another HCP. Answer any questions or address any concerns voiced by the patient or family.
- Instruct the patient in the use of any ordered medications. Explain the importance of adhering to the therapy regimen. As appropriate, instruct the patient in significant adverse effects associated with the prescribed medication. Encourage him or her to review corresponding literature provided by a pharmacist.
- Depending on the results of this procedure, additional testing may be performed to evaluate or monitor progression of the disease process and determine the need for a change in therapy. Evaluate test results in relation to the patient's symptoms and other tests performed.

RELATED STUDIES:

- Related tests include albumin, antibodies gliadin, calcium, cancer antigens, capsule endoscopy, colonoscopy, D-xylose tolerance, fecal analysis, fecal fat, folic acid, iron/TIBC, LTT, ova and parasite, potassium, PT/INR, sodium, US abdomen, vitamin B_{12}, and vitamin D.
- Refer to the Gastrointestinal and Immune systems tables online at Davis*Plus* for related tests by body system.

B

Biopsy, Kidney

SYNONYM/ACRONYM: Renal biopsy.

COMMON USE: To assist in diagnosing cancer of the kidney and other kidney disorders.

SPECIMEN: Kidney tissue or cells.

NORMAL FINDINGS: (Method: Macroscopic and microscopic examination of tissue) No abnormal cells or tissue.

DESCRIPTION: Kidney or renal biopsy is the excision of a tissue sample from the kidney for microscopic analysis to determine cell morphology and the presence of tissue abnormalities. This test assists in confirming a diagnosis of cancer found on x-ray or ultrasound or to diagnose certain inflammatory or immunological conditions. Biopsy specimen is usually obtained either percutaneously or after surgical incision.

This procedure is contraindicated for

Patients with bleeding disorders ***(related to the potential for prolonged bleeding from the biopsy site)***, advanced kidney disease, uncontrolled hypertension, or solitary kidney ***(except transplanted kidney as the biopsy may be required to determine whether rejection or other damage is occurring)***.

INDICATIONS

- Assist in confirming suspected kidney malignancy.
- Assist in the diagnosis of the cause of kidney disease.
- Determine extent of involvement in systemic lupus erythematosus or other immunological disorders.
- Monitor progression of nephrotic syndrome.
- Monitor kidney function after transplantation.

POTENTIAL MEDICAL DIAGNOSIS

Positive Findings in

- Acute and chronic poststreptococcal glomerulonephritis
- Amyloidosis infiltration
- Cancer
- Disseminated lupus erythematosus
- Goodpasture's syndrome
- Immunological rejection of transplanted kidney
- Nephrotic syndrome
- Pyelonephritis
- Renal venous thrombosis

CRITICAL FINDINGS:
- Assessment of clear margins after tissue excision
- Classification or grading of tumor
- Identification of malignancy

Note and immediately report to the requesting health-care provider (HCP) any critical findings and related symptoms. A listing of these findings varies among facilities. Timely notification of a critical finding for laboratory or diagnostic studies is a role expectation of the professional nurse. The notification processes vary among facilities. Upon receipt of the critical, finding the information should be read back to the caller to verify accuracy.

INTERFERING FACTORS
- Obesity and severe spinal deformity can make percutaneous biopsy impossible.
- Failure to follow dietary restrictions before the procedure may cause the procedure to be canceled or repeated.

NURSING IMPLICATIONS AND PROCEDURE

POTENTIAL NURSING PROBLEMS:

Problem	Signs & Symptoms	Interventions
Fear ***(related to lack of understanding of disease process and management; potential death)***	Anxiety; apprehension; stated fear; restlessness; increased tension; continuous questioning; increased blood pressure, heart rate, and respiratory rate	Evaluate both verbal and nonverbal cues of fear; assess for the cause of the fear; acknowledge the patient's awareness of his or her fear; explain all procedures in simple-to-understand, culturally and age-appropriate terms; administer ordered tranquilizer; maintain a confident, assured, professional manner in all patient interactions
Insufficient knowledge ***(related to postoperative care and treatment secondary to surgical intervention associated with cancer, glomerulonephritis, lupus, nephrotic syndrome, infection, thrombus)***	Lack of interest or multiple questions; anxiety in relation to disease process and management; verbalization of inaccurate information	Assess the patient's understanding of the need for further treatment (radiation therapy, chemotherapy); discuss postoperative care and potential complications; review the signs and symptoms of infection

(table continues on page 236)

Problem	Signs & Symptoms	Interventions
Inadequate coping ***(related to new disease process; fear of prognosis [death]; loss of kidney; effects on endocrine functionality)***	Verbal expression of fear; restlessness; anxiety; withdrawal; crying; apparent emotional distress	Assess coping mechanism; support positive coping mechanism; recommend support group; provide clear, concise, appropriate information; administer ordered antianxiety medication; provide contact information for spiritual leader; provide information related to advance directives; maintain a calm, quiet environment

PRETEST:

- Positively identify the patient using at least two person-specific identifiers before services, treatments, or procedures are performed.
- ***Patient Teaching:*** Inform the patient this procedure can assist in establishing a diagnosis of kidney disease.
- Obtain a history of the patient's health concerns (especially any bleeding disorders), symptoms, surgical procedures, and results of previously performed laboratory and diagnostic studies. Include a list of known allergens, especially allergies or sensitivities to latex or anesthetics.
- Record the date of the last menstrual period and determine the possibility of pregnancy in perimenopausal women.
- Note any recent procedures that can interfere with test results.
- Obtain a list of the patient's current medications, including over-the-counter medications, dietary supplements, anticoagulants, aspirin and other salicylates (see Effects of Natural Products on Laboratory Values online at Davis*Plus*). Such products should be discontinued by medical direction for the appropriate number of days prior to a surgical procedure. Note the last time and dose of medication taken.
- Review the procedure with the patient. Inform the patient that it may be necessary to remove hair from the site before the procedure. Instruct the patient that prophylactic antibiotics may be administered before the procedure. Address concerns about pain and explain that a sedative and/or analgesia will be administered before the percutaneous biopsy to promote relaxation and reduce discomfort; general anesthesia will be administered before the open biopsy. Explain to the patient that no pain will be experienced during the test when general anesthesia is used but that any discomfort with a needle biopsy will be minimized with local anesthetics and systemic analgesics. Inform the patient that the biopsy is performed under sterile conditions by an HCP specializing in this procedure. The surgical procedure usually takes about 60 min to complete, and sutures may be necessary to close the site. A needle biopsy usually takes about 40 min to complete.
- ***Sensitivity to social and cultural issues,*** as well as concern for modesty, is important in providing psychological support before, during, and after the procedure.
- Explain that an intravenous (IV) line will be inserted to allow infusion of fluids such as saline, antibiotics, anesthetics, analgesics, or IV sedation.
- Instruct the patient that to reduce the risk of aspiration related to nausea

and vomiting, solid food and milk or milk products are restricted for at least 6 hr, and clear liquids are restricted for at least 2 hr prior to general anesthesia, regional anesthesia, or sedation/analgesia (monitored anesthesia). The American Society of Anesthesiologists has fasting guidelines for risk levels according to patient status. More information can be located at www.asahq.org ✦. Patients on beta blockers before the surgical procedure should be instructed to take their medication as ordered during the perioperative period. Protocols may vary among facilities.

- *Make sure a written and informed consent has been signed prior to the procedure and before administering any medications.*

INTRATEST:

Potential Complications:

Bleeding ***(related to a bleeding disorder, or the effects of natural products and medications with known anticoagulant, antiplatelet, or thrombolytic properties)*** or seeding of the biopsy tract with tumor cells.

- Ensure that the patient has complied with dietary restrictions prior to the study, as instructed.
- Ensure that anticoagulant therapy has been withheld for the appropriate number of days prior to the procedure. Number of days to withhold medication is dependent on the type of anticoagulant. Notify the HCP if patient anticoagulant therapy has not been withheld. Ensure that patients on beta-blocker therapy have continued their medication regimen as ordered.
- Avoid the use of equipment containing latex if the patient has a history of allergic reaction to latex.
- Have emergency equipment readily available.
- Have the patient void before the procedure.
- Observe standard precautions, and follow the general guidelines in Patient Preparation and Specimen Collection online at Davis*Plus*. Positively identify the patient, and label the appropriate specimen containers with the corresponding patient demographics, initials of the person collecting the specimen, date and time of collection, and site location, especially right or left kidney.
- Assist the patient to the desired position depending on the test site to be used, and direct the patient to breathe normally during the beginning of the general anesthetic. Instruct the patient to cooperate fully and to follow directions. Direct the patient to avoid unnecessary movement.
- Record baseline vital signs, and continue to monitor throughout the procedure. Protocols may vary among facilities.
- After the administration of general or local anesthetics, use clippers to remove hair from the surgical site if appropriate, cleanse the site with an antiseptic solution, and drape the area with sterile towels.

Open Biopsy

- Adhere to Surgical Care Improvement Project (SCIP) quality measures. Administer ordered prophylactic antibiotics 1 hr before incision, and use antibiotics that are consistent with current guidelines specific to the procedure.
- After administration of general anesthetics and surgical preparation are completed, an incision is made, suspicious area(s) are located, and tissue samples are collected.

Needle Biopsy

- A sandbag may be placed under the abdomen to aid in moving the kidneys to the desired position. Direct the patient to take slow deep breaths when the local anesthetic is injected. Protect the site with sterile drapes. Instruct the patient to take a deep breath, exhale forcefully, and hold the breath while the biopsy needle is inserted and rotated to obtain a core of renal tissue. Once the needle is removed, the patient may breathe. Pressure is applied to the site for 5 to 20 min, then a sterile pressure dressing is applied.

B

General

- Monitor the patient for complications related to the procedure (e.g., allergic reaction, anaphylaxis).
- Place tissue samples in formalin solution. Label the specimen, indicating site location, and promptly transport the specimen to the laboratory for processing and analysis.

POST-TEST:

- Inform the patient that a report of the results will be made available to the requesting HCP, who will discuss the results with the patient.
- Instruct the patient to resume preoperative diet, as directed by the HCP. Assess the patient's ability to swallow before allowing the patient to attempt liquids or solid foods.
- Monitor vital signs and neurological status every 15 min for 1 hr, then every 2 hr for 4 hr, and then as ordered by the HCP. Monitor temperature every 4 hr for 24 hr. Monitor intake and output at least every 8 hr. Compare with baseline values. Notify the HCP if temperature is elevated. Discontinue prophylactic antibiotics within 24 hr after the conclusion of the procedure. Protocols may vary among facilities.
- Observe/assess for delayed allergic reactions, such as rash, urticaria, tachycardia, hyperpnea, hypertension, palpitations, nausea, or vomiting.
- Instruct the patient to immediately report symptoms such as fast heart rate, difficulty breathing, skin rash, itching, chest pain, persistent right shoulder pain, or abdominal pain. Immediately report symptoms to the appropriate HCP.
- Observe/assess the biopsy site for bleeding, inflammation, or hematoma formation.
- Instruct the patient in the care and assessment of the site.
- Instruct the patient to report any redness, edema, bleeding, or pain at the biopsy site. Instruct the patient to immediately report chills or fever.
- Observe/assess the biopsy site for bleeding, inflammation, or hematoma formation.
- Inform the patient that blood may be seen in the urine after the first or second postprocedural voiding.
- Monitor fluid intake and output for 24 hr. Instruct the patient on intake and output recording and provide appropriate measuring containers.
- Instruct the patient to report any changes in urinary pattern or volume or any unusual appearance of the urine. If urinary volume is less than 200 mL in the first 8 hr, encourage the patient to increase fluid intake unless contraindicated by another medical condition.
- Assess for nausea and pain. Administer antiemetic and analgesic medications as needed and as directed by the HCP.
- Administer antibiotic therapy if ordered. Remind the patient of the importance of completing the entire course of antibiotic therapy, even if signs and symptoms disappear before completion of therapy.
- Recognize anxiety related to test results. Discuss the implications of abnormal test results on the patient's lifestyle. Provide teaching and information regarding the clinical implications of the test results, as appropriate. Educate the patient regarding access to counseling services.
- Reinforce information given by the patient's HCP regarding further testing, treatment, or referral to another HCP. Inform the patient of a follow-up appointment for removal of sutures, if indicated. Answer any questions or address any concerns voiced by the patient or family.
- Instruct the patient in the use of any ordered medications. Explain the importance of adhering to the therapy regimen. As appropriate, instruct the patient in significant adverse effects associated with the prescribed medication. Encourage him or her to review corresponding literature provided by a pharmacist.
- Depending on the results of this procedure, additional testing may be performed to evaluate or monitor progression of the disease process

and determine the need for a change in therapy. Evaluate test results in relation to the patient's symptoms and other tests performed.

Patient Education:

- Teach the patient the pathophysiology associated with cancer, disease, as well as ongoing treatment and screenings.
- Explain that a health-care specialist may need to be consulted to manage the disease and therapeutic interventions.

Expected Patient Outcomes:

Understanding

- The patient and family discuss the medical versus surgical options for disease management.
- The patient and family acknowledge end-of-life treatment options as appropriate.

Ability

- The patient and family demonstrate positive coping strategies.
- The patient and family demonstrate care of surgical site, biopsy site.

Response

- The patient and family agree to attend disease-specific support group meetings.
- The patient and family agree to seek psychological counseling to adjust to lifestyle changes associated with positive therapeutic management strategies.

RELATED STUDIES:

- Related tests include albumin, aldosterone, angiography kidneys, antibodies antiglomerular basement membrane, β_2-microglobulin, BUN, CT kidneys, creatinine, creatinine clearance, cytology urine, cystoscopy, IVP, KUB studies, osmolality, PTH, potassium, protein, renin, renogram, sodium, US kidney, and UA.
- Refer to the Genitourinary and Immune systems tables online at Davis*Plus* for related tests by body system.

Biopsy, Liver

SYNONYM/ACRONYM: N/A

COMMON USE: To assist in diagnosing liver cancer, and other liver disorders such as cirrhosis and hepatitis.

SPECIMEN: Liver tissue or cells.

NORMAL FINDINGS: (Method: Macroscopic and microscopic examination of tissue) No abnormal cells or tissue.

DESCRIPTION: Liver biopsy is the excision of a tissue sample from the liver for microscopic analysis to determine cell morphology and the presence of tissue abnormalities. This test is used to assist in confirming a diagnosis of cancer or certain disorders of the hepatic parenchyma. Biopsy specimen is usually obtained either percutaneously or after surgical incision.

This procedure is contraindicated for

- Patients with bleeding disorders ***(related to the potential for prolonged bleeding from the biopsy site)***, suspected vascular tumor of the liver, ascites that may obscure proper insertion site for needle biopsy, subdiaphragmatic or right hemothoracic infection, or biliary tract infection.

B

INDICATIONS

- Assist in confirming suspected hepatic malignancy.
- Assist in confirming suspected hepatic parenchymal disease.
- Assist in diagnosing the cause of persistently elevated liver enzymes, hepatomegaly, or jaundice.

POTENTIAL MEDICAL DIAGNOSIS

Positive Findings in

- Benign tumor
- Cancer
- Cholesterol ester storage disease
- Cirrhosis
- Galactosemia
- Hemochromatosis
- Hepatic involvement with systemic lupus erythematosus, sarcoidosis, or amyloidosis
- Hepatitis
- Parasitic infestations (e.g., amebiasis, malaria, visceral larva migrans)
- Reye's syndrome
- Wilson's disease

CRITICAL FINDINGS:

- Assessment of clear margins after tissue excision
- Classification or grading of tumor
- Identification of malignancy

Note and immediately report to the requesting health-care provider (HCP) any critical findings and related symptoms. A listing of these findings varies among facilities. Timely notification of a critical finding for laboratory or diagnostic studies is a role expectation of the professional nurse. The notification processes vary among facilities. Upon receipt of the critical finding, the information should be read back to the caller to verify accuracy.

INTERFERING FACTORS

- Failure to follow dietary restrictions before the procedure may cause the procedure to be canceled or repeated.

NURSING IMPLICATIONS AND PROCEDURE

POTENTIAL NURSING PROBLEMS:

Problem	Signs & Symptoms	Interventions
Fear ***(related to lack of understanding of disease process and management; potential death)***	Anxiety; apprehension; stated fear; restlessness; increased tension; continuous questioning; increased blood pressure, heart rate, and respiratory rate	Evaluate both verbal and nonverbal cues of fear; assess for the cause of the fear; acknowledge the patient's awareness of his or her fear; explain all procedures in simple-to-understand, culturally and age-appropriate terms; administer ordered tranquilizer; maintain a confident, assured, professional manner in all patient interactions

Problem	Signs & Symptoms	Interventions
Inadequate coping ***(related to new disease process; fear of prognosis [death]; lifestyle changes; tumor; chronic disease)***	Verbal expression of fear; restlessness; anxiety; withdrawal; crying; apparent emotional distress	Assess coping mechanism; support positive coping mechanism; recommend support group; provide clear, appropriate information; administer ordered antianxiety medication; provide contact information for spiritual advisor; provide information related to advance directives; maintain a calm quiet environment
Insufficient knowledge ***(related to chronic disease [lupus, cirrhosis, hepatitis]; treatment modalities; parasites)***	Lack of interest or multiple questions; anxiety in relation to disease process and management; verbalization of inaccurate information	Assess the patient's understanding of the need for further treatment; assess the patient's understanding of required lifestyle changes and health restrictions (hepatitis); review the signs and symptoms of disease process; discuss special treatment of body fluids

PRETEST:

- Positively identify the patient using at least two person-specific identifiers before services, treatments, or procedures are performed.
- *Patient Teaching:* Inform the patient this procedure can assist in establishing a diagnosis of liver disease.
- Obtain a history of the patient's health concerns (especially fatigue and pain related to inflammation and swelling of the liver, or any bleeding disorders), symptoms, surgical procedures, and results of previously performed laboratory and diagnostic studies. Include a list of known allergens, especially allergies or sensitivities to latex or anesthetics.
- Record the date of the last menstrual period and determine the possibility of pregnancy in perimenopausal women.
- Note any recent procedures that can interfere with test results.
- Obtain a list of the patient's current medications, including over-the-counter medications, dietary supplements, anticoagulants, aspirin and other salicylates (see Effects of Natural Products on Laboratory Values online at Davis*Plus*). Such products should be discontinued by medical direction for the appropriate number of days prior to a surgical procedure. Note the last time and dose of medication taken.

B

- Review the procedure with the patient. Inform the patient that it may be necessary to remove hair from the site before the procedure. Instruct the patient that prophylactic antibiotics may be administered before the procedure. Address concerns about pain and explain that a sedative and/or analgesia will be administered before the percutaneous biopsy to promote relaxation and reduce discomfort; general anesthesia will be administered before the open biopsy. Explain to the patient that no pain will be experienced during the test when general anesthesia is used but that any discomfort with a needle biopsy will be minimized with local anesthetics and systemic analgesics. Inform the patient that the biopsy is performed under sterile conditions by an HCP specializing in this procedure. The surgical procedure usually takes about 90 min to complete, and sutures may be necessary to close the site. A needle biopsy usually takes about 15 min to complete.
- ***Sensitivity to social and cultural issues,*** as well as concern for modesty, is important in providing psychological support before, during, and after the procedure.
- Explain that an intravenous line will be inserted to allow infusion of fluids such as saline, antibiotics, anesthetics, analgesics, or sedation.
- Instruct the patient that to reduce the risk of aspiration related to nausea and vomiting, solid food and milk or milk products are restricted for at least 6 hr, and clear liquids are restricted for at least 2 hr prior to general anesthesia, regional anesthesia, or sedation/analgesia (monitored anesthesia). The American Society of Anesthesiologists has fasting guidelines for risk levels according to patient status. More information can be located at www.asahq.org 🍁. Patients on beta blockers before the surgical procedure should be instructed to take their medication as ordered during the perioperative period. Protocols may vary among facilities.
- *Make sure a written and informed consent has been signed prior to the procedure and before administering any medications.*

INTRATEST:

Potential Complications:

Bleeding ***(related to a bleeding disorder, bleeding initiated by surgical invasion of a vascular tumor of the liver, or the effects of natural products and medications with known anticoagulant, antiplatelet, or thrombolytic properties)*** or seeding of the biopsy tract with tumor cells.

- Ensure that the patient has complied with dietary restrictions prior to the study, as instructed.
- Ensure that anticoagulant therapy has been withheld for the appropriate number of days prior to the procedure. Number of days to withhold medication is dependent on the type of anticoagulant. Notify the HCP if patient anticoagulant therapy has not been withheld. Ensure that patients on beta-blocker therapy have continued their medication regimen as ordered.
- Avoid the use of equipment containing latex if the patient has a history of allergic reaction to latex.
- Have emergency equipment readily available.
- Have the patient void before the procedure.
- Observe standard precautions, and follow the general guidelines in Patient Preparation and Specimen Collection online at Davis*Plus*. Positively identify the patient, and label the appropriate specimen containers with the corresponding patient demographics, initials of the person collecting the specimen, date and time of collection, and site location.
- Assist the patient to the desired position depending on the test site to be used and direct the patient to breathe normally during the beginning of the general anesthetic. Instruct the patient to cooperate fully and to follow directions. For the patient undergoing local anesthesia, direct him or her to breathe normally

and to avoid unnecessary movement during the procedure. Instruct the patient to avoid coughing or straining, which may increase intra-abdominal pressure.

- Record baseline vital signs, and continue to monitor throughout the procedure. Protocols may vary among facilities.
- After the administration of general or local anesthetics, use clippers to remove hair from the surgical site if appropriate, cleanse the site with an antiseptic solution, and drape the area with sterile towels.

Open Biopsy

- Adhere to Surgical Care Improvement Project (SCIP) quality measures. Administer ordered prophylactic antibiotics 1 hr before incision, and use antibiotics that are consistent with current guidelines specific to the procedure.
- After administration of general anesthetics and surgical preparation are completed, an incision is made, suspicious area(s) are located, and tissue samples are collected.

Needle Biopsy

- Direct the patient to take slow deep breaths when the local anesthetic is injected. Protect the site with sterile drapes. Instruct the patient to take a deep breath, exhale forcefully, and hold the breath while the biopsy needle is inserted and rotated to obtain a core of liver tissue. Once the needle is removed, the patient may breathe. Pressure is applied to the site for 3 to 5 min, then a sterile pressure dressing is applied.

General

- Monitor the patient for complications related to the procedure (e.g., allergic reaction, anaphylaxis).
- Place tissue samples in formalin solution. Label the specimen, indicating site location, and promptly transport the specimen to the laboratory for processing and analysis.

POST-TEST:

- Inform the patient that a report of the results will be made available to the requesting HCP, who will discuss the results with the patient.
- Instruct the patient to resume preoperative diet, as directed by the HCP. Assess the patient's ability to swallow before allowing the patient to attempt liquids or solid foods.
- Monitor vital signs and neurological status every 15 min for 1 hr, then every 2 hr for 4 hr, and then as ordered by the HCP. Monitor temperature every 4 hr for 24 hr. Monitor intake and output at least every 8 hr. Compare with baseline values. Notify the HCP if temperature is elevated. Discontinue prophylactic antibiotics within 24 hr after the conclusion of the procedure. Protocols may vary among facilities.
- Observe/assess for delayed allergic reactions, such as rash, urticaria, tachycardia, hyperpnea, hypertension, palpitations, nausea, or vomiting.
- Instruct the patient to immediately report symptoms such as fast heart rate, difficulty breathing, skin rash, itching, chest pain, persistent right shoulder pain, or abdominal pain. Immediately report symptoms to the appropriate HCP.
- Observe/assess the biopsy site for bleeding, inflammation, or hematoma formation.
- Instruct the patient in the care and assessment of the site.
- Instruct the patient to report any redness, edema, bleeding, or pain at the biopsy site. Instruct the patient to immediately report chills or fever.
- Assess for nausea and pain. Administer antiemetic and analgesic medications as needed and as directed by the HCP.
- Administer antibiotic therapy if ordered. Remind the patient of the importance of completing the entire course of antibiotic therapy, even if signs and symptoms disappear before completion of therapy.
- Recognize anxiety related to test results. Discuss the implications of abnormal test results on the patient's lifestyle. Provide teaching and

information regarding the clinical implications of the test results, as appropriate. Educate the patient regarding access to counseling services.

- Reinforce information given by the patient's HCP regarding further testing, treatment, or referral to another HCP. Inform the patient of a follow-up appointment for removal of sutures, if indicated. Answer any questions or address any concerns voiced by the patient or family.
- Instruct the patient in the use of any ordered medications. Explain the importance of adhering to the therapy regimen. As appropriate, instruct the patient in significant adverse effects associated with the prescribed medication. Encourage him or her to review corresponding literature provided by a pharmacist.
- Depending on the results of this procedure, additional testing may be performed to evaluate or monitor progression of the disease process and determine the need for a change in therapy. Evaluate test results in relation to the patient's symptoms and other tests performed.

Patient Education:

- Teach the patient the pathophysiology associated with cancer, disease as well as ongoing treatment and screenings.
- Explain that a health-care specialist may need to be consulted to manage the disease process and therapeutic interventions.

Expected Patient Outcomes:

Understanding

- The patient and family discuss the medical versus surgical options for disease management.
- The patient and family acknowledge end-of-life treatment options as appropriate.

Ability

- The patient and family demonstrate positive coping strategies.
- The patient and family successfully demonstrate care of surgical site, biopsy site.

Response

- The patient and family agree to attend disease-specific support group meetings.
- The patient and family agree to seek psychological counseling to adjust to lifestyle changes associated with positive therapeutic management strategies.

RELATED STUDIES:

- Related tests include ALT, albumin, ALP, ammonia, amylase, AMA/ASMA, α_1-antitrypsin/phenotyping, AST, bilirubin, cholesterol, coagulation factors, CBC, copper, GGT, hepatitis antigens and antibodies, infectious mononucleosis screen, laparoscopy abdominal, lipase, liver and spleen scan, MRI liver, PT/INR, radiofrequency ablation liver, UA, US abdomen, and US liver.
- Refer to the Hepatobiliary and Immune systems tables online at Davis*Plus* for related tests by body system.

Biopsy, Lung

SYNONYM/ACRONYM: Transbronchial lung biopsy, open lung biopsy.

COMMON USE: To assist in diagnosing lung cancer and other lung tissue disease.

SPECIMEN: Lung tissue or cells.

NORMAL FINDINGS: (Method: Macroscopic and microscopic examination of tissue) No abnormal tissue or cells; no growth in culture.

DESCRIPTION: A biopsy of the lung is performed to obtain lung tissue for examination of pathological features. The specimen can be obtained transbronchially or by open lung biopsy. In a transbronchial biopsy, forceps pass through the bronchoscope to obtain the specimen. In a transbronchial needle aspiration biopsy, a needle passes through a bronchoscope to obtain the specimen. In a transcatheter bronchial brushing, a brush is inserted through the bronchoscope. In an open lung biopsy, the chest is opened and a small thoracic incision is made to remove tissue from the chest wall. Lung biopsies are used to differentiate between infection and other sources of disease indicated by initial radiology studies, computed tomography scans, or sputum analysis. Specimens are cultured to detect pathogenic organisms or directly examined for the presence of malignant cells.

This procedure is contraindicated for

Patients with bleeding disorders ***(related to the potential for prolonged bleeding from the biopsy site).***

INDICATIONS

- Assist in the diagnosis of lung cancer.
- Assist in the diagnosis of fibrosis and degenerative or inflammatory diseases of the lung.
- Assist in the diagnosis of sarcoidosis.

POTENTIAL MEDICAL DIAGNOSIS

Abnormal findings related to

- Amyloidosis
- Cancer
- Granulomas
- Infections caused by *Blastomyces, Histoplasma, Legionella* spp., and *Pneumocystis jiroveci*
- Sarcoidosis
- Systemic lupus erythematosus
- Tuberculosis

CRITICAL FINDINGS:

- Any postprocedural decrease in breath sounds noted at the biopsy site should be reported immediately
- Assessment of clear margins after tissue excision
- Classification or grading of tumor
- Identification of malignancy
- Shortness of breath, cyanosis, or rapid pulse during the procedure must be reported immediately

Note and immediately report to the requesting health-care provider (HCP) any critical findings and related symptoms. A listing of these findings varies among facilities. Timely notification of a critical finding for laboratory or diagnostic studies is a role expectation of the professional nurse. The notification processes vary among facilities. Upon receipt of the critical finding, the information should be read back to the caller to verify accuracy.

INTERFERING FACTORS

- Conditions such as vascular anomalies of the lung, bleeding abnormalities, or pulmonary hypertension may increase the risk of bleeding.
- Conditions such as bullae or cysts and respiratory insufficiency increase the risk of pneumothorax.
- Failure to follow dietary restrictions before the procedure may cause the procedure to be canceled or repeated.

NURSING IMPLICATIONS AND PROCEDURE

B

POTENTIAL NURSING PROBLEMS:

Problem	Signs & Symptoms	Interventions
Fear ***(related to lack of understanding of disease process and management; potential death)***	Anxiety; apprehension; stated fear; restlessness; increased tension; continuous questioning; increased blood pressure, heart rate, and respiratory rate	Evaluate both verbal and nonverbal cues of fear; assess for the cause of the fear; acknowledge the patient's awareness of their fear; explain all procedures in simple-to-understand, culturally and age-appropriate terms; administer ordered tranquilizer; maintain a confident, assured, professional manner in all patient interactions
Inadequate coping ***(related to new disease process; fear of prognosis [death]; difficulty breathing; lifestyle changes)***	Verbal expression of fear; restlessness; anxiety; withdrawal; crying; apparent emotional distress	Assess coping mechanism; support positive coping mechanism; recommend support group; provide clear, concise appropriate information; administer ordered antianxiety medication; provide contact information for spiritual advisor; provide information related to advance directives; maintain a calm quiet environment
Insufficient knowledge ***(related to postoperative care and treatment secondary to surgical intervention associated with lung cancer; chronic disease [lupus, tuberculosis, sarcoidosis]; tumor; infection)***	Lack of interest or multiple questions; anxiety in relation to disease process and management; verbalization of inaccurate information	Assess the patient's understanding of the need for further treatment (radiation therapy, chemotherapy); discuss postoperative care and potential complications; review the signs and symptoms of infection; review treatment options associated with disease process or tumor

PRETEST:

- Positively identify the patient using at least two person-specific identifiers before services, treatments, or procedures are performed.
- ***Patient Teaching:*** Inform the patient this procedure can assist in establishing a diagnosis of lung disease.
- Obtain a history of the patient's health concerns, symptoms, surgical procedures, and results of previously performed laboratory and diagnostic studies. Include a list of known allergens, especially allergies or sensitivities to latex and anesthetics.
- Note any recent procedures that can interfere with test results.
- Record the date of the last menstrual period and determine the possibility of pregnancy in perimenopausal women.
- Obtain a list of the patient's current medications, including over-the-counter medications, dietary supplements, anticoagulants, aspirin and other salicylates (see Effects of Natural Products on Laboratory Values online at Davis*Plus*). Such products should be discontinued by medical direction for the appropriate number of days prior to a surgical procedure. Note the last time and dose of medication taken.
- Review the procedure with the patient. Inform the patient that it may be necessary to remove hair from the site before the procedure. Instruct the patient that prophylactic antibiotics may be administered before the procedure. Address concerns about pain and explain that a sedative and/or analgesia will be administered before the percutaneous biopsy to promote relaxation and reduce discomfort; general anesthesia will be administered before the open biopsy. Explain to the patient that no pain will be experienced during the test when general anesthesia is used but that any discomfort with a needle biopsy will be minimized with local anesthetics and systemic analgesics. Atropine is usually given before bronchoscopy examinations to reduce bronchial secretions and prevent vagally induced bradycardia. A sedative and/or analgesia may be administered to promote relaxation and reduce discomfort during the procedure. A local anesthetic such as lidocaine is sprayed in the patient's throat to reduce discomfort caused by the presence of the tube. Inform the patient that the biopsy is performed under sterile conditions by an HCP specializing in this procedure. The surgical procedure usually takes about 30 min to complete, and sutures may be necessary to close the site. A needle biopsy usually takes about 15 to 30 min to complete.
- ***Sensitivity to social and cultural issues,*** as well as concern for modesty, is important in providing psychological support before, during, and after the procedure.
- Explain that an intravenous line will be inserted to allow infusion of fluids such as saline, antibiotics, anesthetics, and analgesics.
- Instruct the patient that to reduce the risk of aspiration related to nausea and vomiting, solid food and milk or milk products are restricted for at least 6 hr, and clear liquids are restricted for at least 2 hr prior to general anesthesia, regional anesthesia, or sedation/analgesia (monitored anesthesia). The American Society of Anesthesiologists has fasting guidelines for risk levels according to patient status. More information can be located at www.asahq.org 🍁. Patients on beta blockers before the surgical procedure should be instructed to take their medication as ordered during the perioperative period. Protocols may vary among facilities.
- Have the patient void before the procedure.
- *Make sure a written and informed consent has been signed prior to the procedure and before administering any medications.*

INTRATEST:

Potential Complications:

Bleeding ***(related to a bleeding disorder, or the effects of natural products***

B

and medications with known anticoagulant, antiplatelet, or thrombolytic properties), pneumothorax ***(increased risk for pneumothorax is related to the presence of bullae or cysts and respiratory insufficiency),*** hemoptysis, air embolism, or seeding of the biopsy tract with tumor cells.

- Ensure that the patient has complied with dietary restrictions prior to the study, as instructed.
- Ensure that anticoagulant therapy has been withheld for the appropriate number of days prior to the procedure. Number of days to withhold medication is dependent on the type of anticoagulant. Notify the HCP if patient anticoagulant therapy has not been withheld. Ensure that patients on beta-blocker therapy have continued their medication regimen as ordered.
- Avoid the use of equipment containing latex if the patient has a history of allergic reaction to latex.
- Have emergency equipment readily available. Keep resuscitation equipment on hand in the case of respiratory impairment or laryngospasm after the procedure.
- Avoid using morphine sulfate in those with asthma or other pulmonary disease. This drug can further exacerbate bronchospasms and respiratory impairment.
- Observe standard precautions, and follow the general guidelines in Patient Preparation and Specimen Collection online at Davis*Plus*. Positively identify the patient, and label the appropriate specimen containers with the corresponding patient demographics, initials of the person collecting the specimen, date and time of collection, and site location, especially right or left lung.
- Have patient remove dentures and notify the HCP if the patient has permanent crowns on teeth. Have the patient remove clothing and change into a gown for the procedure.
- Assist the patient to a comfortable position and direct the patient to breathe normally during the beginning of the general anesthetic. Instruct the patient to cooperate fully and to follow directions. For the patient undergoing local anesthesia, direct him or her to breathe normally and to avoid unnecessary movement during the procedure.
- Record baseline vital signs and continue to monitor throughout the procedure. Protocols may vary among facilities.
- After the administration of general or local anesthetics, use clippers to remove hair from the surgical site if appropriate, cleanse the site with an antiseptic solution, and drape the area with sterile towels.

Open Biopsy

- Adhere to Surgical Care Improvement Project (SCIP) quality measures. Administer ordered prophylactic antibiotics 1 hr before incision, and use antibiotics that are consistent with current guidelines specific to the procedure.
- The patient is prepared for thoracotomy under general anesthesia in the operating room. Tissue specimens are collected from suspicious sites. Place specimen from needle aspiration or brushing on clean glass microscope slides. Place tissue or aspirate specimens in appropriate sterile container for culture or appropriate fixative container for histological studies.
- Carefully observe/assess the patient for any signs of respiratory distress during the procedure.
- A chest tube is inserted after the procedure.

Needle Biopsy

- Instruct the patient to take slow, deep breaths when the local anesthetic is injected. Protect the site with sterile drapes. Assist patient to a sitting position with arms on a pillow over a bed table. Instruct patient to avoid coughing during the procedure. The needle is inserted through the posterior chest wall and into the intercostal space. The needle is rotated to obtain the sample and then withdrawn. Pressure is applied to the site with a petroleum jelly gauze, and a pressure dressing is applied over the petroleum jelly gauze.

Bronchoscopy

- Provide mouth care to reduce oral bacterial flora.
- After administration of general anesthetics, position the patient in a supine position with the neck hyperextended. If a local anesthetic is used, the patient is seated while the tongue and oropharynx are sprayed and swabbed with anesthetic. Provide an emesis basin for the increased saliva and encourage the patient to spit out the saliva because the gag reflex may be impaired. When loss of sensation is adequate, the patient is placed in a supine or side-lying position. The fiberoptic scope can be introduced through the nose, the mouth, an endotracheal tube, a tracheostomy tube, or a rigid bronchoscope. Most common insertion is through the nose. Patients with copious secretions or massive hemoptysis, or in whom airway complications are more likely, may be intubated before the bronchoscopy. Additional local anesthetic is applied through the scope as it approaches the vocal cords and the carina, eliminating reflexes in these sensitive areas. The fiberoptic approach allows visualization of airway segments without having to move the patient's head through various positions.
- After visual inspection of the lungs, tissue samples are collected from suspicious sites by bronchial brush or biopsy forceps to be used for cytological and microbiological studies.
- After the procedure, the bronchoscope is removed. Patients who had local anesthesia are placed in a semi-Fowler's position to recover.

General

- Monitor the patient for complications related to the procedure (e.g., allergic reaction, anaphylaxis).
- Place tissue samples in properly labelled specimen containers containing formalin solution, and promptly transport the specimen to the laboratory for processing and analysis.

POST-TEST:

- Inform the patient that a report of the results will be made available to the requesting HCP, who will discuss the results with the patient.
- Instruct the patient to resume preoperative diet, as directed by the HCP. Assess the patient's ability to swallow before allowing the patient to attempt liquids or solid foods.
- Inform the patient that he or she may experience some throat soreness and hoarseness. Instruct patient to treat throat discomfort with lozenges and warm gargles when the gag reflex returns.
- Monitor vital signs and neurological status every 15 min for 1 hr, then every 2 hr for 4 hr, and then as ordered by the HCP. Monitor temperature every 4 hr for 24 hr. Monitor intake and output at least every 8 hr. Compare with baseline values. Notify the HCP if temperature is elevated. Discontinue prophylactic antibiotics within 24 hr after the conclusion of the procedure. Protocols may vary among facilities.
- Emergency resuscitation equipment should be readily available if the vocal cords become spastic after intubation.
- Observe/assess for delayed allergic reactions, such as rash, urticaria, tachycardia, hyperpnea, hypertension, palpitations, nausea, or vomiting.
- Observe/assess the biopsy site for bleeding, inflammation, or hematoma formation.
- Instruct the patient in the care and assessment of the biopsy site.
- Instruct the patient to report any redness, edema, bleeding, difficulty breathing, or pain at the biopsy site.
- Observe/assess the patient for hemoptysis, dyspnea, cough, air hunger, excessive coughing, pain, or absent breath sounds over the affected area. Monitor chest tube patency and drainage after a thoracotomy.
- Evaluate the patient for symptoms indicating the development of

B

pneumothorax, such as dyspnea, tachypnea, anxiety, decreased breathing sounds, or restlessness. A chest x-ray may be ordered to check for the presence of this complication.

- Evaluate the patient for symptoms of empyema, such as fever, tachycardia, malaise, or elevated white blood cell count.
- Observe/assess the patient's sputum for blood if a biopsy was taken, because large amounts of blood may indicate the development of a problem; a small amount of streaking is expected. Evaluate the patient for signs of bleeding, such as tachycardia, hypotension, or restlessness.
- Instruct the patient to remain in a semi-Fowler's position after bronchoscopy or fine-needle aspiration to maximize ventilation. Semi-Fowler's position is a semisitting position with the knees flexed and supported by pillows on the bed or examination table. Instruct the patient to stay in bed lying on the affected side for at least 2 hr with a pillow or rolled towel under the site to prevent bleeding. The patient will also need to remain on bedrest for 24 hr.
- Assess for nausea and pain. Administer antiemetic and analgesic medications as needed and as directed by the HCP.
- Administer antibiotic therapy if ordered. Remind the patient of the importance of completing the entire course of antibiotic therapy, even if signs and symptoms disappear before completion of therapy.
- Recognize anxiety related to test results. Discuss the implications of abnormal test results on the patient's lifestyle. Provide teaching and information regarding the clinical implications of the test results, as appropriate. Educate the patient regarding access to counseling services.
- Reinforce information given by the patient's HCP regarding further testing, treatment, or referral to another HCP. Instruct the patient to use lozenges or gargle for throat discomfort. Inform the patient of smoking cessation programs as appropriate. Malnutrition is commonly seen in patients with severe respiratory disease for numerous reasons, including fatigue, lack of appetite, and gastrointestinal distress. Adequate intake of vitamins A and C are also important to prevent pulmonary infection and to decrease the extent of lung tissue damage. The importance of following the prescribed diet should be stressed to the patient/caregiver. Educate the patient regarding access to counseling services, as appropriate. Answer any questions or address any concerns voiced by the patient or family.
- Instruct the patient in the use of any ordered medications. Explain the importance of adhering to the therapy regimen. As appropriate, instruct the patient in significant adverse effects associated with the prescribed medication. Encourage him or her to review corresponding literature provided by a pharmacist.
- Depending on the results of this procedure, additional testing may be performed to evaluate or monitor progression of the disease process and determine the need for a change in therapy. Evaluate test results in relation to the patient's symptoms and other tests performed.

Patient Education:

- Teach the patient the pathophysiology associated with cancer, disease, as well as ongoing treatment and screenings.
- Explain that a health-care specialist may need to be consulted to manage the disease process and therapeutic interventions.

Expected Patient Outcomes:

Understanding

- The patient and family discuss the medical versus surgical options for disease management.
- The patient and family acknowledge end-of-life treatment options as appropriate.

Ability

- The patient and family demonstrate positive coping strategies.
- The patient and family successfully demonstrate care of surgical site, biopsy site.

Response

- The patient and family agree to attend disease-specific support group meetings.
- The patient and family agree to seek psychological counseling to adjust to lifestyle changes associated with positive therapeutic management strategies.

RELATED STUDIES:

- Related tests include arterial/alveolar oxygen ratio, antibodies antiglomerular basement membrane, blood gases, bronchoscopy, chest x-ray, CBC, CT thoracic, culture sputum, cytology sputum, gallium scan, Gram/acid fast stain, lung perfusion scan, lung ventilation scan, MRI chest, mediastinoscopy, pleural fluid analysis, PFT, and TB skin tests.
- Refer to the Immune and Respiratory systems tables online at Davis*Plus* for related tests by body system.

B

Biopsy, Lymph Node

SYNONYM/ACRONYM: N/A

COMMON USE: To assist in diagnosing cancer such as lymphoma and leukemia as well as other systemic disorders.

SPECIMEN: Lymph node tissue or cells.

NORMAL FINDINGS: (Method: Macroscopic and microscopic examination of tissue) No abnormal tissue or cells.

DESCRIPTION: Lymph node biopsy is the excision of a tissue sample from one or more lymph nodes for microscopic analysis to determine cell morphology and the presence of tissue abnormalities. This test assists in confirming a diagnosis of cancer, diagnosing disorders causing systemic illness, or determining the stage of metastatic cancer. A biopsy specimen is usually obtained either by needle biopsy or after surgical incision. Biopsies are most commonly performed on the following types of lymph nodes: cervical nodes, which drain the face and scalp; axillary nodes, which drain the arms, breasts, and upper chest; and inguinal nodes, which drain the legs, external genitalia, and lower abdominal wall.

This procedure is contraindicated for

- Patients with bleeding disorders ***(related to the potential for prolonged bleeding from the biopsy site).***

INDICATIONS

- Assist in confirming suspected fungal or parasitic infections of the lymphatics.
- Assist in confirming suspected malignant involvement of the lymphatics.
- Determine the stage of metastatic cancer.

- Differentiate between benign and malignant disorders that may cause lymph node enlargement.
- Evaluate persistent enlargement of one or more lymph nodes for unknown reasons.

B

POTENTIAL MEDICAL DIAGNOSIS

Abnormal findings related to

- Chancroid
- Fungal infection (e.g., cat scratch disease)
- Immunodeficiency
- Infectious mononucleosis
- Lymph involvement of systemic diseases (e.g., systemic lupus erythematosus, sarcoidosis)
- Lymphangitis
- Lymphogranuloma venereum
- Malignancy (e.g., lymphomas, leukemias)
- Metastatic disease
- Parasitic infestation (e.g., pneumoconiosis)

CRITICAL FINDINGS:

- Assessment of clear margins after tissue excision
- Classification or grading of tumor
- Identification of malignancy

Note and immediately report to the requesting health-care provider (HCP) any critical findings and related symptoms. A listing of these findings varies among facilities. Timely notification of a critical finding for laboratory or diagnostic studies is a role expectation of the professional nurse. The notification processes vary among facilities. Upon receipt of the critical finding, the information should be read back to the caller to verify accuracy.

INTERFERING FACTORS

- Failure to follow dietary restrictions before the procedure may cause the procedure to be canceled or repeated.

NURSING IMPLICATIONS AND PROCEDURE

POTENTIAL NURSING PROBLEMS:

Problem	Signs & Symptoms	Interventions
Fear ***(related to lack of understanding of disease process and management; potential death)***	Anxiety; apprehension; stated fear; restlessness; increased tension; continuous questioning; increased blood pressure, heart rate, and respiratory rate	Evaluate both verbal and nonverbal cues of fear; assess for the cause of the fear; acknowledge the patient's awareness of his or her fear; explain all procedures in simple-to-understand, culturally and age-appropriate terms; administer ordered tranquilizer; maintain a confident, assured, professional manner in all patient interactions

Problem	Signs & Symptoms	Interventions
Inadequate coping ***(related to new disease process; fear of prognosis [death])***	Verbal expression of fear; restlessness; anxiety; withdrawal; crying; apparent emotional distress	Assess coping mechanism; support positive coping mechanism; recommend support group; provide clear, concise, appropriate information; administer ordered antianxiety medication; provide contact information for spiritual advisor; provide information related to advance directives; maintain a calm, quiet environment
Insufficient knowledge ***(related to postoperative care and treatment secondary to surgical intervention associated with cancer [leukemia, lymphoma]; related to tumor; chronic disease [lupus, sarcoidosis]; infections [cat scratch, fungal, parasitic, bacterial])***	Lack of interest or multiple questions; anxiety in relation to disease process and management; verbalization of inaccurate information	Assess the patient's understanding of the need for further treatment (radiation therapy, chemotherapy); discuss postoperative care and potential complications; review the signs and symptoms of infection, malignancy, chronic disease

PRETEST:

- Positively identify the patient using at least two person-specific identifiers before services, treatments, or procedures are performed.
- *Patient Teaching:* Inform the patient this procedure can assist in establishing a diagnosis of lymph node disease.
- Obtain a history of the patient's health concerns, symptoms, surgical procedures, and results of previously performed laboratory and diagnostic studies. Include a list of known allergens, especially allergies or sensitivities to latex and anesthetics.
- Record the date of the last menstrual period and determine the possibility of pregnancy in perimenopausal women.
- Note any recent procedures that can interfere with test results.
- Obtain a list of the patient's current medications, including over-the-counter medications, dietary supplements, anticoagulants, aspirin and other salicylates (see Effects of Natural Products on Laboratory Values online at Davis*Plus*). Such products should be discontinued by medical direction for the appropriate number of days prior to a surgical

B

procedure. Note the last time and dose of medication taken.

- Review the procedure with the patient. Inform the patient that it may be necessary to remove hair from the site before the procedure. Instruct the patient that prophylactic antibiotics may be administered before the procedure. Address concerns about pain and explain that a sedative and/or analgesia will be administered before the percutaneous biopsy to promote relaxation and reduce discomfort; general anesthesia will be administered before the open biopsy. Explain to the patient that no pain will be experienced during the test when general anesthesia is used but that any discomfort with a needle biopsy will be minimized with local anesthetics and systemic analgesics. Inform the patient that the biopsy is performed under sterile conditions by an HCP, with support staff, specializing in this procedure. The surgical procedure usually takes about 30 min to complete, and sutures may be necessary to close the site. A needle biopsy usually takes about 15 min to complete.
- ***Sensitivity to social and cultural issues,*** as well as concern for modesty, is important in providing psychological support before, during, and after the procedure.
- Explain that an intravenous line will be inserted to allow infusion of fluids such as saline, antibiotics, anesthetics, analgesics, or sedation.
- Instruct the patient that to reduce the risk of aspiration related to nausea and vomiting, solid food and milk or milk products are restricted for at least 6 hr, and clear liquids are restricted for at least 2 hr prior to general anesthesia, regional anesthesia, or sedation/analgesia (monitored anesthesia). The American Society of Anesthesiologists has fasting guidelines for risk levels according to patient status. More information can be located at www.asahq.org 🍁. Patients on beta blockers before the surgical procedure should be instructed to take their medication as ordered during the perioperative period. Protocols may vary among facilities.
- *Make sure a written and informed consent has been signed prior to the procedure and before administering any medications.*

INTRATEST:

Potential Complications:

Bleeding ***(related to a bleeding disorder, or the effects of natural products and medications with known anticoagulant, antiplatelet, or thrombolytic properties)*** or seeding of the biopsy tract with tumor cells.

- Ensure that the patient has complied with dietary restrictions prior to the study, as instructed.
- Ensure that anticoagulant therapy has been withheld for the appropriate number of days prior to the procedure. Number of days to withhold medication is dependent on the type of anticoagulant. Notify the HCP if patient anticoagulant therapy has not been withheld. Ensure that patients on beta-blocker therapy have continued their medication regimen as ordered.
- Avoid the use of equipment containing latex if the patient has a history of allergic reaction to latex.
- Have emergency equipment readily available.
- Have the patient void before the procedure.
- Observe standard precautions, and follow the general guidelines in Patient Preparation and Specimen Collection online at Davis*Plus*. Positively identify the patient, and label the appropriate specimen containers with the corresponding patient demographics, initials of the person collecting the specimen, date and time of collection, and site location.
- Assist the patient to the desired position depending on the test site to be used, and direct the patient to breathe normally during the beginning of the general anesthesia. Instruct the patient to cooperate fully and to follow directions. For the patient undergoing local anesthesia, direct him or her to breathe normally

and to avoid unnecessary movement during the procedure.

- Record baseline vital signs, and continue to monitor throughout the procedure. Protocols may vary among facilities.
- After the administration of general or local anesthesia, use clippers to remove hair from the surgical site if appropriate, cleanse the site with an antiseptic solution, and drape the area with sterile towels.

Open Biopsy

- Adhere to Surgical Care Improvement Project (SCIP) quality measures. Administer ordered prophylactic antibiotics 1 hr before incision, and use antibiotics that are consistent with current guidelines specific to the procedure.
- After administration of general anesthetics and surgical preparation are completed, an incision is made, suspicious area(s) are located, and tissue samples are collected.

Needle Biopsy

- Instruct the patient to take slow, deep breaths when the local anesthetic is injected. Protect the site with sterile drapes. The node is grasped with sterile gloved fingers, and a needle (with attached syringe) is inserted directly into the node. The node is aspirated to collect the specimen. Pressure is applied to the site for 3 to 5 min, then a sterile dressing is applied.

General

- Monitor the patient for complications related to the procedure (e.g., allergic reaction, anaphylaxis).
- Place tissue samples in formalin solution. Label the specimen, indicating site location, and promptly transport the specimen to the laboratory for processing and analysis.

POST-TEST:

- Inform the patient that a report of the results will be made available to the requesting HCP, who will discuss the results with the patient.
- Instruct the patient to resume preoperative diet, as directed by the HCP. Assess the patient's ability to swallow before allowing the patient to attempt liquids or solid foods.
- Monitor vital signs and neurological status every 15 min for 1 hr, then every 2 hr for 4 hr, and then as ordered by the HCP. Monitor temperature every 4 hr for 24 hr. Monitor intake and output at least every 8 hr. Compare with baseline values. Notify the HCP if temperature is elevated. Discontinue prophylactic antibiotics within 24 hr after the conclusion of the procedure. Protocols may vary among facilities.
- Observe/assess for delayed allergic reactions, such as rash, urticaria, tachycardia, hyperpnea, hypertension, palpitations, nausea, or vomiting.
- Observe/assess the biopsy site for bleeding, inflammation, or hematoma formation.
- Instruct the patient in the care and assessment of the site.
- Instruct the patient to report any redness, edema, bleeding, or pain at the biopsy site.
- Assess for nausea and pain. Administer antiemetic and analgesic medications as needed and as directed by the HCP.
- Administer antibiotic therapy if ordered. Remind the patient of the importance of completing the entire course of antibiotic therapy, even if signs and symptoms disappear before completion of therapy.
- Recognize anxiety related to test results. Discuss the implications of abnormal test results on the patient's lifestyle. Provide teaching and information regarding the clinical implications of the test results, as appropriate. Educate the patient regarding access to counseling services.
- Reinforce information given by the patient's HCP regarding further testing, treatment, or referral to another HCP. Inform the patient of a follow-up appointment for removal of sutures, if indicated. Answer any questions or address any concerns voiced by the patient or family.
- Instruct the patient in the use of any ordered medications. Explain the

B

importance of adhering to the therapy regimen. As appropriate, instruct the patient in significant adverse effects associated with the prescribed medication. Encourage him or her to review corresponding literature provided by a pharmacist.

- Depending on the results of this procedure, additional testing maybe performed to evaluate or monitor progression of the disease process and determine the need for a change in therapy. Evaluate test results in relation to the patient's symptoms and other tests performed.

Patient Education:

- Teach the patient the pathophysiology associated with cancer, disease, as well as ongoing treatment and screenings.
- Explain that a health-care specialist may need to be consulted to manage the disease process and therapeutic interventions.

Expected Patient Outcomes:

Understanding

- The patient and family discuss the medical versus surgical options for disease management.
- The patient and family acknowledge end-of-life treatment options as appropriate.

Ability

- The patient and family demonstrate positive coping strategies.
- The patient and family successfully demonstrate care of surgical site, biopsy site.

Response

- The patient and family agree to attend disease-specific support group meetings.
- The patient and family agree to seek psychological counseling to adjust to lifestyle changes associated with positive therapeutic management strategies.

RELATED STUDIES:

- Related tests include biopsy bone marrow, CD4/CD8 enumeration, cerebrospinal fluid analysis, *Chlamydia* serology, CBC, CT pelvis, CT thoracic, culture for bacteria/fungus, CMV, Gram stain, HIV-1/HIV-2 serology, immunofixation electrophoresis, immunoglobulins (A, G, and M), infectious mononucleosis screen, lymphangiography, mammogram, mediastinoscopy, PET pelvis, RF, total protein and fractions, toxoplasmosis serology, and US lymph nodes.
- Refer to the Immune System table online at Davis*Plus* for related tests by body system.

Biopsy, Muscle

SYNONYM/ACRONYM: N/A

COMMON USE: To assist in diagnosing muscular disease such as Duchenne's muscular dystrophy as well as other neuropathies and parasitic infections.

SPECIMEN: Muscle tissue or cells.

NORMAL FINDINGS: (Method: Macroscopic and microscopic examination of tissue) No abnormal tissue or cells.

DESCRIPTION: Muscle biopsy is the excision of a muscle tissue sample for microscopic analysis to determine cell morphology and the presence of tissue abnormalities. This test is used to confirm a diagnosis of neuropathy or myopathy and to diagnose parasitic infestation. A biopsy specimen is usually obtained from the deltoid or gastrocnemius muscle after a surgical incision.

This procedure is contraindicated for

Patients with bleeding disorders ***(related to the potential for prolonged bleeding from the biopsy site).***

INDICATIONS

- Assist in confirming suspected fungal infection or parasitic infestation of the muscle.
- Assist in diagnosing the cause of neuropathy or myopathy.
- Assist in the diagnosis of Duchenne's muscular dystrophy.

POTENTIAL MEDICAL DIAGNOSIS

Abnormal findings related to

- Alcoholic myopathy
- Amyotrophic lateral sclerosis
- Duchenne's muscular dystrophy
- Fungal infection
- Myasthenia gravis
- Myotonia congenita
- Parasitic infestation
- Polymyalgia rheumatica
- Polymyositis

CRITICAL FINDINGS:

- Assessment of clear margins after tissue excision
- Classification or grading of tumor
- Identification of malignancy

Note and immediately report to the requesting health-care provider (HCP) any critical findings and related symptoms. A listing of these findings varies among facilities. Timely notification of a critical finding for laboratory or diagnostic studies is a role expectation of the professional nurse. The notification processes vary among facilities. Upon receipt of the critical finding, the information should be read back to the caller to verify accuracy.

INTERFERING FACTORS

- If electromyography is performed before muscle biopsy, residual inflammation may lead to false-positive biopsy results.
- Failure to follow dietary restrictions before the procedure may cause the procedure to be canceled or repeated.

NURSING IMPLICATIONS AND PROCEDURE

POTENTIAL NURSING PROBLEMS:

Problem	Signs & Symptoms	Interventions
Fear ***(related to lack of understanding of disease process and management; potential death)***	Anxiety; apprehension; stated fear; restlessness; increased tension; continuous questioning; increased blood pressure, heart rate, and respiratory rate	Evaluate both verbal and nonverbal cues of fear; assess for the cause of the fear; acknowledge the patient's awareness of his or her fear; explain all procedures in simple-to-understand, culturally and age-appropriate terms; administer ordered tranquilizer; maintain a confident, assured, professional manner in all patient interactions

(table continues on page 258)

B

Problem	Signs & Symptoms	Interventions
Inadequate coping ***(related to new disease process; fear of prognosis [death]; degenerative disease progression; lifestyle changes)***	Verbal expression of fear; restlessness; anxiety; withdrawal; crying; apparent emotional distress	Assess coping mechanism; support positive coping mechanism; recommend support group; provide clear, appropriate information; administer ordered antianxiety medication; provide contact information for spiritual advisor; provide information related to advance directives; maintain a calm, quiet environment
Insufficient knowledge ***(related to infection [fungal, parasitic]; chronic disease [alcoholic effects, sclerosis, muscular dystrophy])***	Lack of interest or multiple questions; anxiety in relation to disease process and management; verbalization of inaccurate information	Assess the patient's understanding of the need for further treatment; review the signs and symptoms of infection and chronic disease progression

PRETEST:

- Positively identify the patient using at least two person-specific identifiers before services, treatments, or procedures are performed.
- *Patient Teaching:* Inform the patient this procedure can assist in establishing a diagnosis of musculoskeletal disease.
- Obtain a history of the patient's health concerns, symptoms, surgical procedures, and results of previously performed laboratory and diagnostic studies. Include a list of known allergens, especially allergies or sensitivities to latex and anesthetics.
- Record the date of the last menstrual period and determine the possibility of pregnancy in perimenopausal women.
- Note any recent procedures that can interfere with test results.
- Obtain a list of the patient's current medications, including over-the-counter medications, dietary supplements, anticoagulants, aspirin and other salicylates (see Effects of Natural Products on Laboratory Values online at Davis*Plus*). Such products should be discontinued by medical direction for the appropriate number of days prior to a surgical procedure. Note the last time and dose of medication taken.
- Review the procedure with the patient. Inform the patient that it may be necessary to remove hair from the site before the procedure. Instruct the patient that prophylactic antibiotics may be administered before the procedure. Address concerns about pain and explain that a sedative and/or analgesia will be administered before the percutaneous biopsy to promote relaxation and reduce discomfort; general anesthesia will be administered before the open biopsy. Explain to the patient that no pain will be experienced during the test when general anesthesia is used but that any discomfort with a needle biopsy will be minimized with local anesthetics and systemic analgesics. Inform the patient that the biopsy is performed under sterile

conditions by an HCP specializing in this procedure. The surgical procedure usually takes about 20 min to complete, and sutures may be necessary to close the site. A needle biopsy usually takes about 15 min to complete.

- ***Sensitivity to social and cultural issues,*** as well as concern for modesty, is important in providing psychological support before, during, and after the procedure.
- Explain that an intravenous line may be inserted to allow infusion of fluids such as saline, antibiotics, anesthetics, or sedatives.
- Instruct the patient that to reduce the risk of aspiration related to nausea and vomiting, solid food and milk or milk products are restricted for at least 6 hr, and clear liquids are restricted for at least 2 hr prior to general anesthesia, regional anesthesia, or sedation/analgesia (monitored anesthesia). The American Society of Anesthesiologists has fasting guidelines for risk levels according to patient status. More information can be located at www.asahq.org 🍁. Patients on beta blockers before the surgical procedure should be instructed to take their medication as ordered during the perioperative period. Protocols may vary among facilities.
- *Make sure a written and informed consent has been signed prior to the procedure and before administering any medications.*

INTRATEST:

Potential Complications:

Bleeding ***(related to a bleeding disorder, or the effects of natural products and medications with known anticoagulant, antiplatelet, or thrombolytic properties).***

- Ensure that the patient has complied with dietary restrictions prior to the study, as instructed.
- Ensure that anticoagulant therapy has been withheld for the appropriate number of days prior to the procedure. Number of days to withhold medication is dependent on the type of anticoagulant. Notify the HCP if patient anticoagulant therapy has not been withheld. Ensure that patients on beta-blocker therapy have continued their medication regimen as ordered.
- Avoid the use of equipment containing latex if the patient has a history of allergic reaction to latex.
- Have emergency equipment readily available.
- Have the patient void before the procedure.
- Observe standard precautions, and follow the general guidelines in Patient Preparation and Specimen Collection online at Davis*Plus*. Positively identify the patient, and label the appropriate specimen containers with the corresponding patient demographics, initials of the person collecting the specimen, date and time of collection, and site location.
- Assist the patient to a comfortable position: a supine position (for deltoid biopsy) or prone position (for gastrocnemius biopsy). Instruct the patient to cooperate fully and to follow directions. Direct the patient to breathe normally and to avoid unnecessary movement during the local anesthetic and the procedure.
- Record baseline vital signs, and continue to monitor throughout the procedure. Protocols may vary among facilities.
- After the administration of general or local anesthetics, use clippers to remove hair from the surgical site if appropriate, cleanse the site with an antiseptic solution, and drape the area with sterile towels.

Open Biopsy

- Adhere to Surgical Care Improvement Project (SCIP) quality measures. Administer ordered prophylactic antibiotics 1 hr before incision, and use antibiotics that are consistent with current guidelines specific to the procedure.
- After administration of general anesthetics and surgical preparation are completed, an incision is made,

suspicious areas are located, and tissue samples are collected.

Needle Biopsy

- Instruct the patient to take slow deep breaths when the local anesthetic is injected. Protect the site with sterile drapes.
- After infiltration of the site with local anesthetic, a cutting biopsy needle is introduced through a small skin incision and bored into the muscle. A core needle is introduced through the cutting needle, and a plug of muscle is removed. The needles are withdrawn, and the specimen is placed in a preservative solution. Pressure is applied to the site for 3 to 5 min, and then a pressure dressing is applied.

General

- Monitor the patient for complications related to the procedure (e.g., allergic reaction, anaphylaxis).
- Place tissue samples in properly labelled specimen container containing formalin solution, and promptly transport the specimen to the laboratory for processing and analysis.

POST-TEST:

- Inform the patient that a report of the results will be made available to the requesting HCP, who will discuss the results with the patient.
- Instruct the patient to resume preoperative diet, as directed by the HCP.
- Monitor vital signs and neurological status every 15 min for 1 hr, then every 2 hr for 4 hr, and then as ordered by the HCP. Monitor temperature every 4 hr for 24 hr. Compare with baseline values. Notify the HCP if temperature is elevated. Discontinue prophylactic antibiotics within 24 hr after the conclusion of the procedure. Protocols may vary among facilities.
- Observe/assess for delayed allergic reactions, such as rash, urticaria, tachycardia, hyperpnea, hypertension, palpitations, nausea, or vomiting.
- Observe/assess the biopsy site for bleeding, inflammation, or hematoma formation.
- Instruct the patient in the care and assessment of the site.
- Instruct the patient to report any redness, edema, bleeding, or pain at the biopsy site.
- Assess for nausea and pain. Administer antiemetic and analgesic medications as needed and as directed by the HCP.
- Administer antibiotic therapy if ordered. Remind the patient of the importance of completing the entire course of antibiotic therapy, even if signs and symptoms disappear before completion of therapy.
- Recognize anxiety related to test results. Discuss the implications of abnormal test results on the patient's lifestyle. Provide teaching and information regarding the clinical implications of the test results, as appropriate. Educate the patient regarding access to counseling services.
- Reinforce information given by the patient's HCP regarding further testing, treatment, or referral to another HCP. Inform the patient of a follow-up appointment for removal of sutures, if indicated. Answer any questions or address any concerns voiced by the patient or family.
- Instruct the patient in the use of any ordered medications. Explain the importance of adhering to the therapy regimen. As appropriate, instruct the patient in significant adverse effects associated with the prescribed medication. Encourage him or her to review corresponding literature provided by a pharmacist.
- Depending on the results of this procedure, additional testing may be performed to evaluate or monitor progression of the disease process and determine the need for a change in therapy. Evaluate test results in relation to the patient's symptoms and other tests performed.

Patient Education:

- Teach the patient the pathophysiology associated with cancer, disease

as well as ongoing treatment and screenings.
- Explain that a health-care specialist may need to be consulted to manage the disease process and therapeutic interventions.

Expected Patient Outcomes:

Understanding
- The patient and family discuss the medical versus surgical options for disease management.
- The patient and family acknowledge end-of-life treatment options as appropriate.

Ability
- The patient and family demonstrate positive coping strategies.
- The patient and family successfully demonstrate care of surgical site, biopsy site.

Response
- The patient and family agree to attend disease-specific support group meetings.
- The patient and family agree to seek psychological counseling to adjust to lifestyle changes associated with positive therapeutic management strategies.

RELATED STUDIES:
- Related tests include acetylcholinesterase receptor antibody, aldolase, antinuclear antibody (ANA), antibody Jo-1, antithyroglobulin antibodies, CK and isoenzymes, EMG, ENG, myoglobin, and RF.
- Refer to the Immune and Musculoskeletal systems tables online at Davis*Plus* for related tests by body system.

B

Biopsy, Prostate

SYNONYM/ACRONYM: N/A

COMMON USE: To assist in diagnosing prostate cancer.

SPECIMEN: Prostate tissue.

NORMAL FINDINGS: (Method: Microscopic examination of tissue cells) No abnormal cells or tissue.

DESCRIPTION: Biopsy of the prostate gland is performed to identify cancerous cells, especially if serum prostate-specific antigen (PSA) is increased. New technology makes it possible to combine data such as analysis of molecular biomarkers and cellular structure specific to the individual's biopsy tissue, standard tissue biopsy results, Gleason's score, number of positive tumor cores, tumor stage, presurgical and postsurgical PSA levels, and postsurgical margin status with computerized mathematical programs to create a personalized report that predicts the likelihood of post-prostatectomy disease progression. Serial measurements of PSA in the blood are often performed before and after surgery. Approximately 15% to 40% of patients who have had their prostate removed will encounter an increase in PSA. Patients treated for prostate cancer and who have had a PSA recurrence can still develop a metastasis as much as 8 yr after the post-surgical PSA level increased. The majority of tumors develop slowly and require minimal intervention, but patients with an increase in PSA greater than 2 ng/mL in a year are more likely to have an aggressive form of prostate cancer with a greater risk of death. The Prostate Health Index (PHI) is another multi-marker strategy used to improve the positive prediction rate of prostate cancer, especially when PSA levels are considered to be moderately increased (between 4–10 ng/mL). The PHI applies information provided by the results of prostate marker blood tests to a mathematical formula and offers additional information for clinical decision making. The three tests used in the formula are the total PSA, free PSA, and p2PSA (an isoform of PSA, where PHI = p2PSA/[free PSA × total PSA]). Personalized medicine provides a technology to predict the progression of prostate cancer, likelihood of recurrence, or development of related metastatic disease. New technology makes it possible to combine data such as analysis of molecular biomarkers and cellular structure specific to the individual's biopsy tissue, standard tissue biopsy results, Gleason score, number of positive tumor cores, tumor stage, presurgical and postsurgical PSA levels, and postsurgical margin status with computerized mathematical programs to create a personalized report that predicts the likelihood of post-prostatectomy disease progression.

This procedure is contraindicated for

Patients with bleeding disorders ***(related to the potential for prolonged bleeding from the biopsy site).***

INDICATIONS

- Evaluate prostatic hyperplasia of unknown etiology.
- Investigate suspected cancer of the prostate.

POTENTIAL MEDICAL DIAGNOSIS

Positive findings in prostate cancer

CRITICAL FINDINGS:

- Assessment of clear margins after tissue excision
- Classification or grading of tumor
- Identification of malignancy

Note and immediately report to the requesting health-care provider (HCP) any critical findings and related symptoms. A listing of these findings varies among facilities. Timely notification of a critical finding for laboratory or diagnostic studies is a role expectation of the professional nurse. The notification processes vary among facilities. Upon receipt of the critical finding, the information should be read back to the caller to verify accuracy.

INTERFERING FACTORS

- Failure to follow dietary restrictions before the procedure may cause the procedure to be canceled or repeated.
- The various sampling approaches have individual drawbacks that should be considered: Transurethral sampling does not always ensure that malignant cells will be included in the specimen, whereas transrectal sampling carries the risk of perforating the rectum and creating a channel through which malignant cells can seed normal tissue.

NURSING IMPLICATIONS AND PROCEDURE

POTENTIAL NURSING PROBLEMS:

Problem	Signs & Symptoms	Interventions
Fear ***(related to lack of understanding of disease process and management; potential death)***	Anxiety; apprehension; stated fear; restlessness; increased tension; continuous questioning; increased blood pressure, heart rate, and respiratory rate	Evaluate both verbal and nonverbal cues of fear; assess for the cause of the fear; acknowledge the patient's awareness of his fear; explain all procedures in simple-to-understand, culturally and age-appropriate terms; administer ordered tranquilizer; maintain a confident, assured, professional manner in all patient interactions
Inadequate coping ***(related to new disease process; fear of prognosis [death]; sexuality changes)***	Verbal expression of fear; restlessness; anxiety; withdrawal; crying; apparent emotional distress	Assess coping mechanism; support positive coping mechanism; recommend support group; provide clear, concise, appropriate information; administer ordered antianxiety medication; provide contact information for spiritual advisor; provide information related to advance directives; maintain a calm quiet environment
Insufficient knowledge ***(related to postoperative care and treatment secondary to surgical intervention associated with cancer, tumor)***	Lack of interest or multiple questions; anxiety in relation to disease process and management; verbalization of inaccurate information	Assess the patient's understanding of the need for further treatment (radiation therapy, chemotherapy); discuss postoperative care and potential complications; review the signs and symptoms of infection; discuss the possibility of postoperative self-image dysfunction due to changes in sexual function

B

PRETEST:

- Positively identify the patient using at least two person-specific identifiers before services, treatments, or procedures are performed.
- ***Patient Teaching:*** Inform the patient this procedure can assist in establishing a diagnosis of prostate disease.
- Obtain a history of the patient's health concerns, symptoms, surgical procedures, and results of previously performed laboratory and diagnostic studies. Include a list of known allergens, especially allergies or sensitivities to latex and anesthetics.
- Note any recent procedures that can interfere with test results.
- Obtain a list of the patient's current medications, including over-the-counter medications, dietary supplements, anticoagulants, aspirin and other salicylates (see Effects of Natural Products on Laboratory Values online at Davis*Plus*). Such products should be discontinued by medical direction for the appropriate number of days prior to a surgical procedure. Note the last time and dose of medication taken.
- Review the procedure with the patient. Inform the patient that it may be necessary to remove hair from the site before the procedure. Instruct the patient that prophylactic antibiotics may be administered before the procedure. Address concerns about pain and explain that a sedative and/or analgesia will be administered to promote relaxation and reduce discomfort before the percutaneous biopsy; general anesthesia will be administered before the open biopsy. Explain to the patient that no pain will be experienced during the test when general anesthesia is used but that any discomfort with a needle biopsy will be minimized with local anesthetics and systemic analgesics. Inform the patient that the biopsy is performed under sterile conditions by an HCP, with support staff, specializing in this procedure. The surgical procedure usually takes about 30 min to complete, and sutures may be necessary to close the site. A needle biopsy usually takes about 20 min to complete. Instructions regarding the appropriate transport container for molecular diagnostic studies should be obtained from the laboratory prior to the procedure.
- ***Sensitivity to social and cultural issues,*** as well as concern for modesty, is important in providing psychological support before, during, and after the procedure.
- Explain that an intravenous line will be inserted to allow infusion of fluids such as saline, antibiotics, anesthetics, and analgesics.
- Instruct the patient that to reduce the risk of aspiration related to nausea and vomiting, solid food and milk or milk products are restricted for at least 6 hr, and clear liquids are restricted for at least 2 hr prior to general anesthesia, regional anesthesia, or sedation/analgesia (monitored anesthesia). The American Society of Anesthesiologists has fasting guidelines for risk levels according to patient status. More information can be located at www.asahq.org 🍁. Patients on beta blockers before the surgical procedure should be instructed to take their medication as ordered during the perioperative period. Protocols may vary among facilities.
- *Make sure a written and informed consent has been signed prior to the procedure and before administering any medications.*

INTRATEST:

Potential Complications:

Bleeding ***(related to a bleeding disorder, or the effects of natural products and medications with known anticoagulant, antiplatelet, or thrombolytic properties)*** or seeding of the biopsy tract with tumor cells.

- Ensure that the patient has complied with dietary restrictions prior to the study, as instructed.
- Ensure that anticoagulant therapy has been withheld for the appropriate number of days before the procedure. The number of days to withhold medication depends on the type

of anticoagulant. Notify the HCP if patient anticoagulant therapy has not been withheld. Ensure that patients on beta-blocker therapy have continued their medication regimen as ordered.

- Avoid the use of equipment containing latex if the patient has a history of allergic reaction to latex.
- Have emergency equipment readily available.
- Have the patient void before the procedure. Administer enemas if ordered.
- Observe standard precautions, and follow the general guidelines in Patient Preparation and Specimen Collection online at Davis*Plus*. Positively identify the patient, and label the appropriate specimen containers with the corresponding patient demographics, initials of the person collecting the specimen, date and time of collection, and site location.
- Assist the patient to a comfortable position, and direct the patient to breathe normally during the beginning of the general anesthesia.
- Cleanse the biopsy site with an antiseptic solution, use clippers to remove hair from the surgical site if appropriate, and drape the area with sterile towels.
- Record baseline vital signs, and continue to monitor throughout the procedure. Protocols may vary among facilities.

Transurethral Approach

- After administration of the general anesthetic, position the patient on a urological examination table with the feet in stirrups. The endoscope is inserted into the urethra. The tissue is excised with a cutting loop and is placed in formalin solution.

Transrectal Approach

- Adhere to Surgical Care Improvement Project (SCIP) quality measures. Administer ordered prophylactic antibiotics 1 hr before incision, and use antibiotics that are consistent with current guidelines specific to the procedure.
- After administration of the general anesthetic, position the patient in the Sims' position (left lateral). A rectal examination is performed to locate suspicious nodules. A biopsy needle guide is placed at the biopsy site, and the biopsy needle is inserted through the needle guide. The cells are aspirated, the needle is withdrawn, and the sample is placed in formalin solution.

Perineal Approach

- Adhere to Surgical Care Improvement Project (SCIP) quality measures. Administer ordered prophylactic antibiotics 1 hr before incision, and use antibiotics that are consistent with current guidelines specific to the procedure.
- After administration of the general anesthetic, position the patient in the lithotomy position. Clean the perineum with an antiseptic solution, and protect the biopsy site with sterile drapes. A small incision is made, and the sample is removed by needle biopsy or biopsy punch and placed in formalin solution.

General

- Monitor the patient for complications related to the procedure (e.g., allergic reaction, anaphylaxis).
- Apply digital pressure to the biopsy site. If there is no bleeding after the perineal approach, place a sterile dressing on the biopsy site. Immediately notify the HCP if there is significant bleeding.
- Place tissue samples for standard biopsy examination in properly labelled specimen containers containing formalin solution, place tissue samples for molecular diagnostic studies in properly labelled specimen containers, and promptly transport the specimen to the laboratory for processing and analysis.

POST-TEST:

- Inform the patient that a report of the results will be made available to the requesting HCP, who will discuss the results with the patient.
- Instruct the patient to resume preoperative diet, as directed by the HCP. Assess the patient's ability to swallow

B

before allowing the patient to attempt liquids or solid foods.

- *Nutritional Considerations:* There is growing evidence that inflammation and oxidation play key roles in the development of numerous diseases, including prostate cancer. Research also shows that diets containing dried beans, fresh fruits and vegetables, nuts, spices, whole grains, and smaller amounts of red meats can increase the amount of protective antioxidants. Regular exercise, especially in combination with a healthy diet, can bring about changes in the body's metabolism that decrease inflammation and oxidation.
- Monitor vital signs and neurological status every 15 min for 1 hr, then every 2 hr for 4 hr, and then as ordered by the HCP. Monitor temperature every 4 hr for 24 hr. Monitor intake and output at least every 8 hr. Compare with baseline values. Notify the HCP if temperature is elevated. Discontinue prophylactic antibiotics within 24 hr after the conclusion of the procedure. Protocols may vary among facilities.
- Instruct the patient on intake and output recording and provide appropriate measuring containers.
- Encourage fluid intake of 3,000 mL unless contraindicated.
- Observe/assess for delayed allergic reactions, such as rash, urticaria, tachycardia, hyperpnea, hypertension, palpitations, nausea, or vomiting.
- Instruct the patient in the care and assessment of the site.
- Instruct the patient to report any chills, fever, redness, edema, bleeding, or pain at the biopsy site.
- Assess for infection, hemorrhage, or perforation of the urethra or rectum.
- Inform the patient that blood may be seen in the urine after the first or second postprocedural voiding.
- Instruct the patient to report any further changes in urinary pattern, volume, or appearance.
- Assess for nausea, pain, and bladder spasms. Administer antiemetic, analgesic, and antispasmodic medications as needed and as directed by the HCP.
- Administer antibiotic therapy if ordered. Remind the patient of the importance of completing the entire course of antibiotic therapy, even if signs and symptoms disappear before completion of therapy.
- Recognize anxiety related to test results. Discuss the implications of abnormal test results on the patient's lifestyle. Provide teaching and information regarding the clinical implications of the test results, as appropriate. Educate the patient regarding access to counseling services. Provide contact information, if desired, for the Prostate Cancer Foundation (www.prostatecancerfoundation.org) 🍁.
- Reinforce information given by the patient's HCP regarding further testing, treatment, or referral to another HCP. Decisions regarding the need for and frequency of routine PSA testing or other cancer screening procedures should be made after consultation between the patient and HCP. Recommendations made by various medical associations and national health organizations regarding prostate cancer screening are moving away from routine PSA screening and toward informed decision making. The American Cancer Society's (ACS) guidelines recommend that discussions about screening should begin at age 50 yr for men at average risk, 45 yr for men at high risk, and 40 yr for men at the highest risk of developing prostate cancer. 🍁 The most current guidelines for prostate cancer screening of the general population as well as of individuals with increased risk are available from the ACS (www.cancer.org) and the American Urological Association (www.aua.org). 🍁 Counsel the patient, as appropriate, that sexual dysfunction related to altered body function, drugs, or radiation may occur. Answer any questions or address any concerns voiced by the patient or family.
- Instruct the patient in the use of any ordered medications. Explain the

importance of adhering to the therapy regimen. As appropriate, instruct the patient in significant adverse effects associated with the prescribed medication. Encourage him to review corresponding literature provided by a pharmacist.

- Depending on the results of this procedure, additional testing may be performed to evaluate or monitor progression of the disease process and determine the need for a change in therapy. Evaluate test results in relation to the patient's symptoms and other tests performed.

Patient Education:

- Teach the patient the pathophysiology associated with cancer, disease, as well as ongoing treatment and screenings.
- Explain that a health-care specialist may need to be consulted to manage the disease process and therapeutic interventions.

Understanding

- The patient and family discuss the medical versus surgical options for disease management.
- The patient and family acknowledge end-of-life treatment options as appropriate.

Ability

- The patient and family demonstrate positive coping strategies.
- The patient and family successfully demonstrate care of surgical site, biopsy site.

Response

- The patient and family agree to attend disease-specific support group meetings.
- The patient and family agree to seek psychological counseling to adjust to lifestyle changes associated with positive therapeutic management strategies.

RELATED STUDIES:

- Related tests include cystoscopy, cystourethrography voiding, PSA, retrograde ureteropyelography, semen analysis, and US prostate.
- Refer to the Genitourinary System table online at Davis*Plus* for related tests by body system.

Biopsy, Skin

SYNONYM/ACRONYM: N/A

COMMON USE: To assist in diagnosing skin cancer.

SPECIMEN: Skin tissue or cells.

NORMAL FINDINGS: (Method: Macroscopic and microscopic examination of tissue) No abnormal tissue or cells.

DESCRIPTION: Skin biopsy is the excision of a tissue sample from suspicious skin lesions. The microscopic analysis can determine cell morphology and the presence of tissue abnormalities. This test assists in confirming the diagnosis of malignant or benign skin lesions. A skin biopsy can be obtained by any of these four methods: curettage, shaving, excision, or punch. A Tzanck smear may be prepared from vesicles (blisters) present on the skin. Skin cells in the vesicles can be evaluated microscopically to indicate the presence of certain viruses, especially herpes, that cause cells to become enlarged and otherwise abnormal in appearance.

This procedure is contraindicated for

- Patients with bleeding disorders ***(related to the potential for prolonged bleeding from the biopsy site).***

INDICATIONS

- Assist in the diagnosis of keratoses, warts, moles, keloids, fibromas, cysts, or inflamed lesions.
- Assist in the diagnosis of inflammatory process of the skin, especially herpes infection.
- Assist in the diagnosis of skin cancer.
- Evaluate suspicious skin lesions.

POTENTIAL MEDICAL DIAGNOSIS

Abnormal findings related to

- Basal cell carcinoma
- Cysts
- Dermatitis
- Dermatofibroma
- Keloids
- Malignant melanoma
- Neurofibroma
- Pemphigus
- Pigmented nevi
- Seborrheic keratosis
- Skin involvement in systemic lupus erythematosus, discoid lupus erythematosus, and scleroderma
- Squamous cell carcinoma
- Viral infection (herpes, varicella)
- Warts

CRITICAL FINDINGS:

- Assessment of clear margins after tissue excision
- Classification or grading of tumor
- Identification of malignancy

Note and immediately report to the requesting health-care provider (HCP) any critical findings and related symptoms. A listing of these findings varies among facilities. Timely notification of a critical finding for laboratory or diagnostic studies is a role expectation of the professional nurse. The notification processes vary among facilities. Upon receipt of the critical finding, the information should be read back to the caller to verify accuracy.

INTERFERING FACTORS

- Failure to follow dietary restrictions before the procedure may cause the procedure to be canceled or repeated.

NURSING IMPLICATIONS AND PROCEDURE

PRETEST:

- Positively identify the patient using at least two person-specific identifiers before services, treatments, or procedures are performed.
- ***Patient Teaching:*** Inform the patient this procedure can assist in establishing a diagnosis of skin disease.
- Obtain a history of the patient's health concerns, symptoms, surgical procedures, and results of previously performed laboratory and diagnostic studies. Include a list of known allergens, especially allergies or sensitivities to latex and anesthetics.
- Record the date of the last menstrual period and determine the possibility of pregnancy in perimenopausal women.
- Note any recent procedures that can interfere with test results.
- Obtain a list of the patient's current medications, including over-the-counter medications, dietary supplements, anticoagulants, aspirin and other salicylates (see Effects of Natural Products on Laboratory Values online at Davis*Plus*). Such products should be discontinued by medical direction for the appropriate number of days prior to a surgical procedure. Note the last time and dose of medication taken.

- Review the procedure with the patient. Inform the patient that it may be necessary to remove hair from the site before the procedure. Instruct that prophylactic antibiotics may be administered before the procedure. Address concerns about pain and explain that a sedative and/or analgesia will be administered before the punch biopsy to promote relaxation and reduce discomfort. Explain that any discomfort will be minimized with local anesthetics and systemic analgesics. Inform the patient the biopsy is performed under sterile conditions by an HCP, with support staff, specializing in this procedure. The procedure usually takes about 20 min to complete, and sutures may be necessary to close the site.
- ***Sensitivity to social and cultural issues,*** as well as concern for modesty, is important in providing psychological support before, during, and after the procedure.
- Explain that an intravenous line may be inserted to allow infusion of fluids such as saline, anesthetics, or sedatives, depending on the type of biopsy.
- Note that there are no food, fluid, or medication restrictions unless by medical direction.
- *Make sure a written and informed consent has been signed prior to the procedure and before administering any medications.*

INTRATEST:

Potential Complications:

Bleeding ***(related to a bleeding disorder, or the effects of natural products and medications with known anticoagulant, antiplatelet, or thrombolytic properties)*** or seeding of the biopsy tract with tumor cells.

- Ensure that anticoagulant therapy has been withheld for the appropriate number of days prior to the procedure. Number of days to withhold medication is dependent on the type of anticoagulant. Notify the HCP if patient anticoagulant therapy has not been withheld.
- Avoid the use of equipment containing latex if the patient has a history of allergic reaction to latex.
- Have emergency equipment readily available.
- Have the patient void before the procedure.
- Observe standard precautions, and follow the general guidelines in Patient Preparation and Specimen Collection online at Davis*Plus*. Positively identify the patient, and label the appropriate specimen containers with the corresponding patient demographics, initials of the person collecting the specimen, date and time of collection, and site location.
- Assist the patient to the desired position depending on the test site to be used, and direct the patient to breathe normally during administration of the local anesthetic and the procedure. Instruct the patient to cooperate fully, follow directions, and avoid unnecessary movement.
- Record baseline vital signs, and continue to monitor throughout the procedure. Protocols may vary among facilities.
- After administration of the local anesthetic, use clippers to remove hair from the site if appropriate, cleanse the site with an antiseptic solution, and drape the area with sterile towels.

Curettage

- The skin is scraped with a curette to obtain specimen.

Shaving or Excision

- A scalpel is used to remove a portion of the lesion that protrudes above the epidermis. If the lesion is to be excised, the incision is made as wide and as deep as needed to ensure that the entire lesion is removed. Bleeding is controlled with external pressure to the site. Large wounds are closed with sutures. An adhesive bandage is applied when excision is complete.

Punch Biopsy

- A small, round punch about 4 to 6 mm in diameter is rotated into the skin to the desired depth. The cylinder of skin is pulled upward with

B

forceps and separated at its base with a scalpel or scissors. If needed, sutures are applied. A sterile dressing is applied over the site.
- Monitor the patient for complications related to the procedure (e.g., allergic reaction, anaphylaxis).
- Place tissue samples in properly labelled specimen container containing formalin solution, and promptly transport the specimen to the laboratory for processing and analysis.

POST-TEST:

- Inform the patient that a report of the results will be made available to the requesting HCP, who will discuss the results with the patient.
- Monitor vital signs and neurological status every 15 min for 1 hr, then every 2 hr for 4 hr, and then as ordered by the HCP. Monitor temperature every 4 hr for 24 hr. Compare with baseline values. Notify the HCP if temperature is elevated. Protocols may vary among facilities.
- Observe/assess for delayed allergic reactions, such as rash, urticaria, tachycardia, hyperpnea, hypertension, palpitations, nausea, or vomiting.
- Observe/assess the biopsy site for bleeding, inflammation, or hematoma formation.
- Instruct the patient in the care and assessment of the site.
- Instruct the patient to report any redness, edema, bleeding, or pain at the biopsy site.
- Assess for nausea and pain. Administer antiemetic and analgesic medications as needed and as directed by the HCP.
- Administer antibiotic therapy if ordered. Remind the patient of the importance of completing the entire course of antibiotic therapy, even if signs and symptoms disappear before completion of therapy.
- Recognize anxiety related to test results. Discuss the implications of abnormal test results on the patient's lifestyle. Provide teaching and information regarding the clinical implications of the test results, as appropriate. Provide contact information, if desired, for the American Cancer Society (www.cancer.org) 🍁. Educate the patient regarding access to counseling services.
- Reinforce information given by the patient's HCP regarding further testing, treatment, or referral to another HCP. Inform the patient of a follow-up appointment for the removal of sutures, if indicated. Answer any questions or address any concerns voiced by the patient or family.
- Instruct the patient in the use of any ordered medications. Explain the importance of adhering to the therapy regimen. As appropriate, instruct the patient in significant adverse effects associated with the prescribed medication. Encourage him or her to review corresponding literature provided by a pharmacist.
- Depending on the results of this procedure, additional testing may be performed to evaluate or monitor progression of the disease process and determine the need for a change in therapy. DNA testing for mutations in the CDKN2A, CDK4, or BRAF V600 genes may be requested to identify those at high risk for developing cutaneous melanoma. The test for TA90 (melanoma-associated antigen) is used to evaluate the status of postoperative patients who have had localized areas of melanoma removed. Methods for these genetic markers include microarray, reverse transcriptase polymerase chain reaction (RT-PCR), and enzyme—linked immunosorbent assay (ELISA). Evaluate test results in relation to the patient's symptoms and other tests performed.

RELATED STUDIES:

- Related tests include allergen-specific IgE, ANA, culture skin, eosinophil count, ESR, genetic testing, and IgE.
- Refer to the Immune and Musculoskeletal systems tables online at Davis*Plus* for related tests by body system.

Biopsy, Thyroid

SYNONYM/ACRONYM: N/A

COMMON USE: To assist in diagnosing thyroid cancer.

SPECIMEN: Thyroid gland tissue or cells.

NORMAL FINDINGS: (Method: Macroscopic and microscopic examination of tissue) No abnormal tissue or cells.

DESCRIPTION: Thyroid biopsy is the excision of a tissue sample for microscopic analysis to determine cell morphology and the presence of tissue abnormalities. This test assists in confirming a diagnosis of cancer or determining the cause of persistent thyroid symptoms. A biopsy specimen can be obtained by needle aspiration or by surgical excision.

This procedure is contraindicated for

Patients with bleeding disorders ***(related to the potential for prolonged bleeding from the biopsy site).***

INDICATIONS

- Assist in the diagnosis of thyroid cancer or benign cysts or tumors.
- Determine the cause of inflammatory thyroid disease.
- Determine the cause of hyperthyroidism.
- Evaluate enlargement of the thyroid gland.

POTENTIAL MEDICAL DIAGNOSIS

Positive Findings in

- Benign thyroid cyst
- Granulomatous thyroiditis
- Hashimoto's thyroiditis
- Nontoxic nodular goiter
- Thyroid cancer

CRITICAL FINDINGS:

- Assessment of clear margins after tissue excision
- Classification or grading of tumor
- Identification of malignancy

Note and immediately report to the requesting health-care provider (HCP) any critical findings and related symptoms. A listing of these findings varies among facilities. Timely notification of a critical finding for laboratory or diagnostic studies is a role expectation of the professional nurse. The notification processes vary among facilities. Upon receipt of the critical finding, the information should be read back to the caller to verify accuracy.

INTERFERING FACTORS

- Failure to follow dietary restrictions before the procedure may cause the procedure to be canceled or repeated.

NURSING IMPLICATIONS AND PROCEDURE

PRETEST:

- Positively identify the patient using at least two person-specific identifiers before services, treatments, or procedures are performed.
- *Patient Teaching:* Inform the patient this procedure can assist in establishing a diagnosis of thyroid disease.
- Obtain a history of the patient's health concerns, symptoms, surgical

procedures, and results of previously performed laboratory and diagnostic studies. Include a list of known allergens, especially allergies or sensitivities to latex.

B

- Record the date of the last menstrual period and determine possibility of pregnancy in perimenopausal women.
- Note any recent procedures that can interfere with test results.
- Obtain a list of the patient's current medications, including over-the-counter medications, dietary supplements, anticoagulants, aspirin and other salicylates (see Effects of Natural Products on Laboratory Values online at Davis*Plus*). Such products should be discontinued by medical direction for the appropriate number of days prior to a surgical procedure. Note the last time and dose of medication taken.
- Review the procedure with the patient. Inform the patient that it may be necessary to remove hair from the site before the procedure. Instruct the patient that prophylactic antibiotics may be administered before the procedure. Address concerns about pain and explain that a sedative and/or analgesia will be administered before the percutaneous biopsy to promote relaxation and reduce discomfort; general anesthesia will be administered before the open biopsy. Explain to the patient that no pain will be experienced during the test when general anesthesia is used but that any discomfort with a needle biopsy will be minimized with local anesthetics and systemic analgesics. Inform the patient that the biopsy is performed under sterile conditions by an HCP, with support staff, specializing in this procedure. The surgical procedure usually takes about 30 min to complete, and sutures may be necessary to close the site. A needle biopsy usually takes about 15 min to complete.
- ***Sensitivity to social and cultural issues,*** as well as concern for modesty, is important in providing psychological support before, during, and after the procedure.
- Explain that an intravenous line will be inserted to allow infusion of fluids such as saline, antibiotics, anesthetics, analgesics, or sedation.
- Instruct the patient that to reduce the risk of aspiration related to nausea and vomiting, solid food and milk or milk products are restricted for at least 6 hr, and clear liquids are restricted for at least 2 hr prior to general anesthesia, regional anesthesia, or sedation/analgesia (monitored anesthesia). The American Society of Anesthesiologists has fasting guidelines for risk levels according to patient status. More information can be located at www.asahq.org 🍁. Patients on beta blockers before the surgical procedure should be instructed to take their medication as ordered during the perioperative period. Protocols may vary among facilities.
- Have the patient void before the procedure.
- *Make sure a written and informed consent has been signed prior to the procedure and before administering any medications.*

INTRATEST:

Potential Complications:

Bleeding ***(related to a bleeding disorder, or the effects of natural products and medications with known anticoagulant, antiplatelet, or thrombolytic properties)*** or seeding of the biopsy tract with tumor cells.

- Ensure that the patient has complied with dietary restrictions prior to the study, as instructed.
- Ensure that anticoagulant therapy has been withheld for the appropriate number of days prior to the procedure. Number of days to withhold medication is dependent on the type of anticoagulant. Notify HCP if patient anticoagulant therapy has not been withheld. Ensure that patients on beta-blocker therapy have continued their medication regimen as ordered.

- Avoid the use of equipment containing latex if the patient has a history of allergic reaction to latex.
- Have emergency equipment readily available.
- Observe standard precautions, and follow the general guidelines in Patient Preparation and Specimen Collection online at Davis*Plus*. Positively identify the patient, and label the appropriate specimen containers with the corresponding patient demographics, initials of the person collecting the specimen, date and time of collection, and site location.
- Assist the patient to the desired position depending on the test site to be used, and direct the patient to breathe normally during the beginning of the general anesthetic. Instruct the patient to cooperate fully and to follow directions. For the patient undergoing local anesthesia, direct him or her to breathe normally and to avoid unnecessary movement during the procedure.
- Record baseline vital signs and continue to monitor throughout the procedure. Protocols may vary among facilities.
- After the administration of general or local anesthetics, use clippers to remove hair from the surgical site if appropriate, cleanse the site with an antiseptic solution, and drape the area with sterile towels.

Open Biopsy

- Adhere to Surgical Care Improvement Project (SCIP) quality measures. Administer ordered prophylactic antibiotics 1 hr before incision, use antibiotics that are consistent with current guidelines specific to the procedure.
- After administration of the general anesthetic and surgical preparation is completed, an incision is made, suspicious area(s) are located, and tissue samples are collected.

Needle Biopsy

- Instruct the patient to take slow, deep breaths when the local anesthetic is injected. Protect the site with sterile drapes. Instruct the patient to take a deep breath, exhale forcefully, and hold the breath while the biopsy needle is inserted and rotated to obtain a core of thyroid tissue. Once the needle is removed, the patient may breathe. Pressure is applied to the site for 3 to 5 min, then a sterile pressure dressing is applied.

General

- Monitor the patient for complications related to the procedure (e.g., allergic reaction, anaphylaxis).
- Place tissue samples in properly labelled specimen container containing formalin solution, and promptly transport the specimen to the laboratory for processing and analysis.

POST-TEST:

- Inform the patient that a report of the results will be made available to the requesting HCP, who will discuss the results with the patient.
- Instruct the patient to resume preoperative diet, as directed by the HCP. Assess the patient's ability to swallow before allowing the patient to attempt liquids or solid foods.
- Monitor vital signs and neurological status every 15 min for 1 hr, then every 2 hr for 4 hr, and then as ordered by the HCP. Monitor temperature every 4 hr for 24 hr. Monitor intake and output at least every 8 hr. Compare with baseline values. Notify the HCP if temperature is elevated. Discontinue prophylactic antibiotics within 24 hr after the conclusion of the procedure. Protocols may vary among facilities.
- Observe/assess for delayed allergic reactions, such as rash, urticaria, tachycardia, hyperpnea, hypertension, palpitations, nausea, or vomiting.
- Observe/assess the biopsy site for bleeding, inflammation, or hematoma formation.
- Instruct the patient in the care and assessment of the site.

B

- Instruct the patient to report any redness, edema, bleeding, or pain at the biopsy site.
- Assess for nausea and pain. Administer antiemetic and analgesic medications as needed and as directed by the HCP.
- Administer antibiotic therapy if ordered. Remind the patient of the importance of completing the entire course of antibiotic therapy, even if signs and symptoms disappear before completion of therapy.
- Recognize anxiety related to test. Discuss the implications of the abnormal test results on the patient's lifestyle. Provide teaching and information regarding the clinical implications of the test results, as appropriate. Educate the patient regarding access to counseling services.
- Reinforce information given by the patient's HCP regarding further testing, treatment, or referral to another HCP. Inform the patient of a follow-up appointment for removal of sutures, if indicated. Answer any questions or address any concerns voiced by the patient or family.
- Instruct the patient in the use of any ordered medications. Explain the importance of adhering to the therapy regimen. As appropriate, instruct the patient in significant adverse effects associated with the prescribed medication. Encourage him or her to review corresponding literature provided by a pharmacist.
- Depending on the results of this procedure, additional testing may be performed to evaluate or monitor progression of the disease process and determine the need for a change in therapy. Genetic testing may be conducted to search for mutations in various genes associated with types of thyroid cancer. Markers associated with a significant incidence of thyroid cancers include BRAF (associated with papillary thyroid cancer), RAS (associated with follicular and papillary thyroid cancers), RET/PTC (associated with an increased risk of developing inherited medullary thyroid cancer, also known as multiple endocrine neoplasia or MEN), and PAX8/PPAR (associated with congenital hypothyroidism and thyroid dysgenesis). Evaluate test results in relation to the patient's symptoms and other tests performed.

RELATED STUDIES:

- Related tests include antibodies, antithyroglobulin, calcitonin and stimulation tests, genetic testing, parathyroid scan, radioactive iodine uptake, thyroid-binding inhibitory immunoglobulin, thyroid scan, TSH, free thyroxine, and US thyroid.
- Refer to the Endocrine and Immune systems tables online at Davis*Plus* for related tests by body system.

Bioterrorism and Public Health Safety Concerns: Testing for Toxins and Infectious Agents

B

SYNONYM/ACRONYM: N/A

COMMON USE: To assist in confirming the diagnosis of infection or poisoning in cases of accidental or intentional exposure to agents of high risk to public health safety.

SPECIMEN: The facility or testing laboratory should be contacted regarding specimen collection requirements.

NORMAL FINDINGS: (Method: Disease specific) Negative findings for the organism or toxin of interest; negative serology; negative PCR.

DESCRIPTION: All local and state health departments and the Centers for Disease Control and Prevention (CDC) require health-care providers (HCPs) 🍁 to report specific diseases/pathogens when they are identified by the requesting HCP or the testing laboratory. Information regarding bioterrorism and emergency response plans can be accessed at (http://emergency.cdc.gov/bioterrorism). Information regarding reportable diseases can be accessed at the CDC Web site (www.bt.cdc.bov/agent/agentlist-category.asp). 🍁 This study addresses some of the pathogens and toxins of biological origin that pose a national security risk through unintended exposure or transmission, use in a military action, or to perpetrate terrorist attacks against civilians. The biological agents of most significant concern are grouped into three categories based on the types of impact to public health that include ease of transmission, high mortality or morbidity rates, and level of action required for intervention by public health services. Category A includes infectious organisms and toxins that pose the highest risk, Category B includes the next highest risk group, and Category C includes emerging infectious diseases.

The subspecialty of microbiology has been revolutionized by molecular diagnostics. Molecular diagnostics involves the identification of specific sequences of DNA. The application of molecular diagnostics techniques, such as PCR, has led to the development of automated instruments that can identify a single infectious agent or multiple pathogens from a small amount of specimen in less than 2 hr.

text continues on page 285

B

Infectious Organism/Toxin	Disease	Mode of Transmission and Site of Entry	Incubation Period, Signs, Symptoms, and Treatment	Specimen Required and Test Method
			Category A	
Bacillus anthracis is a gram-positive, aerobic, rod-shaped, spore-forming bacteria; spores are a dormant form of the bacteria. The composition of the spore confers resistance to unfavorable conditions for growth until a suitable environment is attained.	Anthrax	*Bacillus anthracis* is found naturally in soil and causes disease in humans when spores from the bacteria are ingested into the gastrointestinal (GI) system in contaminated water, undercooked meat, or cutaneously by handling meat, wool, or hides from infected animals (usually hoofed animals in close contact with humans); by inhalation of spores or introduction of spores through breaks in the skin from contaminated animal products; or by an intentional and targeted release of spores in a bioterrorist attack. Infected individuals are not contagious; the disease	The incubation period for anthrax infection is between 1 and 7 d and may vary according to the site of entry with inhalation anthrax having the most rapid progression of symptoms. Symptoms may also vary according to the site of entry. General symptoms include fever, malaise, and vomiting. Papules escalating to skin ulceration and eschar formation are associated with cutaneous anthrax; bloody diarrhea is associated with GI anthrax; severe respiratory distress, pulmonary edema, and development of pleural effusions are associated with inhalation anthrax, advancing to shock, coma, and possible death within 1–3 d after inhalation. Treatment for all forms of anthrax with antibiotics (penicillin, doxycycline, and ciprofloxacin) is usually successful, especially if administered early in the course of the disease. Untreated anthrax of any type or late-stage inhaled anthrax may be fatal. Prevention can be enhanced through a veterinary vaccine used for	Specimens considered for testing include blood, stool, skin lesions, sputum, throat culture, body fluids (sputum, ascites, cerebrospinal fluid [CSF], pleural fluid), tissue biopsy, and contaminated food (in the original container if possible). Test methods include culture and gram stain; polymerase chain reaction (PCR); immunochemical techniques (tissue samples); serology; enzyme-linked immunosorbent assays (ELISA). Specimen handling, testing, and culture handling should be performed in a

		is not transmitted directly from person to person.	periodic immunization of livestock, where appropriate. A cell-free culture filtrate vaccine prepared from a non-encapsulated strain of *Bacillus anthracis* is available to individuals in high-risk groups (military personnel and other individuals with high exposure risk due to the nature of their jobs). The vaccine is given in a series of five doses (initial dose and then at 1, 6, 12, and 18 mo after the first dose) followed by a yearly booster dose. 🍁 The effectiveness is not well established, and there is a possibility of significant adverse effects.	Biosafety Level (BSL) 2 environment.
Clostridium botulinum is a gram-positive, anaerobic, rod-shaped, spore-forming bacteria that produces a potent neurotoxin; spores are a dormant form of the bacteria. The	Botulism	*Clostridium botulinum* is found naturally in soil and other types of environments, including the human intestine. There are four forms of botulism. The food-borne disease occurs when the bacteria, toxin, or spores are ingested into the GI system in undercooked, contaminated meat, fish, vegetables, sauces, and home-canned foods,	The most common type of botulism is food borne, and the incubation period is a few hours to 3 d. Incubation periods for other types of botulism may vary according to the site of entry and can extend up to 1 wk for exposure by wound. Neuromuscular symptoms are the hallmark of how the toxin achieves its effect on the body and include blurred vision, difficulty swallowing, and muscle weakness that progresses to paralysis. Irreversible binding of the toxin to sites where neuromuscular activity is normally initiated prevent	Specimens considered for testing include blood, stool, vomitus, and contaminated food (in the original container if possible). Test methods include mouse neutralization test (to detect the toxin), culture. Specimen handling, testing, and culture handling should

(table continues on page 278)

B

Infectious Organism/Toxin	Disease	Mode of Transmission and Site of Entry	Incubation Period, Signs, Symptoms, and Treatment	Specimen Required and Test Method
composition of the spore confers resistance to unfavorable conditions for growth until a suitable environment is attained.		especially when kept at room temperature after cooking. Infants under 1 yr of age are susceptible to a type of botulism linked to ingestion of spores in honey. Wound botulism occurs when the bacteria, toxin, or spores are introduced through breaks in the skin. Botulism can also occur by inhalation of spores from a contaminated source or by an intentional and targeted release of spores in a bioterrorist attack. Infected individuals are not contagious; the disease is not transmitted directly from person to person. Seven distinct botulism neurotoxin types are known to affect humans, identified as A, B, C, D, E, F, and G.	the release of a neurotransmitter called acetylcholine. Normal neuromuscular function halts as the body's muscles are irreversibly paralyzed. Respiratory symptoms may also occur with inhalation botulism. Additional symptoms of infant botulism include other indications of altered neuromuscular function such as poor feeding (due to loss of muscle function related to sucking), constipation (due to loss of muscle function related to elimination), pooled oral secretions (due to loss of muscle function related to swallowing), and loss of head control related to loss of neck muscle strength and function. There is no prescribed treatment for botulism other than palliative care. As the paralysis advances and organ function diminishes, mechanical support is required for breathing and nutrition. A heptavalent vaccine is available for individuals identified as high risk and is effective for clostridial toxin strains A through G. An intravenous botulism immune globulin is available for infant botulism and is approved for the treatment	be performed in a BSL2 environment.

			of botulism types A and B. More information can be obtained from www.infantbotulism.org 🍁.	
Francisella tularensis is a gram-negative, aerobic coccobacillus.	Tularemia	Tularemia can be contracted in a number of different ways: ingestion of the bacteria into the GI system from contaminated water or plants; cutaneously through a break in the skin when handling infected animal products or from the bite of an infected insect, such as a tick or deerfly; or breathing the bacteria into the lungs. Infected individuals are not contagious; the disease is not transmitted directly from person to person.	The incubation period for tularemia averages 3–5 d but can take as long as 2 wk, depending on the site of entry. Symptoms may also vary according to the site of entry. The general symptoms include fever, chills, headache, diarrhea, weakness, muscle aches, and joint pain. Ingestion of the bacteria can cause symptoms that affect the entire alimentary canal, including mouth ulcers, sore throat, swollen and painful lymph glands, intestinal pain, vomiting, and diarrhea. Inhalation of the bacteria can cause symptoms that resemble influenza or pneumonia, such as chest pain from difficulty breathing or bloody sputum. When the infection is introduced cutaneously, skin ulcers and swelling of the associated lymph nodes are evident. The disease can be fatal if it is not treated in a timely manner. Treatment for infection is a 2-wk course of the antibiotic doxycycline or ciprofloxacin. Currently, no vaccine is available in the United States 🍁; there is ongoing research to identify an effective vaccine.	Specimens considered for testing include serum, blood, sputum/throat swab, bronchial/tracheal wash, and stool. Test methods include serology, gram stain, and culture. Specimen handling and testing should be performed in a BSL2 environment; culture handling should be performed in a BSL3 environment.

(table continues on page 280)

B

B

Infectious Organism/Toxin	Disease	Mode of Transmission and Site of Entry	Incubation Period, Signs, Symptoms, and Treatment	Specimen Required and Test Method
Variola major is a severe and potentially lethal strain of the variola DNA virus.	Smallpox	The smallpox virus is transmitted by an infected human through the respiratory system in droplets that become aerosolized and are inhaled by another person in very close proximity. The smallpox virus can also be transmitted by direct contact with contaminated fomites or direct contact with body fluids from an infected person (secretions from rashes, pustules, or scabs), or by an intentional and targeted bioterrorist attack. The disease can be directly transmitted from person to person.	The incubation period for smallpox averages 12–14 d after which general symptoms develop to include fever, headache, and body aches followed by the development of a rash in the mouth and on the skin; the most infectious period is during the first 7–10 d following development of the rash. In the next stage of the infection, the rash becomes pustular. Eventually, the pustules dry up and scab formation occurs. Viable viral particles are present in the scabs; therefore, a person is considered contagious until after the last scab has fallen off. There is no specified treatment for smallpox, and the only prevention is by vaccination. Routine vaccination in the United States ended in 1972 after the disease was eradicated. 🍁	Specimens considered for testing include culture, vesicular fluid, skin scraping, and biopsy specimens. Test methods include viral culture or identification from a sample using electron microscopy. Specimen handling, testing, and culture handling should be performed in a BSL4 environment.
Filoviruses (e.g., Ebola, Marburg), *arenaviruses*	VHF	VHFs are a group of severe infections caused by different RNA viruses. The viruses are transmitted	The incubation period for VHFs varies from 3–21 d. Beginning symptoms include fever, headache, body aches, fatigue, jaundice, and vomiting; some	Specimens considered for testing include serum, blood, sputum, and tissue. Test

(e.g., Lassa, Machupo), *flaviviruses* (including the virus that causes yellow fever), and *Bunyaviridae* (e.g., Haantan). The viruses responsible for viral hemorrhagic fevers (VHFs) are RNA viruses.	to humans cutaneously by way of a bite from an infected reservoir host (e.g., rodent) or infected arthropod vector (e.g., mosquito or tick that has bitten an infected host). Some viruses (e.g., Ebola, Marburg, Lassa) can be directly transmitted from person to person by way of contact with contaminated blood or body fluids. The infection is significant; it can result in multisystem failure and death. Because some viruses have the potential to cause massive numbers of deaths through contagious infection, they are considered possible weapons for use in an intentional and targeted bioterrorist attack.	cases progress with bleeding, shock, and multiorgan failure. There is no prescribed treatment for VHFs, and patients are given supportive treatment for their symptoms. Care should be taken in the selection of medications to reduce fever and pain, avoiding those medications known to increase the risk of bleeding (e.g., salicylates and NSAIDs). Yellow fever is the only VHF for which an effective vaccine is available. Additional preventive measures for yellow fever include avoidance of further exposure to mosquitos by staying indoors during hours when they are most active and using repellents and mosquito netting. Preventive measures decrease the opportunity for uninfected mosquitoes to feed on infected blood, which in turn decreases the spread of the disease.	methods include viral isolation, PCR, ELISA, immunohistochemistry of tissue, and serology. Specimen handling, testing, and culture handling for yellow fever should be performed in a BSL3; for dengue should be performed in a BSL2; for others should be performed in a BSL4 environment.

(*table continues on page 282*)

Infectious Organism/Toxin	Disease	Mode of Transmission and Site of Entry	Incubation Period, Signs, Symptoms, and Treatment	Specimen Required and Test Method
Yersinia pestis is a gram-negative, facultatively anaerobic, obligate intracellular coccobacillus.	Plague	There are three forms of plague. The first and probably best known is bubonic plague. The reservoir host (usually a rodent) carries infected fleas; the fleas spread the disease cutaneously to humans through a bite. The bacteria multiply in the lymph node closest to the site of the flea bite. Septicemic plague occurs when the bacteria is inoculated into the bloodstream by flea bite or by the bite of an infected animal. Pneumonic plague is the most lethal form of plague. It occurs when the infection from either untreated bubonic or septicemic plague spreads to the lungs. Pneumonic is the only	The average incubation period for plague is 1–6 d depending on the site of entry; generally, pneumonic plague has a shorter incubation period. General symptoms include fever, chills, enlarged lymph nodes, malaise, septicemia, hemorrhagic skin changes, pneumonia (pneumonic plague), shock, and death. Early identification and administration of antibiotics (tetracycline or fluoroquinolone) for 7 d, with supportive care, is the most effective treatment for plague.	Specimens considered for testing include serum, blood, sputum/throat swab, bronchial/tracheal wash, and lymph node aspirate. Test methods include serology, gram stain, and culture. Specimen and culture handling should be performed in a BSL2 environment.

		form of plague that can be transmitted person to person from inhalation of aerosolized droplets of contaminated fluid, direct contact with contaminated fomites (for short periods of time), or by an intentional and targeted bioterrorist attack.		
			Category B	
Brucella abortus, *B. suis*, *B. melitensis*, or *B. canis*; the species are gram-negative, aerobic, coccobacilli.	Brucellosis	Infection occurs after ingestion into the GI system from infected meats and contaminated milk products (especially goat's milk), direct puncture of the skin (by butchers and farmers), or by inhalation. It is not a contagious disease that is transmitted from person to person.	The average incubation period for brucellosis infection is 1–2 mo. General symptoms include fever, chills, headache, night sweats, back pain, joint pain, and malaise. The disease is systemic, affecting multiple organs and body systems. Brucellosis can be effectively treated with antibiotics (e.g., doxycycline, tetracycline, streptomycin, Bactrim, rifampin, ciprofloxacin, or gentamicin). Currently, no vaccine is available for use in humans.	Specimens considered for testing include serum, blood, bone marrow, spleen or liver tissue, sputum, and food. Test methods include serology, gram stain, culture, and immunofluorescence. Specimen handling should be performed in a BSL2 environment; culture handling should be performed in a BSL3 environment.

(table continues on page 284)

B

Infectious Organism/Toxin	Disease	Mode of Transmission and Site of Entry	Incubation Period, Signs, Symptoms, and Treatment	Specimen Required and Test Method
Ricinus communis is the name for the castor oil plant. The plant's seeds contain an oil composed mostly of the lipid ricinolein and smaller amounts of ricin, a powerful toxin.	Ricin poisoning. The toxin is released after ingestion of castor beans. It can also be purposely made from a waste product generated in the normal production of castor oil. The manufactured toxin can then be used in an intentional and targeted bioterrorist attack.	Ricin poisoning occurs by ingestion into the GI system or by inhalation into the respiratory system. It is not a contagious disease that is transmitted from person to person, and the likelihood of accidental poisoning is very low. The manufactured toxin can be released as a powder into the air or dissolved in water supplies. Very small amounts could sicken and kill large numbers of people, and for this reason it is considered as a potential weapon for use in an intentional and targeted bioterrorist attack.	Symptoms of ricin poisoning vary according to the site of entry and concentration of the dose. If the toxin is ingested, GI symptoms such as nausea, pain, and vomiting appear in 6–12 hr; if the toxin is inhaled, respiratory symptoms such as difficulty breathing, coughing, and chest pain appear in 4–6 hr. Over the next 12–24 hr, the symptoms rapidly escalate toward organ failure. Ricin affects the body at the cellular level by preventing the production of proteins, an essential process for every living cell, tissue, and organ. Presently there are no methods available for the detection of ricin in biological fluids. Diagnosis of ricin poisoning is made using general laboratory tests for evidence of the effects of the toxin on the body and is arrived at within the context of high suspicion of exposure. Laboratory results of interest might include elevated liver function results, elevated renal function results, abnormal urinalysis findings such as blood in the urine, and moderate to increased WBC count (two to five times normal levels).	Environmental samples can be tested for the presence of ricin by time-resolved fluorescence immunoassay and PCR. Specimen handling should be performed in a BSL2 or BSL3 environment depending on the possibility of aerosolization and concentration of toxin submitted for testing.

This procedure is contraindicated for: N/A

INDICATIONS

- Suspected infection by high-risk pathogen ***(demonstrated by associated signs and symptoms or known exposure).***

POTENTIAL MEDICAL DIAGNOSIS

Positive Findings in

- Positive findings for the organism or toxin of interest; positive serology. Refer to the table in the Description section for details.

CRITICAL FINDINGS:

- Positive findings for a disease listed in Description section leads to a high likelihood of being required for reporting to the appropriate agencies.

Note and immediately report to the requesting health-care provider (HCP) any critical findings and related symptoms. A listing of these findings varies among facilities. Timely notification of a critical finding for laboratory or diagnostic studies is a role expectation of the professional nurse. The notification processes vary among facilities. Upon receipt of the critical finding, the information should be read back to the caller to verify accuracy.

INTERFERING FACTORS

- Failure to follow the appropriate specimen collection and transport procedures may affect the validity of the results.

NURSING IMPLICATIONS AND PROCEDURE

PRETEST:

- Positively identify the patient using at least two person-specific identifiers before services, treatments, or procedures are performed.
- ***Patient Teaching:*** Inform the patient this test can assist in assessing for infection or poisoning.
- Obtain a history of the patient's health concerns, symptoms, surgical procedures, and results of previously performed laboratory and diagnostic studies. Obtain a history of exposure, including all possible sources (e.g., environmental, other individuals who are ill with similar symptoms, food, animals). Include a list of known allergens, especially allergies or sensitivities to latex.
- Obtain a list of the patient's current medications, including over-the-counter medications and dietary supplements (see Effects of Natural Products on Laboratory Values online at Davis*Plus*).
- Review the procedure with the patient. Inform the patient that several tests may be necessary to confirm the diagnosis. Any individual positive serology result may be repeated in 3 wk to monitor a change in detectable level of antibody, as appropriate. Inform the patient that specimen collection takes approximately 5 to 10 min. Address concerns about pain, and explain that there may be some discomfort during the venipuncture.
- ***Sensitivity to social and cultural issues,*** as well as concern for modesty, is important in providing psychological support before, during, and after the procedure.
- Note that there are no food or fluid restrictions unless by medical direction; as a general rule specimens should be collected prior to administration of antibiotics whenever possible. Chain of custody policies may be required in cases of intentional exposure.

INTRATEST:

Potential Complications: N/A

- Avoid the use of equipment containing latex if the patient has a history of allergic reaction to latex.
- Instruct the patient to cooperate fully and to follow directions. Direct the

B

patient to breathe normally and to avoid unnecessary movement.

- Contact the testing laboratory prior to specimen collection in order to obtain accurate information regarding specimen collection containers, sample volumes, and specific transport instructions.
- Observe standard precautions, and follow the general guidelines in Patient Preparation and Specimen Collection online at Davis*Plus*. Positively identify the patient, and label the appropriate specimen container with the corresponding patient demographics, initials of the person collecting the specimen, date, and time of collection. Collect the appropriate specimen as described in the related body fluid analysis or culture study. The facility or testing laboratory should be contacted for guidelines regarding chain of custody, specimen collection requirements, and specimen packaging and shipping instructions.
- Perform a venipuncture if blood is the specimen required for testing. Remove the needle and apply direct pressure with dry gauze to stop bleeding. Observe/assess venipuncture site for bleeding or hematoma formation and secure gauze with adhesive bandage.
- Promptly transport the specimen to the laboratory for processing and analysis.

POST-TEST:

- Inform the patient that a report of the results will be made available to the requesting HCP, who will discuss the results with the patient.
- Recognize anxiety related to test results, and provide emotional support if results are positive. Discuss the implications of abnormal test results on the patient's lifestyle. Provide teaching and information regarding the clinical implications of the test results, as appropriate. Educate the patient regarding access to counseling services.
- Reinforce information given by the patient's HCP regarding further testing, treatment, or referral to another HCP. Instruct the patient in isolation precautions during time of communicability or contagion, as appropriate. Instruct the patient in the proper way to decontaminate solid surfaces with a 1:10 dilution of household bleach:water; to decontaminate clothing; to "cover a cough"; and to perform good hand hygiene.
- Depending on the results of this procedure, additional testing may be performed to evaluate or monitor progression of the disease process and determine the need for a change in therapy. Evaluate test results in relation to the patient's symptoms and other tests performed. Emphasize the need to return to have a convalescent blood sample taken in 3 wk, if ordered. Answer any questions or address any concerns voiced by the patient or family.

RELATED STUDIES:

- Related tests include acetylcholine receptor antibodies, basic metabolic panel, biopsy lung, biopsy lymph node, bronchoscopy, chest x-ray, CSF analysis, comprehensive metabolic panel, CT chest, culture throat, culture blood, culture sputum, culture stool, liver function tests, peritoneal fluid analysis, pleural fluid analysis, and kidney function tests.
- Refer to the Gastrointestinal, Genitourinary, Hematopoietic, Hepatobiliary, Immune, Musculoskeletal, and Respiratory System tables online at Davis*Plus* for related tests by body system.

B

Bladder Cancer Markers, Urine

SYNONYM/ACRONYM: Nuclear matrix protein (NMP) 22, BTA, cytogenic marker for bladder cancer.

COMMON USE: To assist in diagnosing bladder cancer.

SPECIMEN: Urine, unpreserved random specimen collected in a clean plastic collection container for NMP22 and Bard BTA; urine, first void specimen collected in fixative specific for fluorescence in situ hybridization (FISH) testing.

NORMAL FINDINGS: (Method: Enzyme immunoassay for NMP22 and bladder tumor antigen [BTA], FISH for cytogenic marker).

NMP22: Negative: Less than 6 units/mL, borderline: 6 to 10 units/mL, positive: greater than 10 units/mL.

BTA: Negative.

Cytogenic Marker: Negative.

POTENTIAL MEDICAL DIAGNOSIS

Increased in bladder carcinoma

CRITICAL FINDINGS:

- Bladder carcinoma

Note and immediately report to the requesting health-care provider (HCP) any critical findings and related symptoms. A listing of these findings varies among facilities. Timely notification of a critical finding for laboratory or diagnostic studies is a role expectation of the professional nurse. The notification processes vary among facilities. Upon receipt of the critical finding, the information should be read back to the caller to verify accuracy.

Find and print out the full study on Fast Find at davispl.us/vanleeuwen7.

Bleeding Time

SYNONYM/ACRONYM: Mielke bleeding time, Simplate bleeding time, template bleeding time, Surgicutt bleeding time, Ivy bleeding time.

COMMON USE: To evaluate platelet function.

SPECIMEN: Whole blood.

NORMAL FINDINGS: (Method: Timed observation of incision)

Template: 2.5 to 10 min.

Ivy: 2 to 7 min.

Slight differences exist in the disposable devices used to make the incision. Although the Mielke or template bleeding time is believed to offer greater standardization to a fairly subjective procedure, both methods are thought to be of equal sensitivity and reproducibility.

B

POTENTIAL MEDICAL DIAGNOSIS

This test does not predict excessive bleeding during a surgical procedure.

Prolonged In

- Bernard-Soulier syndrome ***(evidenced by a rare hereditary condition in which platelet glycoprotein GP1b is deficient and platelet aggregation is decreased)***
- Fibrinogen disorders ***(related to the role of fibrinogen to help platelets link together)***
- Glanzmann's thrombasthenia ***(evidenced by a rare hereditary condition in which platelet glycoprotein IIb/IIIa is deficient and platelet aggregation is decreased)***
- Hereditary telangiectasia ***(evidenced by fragile blood vessels that do not permit adequate constriction to stop bleeding)***
- Kidney disease ***(related to abnormal platelet function)***
- Liver disease ***(related to decreased production of coagulation proteins that affect bleeding time)***
- Some myeloproliferative disorders ***(evidenced by disorders of decreased platelet production)***
- Thrombocytopenia ***(evidenced by insufficient platelets to stop bleeding)***
- von Willebrand's disease ***(evidenced by deficiency of von Willebrand factor, necessary for normal platelet adhesion)***

Decreased in: N/A

CRITICAL FINDINGS:

Greater than 14 min

Note and immediately report to the requesting health-care provider (HCP) any critical findings and related symptoms. A listing of these findings varies among facilities. Timely notification of a critical finding for laboratory or diagnostic studies is a role expectation of the professional nurse. The notification processes vary among facilities. Upon receipt of the critical finding, the information should be read back to the caller to verify accuracy.

Potential nursing interventions for bleeding include applying pressure to the incision until the bleeding stops and covering the incision site with a bandage. Some people are more prone than others to develop scars or keloids. Generally, they are pink to reddish in color, raised, and shinier than the surrounding skin. They can be itchy, tender, or even painful to the touch. There is no immediate intervention to prevent the formation of scars or keloids. Treatment options for developed scars and keloids range from cortisone injections to a variety of strategies for removal, each of which can vary widely in degree of success. The site should be observed for subsequent bleeding, bruising, or redness. Fever, localized redness, or warmth of the area to the touch may be indications of infection. Potential nursing interventions include monitoring temperature as well as administering antipyretic and antibiotic medications, as ordered.

Find and print out the full study on Fast Find at davispl.us/vanleeuwen7.

Blood Gases

SYNONYM/ACRONYM: Arterial blood gases (ABGs), venous blood gases, capillary blood gases, cord blood gases.

COMMON USE: To assess oxygenation and acid base balance.

SPECIMEN: Whole blood. Specimen volume and collection container may vary with collection method. See Intratest section for specific collection instructions. Specimen should be tightly capped and transported in an ice slurry.

NORMAL FINDINGS: (Method: Selective electrodes for pH, PCO_2 and PO_2)

Blood Gas Value (pH)	Arterial	Venous	Capillary
Scalp	—	—	7.25–7.35
Birth, cord, full term	7.11–7.36	7.25–7.45	7.32–7.49
Adult/child	7.35–7.45	7.32–7.43	7.35–7.45

Note: SI units (conversion factor × 1).

Pco_2	Arterial	SI Units (conventional units × 0.133)	Venous	SI Units (conventional units × 0.133)	Capillary	SI Units (conventional units × 0.133)
Scalp	—	—	—	—	40–50 mm Hg	5.3–6.6 kPa
Birth, cord, full term	32–66 mm Hg	4.3–8.8 kPa	27–49 mm Hg	3.6–6.5 kPa	—	—
Newborn–adult	35–45 mm Hg	4.7–6 kPa	41–51 mm Hg	5.4–6.8 kPa	26–41 mm Hg	3.5–5.4 kPa

Po_2	Arterial	SI Units (conventional units × 0.133)	Venous	SI Units (conventional units × 0.133)	Capillary	SI Units (conventional units × 0.133)
Scalp	—	—	—	—	20–30 mm Hg	2.7–4 kPa
Birth, cord, full term	8–24 mm Hg	1.1–3.2 kPa	17–41 mm Hg	2.3–5.4 kPa	—	—
0–1 hr	33–85 mm Hg	4.4–11.3 kPa	—	—	—	—
Greater than 1 hr–adult	80–95 mm Hg	10.6–12.6 kPa	20–49 mm Hg	2.7–6.5 kPa	80–95 mm Hg	10.6–12.6 kPa

B

HCO_3^-	Arterial Conventional & SI Units	Venous Conventional & SI Units	Capillary Conventional & SI Units
Birth, cord, full term	17–24 mmol/L	17–24 mmol/L	—
2 mo–2 yr	16–23 mmol/L	24–28 mmol/L	18–23 mmol/L
Adult	22–26 mmol/L	24–28 mmol/L	18–23 mmol/L

O_2 Sat	Arterial	Venous	Capillary
Birth, cord, full term	40%–90%	40%–70%	—
Adult/child	95%–99%	70%–75%	95%–98%

Values may be at the lower end of the normal range in older adults

Oxygen Content: Arterial	Oxygen Content: Venous
6.6–9.7 mmol/L	4.9–7.1 mmol/L

Tco$_2$	Arterial Conventional & SI Units mmol/L	Venous Conventional & SI Units mmol/L
Birth, cord, full term	13–22 mmol/L	14–22 mmol/L
Adult/child	22–29 mmol/L	25–30 mmol/L

Base Excess Arterial	Conventional & SI Units
Birth, cord, full term	(−10) – (−2) mmol/L
Adult/child	(−2) – (+3) mmol/L

DESCRIPTION: Blood gas analysis is used to evaluate respiratory function and provide a measure for determining acid-base balance. Respiratory, renal, and cardiovascular system functions are integrated in order to maintain normal acid-base balance. Therefore, respiratory or metabolic disorders may cause abnormal blood gas findings. The blood gas measurements commonly reported are pH, partial pressure of carbon dioxide in the blood (PCO_2), partial pressure of oxygen in the blood (PO_2), bicarbonate (HCO_3^-), O_2 saturation, and base excess (BE) or base deficit (BD). pH reflects the number of free hydrogen ions (H^+) in the body. A pH less than 7.35 indicates acidosis. A pH greater than 7.45 indicates alkalosis. Changes in the ratio of free H^+ to HCO_3 will result in a compensatory response from the lungs or kidneys to restore proper acid-base balance.

PCO_2 is an important indicator of ventilation. The level of PCO_2 is controlled primarily by the lungs and is referred to as the respiratory component of acid-base balance. The main buffer system in the body is the

B

bicarbonate–carbonic acid system. Bicarbonate is an important alkaline ion that participates along with other anions, such as hemoglobin, proteins, and phosphates, to neutralize acids. For the body to maintain proper balance, there must be a ratio of 20 parts bicarbonate to one part carbonic acid (20:1). Carbonic acid level is indirectly measured by PCO_2. Bicarbonate level is indirectly measured by the total carbon dioxide content (TCO_2). The carbonic acid level is not measured directly but can be estimated because it is 3% of the PCO_2. Bicarbonate can also be calculated from these numbers once the carbonic acid value has been obtained because of the 20:1 ratio. For example, if the PCO_2 were 40, the carbonic acid would be calculated as (3% × 40) or 1.2, and the HCO_3^- would be calculated as (20 × 1.2) or 24. The main acid in the acid-base system is carbonic acid. It is the metabolic or nonrespiratory component of the acid-base system and is controlled by the kidney. Bicarbonate levels can either be measured directly or estimated from the TCO_2 in the blood. BE/BD reflects the number of anions available in the blood to help buffer changes in pH. A BD (negative BE) indicates metabolic acidosis, whereas a positive BE indicates metabolic alkalosis.

Extremes in acidosis are generally more life threatening than alkalosis. Acidosis can develop either very quickly (e.g., cardiac arrest) or over a longer period of time (e.g., kidney failure). Infants can develop acidosis very quickly if they are not kept warm and given enough calories. Children with diabetes tend to go into acidosis more quickly than do adults who have been dealing with the disease over a longer period of time. In many cases, a venous or capillary specimen is satisfactory to obtain the necessary information regarding acid-base balance without subjecting the patient to an arterial puncture with its associated risks.

As seen in the table of reference ranges, PO_2 is lower in infants than in children and adults owing to the respective level of maturation of the lungs at birth. PO_2 tends to trail off after age 30, decreasing by approximately 3 to 5 mm Hg per decade as the organs age and begin to lose elasticity. The formula used to approximate the relationship between age and PO_2 is $PO_2 = 104 - (\text{age} \times 0.27)$.

The oxygen-carrying capacity of the blood indicates how much oxygen could be carried if all the hemoglobin were saturated with oxygen. Percentage of oxygen saturation is [oxyhemoglobin concentration ÷ (oxyhemoglobin concentration + deoxyhemoglobin concentration)] × 100.

Like carbon dioxide, oxygen is carried in the body in a dissolved and combined (oxyhemoglobin) form. Most of the oxygen circulating in the body (98%) is bound to hemoglobin; the rest is dissolved. One gram of hemoglobin can bind 1.34 mL of oxygen, whereas plasma is capable of carrying much less—0.3 mL of dissolved oxygen. Oxygen content is the sum of the dissolved and combined oxygen. Because circulating blood may contain less oxygen than it is capable of carrying, it is useful to know the actual oxygen content. Oxygen content can be calculated on the basis of measured parameters (oxygen saturation, hemoglobin, and PO_2) and a solubility factor (0.003 is the Bunsen solubility factor for dissolved oxygen in blood). The oxygen content in arterial blood is calculated as CAO_2 = 1.34 (SAO_2 × Hgb) + 0.003 (PAO_2). The oxygen content of venous blood is calculated as CVO_2 = 1.34 (SVO_2 × Hgb) + 0.003 (PVO_2).

Testing on specimens other than arterial blood is often ordered when oxygen measurements are not needed or when the information regarding oxygen can be obtained by noninvasive techniques such as pulse oximetry. Capillary blood is satisfactory for most purposes for pH and PCO_2; the use of capillary PO_2 is limited to the exclusion of hypoxia. Measurements involving oxygen are usually not useful when performed on venous samples; arterial blood is required to accurately measure PO_2 and oxygen saturation. Considerable evidence indicates that prolonged exposure to high levels of oxygen can result in injury, such as retinopathy of prematurity in infants or the drying of airways in any patient. Monitoring PO_2 from blood gases is especially appropriate under such circumstances.

This procedure is contraindicated for

Arterial puncture in any of the following circumstances:

- Inadequate circulation ***as evidenced by an abnormal (negative) Allen test or the absence of a radial artery pulse.***
- Significant or uncontrolled bleeding disorder ***as the procedure may cause excessive bleeding;*** caution should be used when performing an arterial puncture on patients receiving anticoagulant therapy or thrombolytic medications.
- Infection at the puncture site ***carries the potential for introducing bacteria from the skin surface into the blood stream.***
- Congenital or acquired abnormalities of the skin or blood vessels in the area of the anticipated puncture site such as arteriovenous fistulas, burns, tumors, vascular grafts.

INDICATIONS

This group of tests is used to assess conditions such as asthma, chronic obstructive pulmonary disease (COPD), embolism (e.g., fatty or other embolism) during coronary arterial bypass surgery, and hypoxia. It is also used to assist in the diagnosis of respiratory failure, which is defined as a PO_2 less than 50 mm Hg and PCO_2 greater than 50 mm Hg. Blood gases can be valuable in the management of patients on ventilators or being weaned from ventilators. Blood gas values are used to determine acid-base status, the type of imbalance, and the degree of compensation as summarized in the following section. Restoration of pH to near-normal values is referred to as fully compensated balance. When pH values are moving in the same direction (i.e., increasing or decreasing) as the PCO_2 or HCO_3^-, the imbalance is metabolic. When the pH values are moving in the opposite direction from the PCO_2 or HCO_3^-, the imbalance is caused by respiratory disturbances. To remember this concept, the following mnemonic can be useful: MeTRO = **Metabolic Together, Respiratory Opposite.**

B

Acid-Base Disturbance	pH	Pco_2	Po_2	HCO_3^-
Respiratory Acidosis				
Uncompensated	Decreased	Increased	Normal	Normal
Compensated	Normal	Increased	Increased	Increased
Respiratory Alkalosis				
Uncompensated	Increased	Decreased	Normal	Normal
Compensated	Normal	Decreased	Decreased	Decreased
Uncompensated	Decreased	Normal	Decreased	Decreased
Compensated	Normal	Decreased	Decreased	Decreased
Metabolic (Nonrespiratory) Acidosis				
Uncompensated	Increased	Normal	Increased	Increased
Compensated	Normal	Increased	Increased	Increased

POTENTIAL MEDICAL DIAGNOSIS

Acid-base imbalance is determined by evaluating pH, Pco_2, and HCO_3^- values. pH less than 7.35 reflects an acidic state, whereas pH greater than 7.45 reflects alkalosis. Pco_2 and HCO_3^- determine whether the imbalance is respiratory or nonrespiratory (metabolic). Because a patient may have more than one imbalance and may also be in the process of compensating, the interpretation of blood gas values may not always seem straightforward.

Respiratory conditions that interfere with normal breathing cause CO_2 to be retained in the blood. This results in an increase of circulating carbonic acid and a corresponding decrease in pH (respiratory acidosis). Acute respiratory acidosis can occur in acute pulmonary edema, severe respiratory infections, bronchial obstruction, pneumothorax, hemothorax, open chest wounds, opiate poisoning, respiratory depressant drug therapy, and inhalation of air with a high CO_2 content. Chronic respiratory acidosis can be seen in patients with asthma, pulmonary fibrosis, COPD, bronchiectasis, and respiratory depressant drug therapy. Respiratory conditions that increase the breathing rate cause CO_2 to be removed from the alveoli more rapidly than it is being produced. This results in an alkaline pH. Acute respiratory alkalosis may be seen in anxiety, hysteria, hyperventilation, and pulmonary embolus and with an increase in artificial ventilation. Chronic respiratory alkalosis may be seen in high fever, administration of drugs (e.g., salicylate and sulfa) that stimulate the respiratory system, hepatic coma, hypoxia of high altitude, and central nervous system (CNS) lesions or injury that result in stimulation of the respiratory center.

Metabolic (nonrespiratory) conditions that cause the excessive formation or decreased excretion of organic or inorganic acids result in metabolic acidosis. Some of these conditions include ingestion of salicylates, ethylene glycol, and methanol, as well as uncontrolled diabetes, starvation, shock, kidney disease, and biliary or pancreatic fistula. Metabolic alkalosis results from conditions that increase pH, as can be seen in excessive intake of antacids to treat gastritis or peptic ulcer, excessive administration of HCO_3^-, loss of stomach acid caused by protracted vomiting, cystic fibrosis, or potassium and chloride deficiencies.

Respiratory Acidosis

- Decreased pH
- Decreased O_2 saturation
- Increased P_{CO_2}:
  Acute intermittent porphyria
  Acute respiratory distress syndrome (adult and neonatal)
  Anemia (severe)
  Anorexia
  Anoxia
  Asthma
  Atelectasis
  Bronchitis (chronic)
  Bronchoconstriction
  Carbon monoxide poisoning
  Cardiac disorders
  Congenital heart defects
  COPD
  Cystic fibrosis
  Depression of respiratory center
  Drugs depressing the respiratory system
  Electrolyte disturbances (severe)
  Fever
  Head injury
  Heart failure
  Hypercapnia
  Hypothyroidism (severe)
  Near drowning
  Pleural effusion
  Pneumonia
  Pneumothorax
  Poisoning
  Poliomyelitis
  Pulmonary edema
  Pulmonary embolism
  Pulmonary tuberculosis
  Respiratory failure
  Sarcoidosis
  Smoking
  Tumor (lung, brain)
- A decreased P_{O_2} that increases P_{CO_2}:
  Decreased alveolar gas exchange: acute respiratory distress syndrome (newborns), cancer, compression or resection of lung, sarcoidosis
  Decreased ventilation or perfusion: asthma, bronchiectasis, bronchitis (chronic), cancer, croup, cystic fibrosis (mucoviscidosis), COPD, granulomata, pneumonia, pulmonary infarction, shock
  Hypoxemia: anesthesia, carbon monoxide exposure, cardiac disorders, high altitudes, near drowning, presence of abnormal hemoglobins
  Hypoventilation: cerebrovascular incident, drugs depressing the respiratory system, head injury
  Right-to-left shunt: congenital heart disease, intrapulmonary venoarterial shunting

Compensation

- Increased P_{O_2}:
  Hyperbaric oxygenation
  Hyperventilation
- Increased base excess:
  Increased HCO_3^- to bring pH to (near) normal

Respiratory Alkalosis

- Increased pH
- Decreased P_{CO_2}:
  Anxiety
  CNS lesions or injuries that cause stimulation of the respiratory center
  Excessive artificial ventilation
  Fever
  Head injury
  Hyperthermia
  Hyperventilation
  Hysteria
  Salicylate intoxication

Compensation

- Decreased P_{O_2}:
  Rebreather mask
- Decreased base excess:
  Decreased HCO_3^- to bring pH to (near) normal

Metabolic Acidosis

- Decreased pH
- Decreased HCO_3^-
- Decreased base excess
- Decreased T_{CO_2}:
  Decreased excretion of H^+: acute kidney injury, acquired (e.g., drugs, hypercalcemia), Addison's disease, chronic kidney disease, diabetic ketoacidosis, Fanconi's syndrome, inherited (e.g., cystinosis, Wilson's disease), renal tubular acidosis

Increased acid intake
Increased formation of acids: diabetic ketoacidosis, high-fat/low-carbohydrate diets
Increased loss of alkaline body fluids: diarrhea, excess potassium, fistula
Salicylate intoxication
Shock
Vomiting

Compensation

- Increased Tco_2: Hypoventilation

Compensation

- Decreased Pco_2: Hyperventilation

Metabolic Alkalosis

- Increased pH
- Increased HCO_3^-
- Increased base excess
- Increased Tco_2:

Alkali ingestion (excessive)
Anoxia
Gastric suctioning
Hypochloremic states
Hypokalemic states
Potassium depletion: Cushing's disease, diarrhea, diuresis, excessive vomiting, excessive ingestion of licorice, inadequate potassium intake, potassium-losing nephropathy, steroid administration

CRITICAL FINDINGS:

Note and immediately report to the requesting health-care provider (HCP) any critical findings and related symptoms. A listing of these findings varies among facilities. Timely notification of a critical finding for laboratory or diagnostic studies is a role expectation of the professional nurse. The notification processes vary among facilities. Upon receipt of the critical finding, the information should be read back to the caller to verify accuracy.

Consideration may be given to verification of critical findings before action is taken. Policies vary among facilities and may include requesting recollection and retesting by the laboratory.

	Arterial Blood Gas Parameter	Less Than	Greater Than
Adult/child	pH	7.2	7.6
Adult/child	HCO_3^-	10 mmol/L	40 mmol/L
Adult/child	Pco_2	20 mm Hg (SI: 2.7 kPa)	67 mm Hg (SI: 8.9 kPa)
Adult/child	Po_2	45 mm Hg (SI: 6 kPa)	
Newborns	Po_2	37 mm Hg (SI: 4.9 kPa)	92 mm Hg (SI: 12.2 kPa)

INTERFERING FACTORS

- Drugs and other substances that may cause an increase in HCO_3^- include acetylsalicylic acid (initially), antacids, carbenicillin, ethacrynic acid, glycyrrhiza (licorice), laxatives, mafenide, and sodium bicarbonate.
- Drugs that may cause a decrease in HCO_3^- include acetazolamide, acetylsalicylic acid (long term or high doses), citrates, dimethadione, ether, ethylene glycol, fluorides, mercury compounds (laxatives), methylenedioxyamphetamine, paraldehyde, and xylitol.
- Drugs and other substances that may cause an increase in Pco_2 include acetylsalicylic acid, aldosterone, bicarbonate, carbenicillin,

corticosteroids, dexamethasone, ethacrynic acid, laxatives (chronic misuse), and x-ray contrast medium.

- Drugs and other substances that may cause a decrease in Pco_2 include acetazolamide, acetylsalicylic acid, ethamivan, neuromuscular relaxants (secondary to postoperative hyperventilation), theophylline, tromethamine, and xylitol.
- Drugs and other substances that may cause an increase in Po_2 include theophylline and urokinase.
- Drugs and other substances that may cause a decrease in Po_2 include barbiturates, granulocyte-macrophage colony-stimulating factor, isoproterenol, and meperidine.
- Samples for blood gases are obtained by arterial puncture, which carries a risk of bleeding, especially in patients who have bleeding disorders or are taking anticoagulants or other blood thinning medications.
- Recent blood transfusion may produce misleading values.
- Specimens with extremely elevated white blood cell counts will undergo misleading decreases in pH resulting from cellular metabolism, if transport to the laboratory is delayed.
- Specimens collected soon after a change in inspired oxygen has occurred will not accurately reflect the patient's oxygenation status.
- Specimens collected within 20 to 30 min of respiratory passage suctioning or other respiratory therapy will not be accurate.
- Excessive differences in actual body temperature relative to normal body temperature will not be reflected in the results. Temperature affects the amount of gas in solution. Blood gas analyzers measure samples at 37°C (98.6°F); therefore, if the patient is hyperthermic or hypothermic, it is important to notify the laboratory of the patient's actual body temperature at the time the specimen was collected. Fever will increase actual Po_2 and Pco_2 values; therefore, the uncorrected values measured at 37°C will be falsely decreased. Hypothermia decreases actual Po_2 and Pco_2 values; therefore, the uncorrected values measured at 37°C will be falsely increased.
- A falsely increased O_2 saturation may occur because of elevated levels of carbon monoxide in the blood.
- O_2 saturation is a calculated parameter based on an assumption of 100% hemoglobin A. Values may be misleading when hemoglobin variants with different oxygen dissociation curves are present. Hemoglobin S will cause a shift to the right, indicating decreased oxygen binding. Fetal hemoglobin and methemoglobin will cause a shift to the left, indicating increased oxygen binding.
- Excessive amounts of heparin in the sample may falsely decrease pH, Pco_2, and Po_2.
- Citrates should never be used as an anticoagulant in evacuated collection tubes for venous blood gas determinations because citrates will cause a marked analytic decrease in pH.
- Air bubbles or blood clots in the specimen are cause for rejection. Air bubbles in the specimen can falsely elevate or decrease the results depending on the patient's blood gas status. If an evacuated tube is used for venous blood gas specimen collection, the tube must be removed from the needle before the needle is withdrawn from the arm or else the sample will be contaminated with room air.

B

- Specimens should be placed in ice slurry immediately after collection because blood cells continue to carry out metabolic processes in the specimen after it has been removed from the patient. These natural life processes can affect pH, Po_2, Pco_2, and the other calculated values in a short period of time. The cold temperature provided by the ice slurry will slow down, but not completely stop, metabolic changes occurring in the sample over time. Iced specimens not analyzed within 60 min of collection should be rejected for analysis. Electrolyte analysis from iced specimens should be carried out within 30 min of collection to avoid falsely elevated potassium values.

B

NURSING IMPLICATIONS AND PROCEDURE

POTENTIAL NURSING PROBLEMS:

Problem	Signs & Symptoms	Interventions
Gas exchange ***(related to altered alveolar and capillary exchange; ventilation-perfusion mismatch; compromised oxygen supply; inadequate oxygen-carrying capacity of the blood)***	Confusion; restlessness; hypoxia; irritability; shortness of breath; altered blood gases; orthopnea; cyanosis; increased heart rate, respiratory rate; use of respiratory accessory muscles; elevated blood pressure	Auscultate and trend breath sounds (adventitious breath sound); assess respiratory rate, rhythm, depth, and accessory muscle use; assess for symptoms of infection, atelectasis, consolidation, and pleural effusion; assess for restlessness, dizziness, lethargy, disorientation, and confusion; monitor and trend Hgb; monitor chest x-ray reports; use pulse oximetry to monitor oxygenation; administer oxygen as ordered; collaborate with HCP to consider intubation and/or mechanical ventilation; place the head of the bed in high Fowler's position; administer diuretics, vasodilators as ordered; monitor arterial blood gas results
Tissue perfusion ***(related to compromised cardiac contractility; interrupted***	Hypotension; dizziness; cool extremities; capillary refill greater than 3 sec; weak pedal pulses; altered level of consciousness;	Monitor blood pressure (orthostatic); assess for dizziness; check skin temperature for warmth; assess capillary refill; assess pedal pulses; monitor

Problem	Signs & Symptoms	Interventions
blood flow; inadequate oxygen transportation; decreased Hgb; hypoventilation; hypovolemia)	weak or absent peripheral pulses; compromised sensation; poor healing; cool, clammy skin	level of consciousness; administer prescribed intravenous fluids; administer prescribed vasodilator, antiplatelet, anticoagulant, and inotropic drugs; administer oxygen as required
Breathing ***(related to inflammation; viral or bacterial infection; muscular impairment; tracheal or bronchial obstruction; compromised neuromuscular function; spinal cord injury)***	Shortness of breath, rapid breathing, slow breathing, nasal flare; use of accessory muscles; changes in respiratory effort and depth; cyanosis; pursed lip breathing; bending forward to breathe easier	Assess respiratory rate, rhythm, and depth; assess for use of accessory muscles; monitor for nasal flare with ventilation; assess for adventitious breath sounds; monitor for anxiety; monitor and trend blood gas results; pulse oximetry to monitor and trend oxygenation; administer of prescribed oxygen; administer of ordered antibiotics or antivirals; discuss positions that will improve ventilation and oxygenation; pace activities to match patient energy stores; consider future need for mechanical ventilation
Cardiac output ***(related to altered ventricular filling; impaired contractility; increased afterload; altered conductivity; deceased oxygenation; cardiac disease)***	Hypotension; increased heart rate; decreased cardiac output; decreased oxygen saturation; decreased peripheral pulses; decreased urinary output; cool, clammy skin; tachypnea; dyspnea; edema; altered level of consciousness; abnormal heart sounds; crackles in lungs; decreased activity tolerance; weight gain; fatigue; hypoxia; deceased ejection fraction (less than 55%)	Assess peripheral pulses and capillary refill; monitor blood pressure and check for orthostatic changes; assess respiratory rate, breath sounds, and orthopnea; assess skin color and temperature; assess level of consciousness; monitor urinary output; use pulse oximetry to monitor oxygenation; monitor sodium and potassium levels; monitor BNP levels; administer ordered ACE inhibitors, antidysrhythmics; diuretics, vasodilators, inotropics; provide oxygen administration

B

PRETEST:

- Positively identify the patient using at least two person-specific identifiers before services, treatments, or procedures are performed.
- ***Patient Teaching:*** Inform the patient this test can assist in assessing blood oxygen balance and oxygenation level.
- Obtain a history of the patient's health concerns, symptoms, surgical procedures, and results of previously performed laboratory and diagnostic studies. Include a list of known allergens, especially allergies or sensitivities to latex and anesthetics.
- Note any recent procedures that can interfere with test results.
- Obtain a list of the patient's current medications, including over-the-counter medications, dietary supplements, anticoagulants, aspirin and other salicylates (see Effects of Natural Products on Laboratory Values online at Davis*Plus*). Such products should be discontinued by medical direction for the appropriate number of days prior to a surgical procedure. Note the last time and dose of medication taken.
- Record the patient's temperature.
- Indicate the type of oxygen, mode of oxygen delivery, and delivery rate as part of the test requisition process. Wait 30 min after a change in type or mode of oxygen delivery or rate for specimen collection.
- Review the procedure with the patient and advise rest for 30 min before specimen collection. Explain to the patient that an arterial puncture may be painful. The site may be anesthetized with 1% to 2% lidocaine before puncture. Inform the patient that specimen collection and postprocedure care of the puncture site usually take 10 to 15 min. The person collecting the specimen should be notified beforehand if the patient is receiving anticoagulant therapy or taking aspirin or other natural products that may prolong bleeding from the puncture site.
- ✹ If the sample is to be collected by radial artery puncture, perform an Allen test before puncture to ensure that the patient has adequate collateral circulation to the hand if thrombosis of the radial artery occurs after arterial puncture. The modified Allen test is performed as follows: Extend the patient's wrist over a rolled towel. Ask the patient to make a fist with the hand extended over the towel. Use the second and third fingers to locate the pulses of the ulnar and radial arteries on the palmar surface of the wrist. (The thumb should not be used to locate these arteries because it has a pulse.) Compress both arteries and ask the patient to open and close the fist several times until the palm turns pale. Release pressure on the ulnar artery only. Color should return to the palm within 5 sec if the ulnar artery is functioning. This is a positive Allen test, and blood gases may be drawn from the radial artery site. The Allen test should then be performed on the opposite hand. The hand to which color is restored fastest has better circulation and should be selected for specimen collection.
- ***Sensitivity to social and cultural issues,*** as well as concern for modesty, is important in providing psychological support before, during, and after the procedure.
- Note that there are no food, fluid, or medication restrictions unless by medical direction.
- Prepare an ice slurry in a cup or plastic bag to have ready for immediate transport of the specimen to the laboratory.

INTRATEST:

Potential Complications: Bleeding, pain, hematoma

- Avoid the use of equipment containing latex if the patient has a history of allergic reaction to latex.
- Instruct the patient to cooperate fully and to follow directions. Direct the patient to breathe normally and to avoid unnecessary movement.
- Observe standard precautions, and follow the general guidelines

in Patient Preparation and Specimen Collection online at Davis*Plus*. Positively identify the patient, and label the appropriate specimen container with the corresponding patient demographics, initials of the person collecting the specimen, date, and time of collection. Perform an arterial puncture.

Arterial

- Perform an arterial puncture and collect the specimen in an air-free heparinized syringe. There is no demonstrable difference in results between samples collected in plastic syringes and samples collected in glass syringes. It is very important that no room air be introduced into the collection container because the gases in the room and in the sample will begin equilibrating immediately. The end of the syringe must be stoppered immediately after the needle is withdrawn and removed. Apply a pressure dressing over the puncture site. Samples should be mixed by gently rolling the syringe to ensure proper mixing of the heparin with the sample, which prevents the formation of small clots leading to rejection of the sample. The tightly capped sample should be placed in an ice slurry immediately after collection. Information on the specimen label should be protected from water in the ice slurry by first placing the specimen in a protective plastic bag. Promptly transport the specimen to the laboratory for processing and analysis.

Venous

- Central venous blood is collected in a heparinized syringe.
- Venous blood is collected percutaneously by venipuncture in a 5-mL green-top (heparin) tube (for adult patients) or a heparinized Microtainer (for pediatric patients). The vacuum collection tube must be removed from the needle before the needle is removed from the patient's arm. Apply a pressure dressing over the puncture site. Samples should be mixed by gently rolling the syringe to ensure proper mixing of the heparin with the sample, which prevents the formation of small clots leading to rejection of the sample. The tightly capped sample should be placed in an ice slurry immediately after collection. Information on the specimen label should be protected from water in the ice slurry by first placing the specimen in a protective plastic bag. Promptly transport the specimen to the laboratory for processing and analysis.

Capillary

- Perform a capillary puncture and collect the specimen in two 250-μL heparinized capillaries (scalp or heel for neonatal patients) or a heparinized Microtainer (for pediatric patients). Observe standard precautions, and follow the general guidelines in Patient Preparation and Specimen Collection online at Davis*Plus*. The capillary tubes should be filled as much as possible and capped on both ends. Some hospitals recommend that metal "fleas" be added to the capillary tube before the ends are capped. During transport, a magnet can be moved up and down the outside of the capillary tube to facilitate mixing and prevent the formation of clots, which would cause rejection of the sample. It is important to inform the laboratory or respiratory therapy staff of the number of fleas used so the fleas can be accounted for and removed before the sample is introduced into the blood gas analyzers. Fleas left in the sample may damage the blood gas equipment if allowed to enter the analyzer. Microtainer samples should be mixed by gently rolling the capillary tube to ensure proper mixing of the heparin with the sample, which prevents the formation of small clots leading to rejection of the sample. Promptly transport the specimen to the laboratory for processing and analysis.

Cord Blood

- The sample may be collected immediately after delivery from the clamped cord, using a heparinized syringe. The tightly capped sample should be placed in an ice slurry immediately after collection. Information on the specimen label should be protected from water in the ice slurry by first placing the specimen in a protective plastic bag. Promptly transport the specimen to the laboratory for processing and analysis.

Scalp Sample

- Samples for scalp pH may be collected anaerobically before delivery in special scalp-sample collection capillaries and transported immediately to the laboratory for analysis. The procedure takes approximately 5 min. Place the patient on her back with her feet in stirrups. The cervix must be dilated at least 3 to 4 cm. A plastic cone is placed in the vagina and fit snugly against the scalp of the fetus. The cone provides access for visualization using an endoscope and to cleanse the site. The site is pierced with a sharp blade. Containment of the blood droplet can be aided by smearing a small amount of silicone cream on the fetal skin site. The blood sample is collected in a thin, heparinized tube. Some hospitals recommend that small metal fleas be added to the scalp tube before the ends are capped. See preceding section on capillary collection for discussion of fleas.

POST-TEST:

- Inform the patient that a report of the results will be made available to the requesting HCP, who will discuss the results with the patient.
- Apply pressure to the puncture site for at least 5 min in the unanticoagulated patient and for at least 15 min in the case of a patient receiving anticoagulant therapy. Observe/assess puncture site for bleeding or hematoma formation. Apply pressure bandage.
- Observe/assess the patient for signs or symptoms of respiratory acidosis, such as dyspnea, headache, tachycardia, pallor, diaphoresis, apprehension, drowsiness, coma, hypertension, or disorientation.
- Teach the patient breathing exercises to assist with the appropriate exchange of oxygen and carbon dioxide.
- Administer oxygen, if appropriate.
- Teach the patient how to properly use the incentive spirometer device or mininebulizer if ordered.
- Observe/assess the patient for signs or symptoms of respiratory alkalosis, such as tachypnea, restlessness, agitation, tetany, numbness, seizures, muscle cramps, dizziness, or tingling fingertips.
- Instruct the patient to breathe deeply and slowly; performing this type of breathing exercise into a paper bag decreases hyperventilation and quickly helps the patient's breathing return to normal.
- Observe/assess the patient for signs or symptoms of metabolic acidosis, such as rapid breathing, flushed skin, nausea, vomiting, dysrhythmias, coma, hypotension, hyperventilation, and restlessness.
- Observe/assess the patient for signs or symptoms of metabolic alkalosis, such as shallow breathing, weakness, dysrhythmias, tetany, hypokalemia, hyperactive reflexes, and excessive vomiting.
- ***Nutritional Considerations:*** Abnormal blood gas values may be associated with diseases of the respiratory system. Malnutrition is commonly seen in patients with severe respiratory disease for reasons including fatigue, lack of appetite, and gastrointestinal distress. Research has estimated that the daily caloric intake required for respiration of patients with COPD is 10 times higher than that of normal individuals. Inadequate nutrition can result in hypophosphatemia, especially in the respirator-dependent patient. During periods of starvation, phosphorus leaves the intracellular space and moves outside the tissue, resulting in dangerously decreased phosphorus levels. Adequate intake of vitamins A and C is also important to prevent pulmonary infection

and to decrease the extent of lung tissue damage. The importance of following the prescribed diet should be stressed to the patient and/or caregiver.
- Water balance needs to be closely monitored in COPD patients. Fluid retention can lead to pulmonary edema.
- Depending on the results of this procedure, additional testing may be performed to evaluate or monitor progression of the disease process and determine the need for a change in therapy. Evaluate test results in relation to the patient's symptoms and other tests performed.

Patient Education:
- Reinforce information given by the patient's HCP regarding further testing, treatment, or referral to another HCP.
- Answer any questions or address any concerns voiced by the patient or family.
- Teach the patient cough and breathing techniques with splinting to improve ventilation.
- Teach the patient to pace activities to avoid becoming short of breath.
- Teach the patent the appropriate use of oxygen therapy.

Expected Patient Outcomes:

Understanding
- The patient and family state that additional diagnostic studies may need to be completed to identify the underlying cause of the altered blood gas results.
- The patient and family state that oxygen therapy can improve blood oxygen levels.

Ability
- The patient demonstrates proficiency in the self-administration of medication to treat the underlying cause of the altered blood gas results.
- The patient demonstrates the ability to position himself or herself in an upright position to improve oxygenation.

Response
- The patient and family comply with the request to change position every 2 hr to decrease the risk of atelectasis.
- The patient and family comply with the request to use ordered oxygen to support and improve oxygenation.

RELATED STUDIES:
- Related tests include α_1-AT, anion gap, arterial/alveolar oxygen ratio, biopsy lung, bronchoscopy, carboxyhemoglobin, chest x-ray, chloride sweat, CBC hemoglobin, CBC WBC and diff, culture and smear for mycobacteria, culture bacterial sputum, culture viral, cytology sputum, electrolytes, Gram stain, IgE, lactic acid, lung perfusion scan, lung ventilation scan, MRI venography, osmolality, phosphorus, plethysmography, pleural fluid analysis, pulse oximetry, PFT, and TB skin tests.
- Refer to the Cardiovascular, Genitourinary, and Respiratory systems tables online at Davis*Plus* for related tests by body system.

Blood Groups and Antibodies

SYNONYM/ACRONYM: ABO group and Rh typing, blood group antibodies, type and screen, type and crossmatch.

COMMON USE: To identify ABO blood group and Rh type, typically for prenatal screen and transfusion purposes. These tests are also used to help establish compatibility for cellular therapy and solid organ transplantation (in addition to human leukocyte antigen [HLA] and HLA antibody typing).

SPECIMEN: Serum collected in a red-top tube or whole blood collected in a lavender-top (EDTA) tube.

NORMAL FINDINGS: (Method: FDA ✱ -approved reagents with glass slides, glass tubes, gel, or automated systems) Compatibility (no clumping or hemolysis).

DESCRIPTION: Blood typing is a series of tests that include the ABO and Rh blood-group system performed to detect surface antigens on red blood cells (RBCs) by an agglutination test and compatibility tests to determine antibodies against these antigens. The major antigens in the ABO system are A and B, although AB and O are also common phenotypes. The patient with A antigens has group A blood; the patient with B antigens has group B blood. The patient with both A and B antigens has group AB blood (universal recipient); the patient with neither A nor B antigens has group O blood (universal donor). Blood group and type is genetically determined. After 6 mo of age, individuals develop serum antibodies that react with A or B antigen absent from their own RBCs. These are called *anti-A* and *anti-B* antibodies.

In ABO blood typing, the patient's RBCs mix with anti-A and anti-B sera, a process known as *forward grouping*. The process then reverses, and the patient's serum mixes with type A and B cells in *reverse grouping*.

Generally, only blood with the same ABO group and Rh type as the recipient is transfused because the anti-A and anti-B antibodies are strong agglutinins that cause a rapid, complement-mediated destruction of incompatible cells. However, blood donations have decreased nationwide, creating shortages in the available supply. Safe substitutions with blood of a different group and/or Rh type may occur depending on the inventory of available units. Many laboratories require consultation with the requesting health-care provider (HCP) prior to issuing Rh-positive units to an Rh-negative individual.

ABO and Rh testing is also performed as a prenatal screen in pregnant women to identify the risk of hemolytic disease of the newborn. Although most of the anti-A and anti-B activity resides in the immunoglobulin M (IgM) class of immunoglobulins, some activity rests with immunoglobulin G (IgG). Anti-A and anti-B antibodies of the IgG class coat the RBCs without immediately affecting their viability and can readily cross the placenta, resulting in hemolytic disease of the newborn. Individuals with type O blood frequently have more IgG anti-A and anti-B than other people; thus, ABO hemolytic disease of the newborn will affect infants of type O mothers almost exclusively (unless the newborn is also type O).

Major antigens of the Rh system are D (or Rh_o), C, E, c, and e. Individuals whose RBCs possess D antigen are called Rh-positive; those who lack D antigen are called Rh-negative, no matter what other Rh antigens are present. Individuals who are Rh-negative produce anti-D antibodies when exposed to Rh-positive cells by either transfusions or pregnancy. These anti-D antibodies cross the placenta to the fetus and can cause hemolytic disease of the newborn or transfusion reactions if Rh-positive blood is administered.

The type and screen (T&S) procedure is performed to determine the ABO/Rh and identify any antibodies that may react with transfused blood products. The T&S may take from 30 to 45 min or longer to complete depending on whether unexpected or unusual antibodies are detected. Every unit of product must be crossmatched against the intended recipient's serum and red blood cells for compatibility before transfusion. Knowing the ABO/Rh and antibody status saves time when the patient's sample is crossmatched against units of donated blood products. There are three crossmatch procedures. If no antibodies are identified in the T&S, it is permissible to use either an immediate spin crossmatch or an electronic crossmatch, either of which may take 5 to 10 min to complete. If antibodies are detected, the antiglobulin crossmatch procedure is performed, along with antibody identification testing, or the process is repeated, beginning with the selection of other units for compatibility testing. Typically, specimens for T&S can be held for 72 hr from the time of collection for use in future crossmatch procedures. This time frame may be extended for up to 14 days for patients with a reliably known history of no prior transfusions or pregnancy within the previous 3 mo. Donated blood products are tested for ABO group, Rh type, unexpected RBC antibodies, and transmissible infectious diseases that include the presence of hepatitis B core antibody (antibodies directed against the hepatitis B core antigen), hepatitis B surface antigen, hepatitis B virus (viral DNA by nucleic acid testing [NAT]), hepatitis C antibody (viral RNA by NAT), HTLV I and II antibody, HIV 1 (viral RNA by NAT) and 2 antibody, and syphilis. Additional testing may be performed in cases of specific need and include cytomegalovirus antibody and IgA deficiency. Additional testing may also be performed for the presence of West Nile virus (viral RNA by NAT) or antibodies to *Trypanosoma cruzi* or Chagas disease when increased risk for transmission from a particular donor is suspected. All donated units receiving additional testing will be labelled with the results (positive or negative). Testing for emerging transmissible pathogens (e.g., Zika virus) is not always available when the pathogens are identified. Therefore, blood component collection facilities implement a variety of strategies to help ensure the safety of the blood supply. Recommendations may include the addition of specific questions to the donor history questionnaire to evaluate risk of infection, implementation of a waiting period prior to donation, or deferral of donation. Decisions regarding donor eligibility are based on criteria and recommendations developed by national (e.g., AABB, FDA, CDC) 🍁 and international scientific communities (e.g., World Health Organization). Educational material is also available at collection facilities for potential donors to review and determine whether they should self-defer from donation.

Febrile nonhemolytic reaction and urticarial/allergic reaction are the two most common types of reactions that occur in blood product transfusions. Many institutions have a policy that provides for premedication with acetaminophen and diphenhydramine ✤ to avoid initiation of mild transfusion reactions, where appropriate.

Many of the same tests used to determine the compatibility and safety of blood products (ABO, Rh, antibody screen, and infectious disease markers) are also used to establish a safe, compatible transplantation between donors and recipients of cellular therapy and solid organs. Cellular therapy uses human cells, such as bone marrow or stem cells, from a donated source to replace or repair damaged cells in a human recipient; solid organ transplantation serves a similar purpose, most commonly with heart, kidney, liver, lungs, pancreas, and skin. Tissue typing, also called *HLA typing,* is additional testing performed to match a compatible donor and recipient for cellular therapy or solid organ transplantation. Blood cell antigens and tissue type are inherited, half from each of the biological parents. The individual antigens and tissue surface antigen patterns are specific for each person and are unique except in the case of identical twins. HLA typing is also performed to identify antibodies the recipient may develop against the donor's foreign tissue cells in order to prevent graft versus host rejection. Although it is possible to find a compatible, nonrelated, donor-recipient pair in the general population, donor compatibility is best matched to a recipient who shares some of the same genetic markers—in other words, a person who is a blood relative.

This procedure is contraindicated for: N/A

INDICATIONS

- Determine ABO and Rh compatibility of donor and recipient before transfusion (type and screen or crossmatch).
- Determine anti-D antibody titer of Rh-negative mothers after sensitization by pregnancy with an Rh-positive fetus.
- Determine the need for a microdose of immunosuppressive therapy (e.g., with Rh(D) immune globulin RhoGAM intramuscular (IM) or Rhophylac IM or intravenous) during the first 12 wk of gestation or a standard dose after 12 wk of gestation for complications such as abortion, miscarriage, vaginal hemorrhage, ectopic pregnancy, or abdominal trauma.
- Determine Rh blood type and perform antibody screen of prenatal patients on initial visit to determine maternal Rh type and to indicate whether maternal RBCs have been sensitized by any antibodies known to cause hemolytic disease of the newborn, especially anti-D antibody. Rh blood type, antibody screen, and antibody titration (if an antibody has been identified) will be rechecked at 28 wk of gestation and prior to injection of prophylactic standard dose of RhoGAM for Rh-negative mothers. These tests will also be repeated after delivery of an Rh-positive fetus to an Rh-negative mother and prior to injection of prophylactic standard dose of RhoGAM (if maternal Rh-negative blood has not been previously sensitized with Rh-positive cells resulting in a positive anti-D antibody titer). A postpartum blood sample must be evaluated for fetal-maternal bleed on all Rh-negative

mothers to determine the need for additional doses of Rh immune globulin. One in 300 cases will demonstrate hemorrhage greater than 15 mL of blood and require additional RhoGAM.
- Identify donor ABO and Rh blood type for stored blood.
- Identify maternal and infant ABO and Rh blood types to predict risk of hemolytic disease of the newborn.
- Identify the patient's ABO and Rh blood type, especially before a procedure in which blood loss is a threat or blood replacement may be needed.
- Identify any unusual transfusion related antibodies in the patient's blood, especially before a procedure in which blood replacement may be needed.

POTENTIAL MEDICAL DIAGNOSIS

- ***Agglutination is graded from 1+ to 4+ in manual testing systems; with 4+ being the strongest degree of agglutination. Automated testing systems are capable of reporting 1+ to 4+ graded results, or providing images of the tested material so laboratory professionals can interpret the results, or providing computer assisted interpretation of the test results as positive or negative findings.***
- ABO system: A, B, AB, or O specific to person
- Rh system: positive or negative specific to person
- Crossmatching: compatibility between donor and recipient
- Incompatibility indicated by clumping (agglutination) of red blood cells

Group and Type	Incidence (%)	Alternative Transfusion Group and Type of Packed Cell Units in Order of Preference If Patient's Own Group and Type Not Available
O positive	37.4	O negative
O negative	6.6	O positive*
A positive	35.7	A negative, O positive, O negative
A negative	6.3	O negative, A positive,* **O positive***
B positive	8.5	B negative, O positive, O negative
B negative	1.5	O negative, B positive,* **O positive***
AB positive	3.4	AB negative, A positive, B positive, A negative, B negative, O positive, O negative
AB negative	0.6	A negative, B negative, O negative, AB positive,* **A positive,* B positive,* O positive***
Rh Type		
Rh positive	85–90	
Rh negative	10–15	

*If blood units of exact match to the patient's group and type are not available, a switch in ABO blood group is preferable to a change in Rh type. However, in extreme circumstances, Rh-positive blood can be issued to an Rh-negative recipient. It is very likely that the recipient will develop antibodies as the result of receiving Rh-positive red blood cells. Rh antibodies are highly immunogenic, and, once the antibodies are developed, the recipient can only receive Rh-negative blood for subsequent red blood cell transfusion.

CRITICAL FINDINGS:

Note and immediately report to the requesting health-care provider (HCP) any critical findings and any signs and symptoms associated with a blood transfusion reaction. A listing of these

B

findings varies among facilities. Timely notification of a critical finding for laboratory or diagnostic studies is a role expectation of the professional nurse. The notification processes vary among facilities. Upon receipt of the critical finding, the information should be read back to the caller to verify accuracy.

Signs and symptoms of blood transfusion reaction range from mildly febrile to anaphylactic and may include chills, dyspnea, fever, headache, nausea, vomiting, palpitations and tachycardia, chest or back pain, apprehension, flushing, hives, angioedema, diarrhea, hypotension, oliguria, hemoglobinuria, acute kidney injury, sepsis, shock, and jaundice. Complications from disseminated intravascular coagulation (DIC) may also occur.

Possible interventions in mildly febrile reactions include slowing the rate of infusion, then verifying and comparing patient identification, transfusion requisition, and blood bag label. The patient should be monitored closely for further development of signs and symptoms. Administration of epinephrine may be ordered.

Possible interventions in a more severe transfusion reaction may include immediate cessation of infusion, notification of the HCP, keeping the intravenous (IV) line open with saline or lactated Ringer's solution, collection of red- and lavender-top tubes for post-transfusion work-up, collection of urine, monitoring vital signs every 5 min, ordering additional testing if DIC is suspected, maintaining patent airway and blood pressure, and administering mannitol. See Transfusion Reactions: Laboratory Findings and Potential online at Davis*Plus* for a more detailed description of transfusion reactions and potential nursing interventions.

INTERFERING FACTORS

- Drugs and other substances, including cephalexin, levodopa, methyldopa, and methyldopate hydrochloride, may cause a false-positive result in Rh typing and in antibody screens.
- Recent administration of blood, blood products, dextran, or IV contrast medium causes cellular aggregation resembling agglutination in ABO typing.
- Contrast material such as iodine, barium, and gadolinium may interfere with testing.
- Abnormal proteins, cold agglutinins, and bacteremia may interfere with testing.
- Testing does not detect every antibody and may miss the presence of a weak antibody.
- History of bone marrow transplant, cancer, or leukemia may cause discrepancy in ABO typing.

NURSING IMPLICATIONS AND PROCEDURE

POTENTIAL NURSING PROBLEMS:

Problem	Signs & Symptoms	Interventions
Injury risk ***(related to possible transfusion reaction secondary to protein***	Fever, chills, rash, itching, decreased blood flow to organs, acute kidney injury	Take vital signs prior to transfusion; take vital signs within 15 min after the transfusion has started and assess for fever and chills; monitor for fever, chills,

B

Problem	Signs & Symptoms	Interventions
hypersensitivity; WBC febrile reaction; hemolytic incompatibility)		itching, and rash during transfusion; administer ordered premedication to prevent fever and itching; consider the use of a leukocyte filter; follow standard hospital procedure to ensure a correct match prior to transfusion; immediately stop transfusion if reaction is noted; follow institutional process for assessing for transfusion reaction; collect urine and blood sample for analysis per institutional policy
Gas exchange ***(related to insufficient oxygen supply secondary to blood loss)***	Decreased activity tolerance; increased shortness of breath with activity; weakness; orthopnea; cyanosis; cough; increased heart rate; weight gain; edema in the lower extremities; weakness; increased respiratory rate; use of respiratory accessory muscles	Auscultate and trend breath sounds; perform pulse oximetry to monitor oxygenation; administer oxygen as ordered; collaborate with HCP to consider intubation and/or mechanical ventilation; place the head of the bed in high Fowler's position; administer diuretics, vasodilators as ordered; administer ordered blood or blood products; monitor Hgb/Hct
Cardiac output ***(related to inadequate circulating blood supply secondary to blood loss)***	Decreased peripheral pulses; decreased urinary output; cool, clammy skin; tachypnea; dyspnea; edema; altered level of consciousness; abnormal heart sounds; crackles in lungs; decreased activity tolerance; weight gain; fatigue; hypoxia	Assess peripheral pulses and capillary refill; monitor blood pressure and check for orthostatic changes; assess respiratory rate, breath sounds, and orthopnea; assess skin color and temperature; assess level of consciousness; monitor urinary output; use pulse oximetry to monitor oxygenation; monitor sodium and potassium levels; monitor Hgb/Hct; administer ordered oxygen

(table continues on page 310)

B

Problem	Signs & Symptoms	Interventions
Fluid volume ***(related to increased circulatory volume secondary to blood transfusion and normal saline IV fluids)***	**Excess:** Edema, shortness of breath, increased weight, ascites, rales, rhonchi, and diluted laboratory values	Monitor transfusion rate, transfuse according to standards of care; monitor respiratory status with establishment of baseline assessment data; administer ordered diuretic

PRETEST:

- Positively identify the patient using at least two person-specific identifiers before services, treatments, or procedures are performed.
- ***Patient Teaching:*** Inform the patient this test can assist in identification of blood type.
- Obtain a history of the patient's health concerns, symptoms, surgical procedures, and results of previously performed laboratory and diagnostic studies. Include a list of known allergens, especially allergies or sensitivities to latex.
- Note any recent or past procedures, especially blood or blood product transfusion or bone marrow transplantation, that could complicate or interfere with test results.
- Obtain a list of the patient's current medications, including over-the-counter medications and dietary supplements (see Effects of Natural Products on Laboratory Values online at Davis*Plus*).
- Review the procedure with the patient. Inform the patient that specimen collection takes approximately 5 to 10 min. Address concerns about pain and explain that there may be some discomfort during the venipuncture.
- ***Sensitivity to social and cultural issues,*** as well as concern for modesty, is important in providing psychological support before, during, and after the procedure.
- Note that there are no food, fluid, or medication restrictions unless by medical direction.
- *Make sure a written and informed consent has been signed prior to any transfusion blood products.*

INTRATEST:

Potential Complications:

A transfusion reaction may occur in some patients. A transfusion reaction is also a critical finding. Signs, symptoms, and possible interventions are described in the Critical Findings section.

- Avoid the use of equipment containing latex if the patient has a history of allergic reaction to latex.
- Instruct the patient to cooperate fully and to follow directions. Direct the patient to breathe normally and to avoid unnecessary movement.
- Observe standard precautions, and follow the general guidelines in Patient Preparation and Specimen Collection online at Davis*Plus*. Positively identify the patient, and label the appropriate specimen container with the corresponding patient demographics, initials of the person collecting the specimen, date, and time of collection. Perform a venipuncture.
- Although correct patient identification is important for test specimens, it is crucial when blood is collected for type and crossmatch because clerical error is the most frequent cause of life-threatening ABO incompatibility. Therefore, additional requirements are necessary, including the verification of two unique identifiers that could include any two unique patient

demographics such as name, date of birth, Social Security number, hospital number, date, or blood bank number on requisition and specimen labels; completing and applying a wristband on the arm with the same information; and placing labels with the same information and blood bank number on blood sample tubes.

- Remove the needle and apply direct pressure with dry gauze to stop bleeding. Observe/assess venipuncture site for bleeding or hematoma formation and secure gauze with adhesive bandage.
- Promptly transport the specimen to the laboratory for processing and analysis.

POST-TEST:

- Inform the patient that a report of the results will be made available to the requesting HCP, who will discuss the results with the patient.
- Depending on the results of this procedure, additional testing may be performed to evaluate or monitor progression of the disease process and determine the need for a change in therapy. Evaluate test results in relation to the patient's symptoms and other tests performed.

Patient Education:

- Inform the patient of ABO blood and Rh type, and advise him or her to record the information on a card or other document routinely carried.
- Inform women who are Rh-negative to inform the HCP of their Rh-negative status if they become pregnant or need a transfusion.
- Reinforce information given by the patient's HCP regarding further testing, treatment, or referral to another HCP.
- Answer any questions or address any concerns voiced by the patient or family.

Expected Patient Outcomes:

Understanding

- The patient and family verbalize the risks and benefits of blood transfusion.
- The patient and family discuss possible transfusion alternatives other than donor blood.

Ability

- The patient and family identify transfusion reaction symptoms that should be immediately reported.
- The patient and family state that the purpose of the transfusion is to replace lost circulating blood stores.

Response

- The patient and family discuss and resolve anxiety related to blood transfusion.
- The patient and family voice any religious or cultural objections to the ordered transfusion.

RELATED STUDIES:

- Related tests include Coomb's antiglobulin, bilirubin, CBC, CBC hematocrit, CBC hemoglobin, CBC platelet count, CBC RBC count, cold agglutinin, FDP, fecal analysis, GI blood loss scan, haptoglobin, IgA, iron, Kleihauer-Betke, laparoscopy abdominal, Meckel's diverticulum scan, and UA.
- Refer to Transfusion Reactions: Laboratory Findings and Potential online at Davis*Plus* for further information regarding laboratory studies used in the investigation of transfusion reactions, findings, and potential nursing interventions associated with types of transfusion reactions.
- Refer to the Immune and Hematopoietic systems tables online at Davis*Plus* for related tests by body system.

Blood Pool Imaging

SYNONYM/ACRONYM: Cardiac blood pool scan, cardiac flow studies, ejection fraction study, gated cardiac scan, multigated acquisition (MUGA) scan, radionuclide ventriculogram, wall motion study.

Access Canadian content on Fast Find: Lab and Dx at davispl.us/vanleeuwen7

COMMON USE: To evaluate blood flow through the ventricles of the heart.

AREA OF APPLICATION: Heart.

B

DESCRIPTION: Two main types of cardiac blood scans are performed on adults and children. They are used to evaluate the direction of blood flow in the major blood vessels, to provide information regarding patency of vessels after vascular surgery, and to evaluate the ejection fraction of the right and left ventricles. First-pass or shunt imaging scans are commonly performed on pediatric patients to measure left-to-right shunts and assess for congenital heart defects. MUGA blood pool imaging, also known as *radionuclide ventriculogram (RVG),* provides information about cardiac function such as ejection fraction, ventricular wall motion, ventricular dilation, stroke volume, and cardiac output. Heart shunt imaging is sometimes done in conjunction with a resting MUGA scan to obtain ejection fraction and assess regional wall motion.

The radionuclide is prepared by one of several in vitro or in vivo methods. One commonly used in vitro method of preparation is performed by adding a radioactive tracer, technetium-99m (Tc-99m), to a sample of the patient's blood and reinjecting the labelled blood. The in vivo method involves two steps: first an injection of stannous pyrophosphate (PyP), a "sticky" substance that adheres to the circulating RBCs, followed 20 min later by an injection of radioactive tracer that adheres to the PyP. The radionuclide is injected into a jugular or antecubital vein. The ventricular blood pool can be imaged during the initial transit of a peripherally injected, intravenous bolus of radionuclide (first-pass technique) or when the radionuclide has reached equilibrium concentration. For multigated studies, the patient's heartbeat, as measured with an electrocardiogram (ECG), is synchronized to the gamma camera imager and computer and therefore termed *gated*.

MUGA scans can be performed with the heart at rest or additionally as part of a stress test. The MUGA procedure, performed with the heart in motion, is used to obtain multiple images of the heart in contraction and relaxation during an R-to-R cardiac cycle. The resulting images can be displayed in a cinematic mode to visualize cardiac function. They can also be compared to MUGA scans performed at rest. Repetitive data acquisitions are possible during graded levels of exercise, usually a bicycle ergometer or handgrip, to assess ventricular functional response to exercise. The MUGA scan can also be used to evaluate the effectiveness of sublingual nitroglycerin on ventricular function; nitroglycerin is a strong vasodilator used to treat angina.

A related cardiac nuclear study is the myocardial perfusion scan (MPS). The MPS evaluates myocardial tissue perfusion, as demonstrated by presence of the radionuclide in the myocardium, whereas the MUGA scan evaluates blood flow and the pumping action of the heart by following the movement of a radionuclide in the circulating blood.

This procedure is contraindicated for

- Patients who are pregnant or suspected of being pregnant, unless the potential benefits of a procedure using radiation far outweigh the risk of radiation exposure to the fetus and mother.
- Patients with anginal pain at rest or in patients with severe atherosclerotic coronary vessels; dipyridamole testing is not performed in these circumstances.
- Chemical stress with vasodilators in patients having asthma ***(because bronchospasm can occur).***

INDICATIONS

Adult

- Aid in the diagnosis of true or false ventricular aneurysms.
- Aid in the diagnosis of valvular heart disease and determining the optimal time for valve replacement surgery.
- Detect left-to-right shunts and determine pulmonary-to-systemic blood flow ratios.
- Determine cardiomyopathy.
- Determine drug cardiotoxicity to stop therapy before development of heart failure ***related to chemotherapy drugs or other medications known to cause cardiac damage.***
- Determine ischemic coronary artery disease.
- Differentiate between chronic obstructive pulmonary disease and left ventricular failure.
- Evaluate ventricular size, function, and wall motion after an acute episode or in chronic heart disease.
- Quantitate cardiac output by calculating global or regional ejection fraction.

Pediatric

- Detect left-to-right and right-to-left shunts; determine pulmonary-to-systemic blood flow ratios.
- Evaluate for cardiac dysfunction related to diagnosed or undiagnosed congenital heart defects (chambers, valves, or vessels).
- Quantitatively assess valvular regurgitation.

POTENTIAL MEDICAL DIAGNOSIS

Normal findings

- Normal wall motion, ejection fraction (55% to 70%), coronary blood flow, ventricular size and function, and symmetry in contractions of the left ventricle

Abnormal findings related to

Measurements of blood volume and flow are recorded as the concentration of radionuclide is detected by the imaging equipment. The measurements are used to indicate abnormalities identified in the ventricles during different periods of the cardiac cycle. The scan also provides moving images of the heart to assess abnormalities in the size and function of the heart.

- Abnormal wall motion (akinesia or dyskinesia)
- Cardiac hypertrophy
- Cardiac ischemia
- Heart failure
- Enlarged left ventricle
- Infarcted areas are akinetic
- Ischemic areas are hypokinetic

CRITICAL FINDINGS: N/A

INTERFERING FACTORS: N/A

Factors that may alter the results of the study

- Inability of the patient to cooperate or remain still during the procedure because of age, significant pain, or mental status.
- Metallic objects within the examination field (e.g., jewelry, body rings), which may inhibit organ

visualization and can produce unclear images.

Other considerations

- **Conditions such as chest wall trauma, cardiac trauma, angina that is difficult to control, significant cardiac dysrhythmias, or a recent cardioversion procedure may affect test results.**
- **Atrial fibrillation and extrasystoles invalidate the procedure.**
- **Suboptimal cardiac stress or patient exhaustion, preventing maximum heart rate testing, will affect results when the procedure is done in conjunction with exercise testing.**

B

NURSING IMPLICATIONS AND PROCEDURE

See Potential Nursing Problems on Fast Find at davispl.us/vanleeuwen7.

PRETEST:

- Positively identify the patient using at least two person-specific identifiers before services, treatments, or procedures are performed.
- *Patient Teaching:* Inform the patient this procedure can assist in assessing the pumping action of the heart.
- Obtain a history of the patient's health concerns, symptoms, surgical procedures, and results of previously performed laboratory and diagnostic studies. Include a list of known allergens, especially allergies or sensitivities to latex, anesthetics, sedatives, radionuclides, or medications used in the procedure.
- Note any recent procedures that can interfere with test results, including examinations using iodine-based contrast medium.
- Record the date of the last menstrual period and determine the possibility of pregnancy in perimenopausal women.
- Obtain a list of the patient's current medications, including over-the-counter medications and dietary supplements (see Effects of Natural Products on Laboratory Values online at Davis*Plus*).
- Review the procedure with the patient. Address concerns about pain related to the procedure and explain that some pain may be experienced during the test, or there may be moments of discomfort. Reassure the patient that the radionuclide poses no radioactive hazard and rarely produces adverse effects. Inform the patient that the procedure is performed in a nuclear medicine department by an HCP specializing in this procedure and takes approximately 60 min.
- *Sensitivity to social and cultural issues,* as well as concern for modesty, is important in providing psychological support before, during, and after the procedure.
- Explain that an intravenous (IV) line may be inserted to allow infusion of fluids such as normal saline, anesthetics, sedatives, radionuclides, medications used in the procedure, or emergency medications.
- Instruct the patient to wear walking shoes for the treadmill or bicycle exercise. Emphasize to the patient the importance of reporting fatigue, pain, or shortness of breath.
- Instruct the patient to remove external metallic objects from the area to be examined prior to the procedure.
- Instruct the patient to fast, restrict fluids (especially those containing caffeine), and abstain from the use of tobacco products for 4 hr prior to the procedure. Instruct the patient to withhold medications for 24 hr before the test as ordered by the HCP. Protocols may vary among facilities.
- *Make sure a written and informed consent has been signed prior to the procedure and before administering any medications.*

INTRATEST:

Potential Complications:

Although it is rare, there is the possibility of allergic reaction to the radionuclide. Have emergency equipment and medications readily available. If the patient has a history of allergic reactions to any substance or drug, administer ordered prophylactic steroids or antihistamines before the procedure.

Establishing an IV site and injection of radionuclides is an invasive procedure. Complications are rare but do include bleeding from the puncture site ***(related to a bleeding disorder, or the effects of natural products and medications with known anticoagulant, antiplatelet, or thrombolytic properties),*** hematoma ***(related to blood leakage into the tissue following needle insertion),*** infection ***(that might occur if bacteria from the skin surface is introduced at the puncture site),*** or nerve injury ***(that might occur if the needle strikes a nerve).***

- Observe standard precautions, and follow the general guidelines in Patient Preparation and Specimen Collection online at Davis*Plus*. Positively identify the patient.
- Ensure that the patient has complied with dietary and medication restrictions prior to the study, as instructed.
- Ensure that the patient has removed external metallic objects from the area to be examined prior to the procedure.
- Administer ordered prophylactic steroids or antihistamines before the procedure if the patient has a history of allergic reactions to any substance or drug.
- Avoid the use of equipment containing latex if the patient has a history of allergic reaction to latex.
- Have emergency equipment readily available.
- Record baseline vital signs and assess neurological status. Protocols may vary among facilities.
- Establish an IV fluid line for the injection of saline, anesthetics, sedatives, radionuclides, or emergency medications.
- Instruct the patient to cooperate fully and to follow directions. Instruct the patient to remain still throughout the procedure because movement produces unreliable results.
- The patient is placed at rest in the supine position on the scanning table.
- Expose the chest and attach the ECG leads. Record baseline readings.
- IV radionuclide is administered and the heart is scanned with images taken in various positions over the entire cardiac cycle.
- When the scan is to be done under exercise conditions, the patient is assisted onto the treadmill or bicycle ergometer and is exercised to a calculated 80% to 85% of the maximum heart rate as determined by the protocol selected. Images are done at each exercise level and begun immediately after injection of the radionuclide.
- If nitroglycerin is given, an HCP assessing the baseline MUGA scan injects the medication. Additional scans are repeated until blood pressure reaches the desired level.
- Patients who cannot exercise are given dipyridamole before the radionuclide is injected.
- Monitor the patient for complications related to the procedure (e.g., allergic reaction, anaphylaxis, bronchospasm).
- Remove the needle or catheter and apply a pressure dressing over the puncture site.
- Observe/assess the needle/catheter site for bleeding, hematoma formation, or inflammation.

POST-TEST:

- Inform the patient that a report of the results will be made available to the requesting HCP, who will discuss the results with the patient.
- Unless contraindicated, advise patient to drink increased amounts of fluids for 24 to 48 hr to eliminate the radionuclide from the body. Inform the patient that radionuclide is eliminated from the body within 6 to 24 hr.
- No other radionuclide tests should be scheduled for 24 to 48 hr after this procedure.
- Evaluate the patient's vital signs. Monitor vital signs and neurological

B

status every 15 min for 1 hr, then every 2 hr for 4 hr, and then as ordered by HCP. Monitor intake and output at least every 8 hr. Compare with baseline values. Protocols may vary among facilities.

- Instruct the patient to resume usual dietary, medication, and activity, as directed by the HCP.
- Observe for delayed allergic reactions, such as rash, urticaria, tachycardia, hyperpnea, hypertension, palpitations, nausea, or vomiting.
- Instruct the patient to immediately report symptoms such as fast heart rate, difficulty breathing, skin rash, itching, chest pain, persistent right shoulder pain, or abdominal pain. Immediately report symptoms to the appropriate HCP.
- Monitor ECG tracings and compare with baseline readings until stable.
- Observe/assess the needle/catheter site for bleeding, hematoma formation, or inflammation.
- Instruct the patient in the care and assessment of the injection site.
- If a woman who is breastfeeding must have a nuclear scan, she should not breastfeed the infant until the radionuclide has been eliminated. This could take as long as 3 days. She should be instructed to express the milk and discard it during the 3-day period to prevent cessation of milk production.
- Instruct the patient to immediately flush the toilet and to meticulously wash hands with soap and water after each voiding for 24 hr after the procedure.
- Instruct all caregivers to wear gloves when discarding urine for 24 hr after the procedure. Wash gloved hands with soap and water before removing gloves; then wash ungloved hands.
- Recognize anxiety related to test results, and be supportive of fear of shortened life expectancy. Discuss the implications of abnormal test results on the patient's lifestyle. Provide teaching and information regarding the clinical implications of the test results, as appropriate. Educate the patient regarding access to counseling services. Provide contact information, if desired, for the American Heart Association (www.americanheart.org) or the NHLBI (www.nhlbi.nih.gov) 🍁.
- Recognize anxiety related to test results, and be supportive of perceived loss of independent function. Discuss the implications of abnormal test results on the patient's lifestyle. Provide teaching and information regarding the clinical implications of the test results, as appropriate.
- Reinforce information given by the patient's HCP regarding further testing, treatment, or referral to another HCP. Answer any questions or address any concerns voiced by the patient or family.
- Depending on the results of this procedure, additional testing may be needed to evaluate and determine the need for a change in therapy or progression of the disease process. Evaluate test results in relation to the patient's symptoms and other tests performed.

Patient Education:

- Teach the patient basic pathophysiology of the pumping action of the heart in simple, understandable terms.
- Teach the patient about the recommended treatment and expected outcomes in relation to their cardiac status.

Expected Patient Outcomes:

Understanding

- The patient and family state the purpose of the medications that are being administered related to cardiac status.
- The patient and family describe the lifestyle changes that will need to be made to support positive cardiac health.

Ability

- The patient and family work collaboratively with a registered dietician to make heart healthy changes that are culturally congruent.
- The patient and family recognize the importance of cardiac rehabilitation and are able to identify their role in meeting therapeutic goals.

Response

- The patient and family are willing to make lifestyle changes that will support positive cardiac health.
- The patient and family agree to meet with a support group to decrease risk of depression.

RELATED STUDIES:

- Related tests include antidysrhythmic drugs, ANP, blood gases, BNP, calcium (total and ionized), culture viral, echocardiography, echocardiography transesophageal, ECG, exercise stress test, Holter monitor, magnesium, MRI chest, myocardial perfusion heart scan, myoglobin, pericardial fluid analysis, PET heart scan, potassium.
- Refer to the Cardiovascular System table online at Davis*Plus* for related tests by body system.

Bone Mineral Densitometry

SYNONYM/ACRONYM: BMD, DEXA, DXA, SXA, QCT, RA, ultrasound densitometry.

Dual-energy x-ray absorptiometry (DEXA, DXA): Two x-rays of different energy levels measure bone mineral density and predict risk of fracture.

Single-energy x-ray absorptiometry (SXA): A single-energy x-ray measures bone density at peripheral sites.

Quantitative computed tomography (QCT): QCT is used to examine the lumbar vertebrae. It measures trabecular and cortical bone density. Results are compared to a known standard. This test is the most expensive and involves the highest radiation dose of all techniques.

Radiographic absorptiometry (RA): A standard x-ray of the hand. Results are compared to a known standard.

Ultrasound densitometry: Studies bone mineral content in peripheral densitometry sites such as the heel or wrist. It is not as precise as x-ray techniques but is less expensive than other techniques.

COMMON USE: To evaluate bone density related to osteoporosis.

AREA OF APPLICATION: Lumbar spine, heel, hip, wrist, whole body.

DESCRIPTION: Bone mineral density (BMD) can be measured at any of several body sites, including the spine, hip, wrist, and heel. Equipment used to measure BMD include computed tomography (CT), radiographic absorptiometry, ultrasound, SXA, and most commonly, DEXA. The radiation exposure from SXA and DEXA machines is approximately one-tenth that of a standard chest x-ray.

Osteoporosis is a condition characterized by low BMD, which results in increased risk of fracture. The National Osteoporosis Foundation estimates that 4 to 6 million postmenopausal women in the United States have osteoporosis, and an additional 13 to 17 million (30%–50%) have low bone density at the hip. It is estimated that one of every two women will experience a fracture as a result of low bone mineral content in her lifetime. 🍁 The measurement of BMD gives the best indication of risk for a fracture. The lower the BMD, the

B

greater is the risk of fracture. The most common fractures are those of the hip, vertebrae, and distal forearm. Bone mineral loss is a disease of the entire skeleton and is not restricted to the areas listed. The effect of the fractures has a wide range, from complete recovery to chronic pain, disability, and possible death.

The BMD values measured by the various techniques cannot be directly compared. Therefore, they are stated in terms of standard deviation (SD) units. The patient's T-score is the number of SD units above or below the average BMD in young adults. A Z-score is the number of SD units above or below the average value for a person of the same age as the measured patient. Since bone loss occurs naturally as part of the aging process, using a patient's Z-score in comparison to a person of the same age could be misleading, especially in the early development of osteoporosis. The World Health Organization has defined normal bone density as being within (above or below) 1 SD of the mean for young adults. Low bone density is defined as density below 1 SD and 2.5 SD the mean for young adults, bone density 2.5 SD or more below the mean for young adults is indicative of osteoporosis (osteopenia), and bone density more than 2.5 SD below the mean for young adults is defined as severe (established) osteoporosis. The baseline age for young adults is approximately 30 years of age. For most BMD readings, 1 SD is equivalent to 10% to 12% of the average young-normal BMD value. A T-score of −2.5 is therefore equivalent to a bone mineral loss of 30% when compared to a young adult.

This procedure is contraindicated for

Patients who are pregnant or suspected of being pregnant, unless the potential benefits of a procedure using radiation far outweigh the risk of radiation exposure to the fetus and mother.

INDICATIONS

- Determine the mineral content of bone.
- Determine a possible cause of amenorrhea.
- Establish a diagnosis of osteoporosis.
- Estimate the actual fracture risk compared to young adults.
- Evaluate bone demineralization associated with chronic conditions (e.g., chronic kidney disease) or long term use of corticosteroids.
- Evaluate bone demineralization associated with immobilization.
- Evaluate secondary causes of bone demineralization associated with endocrine disorders (e.g., Cushing syndrome, diabetes, eating disorders, hyperparathyroidism, hyperprolactinemia).
- Monitor changes in BMD due to medical problems (e.g., malabsorption, multiple myeloma) or therapeutic intervention.
- Predict future fracture risk.

POTENTIAL MEDICAL DIAGNOSIS

Normal findings

- Normal bone mass with T-score value not less than −1.

Abnormal findings related to

- Osteoporosis is defined as T-score value less than −2.5.
- Low bone mass or osteopenia has T-scores from −1 to −2.5.

- Fracture risk increases as BMD declines from young-normal levels (low T-scores).
- Low Z-scores in older adults can be misleading because low BMD is very common.
- Z-scores estimate fracture risk compared to others of the same age (versus young-normal adults).

CRITICAL FINDINGS: N/A

INTERFERING FACTORS

- BMD test results may be lower in individuals receiving corticosteroid therapy; ideally BMD testing should be performed before a patient is placed on a regimen of chronic steroid therapy to obtain a valid baseline.

Factors that may alter the results of the study

- Inability of the patient to cooperate or remain still during the procedure because of age, significant pain, or mental status.
- Metallic objects within the examination field (e.g., jewelry, earrings, and/or dental amalgams), which may inhibit organ visualization and can produce unclear images.

Other considerations

- The use of anticonvulsant drugs, cytotoxic drugs, tamoxifen, glucocorticoids, lithium, or heparin, as well as increased alcohol intake, increased aluminum levels, excessive thyroxin, hemodialysis, or smoking, may affect the test results by either increasing or decreasing the bone mineral content.

Other Considerations as a Result of Altered BMD, Not the BMD Testing Process

- Vertebral fractures may cause complications including back pain, height loss, and kyphosis.
- Limited activity, including difficulty bending and reaching, may result.
- Patient may have poor self-esteem resulting from the cosmetic effects of kyphosis.
- Potential restricted lung function may result from fractures.
- Fractures may alter abdominal anatomy, resulting in constipation, pain, distention, and diminished appetite.
- Potential for a restricted lifestyle may result in depression and other psychological symptoms.
- Possible increased dependency on family for basic care may occur.

NURSING IMPLICATIONS AND PROCEDURE

PRETEST:

- Positively identify the patient using at least two person-specific identifiers before services, treatments, or procedures are performed.
- *Patient Teaching:* Inform the patient this procedure can assist in assessing bone density.
- Obtain a history of the patient's health concerns, symptoms, surgical procedures, and results of previously performed laboratory and diagnostic studies. Include a list of known allergens, especially allergies or sensitivities to latex, contrast medium, or anesthetics.
- Note any recent procedures that can interfere with test results, including examinations using iodine-based contrast medium.
- Record the date of the last menstrual period and determine the possibility of pregnancy in perimenopausal women.
- Obtain a list of the patient's current medications, including over-the-counter medications and dietary supplements (see Effects of Natural Products on Laboratory Values online at Davis*Plus*).
- Review the procedure with the patient. Address concerns about pain related to the procedure and explain that

some pain may be experienced during the test, or there may be moments of discomfort. Inform the patient that the procedure is usually performed in a radiology department by an HCP, and staff, specializing in this procedure and takes approximately 60 min.

- Instruct the patient to remove jewelry and other metallic objects from the area to be examined.
- Note that there are no food, fluid, or medication restrictions unless by medical direction.
- ***Sensitivity to social and cultural issues,*** as well as concern for modesty, is important in providing psychological support before, during, and after the procedure.

INTRATEST:

Potential Complications: N/A

- Observe standard precautions, and follow the general guidelines in Patient Preparation and Specimen Collection online at Davis*Plus*. Positively identify the patient.
- Ensure that the patient has removed all external metallic objects from the area to be examined prior to the procedure.
- Instruct the patient to void prior to the procedure and to change into the gown, robe, and foot coverings provided. Patient's clothing may not need to be removed unless it contains metal that would interfere with the test.
- Avoid the use of equipment containing latex if the patient has a history of allergic reaction to latex.
- Instruct the patient to cooperate fully and to follow directions. Instruct the patient to remain still throughout the procedure because movement produces unreliable results.
- Place the patient in a supine position on a flat table with foam wedges, which help maintain position and immobilization.

POST-TEST:

- Inform the patient that a report of the results will be made available to the requesting HCP, who will discuss the results with the patient.
- ***Nutritional Considerations:*** Educate the patient with vitamin D deficiency, as appropriate, that foods high in calcium and vitamin D should be included in the diet. Examples of foods rich in calcium and vitamin D are yogurt, cheese, cottage cheese, canned sardines with bones, flounder, salmon, dried figs, and dark-green leafy vegetables such as spinach and broccoli. Processed foods with added calcium, such as breads and cereals, can also be included. Avoiding red meat and high-fat foods that bind calcium in the intestine can reduce loss. The excess use of alcohol, salt, or caffeine can also decrease absorption. Explain to the patient that vitamin D is also synthesized by the body, in the skin, and is activated by sunlight. Daily recommendations for calcium and vitamin D intake are based on age. Calcium and vitamin D supplements may be used if dietary intake is insufficient. Provide contact information, if desired, for the Institute of Medicine of the National Academies (www.iom.edu) or the USDA's resource for nutrition (www.choosemyplate.gov) 🍁
- Recognize anxiety related to test results, and be supportive of perceived loss of independent function. Discuss the implications of abnormal test results on the patient's lifestyle. Provide teaching and information regarding the clinical implications of the test results, as appropriate. Provide contact information, if desired, for the National Osteoporosis Foundation (www.nof.org) 🍁.
- Reinforce information given by the patient's HCP regarding further testing, treatment, or referral to another HCP. Answer any questions or address any concerns voiced by the patient or family.
- Depending on the results of this procedure, additional testing may be needed to evaluate or monitor progression of the disease process and determine the need for a change in therapy. Evaluate test results in relation to the patient's symptoms, previous BMD values, and other tests performed.

RELATED STUDIES:

- Related tests include ALP, antibodies anticyclic citrullinated peptide, ANA, arthrogram, arthroscopy, biopsy bone, bone scan, calcium, CRP, collagen cross-linked telopeptides, CT pelvis, CT spine, ESR, MRI musculoskeletal, MRI pelvis, osteocalcin, PTH, phosphorus, radiography bone, RF, synovial fluid analysis, and vitamin D.
- Refer to the Musculoskeletal System table online at Davis*Plus* for related tests by body system.

B

Bone Scan

SYNONYM/ACRONYM: Bone imaging, radionuclide bone scan, bone scintigraphy, whole-body bone scan.

COMMON USE: To assist in diagnosing bone disease such as cancer or other degenerative bone disorders.

AREA OF APPLICATION: Bone/skeleton.

DESCRIPTION: This nuclear medicine scan assists in diagnosing and determining the extent of primary and metastatic bone disease and bone trauma and monitors the progression of degenerative disorders. Abnormalities are identified by scanning 1 to 3 hr after the intravenous injection of a radionuclide such as technetium-99m methylene diphosphonate. Areas of increased uptake and activity on the bone scan represent abnormalities unless they occur in normal areas of increased activity, such as the sternum, sacroiliac, clavicle, and scapular joints in adults, and growth centers and cranial sutures in children. A number of types of cancer, such as breast, lung, lymphomas, and prostate, are known to metastasize to bone. The radionuclide mimics calcium physiologically and therefore localizes in bone with an intensity proportional to the degree of metabolic activity. Bone scan is very sensitive; abnormalities can be identified weeks or months before they might be detected by x-ray. Gallium, magnetic resonance imaging (MRI), or white blood cell scanning may be performed after a bone scan to obtain a more sensitive study if acute inflammatory conditions such as osteomyelitis or septic arthritis are suspected. In addition, bone scan can detect fractures in patients who continue to have pain even though x-rays have proved negative. A gamma camera detects the radiation emitted from the injected radioactive material. Whole-body or representative images of the skeletal system can be obtained. Single-photon emission computed tomography (SPECT) has significantly improved the resolution and accuracy of bone scanning and may or may not be included as part of the examination. SPECT enables images to be recorded from multiple angles around the body and reconstructed by a computer to produce images or "slices" representing the area of interest at different levels.

This procedure is contraindicated for

Patients who are pregnant or suspected of being pregnant, unless the potential benefits of a procedure using radiation far outweigh the risk of radiation exposure to the fetus and mother.

B

INDICATIONS

- Aid in the diagnosis of benign tumors or cysts.
- Aid in the diagnosis of metabolic bone diseases.
- Aid in the diagnosis of osteomyelitis.
- Aid in the diagnosis of primary malignant bone tumors (e.g., osteogenic sarcoma, chondrosarcoma, Ewing's sarcoma, metastatic malignant tumors).
- Aid in the detection of traumatic or stress fractures.
- Assess degenerative joint changes or acute septic arthritis.
- Assess suspected child abuse.
- Confirm temporomandibular joint derangement.
- Detect Legg-Calvé-Perthes disease.
- Determine the cause of unexplained bone or joint pain.
- Evaluate the healing process following fracture, especially if an underlying bone disease is present.
- Evaluate prosthetic joints for infection, loosening, dislocation, or breakage.
- Evaluate tumor response to radiation or chemotherapy.
- Identify appropriate site for bone biopsy, lesion excision, or débridement.

POTENTIAL MEDICAL DIAGNOSIS

Normal findings

- No abnormalities, as indicated by homogeneous and symmetric distribution of the radionuclide throughout all skeletal structures

Abnormal findings related to

Uneven distribution of the radionuclide, deposited in concentrated "hot spots," indicate areas where lesions, trauma, or degeneration in bone tissue are located.

- Bone necrosis
- Degenerative arthritis
- Fracture
- Legg-Calvé-Perthes disease
- Metastatic bone neoplasm
- Osteomyelitis
- Paget's disease
- Primary metastatic bone tumors
- Renal osteodystrophy
- Rheumatoid arthritis

CRITICAL FINDINGS: N/A

INTERFERING FACTORS: N/A

Factors that may alter the results of the study

- Inability of the patient to cooperate or remain still during the procedure because of age, significant pain, or mental status.
- Metallic objects within the examination field (e.g., jewelry, earrings, and/or dental amalgams), which may inhibit organ visualization and can produce unclear images.
- Retained barium from a previous radiological procedure may affect the image.
- A distended bladder may obscure pelvic detail.
- Other nuclear scans done within the previous 24 to 48 hr may alter images.

Other considerations

- The existence of multiple myeloma or cancers that have metastasized to the bones (e.g., thyroid cancer) can result in a false-negative scan for bone abnormalities until a significant amount of bone and bone marrow destruction has occurred; these conditions are better

detected using other imaging techniques (radiography for multiple myeloma and radioactive iodine uptake for thyroid cancer).
- Improper injection of the radionuclide may allow the tracer to seep deep into the muscle tissue, producing erroneous hot spots.

NURSING IMPLICATIONS AND PROCEDURE

See Potential Nursing Problems on Fast Find at davispl.us/vanleeuwen7.

PRETEST:

- Positively identify the patient using at least two person-specific identifiers before services, treatments, or procedures are performed.
- ***Patient Teaching:*** Inform the patient this procedure can assist in identification of bone disease before it can be detected with plain x-ray images.
- Obtain a history of the patient's health concerns, symptoms, surgical procedures, and results of previously performed laboratory and diagnostic studies. Include a list of known allergens, especially allergies or sensitivities to latex, anesthetics, sedatives, or radionuclides.
- Note any recent procedures that can interfere with test results, including examinations using iodine-based contrast medium.
- Record the date of the last menstrual period and determine the possibility of pregnancy in perimenopausal women.
- Obtain a list of the patient's current medications, including over-the-counter medications and dietary supplements (see Effects of Natural Products on Laboratory Values online at Davis*Plus*).
- Review the procedure with the patient. Address concerns about pain related to the procedure and explain to the patient that some pain may be experienced during the test, or there may be moments of discomfort. Reassure the patient that the radionuclide poses no radioactive hazard and rarely produces adverse effects. Inform the patient the procedure is performed in a nuclear medicine department by an HCP specializing in this procedure, and takes approximately 30 to 60 min. **Pediatric Considerations:** Preparing children for a bone scan depends on the age of the child. Encourage parents to be truthful about what the child may experience during the procedure (e.g., there may be a pinch or minor discomfort when the intravenous (IV) needle is inserted) and to use words that they know their child will understand. Toddlers and preschool-age children have a very short attention span, so the best time to talk about the test is right before the procedure. The child should be assured that he or she will be allowed to bring a favorite comfort item into the examination room, and if appropriate, that a parent will be with the child during the procedure. Explain the importance of remaining still while the images are taken.
- ***Sensitivity to social and cultural issues,*** as well as concern for modesty, is important in providing psychological support before, during, and after the procedure.
- Explain that an IV line may be inserted to allow infusion of fluids such as saline, anesthetics, sedatives, radionuclides, medications used in the procedure, or emergency medications.
- Note that there are no food, fluid, or medication restrictions unless by medical direction.
- Instruct the patient to remove jewelry and other metallic objects in the area to be examined.
- *Make sure a written and informed consent has been signed prior to the procedure and before administering any medications.*

INTRATEST:

Potential Complications:

Although it is rare, there is the possibility of allergic reaction to the radionuclide. Have emergency equipment and medications readily available. If the patient has a history of allergic

B

reactions to any substance or drug, administer ordered prophylactic steroids or antihistamines before the procedure.

Establishing an IV site and injection of radionuclides is an invasive procedure. Complications are rare but do include bleeding from the puncture site ***(related to a bleeding disorder, or the effects of natural products and medications with known anticoagulant, antiplatelet, or thrombolytic properties),*** hematoma ***(related to blood leakage into the tissue following needle insertion),*** infection ***(that might occur if bacteria from the skin surface is introduced at the puncture site),*** or nerve injury ***(that might occur if the needle strikes a nerve).***

- Observe standard precautions, and follow the general guidelines in Patient Preparation and Specimen Collection online at Davis*Plus*. Positively identify the patient.
- Ensure that the patient has removed all external metallic objects from the area to be examined prior to the procedure.
- Administer ordered prophylactic steroids or antihistamines before the procedure if the patient has a history of allergic reactions to any substance or drug to be used in the study.
- Avoid the use of equipment containing latex if the patient has a history of allergic reaction to latex.
- Have emergency equipment readily available.
- Instruct the patient to void prior to the procedure as a full bladder may obscure pelvic bones, and to change into the gown, robe, and foot coverings provided.
- Record baseline vital signs and assess neurological status. Protocols may vary among facilities.
- Establish an IV fluid line for the injection of saline, anesthetics, sedatives, radionuclides, or emergency medications.
- Instruct the patient to cooperate fully and to follow directions. Instruct the patient to remain still throughout the procedure because movement produces unreliable results.
- Administer sedative to a child or to an uncooperative adult, as ordered.
- Place the patient in a supine position on a flat table with foam wedges to help maintain position and immobilization.
- IV radionuclide is administered and images are taken immediately to assess blood flow to the bones.
- After a delay of 2 to 3 hr to allow the radionuclide to be taken up by the bones, multiple images are obtained over the complete skeleton. Delayed views may be taken up to 24 hr after the injection.
- The needle or catheter is removed, and a pressure dressing is applied over the puncture site.
- Observe/assess the needle/catheter insertion site for bleeding, inflammation, or hematoma formation.
- The patient may be imaged by single-photon emission computed tomography (SPECT) techniques to further clarify areas of suspicious radionuclide localization.

POST-TEST:

- Inform the patient that a report of the results will be made available to the requesting HCP, who will discuss the results with the patient.
- Unless contraindicated, advise patient to drink increased amounts of fluids for 24 to 48 hr to eliminate the radionuclide from the body. Inform the patient that radionuclide is eliminated from the body within 6 to 24 hr.
- No other radionuclide tests should be scheduled for 24 to 48 hr after this procedure.
- Instruct the patient to resume medication and activity as directed by the HCP.
- Observe/assess the needle/catheter insertion site for bleeding, inflammation, or hematoma formation.
- Instruct the patient in the care and assessment of the injection site.
- If a woman who is breastfeeding must have a nuclear scan, she should not breastfeed the infant until the radionuclide has been eliminated. This could take as long as 3 days. She should be instructed to express the milk and

discard it during the 3-day period to prevent cessation of milk production.

- Instruct the patient to immediately flush the toilet and to meticulously wash hands with soap and water after each voiding for 24 hr after the procedure.
- Instruct all caregivers to wear gloves when discarding urine for 24 hr after the procedure. Wash gloved hands with soap and water before removing gloves; then wash ungloved hands.
- Recognize anxiety related to test results, and be supportive of perceived loss of independent function. Discuss the implications of abnormal test results on the patient's lifestyle. Provide teaching and information regarding the clinical implications of the test results, as appropriate. Provide contact information, if desired, for the American Cancer Society (www.cancer.org), American College of Rheumatology (www.rheumatology.org), or Arthritis Foundation (www.arthritis.org) 🍁.
- Reinforce information given by the patient's HCP regarding further testing, treatment, or referral to another HCP. Answer any questions or address any concerns voiced by the patient or family.
- Depending on the results of this procedure, additional testing may be needed to evaluate or monitor progression of the disease process and determine the need for a change in therapy. Evaluate test results in relation to the patient's symptoms and other tests performed.

Patient Education:

- Teach the patient that some fatigue associated with chemotherapy and radiation therapy is normal.
- Teach the patient that nausea may be better controlled by taking antiemetics around the clock rather that with each individual episode of nausea.

Expected Patient Outcomes:

Understanding

- The patient and family state that eating in small amounts can decrease nausea.
- The patient and family state that spicy, greasy, fried, strong-odor foods can precipitate nausea and agree to avoid these foods.

Ability

- The patient and family select activities that can be bundled to conserve energy and decrease fatigue.
- The patient and family select foods that are least likely to cause nausea.

Response

- The patient and family agree to attend a support group to provide emotional support related to diagnosis and prognosis.
- The patient and family demonstrate willingness to review the pathophysiology of the disease process to better make informed decisions involving intervention choices.

RELATED STUDIES:

- Related tests include antibodies, anticyclic citrullinated peptide, ANA, arthroscopy, BMD, calcium, CRP, collagen cross-linked telopeptide, CT pelvis, CT spine, culture blood, ESR, MRI musculoskeletal, MRI pelvis, osteocalcin, radiography bone, RF, synovial fluid analysis, and white blood cell scan.
- Refer to the Musculoskeletal System table online at Davis*Plus* for related tests by body system.

Bronchoscopy

SYNONYM/ACRONYM: Flexible bronchoscopy.

COMMON USE: To visualize and assess bronchial structure for disease such as cancer and infection.

AREA OF APPLICATION: Bronchial tree, larynx, trachea.

DESCRIPTION: This procedure provides direct visualization of the larynx, trachea, and bronchial tree by means of either a rigid or a flexible bronchoscope. A bronchoscope with a light incorporated is guided into the tracheobronchial tree. A local anesthetic may be used to allow the scope to be inserted through the mouth or nose into the trachea and into the bronchi. The patient must breathe during insertion and with the scope in place. The purpose of the procedure is both diagnostic and therapeutic.

The rigid bronchoscope allows visualization of the larger airways, including the lobar, segmental, and subsegmental bronchi, while maintaining effective gas exchange. Rigid bronchoscopy is preferred when large volumes of blood or secretions need to be aspirated, foreign bodies are to be removed, large-sized biopsy specimens are to be obtained, and for most bronchoscopies in children. The flexible bronchoscope has a smaller lumen that is designed to allow for visualization of all segments of the bronchial tree. The accessory lumen of the bronchoscope is used for tissue biopsy, bronchial washings, instillation of anesthetic drugs and medications, and to obtain specimens with brushes for cytological examination. In general, flexible bronchoscopy is less traumatic to the surrounding tissues than the larger rigid bronchoscopes. Flexible bronchoscopy is performed under local anesthesia; patient tolerance is better for flexible bronchoscopy than for rigid bronchoscopy.

This procedure is contraindicated for

- Patients with bleeding disorders, especially those associated with uremia and cytotoxic chemotherapy.
- Patients with pulmonary hypertension.
- Patients with cardiac conditions or dysrhythmias.
- Patients with disorders that limit extension of the neck.
- Patients with severe obstructive tracheal conditions.
- Patients with or having the potential for respiratory failure; ***(introduction of the bronchoscope alone may cause a 10 to 20 mm Hg drop in Pao_2).***

INDICATIONS

- Detect end-stage bronchogenic cancer.
- Detect lung infections and inflammation.
- Determine etiology of persistent cough, hemoptysis, hoarseness, unexplained chest x-ray abnormalities, and/or abnormal cytological findings in sputum.
- Determine extent of smoke-inhalation or other traumatic injury.
- Evaluate airway patency; aspirate deep or retained secretions.
- Evaluate endotracheal tube placement or possible adverse sequelae to tube placement.
- Evaluate possible airway obstruction in patients with known or suspected sleep apnea.
- Evaluate respiratory distress and tachypnea in an infant to rule out tracheoesophageal fistula or other congenital anomaly.
- Identify bleeding sites and remove clots within the tracheobronchial tree.

- Identify hemorrhagic and inflammatory changes in Kaposi's sarcoma.
- Intubate patients with cervical spine injuries or massive upper airway edema.
- Remove foreign body.
- Treat lung cancer through instillation of chemotherapeutic drugs, implantation of radioisotopes, or laser palliative therapy.

POTENTIAL MEDICAL DIAGNOSIS

Normal findings

- Normal larynx, trachea, bronchi, bronchioles, and alveoli

Abnormal findings related to

- Abscess
- Bronchial diverticulum
- Bronchial stenosis
- Bronchogenic cancer
- Coccidioidomycosis, histoplasmosis, blastomycosis, phycomycosis
- Foreign bodies
- Inflammation
- Interstitial pulmonary disease
- Opportunistic lung infections (e.g., pneumocystitis, nocardia, cytomegalovirus)
- Strictures
- Tuberculosis
- Tumors

CRITICAL FINDINGS: N/A

INTERFERING FACTORS

Factors that may impair the results of the examination

- Inability of the patient to cooperate or remain still during the procedure because of age, significant pain, or mental status.
- Metallic objects within the examination field (e.g., jewelry, earrings, and/or dental amalgams), which may inhibit organ visualization and can produce unclear images.

Other considerations

- Hypoxemic or hypercapnic states require continuous oxygen administration.
- Failure to follow dietary restrictions before the procedure may cause the procedure to be canceled or repeated.

NURSING IMPLICATIONS AND PROCEDURE

See Potential Nursing Problems on Fast Find at davispl.us/vanleeuwen7.

PRETEST:

- Positively identify the patient using at least two person-specific identifiers before services, treatments, or procedures are performed.
- *Patient Teaching:* Inform the patient this procedure can assess the lungs and respiratory system.
- Obtain a history of the patient's health concerns, including a list of known allergens, especially allergies or sensitivities to latex, sedatives, or anesthetics.
- Obtain a history of the patient's immune and respiratory systems, symptoms, and results of previously performed laboratory tests and diagnostic and surgical procedures.
- Note any recent procedures that can interfere with test results. Ensure that this procedure is performed before an upper gastrointestinal study or barium swallow.
- Record the date of the last menstrual period and determine the possibility of pregnancy in perimenopausal women.
- Obtain a list of the patient's current medications, including over-the-counter medications, anticoagulants, aspirin and other salicylates, and dietary supplements (see Effects of Natural Products on Laboratory Values online at Davis*Plus*). Such products should be discontinued by medical direction for the appropriate number of days prior to a surgical procedure. Note the last time and dose of medication taken.

B

- Review the procedure with the patient. Instruct that prophylactic antibiotics may be administered prior to the procedure. Address concerns about pain related to the procedure and explain that some pain may be experienced during the test, and there may be moments of discomfort. Explain that a sedative and/or analgesia may be administered to promote relaxation and reduce discomfort prior to the bronchoscopy. Atropine is usually given before bronchoscopy examinations to reduce bronchial secretions and prevent vagally induced bradycardia. A local anesthetic such as lidocaine is sprayed in the patient's throat to reduce discomfort caused by the presence of the tube. Inform the patient that the procedure is performed in a gastrointestinal laboratory or radiology department, under sterile conditions, by a health-care provider (HCP) specializing in this procedure. The procedure usually takes about 30 to 60 min to complete.
- ***Sensitivity to social and cultural issues,*** as well as concern for modesty, is important in providing psychological support before, during, and after the procedure.
- Explain that an intravenous (IV) line may be inserted to allow infusion of fluids such as saline, antibiotics, anesthetics, analgesics, sedatives, or emergency medications.
- Instruct the patient that to reduce the risk of aspiration related to nausea and vomiting, solid food and milk or milk products are restricted for at least 6 hr, and clear liquids are restricted for at least 2 hr prior to general anesthesia, regional anesthesia, or sedation/analgesia (monitored anesthesia). The American Society of Anesthesiologists has fasting guidelines for risk levels according to patient status. More information can be located at www.asahq.org 🍁. Patients on beta blockers before the surgical procedure should be instructed to take their medication as ordered during the perioperative period. Protocols may vary among facilities.
- Instruct the patient to avoid taking anticoagulant medication or to reduce dosage as ordered prior to the procedure. Number of days to withhold medication is dependent on the type of anticoagulant. Protocols may vary among facilities.
- *Make sure a written and informed consent has been signed prior to the procedure and before administering any medications.*

INTRATEST:

Potential Complications:

Complications from the procedure are rare but may include infection ***(related to the use of an endoscope),*** hypoxemia, pneumothorax, or bleeding ***(related to a bleeding disorder, or the effects of natural products and medications with known anticoagulant, antiplatelet, or thrombolytic properties).***

Establishing an IV site is an invasive procedure. Complications are rare but do include risk for bleeding from the puncture site ***(related to a bleeding disorder, or the effects of natural products and medications with known anticoagulant, antiplatelet, or thrombolytic properties),*** hematoma ***(related to blood leakage into the tissue following needle insertion),*** infection ***(that might occur if bacteria from the skin surface is introduced at the puncture site),*** or nerve injury ***(that might occur if the needle strikes a nerve).***

- Ensure that the patient has complied with food, fluid, and medication restrictions for 6 hr prior to the procedure.
- Ensure that the patient has removed dentures, jewelry, and external metallic objects in the area to be examined prior to the procedure.
- Avoid the use of equipment containing latex if the patient has a history of allergic reaction to latex.
- Have emergency equipment readily available.
- Instruct the patient to void prior to the procedure and change into the gown, robe, and foot coverings provided.

- Avoid using morphine for sedation in patients with asthma or other pulmonary disease. This drug can further exacerbate bronchospasms and respiratory impairment.
- Observe standard precautions, and follow the general guidelines in Patient Preparation and Specimen Collection online at Davis*Plus*. Positively identify the patient, and label the appropriate specimen container with the corresponding patient demographics, initials of the person collecting the specimen, date and time of collection, and site location, especially right or left lung.
- Assist the patient to a comfortable position, and direct the patient to breathe normally during the beginning of the general anesthesia. Instruct the patient to cooperate fully and to follow directions. Direct the patient to breathe normally and to avoid unnecessary movement during the local anesthetic and the procedure.
- Record baseline vital signs and continue to monitor throughout the procedure. Protocols may vary among facilities.
- Establish an IV fluid line for the injection of saline, antibiotics, anesthetics, analgesics, sedatives, or emergency medications.

Rigid Bronchoscopy

- The patient is placed in the supine position and a general anesthetic is administered. The patient's neck is hyperextended, and the lightly lubricated bronchoscope is inserted orally and passed through the glottis. The patient's head is turned or repositioned to aid visualization of various segments.
- After inspection, the bronchial brush, suction catheter, biopsy forceps, laser, and electrocautery devices are introduced to obtain specimens for cytological or microbiological study or for therapeutic procedures.
- If a bronchial washing is performed, small amounts of solution are instilled into the airways and removed.
- After the procedure, the bronchoscope is removed and the patient is placed in a side-lying position with the head slightly elevated to promote recovery.

Flexible Bronchoscopy

- Provide mouth care to reduce oral bacterial flora.
- The patient is placed in a sitting position while the tongue and oropharynx are sprayed or swabbed with local anesthetic. Provide an emesis basin for the increased saliva and encourage the patient to spit out the saliva because the gag reflex may be impaired. When loss of sensation is adequate, the patient is placed in a supine or side-lying position. The flexible scope can be introduced through the nose, the mouth, an endotracheal tube, a tracheostomy tube, or a rigid bronchoscope. Most common insertion is through the nose. Patients with copious secretions or massive hemoptysis, or in whom airway complications are more likely, may be intubated before the bronchoscopy. Additional local anesthetic is applied through the scope as it approaches the vocal cords and the carina, eliminating reflexes in these sensitive areas. The flexible broncoscopy approach allows visualization of airway segments without having to move the patient's head through various positions.
- After visual inspection of the lungs, tissue samples are collected from suspicious sites by bronchial brush or biopsy forceps to be used for cytological and microbiological studies.
- After the procedure, the bronchoscope is removed. Patients who had local anesthesia are placed in a semi-Fowler's position to recover.

General

- Monitor the patient for complications related to the procedure (e.g., allergic reaction, anaphylaxis).
- Place tissue samples in properly labelled specimen containers containing formalin solution, and promptly transport the specimen to the laboratory for processing and analysis.

B

POST-TEST:

- Inform the patient that a report of the results will be made available to the requesting HCP, who will discuss the results with the patient.
- Instruct the patient to resume preoperative diet, as directed by the HCP. Assess the patient's ability to swallow before allowing the patient to attempt liquids or solid foods.
- Inform the patient that he or she may experience some throat soreness and hoarseness. Instruct patient to treat throat discomfort with lozenges and warm gargles when the gag reflex returns.
- Monitor vital signs and neurological status every 15 min for 1 hr, then every 2 hr for 4 hr, and then as ordered by the HCP. Monitor temperature every 4 hr for 24 hr. Monitor intake and output at least every 8 hr. Compare with baseline values. Notify the HCP if temperature changes. Protocols may vary among facilities.
- Emergency resuscitation equipment should be readily available if the vocal cords become spastic after intubation.
- Observe for delayed allergic reactions, such as rash, urticaria, tachycardia, hyperpnea, hypertension, palpitations, nausea, or vomiting.
- Observe the patient for hemoptysis, dyspnea, cough, air hunger, excessive coughing, pain, or absent breathing sounds over the affected area. Immediately report symptoms to the appropriate HCP.
- Evaluate the patient for symptoms indicating the development of pneumothorax, such as dyspnea, tachypnea, anxiety, decreased breathing sounds, or restlessness. A chest x-ray may be ordered to check for the presence of this complication.
- Evaluate the patient for symptoms of empyema, such as fever, tachycardia, malaise, or elevated white blood cell count.
- Observe the patient's sputum for blood if a biopsy was taken, because large amounts of blood may indicate the development of a problem; a small amount of streaking is expected. Evaluate the patient for signs of bleeding such as tachycardia, hypotension, or restlessness.
- Assess for nausea and pain. Administer antiemetic and analgesic medications as needed and as directed by the HCP.
- Administer antibiotic therapy if ordered. Remind the patient of the importance of completing the entire course of antibiotic therapy even if signs and symptoms disappear before completion of therapy.
- Recognize anxiety related to test results. Discuss the implications of abnormal test results on the patient's lifestyle. Provide teaching and information regarding the clinical implications of the test results, as appropriate. Educate the patient regarding access to counseling services.
- Instruct the patient to use lozenges or gargle for throat discomfort. Inform the patient of smoking cessation programs as appropriate. Malnutrition is commonly seen in patients with severe respiratory disease for numerous reasons, including fatigue, lack of appetite, and gastrointestinal distress. Adequate intake of vitamins A and C is also important to prevent pulmonary infection and to decrease the extent of lung tissue damage. The importance of following the prescribed diet should be stressed to the patient/caregiver. Educate the patient regarding access to counseling services, as appropriate.
- Reinforce information given by the patient's HCP regarding further testing, treatment, or referral to another HCP. Answer any questions or address any concerns voiced by the patient or family.
- Depending on the results of this procedure, additional testing may be needed to evaluate or monitor progression of the disease process and determine the need for a change in therapy. Evaluate test results in relation to the patient's symptoms and other tests performed.

Patient Education:
- Teach the patient the pathophysiology behind diminished oxygenation and disease process.
- Explain that a health-care specialist may need to be consulted to assist managing the disease.

Expected Patient Outcomes:

Understanding
- The patient and family state the importance of keeping oxygen on at all times.
- The patient and family describe the reportable signs and symptoms of poor oxygenation.

Ability
- The patient demonstrates how to use controlled breathing to improve breathing patterns.
- The patient and family demonstrate how to pace and bundle activities to improve activity tolerance.

Response
- The patient and family agree to make required lifestyle changes to support positive health.
- The patient and family agree to work with the health-care team to discuss treatment options and expected outcomes.

RELATED STUDIES:
- Related tests include arterial/alveolar oxygen ratio, antibodies, antiglomerular basement membrane, biopsy lung, blood gases, chest x-ray, complete blood count, CT thorax, culture and smear mycobacteria, culture sputum, culture viral, cytology sputum, Gram stain, lung perfusion scan, lung ventilation scan, MRI chest, mediastinoscopy, and pulse oximetry.
- Refer to the Immune and Respiratory systems tables online at Davis*Plus* for related tests by body system.

B-Type Natriuretic Peptide and Pro-B-Type Natriuretic Peptide

SYNONYM/ACRONYM: BNP and proBNP.

COMMON USE: To assist in diagnosing heart failure (HF).

SPECIMEN: Plasma collected in a plastic, lavender-top (EDTA) tube.

NORMAL FINDINGS: (Method: Chemiluminescent immunoassay for BNP; electrochemiluminescent immunoassay for proBNP)

BNP	Conventional Units	SI Units (Conventional Units × 1)
Male & Female	Less than 100 pg/mL	Less than 100 ng/L
proBNP (N-terminal)		
0–74 yr	Less than 125 pg/mL	Less than 125 ng/L
Greater than 75 yr	Less than 449 pg/mL	Less than 449 ng/L

BNP levels are increased in older adults.

DESCRIPTION: The peptides B-type natriuretic peptide (BNP) and atrial natriuretic peptide (ANP) are antagonists of the renin-angiotensin-aldosterone system, which assist in the regulation of electrolytes, fluid balance, and blood pressure. BNP, proBNP, and

ANP are useful markers in the diagnosis of heart failure HF. BNP, first isolated in the brain of pigs, is a neurohormone synthesized primarily in the ventricles of the human heart in response to increases in ventricular pressure and volume. Circulating levels of BNP and proBNP increase in proportion to the severity of heart failure. A rapid BNP point-of-care immunoassay may be performed, in which a venous blood sample is collected, placed on a strip, and inserted into a device that measures BNP. Results are completed in 10 to 15 min.

This procedure is contraindicated for

Patients receiving nesiritide. Nesiritide (Natrecor) is a recombinant form of BNP that may be given therapeutically by intravenous to patients in acutely decompensated heart failure; with some assays, BNP levels may be transiently and significantly elevated at the time of administration and must be interpreted with caution. The testing laboratory should be consulted to verify whether test measurements are affected by nesiritide.

INDICATIONS

- Assist in determining the prognosis and therapy of patients with heart failure.
- Assist in the diagnosis of heart failure.
- Assist in differentiating heart failure from pulmonary disease.
- Cost-effective screen for left ventricular dysfunction; positive findings would point to the need for echocardiography and further assessment.

POTENTIAL MEDICAL DIAGNOSIS

Increased in:

BNP is secreted in response to increased hemodynamic load caused by physiological stimuli, as with ventricular stretch or endocrine stimuli from the aldosterone/renin system.

- Acute kidney injury
- Cardiac inflammation (myocarditis, cardiac allograft rejection)
- Chronic kidney disease
- Cirrhosis
- Cushing's syndrome
- Heart failure
- Kawasaki's disease
- Left ventricular hypertrophy
- Myocardial infarction
- Primary hyperaldosteronism
- Primary pulmonary hypertension
- Ventricular dysfunction

Decreased in: N/A

CRITICAL FINDINGS: N/A

INTERFERING FACTORS: N/A

NURSING IMPLICATIONS AND PROCEDURE

POTENTIAL NURSING PROBLEMS:

Problem	Signs & Symptoms	Interventions
Gas exchange ***(related to altered alveolar and capillary exchange***	Decreased activity tolerance; increased shortness of breath with activity; weakness; orthopnea;	Auscultate and trend breath sounds; perform pulse oximetry to monitor oxygenation; administer oxygen as ordered;

Problem	Signs & Symptoms	Interventions
secondary to fluid in the alveoli)	cyanosis; cough; increased heart rate; weight gain; edema in the lower extremities; weakness; increased respiratory rate; use of respiratory accessory muscles	collaborate with health-care provider (HCP) to consider intubation and/or mechanical ventilation; place the head of the bed in high Fowler's position; administer diuretics, vasodilators as ordered; monitor potassium levels
Tissue perfusion ***(related to compromised cardiac contractility; interrupted blood flow)***	Hypotension; dizziness; cool extremities; capillary refill greater than 3 sec; weak pedal pulses; altered level of consciousness	Monitor blood pressure; assess for dizziness; check skin temperature for warmth; assess capillary refill; assess pedal pulses; monitor level of consciousness; administer prescribed vasodilators and inotropic drugs
Cardiac output ***(related to increased preload; increased afterload; impaired cardiac contractility; cardiac muscle disease; altered cardiac conduction)***	Decreased peripheral pulses; decreased urinary output; cool, clammy skin; tachypnea; dyspnea; edema; altered level of consciousness; abnormal heart sounds; crackles in lungs; decreased activity tolerance; weight gain; fatigue; hypoxia	Assess peripheral pulses and capillary refill; monitor blood pressure and check for orthostatic changes; assess respiratory rate, breath sounds, and orthopnea; assess skin color and temperature; assess level of consciousness; monitor urinary output; use pulse oximetry to monitor oxygenation; monitor sodium and potassium levels; monitor BNP levels; administer ordered angiotensin-converting enzyme (ACE) inhibitors, beta blockers, diuretics, aldosterone antagonists, and vasodilators; provide oxygen administration
Fluid volume (water) ***(related to altered cardiac output)***	**Overload:** Edema; shortness of breath; increased weight; ascites; rales; rhonchi; diluted laboratory	Daily weight with monitoring of trends; fluid limit as appropriate; assess for peripheral edema; assess for

(table continues on page 334)

Problem	Signs & Symptoms	Interventions
	values; increased blood pressure; positive jugular venous distention (JVD); orthopnea; cough; restlessness; tachycardia; pulmonary congestion with x-ray; restlessness	adventitious lung sounds such as crackles; monitor blood pressure and heart rate; assess for JVD; monitor intake versus output; administer prescribed diuretics; restrict sodium intake; order low sodium diet; monitor laboratory values that reflect alterations in fluid status; manage underlying cause of fluid alteration

PRETEST:

- Positively identify the patient using at least two person-specific identifiers before services, treatments, or procedures are performed.
- ***Patient Teaching:*** Inform the patient this test can assist in diagnosing heart failure.
- Obtain a history of the patient's health concerns, symptoms, surgical procedures, and results of previously performed laboratory and diagnostic studies. Include a list of known allergens, especially allergies or sensitivities to latex.
- Obtain a list of the patient's current medications, including over-the-counter medications and dietary supplements (see Effects of Natural Products on Laboratory Values online at Davis*Plus*).
- Review the procedure with the patient. Inform the patient that specimen collection takes approximately 5 to 10 min. Address concerns about pain and explain to the patient that there may be some discomfort during the venipuncture.
- ***Sensitivity to social and cultural issues,*** as well as concern for modesty, is important in providing psychological support before, during, and after the procedure.
- Note that there are no food, fluid, or medication restrictions unless by medical direction.

INTRATEST:

Potential Complications: N/A

- Avoid the use of equipment containing latex if the patient has a history of allergic reaction to latex.
- Instruct the patient to cooperate fully and to follow directions. Direct the patient to breathe normally and to avoid unnecessary movement.
- Observe standard precautions, and follow the general guidelines in Patient Preparation and Specimen Collection online at Davis*Plus*. Positively identify the patient, and label the appropriate specimen container with the corresponding patient demographics, initials of the person collecting the specimen, date, and time of collection. Perform a venipuncture.
- Remove the needle and apply direct pressure with dry gauze to stop bleeding. Observe/assess venipuncture site for bleeding or hematoma formation and secure gauze with adhesive bandage.
- Promptly transport the specimen to the laboratory for processing and analysis.

POST-TEST:

- Inform the patient that a report of the results will be made available to the requesting HCP, who will discuss the results with the patient.

- ***Treatment Considerations for HF:*** Recognize anxiety related to test results, and ensure that the patient (if not currently taking) is placed on an ACE inhibitor, β blocker, and diuretic, and is monitored with daily weight measurement. Discuss risk factors. Teach the patient to safely administer ordered oxygen, as appropriate.
- *Nutritional Considerations:* Instruct patients to consume a variety of foods within the basic food groups, eat foods high in potassium when taking diuretics, eat a diet high in fiber (25–35 g/day), maintain a healthy weight, be physically active, limit salt intake to 2,000 mg/day, limit alcohol intake, and be a nonsmoker.
- *Nutritional Considerations:* Foods high in potassium include fruits such as bananas, strawberries, oranges; cantaloupes; green leafy vegetables such as spinach and broccoli; dried fruits such as dates, prunes, and raisins; legumes such as peas and pinto beans; nuts and whole grains.
- Depending on the results of this procedure, additional testing may be performed to evaluate or monitor progression of the disease process and determine the need for a change in therapy. Evaluate test results in relation to the patient's symptoms and other tests performed.

Patient Education:

- Reinforce information given by the patient's HCP regarding further testing, treatment, or referral to another HCP.
- Answer any questions or address any concerns voiced by the patient or family.
- Explain to the patient and family the importance of reporting life-threatening changes such as cool extremities, pallor, and diaphoresis to HCP immediately.
- Ensure family understands to report any changes in mental status such as confusion.

Expected Patient Outcomes:

Understanding

- The patient and family recite the importance of limiting fluids to decrease cardiac stress.
- The patient and family describe the purpose of taking the prescribed diuretic.

Ability

- The patient and family accurately describe strategies to limit fluid intake and decrease cardiac stress.
- The patient and family accurately demonstrate how to keep an accurate intake and output.

Response

- The patient complies with taking all medications as prescribed to support cardiac health.
- The patient and family adhere to treatment recommendations that can help to prevent a potentially life-threatening situation.

RELATED STUDIES:

- Related tests include angiography pulmonary, ANF, calcium, CRP, CK and isoenzymes, CT scoring, echocardiography, glucose, homocysteine, Holter monitor, LDH and isoenzymes, magnesium, MRI chest, MI scan, myocardial perfusion heart scan, myoglobin, PET heart, potassium, and troponin.
- Refer to the Cardiovascular System table online at Davis*Plus* for related tests by body system.

Calcitonin and Calcitonin Stimulation Tests

SYNONYM/ACRONYM: Thyrocalcitonin.

COMMON USE: To diagnose and monitor the effectiveness of treatment for medullary thyroid cancer.

SPECIMEN: Serum collected in a gold-, red-, or red/gray-top tube. Place separated serum in a plastic transport tube within 2 hr of collection.

NORMAL FINDINGS: (Method: Chemiluminescent immunoassay)

Procedure	Medication Administered	Recommended Collection Times
Calcium and pentagastrin stimulation	Calcium, 2 mg/kg IV for 1 min, followed by pentagastrin 0.5 mcg/kg	4 calcitonin levels—baseline immediately before bolus; and 1 min, 2 min, and 5 min postbolus
Calcium stimulation	Calcium, 2 mg/kg IV for 1 min or 2.4 mg/kg IV push	4 calcitonin levels—baseline immediately before bolus; and 1 min, 2 min, and 5 min postbolus
Pentagastrin stimulation	Pentagastrin 0.5 mcg/kg	4 calcitonin levels—baseline immediately before bolus; and 1 min, 2 min, and 5 min postbolus

IV = intravenous.

	Conventional Units	SI Units (Conventional Units × 1)
Calcitonin *Baseline*		
Male	Less than 10 pg/mL	Less than 10 ng/L
Female	Less than 5 pg/mL	Less than 5 ng/L
Maximum Response		
5 min after calcium and pentagastrin stimulation		
Male	8–343 pg/mL	8–343 ng/L
Female	Less than 39 pg/mL	Less than 39 ng/L
5 min after calcium stimulation		
Male	Less than 190 pg/mL	Less than 190 ng/L
Female	Less than 130 pg/mL	Less than 130 ng/L
5 min after pentagastrin stimulation		
Male	Less than 110 pg/mL	Less than 110 ng/L
Female	Less than 30 pg/mL	Less than 30 ng/L

POTENTIAL MEDICAL DIAGNOSIS

Increased in:

- Alcoholic cirrhosis ***(related to release of calcium from body stores associated with acute instances of malnutrition)***
- Cancer of the breast, lung, and pancreas ***(related to metastasis of calcitonin-producing cells to other organs)***
- Carcinoid syndrome ***(related to calcitonin-producing tumor cells)***
- C-cell hyperplasia ***(related to increased production due to hyperplasia)***
- Chronic kidney disease ***(related to increased excretion of calcium and retention of phosphorus resulting in release of calcium from body stores; C cells respond to an increase in serum calcium levels)***
- Ectopic secretion ***(especially neuroendocrine origins)***
- Hypercalcemia (any cause) ***(related to increased production by C cells in response to increased calcium levels)***
- Medullary thyroid cancer ***(related to overproduction by cancerous cells)***
- MEN type II ***(related to calcitonin-producing tumor cells)***
- Pancreatitis ***(related to alcoholism or hypercalcemia)***
- Pernicious anemia ***(related to hypergastrinemia)***
- Pheochromocytoma ***(related to calcitonin-producing tumor cells)***
- Pregnancy (late) ***(related to increased maternal loss of circulating calcium to developing fetus; release of calcium from maternal stores stimulates increased release of calcitonin)***
- Pseudohypoparathyroidism ***(related to release of calcium from body stores initiates feedback response from C cells)***
- Thyroiditis ***(related to calcitonin-producing tumor cells)***
- Zollinger-Ellison syndrome ***(related to hypergastrinemia)***

Decreased in: N/A

CRITICAL FINDINGS: N/A

Find and print out the full study on Fast Find at davispl.us/vanleeuwen7.

Calcium, Blood, Total and Ionized

SYNONYM/ACRONYM: Total and free calcium, Ca (total), unbound calcium (ionized), Ca^{++} (ionized), Ca^{2+} (ionized).

COMMON USE: To investigate various conditions, such as hypercalcemia and hypocalcemia, related to abnormally increased or decreased calcium levels.

SPECIMEN: Serum collected in a red- or red/gray-top tube. Plasma collected in a green-top (heparin) tube is also acceptable.

NORMAL FINDINGS: (Method: Spectrophotometry for total calcium; ion-selective electrode for ionized calcium)

Calcium, total

Age	Conventional Units	SI Units (Conventional Units × 0.25)
Cord	8.2–11.2 mg/dL	2.1–2.8 mmol/L
0–10 d	7.6–10.4 mg/dL	1.9–2.6 mmol/L
11 d–2 yr	9–11 mg/dL	2.2–2.8 mmol/L
3–12 yr	8.8–10.8 mg/dL	2.2–2.7 mmol/L
13–18 yr	8.4–10.2 mg/dL	2.1–2.6 mmol/L
Adult	8.2–10.2 mg/dL	2.1–2.6 mmol/L
Adult older than 90 yr	8.2–9.6 mg/dL	2.1–2.4 mmol/L

Calcium, ionized

Age	Conventional Units	SI Units (Conventional Units × 0.25)
Whole blood		
0–11 mo	4.2–5.84 mg/dL	1.05–1.46 mmol/L
1 yr–adult	4.6–5.08 mg/dL	1.15–1.27 mmol/L
Plasma		
Adult	4.12–4.92 mg/dL	1.03–1.23 mmol/L
Serum		
1–18 yr	4.8–5.52 mg/dL	1.2–1.38 mmol/L
Adult and older adult	4.64–5.28 mg/dL	1.16–1.32 mmol/L

DESCRIPTION: Calcium, the most abundant cation in the body, participates in almost all of the body's vital processes. Calcium concentration is largely regulated by the parathyroid glands and by the action of vitamin D. Of the body's calcium reserves, 98% to 99% is stored in the teeth and skeleton. Calcium values are higher in children because of growth and active bone formation. About 45% of the total amount of blood calcium circulates as free ions that participate in numerous regulatory functions to include bone development and maintenance, blood coagulation, transmission of nerve impulses, activation of enzymes, stimulating the glandular secretion of hormones, and control of skeletal and cardiac muscle contractility. The remaining calcium is bound to circulating proteins (40% bound mostly to albumin) and anions (15% bound to anions such as bicarbonate, citrate, phosphate, and lactate) and plays no physiological role. Calcium values can be adjusted up or down by 0.8 mg/dL (0.2 mmol/L) for every 1 g/dL (10 g/L) that albumin is greater than or less than 4 g/dL (40 g/L). Calcium levels are regulated largely by the parathyroid glands and by vitamin D; calcium levels are inversely proportional to parathyroid hormone (PTH) levels. Vitamin D enhances gastrointestinal (GI) absorption of calcium. Calcium and phosphorus levels are inversely proportional.

Fluid and electrolyte imbalances are often seen in patients

with serious illness or injury; in these clinical situations, the normal homeostatic balance of the body is altered. During surgery or in the case of a critical illness, bicarbonate, phosphate, and lactate concentrations can change dramatically. Therapeutic treatments may also cause or contribute to electrolyte imbalance. This is why total calcium values can sometimes be misleading. Abnormal calcium levels are used to indicate general malfunctions in various body systems. Compared to total calcium level, ionized calcium is a better measurement of calcium metabolism. Ionized calcium levels are not influenced by protein concentrations, as seen in patients with hypoalbuminemia, chronic kidney disease, nephrotic syndrome, malabsorption, and multiple myeloma. Levels are also not affected in patients with metabolic acid-base balance disturbances. Elevations in ionized calcium may be seen when the total calcium is normal. Measurement of ionized calcium is useful to monitor patients undergoing cardiothoracic surgery or organ transplantation. It is also useful in the evaluation of patients in cardiac arrest.

Calcium values should be interpreted in conjunction with results of other tests. Normal calcium with an abnormal phosphorus value indicates impaired calcium absorption (possibly because of altered parathyroid hormone level or activity). Normal calcium with an elevated urea nitrogen value indicates possible hyperparathyroidism (primary or secondary). Normal calcium with decreased albumin value is an indication of hypercalcemia. The most common cause of hypocalcemia is hypoalbuminemia. The most common causes of hypercalcemia are hyperparathyroidism and cancer (with or without bone metastases).

This procedure is contraindicated for: N/A

INDICATIONS

- Detect ectopic PTH-producing neoplasms.
- Detect parathyroid gland loss after thyroid or other neck surgery, as indicated by decreased levels.
- Evaluate cardiac arrhythmias and coagulation disorders to determine if altered serum calcium level is contributing to the problem.
- Evaluate the effect of protein on calcium levels.
- Evaluate the effects of various disorders on calcium metabolism, especially diseases involving bone.
- Identify individuals with hypo- or hypercalcemia.
- Identify individuals with toxic levels of vitamin D.
- Investigate suspected hyperparathyroidism.
- Monitor the effectiveness of therapy being administered to correct abnormal calcium levels, especially calcium deficiencies.
- Monitor patients with chronic kidney disease or organ transplantation in whom secondary hyperparathyroidism may be a complication.
- Monitor patients with sepsis or magnesium deficiency.

POTENTIAL MEDICAL DIAGNOSIS

Increased in:

- Acidosis ***(related to imbalance in electrolytes; longstanding acidosis can result in osteoporosis and release of calcium into circulation)***

- Acromegaly ***(related to alteration in vitamin D metabolism, resulting in increased calcium)***
- Addison's disease ***(related to adrenal gland dysfunction; decreased blood volume and dehydration occur in the absence of aldosterone)***
- Cancers (bone, Burkitt's lymphoma, Hodgkin's lymphoma, leukemia, myeloma, and metastases from other organs)
- Dehydration ***(related to a decrease in the fluid portion of blood, causing an overall increase in the concentration of most plasma constituents)***
- Hyperparathyroidism ***(related to increased PTH and vitamin D levels, which increase circulating calcium levels)***
- Idiopathic hypercalcemia of infancy
- Kidney transplant ***(related to imbalances in electrolytes; a common post-transplant issue)***
- Lung disease (tuberculosis, histoplasmosis, coccidioidomycosis, berylliosis) ***(related to activity by macrophages in the epithelium that interfere with vitamin D regulation by converting it to its active form; vitamin D increases circulating calcium levels)***
- Malignant disease without bone involvement ***(some cancers [e.g., squamous cell carcinoma of the lung and kidney cancer] produce PTH-related peptide that increases calcium levels)***
- Milk-alkali syndrome (Burnett's syndrome) ***(related to excessive intake of calcium-containing milk or antacids, which can increase calcium levels)***
- PTH-producing neoplasms ***(PTH increases calcium levels)***
- Paget's disease ***(related to calcium released from bone)***
- Pheochromocytoma ***(hyperparathyroidism related to multiple endocrine neoplasia type 2A [MEN2A] syndrome associated with some pheochromocytomas; PTH increases calcium levels)***
- Polycythemia vera ***(related to dehydration; decreased blood volume due to excessive production of red blood cells)***
- Sarcoidosis ***(related to activity by macrophages in the granulomas that interfere with vitamin D regulation by converting it to its active form; vitamin D increases circulating calcium levels)***
- Thyrotoxicosis ***(related to increased bone turnover and release of calcium into the blood)***
- Vitamin D toxicity ***(vitamin D increases circulating calcium levels)***

Decreased in:

- Acute pancreatitis ***(complication of pancreatitis related to hypoalbuminemia and calcium binding by excessive fats)***
- Alcoholism ***(related to insufficient nutrition)***
- Alkalosis ***(increased blood pH causes intracellular uptake of calcium to increase)***
- Burns, severe ***(related to increased amino acid release)***
- Chronic kidney disease ***(related to decreased synthesis of vitamin D)***
- Cystinosis ***(hereditary disorder of the renal tubules that results in excessive calcium loss)***
- Hepatic cirrhosis ***(related to impaired metabolism of vitamin D and calcium)***
- Hyperphosphatemia ***(phosphorus and calcium have an inverse relationship)***
- Hypoalbuminemia ***(related to insufficient levels of albumin, an important carrier protein)***

- Hypomagnesemia ***(lack of magnesium inhibits PTH and thereby decreases calcium levels)***
- Hypoparathyroidism (congenital, idiopathic, surgical) ***(related to lack of PTH)***
- Inadequate nutrition
- Leprosy ***(related to increased bone retention)***
- Long-term anticonvulsant therapy ***(these medications block calcium channels and interfere with calcium transport)***
- Magnesium deficiency ***(inhibits release of PTH)***
- Malabsorption (celiac disease, tropical sprue, pancreatic insufficiency) ***(related to insufficient absorption)***
- Massive blood transfusion ***(related to the presence of citrate preservative in blood product that chelates or binds calcium and removes it from circulation)***
- Multiple organ failure
- Osteomalacia (advanced) ***(bone loss is so advanced there is little calcium remaining to be released into circulation)***
- Premature infants with hypoproteinemia and acidosis ***(related to alterations in transport protein levels)***
- Pseudohypoparathyroidism ***(related to decreased PTH)***
- Sepsis ***(related to decreased PTH)***
- The postdialysis period ***(result of low-calcium dialysate administration)***
- Trauma (i.e., major surgeries) ***(related to decreased PTH)***
- Renal tubular disease ***(related to decreased synthesis of vitamin D)***
- Vitamin D deficiency (rickets) ***(related to insufficient amounts of vitamin D, resulting in decreased calcium metabolism)***

CRITICAL FINDINGS:

Calcium, total

- Less than 7 mg/dL (SI: Less than 1.8 mmol/L)
- Greater than 12 mg/dL (SI: Greater than 3 mmol/L) (some patients can tolerate higher concentrations)

Calcium, ionized

- Less than 3.2 mg/dL (SI: Less than 0.8 mmol/L)
- Greater than 6.2 mg/dL (SI: Greater than 1.6 mmol/L)

Note and immediately report to the requesting health-care provider (HCP) any critical findings and related symptoms. A listing of these findings varies among facilities. Timely notification of a critical finding for laboratory or diagnostic studies is a role expectation of the professional nurse. The notification processes vary among facilities. Upon receipt of the critical finding, the information should be read back to the caller to verify accuracy.

Consideration may be given to verification of critical findings before action is taken. Policies vary among facilities and may include requesting immediate recollection and retesting by the laboratory or retesting using a rapid point-of-care testing instrument at the bedside, if available.

Observe the patient for symptoms of critically decreased or elevated calcium levels. Hypocalcemia is evidenced by convulsions, nervousness, dysrhythmias, changes in electrocardiogram (ECG) in the form of prolonged ST segment and Q-T interval, facial spasms (positive Chvostek's sign), tetany, lethargy, muscle cramps, tetany, numbness in extremities, tingling, and muscle twitching (positive Trousseau's sign). Possible interventions include seizure precautions, increased frequency of ECG monitoring, and administration of calcium or magnesium.

Severe hypercalcemia is manifested by excessive thirst, polyuria, constipation, changes in ECG (shortened QT interval due to shortening of the ST segment and prolonged PR interval), lethargy, confusion, muscle weakness, joint aches, apathy, anorexia, headache, nausea, vomiting, and ultimately may result in coma. Possible interventions include the administration of normal saline and diuretics to speed up dilution and excretion or administration of calcitonin or steroids to force the circulating calcium into the cells.

INTERFERING FACTORS

- Drugs and other substances that may increase calcium levels include anabolic steroids, some antacids, calcitriol, calcium salts, danazol, diuretics (long-term), ergocalciferol, hydralazine, isotretinoin, lithium, oral contraceptives, parathyroid extract, parathyroid hormone, prednisone, progesterone, tamoxifen, vitamin A, and vitamin D.
- Drugs and other substances that may decrease calcium levels include acetazolamide, albuterol, alprostadil, aminoglycosides, anticonvulsants, asparaginase, aspirin, calcitonin, cisplatin, citrates, diuretics (initially), estrogens, foscarnet, gastrin, glucagon, glucocorticoids, glucose, heparin, insulin, laxatives (excessive use), magnesium salts, methicillin, phosphates, plicamycin, sodium sulfate (given intravenous (IV)), tetracycline (in pregnancy), trazodone, and viomycin.
- Calcium exhibits diurnal variation; serial samples should be collected at the same time of day for comparison.
- Venous hemostasis caused by prolonged use of a tourniquet during venipuncture can falsely elevate calcium levels.
- Patients on ethylenediaminetetraacetic acid (EDTA) therapy (chelation) may show falsely decreased calcium values.
- Patients receiving massive blood transfusions may experience decreased ionized calcium values related to chelation of the free calcium by the anticoagulant in the blood products.
- Patients with low albumin levels (e.g., in cases of malnutrition or dilutional effect of IV fluid overload) will have low total calcium levels.
- Patients who ingest large amounts of milk, calcium or vitamin D supplements, or antacid tablets shortly before specimen collection will have increased calcium values.
- Patients with chronic kidney disease, especially those on hemodialysis, may have low calcium levels. The inability of the kidneys to filter excess phosphorus from the blood into urine stimulates abnormal excretion of calcium, resulting in lower circulating calcium levels. If the calcium concentration in the dialysate fluid is not adjusted to correct the blood levels, the parathyroid glands secrete PTH, which causes calcium to be lost from the bones. Over time, bone loss results in deformities and loss of function.
- Hemolysis and icterus cause false-positive results because of interference from biological pigments.
- Specimens should never be collected above an IV line because of the potential for dilution when the specimen and the IV solution combine in the collection container, falsely decreasing the result. There is also the potential of contaminating the sample with the substance of interest if it is present in the IV solution, falsely increasing the result.

C

NURSING IMPLICATIONS AND PROCEDURE

POTENTIAL NURSING PROBLEMS:

Problem	Signs & Symptoms	Interventions
Pain ***(related to organ inflammation and surrounding tissues; excessive alcohol intake; infection; bone deformity)***	Emotional symptoms of distress; crying; agitation; facial grimace; moaning; verbalization of pain; rocking motions; irritability; disturbed sleep; diaphoresis; altered blood pressure and heart rate; nausea; vomiting; self-report of pain	Collaborate with the patient and HCP to identify the best pain management modality to provide relief; refrain from activities that may aggravate pain; use the application of heat or cold to the best effect in managing the pain; monitor pain severity
Health management ***(related to failure to regulate diet; lack of exercise; alcohol use; smoking)***	Inability or failure to recognize or process information toward improving health and preventing illness with associated mental and physical effects	Encourage regular participation in weight-bearing exercise; assess diet, smoking, and alcohol use; teach the importance of adequate calcium intake with diet and supplements; refer to smoking cessation and alcohol treatment programs; collaborate with HCP for bone density evaluation
Nutrition ***(related to inability to digest foods, metabolize foods, ingest foods; refusal to eat; increased metabolic needs associated with disease process; lack of understanding; inability to obtain healthy foods)***	Unintended weight loss; current weight 20% below ideal weight; pale, dry skin; dry mucous membranes; documented inadequate caloric intake; subcutaneous tissue loss; hair pulls out easily; paresthesia	Obtain accurate daily weight at the same time each day with the same scale; obtain an accurate nutritional history; assess attitude toward eating; promote a dietary consult to evaluate current eating habits and best method of nutritional supplementation; develop short-term and long-term eating strategies; monitor nutritional laboratory values such as albumin, transferrin, red blood cells (RBC), white blood cells (WBC), and serum electrolytes; discourage caffeinated and carbonated

(table continues on page 344)

Problem	Signs & Symptoms	Interventions
		beverages; assess swallowing ability; encourage cultural home foods; provide a pleasant environment for eating; alter food seasoning to enhance flavor; provide parenteral or enteral nutrition as prescribed
Injury risk ***(related to phosphorous retention; bone resorption; inadequate calcium resorption; acute kidney injury or chronic kidney disease; lack of dietary vitamin D; decreased sun exposure; eating disorders)***	Tingling sensation in the fingertips and around the mouth; muscle cramps; tetany; seizures; bone pain; weakness; unsteady gait; laryngospasm; cardiac dysrhythmias; hyperactive tendon reflexes	Assess for signs and symptoms of hypocalcemia; monitor calcium and phosphorus levels; provide medication replacement therapy as prescribed; assess for bone pain; assess for alterations in mobility; increase the calcium in the diet; encourage the minimum recommended sun exposure

PRETEST:

- Positively identify the patient using at least two person-specific identifiers before services, treatments, or procedures are performed.
- *Patient Teaching:* Inform the patient this test can assist as a general indicator in diagnosing health concerns.
- Obtain a history of the patient's health concerns, symptoms, surgical procedures, and results of previously performed laboratory and diagnostic studies. Include a list of known allergens, especially allergies or sensitivities to latex.
- Note any recent procedures that can interfere with test results.
- Obtain a list of the patient's current medications, including over-the-counter medications and dietary supplements (see Effects of Natural Products on Laboratory Values online at Davis*Plus*).
- Review the procedure with the patient. Inform the patient that specimen collection takes approximately 5 to 10 min. Address concerns about pain and explain that there may be some discomfort during the venipuncture.
- *Sensitivity to social and cultural issues,* as well as concern for modesty, is important in providing psychological support before, during, and after the procedure.
- Note that there are no food, fluid, or medication restrictions unless by medical direction.

INTRATEST:

Potential Complications: N/A

- Avoid the use of equipment containing latex if the patient has a history of allergic reaction to latex.
- Instruct the patient to cooperate fully and to follow directions. Direct the patient to breathe normally and to avoid unnecessary movement.
- Observe standard precautions, and follow the general guidelines in Patient Preparation and Specimen Collection online at Davis*Plus*. Positively identify the patient, and label

the appropriate specimen container with the corresponding patient demographics, initials of the person collecting the specimen, date, and time of collection. Perform a venipuncture.
- Remove the needle and apply direct pressure with dry gauze to stop bleeding. Observe/assess venipuncture site for bleeding or hematoma formation and secure gauze with adhesive bandage.
- Promptly transport the specimen to the laboratory for processing and analysis.

POST-TEST:

- Inform the patient that a report of the results will be made available to the requesting HCP, who will discuss the results with the patient.
- Recognize anxiety related to test results, and assess the patient for signs and symptoms of calcium imbalance. Teach the patient the signs and symptoms associated with a calcium imbalance. Assess associated studies such as ECG, phosphorus, and albumin so the correct therapeutic measures can be taken. Hypoalbuminemia may initiate symptoms of hypocalcemia in the presence of near-normal calcium levels.
- ***Nutritional Considerations:*** Patients with abnormal calcium values should be informed that daily intake of calcium is important even though body stores in the bones can be called on to supplement circulating levels. Dietary calcium can be obtained from animal or plant sources. Almonds (milk, nuts), beet greens, broccoli, cheese, clams, kale, legumes, milk and milk products, oysters, rhubarb, salmon (canned), sardines (canned), spinach, tofu, yogurt, and calcium fortified foods such as orange juice are high in calcium. Milk and milk products also contain vitamin D and lactose, which assist calcium absorption.
- Depending on the results of this procedure, additional testing may be performed to evaluate or monitor progression of the disease process and determine the need for a change in therapy. Evaluate test results in relation to the patient's symptoms and other tests performed.

Patient Education:

- Reinforce information given by the patient's HCP regarding further testing, treatment, or referral to another HCP.
- Answer any questions or address any concerns voiced by the patient or family.
- Educate the patient regarding access to nutritional counseling services.
- Provide contact information, if desired, for the Institute of Medicine of the National Academies (www.iom.edu) or the USDA's resource for nutrition (www.choosemyplate.gov). 🍁
- Teach the patient and family the importance of adequate dietary calcium intake to maintain health.
- Teach the patient that good oral hygiene prior to eating can improve the food's flavor.

Expected Patient Outcomes:

Understanding

- The patient and family verbalize that eating in a pleasant environment with companionship can enhance the appetite.
- States that parenteral or enteral nutrition may be used if oral intake is insufficient to support caloric needs.

Ability

- Performs an accurate daily self-weight and records the results correctly.
- Accurately self-administers prescribed dietary supplements.

Response

- The patient complies with the request to take prescribed calcium replacement therapy.
- The patient and family arrange consultation with the speech therapist to evaluate swallowing ability.

RELATED STUDIES:

- Related tests include ACTH, albumin, aldosterone, ALP, biopsy bone marrow, BMD, bone scan, calcitonin, urine calcium, calculus kidney stone analysis, catecholamines, chloride, collagen cross-linked telopeptides,

CBC, CT pelvis, CT spine, cortisol, CK and isoenzymes, DHEA, fecal fat, glucose, HVA, magnesium, metanephrines, osteocalcin, PTH, phosphorus, potassium, protein total, radiography bone, renin, sodium, thyroid scan, thyroxine, US abdomen, US thyroid and parathyroid, UA, and vitamin D.

- Refer to the Cardiovascular, Gastrointestinal, Genitourinary, Hematopoietic, Hepatobiliary, and Musculoskeletal systems tables online at Davis*Plus* for related tests by body system.

C

Calcium, Urine

SYNONYM/ACRONYM: N/A

COMMON USE: To indicate sufficiency of dietary calcium intake and rate of absorption. Urine calcium levels are also used to assess bone resorption, kidney stones, and renal loss of calcium.

SPECIMEN: Urine from an unpreserved random or timed specimen collected in a clean plastic collection container.

NORMAL FINDINGS: (Method: Spectrophotometry)

Age	Conventional Units*	SI Units (Conventional Units × 0.025)*
Infant and child	Up to 6 mg/kg per 24 hr	Up to 0.15 mmol/kg per 24 hr
Adult on average diet	100–300 mg/24 hr	2.5–7.5 mmol/24 hr

*Values depend on diet.

POTENTIAL MEDICAL DIAGNOSIS

Increased in:

- Acromegaly ***(related to imbalance in vitamin D metabolism)***
- Diabetes ***(related to increased loss from damaged kidneys)***
- Fanconi's syndrome ***(evidenced by hereditary or acquired disorder of the renal tubules that results in excessive calcium loss)***
- Glucocorticoid excess ***(related to action of glucocorticoids, which is to decrease the gastrointestinal absorption of calcium and increase urinary excretion)***
- Hepatolenticular degeneration (Wilson's disease) ***(related to excessive electrolyte loss due to renal damage)***
- Hyperparathyroidism ***(related to increased levels of parathyroid hormone [PTH], which result in increased calcium levels)***
- Hyperthyroidism ***(related to increased bone turnover; excess circulating calcium is excreted by the kidneys)***
- Idiopathic hypercalciuria
- Immobilization ***(related to disruption in calcium homeostasis and bone loss)***
- Kidney stones ***(evidenced by excessive urinary calcium; contributes to the formation of kidney stones)***
- Leukemia and lymphoma (some instances)
- Myeloma ***(calcium is released from damaged bone; excess***

circulating calcium is excreted by the kidneys)
- Neoplasm of the breast or bladder ***(some cancers secrete PTH or PTH-related peptide that increases calcium levels)***
- Osteitis deformans ***(calcium is released from damaged bone; excess circulating calcium is excreted by the kidneys)***
- Osteolytic bone metastases (carcinoma, sarcoma) ***(calcium is released from damaged bone; excess circulating calcium is excreted by the kidneys)***
- Osteoporosis ***(calcium is released from damaged bone; excess circulating calcium is excreted by the kidneys)***
- Paget's disease ***(calcium is released from damaged bone; excess circulating calcium is excreted by the kidneys)***
- Renal tubular acidosis ***(metabolic acidosis resulting in loss of calcium by the kidneys)***
- Sarcoidosis ***(macrophages in the granulomas interfere with vitamin D regulation by converting it to its active form; vitamin D increases circulating calcium levels, and excess is excreted by the kidneys)***
- Schistosomiasis
- Thyrotoxicosis ***(increased bone turnover; excess circulating calcium is excreted by the kidneys)***
- Vitamin D intoxication ***(increases calcium metabolism; excess is excreted by the kidneys)***

Decreased in:
- Hypocalcemia (other than renal disease)
- Hypocalciuric hypercalcemia (familial, nonfamilial)
- Hypoparathyroidism ***(PTH instigates release of calcium; if PTH levels are low, calcium levels will be decreased)***
- Hypothyroidism
- Malabsorption (celiac disease, tropical sprue) ***(related to insufficient levels of calcium)***
- Malignant bone neoplasm
- Nephrosis and acute nephritis ***(related to decreased synthesis of vitamin D)***
- Osteoblastic metastases
- Osteomalacia ***(related to vitamin D deficiency)***
- Pre-eclampsia
- Pseudohypoparathyroidism
- Renal osteodystrophy
- Rickets ***(related to deficiency in vitamin D)***
- Vitamin D deficiency ***(deficiency in vitamin D results in decreased calcium levels)***

CRITICAL FINDINGS: N/A

Find and print out the full study on Fast Find at davispl.us/vanleeuwen7.

Calculus, Kidney Stone Panel

SYNONYM/ACRONYM: Kidney stone analysis, nephrolithiasis analysis.

COMMON USE: To identify the presence of kidney stones.

SPECIMEN: Kidney stones.

NORMAL FINDINGS: (Method: Infrared spectrometry) None detected.

DESCRIPTION: Renal calculi (kidney stones) are formed by the crystallization of calcium oxalate (most common), magnesium ammonium phosphate, calcium phosphate, uric acid, and cystine. Formation of stones may be hereditary, related to diet or poor hydration, urinary tract infections caused by urease-producing bacteria, conditions resulting in reduced urine flow, or excessive amounts of the previously mentioned insoluble substances due to other predisposing conditions. The presence of stones is confirmed by diagnostic visualization or passing of the stones in the urine. The chemical nature of the stones is confirmed qualitatively. Analysis also includes a description of color, size, and weight.

This procedure is contraindicated for: N/A

INDICATIONS

- Identify substances present in renal calculi

POTENTIAL MEDICAL DIAGNOSIS

Positive findings in

Presence of calcium calculi (75%–85%)

- Decreased levels of citric acid, which creates an imbalance of mineral salts ***(related to conditions such as enteric hyperoxaluria, enterocystoplasty, or small bowel resection)***
- Distal renal tubular acidosis ***(related to accumulation of calcium in the kidneys)***
- Etiology unknown
- Increased levels of calcium with or without alkaline pH, which creates an imbalance of mineral salts ***(related to conditions such as Cushing's disease, Dent's disease, enterocystoplasty, ileostomy, immobilization, medullary sponge kidney, metabolic syndrome, milk alkali syndrome, primary biliary cirrhosis, primary hyperparathyroidism, sarcoidosis, Sjörgren's syndrome, use of calcium carbonate–containing antacids, use of corticosteroids, or vitamin D intoxication)***
- Increased levels of oxalic acid, which creates an imbalance of mineral salts ***(related to conditions such as bariatric surgery, enteric hyperoxaluria, enterocystoplasty, hereditary hyperoxaluria, hypomagnesemia, jejunal-ileal bypass, metabolic syndrome, pancreatitis, or small bowel resection)***
- Increased levels of uric acid, which creates an imbalance of mineral salts (uric acid crystals sometimes provide the base upon which calcium oxalate crystals grow)

Presence of magnesium ammonium phosphate (struvite or triple phosphate) calculi (10%–15%)

- Urinary tract infection ***(related to chronic indwelling catheter, neurogenic bladder dysfunction, obstruction, or urinary diversion)***
- Gram-positive bacteria associated with development of struvite calculi include *Bacillus* species, *Corynebacterium* species, *Peptococcus asaccharolyticus*, *Staphylococcus aureus*, and *Staphylococcus epidermidis*
- Gram-negative bacteria associated with development of struvite calculi include *Bacteroides corrodens*, *Flavobacterium* species, *Klebsiella* species, *Pasteurella* species, *Proteus* species, *Providencia stuartii*, *Pseudomonas aeruginosa*, *Serratia marcescens*, *Ureaplasma urealyticum*, and *Yersinia enterocolitica*

- Yeast associated with development of struvite calculi include *Candida humicola*, *Cryptococcus* species, *Rhodotorula* species, *Sporobolomyces* species, and *Trichosporon cutaneum*

Presence of uric acid calculi (5%–8%)

- Increased levels of uric acid or increased urinary excretion of uric acid
- Anemias (pernicious, lead poisoning) ***(related to cellular destruction and turnover)***
- Chemotherapy and radiation therapy ***(related to high cell turnover)***
- Gout ***(usually related to excess dietary intake)***
- Glycogen storage disease type I (von Gierke's disease) ***(related to a genetic deficiency of the enzyme G-6-P-D, ultimately resulting in hyperuricemia, increased production of uric acid via the pentose phosphate pathway, and increased purine catabolism)***
- Hemoglobinopathies (sickle cell anemia, thalassemias) ***(related to cellular destruction and turnover)***
- Ileostomy ***(related to imbalances in mineral salts)***
- Lesch-Nyhan syndrome ***(related to a disorder of uric acid metabolism)***
- Metabolic syndrome ***(elevated uric acid levels are associated with metabolic syndrome; there is evidence that uric acidemia is a risk factor for cardiovascular and renal disease)***
- Polycythemia ***(related to increased cellular destruction)***
- Psoriasis ***(related to increased skin cell turnover)***
- Tumors ***(related to high cell turnover)***

Presence of cystine calculi (approximately 1%)

- Fanconi's syndrome (hereditary hypercistinuria) ***(related to increased excretion of cystine)***

Negative findings in: N/A

CRITICAL FINDINGS: N/A

INTERFERING FACTORS

- Drugs and other substances that may increase the formation of urine calculi include probenecid and vitamin D.
- Adhesive tape should not be used to attach stones to any transportation or collection container, because the adhesive interferes with infrared spectrometry.

NURSING IMPLICATIONS AND PROCEDURE

POTENTIAL NURSING PROBLEMS:

Problem	Signs & Symptoms	Interventions
Pain ***(related to obstruction of urinary flow by stone, presence of stone, movement of stone)***	Report of pain, restlessness, grimace, moan, sleeplessness, diaphoresis, nausea, vomiting; elevated blood pressure	Administer prescribed medication for pain; assesses effectiveness of pain medication and trend outcome; assess characteristics of pain (location, duration); consider nonpharmacological pain interventions that have worked for the patient in the past

(table continues on page 350)

Problem	Signs & Symptoms	Interventions
Infection ***(related to stasis; interrupted urinary flow; gravel; urinary tract instrumentation)***	Elevated temperature; elevated white blood cell (WBC) count; cloudy urine; sediment in urine; blood in urine	Monitor urinary output; assess urine color, odor, presence of blood; monitor and trend temperature and WBC count; obtain urine for culture and sensitivity as required; encourage fluid intake in excess of 3,000 mL/day; administer prescribed antibiotics
Knowledge ***(related to unfamiliarity of factors related to the development of kidney stones; unfamiliarity with disease management; methods of disease prevention)***	Lack of interest or questions; multiple questions; anxiety in relation to disease process and management; renal stone reoccurrence	Assess understanding of kidney stone formation; assess for a family history of kidney stones; assess patient's understanding of the relationship between fluid intake and stone formation; strain urine; limit protein intake to decrease risk of stone formation; add cranberry juice to dietary intake; administer prescribed medications to decrease stone formation (cholestyramine, thiazide, allopurinol)
Elevated temperature ***(related to infection secondary to stone formation)***	Elevated temperature; flushed; warm skin; diaphoresis	Assess the patient's temperature frequently; encourage the use of light bedding and lightweight clothing to prevent overheating; increase fluid intake to offset insensible fluid loss; encourage bathing with tepid water for comfort and promotion of cooling; administer prescribed medication for elevated temperature

PRETEST:

- Positively identify the patient using at least two person-specific identifiers before services, treatments, or procedures are performed.
- ***Patient Teaching:*** Inform the patient this test can assist in identification of the presence of kidney stones.
- Obtain a history of the patient's health concerns, symptoms, surgical procedures, and results of previously performed laboratory and diagnostic studies. Include a list of known allergens, especially allergies or sensitivities to latex.
- Obtain a list of the patient's current medications, including over-the-counter medications and dietary supplements (see Effects of Natural Products on Laboratory Values online at Davis*Plus*).
- Review the procedure with the patient. Address concerns about pain

and explain that there may be some discomfort during the procedure.
- ***Sensitivity to social and cultural issues,*** as well as concern for modesty, is important in providing psychological support before, during, and after the procedure.
- Note that there are no food, fluid, or medication restrictions unless by medical direction.

INTRATEST:

Potential Complications: N/A

- Instruct the patient to cooperate fully and to follow directions.
- Observe standard precautions, and follow the general guidelines in Patient Preparation and Specimen Collection online at Davis*Plus*. Positively identify the patient, and label the appropriate specimen container with the corresponding patient demographics, initials of the person collecting the specimen, date, and time of collection.
- The patient presenting with symptoms indicating the presence of kidney stones may be provided with a device to strain the urine. The patient should be informed to transfer any particulate matter remaining in the strainer into the specimen collection container provided. Stones removed by the health-care provider (HCP) should be placed in the appropriate collection container.
- Promptly transport the specimen to the laboratory for processing and analysis.

POST-TEST:

- Inform the patient that a report of the results will be made available to the requesting HCP, who will discuss the results with the patient.
- Inform the patient with kidney stones that the likelihood of recurrence is high. Educate the patient regarding risk factors that contribute to the likelihood of kidney stone formation, including family history, osteoporosis, urinary tract infections, gout, magnesium deficiency, Crohn's disease with prior resection, age, gender (males are two to three times more likely than females to develop stones), ethnicity (Caucasians are three to four times more likely than African Americans to develop stones), and climate.
- ***Nutritional Considerations:*** Nutritional therapy is indicated for individuals identified as being at high risk for developing kidney stones. Educate the patient that diets rich in protein, salt, and oxalates increase the risk of stone formation. Adequate fluid intake should be encouraged.
- Recognize anxiety related to test results.
- Follow-up testing of urine may be requested, but usually not for 1 mo after the stones have passed or been removed. Answer any questions or address any concerns voiced by the patient or family.
- Depending on the results of this procedure, additional testing may be performed to evaluate or monitor progression of the disease process and determine the need for a change in therapy. Evaluate test results in relation to the patient's symptoms and other tests performed.

Patient Education:

- Discuss the implications of abnormal test results on the patient's lifestyle.
- Provide teaching and information regarding the clinical implications of the test results, as appropriate.
- Reinforce information given by the patient's HCP regarding further testing, treatment, or referral to another HCP.
- Teach patient to report worsening symptoms of infection such as fever, chills, and pain.

Expected Patient Outcomes:

Understanding

- The patient and family state the process and importance of straining all urine.
- The patient and family state the importance of increasing fluid intake and adding cranberry juice to their diet.

Ability

- The patient accurately self-administers prescribed medication.

- The patient demonstrates proficiency in straining urine to check for stones.

Response

- The patient complies with the recommendation to increase fluid intake to more than 3,000 mL/day.
- The patient and family discuss the importance in reporting changes in the characteristics of the urine in relation to infection risk.

RELATED STUDIES:

- Related tests include CT abdomen, calcium, creatinine clearance, culture bacterial urine, cystoscopy, IVP, KUB, magnesium, oxalate, phosphorus, potassium, renogram, retrograde ureteropyelography, US abdomen, US kidney, uric acid, and UA.
- Refer to the Genitourinary System table online at Davis*Plus* for related tests by body system.

Cancer Antigens: CA 15-3, CA 19-9, CA 125, and Carcinoembryonic

SYNONYM/ACRONYM: Carcinoembryonic antigen (CEA), cancer antigen 125 (CA 125), cancer antigen 15-3 (CA 15-3), cancer antigen 19-9 (CA 19-9), cancer antigen 27.29 (CA 27.29).

COMMON USE: To identify the presence of various cancers, such as breast and ovarian, as well as to evaluate the effectiveness of cancer treatment.

SPECIMEN: Serum collected in a red-top tube. Care must be taken to use the same assay method if serial measurements are to be taken.

NORMAL FINDINGS: (Method: Electrochemiluminometric immunoassay)

Smoking Status	Conventional Units	SI Units (Conventional Units × 1)
CEA		
Smoker	Less than 5 ng/mL	Less than 5 mcg/L
Nonsmoker	Less than 2.5 ng/mL	Less than 2.5 mcg/L

Conventional Units	SI Units (Conventional Units × 1)
CA 125	
Less than 35 units/mL	Less than 35 kilo units/L
CA 15-3	
Less than 25 units/mL	Less than 25 kilo units/L
CA 19-9	
Less than 35 units/mL	Less than 35 kilo units/L
CA 27.29	
Less than 38.6 units/mL	Less than 38.6 kilo units/L

DESCRIPTION: Carcinoembryonic antigen (CEA) is a family of 36 different glycoproteins whose function is believed to be involved in cell adhesion. These structurally related proteins are part of the immunoglobulin superfamily. CEA is normally produced during fetal development and rapid multiplication of epithelial cells, especially those of the digestive system. A small amount of circulating CEA is detectable in the blood of normal adults; normal half-life is 7 days. The liver is the main site for metabolism of CEA. Because of the variability in CEA molecules the test is not diagnostic for any specific disease and is not useful as a screening test for cancer. However, it is very useful for monitoring response to therapy in breast, liver, colon, and gastrointestinal cancer. Serial monitoring is also a useful indicator of recurrence or metastasis in colon or liver carcinoma. CEA levels are higher in the blood of individuals who smoke than in those who do not smoke, so most laboratories will have a normal range for each group.

CA 125 or Muc16 is a glycoprotein member of the mucin family and is present in normal endometrial tissue. It appears in the blood when natural endometrial protective barriers are destroyed, as occurs in cancer or endometriosis. CA 125 is most useful in monitoring the progression or recurrence of known ovarian cancer. It is not useful as a screening test because elevations can occur with numerous other conditions such as endometriosis, other diseases of the ovary, menstruation, pregnancy, and uterine fibroids. Persistently rising levels indicate a poor prognosis. Levels may also rise in pancreatic, liver, colon, breast, and lung cancers. Absence of detectable levels of CA 125 does not rule out the presence of tumor Human epididymis protein 4 (HE4) is a newer protein marker associated with various types of cancer including ovarian cancer. Significant or persistent elevations of HE4 may indicate the appearance, recurrence, or progression of epithelial ovarian cancer. A significant elevation would be an increase of greater than 25% over normal findings. Normal findings for HE4 in females who are premenopausal is less than 70 pmol/L and less than 140 pmol/L in females who are postmenopausal.

CA 15-3 monitors patients for recurrence or metastasis of breast carcinoma.

CA 19-9 is a carbohydrate antigen used for post-therapeutic monitoring of patients with gastrointestinal, pancreatic, liver, and colorectal cancer.

CA 27.29 is a glycoprotein product of the muc-1 gene. It is most useful as a serial monitor for response to therapy or recurrence of breast carcinoma.

This procedure is contraindicated for: N/A

INDICATIONS

CEA

- Determine stage of colorectal cancer and test for recurrence or metastasis.
- Monitor response to treatment of breast and gastrointestinal cancers.

CA 125
- Assist in the diagnosis of carcinoma of the cervix and endometrium.
- Assist in the diagnosis of ovarian cancer.
- Monitor response to treatment of ovarian cancer.

C

CA 15-3 and CA 27.29
- Monitor recurrent carcinoma of the breast.

CA 19-9
- Monitor effectiveness of therapy.
- Monitor gastrointestinal, head and neck, and gynecological carcinomas.
- Predict recurrence of cholangiocarcinoma.
- Predict recurrence of stomach, pancreatic, colorectal, gallbladder, liver, and urothelial carcinomas.

POTENTIAL MEDICAL DIAGNOSIS

Increased in:

CEA
- Benign tumors, including benign breast disease
- Chronic tobacco smoking
- Cirrhosis
- Colorectal, pulmonary, gastric, pancreatic, breast, head and neck, esophageal, ovarian, and prostate cancer
- Inflammatory bowel disease
- Pancreatitis
- Radiation therapy (transient)

CA 125
- Breast, colon, endometrial, liver, lung, ovarian, and pancreatic cancer
- Endometriosis
- First-trimester pregnancy
- Menses
- Ovarian abscess
- Pelvic inflammatory disease
- Peritonitis

CA 15-3 and CA 27.29
- Recurrence of breast carcinoma

CA 19-9
- Gastrointestinal, head and neck, and gynecologic carcinomas
- Recurrence of stomach, pancreatic, colorectal, gallbladder, liver, and urothelial carcinomas
- Recurrence of cholangiocarcinoma

Decreased in:
- Effective therapy or removal of the tumor

CRITICAL FINDINGS: N/A

INTERFERING FACTORS: N/A

NURSING IMPLICATIONS AND PROCEDURE

PRETEST:

- Positively identify the patient using at least two person-specific identifiers before services, treatments, or procedures are performed.
- *Patient Teaching:* Inform the patient this test can assist in monitoring the progress of various types of disease and evaluate response to therapy.
- Obtain a history of the patient's health concerns, symptoms, surgical procedures, and results of previously performed laboratory and diagnostic studies. Include a list of known allergens, especially allergies or sensitivities to latex.
- Obtain a list of the patient's current medications, including over-the-counter medications and dietary supplements (see Effects of Natural Products on Laboratory Values online at Davis*Plus*).
- Determine if the patient smokes, because people who smoke may have false elevations of CEA.
- Review the procedure with the patient. Inform the patient that specimen collection takes approximately 5 to 10 minutes. Address concerns about pain and explain that there may be some discomfort during the venipuncture.
- ***Sensitivity to social and cultural issues,*** as well as concern for modesty, is important in providing psychological

support before, during, and after the procedure.

- Note that there are no food, fluid, or medication restrictions unless by medical direction.

INTRATEST:

Potential Complications: N/A

- Avoid the use of equipment containing latex if the patient has a history of allergic reaction to latex.
- Instruct the patient to cooperate fully and to follow directions. Direct the patient to breathe normally and to avoid unnecessary movement.
- Observe standard precautions, and follow the general guidelines in Patient Preparation and Specimen Collection online at Davis*Plus*. Positively identify the patient, and label the appropriate specimen container with the corresponding patient demographics, initials of the person collecting the specimen, date, and time of collection. Perform a venipuncture.
- Remove the needle and apply direct pressure with dry gauze to stop bleeding. Observe/assess venipuncture site for bleeding or hematoma formation and secure gauze with adhesive bandage.
- Promptly transport the specimen to the laboratory for processing and analysis.

POST-TEST:

- Inform the patient that a report of the results will be made available to the requesting health-care provider (HCP), who will discuss the results with the patient.
- Recognize anxiety related to test results, and be supportive of perceived loss of independence and fear of shortened life expectancy. Discuss the implications of abnormal test results on the patient's lifestyle. Provide teaching and information regarding the clinical implications of the test results, as appropriate. Educate the patient regarding access to counseling services. Provide contact information, if desired, for the American Cancer Association (ACS) (www.cancer.org). 🍁 Reinforce information given by the patient's HCP regarding further testing, treatment, or referral to another HCP.
- Decisions regarding the need for and frequency of breast self-examination, mammography, MRI breast, or other cancer screening procedures should be made after consultation between the patient and HCP. The most current guidelines for breast cancer screening of the general population as well as of individuals with increased risk are available from the ACS (www.cancer.org), American College of Obstetricians and Gynecologists (ACOG) (www.acog.org), and American College of Radiology (www.acr.org). The ACS recommends breast examinations be performed every 3 yr for women between the ages of 20 and 39 yr and annually for women over 40 yr; annual mammograms should be performed on women 40 yr and older as long as they are in good health. The ACS also recommends annual MRI testing, in addition to an annual mammogram, for women at high risk of developing breast cancer. 🍁 Genetic testing for inherited mutations (BRCA1 and BRCA2) associated with increased risk of developing breast cancer may be ordered for women at risk. The test is performed on a blood specimen. Answer any questions or address any concerns voiced by the patient or family.
- Decisions regarding the need for and frequency of occult blood testing, colonoscopy, or other cancer screening procedures should be made after consultation between the patient and HCP. The ACS recommends regular screening for colon cancer beginning at age 50 yr for individuals without identified risk factors and sooner for those with identified risk factors. Their recommendations for frequency of screening are to use one of the following: (1) annual for occult blood testing (fecal occult blood testing or fecal immunochemical testing); (2) every 5 yr for flexible sigmoidoscopy, double contrast barium

enema, or computed tomography (CT) colonography; (3) every 10 yr for colonoscopy; or (4) every 3 yr for stool DNA testing. Abnormal findings should be followed up by colonoscopy. There are advantages and disadvantages to the screening tests that are available today. Methods to use DNA testing of stool are being investigated and are designed to identify abnormal changes in DNA from the cells in the lining of the colon that are normally shed and excreted in stool. The DNA tests under development use multiple markers to identify colon cancers that demonstrate different, abnormal DNA changes. Unlike some of the current screening methods, the DNA tests would be able to detect precancerous polyps. The most current guidelines for colon cancer screening of the general population as well as of individuals with increased risk are available from the ACS (www.cancer.org), U.S. Preventive Services Task Force (www.uspreventiveservicestaskforce.org), and American College of Gastroenterology (www.gi.org).

- Depending on the results of this procedure, additional testing may be performed to evaluate or monitor progression of the disease process and determine the need for a change in therapy. Evaluate test results in relation to the patients symptoms and other tests performed.

RELATED STUDIES:

- Related tests include barium enema, biopsy breast, biopsy cervical, biopsy intestinal, biopsy liver, capsule endoscopy, colonoscopy, colposcopy, fecal analysis, genetic testing, HCG, liver and spleen scan, MRI breast, MRI liver, mammogram, stereotactic breast biopsy, proctosigmoidoscopy, radiofrequency ablation liver, US abdomen, US breast, and US liver.
- Refer to the Gastrointestinal, Immune, and Reproductive systems tables online at Davis*Plus* for related tests by body system.

Capsule Endoscopy

SYNONYM/ACRONYM: Pill GI endoscopy.

COMMON USE: To assist in visualization of the gastrointestinal (GI) tract to identify disease such as tumor and inflammation.

AREA OF APPLICATION: Esophagus, stomach, upper duodenum, and small bowel.

DESCRIPTION: This outpatient procedure involves ingesting a small (size of a large vitamin pill) capsule that is wireless and contains a small video camera that will pass naturally through the digestive system while taking pictures of the intestine. The capsule is 11 mm by 30 mm and contains a camera, light source, radio transmitter, and battery. The patient swallows the capsule, and the camera takes and transmits two images per second. The images are transmitted to a recording device, which saves all images for review later by a health-care provider (HCP). This device is approximately the size of a personal compact disk player. The recording device is worn on a belt around the patient's waist, and the video images are transmitted to aerials taped to the body and stored on the device. After 8 hr, the device is removed and returned to the HCP for processing. Thousands of images are downloaded onto a computer for viewing by an HCP specialist. The capsule is disposable and will be excreted naturally in the patient's bowel movements. In the rare case that it is not excreted naturally, it will need to be removed endoscopically or surgically.

This procedure is contraindicated for

- Patients who have had surgery involving the stomach or duodenum, ***which can make locating the duodenal papilla difficult.***
- Patients with a bleeding disorder.
- Patients with unstable cardiopulmonary status, blood coagulation defects, or cholangitis, unless the patient received prophylactic antibiotic therapy before the test (otherwise, the examination must be rescheduled).
- Patients with unstable cardiopulmonary status, blood coagulation defects, known aortic arch aneurysm, large esophageal Zenker's diverticulum, recent gastrointestinal (GI) surgery, esophageal varices, or known esophageal perforation.
- Patients with swallowing disorders.
- Patients with intestinal blockages or obstructions that may prevent passage of the capsule through the GI tract.
- Patients who are unable to have surgery in the case of recovering a retained capsule.
- Patients with implanted electronic devices such as pacemakers or cardiac defibrillators ***because normal function of the implanted device may be affected by the capsule device's electromagnetic field.***

INDICATIONS

- Assist in differentiating between benign and neoplastic tumors.
- Detect gastric or duodenal ulcers.
- Detect GI inflammatory disease.
- Determine the presence and location of GI bleeding and vascular abnormalities.
- Evaluate the extent of esophageal injury after ingestion of chemicals.
- Evaluate stomach or duodenum after surgical procedures.
- Evaluate suspected gastric obstruction.
- Identify Crohn's disease, infectious enteritis, and celiac sprue.
- Identify source of chronic diarrhea.
- Investigate the cause of abdominal pain, celiac syndrome, and other malabsorption syndromes.

POTENTIAL MEDICAL DIAGNOSIS

Normal findings

- Esophageal mucosa is normally yellow-pink. At about 9 in. from the incisor teeth, a pulsation indicates the location of the aortic arch. The gastric mucosa is orange-red and contains rugae. The proximal duodenum is reddish and contains a few longitudinal folds, whereas the distal duodenum has circular folds lined with villi. No abnormal structures or functions are observed in the esophagus, stomach, or duodenum.

Abnormal findings related to

- Achalasia
- Acute and chronic gastric and duodenal ulcers
- Crohn's disease, infectious enteritis, and celiac sprue
- Diverticular disease
- Duodenal cancer, diverticula, and ulcers
- Duodenitis
- Esophageal or pyloric stenosis

- Esophageal varices
- Esophagitis or strictures
- Gastric cancer, tumors, and ulcers
- Gastritis
- Hiatal hernia
- Mallory-Weiss syndrome
- Perforation of the esophagus, stomach, or small bowel
- Polyps
- Small bowel tumors
- Strictures
- Tumors (benign or malignant)

CRITICAL FINDINGS: N/A

INTERFERING FACTORS

Factors that may alter the results of the study

- Gas or feces in the GI tract resulting from inadequate cleansing or failure to restrict food intake before the study.
- Retained barium from a previous radiological procedure.

Other considerations

- The patient should not be near any strong electromagnetic source, such as magnetic resonance imaging (MRI) or amateur (ham) radio equipment until the capsule has been eliminated from the body; magnetic fields can disrupt the function of the capsule device and serious damage could be caused to the patient's GI tract if he or she is exposed to the strong magnetic force of MRI equipment.
- The patient with an implanted cardiac device should contact his or her HCP for evaluation regarding compatibility with the capsule device prior to the procedure.
- Delayed capsule transit times may be a result of narcotic use, somatostatin use, gastroparesis, or drugs used to treat psychiatric illness.

NURSING IMPLICATIONS AND PROCEDURE

PRETEST:

- Positively identify the patient using at least two person-specific identifiers before services, treatments, or procedures are performed.
- ***Patient Teaching:*** Inform the patient this procedure can assist in assessing the esophagus, stomach, and upper intestines for disease.
- Obtain a history of the patient's health concerns, symptoms, surgical procedures, and results of previously performed laboratory and diagnostic studies. Include a list of known allergens, especially allergies or sensitivities to latex.
- Ensure that this procedure is performed before an upper GI series or barium swallow.
- Record the date of the last menstrual period and determine the possibility of pregnancy in perimenopausal women.
- Obtain a list of the patient's current medications, including over-the-counter medications, dietary supplements, anticoagulants, aspirin and other salicylates (see Effects of Natural Products on Laboratory Values online at Davis*Plus*). Such products should be discontinued by medical direction for the appropriate number of days prior to a surgical procedure. Note the last time and dose of medication taken.
- Review the procedure with the patient. Address concerns about pain and explain that no pain will be experienced during the procedure. Inform the patient that the procedure is begun in a GI laboratory or office, usually by an HCP or support staff, and that it takes approximately 30 to 60 min to begin the procedure.
- ***Sensitivity to social and cultural issues,*** as well as concern for modesty, is important in providing psychological support before, during, and after the procedure.
- Instruct the patient to stop taking medications that have a coating effect, such as sucralfate and

Pepto-Bismol, 3 days before the procedure; they may prevent the camera from providing clear images.
- Instruct the patient to abstain from the use of tobacco products for 24 hr prior to the procedure.
- Instruct the patient to start a liquid diet on the day before the procedure. From 2200 the evening before the procedure, the patient should not eat or drink except for necessary medication with a sip of water. Instruct the patient to take a standard bowel prep the night before the procedure. Protocols may vary among facilities.
- Instruct the patient not to take any medication for 2 hr prior to the procedure.
- Inform the patient that there is a chance of intestinal obstruction associated with the procedure.
- Instruct the patient to wear loose, two-piece clothing on the day of the procedure. This assists with the placement of the sensors on the patient's abdomen.
- Inform the patient that after ingesting the capsule and until it is excreted, he or she should not be near any source of powerful electromagnetic fields, such as MRI or amateur (ham) radio equipment.
- Make sure a written and informed consent has been signed prior to the procedure.

INTRATEST:

Potential Complications: N/A

- Observe standard precautions, and follow the general guidelines in Patient Preparation and Specimen Collection online at Davis*Plus*. Positively identify the patient.
- Ensure that the patient has complied with dietary and medication restrictions and pretesting preparations prior to the study, as instructed.
- Ensure that the patient with an implanted cardiac device has been cleared to have the procedure.
- Obtain accurate height, weight, and abdominal girth measurements prior to beginning the examination.
- Instruct the patient to cooperate fully and to follow directions.
- Ask the patient to ingest the capsule with a full glass of water. The water may have simethicone in it to reduce gastric and bile bubbles.
- After ingesting the capsule, the patient should not eat or drink for at least 2 hr. After 4 hr, the patient may have a light snack.
- The procedure lasts approximately 8 hr.
- Instruct the patient not to disconnect the equipment or remove the belt at any time during the test.
- If the data recorder stops functioning, instruct the patient to record the time and the nature of any event such as eating or drinking.
- Instruct the patient to keep a timed diary for the day detailing the food and liquids ingested and symptoms during the recording period.
- Instruct the patient to avoid any strenuous physical activity, bending, or stooping during the test.

POST-TEST:

- Instruct the patient to resume normal activity, medication, and diet after the test is ended or as tolerated after the examination, as directed by the HCP.
- Instruct the patient to remove the recorder and return it to the HCP.
- Patients are asked to verify the elimination of the capsule but not to retrieve the capsule.
- Inform the patient that the capsule is a single-use device that does not harbor any environmental hazards.
- Emphasize that any abdominal pain, fever, nausea, vomiting, or difficulty breathing must be immediately reported to the HCP.
- Inform the patient that a report of the results will be made available to the requesting HCP, who will discuss the results with the patient.
- Recognize anxiety related to test results. Discuss the implications of abnormal test results on the patient's lifestyle. Provide teaching and information regarding the clinical implications of the test results, as appropriate.
- Reinforce information given by the patient's HCP regarding further

testing, treatment, or referral to another HCP. Decisions regarding the need for and frequency of occult blood testing, colonoscopy, or other cancer screening procedures should be made after consultation between the patient and HCP. The ACS recommends regular screening for colon cancer beginning at age 50 yr for individuals without identified risk factors and sooner for those with identified risk factors. Their recommendations for frequency of screening are to use one of the following: (1) annual for occult blood testing (fecal occult blood testing or fecal immunochemical testing); (2) every 5 yr for flexible sigmoidoscopy, double contrast barium enema, or computed tomography (CT) colonography; (3) every 10 yr for colonoscopy; or (4) every 3 yr for stool DNA testing. ✦ Abnormal findings should be followed up by colonoscopy. There are both advantages and disadvantages to the screening tests that are available today. Methods to use DNA testing of stool are being investigated and await FDA approval. The DNA test is designed to identify abnormal changes in DNA from the cells in the lining of the colon that are normally shed and excreted in stool. The DNA tests under development use multiple markers to identify colon cancers that demonstrate different, abnormal DNA changes. Unlike some of the current screening methods, the DNA tests would be able to detect precancerous polyps. The most current guidelines for colon cancer screening of the general population as well as of individuals with increased risk are available from the ACS (www.cancer.org), U.S. Preventive Services Task Force (www.uspreventiveservicestaskforce.org), and American College of Gastroenterology (www.gi.org). ✦ Answer any questions or address any concerns voiced by the patient or family.

- Depending on the results of this procedure, additional testing may be needed to evaluate or monitor progression of the disease process and determine the need for a change in therapy. Evaluate test results in relation to the patient's symptoms and other tests performed.

RELATED STUDIES:

- Related tests include barium enema, barium swallow, biopsy intestinal, cancer antigens, colonoscopy, CT abdomen, CT colonoscopy, esophageal manometry, esophagogastroduodenoscopy, fecal analysis, folate, gastric acid emptying scan, gastric acid stimulation test, gastrin, Helicobacter pylori, KUB studies, MRI abdomen, PET pelvis, proctosigmoidoscopy, upper GI and small bowel series, US abdomen, and vitamin B_{12}.
- Refer to the Gastrointestinal System table online at Davis*Plus* for related tests by body system.

Carbon Dioxide

SYNONYM/ACRONYM: CO_2 combining power, CO_2, Tco_2.

COMMON USE: To assess the effect of total carbon dioxide levels on respiratory and metabolic acid-base balance.

SPECIMEN: Serum collected in a gold-, red-, or red/gray-top tube, plasma collected in a green-top (lithium or sodium heparin) tube; or whole blood collected in a green-top (lithium or sodium heparin) tube or heparinized syringe.

NORMAL FINDINGS: (Method: Colorimetry, enzyme assay, or Pco_2 electrode)

Carbon Dioxide	Conventional & SI Units
Plasma or serum (venous)	
Infant–2 yr	13–29 mEq/L or mmol/L
2 yr–older adult	23–29 mEq/L or mmol/L
Whole blood (venous)	
Infant–2 yr	18–28 mEq/L or mmol/L
2 yr–older adult	22–26 mEq/L or mmol/L

C

DESCRIPTION: Serum or plasma carbon dioxide (CO_2) measurement is usually done as part of an electrolyte panel. Total CO_2 (Tco_2) is an important component of the body's buffering capability, and measurements are used mainly in the evaluation of acid-base balance. It is important to understand the differences between Tco_2 (CO_2 content) and CO_2 gas (Pco_2). Total CO_2 reflects the majority of CO_2 in the body, mainly in the form of bicarbonate (HCO_3^-); is present as a base; and is regulated by the kidneys. CO_2 gas contributes little to the Tco_2 level, is acidic, and is regulated by the lungs (see study titled "Blood Gases").

CO_2 provides the basis for the principal buffering system of the extracellular fluid system, which is the bicarbonate–carbonic acid buffer system. CO_2 circulates in the body either bound to protein or physically dissolved. Constituents in the blood that contribute to Tco_2 levels are bicarbonate, carbamino compounds, and carbonic acid (carbonic acid includes undissociated carbonic acid and dissolved CO_2). Bicarbonate is the second-largest group of anions in the extracellular fluid (chloride is the largest). Tco_2 levels closely reflect bicarbonate levels in the blood, because 90% to 95% of CO_2 circulates as HCO_3^-.

This procedure is contraindicated for: N/A

INDICATIONS
- Evaluate decreased venous CO_2 in the case of compensated metabolic acidosis
- Evaluate increased venous CO_2 in the case of compensated metabolic alkalosis
- Monitor decreased venous CO_2 as a result of compensated respiratory alkalosis
- Monitor increased venous CO_2 as a result of compensation for respiratory acidosis secondary to significant respiratory system infection or cancer; decreased respiratory rate

POTENTIAL MEDICAL DIAGNOSIS

Increased in:
- ***Interpretation requires clinical information and evaluation of other electrolytes***
- Acute intermittent porphyria ***(related to severe vomiting associated with acute attacks)***
- Airway obstruction ***(related to impaired elimination from weak breathing responses)***
- Asthmatic shock ***(related to impaired elimination from abnormal breathing responses)***
- Brain tumor ***(related to abnormal blood circulation)***
- Bronchitis (chronic) ***(related to impaired elimination from weak breathing responses)***

- Cardiac disorders ***(related to lack of blood circulation)***
- Chronic obstructive pulmonary disease (COPD) ***(related to impaired elimination from weak breathing responses)***
- Depression of respiratory center ***(related to impaired elimination from weak breathing responses)***
- Electrolyte disturbance (severe) ***(response to maintain acid-base balance)***
- Hypothyroidism ***(related to impaired elimination from weak breathing responses)***
- Hypoventilation ***(related to impaired elimination from weak breathing responses)***
- Metabolic alkalosis ***(various causes; excessive vomiting)***
- Myopathy ***(related to impaired ventilation)***
- Pneumonia ***(related to impaired elimination from weak breathing responses)***
- Poliomyelitis ***(related to impaired elimination from weak breathing responses)***
- Respiratory acidosis ***(related to impaired elimination)***
- Tuberculosis (pulmonary) ***(related to impaired elimination from weak breathing responses)***

Decreased in:

- ***Interpretation requires clinical information and evaluation of other electrolytes***
- Acute kidney injury ***(response to buildup of ketoacids)***
- Anxiety ***(related to hyperventilation; too much CO_2 is exhaled)***
- Dehydration ***(response to metabolic acidosis that develops)***
- Diabetic ketoacidosis ***(response to buildup of ketoacids)***
- Diarrhea (severe) ***(acidosis related to loss of base ions like HCO_3^-; most of CO_2 content is in this form)***
- High fever ***(response to neutralize acidosis present during fever)***
- Metabolic acidosis ***(response to neutralize acidosis)***
- Respiratory alkalosis ***(hyperventilation; too much CO_2 is exhaled)***
- Salicylate intoxication ***(response to neutralize related metabolic acidosis)***
- Starvation ***(CO_2 buffer system used to neutralize buildup of ketoacids)***

CRITICAL FINDINGS:

- Less than 15 mEq/L or mmol/L (SI: Less than 15 mmol/L)
- Greater than 40 mEq/L or mmol/L (SI: Greater than 40 mmol/L)

Note and immediately report to the requesting health-care provider (HCP) any critical findings and related symptoms. A listing of these findings varies among facilities. Timely notification of a critical finding for laboratory or diagnostic studies is a role expectation of the professional nurse. The notification processes vary among facilities. Upon receipt of the critical finding, the information should be read back to the caller to verify accuracy.

Consideration may be given to verification of critical findings before action is taken. Policies vary among facilities and may include requesting immediate recollection and retesting by the laboratory or retesting using a rapid point-of-care testing instrument at the bedside, if available.

Observe the patient for signs and symptoms of excessive or insufficient CO_2 levels, and report these findings to the HCP. If the patient has been vomiting for several days and is breathing shallowly, or if the patient has had gastric suctioning and is breathing shallowly, this may indicate elevated CO_2 levels. Decreased CO_2 levels are evidenced by deep, vigorous breathing and flushed skin.

INTERFERING FACTORS

- Drugs and other substances that may cause an increase in Tco_2 levels include acetylsalicylic acid, aldosterone, bicarbonate, carbenicillin, corticosteroids, dexamethasone, ethacrynic acid, laxatives (chronic misuse), and x-ray contrast .
- Drugs and other substances that may cause a decrease in Tco_2 levels include acetazolamide, acetylsalicylic acid (initially), amiloride, ammonium chloride, fluorides, metformin, methicillin, nitrofurantoin, paraldehyde, tetracycline, triamterene and xylitol.
- Prompt and proper specimen processing, storage, and analysis are important to achieve accurate results. The specimen should be stored under anaerobic conditions after collection to prevent the diffusion of CO_2 gas from the specimen. Falsely decreased values result from uncovered specimens. It is estimated that CO_2 diffuses from the sample at the rate of 6 mmol/hr.

NURSING IMPLICATIONS AND PROCEDURE

PRETEST:

- Positively identify the patient using at least two person-specific identifiers before services, treatments, or procedures are performed.
- ***Patient Teaching:*** Inform the patient this test can assist in measuring the amount of carbon dioxide in the body.
- Obtain a history of the patient's health concerns, symptoms, surgical procedures, and results of previously performed laboratory and diagnostic studies. Include a list of known allergens, especially allergies or sensitivities to latex.
- Note any recent procedures that can interfere with test results.
- Obtain a list of the patient's current medications, including over-the-counter medications and dietary supplements (see Effects of Natural Products on Laboratory Values online at Davis*Plus*).
- Review the procedure with the patient. Inform the patient that specimen collection takes approximately 5 to 10 min. Address concerns about pain and explain that there may be some discomfort during the venipuncture.
- ***Sensitivity to social and cultural issues,*** as well as concern for modesty, is important in providing psychological support before, during, and after the procedure.
- Note that there are no food, fluid, or medication restrictions unless by medical direction.

INTRATEST:

Potential Complications: N/A

- Avoid the use of equipment containing latex if the patient has a history of allergic reaction to latex.
- Instruct the patient to cooperate fully and to follow directions. Direct the patient to breathe normally and to avoid unnecessary movement.
- Observe standard precautions, and follow the general guidelines in Patient Preparation and Specimen Collection online at Davis*Plus*. Positively identify the patient, and label the appropriate specimen container with the corresponding patient demographics, initials of the person collecting the specimen, date, and time of collection. Perform a venipuncture.
- Remove the needle and apply direct pressure with dry gauze to stop bleeding. Observe/assess venipuncture site for bleeding or hematoma formation and secure gauze with adhesive bandage.
- Promptly transport the specimen to the laboratory for processing and analysis.

POST-TEST:

- Inform the patient that a report of the results will be made available to the requesting HCP, who will discuss the results with the patient.
- ***Nutritional Considerations:*** Abnormal CO_2 values may be associated with

diseases of the respiratory system. Malnutrition is commonly seen in patients with severe respiratory disease for reasons including fatigue, lack of appetite, and gastrointestinal distress. Research has estimated that the daily caloric intake required for respiration of patients with chronic obstructive pulmonary disease is 10 times higher than that of normal individuals. Adequate intake of vitamins A and C is also important to prevent pulmonary infection and to decrease the extent of lung tissue damage. The importance of following the prescribed diet should be stressed to the patient and/or caregiver.

- Reinforce information given by the patient's HCP regarding further testing, treatment, or referral to another HCP. Answer any questions or address any concerns voiced by the patient or family.
- Depending on the results of this procedure, additional testing may be performed to evaluate or monitor progression of the disease process and determine the need for a change in therapy. Evaluate test results in relation to the patient's symptoms and other tests performed.

RELATED STUDIES:

- Related tests include anion gap, arterial/alveolar oxygen ratio, biopsy lung, blood gases, chest x-ray, chloride, cold agglutinin titer, CBC white blood cell count and differential, culture bacterial blood, culture bacterial sputum, culture mycobacterium, culture viral, cytology sputum, eosinophil count, ESR, gallium scan, Gram stain, IgE, ketones, lung perfusion scan, osmolality, phosphorus, plethysmography, pleural fluid analysis, potassium, PFT, pulse oximetry, salicylate, and US abdomen.
- Refer to the Cardiovascular, Genitourinary, and Respiratory systems tables online at Davis*Plus* for related tests by body system.

Carboxyhemoglobin

SYNONYM/ACRONYM: Carbon monoxide, CO, COHb, COH.

COMMON USE: To identify the amount of carbon monoxide in the blood related to poisoning, toxicity from smoke inhalation, or exhaust from cars.

SPECIMEN: Whole blood collected in a green-top (heparin) or lavender-top (EDTA) tube, depending on laboratory requirement. Specimen should be transported tightly capped (anaerobic) and in an ice slurry if blood gases are to be performed simultaneously. Carboxyhemoglobin is stable at room temperature.

NORMAL FINDINGS: (Method: Spectrophotometry, co-oximetry)

	% Saturation of Hemoglobin
Newborns	10%–12%
Nonsmokers	Up to 2%
Smokers	Up to 10%

DESCRIPTION: Exogenous carbon monoxide (CO) is a colorless, odorless, tasteless by-product of incomplete combustion derived from the exhaust of automobiles, coal and gas burning, and tobacco smoke. Endogenous CO is produced as a result of red blood cell catabolism. CO levels are elevated in newborns as a result of the combined effects of high hemoglobin turnover and the inefficiency of the infant's respiratory system. CO binds tightly to hemoglobin with an affinity 250 times greater than oxygen, competitively and dramatically reducing the oxygen-carrying capacity of hemoglobin. The increased percentage of bound CO reflects the extent to which normal transport of oxygen has been negatively affected. Overexposure causes hypoxia, which results in headache, nausea, vomiting, vertigo, collapse, or convulsions. Toxic exposure causes anoxia, increased levels of lactic acid, and irreversible tissue damage, which can result in coma or death. Acute exposure may be evidenced by a cherry red color to the lips, skin, and nail beds; this observation may not be apparent in cases of chronic exposure. A direct correlation has been implicated between carboxyhemoglobin levels and symptoms of atherosclerotic disease, angina, and myocardial infarction.

This procedure is contraindicated for: N/A

INDICATIONS

- Assist in the diagnosis of suspected CO poisoning.
- Evaluate the effect of smoking on the patient.
- Evaluate exposure to fires and smoke inhalation.

POTENTIAL MEDICAL DIAGNOSIS

Increased in:

- CO poisoning
- Hemolytic disease ***(CO released during red blood cell catabolism)***
- Tobacco smoking

Decreased in: N/A

CRITICAL FINDINGS:

% Total Hemoglobin	Symptoms
10%–20%	Asymptomatic
10%–30%	Disturbance of judgment, headache, dizziness
30%–40%	Dizziness, muscle weakness, vision problems, confusion, increased heart rate, increased breathing rate
50%–60%	Loss of consciousness, coma
Greater than 60%	Death

Note and immediately report to the requesting health-care provider (HCP) any critical findings and related symptoms. A listing of these findings varies among facilities. Timely notification of a critical finding for laboratory or diagnostic studies is a role expectation of the professional nurse. The notification processes vary among facilities. Upon receipt of the critical finding, the information should be read back to the caller to verify accuracy.

Consideration may be given to verification of critical findings before action is taken. Policies vary among facilities and may include requesting immediate recollection and retesting by the laboratory or retesting using a rapid point-of-care testing instrument at the bedside, if available.

Women and children may suffer more severe symptoms of carbon monoxide poisoning at lower levels of carbon monoxide than men because women and children usually have lower red blood cell counts.

A possible intervention in moderate CO poisoning is the administration of supplemental oxygen given at atmospheric pressure. In severe CO poisoning, hyperbaric oxygen treatments may be used.

C

INTERFERING FACTORS

Specimen should be collected before administration of oxygen therapy.

NURSING IMPLICATIONS AND PROCEDURE

PRETEST:

- Positively identify the patient using at least two person-specific identifiers before services, treatments, or procedures are performed.
- ***Patient Teaching:*** Inform the patient this test can assist in evaluating the extent of carbon monoxide poisoning or toxicity.
- Obtain a history of the patient's health concerns, symptoms, surgical procedures, and results of previously performed laboratory and diagnostic studies. Include a list of known allergens, especially allergies or sensitivities to latex.
- Note any recent procedures that can interfere with test results.
- Obtain a list of the patient's current medications, including over-the-counter medications and dietary supplements (see Effects of Natural Products on Laboratory Values online at Davis*Plus*).
- Review the procedure with the patient. Explain to the patient or family members that the cause of the headache, vomiting, dizziness, convulsions, or coma could be related to CO exposure. Inform the patient that specimen collection takes approximately 5 to 10 min. Address concerns about pain and explain to the patient that there may be some discomfort during the venipuncture.
- ***Sensitivity to social and cultural issues,*** as well as concern for modesty, is important in providing psychological support before, during, and after the procedure.
- If carboxyhemoglobin measurement will be performed simultaneously with arterial blood gases, prepare an ice slurry in a cup or plastic bag and have it on hand for immediate transport of the specimen to the laboratory.
- Note that there are no food, fluid, or medication restrictions unless by medical direction.

INTRATEST:

Potential Complications: N/A

- Avoid the use of equipment containing latex if the patient has a history of allergic reaction to latex.
- Instruct the patient to cooperate fully and to follow directions. Direct the patient to breathe normally and to avoid unnecessary movement.
- Observe standard precautions, and follow the general guidelines in Patient Preparation and Specimen Collection online at Davis*Plus*. Positively identify the patient, and label the appropriate specimen container with the corresponding patient demographics, initials of the person collecting the specimen, date, and time of collection. Perform a venipuncture. The tightly capped sample should be placed in an ice slurry immediately after collection. Information on the specimen label should be protected from water in the ice slurry by first placing the specimen in a protective plastic bag.
- Remove the needle and apply direct pressure with dry gauze to stop bleeding. Observe/assess venipuncture site for bleeding or hematoma formation and secure gauze with adhesive bandage.
- Promptly transport the specimen to the laboratory for processing and analysis.

POST-TEST:

- Inform the patient that a report of the results will be made available to the requesting HCP, who will discuss the results with the patient.
- Recognize anxiety related to test results, and be supportive of impaired activity related to fear of shortened life expectancy. Discuss the implications of abnormal test results on the patient's lifestyle. Provide teaching and information regarding the clinical implications of the test results, as appropriate. Educate the patient regarding access to counseling services. Educate the patient regarding avoiding gas heaters and indoor cooking fires without adequate ventilation and the need to have gas furnaces checked yearly for CO leakage. Inform the patient of smoking cessation programs, as appropriate.
- Reinforce information given by the patient's HCP regarding further testing, treatment, or referral to another HCP. Answer any questions or address any concerns voiced by the patient or family.
- Depending on the results of this procedure, additional testing may be performed to evaluate or monitor progression of the disease process and determine the need for a change in therapy. Evaluate test results in relation to the patient's symptoms and other tests performed.

RELATED STUDIES:

- Related tests include angiography pulmonary, arterial/alveolar oxygen ratio, blood gases, carbon dioxide, CBC, lung perfusion scan, lung ventilation scan, plethysmography, and PFT.
- Refer to the Respiratory System table online at Davis*Plus* for related tests by body system.

Catecholamines, Blood and Urine

SYNONYM/ACRONYM: Epinephrine, norepinephrine, dopamine.

COMMON USE: To assist in diagnosing catecholamine-secreting tumors, such as those found in the adrenal medulla, and in the investigation of hypertension. The urine test is used to assist in diagnosing pheochromocytoma and as a work-up of neuroblastoma.

SPECIMEN: Plasma collected in green-top (heparin) tube. Urine from a timed specimen collected in a clean, plastic, amber collection container with 6N hydrochloric acid as a preservative.

NORMAL FINDINGS: (Method: High-performance liquid chromatography)

Blood	Conventional Units	SI Units (Conventional Units × 5.46)
Epinephrine		
Newborn–1 yr	0–34 pg/mL	0–186 pmol/L
1–18 yr	0–80 pg/mL	0–437 pmol/L
Adult		
Supine, 30 min	0–110 pg/mL	0–600 pmol/L
Standing, 30 min	0–140 pg/mL	0–764 pmol/L

(table continues on page 368)

Blood	Conventional Units	SI Units
		(Conventional Units × 5.91)
Norepinephrine		
Newborn–1 yr	0–659 pg/mL	0–3,895 pmol/L
1–18 yr	0–611 pg/mL	0–3,611 pmol/L
Adult		
Supine, 30 min	70–750 pg/mL	414–4,432 pmol/L
Standing, 30 min	200–1,700 pg/mL	1,182–10,047 pmol/L
		(Conventional Units × 6.53)
Dopamine		
Newborn–1 yr	0–42 pg/mL	0–274 pmol/L
1–18 yr	0–32 pg/mL	0–209 pmol/L
Adult		
Supine or standing	0–48 pg/mL	0–313 pmol/L

Urine	Conventional Units	SI Units
		(Conventional Units × 5.46)
Epinephrine		
Newborn–9 yr	0–11 mcg/24 hr	0–60 nmol/24 hr
10–19 yr	0–18 mcg/24 hr	0–98 nmol/24 hr
20 yr–older adult	0–20 mcg/24 hr	0–109 nmol/24 hr
		(Conventional Units × 5.91)
Norepinephrine		
Newborn–9 yr	0–59 mcg/24 hr	0–349 nmol/24 hr
10–19 yr	0–90 mcg/24 hr	0–532 nmol/24 hr
20 yr–older adult	0–135 mcg/24 hr	0–798 nmol/24 hr
		(Conventional Units × 6.53)
Dopamine		
Newborn–9 yr	0–414 mcg/24 hr	0–2,703 nmol/24 hr
10–19 yr	0–575 mcg/24 hr	0–3,755 nmol/24 hr
20 yr–older adult	0–510 mcg/24 hr	0–3,330 nmol/24 hr

DESCRIPTION: Catecholamines are produced by the chromaffin tissue of the adrenal medulla. They also are found in sympathetic nerve endings and in the brain. The major catecholamines are epinephrine, norepinephrine, and dopamine. They prepare the body for the fight-or-flight stress response, help to regulate metabolism, and are excreted from the body by the kidneys. Levels are affected by diurnal variations, fluctuating in response to stress, postural changes, diet, smoking, drugs, and temperature changes. As a result, blood measurement is not as reliable as a 24-hr timed urine test. For test results to be valid, all of the previously mentioned environmental variables must be controlled when the test is performed. Results of blood specimens are most reliable when the specimen is collected during a hypertensive episode. Catecholamines are measured when there is high suspicion of pheochromocytoma but urine results are normal or borderline. Use of a clonidine suppression test with measurement of plasma catecholamines may be requested. Failure to suppress production of catecholamines after administration of clonidine supports the diagnosis of pheochromocytoma. Elevated homovanillic acid levels rule out pheochromocytoma because this tumor primarily secretes epinephrine. Elevated catecholamines without hypertension suggest neuroblastoma or ganglioneuroma. Findings should be compared with metanephrines and vanillylmandelic acid, which are the metabolites of epinephrine and norepinephrine. Findings should also be compared with homovanillic acid, which is the product of dopamine metabolism.

This procedure is contraindicated for: N/A

INDICATIONS

- Assist in the diagnosis of neuroblastoma, ganglioneuroma, or dysautonomia.
- Assist in the diagnosis of pheochromocytoma.
- Evaluate acute hypertensive episode.
- Evaluate hypertension of unknown origin.
- Screen for pheochromocytoma among family members with an autosomal dominant inheritance pattern for Lindau–von Hippel disease or multiple endocrine neoplasia.

POTENTIAL MEDICAL DIAGNOSIS

Increased in:

- Diabetic acidosis (epinephrine and norepinephrine) ***(related to metabolic stress; are released to initiate glycogenolysis, gluconeogenesis, and lipolysis)***
- Ganglioblastoma (epinephrine, slight increase; norepinephrine, large increase) ***(related to production by the tumor)***
- Ganglioneuroma (all are increased; norepinephrine, largest increase) ***(related to production by the tumor)***
- Hypothyroidism (epinephrine and norepinephrine) ***(possibly related to interactions among the immune, endocrine, and nervous systems)***
- Long-term bipolar disorder (epinephrine and norepinephrine) ***(some studies indicate a relationship between decreased catecholamine levels and bipolar disorder; the pathophysiology is not well understood)***
- Myocardial infarction (epinephrine and norepinephrine) ***(related to physical stress)***
- Neuroblastoma (all are increased, norepinephrine and dopamine, largest increase) ***(related to production by the tumor)***
- Pheochromocytoma (epinephrine, continuous or intermittent increase; norepinephrine, slight increase) ***(related to production by the tumor)***
- Shock (epinephrine and norepinephrine) ***(related to physical stress)***
- Strenuous exercise (epinephrine and norepinephrine) ***(related to physical stress)***

Decreased in:

- Autonomic nervous system dysfunction (norepinephrine)
- Orthostatic hypotension caused by central nervous system disease (norepinephrine) ***(related to inability of sympathetic nervous system to activate postganglionic neuron)***

- Parkinson's disease (dopamine) ***(some studies indicate a relationship between decreased catecholamine levels and Parkinson's disease; the pathophysiology is not well understood)***

CRITICAL FINDINGS: N/A

INTERFERING FACTORS

- Drugs and other substances that may increase plasma catecholamine levels include ajmaline, chlorpromazine, cyclopropane, diazoxide, ether, monoamine oxidase inhibitors, nitroglycerin, pentazocine, perphenazine, phenothiazines, promethazine, and theophylline.
- Drugs and other substances that may decrease plasma catecholamine levels include captopril, and reserpine.
- Drugs and other substances that may increase urine catecholamine levels include atenolol, isoproterenol, methyldopa, niacin, nitroglycerin, prochlorperazine, rauwolfia, reserpine, and theophylline.
- Drugs and other substances that may decrease urine catecholamine levels include bretylium tosylate, clonidine, decaborane, guanethidine, guanfacine, methyldopa, ouabain, radiographic substances, and reserpine.
- Stress, hypoglycemia, smoking, and drugs can produce elevated catecholamines.
- Secretion of catecholamines exhibits diurnal variation, with the lowest levels occurring at night.
- Secretion of catecholamines varies during the menstrual cycle, with higher levels excreted during the luteal phase and lowest levels during ovulation.
- Diets high in amines (e.g., bananas, avocados, beer, aged cheese, chocolate, cocoa, coffee, fava beans, grains, tea, vanilla, walnuts, Chianti wine) can produce elevated catecholamine levels.
- Failure to collect all urine and store 24-hr specimen properly will yield a falsely low result.
- Failure to follow dietary restrictions before the procedure may cause the procedure to be canceled or repeated.

NURSING IMPLICATIONS AND PROCEDURE

PRETEST:

- Positively identify the patient using at least two person-specific identifiers before services, treatments, or procedures are performed.
- ***Patient Teaching:*** Inform the patient this test can assist in the diagnosis of a type of tumor that produces excessive amounts of hormones related to physical and emotional stress.
- Obtain a history of the patient's health concerns, symptoms, surgical procedures, and results of previously performed laboratory and diagnostic studies. Include a list of known allergens, especially allergies or sensitivities to latex.
- Record the date of the patient's last menstrual period.
- Obtain a list of the patient's current medications, including over-the-counter medications and dietary supplements (see Effects of Natural Products on Laboratory Values online at Davis*Plus*).
- Review the procedure with the patient.

Blood

- Inform the patient that he or she may be asked to keep warm and to rest for 45 to 60 min before the test. Inform the patient that multiple specimens may be required. Inform the patient that specimen collection takes approximately 5 to 10 min. Address concerns about pain and explain that there may be some discomfort during the venipuncture. Inform the patient that a saline lock for blood sample collection may be inserted before the test because the stress of repeated venipunctures may increase catecholamine levels.

Urine

- Provide a nonmetallic urinal, bedpan, or toilet-mounted collection device. Address concerns about pain related to the procedure. Explain to the patient that there should be no discomfort during the procedure. Usually a 24-hr time frame for urine collection is ordered. Inform the patient that all urine over a 24-hr period must be saved; if a preservative has been added to the container, instruct the patient not to discard the preservative. Instruct the patient not to void directly into the laboratory collection container. Instruct the patient to avoid defecating in the collection device and to keep toilet tissue out of the collection device to prevent contamination of the specimen. Place a sign in the bathroom as a reminder to save all urine. Instruct the patient to void all urine into the collection device, then pour the urine into the laboratory collection container. Alternatively, the specimen can be left in the collection device for a health-care staff member to add to the laboratory collection container.

Blood and Urine

- ***Sensitivity to social and cultural issues,*** as well as concern for modesty, is important in providing psychological support before, during, and after the procedure.
- Instruct the patient to follow a normal-sodium diet for 3 days before testing, abstain from smoking tobacco for 24 hr before testing, and avoid consumption of foods high in amines for 48 hr before testing.
- Instruct the patient to avoid self-prescribed medications for 2 wk before testing (especially appetite suppressants and cold and allergy medications, such as nose drops, cough suppressants, and bronchodilators).
- Instruct the patient to withhold prescribed medication (especially methyldopa, epinephrine, levodopa, and methenamine mandelate) if directed by the health-care provider (HCP).
- Instruct the patient to withhold food and fluids for 10 to 12 hr before the test. Protocols may vary from facility to facility.
- Instruct the patient collecting a 24-hr urine specimen to avoid excessive stress and exercise during the test collection period.
- Prior to blood specimen collection, prepare an ice slurry in a cup or plastic bag to have ready for immediate transport of the specimen to the laboratory. Prechill the collection tube in the ice slurry.

INTRATEST:

Potential Complications: N/A

- Ensure that the patient has complied with dietary, medication, and activity restrictions and with pretesting preparations prior to the study, as instructed. Instruct the patient to continue to avoid excessive exercise and stress during the 24-hr collection of urine.
- Avoid the use of equipment containing latex if the patient has a history of allergic reaction to latex.
- Instruct the patient to cooperate fully and to follow directions.
- Observe standard precautions, and follow the general guidelines in Patient Preparation and Specimen Collection online at Davis*Plus*. Positively identify the patient, and label the appropriate specimen container with the corresponding patient demographics, initials of the person collecting the specimen, date, and time of collection. Perform a venipuncture as appropriate.

Blood

- Perform a venipuncture between 0600 and 0800; collect the specimen in a prechilled tube.

- Remove the needle and apply direct pressure with dry gauze to stop bleeding. Observe/assess venipuncture site for bleeding or hematoma formation and secure gauze with adhesive bandage.
- Ask the patient to stand for 10 min, and then perform a second venipuncture and obtain a sample as previously described.
- Each sample should be placed in an ice slurry immediately after collection. Information on the specimen labels should be protected from water in the ice slurry by first placing the specimens in a protective plastic bag. Promptly transport the specimens to the laboratory for processing and analysis.

Urine

- Obtain a clean 3-L urine specimen container, toilet-mounted collection device, and plastic bag (for transport of the specimen container). The specimen must be refrigerated or kept on ice throughout the collection period. If an indwelling urinary catheter is in place, the drainage bag must be kept on ice.
- Begin the test between 0600 and 0800 if possible. Collect first voiding and discard. Record the time the specimen was discarded as the beginning of the timed collection period. The next morning, ask the patient to void at the same time the collection was started and add this last voiding to the container.
- If an indwelling catheter is in place, replace the tubing and container system at the start of the collection time. Keep the container system on ice during the collection period or empty the urine into a larger container periodically during the collection period; monitor to ensure continued drainage, and conclude the test the next morning at the same hour the collection was begun.
- At the conclusion of the test, compare the quantity of urine with the urinary output record for the collection; if the specimen contains less than what was recorded as output, some urine may have been discarded, invalidating the test.

Blood and Urine

- Include on the collection container's label the amount of urine, test start and stop times, and ingestion of any foods or medications that can affect test results.
- Promptly transport the specimen to the laboratory for processing and analysis.

POST-TEST:

- Inform the patient that a report of the results will be made available to the requesting HCP, who will discuss the results with the patient.
- Instruct the patient to resume usual diet, fluids, medications, and activity, as directed by the HCP.
- Recognize anxiety related to test results. Discuss the implications of abnormal test results on the patient's lifestyle. Provide teaching and information regarding the clinical implications of the test results, as appropriate.
- Reinforce information given by the patient's HCP regarding further testing, treatment, or referral to another HCP. Answer any questions or address any concerns voiced by the patient or family.
- Depending on the results of this procedure, additional testing may be performed to evaluate or monitor progression of the disease process and determine the need for a change in therapy. Evaluate test results in relation to the patient's symptoms and other tests performed.

RELATED STUDIES:

- Related tests include angiography adrenal, calcitonin, CT renal, HVA, metanephrines, renin, and VMA.
- Refer to the Endocrine System table online at Davis*Plus* for related tests by body system.

CD4/CD8 Enumeration and Viral Load Testing

SYNONYM/ACRONYM: T-cell profile.

COMMON USE: To monitor HIV disease progression and the effectiveness of retroviral therapy.

SPECIMEN: Whole blood collected in a green-top (heparin) tube.

NORMAL FINDINGS: (Method: Flow cytometry)

	Mature T cells (CD3)		Helper T cells (CD4)		Suppressor T cells (CD8)	
Age	Absolute (cells/microL)	%	Absolute (cells/microL)	%	Absolute (cells/microL)	%
0–3 mo	2,500–5,500	53–84	1,600–4,000	35–64	560–1,700	12–28
3–6 mo	2,500–5,600	51–77	1,800–4,000	35–56	590–1,600	12–23
6–12 mo	1,900–5,900	49–76	1,400–4,300	31–56	500–1,700	12–24
12–24 mo	2,100–6,200	53–75	1,300–3,400	32–51	620–2,000	14–30
2–56 yr	1,400–3,700	56–75	700–2,200	28–47	490–1,300	16–30
6–12 yr	1,200–2,600	60–76	650–1,500	31–47	370–1,100	18–35
12–18 yr	1,000–2,200	56–84	530–1,300	31–52	330–920	18–35
Adult	527–2,846	49–81	332–1,642	28–51	170–811	12–38

Pediatric values adapted with permission by Elsevier from Shearer, W., et al. (November 2003). Lymphocyte subsets in healthy children from birth through 18 years of age: The pediatric AIDS clinical trials group P1009 study. *Journal of Allergy and Clinical Immunology*, 112(5): 973–980.

DESCRIPTION: Enumeration of lymphocytes, identification of cell lineage, and identification of cellular stage of development are used to diagnose and classify malignant myeloproliferative diseases and to plan treatment. T-cell enumeration is also useful in the evaluation and management of immunodeficiency and autoimmune disease. The CD4 count is a reflection of immune status. It is used to make decisions regarding initiation of antiretroviral therapy (ART) and is also an excellent predictor of imminent opportunistic infection. A sufficient response for patients receiving ART is defined as an increase of 50 to 150 (cells/microL) per year with rapid response during the first 3 mo of treatment followed by an annual increase of 50 to 100 (cells/microL) until stabilization is achieved. HIV viral load is another important test used to establish a baseline for viral activity when a person is first diagnosed with HIV and then afterward to monitor response to ART. Viral load testing, also called plasma HIV RNA, is performed on plasma from a whole blood sample. The viral load demonstrates how actively the virus is reproducing and helps determine whether treatment is necessary. Optimal viral load is considered to be less than 20 to 75 copies/mL or below the level of detection, but the actual level of detection varies somewhat by test method. Methods commonly used to perform viral load testing include branched DNA (bDNA) or reverse transcriptase polymerase chain reaction (RT-PCR). Results are not interchangeable from method to method. Therefore, it is important to use the same viral load method for serial testing. Public health guidelines recommend CD4 counts and viral load testing upon initiation of care for HIV; 3 to 4 mo before commencement of ART; every 3 to 4 mo, but no later than 6 mo, thereafter; and if treatment failure is suspected or otherwise when clinically indicated. Additionally, viral load testing should be requested 2 to 4 wk, but no later than 8 wk, after initiation of ART to verify success of therapy. In clinically stable patients, CD4 testing may be recommended every 6 to 12 mo rather than every 3 to 6 mo. Guidelines also state that treatment of asymptomatic patients should begin when CD4 count is less than 350 cells/microL; treatment is recommended when the patient is symptomatic regardless of test results or when the patient is asymptomatic and CD4 count is between 350 and 500 cells/microL. Failure to respond to therapy is defined as a viral load greater than 200 copies/mL. Increased viral load may be indicative of viral mutations, drug resistance, or noncompliance to the therapeutic regimen. Testing for drug resistance is recommended if viral load is greater than 1,000 copies/mL.

This procedure is contraindicated for: N/A

INDICATIONS

- Assist in the diagnosis of AIDS and plan treatment.
- Evaluate malignant myeloproliferative diseases and plan treatment.
- Evaluate thymus-dependent or cellular immunocompetence.

POTENTIAL MEDICAL DIAGNOSIS

Increased in:

- Malignant myeloproliferative diseases (e.g., acute and chronic lymphocytic leukemia, lymphoma)

Decreased in:

- AIDS
- Aplastic anemia
- Hodgkin's disease

CRITICAL FINDINGS: N/A

INTERFERING FACTORS

- Drugs and other substances that may increase T-cell count include interferon.
- Drugs and other substances that may decrease T-cell count include chlorpromazine and prednisone.
- Specimens should be stored at room temperature.
- Recent radioactive scans or radiation can decrease T-cell counts.
- Values may be abnormal in patients with severe recurrent illness or after recent surgery requiring general anesthesia.

C

NURSING IMPLICATIONS AND PROCEDURE

POTENTIAL NURSING PROBLEMS:

Problem	Signs & Symptoms	Interventions
Gas exchange ***(related to insufficient oxygen supply secondary to pulmonary infiltrates; sepsis; hyperventilation)***	Decreased activity tolerance; increased shortness of breath with activity; weakness; orthopnea; cyanosis; cough; increased heart rate; weight gain; edema in the lower extremities; weakness; increased respiratory rate; use of respiratory accessory muscles	Auscultate and trend breath sounds; use pulse oximetry to monitor oxygenation; administer oxygen as ordered; collaborate with health-care provider (HCP) to consider intubation and/or mechanical ventilation; place the head of the bed in high Fowler's position; administer diuretics, vasodilators as ordered; monitor arterial blood gas (ABG) results; monitor color and character of sputum; encourage periods of rest; administer prescribed medications for *Pneumocystis jiroveci*; administer prescribed steroids
Infection ***(related to altered immune system; malnutrition; chemotherapy)***	Symptoms of infection (increased temperature, increased heart rate, increased blood pressure, shaking, chills, mottled skin, lethargy, fatigue, swelling, edema, pain, localized pressure, diaphoresis, night sweats, confusion, vomiting, nausea, headache); night sweats; persistent cough; adventitious breath sounds (crackles, course, diminished)	Decrease exposure to environment by placing the patient in a private room; monitor and trend vital signs; monitor and trend laboratory values that would indicate an infection (white blood cells [WBC], C-reactive protein [CRP]); promote good hygiene; assist with hygiene as needed; administer prescribed antibiotics, antipyretics; provide cooling measures; administer prescribed intravenous fluids; monitor vital signs and trend temperatures; encourage oral fluids; adhere to standard or universal precautions; provide isolation as

(table continues on page 376)

C

Problem	Signs & Symptoms	Interventions
		appropriate; obtain cultures as ordered; provide lightweight clothing and bedding; assess for night sweats; assess for cough and sputum color (if productive, check for blood in sputum); use isolation as appropriate (TB); encourage use of incentive spirometer
Nutrition ***(related to fatigue; malabsorption; nausea [adverse effects of medication]; effects of chemotherapy)***	Unintended weight loss; current weight 20% below ideal weight; skin tone loss and pale dry skin; dry mucous membranes; documented inadequate caloric intake; subcutaneous tissue loss; hair pulls out easily; paresthesia; muscle wasting	Obtain accurate daily weight at the same time each day with the same scale; obtain an accurate nutritional history; assess attitude toward eating; promote a dietary consult to evaluate current eating habits and best method of nutritional supplementation; develop short-term and long-term eating strategies; monitor nutritional laboratory values such as albumin, transferrin, red blood cells [RBC], WBC, and serum electrolytes; discourage caffeinated and carbonated beverages; assess swallowing ability; encourage cultural home foods; provide a pleasant environment for eating; alter food seasoning to enhance flavor; provide parenteral or enteral nutrition as prescribed, if used check gastric residual every 4 hr; encourage good oral hygiene; provide frequent small meals; administer prescribed antiemetics
Tissue integrity ***(related to insufficient nutrition; vomiting and***	Area on the skin that is warm or tender to touch; skin that turns red, purple, or black; localized pain;	Conduct baseline skin assessment and frequent reassessment using a standardized scale (Braden); monitor and note

Problem	Signs & Symptoms	Interventions
diarrhea secondary to adverse effects of medications, chemotherapy; altered mobility)	swelling of affected area	the presence of herpes lesions; encourage the use of hypoallergenic soap and lanolin products, pat rather than rub skin dry; avoid bed wrinkles; ensure sheets are soft and gentle on skin; encourage adequate nutrition; administer prescribed vitamin supplements; encourage and assist range of motion; assess the characteristics of a wound (color, size, length, width, depth, drainage, and odor); monitor for fever; identify the cause of the tissue damage

C

PRETEST:

- Positively identify the patient using at least two person-specific identifiers before services, treatments, or procedures are performed.
- ***Patient Teaching:*** Inform the patient this test can assist in diagnosing disease and monitoring the effectiveness of disease therapy.
- Obtain a history of the patient's health concerns, symptoms, surgical procedures, and results of previously performed laboratory and diagnostic studies. Include a list of known allergens, especially allergies or sensitivities to latex.
- Note any recent procedures that can interfere with test results.
- Obtain a list of the patient's current medications, including over-the-counter medications and dietary supplements (see Effects of Natural Products on Laboratory Values online at Davis*Plus*).
- Review the procedure with the patient. Inform the patient that specimen collection takes approximately 5 to 10 min. Address concerns about pain and explain that there may be some discomfort during the venipuncture.
- ***Sensitivity to social and cultural issues,*** as well as concern for modesty, is important in providing psychological support before, during, and after the procedure.
- Note that there are no food, fluid, or medication restrictions unless by medical direction.

INTRATEST:

Potential Complications: N/A

- Avoid the use of equipment containing latex if the patient has a history of allergic reaction to latex.
- Instruct the patient to cooperate fully and to follow directions. Direct the patient to breathe normally and to avoid unnecessary movement.
- Observe standard precautions, and follow the general guidelines in Patient Preparation and Specimen Collection online at Davis*Plus*. Positively identify the patient, and label the appropriate specimen container with the corresponding patient demographics, initials of the person collecting the specimen, date, and time of collection. Perform a venipuncture.
- Remove the needle and apply direct pressure with dry gauze to stop

bleeding. Observe/assess venipuncture site for bleeding or hematoma formation and secure gauze with adhesive bandage.
- Promptly transport the specimen to the laboratory for processing and analysis.

C

POST-TEST:

- Inform the patient that a report of the results will be made available to the requesting HCP, who will discuss the results with the patient.
- ***Nutritional Considerations:*** As appropriate, stress the importance of good nutrition and suggest that the patient meet with a nutritional specialist. Stress the importance of following the care plan for medications and follow-up visits. Inform the patient that subsequent requests for follow-up blood work at regular intervals should be anticipated.
- Recognize anxiety related to test results, and be supportive of impaired activity related to perceived loss of independence and fear of shortened life expectancy. Discuss the implications of abnormal test results on the patient's lifestyle. Provide teaching and information regarding the clinical implications of the test results, as appropriate. Educate the patient as to the risk of infection related to immunosuppressed inflammatory response and fatigue related to decreased energy production. Educate the patient regarding access to counseling services.
- Depending on the results of this procedure, additional testing may be performed to evaluate or monitor progression of the disease process and determine the need for a change in therapy. Evaluate test results in relation to the patient's symptoms and other tests performed.

Patient Education:

- Counsel the patient, as appropriate, regarding risk of transmission and proper prophylaxis, and reinforce the importance of strict adherence to the treatment regimen, including consultation with a pharmacist.
- Reinforce information given by the patient's HCP regarding further testing, treatment, or referral to another HCP.
- Provide contact information, if desired, for the National Institutes of Health (www.aidsinfo.nih.gov), American Congress of Obstetricians and Gynecologists (www.acog.org), or Centers for Disease Control and Prevention (www.cdc.gov). 🍁
- Answer any questions or address any concerns voiced by the patient or family.

Expected Patient Outcomes:

Understanding

- The patient and family state the importance of reporting cough and shortness of breath to ensure early intervention of opportunistic hosts.
- The patient and family state steps that can be taken in the home environment to decease infection risk.

Ability

- The patient and family correctly describe the process for the collection of a sputum specimen.
- The patient demonstrates proficient use of the incentive spirometer.

Response

- The patient takes proactive measures to improve overall health by complying with recommended therapeutic plan.
- The patient complies with the request to refrain from scratching, which causes tissue damage.

RELATED STUDIES:

- Related tests include biopsy bone marrow, bronchoscopy, CBC, CBC platelet count, CBC WBC count and differential, culture and smear mycobacteria, culture viral, cytology sputum, gallium scan, HIV-1/HIV-2 antibodies, laparoscopy abdominal, LAP, lymphangiogram, MRI musculoskeletal, mediastinoscopy, and β_2-microglobulin.
- Refer to the Hematopoietic and Immune systems tables online at Davis*Plus* for related tests by body system.

Cerebrospinal Fluid Analysis

SYNONYM/ACRONYM: CSF analysis (lumbar puncture, spinal tap).

COMMON USE: To assist in the differential diagnosis of infection or hemorrhage of the brain. Also used in the evaluation of other conditions with significant neuromuscular effects, such as multiple sclerosis.

SPECIMEN: Cerebrospinal fluid (CSF) collected in three or four separate plastic conical tubes. Tube 1 is used for chemistry and serology testing, tube 2 is used for microbiology, tube 3 is used for cell count, and tube 4 is used for miscellaneous testing.

NORMAL FINDINGS: (Method: Macroscopic evaluation of appearance; spectrophotometry for glucose, lactic acid, and protein; immunoassay for myelin basic protein; nephelometry for immunoglobulin G [IgG]; electrophoresis for oligoclonal banding; Gram stain, India ink preparation, and culture or PCR for microbiology; microscopic examination of fluid for cell count; flocculation for Venereal Disease Research Laboratory [VDRL])

Lumbar Puncture	Conventional Units	SI Units
Color and appearance	Crystal clear	
		(Conventional Units × 10)
Protein		
0–1 mo	Less than 150 mg/dL	Less than 1,500 mg/L
1–6 mo	30–100 mg/dL	300–1,000 mg/L
7 mo–adult	15–45 mg/dL	150–450 mg/L
Older adult	15–60 mg/dL	150–600 mg/L
		(Conventional Units × 0.0555)
Glucose		
Infant or child	60–80 mg/dL	3.3–4.4 mmol/L
Adult/older adult	40–70 mg/dL	2.2–3.9 mmol/L
		(Conventional Units × 0.111)
Lactic acid		
Neonate	10–60 mg/dL	1.1–6.7 mmol/L
3–10 d	10–40 mg/dL	1.1–4.4 mmol/L
Adult	Less than 25.2 mg/dL	Less than 2.8 mmol/L
		(Conventional Units × 1)
Myelin basic protein		
	Less than 4 ng/mL	Less than 4 mcg/L
Oligoclonal bands	Absent	
		(Conventional Units × 10)
IgG	Less than 3.4 mg/dL	Less than 34 mg/L
Gram stain	Negative	
India ink	Negative	

(table continues on page 380)

Lumbar Puncture	Conventional Units	SI Units
Culture	No growth	
RBC count	0	0 *(Conventional Units × 1)*
WBC count		
Neonate–1 mo	0–30 /microL	$0–30 \times 10^6$/L
1 mo–1 yr	0–10 /microL	$0–10 \times 10^6$/L
1–5 yr	0–8 /microL	$0–8 \times 10^6$/L
5 yr–adult	0–5 /microL	$0–5 \times 10^6$/L
VDRL	Nonreactive	
Cytology	No abnormal cells seen	

CSF glucose should be 60%–70% of plasma glucose level.
RBC = red blood cell; VDRL = Venereal Disease Research Laboratory; WBC = white blood cell.
Color should be assessed after sample is centrifuged.

WBC Differential	Adult	Children
Lymphocytes	40%–80%	5%–13%
Monocytes	15%–45%	50%–90%
Neutrophils	0%–6%	0%–8%

DESCRIPTION: Cerebrospinal fluid (CSF) circulates in the subarachnoid space and has a twofold function: to protect the brain and spinal cord from injury and to transport products of cellular metabolism and neurosecretion. The total volume of CSF is 90 to 150 mL in adults and 60 mL in infants. CSF analysis helps determine the presence and cause of bleeding and assists in diagnosing cancer, infections, and degenerative and autoimmune diseases of the brain and spinal cord. Specimens for analysis are most frequently obtained by lumbar puncture and sometimes by ventricular or cisternal puncture. Lumbar puncture can also have therapeutic uses, including injection of drugs and anesthesia. The subspeciality of microbiology has been revolutionized by molecular diagnostics. Molecular diagnostics involves the identification of specific sequences of DNA. The application of molecular diagnostics techniques, such as PCR, has led to the development of automated instruments that can identify a single infectious organism or multiple pathogens from a cerebrospinal fluid sample in less than 2 hr. The instruments can detect the presence of bacteria, viruses, and yeast commonly associated with meningitis and encephalitis.

This procedure is contraindicated for

- Patients with infection present at the needle insertion site.
- Patients with degenerative joint disease or coagulation defects.
- Patients who are uncooperative during the procedure.
- Patients with increased intracranial pressure; extreme caution should be used ***because overly rapid removal of CSF can result in herniation.***

INDICATIONS

- Assist in the diagnosis and differentiation of subarachnoid or intracranial hemorrhage.
- Assist in the diagnosis and differentiation of viral or bacterial meningitis or encephalitis.
- Assist in the diagnosis of diseases such as multiple sclerosis, autoimmune disorders, or degenerative brain disease.
- Assist in the diagnosis of neurosyphilis and chronic central nervous system (CNS) infections.
- Detect obstruction of CSF circulation due to hemorrhage, tumor, or edema.
- Establish the presence of any condition decreasing the flow of oxygen to the brain.
- Monitor for metastases of cancer into the CNS.
- Monitor severe brain injuries.

POTENTIAL MEDICAL DIAGNOSIS

Increased in:

- Color and appearance ***(xanthochromia is any pink, yellow, or orange color; bloody—hemorrhage; xanthochromic—old hemorrhage, red blood cell [RBC] breakdown, methemoglobin, bilirubin [greater than 6 mg/dL (SI: 102.6 micromol/L)], increased protein [greater than 150 mg/dL (SI: 1,500 mg/L)], melanin [meningeal melanosarcoma], carotene [systemic carotenemia]; hazy—meningitis; pink to dark yellow—aspiration of epidural fat; turbid—cells, microorganisms, protein, fat, or contrast medium; turbidity related to increased cell count is called pleocytosis)***
- Protein ***(related to alterations in blood-brain barrier that allow permeability to proteins):*** Type 2 diabetes ***(related to relative increase in plasma glucose),*** encephalitis, Guillain-Barré syndrome (elevated protein with normal WBC count—also called albuminocytological dissociation), meningitis, trauma, tumors
- Lactic acid ***(related to cerebral hypoxia and correlating anaerobic metabolism):*** Bacterial, tubercular, fungal meningitis
- Myelin basic protein ***(related to accumulation as a result of nerve sheath demyelination):*** Trauma, stroke, tumor, multiple sclerosis, subacute sclerosing panencephalitis
- IgG and oligoclonal banding ***(related to autoimmune or inflammatory response):*** Multiple sclerosis, CNS syphilis, and subacute sclerosing panencephalitis
- Gram stain: ***Meningitis due to Escherichia coli, Streptococcus agalactiae, Streptococcus pneumoniae, Haemophilus influenzae, Mycobacterium avium-intracellulare, Mycobacterium leprae, Mycobacterium tuberculosis, Neisseria meningitidis, Cryptococcus neoformans***
- India ink preparation: ***Meningitis due to C. neoformans***
- Culture: ***Encephalitis or meningitis due to herpes simplex virus, S. pneumoniae, H. influenzae, N. meningitidis, C. neoformans***
- RBC count: ***Hemorrhage***
- White blood cell (WBC) count:

General increase—injection of contrast media or anticancer drugs in subarachnoid space; CSF infarct; metastatic tumor in contact with CSF; reaction to repeated lumbar puncture

Elevated WBC count with a predominance of neutrophils indicative of abscess, bacterial meningitis, tubercular meningitis

Elevated WBC count with a predominance of lymphocytes indicative of viral, tubercular, parasitic, or fungal meningitis; multiple sclerosis

Elevated WBC count with a predominance of monocytes indicative of

chronic bacterial meningitis, amebic meningitis, multiple sclerosis, toxoplasmosis

Increased plasma cells indicative of acute viral infections, demyelinating diseases, multiple sclerosis, neurosyphilis, sarcoidosis, syphilitic meningoencephalitis, subacute sclerosing panencephalitis, tubercular meningitis, parasitic infections, Guillain-Barré syndrome

Presence of eosinophils indicative of parasitic and fungal infections, acute polyneuritis, idiopathic hypereosinophilic syndrome, reaction to drugs or a shunt in CSF

- VDRL: ***Syphilis***

Positive findings in

- Cytology: ***Malignant cells***

Decreased in:

- Glucose: ***Bacterial and tubercular meningitis***

CRITICAL FINDINGS:

- Positive Gram stain, India ink preparation, or culture
- Presence of malignant cells or blasts
- Elevated WBC count
- Adults: Glucose less than 37 mg/dL (SI: Less than 2.1 mmol/L); greater than 440 mg/dL (SI: Greater than 24.4 mmol/L)
- Children: Glucose less than 31 mg/dL (SI: Less than 1.7 mmol/L); greater than 440 mg/dL (SI: Greater than 24.4 mmol/L)

Note and immediately report to the requesting health-care provider (HCP) any critical findings and related symptoms. A listing of these findings varies among facilities. Timely notification of a critical finding for laboratory or diagnostic studies is a role expectation of the professional nurse. The notification processes vary among facilities. Upon receipt of the critical finding, the information should be read back to the caller to verify accuracy.

Important signs to note include allergic or other reaction to the anesthesia, bleeding or CSF drainage at the puncture sight, changes in level of consciousness, changes to or inequality of pupil size, or respiratory failure.

INTERFERING FACTORS

Other considerations

- Drugs and other substances that may decrease CSF protein levels include cefotaxime and dexamethasone.
- Interferon-β may increase myelin basic protein levels.
- Drugs and other substances that may increase CSF glucose levels include cefotaxime and dexamethasone.
- RBC count may be falsely elevated with a traumatic spinal tap.
- Delays in analysis may present a false-positive appearance of xanthochromia due to RBC lysis that begins within 4 hr of a bloody tap.

NURSING IMPLICATIONS AND PROCEDURE

POTENTIAL NURSING PROBLEMS:

Problem	Signs & Symptoms	Interventions
Mobility ***(related to nerve demyelination; spastic muscle movement; weakness; muscle tremors)***	Weak or unsteady gait; uncoordinated movement; difficult purposeful movement; limited range of motion	Assess the patient's muscle strength and coordination; use assistive devices if necessary; encourage self-care; encourage appropriate and safe activity

C

Problem	Signs & Symptoms	Interventions
Skin ***(related to limited mobility; sensory changes)***	Development of pressure ulcers; open sores that are unattended due to lack of sensation and recognition; skin injury from burn	Careful use of heat and cold to prevent skin damage and unintended burns; ensure water used for personal hygiene is tested for temperature prior to use; change position a minimum of every 2 hours
Visual disturbance ***(related to optic nerve demyelination)***	Blurred vision, some visual loss or blind spots; nystagmus; double vision; altered color perception	Check the immediate environment for items that could cause fall and injury; encourage the patient to wear assistive devices such as glasses or contacts to improve vision; provide information for support group related to vision loss; encourage the use of an eye patch as appropriate

PRETEST:

- Positively identify the patient using at least two person-specific identifiers before services, treatments, or procedures are performed.
- *Patient Teaching:* Inform the patient this procedure can assist in evaluating health by providing a sample of fluid from around the spinal cord to be tested for disease and infection.
- Obtain a history of the patient's health concerns, symptoms, surgical procedures, and results of previously performed laboratory and diagnostic studies. Include a list of known allergens, especially allergies or sensitivities to latex or iodine disinfectant solutions. Perform a basic neurological examination; assess the patient's gait and leg muscle strength prior to the procedure.
- Obtain a list of the patient's current medications, including over-the-counter medications and dietary supplements (see Effects of Natural Products on Laboratory Values online at Davis*Plus*).
- Review the procedure with the patient. Inform the patient that the position required may be awkward but that someone will assist during the procedure. Stress the importance of remaining still and breathing normally throughout the procedure. Inform the patient that specimen collection takes approximately 20 min. Address concerns about pain and explain that a stinging sensation may be felt when the local anesthetic is injected. Instruct the patient to report any pain or other sensations that may require repositioning the spinal needle. Explain that there may be some discomfort during the procedure. Inform the patient the procedure will be performed by an HCP.
- ***Sensitivity to social and cultural issues,*** as well as concern for modesty, is important in providing psychological support before, during, and after the procedure.
- Note that there are no food, fluid, or medication restrictions unless by medical direction.
- *Make sure a written and informed consent has been signed prior to the procedure and before administering any medications.*

INTRATEST:

Potential Complications:
Headache is a common minor complication experienced after lumbar puncture and is caused by leakage of the spinal fluid from around the puncture site. On a rare occasion the headache may require treatment with an epidural blood patch in which an anesthesiologist or pain management specialist injects a small amount of the patient's blood in the epidural space of the puncture site. The blood patch forms a clot and seals the puncture site to prevent further leakage of CSF and provides relief within 30 min. Other complications include lower back pain after the procedure, infection that might occur if bacteria from the skin surface is introduced at the puncture site, bleeding near the puncture site, or brainstem herniation, due to increased intracranial pressure.

- Avoid the use of equipment containing latex if the patient has a history of allergic reaction to latex. If the patient is sensitive to iodine disinfectant solutions, a double alcohol scrub or green soap may be substituted.
- Ensure that anticoagulant therapy has been withheld for the appropriate number of days prior to the procedure. Number of days to withhold medication is dependent on the type of anticoagulant. Notify the HCP if patient anticoagulant therapy has not been withheld.
- Have emergency equipment readily available.
- Instruct the patient to cooperate fully and to follow directions. Direct the patient to breathe normally and to avoid unnecessary movement.
- Observe standard precautions, and follow the general guidelines in Patient Preparation and Specimen Collection online at Davis*Plus*. Positively identify the patient, and label the appropriate tubes with the corresponding patient demographics, date, and time of collection. Collect the specimen in four plastic conical tubes.
- Record baseline vital signs, and assess neurological status.
- To perform a lumbar puncture, position the patient in the knee-chest position at the side of the bed. Provide pillows to support the spine or for the patient to grasp. The sitting position is an alternative. In this position, the patient must bend the neck and chest to the knees.
- Prepare the site—usually between L3 and L4, or between L4 and L5—with povidone-iodine and drape the area.
- A local anesthetic is injected. Using sterile technique, the HCP inserts the spinal needle through the spinous processes of the vertebrae and into the subarachnoid space. Needle size has been shown to play a significant role in predictable incidence of post-puncture headache. However, the smaller the bevel, the more time is required to collect a sufficient volume of fluid; usually a 22-g needle is used. The stylet is removed. If the needle is properly placed, CSF drips from the needle.
- Attach the stopcock and manometer, and measure initial pressure. Normal pressure for an adult in the lateral recumbent position is 60–200 mm H_2O, and 10–100 mm H_2O for children less than 8 yr. These values depend on the body position and are different in a horizontal than in a sitting position.
- CSF pressure may be elevated if the patient is anxious, holding his or her breath, or tensing muscles. It may also be elevated if the patient's knees are flexed too firmly against the abdomen. CSF pressure may be significantly elevated in patients with intracranial tumors or space occupying pockets of infection as seen in meningitis. If the initial pressure is elevated, the HCP may perform Queckenstedt's test. To perform this test, pressure is applied to the jugular vein for about 10 sec. CSF pressure usually rises rapidly in response to the occlusion and then returns to the pretest level within 10 sec after the pressure is released. Sluggish response may indicate CSF obstruction.
- Obtain four (or five) vials of fluid, according to the HCP's request, in separate tubes (1 to 3 mL in each), and label them numerically (1 to 4 or 5) in the order they were filled.

- A final pressure reading is taken, and the needle is removed. Clean the puncture site with an antiseptic solution and apply direct pressure with dry gauze to stop bleeding or CSF leakage. Observe/assess puncture site for bleeding, CSF leakage, or hematoma formation and secure gauze with adhesive bandage.
- Promptly transport the specimen to the laboratory for processing and analysis.

POST-TEST:

- Inform the patient that a report of the results will be made available to the requesting HCP, who will discuss the results with the patient.
- Monitor vital signs and neurological status and for headache every 15 min for 1 hr, then every 2 hr for 4 hr, and then as ordered by the HCP. Monitor temperature every 4 hr for 24 hr. Compare with baseline values. Notify the HCP if temperature is elevated. Protocols may vary among facilities.
- Administer fluids if permitted, especially fluids containing caffeine, to replace lost CSF and help prevent or relieve headache, which is an adverse effect of lumbar puncture. The use of a flexible straw facilitates intake of fluids while the patient remains flat. Advise the patient that headache may begin within a few hours up to 2 days after the procedure and may be associated with dizziness, nausea, and vomiting. The length of time for the headache to resolve varies considerably.
- Observe/assess the puncture site for leakage, and frequently monitor body signs, such as temperature and blood pressure. Position the patient flat, either on the back or abdomen following the HCP's instructions; some HCPs allow 30 degrees of elevation. Maintain this position for 8 hr. Changing position is acceptable as long as the body remains horizontal. Observe/assess the patient for neurological changes, such as altered level of consciousness, change in pupils, reports of tingling or numbness, and irritability.
- Recognize anxiety related to test results. Discuss the implications of abnormal test results on the patient's lifestyle. Provide teaching and information regarding the clinical implications of the test results, as appropriate.
- Reinforce information given by the patient's HCP regarding further testing, treatment, or referral to another HCP. Provide information regarding vaccine-preventable diseases when indicated (encephalitis, influenza, meningococcal diseases). Answer any questions or address any concerns voiced by the patient or family.
- Instruct the patient in the use of any ordered medications. Explain the importance of adhering to the therapy regimen. As appropriate, instruct the patient in significant adverse effects associated with the prescribed medication. Encourage him or her to review corresponding literature provided by a pharmacist.
- Depending on the results of this procedure, additional testing may be performed to evaluate or monitor progression of the disease process and determine the need for a change in therapy. Evaluate test results in relation to the patient's symptoms and other tests performed.

Patient Education:

- Teach the patient to keep frequently used items within easy reach.
- Teach the patient the importance of changing position frequently to prevent pressure ulcers.

Expected Patient Outcomes:

Understanding

- The patient and family state that the disease process may be accompanied by periods of exacerbation.
- The patient and family state the importance of creating a safe home environment to prevent injury due to vision loss.

Ability

- The patient demonstrates the ability to successfully perform activities of daily living.
- The patient demonstrates the ability to use assistive devices safely.

Response

- The patient agrees to use assistive devices to decrease fall risk and associated injury.

- The patient agrees to attend a support group to meet emotional needs associated with vision loss.

RELATED STUDIES:

- Related tests include CBC, CT brain, culture for appropriate organisms (blood, fungal, mycobacteria, sputum, throat, viral, wound), EMG, evoked brain potentials, Gram stain, MRI brain, PET brain, and syphilis serology.
- Refer to the Immune and Musculoskeletal systems tables online at Davis*Plus* for related tests by body system.

C

Ceruloplasmin

SYNONYM/ACRONYM: Copper oxidase, Cp.

COMMON USE: To assist in the evaluation of copper intoxication and liver disease, especially Wilson's disease.

SPECIMEN: Serum collected in a gold-, red-, or red/gray-top tube.

NORMAL FINDINGS: (Method: Nephelometry)

Age	Conventional Units	SI Units (Conventional Units × 10)
Newborn–3 mo	5–18 mg/dL	50–180 mg/L
6–12 mo	33–43 mg/dL	330–430 mg/L
1–3 yr	26–55 mg/dL	260–550 mg/L
4–5 yr	27–56 mg/dL	270–560 mg/L
6–7 yr	24–48 mg/dL	240–480 mg/L
8 yr–older adult	20–54 mg/dL	200–540 mg/L

POTENTIAL MEDICAL DIAGNOSIS

Increased in:

Ceruloplasmin is an acute-phase reactant protein and will be increased in many inflammatory conditions, including cancer

- Acute infections
- Biliary cirrhosis
- Cancer of the bone, lung, stomach
- Copper intoxication
- Hodgkin's disease
- Leukemia
- Pregnancy (last trimester) ***(estrogen increases copper levels)***
- Rheumatoid arthritis
- Tissue necrosis

Decreased in:

- Menkes' disease ***(severe X-linked defect causing failed transport to the liver and tissues)***
- Nutritional deficiency of copper
- Wilson's disease ***(genetic defect causing failed transport to the liver and tissues)***

CRITICAL FINDINGS: N/A

Find and print out the full study on Fast Find at davispl.us/vanleeuwen7.

Chest X-Ray

SYNONYM/ACRONYM: Chest radiography, CXR, lung radiography.

COMMON USE: To assist in the evaluation of cardiac, respiratory, and skeletal structure within the lung cavity and diagnose multiple diseases such as pneumonia and heart failure.

AREA OF APPLICATION: Heart, mediastinum, lungs.

C

DESCRIPTION: Chest radiography, commonly called chest x-ray, is one of the most frequently performed radiological diagnostic studies. This study yields information about the pulmonary, cardiac, and skeletal systems. The lungs, filled with air, are easily penetrated by x-rays and appear black on chest images. A routine chest x-ray includes a posteroanterior projection, in which x-rays pass from the posterior to the anterior, and a left lateral projection. Additional projections that may be requested are obliques, lateral decubitus, or lordotic views. Portable x-rays, done in acute or critical situations, can be done at the bedside and usually include only the anteroposterior projection with additional images taken in a lateral decubitus position if the presence of free pleural fluid or air is in question. Chest images should be taken on full inspiration and erect when possible to minimize heart magnification and demonstrate fluid levels. Expiration images may be added to detect a pneumothorax or locate foreign bodies. Rib detail images may be taken to delineate bone pathology, useful when chest radiographs suggest fractures or metastatic lesions. Fluoroscopic studies of the chest can also be done to evaluate lung and diaphragm movement. In the beginning of the disease process of tuberculosis, asthma, and chronic obstructive pulmonary disease, the results of a chest x-ray may not correlate with the clinical status of the patient and may even be normal.

This procedure is contraindicated for

Patients who are pregnant or suspected of being pregnant, unless the potential benefits of a procedure using radiation far outweigh the risk of radiation exposure to the fetus and mother.

INDICATIONS

- Aid in the diagnosis of diaphragmatic hernia, lung tumors, intravenous devices, and metastasis.
- Evaluate known or suspected pulmonary disorders, chest trauma, cardiovascular disorders, and skeletal disorders.
- Evaluate placement and position of an endotracheal tube, tracheostomy tube, nasogastric feeding tube, pacemaker wires, central venous catheters, Swan-Ganz catheters, chest tubes, and intra-aortic balloon pump.
- Evaluate positive purified protein derivative (PPD) or Mantoux tests.
- Monitor resolution, progression, or maintenance of disease.
- Monitor effectiveness of the treatment regimen.

POTENTIAL MEDICAL DIAGNOSIS

Normal findings

- Normal lung fields, cardiac size, mediastinal structures, thoracic spine, ribs, and diaphragm

Abnormal findings related to

- Atelectasis
- Bronchitis
- Curvature of the spinal column (scoliosis)
- Enlarged heart
- Enlarged lymph nodes
- Flattened diaphragm
- Foreign bodies lodged in the pulmonary system ***as seen by a radiopaque object***
- Fractures of the sternum, ribs, and spine
- Lung pathology, including tumors
- Malposition of tubes or wires
- Mediastinal tumor and pathology
- Pericardial effusion
- Pericarditis
- Pleural effusion
- Pneumonia
- Pneumothorax
- Pulmonary bases, fibrosis, infiltrates
- Tuberculosis
- Vascular abnormalities

CRITICAL FINDINGS:

- Foreign body
- Malposition of tube, line, or postoperative device (pacemaker)
- Pneumonia
- Pneumoperitoneum
- Pneumothorax
- Spine fracture

Note and immediately report to the requesting health-care provider (HCP) any critical findings and related symptoms. A listing of these findings varies among facilities. Timely notification of a critical finding for laboratory or diagnostic studies is a role expectation of the professional nurse. The notification processes vary among facilities. Upon receipt of the critical finding, the information should be read back to the caller to verify accuracy.

INTERFERING FACTORS

Factors that may impair the results of the examination

- Metallic objects within the examination field.
- Improper adjustment of the radiographic equipment to accommodate obese or thin patients, which can cause overexposure or underexposure.
- Incorrect positioning of the patient, which may produce poor visualization of the area to be examined.
- Inability of the patient to cooperate or remain still during the procedure because of age, significant pain, or mental status.

Other considerations

- The procedure may be terminated if chest pain or severe cardiac dysrhythmias occur.

NURSING IMPLICATIONS AND PROCEDURE

See Potential Nursing Problems on Fast Find at davispl.us/vanleeuwen7

PRETEST:

- Positively identify the patient using at least two person-specific identifiers before services, treatments, or procedures are performed.
- ***Patient Teaching:*** Inform the patient this procedure can assist in assessing the heart and lungs for disease.
- Obtain a history of the patient's health concerns, symptoms, surgical procedures, and results of previously performed laboratory and diagnostic studies. Include a list of known allergens, especially allergies or sensitivities to latex.
- Record the date of the last menstrual period and determine the possibility of pregnancy in women who are perimenopausal.

- Obtain a list of the patient's current medications, including over-the-counter medications and dietary supplements (see Effects of Natural Products on Laboratory Values online at Davis*Plus*).
- Review the procedure with the patient. Address concerns about pain and explain that no pain will be experienced during the test. Inform the patient that the procedure is performed in the radiology department or at the bedside by a registered radiological technologist, and takes approximately 5 to 15 min.

Pediatric Considerations: Preparing children for a chest x-ray depends on the age of the child. Encourage parents to be truthful about what the child may experience during the procedure and to use words that they know their child will understand. Toddlers and preschool-age children have a very short attention span, so the best time to talk about the test is right before the procedure. The child should be assured that he or she will be allowed to bring a favorite comfort item into the examination room, and if appropriate, that a parent will be with the child during the procedure. Provide older children with information about the test, and allow them to participate in as many decisions as possible (e.g., choice of clothes to wear to the appointment) in order to reduce anxiety and encourage cooperation. If the child will be asked to maintain a certain position for the test, encourage the child to practice the required position, provide a CD that demonstrates the procedure, and teach strategies to remain calm, such as deep breathing, humming, or counting to himself or herself.

- ***Sensitivity to social and cultural issues,*** as well as concern for modesty, is important in providing psychological support before, during, and after the procedure.
- Instruct the patient to remove all metallic objects from the area to be examined.
- Note that there are no food, fluid, or medication restrictions unless by medical direction.

INTRATEST:

Potential Complications: N/A

- Avoid the use of equipment containing latex if the patient has a history of allergic reaction to latex.
- Observe standard precautions, and follow the general guidelines in Patient Preparation and Specimen Collection online at Davis*Plus*. Positively identify the patient.
- Ensure that the patient has removed all external metallic objects from the area to be examined.
- Patients are given a gown, robe, and foot coverings to wear.
- Instruct the patient to cooperate fully and to follow directions. Instruct the patient to remain still throughout the procedure because movement produces unreliable results.
- Place the patient in the standing position facing the cassette or image detector, with hands on hips, neck extended, and shoulders rolled forward.
- Position the chest with the left side against the image holder for a lateral view.
- For portable examinations, elevate the head of the bed to the high Fowler's position.
- Ask the patient to inhale deeply and hold his or her breath while the x-ray images are taken, and then to exhale after the images are taken.

POST-TEST:

- Inform the patient that a report of the results will be made available to the requesting HCP, who will discuss the results with the patient.
- Recognize anxiety related to test results and be supportive of impaired activity related to respiratory capacity and perceived loss of physical activity. Discuss the implications of abnormal test results on the patient's lifestyle. Provide teaching and information regarding the clinical implications of the test results, as appropriate.
- Reinforce information given by the patient's HCP regarding further testing, treatment, or referral to

another HCP. Answer any questions or address any concerns voiced by the patient or family.

- Depending on the results of this procedure, additional testing may be performed to evaluate and determine the need for a change in therapy or progression of the disease process. Evaluate test results in relation to the patient's symptoms and other tests performed.

Patient Education:

- Teach the patient to weigh self at the same time each day and record the weight to report to his or her HCP.
- Teach the patient how to effectively cough and deep breathe.

Expected Patient Outcomes:

Understanding

- The patient and family state the importance of pacing activities to conserve energy and decrease shortness of breath.
- The patient and family state the importance of maintaining oxygen therapy to support a stable oxygen saturation.

Ability

- The patient and family demonstrate good hand hygiene to decrease infection risk.
- The patient and family choose activities that decrease the risk of fatigue leading to a compromised respiratory status.

Response

- The patient agrees to use effective cough techniques to improve oxygenation.
- The patient agrees complete the full course of antibiotics to treat the infection.

RELATED STUDIES:

- Related tests include biopsy lung, blood gases, bronchoscopy, CT thoracic, CBC, culture mycobacteria, culture sputum, culture viral, electrocardiogram, Gram stain, lung perfusion scan, MRI chest, pulmonary function study, pulse oximetry, and TB tests.
- Refer to the Cardiovascular and Respiratory systems tables online at Davis*Plus* for related tests by body system.

Chlamydia Group Antibody, IgG and IgM

SYNONYM/ACRONYM: N/A

COMMON USE: To diagnose some of the more common chlamydia infections such as community-acquired pneumonia transmitted by *Chlamydophila pneumoniae* and chlamydia disease that is sexually transmitted by *Chlamydia trachomatis*.

SPECIMEN: Serum collected in a red-top tube. Place separated serum into a standard transport tube within 2 hr of collection.

NORMAL FINDINGS: (Method: Enzyme immunofluorescent assay)

IgG	IgM
Less than 1:64	Less than 1:20

DESCRIPTION: *Chlamydia trachomatis* is the cause of one of the most common sexually transmitted infections. These gram-negative bacteria are called *obligate cell parasites* because they require living cells for growth. There are three serotypes of *C. trachomatis*. One group causes lymphogranuloma venereum, with symptoms of the first phase of the disease appearing 2 to 6 wk after infection; another causes a genital tract infection different from lymphogranuloma venereum, in which symptoms in men appear 7 to 28 days after intercourse (women are generally asymptomatic); and the third causes the ocular disease trachoma (incubation period, 7 to 10 days). *C. psittaci* is the cause of psittacosis in birds and humans. It is increasing in prevalence as a pathogen responsible for other significant diseases of the respiratory system. The incubation period for *C. psittaci* infections in humans is 7 to 15 days and is followed by chills, fever, and a persistent nonproductive cough. Another chlamydia, *C. pneumoniae*, is a common cause of community-acquired pneumonia.

Chlamydia is difficult to culture and grow, so antibody testing has become the technology of choice to identify antibodies to *C. psittaci* and *C. pneumoniae*. A limitation of antibody screening is that positive results may not distinguish past from current infection. Antibody testing may also be used to identify sexually transmitted chlamydial disease; however, nucleic acid amplification and DNA probes are more commonly used to identify the Chlamydia species. Assays can specifically identify *C. trachomatis* and require special collection and transport kits. They also have specific collection instructions, and the specimens are collected on swabs. The laboratory performing this testing should be consulted before specimen collection. Culture- or liquid-based Pap test may also be requested for identification of oculogenital chlamydia infections.

This procedure is contraindicated for: N/A

INDICATIONS

- Establish Chlamydia as the cause of atypical pneumonia.
- Establish the presence of chlamydial infection.

POTENTIAL MEDICAL DIAGNOSIS

Positive findings in

- Chlamydial infection
- Community-acquired pneumonia
- Infantile pneumonia ***(related to transmission at birth from an infected mother)***
- Infertility ***(related to scarring of ovaries or fallopian tubes from untreated chlamydial infection)***
- Lymphogranuloma venereum
- Ophthalmia neonatorum ***(related to transmission at birth from an infected mother)***
- Pelvic inflammatory disease
- Urethritis

CRITICAL FINDINGS: N/A

INTERFERING FACTORS

- Hemolysis or lipemia may interfere with analysis.
- Positive results may demonstrate evidence of past infection and not necessarily indicate current infection.

NURSING IMPLICATIONS AND PROCEDURE

POTENTIAL NURSING PROBLEMS:

Problem	Signs & Symptoms	Interventions
Infection ***(related to exposure to bacterial organisms)***	Temperature; increased heart rate; increased blood pressure; shaking; chills; mottled skin; lethargy; fatigue; swelling; elevated white blood cell (WBC) count; sputum culture positive for infecting organism; tachypnea; dyspnea; productive cough; tachycardia	Promote good hygiene; assist with hygiene as needed; administer prescribed antibiotics, antipyretics; provide cooling measures; administer prescribed intravenous fluids; monitor vital signs and trend temperatures; encourage oral fluids; adhere to standard precautions; provide isolation as appropriate; obtain cultures as ordered; provide lightweight clothing and bedding; assess and monitor breath sounds; obtain ordered sputum specimen for culture; monitor and trend WBC results; monitor chest x-ray results
Airway ***(related to congestion; sputum production)***	Ineffective cough; purulent sputum; dyspnea; tachypnea; documented infiltrates; decreased or diminished breath sounds	Assess respiratory characteristics (rate, rhythm, depth, accessory muscle use); assess effectiveness of cough and amount of productivity; monitor sputum characteristics (color, viscosity); assess hydration status, encourage increased fluid intake; auscultate lungs for adventitious breath sounds (crackles); use pulse oximetry; administer prescribed oxygen; suction as needed; humidify oxygen as appropriate;

Problem	Signs & Symptoms	Interventions
		encourage use of incentive spirometer; facilitate chest physiotherapy and nebulized treatments with mucolytic and bronchodilator medications; facilitate ordered bronchoscopy or thoracentesis
Gas exchange ***(related to congestion [fluid in alveoli or mucous in airways]; mucous secretions; ventilation and perfusion mismatch; lung consolidation)***	Decreased activity tolerance; increased shortness of breath with activity; weakness; orthopnea; cyanosis (pale, dusky); cough; increased heart rate; increased respiratory rate; use of respiratory accessory muscles; tachypnea; tachycardia; hypotension; restlessness; irritability; confusion; lethargy; disorientation; hypercapnia	Auscultate and trend breath sounds; use pulse oximetry to monitor oxygenation; administer oxygen as ordered; collaborate with physician to consider intubation and/or mechanical ventilation; place the head of the bed in high Fowler's position; administer diuretics, vasodilators as ordered; assess for hypoxia (nailbeds, mucous membranes); monitor and trend blood pressure and heart rate; monitor for altered level of consciousness
Infection ***(related to sexual exposure to** C. trachomatis**)***	Purulent penile or vaginal drainage; dysuria; lower abdominal pain in women (pelvic inflammatory disease); testicular pain and swelling (epididymitis); pain, bleeding, and discharge from the rectum (proctitis); sometimes there are no symptoms	Provide written information about sexually transmitted infections; complete a thorough history and physical assessment; administer prescribed antibiotics; teach patient to refrain from sexual activity until course of antibiotics is completed; explain that it may be necessary to have repeat testing 3 mo after initial treatment to assess for re-infection from sexual partner

C

PRETEST:

- Positively identify the patient using at least two person-specific identifiers before services, treatments, or procedures are performed.
- ***Patient Teaching:*** Inform the patient this test can assist in diagnosing chlamydial infection.
- Obtain a history of the patient's health concerns, symptoms, surgical procedures, and results of previously performed laboratory and diagnostic studies. Include a list of known allergens, especially allergies or sensitivities to latex.
- Obtain a list of the patient's current medications, including over-the-counter medications and dietary supplements (see Effects of Natural Products on Laboratory Values online at Davis*Plus*).
- Review the procedure with the patient. Inform the patient that specimen collection takes approximately 5 to 10 min. Address concerns about pain and explain that there may be some discomfort during the venipuncture.
- ***Sensitivity to social and cultural issues,*** as well as concern for modesty, is important in providing psychological support before, during, and after the procedure.
- Inform the patient that several tests may be necessary to confirm diagnosis. Any individual positive result should be repeated in 7 to 10 days to monitor a change in titer.
- Note that there are no food, fluid, or medication restrictions unless by medical direction.

INTRATEST:

Potential Complications:

- Avoid the use of equipment containing latex if the patient has a history of allergic reaction to latex.
- Instruct the patient to cooperate fully and to follow directions. Direct the patient to breathe normally and to avoid unnecessary movement.
- Observe standard precautions, and follow the general guidelines in Patient Preparation and Specimen Collection online at Davis*Plus*. Positively identify the patient, and label the appropriate specimen container with the corresponding patient demographics, initials of the person collecting the specimen, date, and time of collection. Perform a venipuncture.
- Remove the needle and apply direct pressure with dry gauze to stop bleeding. Observe/assess venipuncture site for bleeding or hematoma formation and secure gauze with adhesive bandage.
- Promptly transport the specimen to the laboratory for processing and analysis.

POST-TEST:

- Inform that patient that a report of the results will be made available to the requesting health-care provider (HCP), who will discuss the results with the patient.
- Recognize anxiety related to test results, and be supportive. Discuss the implications of abnormal test results on the patient's lifestyle. Provide teaching and information regarding the clinical implications of the test results, as appropriate. Emphasize the need to return to have a convalescent blood sample taken in 7 to 14 days. Educate the patient regarding access to counseling services.
- ***Social and Cultural Considerations:*** Counsel the patient, as appropriate, as to the risk of sexual transmission and educate the patient regarding proper prophylaxis. Reinforce the importance of strict adherence to the treatment regimen.
- ***Social and Cultural Considerations:*** Inform the patient with positive *C. trachomatis* that findings must be reported to a local public health department official, who will question the patient regarding his or her sexual partners.
- ***Social and Cultural Considerations:*** Offer support, as appropriate, to patients who may be the victim of rape or

sexual assault. Educate the patient regarding access to counseling services. Provide a nonjudgmental, nonthreatening atmosphere for a discussion during which you explain the risks of sexually transmitted infections. It is also important to discuss emotions the patient may experience (guilt, depression, anger) as a victim of sexual assault.

- Depending on the results of this procedure, additional testing may be performed to evaluate or monitor progression of the disease process and determine the need for a change in therapy. Evaluate test results in relation to the patient's symptoms and other tests performed.

Patient Education:

- Provide emotional support if the patient is pregnant and if results are positive.
- Inform the patient that chlamydial infection during pregnancy places the newborn at risk for pneumonia and conjunctivitis.
- Reinforce information given by the patient's HCP regarding further testing, treatment, or referral to another HCP.
- Answer any questions or address any concerns voiced by the patient or family.

Expected Patient Outcomes:

Understanding

- The patient states the importance of increasing fluid intake to thin and mobilize secretions.
- The patient states the importance of completing course of antibiotics for chlamydial infection prior to engaging in sexual activity.

Ability

- The patient demonstrates proficiency with cough and deep breathing.
- The patient demonstrates proficient use of incentive spirometer.

Response

- The patient complies with the request to complete retesting for chlamydial infection in 3 mo or as requested.

RELATED STUDIES:

- Related tests include culture bacterial (anal, genital), culture viral, Gram stain, Pap smear, and syphilis serology.
- Refer to the Immune and Reproductive Systems tables online at Davis*Plus* for related tests by body system.

Chloride, Blood

SYNONYM/ACRONYM: Cl^-.

COMMON USE: To evaluate electrolytes, acid-base balance, and hydration level.

SPECIMEN: Serum collected in a gold-, red-, or red/gray-top tube. Plasma collected in a green-top (heparin) tube is also acceptable.

NORMAL FINDINGS: (Method: Ion-selective electrode)

Age	Conventional & SI Units
Premature	95–110 mEq/L or mmol/L
0–1 mo	98–113 mEq/L or mmol/L
2 mo–older	adult 97–107 mEq/L or mmol/L

C

DESCRIPTION: Chloride is the most abundant anion in the extracellular fluid. Its most important function is in the maintenance of acid-base balance, in which it competes with bicarbonate for sodium. Chloride levels generally increase and decrease proportionally to sodium levels and inversely proportional to bicarbonate levels. Chloride also participates with sodium in the maintenance of water balance and aids in the regulation of osmotic pressure. Chloride contributes to gastric acid (hydrochloric acid) for digestion and activation of enzymes. The chloride content of venous blood is slightly higher than that of arterial blood because chloride ions enter red blood cells in response to absorption of carbon dioxide into the cell. As carbon dioxide enters the blood cell, bicarbonate leaves and chloride is absorbed in exchange to maintain electrical neutrality within the cell.

Chloride is provided by dietary intake, mostly in the form of sodium chloride. It is absorbed by the gastrointestinal system, filtered out by the glomeruli, and reabsorbed by the renal tubules. Excess chloride is excreted in the urine. Serum values normally remain fairly stable. A slight decrease may be detectable after meals because chloride is used to produce hydrochloric acid as part of the digestive process. Measurement of chloride levels is not as essential as measurement of other electrolytes such as sodium or potassium. Chloride is usually included in standard electrolyte panels to detect the presence of unmeasured anions via calculation of the anion gap. Chloride levels are usually not interpreted apart from sodium, potassium, carbon dioxide, and anion gap.

The patient's clinical picture needs to be considered in the evaluation of electrolytes. Fluid and electrolyte imbalances are often seen in patients with serious illness or injury because in these cases the clinical situation has affected the normal homeostatic balance of the body. It is also possible that therapeutic treatments being administered are causing or contributing to the electrolyte imbalance. Children and older adults are at high risk for fluid and electrolyte imbalances when chloride levels are depleted. Children are considered to be at high risk during chloride imbalance because a positive serum chloride balance is important for expansion of the extracellular fluid compartment. Anemia, the result of decreased hemoglobin levels, is a frequent issue for older adult patients. Because hemoglobin participates in a major buffer system in the body, depleted hemoglobin levels affect the efficiency of chloride ion exchange for bicarbonate in red blood cells, which in turn affects acid-base balance. Older adult patients are also at high risk because their renal response to change in pH is slower, resulting in a more rapid development of electrolyte imbalance.

This procedure is contraindicated for: N/A

INDICATIONS

- Assist in confirming a diagnosis of disorders associated with abnormal chloride values, as seen in acid-base and fluid imbalances.
- Differentiate between types of acidosis (hyperchloremic versus anion gap).

- Monitor effectiveness of drug therapy to increase or decrease serum chloride levels.

POTENTIAL MEDICAL DIAGNOSIS

Increased in:

- Acute kidney injury ***(related to decreased renal excretion)***
- Cushing's disease ***(related to sodium retention as a result of increased levels of aldosterone; typically, chloride levels follow sodium levels)***
- Dehydration ***(related to hemoconcentration)***
- Diabetes insipidus ***(hemoconcentration related to excessive urine production)***
- Excessive infusion of normal saline ***(related to excessive intake)***
- Head trauma with hypothalamic stimulation or damage
- Hyperparathyroidism (primary) ***(high chloride-to-phosphate ratio is used to assist in diagnosis)***
- Metabolic acidosis ***(associated with prolonged diarrhea)***
- Renal tubular acidosis ***(acidosis related to net retention of chloride ions)***
- Respiratory alkalosis (e.g., hyperventilation) ***(related to metabolic exchange of intracellular chloride replaced by bicarbonate; chloride levels increase)***
- Salicylate intoxication ***(related to acid-base imbalance resulting in a hyperchloremic acidosis)***

Decreased in:

- Addison's disease ***(related to insufficient production of aldosterone; potassium is retained while sodium and chloride are lost)***
- Burns ***(dilutional effect related to sequestration of extracellular fluid)***
- Heart failure ***(related to dilutional effect of fluid buildup)***
- Diabetic ketoacidosis ***(related to acid-base imbalance with accumulation of ketone bodies and increased chloride)***
- Excessive sweating ***(related to excessive loss of chloride without replacement)***
- Gastrointestinal loss from vomiting (severe), diarrhea, nasogastric suction, or fistula
- Metabolic alkalosis ***(related to homeostatic response in which intracellular chloride increases to reduce alkalinity of extracellular fluid)***
- Overhydration ***(related to dilutional effect)***
- Respiratory acidosis (chronic)
- Salt-losing nephritis ***(related to excessive loss)***
- Syndrome of inappropriate antidiuretic hormone secretion ***(related to dilutional effect)***
- Water intoxication ***(related to dilutional effect)***

CRITICAL FINDINGS:

- Less than 80 mEq/L or mmol/L (SI: Less than 80 mmol/L)
- Greater than 115 mEq/L or mmol/L (SI: Greater than 115 mmol/L)

Note and immediately report to the requesting health-care provider (HCP) any critical findings and related symptoms. A listing of these findings varies among facilities. Timely notification of a critical finding for laboratory or diagnostic studies is a role expectation of the professional nurse. The notification processes vary among facilities. Upon receipt of the critical finding, the information should be read back to the caller to verify accuracy.

Consideration may be given to verification of critical findings before action is taken. Policies vary among facilities and may include requesting immediate recollection and retesting by the laboratory or retesting using a rapid point-of-care testing instrument at the bedside, if available.

The following may be seen in hypochloremia: twitching or tremors, which may indicate excitability of the nervous system; slow and shallow breathing; and decreased blood pressure as a result of fluid loss. Possible interventions relate to treatment of the underlying cause.

Signs and symptoms associated with hyperchloremia are weakness; lethargy; and deep, rapid breathing. Proper interventions include treatments that correct the underlying cause.

C

INTERFERING FACTORS

- Drugs or other substances that may cause an increase in chloride levels include acetazolamide, acetylsalicylic acid, ammonium chloride, androgens, bromide, cholestyramine, cyclosporine, hydrochlorothiazide, estrogens, guanethidine, lithium, methyldopa, NSAIDs, phenylbutazone, and triamterene.
- Drugs or other substances that may cause a decrease in chloride levels include aldosterone, bicarbonate, corticosteroids, corticotropin, cortisone, diuretics, ethacrynic acid, furosemide, hydroflumethiazide, laxatives (chronic misuse), mannitol, meralluride, mersalyl, methyclothiazide, metolazone, and triamterene. Many of these drugs can cause a diuretic action that inhibits the tubular reabsorption of chloride. Note: Triamterene has nephrotoxic and azotemic effects, and when organ damage has occurred, increased serum chloride levels result. Potassium chloride (found in salt substitutes) can lower blood chloride levels and raise urine chloride levels.
- Elevated triglyceride or protein levels may cause a volume-displacement error in the specimen, reflecting falsely decreased chloride values when chloride measurement methods employing predilution specimens are used (e.g., indirect ion-selective electrode, flame photometry).
- Specimens should never be collected above an intravenous (IV) line because of the potential for dilution when the specimen and the IV solution combine in the collection container, falsely decreasing the result. There is also the potential of contaminating the sample with the normal saline contained in the IV solution, falsely increasing the result.

NURSING IMPLICATIONS AND PROCEDURE

PRETEST:

- Positively identify the patient using at least two person-specific identifiers before services, treatments, or procedures are performed.
- ***Patient Teaching:*** Inform the patient this test can assist in evaluating the amount of chloride in the blood.
- Obtain a history of the patient's health concerns, symptoms, surgical procedures, and results of previously performed laboratory and diagnostic studies. Include a list of known allergens, especially allergies or sensitivities to latex.
- Obtain a list of the patient's current medications, including over-the-counter medications and dietary supplements (see Effects of Natural Products on Laboratory Values online at Davis*Plus*).
- Review the procedure with the patient. Inform the patient that specimen collection takes approximately 5 to 10 min. Address concerns about pain and explain that there may be some discomfort during the venipuncture.
- ***Sensitivity to social and cultural issues,*** as well as concern for modesty, is important in providing psychological

support before, during, and after the procedure.

- Note that there are no food, fluid, or medication restrictions unless by medical direction.

INTRATEST:

Potential Complications: N/A

- Avoid the use of equipment containing latex if the patient has a history of allergic reaction to latex.
- Specimens should not be collected during hemodialysis.
- Instruct the patient to cooperate fully and to follow directions. Direct the patient to breathe normally and to avoid unnecessary movement. Instruct the patient not to clench and unclench fist immediately before or during specimen collection.
- Observe standard precautions, and follow the general guidelines in Patient Preparation and Specimen Collection online at Davis*Plus*. Positively identify the patient, and label the appropriate specimen container with the corresponding patient demographics, initials of the person collecting the specimen, date, and time of collection. Perform a venipuncture.
- Remove the needle and apply direct pressure with dry gauze to stop bleeding. Observe/assess venipuncture site for bleeding or hematoma formation and secure gauze with adhesive bandage.
- Promptly transport the specimen to the laboratory for processing and analysis.

POST-TEST:

- Inform the patient that a report of the results will be made available to the requesting HCP, who will discuss the results with the patient.
- Observe the patient on saline IV fluid replacement therapy for signs of overhydration, especially in cases in which there is a history of heart or kidney disease. Signs of overhydration include constant, irritable cough; chest rales; dyspnea; or engorgement of neck and hand veins.
- Evaluate the patient for signs and symptoms of dehydration. Check the patient's skin turgor, mucous membrane moisture, and ability to produce tears. Dehydration is a significant and common finding in older adult and other patients in whom kidney function has deteriorated.
- Monitor daily weights as well as intake and output to determine whether fluid retention is occurring because of sodium and chloride excess. Patients at risk for or with a history of fluid imbalance are also at risk for electrolyte imbalance.
- *Nutritional Considerations:* Careful observation of the patient on IV fluid replacement therapy is important. A patient receiving a continuous 5% dextrose solution (D_5W) may not be taking in an adequate amount of chloride to meet the body's needs. The patient, if allowed, should be encouraged to drink fluids such as broths, tomato juice, or colas and to eat foods such as meats, seafood, or eggs, which contain sodium and chloride. The use of table salt may also be appropriate.
- *Nutritional Considerations:* Instruct patients with elevated chloride levels to avoid eating or drinking anything containing sodium chloride salt. The patient or caregiver should also be encouraged to read food labels to determine which products are suitable for a low-sodium diet.
- *Nutritional Considerations:* Instruct patients with low chloride levels that a decrease in iron absorption may occur as a result of less chloride available to form gastric acid, which is essential for iron absorption. In prolonged periods of chloride deficit, iron-deficiency anemia could develop.
- Reinforce information given by the patient's HCP regarding further testing, treatment, or referral to another HCP. Answer any questions or address any concerns voiced by the patient or family. Educate the patient regarding access to nutritional counseling services. Provide contact information, if desired, for the Institute of Medicine of the National

Academies (www.iom.edu) or the USDA's resource for nutrition (www.choosemyplate.gov). 🍁

- Depending on the results of this procedure, additional testing may be performed to evaluate or monitor progression of the disease process and determine the need for a change in therapy. Evaluate test results in relation to the patient's symptoms and other tests performed.

RELATED STUDIES:

- Related tests include ACTH, anion gap, blood gases, carbon dioxide, CBC hematocrit, CBC hemoglobin, osmolality, potassium, protein total and fractions, sodium, and US abdomen.
- Refer to the Cardiovascular, Endocrine, Gastrointestinal, Genitourinary, and Respiratory systems tables online at Davis*Plus* for related test by body system.

Chloride, Sweat

SYNONYM/ACRONYM: Sweat test, pilocarpine iontophoresis sweat test, sweat chloride.

COMMON USE: To assist in diagnosing cystic fibrosis (CF).

SPECIMEN: Sweat collected by pilocarpine iontophoresis.

NORMAL FINDINGS: (Method: Ion-specific electrode or titration)

	Conventional & SI Units	Interpretation
Birth–6 mo		
	0–29 mEq/L or mmol/L	Normal
	30–59 mEq/L or mmol/L	Borderline
	Greater than 60 mEq/L or mmol/L	Consistent with the diagnosis of CF
6 mo–adult		
	0–39 mEq/L or mmol/L	Normal
	40–59 mEq/L or mmol/L	Borderline
	Greater than 60 mEq/L or mmol/L	Consistent with the diagnosis of CF

DESCRIPTION: CF is a genetic disease that affects normal functioning of the exocrine glands, causing them to excrete large amounts of electrolytes. Patients with CF have sweat electrolyte levels two to five times normal. Sweat test values, with family history and signs and symptoms, are required to establish a diagnosis of CF. CF is transmitted as an autosomal recessive trait in which the offspring inherits a copy of the defective cystic fibrosis transmembrane conductance regulator (CFTR) gene from each parent. Mutations of this gene disrupt the regulation of chloride and sodium transport between cells within the lungs, pancreas, small intestine, bile ducts, and skin, and the disease is characterized by abnormal exocrine secretions. Clinical presentation may include chronic problems of the gastrointestinal and/or respiratory system. CF is more common in Caucasians. Sweat conductivity is a screening method that estimates chloride levels. Sweat conductivity values greater than or equal to 50 mmol/L should be referred for quantitative analysis of sweat chloride. Testing of stool samples for decreased trypsin activity has been used as a screen for CF in infants and children, but this is a much less reliable method than the sweat test.

Knowledge of genetics assists the nurse in identifying patients and family members who may benefit from additional education, risk assessment, and counseling. Genetics is the study and identification of genes, genetic mutations, and inheritance. For example, genetics provides some insight into the likelihood of inheriting a trait such as blue eyes or a medical condition such as CF. Every person receives a copy of the CFTR gene from each parent. If each parent provides an abnormal or mutated CFTR gene, the baby will likely develop CF. Babies who inherit a normal and abnormal copy of the CFTR gene are considered "carriers" because they provide the potential for transmitting the condition to the next generation. More than 2,000 mutations of the CFTR gene have been documented. Some conditions are the result of mutations involving a single gene, whereas other conditions may involve multiple genes and/or multiple chromosomes. Further information regarding inheritance of genes can be found in the study titled "Genetic Testing." The American College of Obstetricians and Gynecologists (ACOG) suggests that carrier screening be discussed as an option to patients (and couples) who are pregnant or are considering pregnancy. Laboratories generally offer a panel of the current and most common CF mutations recommended by ACOG and the American College of Medical Genetics. All 50 states include CF in the neonatal screening performed at birth. Genetic testing can also be reliably performed on DNA material harvested from whole blood, amniotic fluid (submitted with maternal blood sample), chorionic villus samples (submitted with maternal blood sample), or buccal swabs to screen for genetic mutations associated with CF and can assist in confirming a diagnosis of CF, but the sweat electrolyte test is still considered the gold standard diagnostic for CF. Genetic testing for confirmation by polymerase chain reaction (PCR) may be indicated when the sweat chloride test results are indeterminate and the patient demonstrates symptoms, especially in the presence of family history for CF. 🍁

The sweat test is a noninvasive study done to assist in the diagnosis of CF when considered with other test results and physical assessments. This test is usually performed on children, although adults may also be tested; it is not usually ordered on adults or infants in the first few weeks of life because results can be highly variable and should be interpreted with caution. Sweat for specimen collection is induced by a small electrical current carrying the drug pilocarpine. The test measures the concentration of chloride produced by the sweat glands of the skin. A high concentration of chloride in the specimen indicates the presence of CF. The sweat test is used less commonly to measure the concentration of sodium ions for the same purpose.

C

This procedure is contraindicated for

- Patients with skin disorders (e.g., rash, erythema, eczema).

INDICATIONS

- Assist in the diagnosis of CF.
- Screen for CF in individuals with a family history of the disease.
- Screen for suspected CF in children with recurring respiratory infections.
- Screen for suspected CF in infants with failure to thrive and infants who pass meconium late.
- Screen for suspected CF in individuals with malabsorption syndrome.

POTENTIAL MEDICAL DIAGNOSIS

Increased in:

Conditions that affect electrolyte distribution and excretion may produce false-positive sweat test results.

- Addison's disease
- Alcoholic pancreatitis ***(dysfunction of CF gene is linked to pancreatic disease susceptibility)***
- CF
- Chronic kidney disease
- Chronic pulmonary infections ***(related to undiagnosed CF)***
- Congenital adrenal hyperplasia
- Diabetes insipidus
- Familial cholestasis
- Familial hypoparathyroidism
- Fucosidosis
- Glucose-6-phosphate dehydrogenase deficiency
- Hypothyroidism
- Mucopolysaccharidosis
- Nephrogenic diabetes insipidus

Decreased in:

Conditions that affect electrolyte distribution and retention may produce false-negative sweat test results.

- Edema
- Hypoaldosteronism
- Hypoproteinemia
- Sodium depletion

CRITICAL FINDINGS:

- Greater than 60 mEq/L or mmol/L (SI greater than 60 mEq/L) is considered diagnostic of CF.

Note and immediately report to the requesting health-care provider (HCP) any critical findings and related symptoms. A listing of these findings varies among facilities. Timely notification of a critical finding for laboratory or diagnostic studies is a role expectation of the professional nurse. The notification processes vary among facilities. Upon receipt of the critical finding, the information should be read back to the caller to verify accuracy.

Consideration may be given to verification of critical findings before action is taken. Policies vary among facilities and may include requesting recollection and retesting by the laboratory.

The validity of the test result is affected tremendously by proper specimen collection and handling. Before proceeding with appropriate patient education and counseling, it is important to perform duplicate testing on patients whose results are in the diagnostic or intermediate ranges. A negative test should be repeated if test results do not support the clinical picture.

INTERFERING FACTORS

- An inadequate amount of sweat may produce inaccurate results.
- Improper cleaning of the skin or improper application of gauze pad or filter paper for collection affects test results.

- **Hot environmental temperatures may reduce the sodium chloride concentration in sweat; cool environmental temperatures may reduce the amount of sweat collected.**
- **If the specimen container that stores the gauze or filter paper is handled without gloves, the test results may show a false increase in the final weight of the collection container.**

NURSING IMPLICATIONS AND PROCEDURE

PRETEST:

- Positively identify the patient using at least two person-specific identifiers before services, treatments, or procedures are performed.
- *Patient Teaching:* Inform the patient this test can assist in diagnosing an inherited disease that affects the lungs.
- Obtain a history of the patient's health concerns (especially failure to thrive or CF in other family members), symptoms, surgical procedures, and results of previously performed laboratory and diagnostic studies. Include a list of known allergens, especially allergies or sensitivities to latex.
- Obtain a list of the patient's current medications, including over-the-counter medications and dietary supplements (see Effects of Natural Products on Laboratory Values online at Davis*Plus*).
- Review the procedure with the patient and caregiver. Encourage the caregiver to stay with and support the child during the test. The iontophoresis and specimen collection usually takes approximately 75 to 90 min. Address concerns about pain and explain that there is no pain associated with the test, but a stinging sensation may be experienced when the low electrical current is applied at the site.
- ***Sensitivity to social and cultural issues,*** as well as concern for modesty, is important in providing psychological support before, during, and after the procedure.
- Note that there are no food, fluid, or medication restrictions unless by medical direction.

INTRATEST:

Potential Complications: N/A

- Avoid the use of equipment containing latex if the patient has a history of allergic reaction to latex.
- Instruct the patient to cooperate fully and to follow directions.
- Observe standard precautions, and follow the general guidelines in Patient Preparation and Specimen Collection online at Davis*Plus*. Positively identify the patient, and label the appropriate specimen container with the corresponding patient demographics, initials of the person collecting the specimen, date, and time of collection.
- The test should not be performed if the patient is receiving oxygen by means of an open system related to the remote possibility of explosion from an electrical spark. If the patient can temporarily receive oxygen via a facemask or nasal cannula, then sweat testing can be done.
- The patient is placed in a position that will allow exposure of the site on the forearm or thigh. To ensure collection of an adequate amount of sweat in a small infant, two sites (right forearm and right thigh) can be used. The patient should be covered to prevent cool environmental temperatures from affecting sweat production. The site selected for iontophoresis should never be the chest or left side because of the risk of cardiac arrest from the electrical current.
- The site is washed with distilled water and dried. A positive electrode is attached to the site on the right forearm or right thigh and covered with a pad that is saturated with pilocarpine, a drug that stimulates sweating. A negative electrode is covered with a pad that is saturated with bicarbonate solution. Iontophoresis is achieved by supplying a low

(4 to 5 mA) electrical current via the electrode for 12 to 15 min. Battery-powered equipment is preferred over an electrical outlet to supply the current.

- The electrodes are removed, revealing a red area at the site, and the site is washed with distilled water and dried to remove any possible contaminants on the skin.
- Preweighed disks made of filter paper are placed on the site with a forceps; to prevent evaporation of sweat collected at the site, the disks are covered with paraffin or plastic and sealed at the edges. The disks are left in place for about 1 hr. Distract the child with books or games to allay fears.
- After 1 hr, the paraffin covering is removed, and disks are placed in a preweighed container with a forceps. Use gloves to handle the specimen container; do not directly handle the preweighed specimen container or filter paper. The container is sealed and sent immediately to the laboratory for weighing and analysis of chloride content. At least 100 mg of sweat is required for accurate results.
- Terminate the test if the patient complains of burning at the electrode site. Reposition the electrode before the test is resumed.
- Promptly transport the specimen to the laboratory for processing and analysis. Do not directly handle the preweighed specimen container or filter paper.

POST-TEST:

- Inform the patient that a report of the results will be made available to the requesting HCP, who will discuss the results with the patient/caregiver.
- Observe/assess the site for unusual color, sensation, or discomfort.
- Inform the patient and caregiver that redness at the site fades in 2 to 3 hr.
- Instruct the patient to resume usual diet, fluids, medications, and activity, as directed by the HCP.
- ***Nutritional Considerations:*** If appropriate, instruct the patient and caregiver that nutrition may be altered because of impaired digestive processes associated with CF. Increased viscosity of exocrine gland secretion may lead to poor absorption of digestive enzymes and fat-soluble vitamins, necessitating oral intake of digestive enzymes with each meal and calcium and vitamin (A, D, E, and K) supplementation. Malnutrition also is seen commonly in patients with chronic, severe respiratory disease for many reasons, including fatigue, lack of appetite, and gastrointestinal distress. Research has estimated that the daily caloric intake needed for children with CF between 4 and 7 yr may be 2,000 to 2,800 and for teens 3,000 to 5,000. Tube feeding may be necessary to supplement regular high-calorie meals. To prevent pulmonary infection and decrease the extent of lung tissue damage, adequate intake of vitamins A and C is also important. Excessive loss of sodium chloride through the sweat glands of a patient with CF may necessitate increased salt intake, especially in environments where increased sweating is induced. The importance of following the prescribed diet should be stressed to the patient and caregiver.
- If appropriate, instruct the patient and caregiver that ineffective airway clearance related to excessive production of mucus and decreased ciliary action may result. Chest physical therapy and the use of aerosolized antibiotics and mucus-thinning drugs are an important part of the daily treatment regimen.
- Recognize anxiety related to test results, and be supportive of impaired activity related to perceived loss of independence and fear of shortened life expectancy. Discuss the implications of abnormal test results on the patient's lifestyle. Provide teaching and information regarding the clinical implications of the test results, as appropriate. Educate the patient regarding access to counseling services. Help the patient and caregiver to cope with long-term implications. Recognize that anticipatory anxiety

and grief related to potential lifestyle changes may be expressed when someone is faced with a chronic disorder. Provide information regarding genetic counseling and possible screening of other family members if appropriate. Provide contact information, if desired, for the Cystic Fibrosis Foundation (www.cff.org) or ACOG (www.acog.org).

- Reinforce information given by the patient's HCP regarding further testing, treatment, or referral to another HCP. Explain that a positive sweat test alone is not diagnostic of CF; repetition of borderline and positive tests is generally recommended. Answer any questions or address any concerns voiced by the patient or family.
- Depending on the results of this procedure, additional testing may be performed to evaluate or monitor progression of the disease process and determine the need for a change in therapy. Evaluate test results in relation to the patient's symptoms and other tests performed.

RELATED STUDIES:

- Related tests include α_1-antitrypsin/phenotype, amylase, anion gap, biopsy chorionic villus, blood gases, fecal analysis, fecal fat, genetic testing, newborn screening, osmolality, phosphorus, potassium, and sodium.
- Refer to the Endocrine and Respiratory systems tables online at Davis*Plus* for related tests by body system.

C

Cholangiography, Percutaneous Transhepatic

SYNONYM/ACRONYM: Percutaneous cholecystogram, PTC, PTHC.

COMMON USE: To visualize and assess biliary ducts for causes of obstruction and jaundice, such as cancer or stones.

AREA OF APPLICATION: Biliary system.

DESCRIPTION: Percutaneous transhepatic cholangiography (PTC) is a test used to visualize the biliary system in order to evaluate persistent upper abdominal pain after cholecystectomy and to determine the presence and cause of obstructive jaundice. The liver is punctured with a thin needle under fluoroscopic guidance, and contrast medium is injected as the needle is slowly withdrawn. This study visualizes the biliary ducts without depending on the gallbladder's concentrating ability. The intrahepatic and extrahepatic biliary ducts, and occasionally the gallbladder, can be visualized to determine possible obstruction. In obstruction of the extrahepatic ducts, a catheter can be placed in the duct to allow external drainage of bile. Endoscopic retrograde cholangiopancreatography (ERCP) and percutaneous transhepatic cholangiography (PTC) are the only methods available to view the biliary tree in the presence of jaundice. ERCP poses less risk and is probably done more often.

This procedure is contraindicated for

- Patients who are pregnant or suspected of being pregnant, unless the potential benefits of a procedure using radiation far outweigh the risk of radiation exposure to the fetus and mother.

- Patients with conditions associated with adverse reactions to contrast medium (e.g., asthma, food allergies, or allergy to contrast medium).

Although patients are asked specifically if they have a known allergy to iodine or shellfish, it has been well established that the reaction is not to iodine, in fact an actual iodine allergy would be problematic because iodine is required for the production of thyroid hormones. In the case of shellfish the reaction is to a muscle protein called tropomyosin; in the case of iodinated contrast medium the reaction is to the noniodinated part of the contrast molecule. Patients with a known hypersensitivity to the medium may benefit from premedication with corticosteroids and diphenhydramine; the use of nonionic contrast or an alternative noncontrast imaging study, if available, may be considered for patients who have severe asthma or who have experienced moderate to severe reactions to ionic contrast medium.

- Patients with conditions associated with preexisting renal insufficiency (e.g., chronic kidney disease, single kidney transplant, nephrectomy, diabetes, multiple myeloma, treatment with aminoglycosides and NSAIDs) ***because iodinated contrast is nephrotoxic.***
- Patients who are chronically dehydrated before the test, especially older adults and patients whose health is already compromised ***because of their risk of contrast-induced acute kidney injury.***
- Patients with bleeding disorders or receiving anticoagulant therapy ***because the puncture site may not stop bleeding.***
- Patients with cholangitis; ***the injection of the contrast medium can increase biliary pressure, leading to bacteremia, septicemia, and shock.***

INDICATIONS

- Aid in the diagnosis of obstruction caused by gallstones, benign strictures, malignant tumors, congenital cysts, and anatomic variations.
- Determine the cause, extent, and location of mechanical obstruction.
- Determine the cause of upper abdominal pain after cholecystectomy.
- Distinguish between obstructive and nonobstructive jaundice.

POTENTIAL MEDICAL DIAGNOSIS

Normal findings

- Biliary ducts are normal in diameter, with no evidence of dilation, filling defects, duct narrowing, or extravasation
- Contrast medium fills the ducts and flows freely
- Gallbladder appears normal in size and shape

Abnormal findings related to

- Anatomic biliary or pancreatic duct variations
- Biliary sclerosis
- Cholangiocarcinoma
- Cirrhosis
- Common bile duct cysts
- Gallbladder carcinoma
- Gallstones
- Hepatitis
- Nonobstructive jaundice
- Pancreatitis
- Sclerosing cholangitis
- Tumors, strictures, inflammation, or gallstones of the common bile duct

CRITICAL FINDINGS: N/A

INTERFERING FACTORS

Factors that may alter the results of the study

- Gas or feces in the gastrointestinal (GI) tract resulting from inadequate

cleansing or failure to restrict food intake before the study.
- Retained barium from a previous radiological procedure.
- Metallic objects within the examination field, which may inhibit organ visualization and cause unclear images.
- Inability of the patient to cooperate or remain still during the procedure because of age, significant pain, or mental status.

Other considerations
- The procedure may be terminated if chest pain or severe cardiac dysrhythmias occur.
- Failure to follow dietary restrictions and other pretesting preparations may cause the procedure to be canceled or repeated.

NURSING IMPLICATIONS AND PROCEDURE

PRETEST:
- Positively identify the patient using at least two person-specific identifiers before services, treatments, or procedures are performed.
- ***Patient Teaching:*** Inform the patient this procedure can assist in assessing the bile ducts of the gallbladder and pancreas.
- Obtain a history of the patient's health concerns, symptoms, surgical procedures, and results of previously performed laboratory and diagnostic studies. Include a list of known allergens, especially allergies or sensitivities to latex, anesthetics, contrast medium, or sedatives.
- Ensure that this procedure is performed before an upper GI study or barium swallow.
- Record the date of the last menstrual period and determine the possibility of pregnancy in perimenopausal women.
- Obtain a list of the patient's current medications, including over-the-counter medications, dietary supplements, anticoagulants, aspirin and other salicylates (see Effects of Natural Products on Laboratory Values online at Davis*Plus*). Such products should be discontinued by medical direction for the appropriate number of days prior to a surgical procedure. Note the last time and dose of medication taken.
- If iodinated contrast medium is scheduled to be used in patients receiving metformin (Glucophage) for type 2 diabetes, the drug should be discontinued on the day of the test and continue to be withheld for 48 hr after the test. Iodinated contrast can temporarily impair kidney function, and failure to withhold metformin may indirectly result in drug-induced lactic acidosis, a dangerous and sometimes fatal adverse effect of metformin ***related to renal impairment that does not support sufficient excretion of metformin.***
- Review the procedure with the patient. Address concerns about pain and explain that there may be moments of discomfort and some pain experienced during the test. Inform the patient that the procedure is usually performed in the radiology department by a health-care provider (HCP), with support staff, and takes approximately 30 to 60 min.
- ***Sensitivity to social and cultural issues,*** as well as concern for modesty, is important in providing psychological support before, during, and after the procedure.
- Explain that an intravenous (IV) line may be inserted to allow infusion of fluids such as saline, antibiotics, anesthetics, sedatives, or emergency medications. Patients who will undergo percutaneous bile drainage may have infected bile and as such should have an antibiotic administered at least 1 hr before the procedure in order to avoid spreading the infection to other parts of the body. Explain that the contrast medium will be injected, by catheter, at a separate site from the IV line.
- Type and screen the patient's blood for possible transfusion.

- Inform the patient that a laxative and cleansing enema may be needed the day before the procedure, with cleansing enemas on the morning of the procedure depending on the institution's policy.
- Instruct the patient to remove all external metallic objects from the area to be examined.
- Instruct the patient that to reduce the risk of aspiration related to nausea and vomiting, solid food and milk or milk products are restricted for at least 6 hr, and clear liquids are restricted for at least 2 hr prior to general anesthesia, regional anesthesia, or sedation/analgesia (monitored anesthesia). The American Society of Anesthesiologists has fasting guidelines for risk levels according to patient status. More information can be located at www.asahq.org. 🍁 Patients on beta blockers before the surgical procedure should be instructed to take their medication as ordered during the perioperative period. Protocols may vary among facilities.
- Instruct the patient to fast and restrict fluids for 6 hr prior to the procedure as ordered and to avoid taking anticoagulant medication or to reduce dosage as ordered prior to the procedure. Protocols may vary among facilities.
- *Make sure a written and informed consent has been signed prior to the procedure and before administering any medications.*

INTRATEST:

Potential Complications:

PTC is an invasive procedure and has potential risks that include allergic reaction ***related to contrast reaction,*** bleeding, septicemia, bile peritonitis, and extravasation of the contrast medium.

- Observe standard precautions, and follow the general guidelines in Patient Preparation and Specimen Collection online at Davis*Plus*. Positively identify the patient.
- Ensure that the patient has complied with dietary, fluid, and medication restrictions prior to the study, as instructed.
- Ensure the patient has removed all external metallic objects from the area to be examined.
- Assess for completion of bowel preparation according to the institution's procedure.
- Administer ordered prophylactic steroids or antihistamines before the procedure. Use nonionic contrast medium for the procedure if the patient has a history of allergic reactions to any relevant substance or drug.
- Avoid the use of equipment containing latex if the patient has a history of allergic reaction to latex.
- Have emergency equipment readily available.
- Instruct the patient to void prior to the procedure and to change into the gown, robe, and foot coverings provided.
- Instruct the patient to cooperate fully and to follow directions. Instruct the patient to remain still throughout the procedure because movement produces unreliable results.
- Record baseline vital signs, and continue to monitor throughout the procedure. Protocols may vary among facilities.
- Establish an IV fluid line for the injection of saline, sedatives, or emergency medications.
- Place the patient in the supine position on an examination table.
- A kidney, ureter, and bladder (KUB) or plain film is taken to ensure that no barium or stool will obscure visualization of the biliary system.
- An area over the abdominal wall is anesthetized, and the needle is inserted and advanced under fluoroscopic guidance. Contrast medium is injected when placement is confirmed by the free flow of bile.
- A specimen of bile may be sent to the laboratory for culture and cytological analysis.
- At the end of the procedure, the contrast medium is aspirated from the biliary ducts, relieving pressure on the dilated ducts.

- If an obstruction is found during the procedure, a catheter is inserted into the bile duct to allow drainage of bile.
- Maintain pressure over the needle insertion site for several hours if bleeding is persistent.
- Observe/assess the needle site for bleeding, inflammation, or hematoma formation.
- Establish a closed and sterile drainage system if a catheter is left in place.

POST-TEST:

- Inform the patient that a report of the results will be made available to the requesting HCP, who will discuss the results with the patient.
- Instruct the patient to resume usual diet, fluids, medications, and activity, as directed by the HCP. Kidney function should be assessed before metformin is restarted.
- Monitor vital signs and neurological status every 15 min for 1 hr, then every 2 hr for 4 hr, and as ordered. Take temperature every 4 hr for 24 hr. Monitor intake and output at least every 8 hr. Compare with baseline values. Notify the HCP if temperature is elevated. Protocols may vary among facilities.
- Monitor for reaction to iodinated contrast medium, including rash, urticaria, tachycardia, hyperpnea, hypertension, palpitations, nausea, or vomiting.
- Observe/assess the puncture site for signs of bleeding, hematoma formation, ecchymosis, or leakage of bile. Notify the HCP if any of these is present.
- Advise the patient to watch for symptoms of infection, such as pain, fever, increased pulse rate, and muscle aches.
- Recognize anxiety related to test results. Discuss the implications of abnormal test results on the patient's lifestyle. Provide teaching and information regarding the clinical implications of the test results, as appropriate.
- Reinforce information given by the patient's HCP regarding further testing, treatment, or referral to another HCP. Answer any questions or address any concerns voiced by the patient or family.
- Depending on the results of this procedure, additional testing may be needed to evaluate or monitor progression of the disease process and determine the need for a change in therapy. Evaluate test results in relation to the patient's symptoms and other tests performed.

RELATED STUDIES:

- Related tests include ALT, amylase, antibodies actin and mitochondrial M2, AST, biopsy liver, cancer antigens, cholangiography postoperative, cholangiopancreatography endoscopic retrograde, CT abdomen, GGT, hepatitis antigens and antibodies (A, B, C), hepatobiliary scan, KUB studies, laparoscopy abdominal, lipase, MRI abdomen, peritoneal fluid analysis, pleural fluid analysis, and US liver and biliary tract.
- Refer to the Gastrointestinal and Hepatobiliary systems tables online at Davis*Plus* for related tests by body system.

Cholangiography, Postoperative

SYNONYM/ACRONYM: T-tube cholangiography.

COMMON USE: A postoperative evaluation to provide ongoing assessment of the effectiveness of bile duct or gall bladder surgery.

AREA OF APPLICATION: Gallbladder, bile ducts.

Access Canadian content on Fast Find: Lab and Dx at davispl.us/vanleeuwen7

C

DESCRIPTION: After cholecystectomy, a self-retaining, T-shaped tube may be inserted into the common bile duct. Postoperative (T-tube) cholangiography is a fluoroscopic and radiographic examination of the biliary tract that involves the injection of a contrast medium through the T-tube inserted during surgery. This test may be performed during surgery and again 5 to 10 days after cholecystectomy to assess the patency of the common bile duct and to detect any remaining calculi. The procedure will also help identify areas of stenosis or the presence of fistulae (as a result of the surgery). T-tube placement may also be done after a liver transplant because biliary duct obstruction or anastomotic leakage is possible. This test should be performed before any gastrointestinal (GI) studies using barium and after any studies involving the measurement of iodinated compounds.

This procedure is contraindicated for

- Patients who are pregnant or suspected of being pregnant, unless the potential benefits of a procedure using radiation far outweigh the risk of radiation exposure to the fetus and mother.
- Patients with conditions associated with adverse reactions to contrast medium (e.g., asthma, food allergies, or allergy to contrast medium).

Although patients are asked specifically if they have a known allergy to iodine or shellfish, it has been well established that the reaction is not to iodine, in fact an actual iodine allergy would be problematic because iodine is required for the production of thyroid hormones. In the case of shellfish the reaction is to a muscle protein called tropomyosin; in the case of iodinated contrast medium the reaction is to the noniodinated part of the contrast molecule. Patients with a known hypersensitivity to the medium may benefit from premedication with corticosteroids and diphenhydramine; the use of nonionic contrast or an alternative noncontrast imaging study, if available, may be considered for patients who have severe asthma or who have experienced moderate to severe reactions to ionic contrast medium.

- Patients with conditions associated with preexisting renal insufficiency (e.g., chronic kidney disease, single kidney transplant, nephrectomy, diabetes, multiple myeloma, treatment with aminoglycosides and NSAIDs) ***because iodinated contrast is nephrotoxic.***

Patients who are chronically dehydrated before the test, especially older adults and patients whose health is already compromised ***because of their risk of contrast-induced acute kidney injury.***

- Patients with bleeding disorders or receiving anticoagulant therapy ***because the puncture site may not stop bleeding.***
- Patients with cholangitis; ***the injection of the contrast medium can increase biliary pressure, leading to bacteremia, septicemia, and shock.***
- Patients with acute cholecystitis or severe liver disease; ***the procedure may worsen the condition.***

INDICATIONS

- Determine biliary duct patency before T-tube removal.
- Identify the cause, extent, and location of obstruction after surgery.

POTENTIAL MEDICAL DIAGNOSIS

Normal findings

- Biliary ducts are normal in size
- Contrast medium fills the ductal system and flows freely

Abnormal findings related to

- Appearance of channels of contrast medium outside of the biliary ducts, indicating a fistula
- Filling defects, dilation, or radiolucent shadows within the biliary ducts, indicating calculi or neoplasm

CRITICAL FINDINGS: N/A

INTERFERING FACTORS

Factors that may alter the results of the study

- Gas or feces in the GI tract resulting from inadequate cleansing or failure to restrict food intake before the study.
- Retained barium from a previous radiological procedure.
- Metallic objects within the examination field, which may inhibit organ visualization and cause unclear images.
- Inability of the patient to cooperate or remain still during the procedure because of age, significant pain, or mental status.

Other considerations

- The procedure may be terminated if chest pain or severe cardiac dysrhythmias occur.
- Air bubbles resembling calculi may be seen if there is inadvertent injection of air.
- Failure to follow dietary restrictions and other pretesting preparations may cause the procedure to be canceled or repeated.

NURSING IMPLICATIONS AND PROCEDURE

PRETEST:

- Positively identify the patient using at least two person-specific identifiers before services, treatments, or procedures are performed.
- *Patient Teaching:* Inform the patient this procedure can assist in assessing the bile ducts of the gallbladder and pancreas.
- Obtain a history of the patient's health concerns, symptoms, surgical procedures, and results of previously performed laboratory and diagnostic studies. Include a list of known allergens, especially allergies or sensitivities to latex.
- Ensure that this procedure is performed before an upper GI study or barium swallow.
- Record the date of the last menstrual period and determine the possibility of pregnancy in perimenopausal women.
- Obtain a list of the patient's current medications, including over-the-counter medications and dietary supplements (see Effects of Natural Products on Laboratory Values online at Davis*Plus*).
- If iodinated contrast medium is scheduled to be used in patients receiving metformin (Glucophage) for type 2 diabetes, the drug should be discontinued on the day of the test and continue to be withheld for 48 hr after the test. Iodinated contrast can temporarily impair kidney function, and failure to withhold metformin may indirectly result in drug-induced lactic acidosis, a dangerous and sometimes fatal adverse effect of metformin ***related to renal impairment that does not support sufficient excretion of metformin.***
- Review the procedure with the patient. Address concerns about pain and explain that there may be moments of discomfort and some pain experienced during the test. Inform the patient that the procedure is usually performed in the radiology department by a health-care provider (HCP) and takes approximately 30 to 60 min.
- *Sensitivity to social and cultural issues,* as well as concern for modesty, is important in providing psychological support before, during, and after the procedure.
- Explain that an intravenous (IV) line may be inserted to allow infusion

of fluids such as saline, anesthetics, sedatives, or emergency medications. Explain that the contrast medium will be injected through the T-tube that was left in place.
- Instruct the patient to remove jewelry and other metallic objects in the area to be examined.
- Note that there are no food or fluid restrictions for a postsurgical study but the patient should follow the standard preoperative restrictions on food and fluids for 6 hr prior to an operative cholangiogram. Protocols may vary among facilities.
- *Make sure a written and informed consent has been signed prior to the procedure and before administering any medications.*

C

INTRATEST:

Potential Complications:

Cholangiography and establishing an IV site are invasive procedures and have potential risks that include allergic reaction ***related to contrast reaction,*** bleeding, septicemia, bile peritonitis, and extravasation of the contrast medium.
- Observe standard precautions, and follow the general guidelines in Patient Preparation and Specimen Collection online at Davis*Plus*. Positively identify the patient.
- Ensure that the patient has complied with dietary, fluid, and medication restrictions prior to the operative cholangiogram study, as instructed.
- Ensure that the patient has removed all external metallic objects from the area to be examined prior to the procedure.
- Administer ordered prophylactic steroids or antihistamines before the procedure if the patient has a history of allergic reactions to any relevant substance or drug.
- Avoid the use of equipment containing latex if the patient has a history of allergic reaction to latex.
- Have emergency equipment readily available.
- Instruct the patient to void prior to the procedure and to change into the gown, robe, and foot coverings provided.
- Instruct the patient to cooperate fully and to follow directions. Instruct the patient to remain still throughout the procedure because movement produces unreliable results.
- Record baseline vital signs, and continue to monitor throughout the procedure. Protocols may vary among facilities.
- Establish an IV fluid line for the injection of saline, sedatives, or emergency medications.
- Clamp the T-tube 24 hr before and during the procedure, if ordered, to help prevent air bubbles from entering the ducts.
- An x-ray of the abdomen is obtained to determine if any residual contrast medium is present from previous studies.
- The patient is placed on an examination table in the supine position.
- The area around the T-tube is draped; the end of the T-tube is cleansed with 70% alcohol. If the T-tube site is inflamed and painful, a local anesthetic (e.g., lidocaine) may be injected around the site. A needle is inserted into the open end of the T-tube, and the clamp is removed.
- Contrast medium is injected, and fluoroscopy is performed to visualize contrast medium moving through the duct system.
- The patient may feel a bloating sensation in the upper right quadrant as the contrast medium is injected. The tube is clamped, and images are taken. A delayed image may be taken 15 min later to visualize passage of the contrast medium into the duodenum.
- For procedures done after surgery, the T-tube is removed if findings are normal; a dry, sterile dressing is applied to the site.
- If retained calculi are identified, the T-tube is left in place for 4 to 6 wk until the tract surrounding the T-tube is healed to perform a percutaneous removal.

POST-TEST:

- Inform the patient that a report of the results will be made available to the requesting HCP, who will discuss the results with the patient.
- Instruct the patient to resume usual diet, fluids, medications, and activity, as directed by the HCP. Kidney function should be assessed before metformin is resumed, if contrast was used.
- Monitor vital signs and neurological status every 15 min for 1 hr, then every 2 hr for 4 hr, and as ordered. Take temperature every 4 hr for 24 hr. Monitor intake and output at least every 8 hr. Compare with baseline values. Notify the HCP if temperature is elevated. Protocols may vary among facilities.
- Monitor T-tube site and change sterile dressing, as ordered.
- Instruct the patient on the care of the site and dressing changes.
- Monitor for reaction to iodinated contrast medium, including rash, urticaria, tachycardia, hyperpnea, hypertension, palpitations, nausea, or vomiting.
- Instruct the patient to immediately report symptoms such as fast heart rate, difficulty breathing, skin rash, itching, chest pain, persistent right shoulder pain, or abdominal pain. Immediately report symptoms to the appropriate HCP.
- Carefully monitor the patient for fatigue and fluid and electrolyte imbalance.
- Recognize anxiety related to test results. Discuss the implications of abnormal test results on the patient's lifestyle. Provide teaching and information regarding the clinical implications of the test results, as appropriate.
- Reinforce information given by the patient's HCP regarding further testing, treatment, or referral to another HCP. Answer any questions or address any concerns voiced by the patient or family.
- Depending on the results of this procedure, additional testing may be needed to evaluate or monitor progression of the disease process and determine the need for a change in therapy. Evaluate test results in relation to the patient's symptoms and other tests performed.

RELATED STUDIES:

- Related tests include CT abdomen, hepatobiliary scan, KUB, MRI abdomen, and US liver and biliary system.
- Refer to the Gastrointestinal and Hepatobiliary systems tables online at Davis*Plus* for tests by related body systems.

Cholangiopancreatography, Endoscopic Retrograde

SYNONYM/ACRONYM: ERCP.

COMMON USE: To visualize and assess the pancreas and common bile ducts for occlusion or stricture.

AREA OF APPLICATION: Gallbladder, bile ducts, pancreatic ducts.

DESCRIPTION: Endoscopic retrograde cholangiopancreatography (ERCP) allows direct visualization of the pancreatic and biliary ducts with a flexible endoscope and, after injection of contrast material, with x-rays. It allows the health-care provider (HCP) performing the

C

procedure to view the pancreatic, hepatic, and common bile ducts and the ampulla of Vater. ERCP and percutaneous transhepatic cholangiography (PTC) are the only procedures that allow direct visualization of the biliary and pancreatic ducts. ERCP is less invasive and has less morbidity than PTC. It is useful in the evaluation of patients with jaundice, because the ducts can be visualized even when the patient's bilirubin level is high. (In contrast, oral cholecystography and intravenous (IV) cholangiography cannot visualize the biliary system when the patient has high bilirubin levels.) With endoscopy, the distal end of the common bile duct can be widened, and gallstones can be removed and stents placed in narrowed bile ducts to allow bile to be drained in jaundiced patients. During the endoscopic procedure, specimens of suspicious tissue can be taken for pathological review, and manometry pressure readings can be obtained from the bile and pancreatic ducts. ERCP is used in the diagnosis and follow-up of pancreatic disease; it can also be used therapeutically to remove small lesions called choleliths, perform sphincterotomy (biliary or pancreatic repair for stenosis), perform stent placement, repair stenosis using dilation balloons, or accomplish the extraction of stones using dilation balloons.

This procedure is contraindicated for

- Patients who are pregnant or suspected of being pregnant, unless the potential benefits of a procedure using radiation far outweigh the risk of radiation exposure to the fetus and mother.

- Patients with conditions associated with adverse reactions to contrast medium (e.g., asthma, food allergies, or allergy to contrast medium).

  Although patients are asked specifically if they have a known allergy to iodine or shellfish, it has been well established that the reaction is not to iodine, in fact an actual iodine allergy would be problematic because iodine is required for the production of thyroid hormones. In the case of shellfish the reaction is to a muscle protein called tropomyosin; in the case of iodinated contrast medium the reaction is to the noniodinated part of the contrast molecule. Patients with a known hypersensitivity to the medium may benefit from premedication with corticosteroids and diphenhydramine; the use of nonionic contrast or an alternative noncontrast imaging study, if available, may be considered for patients who have severe asthma or who have experienced moderate to severe reactions to ionic contrast medium.

- Patients with conditions associated with preexisting renal insufficiency (e.g., chronic kidney disease, single kidney transplant, nephrectomy, diabetes, multiple myeloma, treatment with aminoglycosides and NSAIDs) ***because iodinated contrast is nephrotoxic.***

- Patients who are chronically dehydrated before the test, especially older adults and patients whose health is already compromised, ***because of their risk of contrast-induced acute kidney injury.***

- Patients with bleeding disorders or receiving anticoagulant therapy ***because the puncture site may not stop bleeding.***

- Patients with an acute infection of the biliary system, pharyngeal or esophageal obstruction (e.g., Zenker's diverticulum), or possible pseudocyst of the pancreas.

INDICATIONS

- Assess jaundice of unknown cause to differentiate biliary tract obstruction from liver disease.
- Collect specimens for cytology.
- Identify obstruction caused by calculi, cysts, ducts, strictures, stenosis, and anatomic abnormalities.
- Retrieve calculi from the distal common bile duct and release strictures.
- Perform therapeutic procedures, such as sphincterotomy and placement of biliary drains.

POTENTIAL MEDICAL DIAGNOSIS

Normal findings

- Normal appearance of the duodenal papilla
- Patency of the pancreatic and common bile ducts

Abnormal findings related to

- Anatomical deviations of biliary or pancreatic ducts
- Biliary cirrhosis
- Cancer of the bile ducts
- Duodenal papilla tumors
- Gallstones
- Pancreatic cancer
- Pancreatic cysts or pseudocysts
- Pancreatic fibrosis
- Pancreatitis
- Sclerosing cholangitis
- Stenosis of biliary or pancreatic ducts

CRITICAL FINDINGS: N/A

INTERFERING FACTORS

Factors that may alter the results of the study

- Gas or feces in the gastrointestinal (GI) tract resulting from inadequate cleansing or failure to restrict food intake before the study.
- Retained barium from a previous radiological procedure.
- Previous surgery involving the stomach or duodenum, which can make locating the duodenal papilla difficult.
- Incorrect positioning of the patient, which may produce poor visualization of the area to be examined.
- Inability of the patient to cooperate or remain still during the procedure because of age, significant pain, or mental status.

Other considerations

- The procedure may be terminated if chest pain or severe cardiac dysrhythmias occur.
- A patient with unstable cardiopulmonary status, blood coagulation defects, or cholangitis (test may have to be rescheduled unless the patient received antibiotic therapy before the test).
- Failure to follow dietary restrictions and other pretesting preparations may cause the procedure to be canceled or repeated.
- Blood specimens for bilirubin, amylase, or lipase, if ordered, should be collected before the procedure; results will be elevated after the procedure.
- Risks associated with radiation overexposure can result from frequent x-ray procedures. Personnel in the examination room with the patient should wear a protective lead apron, stand behind a shield, or leave the area while the examination is being done. Personnel working in the examination area should wear badges to record their level of radiation exposure.

NURSING IMPLICATIONS AND PROCEDURE

See Potential Nursing Problems on Fast Find at davispl.us/vanleeuwen7

PRETEST:

- Positively identify the patient using at least two person-specific identifiers

before services, treatments, or procedures are performed.

- ***Patient Teaching:*** Inform the patient this procedure can assist in assessing the bile ducts of the gallbladder and pancreas.
- Obtain a history of the patient's health concerns, symptoms, surgical procedures, and results of previously performed laboratory and diagnostic studies. Include a list of known allergens, especially allergies or sensitivities to latex, anesthetics, contrast medium, or sedatives.
- Ensure that this procedure is performed before an upper GI study or barium swallow.
- Record the date of the last menstrual period and determine the possibility of pregnancy in perimenopausal women.
- Obtain a list of the patient's current medications, including over-the-counter medications, dietary supplements, anticoagulants, aspirin and other salicylates (see Effects of Natural Products on Laboratory Values online at Davis*Plus*). Such products should be discontinued by medical direction for the appropriate number of days prior to a surgical procedure. Note the last time and dose of medication taken.
- If iodinated contrast medium is scheduled to be used in patients receiving metformin (Glucophage) for type 2 diabetes, the drug should be discontinued on the day of the test and continue to be withheld for 48 hr after the test. Iodinated contrast can temporarily impair kidney function, and failure to withhold metformin may indirectly result in drug-induced lactic acidosis, a dangerous and sometimes fatal adverse effect of metformin ***related to renal impairment that does not support sufficient excretion of metformin.***
- Review the procedure with the patient. Address concerns about pain and explain that some pain may be experienced during the test, and there may be moments of discomfort. Inform the patient that the procedure is performed in a GI lab or radiology department, usually by an HCP, with support staff, and takes approximately 30 to 60 min.
- ***Sensitivity to social and cultural issues,*** as well as concern for modesty, is important in providing psychological support before, during, and after the procedure.
- Explain that an IV line may be inserted to allow infusion of fluids such as saline, anesthetics, sedatives, or emergency medications. Explain that the contrast medium will be injected at a separate site from the IV line.
- Instruct the patient to remove jewelry and other metallic objects from the area to be examined.
- Instruct the patient that to reduce the risk of aspiration related to nausea and vomiting, solid food and milk or milk products are restricted for at least 6 hr, and clear liquids are restricted for at least 2 hr prior to general anesthesia, regional anesthesia, or sedation/analgesia (monitored anesthesia). The American Society of Anesthesiologists has fasting guidelines for risk levels according to patient status. More information can be located at www.asahq.org. 🍁 Patients on beta blockers before the surgical procedure should be instructed to take their medication as ordered during the perioperative period. Protocols may vary among facilities.
- Instruct the patient to fast and restrict fluids for 6 hr prior to the procedure as ordered and to avoid taking anticoagulant medication or to reduce dosage as ordered prior to the procedure. Protocols may vary among facilities.
- *Make sure a written and informed consent has been signed prior to the procedure and before administering any medications.*

INTRATEST:

Potential Complications:

Cholangiography is an invasive procedure and has potential risks that include allergic reaction ***related to contrast reaction,*** aspiration, bleeding, pancreatitis, perforation, respiratory depression, and septicemia.

- Observe standard precautions, and follow the general guidelines in Patient Preparation and Specimen Collection online at Davis*Plus*. Positively identify the patient, and label the appropriate specimen container with the corresponding patient demographics, initials of the person collecting the specimen, date, and time of collection.
- Ensure the patient has complied with dietary, fluid, and medication restrictions prior to the study, as instructed.
- Ensure the patient has removed all external metallic objects from the area to be examined.
- Assess for completion of bowel preparation according to the institution's procedure.
- Administer ordered prophylactic steroids or antihistamines before the procedure if the patient has a history of allergic reactions to any relevant substance or drug.
- Avoid the use of equipment containing latex if the patient has a history of allergic reaction to latex.
- Have emergency equipment readily available.
- Instruct the patient to void prior to the procedure and to change into the gown, robe, and foot coverings provided.
- Instruct the patient to cooperate fully and to follow directions. Instruct the patient to remain still throughout the procedure because movement produces unreliable results.
- Record baseline vital signs, and continue to monitor throughout the procedure. Protocols may vary among facilities.
- Establish an IV fluid line for the injection of saline, sedatives, or emergency medications.
- Administer ordered sedation.
- An x-ray of the abdomen is obtained to determine if any residual contrast medium is present from previous studies.
- The oropharynx is sprayed or swabbed with a topical local anesthetic.
- The patient is placed on an examination table in the left lateral position with the left arm behind the back and right hand at the side with the neck slightly flexed. A protective guard is inserted into the mouth to cover the teeth. A bite block can also be inserted to maintain adequate opening of the mouth.
- The endoscope is passed through the mouth with a dental suction device in place to drain secretions. A side-viewing flexible fiberoptic endoscope is passed into the duodenum, and a small cannula is inserted into the duodenal papilla (ampulla of Vater).
- The patient is placed in the prone position. The duodenal papilla is visualized and cannulated with a catheter. Occasionally the patient can be turned slightly to the right side to aid in visualization of the papilla.
- IV glucagon or anticholinergics can be administered to minimize duodenal spasm and to facilitate visualization of the ampulla of Vater.
- ERCP manometry can be done at this time to measure the pressure in the bile duct, pancreatic duct, and sphincter of Oddi at the papilla area via the catheter as it is placed in the area before the contrast medium is injected.
- When the catheter is in place, contrast medium is injected into the pancreatic and biliary ducts via the catheter, and fluoroscopic images are taken. Biopsy specimens for cytological analysis may be obtained.
- Place specimens in appropriate containers, label them properly, and promptly transport them to the laboratory.

POST-TEST:

- Inform the patient that a report of the results will be made available to the requesting HCP, who will discuss the results with the patient.

- Do not allow the patient to eat or drink until the gag reflex returns, after which the patient is permitted to eat lightly for 12 to 24 hr.
- Instruct the patient to resume usual diet, fluids, medications, and activity after 24 hr, or as directed by the HCP. Renal function should be assessed before metformin is resumed, if contrast was used.
- Monitor vital signs and neurological status every 15 min for 1 hr, then every 2 hr for 4 hr, and as ordered. Take temperature every 4 hr for 24 hr. Monitor intake and output at least every 8 hr. Compare with baseline values. Notify the HCP if temperature is elevated. Protocols may vary among facilities.
- Monitor for reaction to iodinated contrast medium, including rash, urticaria, tachycardia, hyperpnea, hypertension, palpitations, nausea, or vomiting.
- Tell the patient to expect some throat soreness and possible hoarseness. Advise the patient to use warm gargles, lozenges, ice packs to the neck, or cool fluids to alleviate throat discomfort.
- Inform the patient that any belching, bloating, or flatulence is the result of air insufflation.
- Instruct the patient to immediately report symptoms such as fast heart rate, difficulty breathing, skin rash, itching, chest pain, persistent right shoulder pain, or abdominal pain. Immediately report symptoms to the appropriate HCP.
- Recognize anxiety related to test results. Discuss the implications of abnormal test results on the patient's lifestyle. Provide teaching and information regarding the clinical implications of the test results, as appropriate.
- Reinforce information given by the patient's HCP regarding further testing, treatment, or referral to another HCP. Answer any questions or address any concerns voiced by the patient or family.
- Depending on the results of this procedure, additional testing may be needed to evaluate or monitor progression of the disease process and determine the need for a change in therapy. Evaluate test results in relation to the patient's symptoms and other tests performed.

Patient Education:

- Teach the patient that a combination of pharmacological and nonpharmacological treatment choices can provide better overall pain relief.
- Teach the patient which foods to avoid to prevent nausea.

Expected Patient Outcomes:

Understanding

- The patient states the importance of accurately communicating the effectiveness of pain relief measures to better adjust therapeutic interventions to individualized needs.
- The patient states that antiemetics can assist to relieve nausea and improve oral intake.

Ability

- The patient identifies pain management strategies that provide the best relief and communicates that to the HCP.
- The patient identifies odors that precipitate nausea and adjusts environment to avoid exposure.

Response

- The patient agrees to collaborate with the HCP to design a pain management plan.
- The patient agrees to discuss fears related to diagnosis to decrease anxiety and better communicate needs to the HCP.

RELATED STUDIES:

- Related tests include amylase, CT abdomen, hepatobiliary scan, KUB studies, lipase, MRI abdomen, peritoneal fluid analysis, pleural fluid analysis, and US liver and biliary system.
- Refer to the Gastrointestinal and Hepatobiliary systems tables online at Davis*Plus* for related tests by body system.

Cholesterol, HDL and LDL

SYNONYM/ACRONYM: α_1-Lipoprotein cholesterol, high-density cholesterol, HDLC, and β-lipoprotein cholesterol, low-density cholesterol, LDLC.

COMMON USE: To assess risk and monitor for coronary artery disease.

SPECIMEN: Serum collected in a gold-, red-, or red/gray-top tube.

NORMAL FINDINGS: (Method: Spectrophotometry)

HDLC	Conventional Units	SI Units (Conventional Units × 0.0259)
Birth	6–56 mg/dL	0.16–1.45 mmol/L
Children, adults, and older adults		
Desirable	Greater than 60 mg/dL	Greater than 1.55 mmol/L
Acceptable	40–60 mg/dL	1–1.55 mmol/L
Low	Less than 40 mg/dL	Less than 1 mmol/L

LDLC	Conventional Units	SI Units (Conventional Units × 0.0259)
Optimal	Less than 100 mg/dL	Less than 2.59 mmol/L
Near optimal	100–129 mg/dL	2.59–3.34 mmol/L
Borderline high	130–159 mg/dL	3.37–4.11 mmol/L
High	160–189 mg/dL	4.14–4.9 mmol/L
Very high	Greater than 190 mg/dL	Greater than 4.92 mmol/L

	NMR LDLC Particle Number	NMR LDLC Small Particle Size
High-risk CAD	Less than 1,000 nmol/L	Less than 528 nmol/L
Moderately high-risk CAD	Less than 1,300 nmol/L	Less than 528 nmol/L

CAD, coronary artery disease; NMR, nuclear magnetic resonance.

DESCRIPTION: High-density lipoprotein cholesterol (HDLC) and low-density lipoprotein cholesterol (LDLC) are the major transport proteins for cholesterol in the body. It is believed that HDLC may have protective properties in that its role includes transporting cholesterol from the arteries to the liver. LDLC is the major transport protein for cholesterol to the arteries from the liver. LDLC can be calculated using total cholesterol, total triglycerides, and HDLC levels. Beyond the total cholesterol, HDL and LDL cholesterol

C

values, other important risk factors must be considered. Guidelines for the prevention of cardiovascular disease (CVD) have been developed by the American College of Cardiology (ACC) and the American Heart Association (AHA) in conjunction with members of the National Heart, Lung, and Blood Institute's (NHLBI) ATP intravenous Expert Panel. The updated, evidence-based guidelines redefine the condition of concern as *atherosclerotic cardiovascular disease (ASCVD)* and expand ASCVD to include CVD, stroke, and peripheral arterial disease. Some of the important highlights include the following:

- Movement away from the use of LDL cholesterol targets in determining treatment with statins. Recommendations that focus on selecting (a) the patients who fall into four groups most likely to benefit from statin therapy and (b) the level of statin intensity most likely to affect or reduce development of ASCVD.
- Development of a new 10-yr risk assessment tool based on findings from a large, diverse population. Evidence-based risk factors include age, sex, ethnicity, total cholesterol, HDLC, blood pressure, blood-pressure treatment status, diabetes, and current use of tobacco products.
- Recommendations for aspects of lifestyle that would encourage prevention of ASCVD to include adherence to a Mediterranean-style or DASH (Dietary Approaches to Stop Hypertension)-style diet; dietary restriction of saturated fats, trans fats, sugar, and sodium; and regular participation in aerobic exercise. The guidelines contain reductions in body mass index (BMI) cutoffs for men and women designed to promote discussions between health-care providers (HCPs) and their patients regarding the benefits of maintaining a healthy weight.
- Recognition that additional biological markers, such as family history, high-sensitivity C-reactive protein, ankle-brachial index (ABI), and coronary artery calcium score, may be selectively used with the assessment tool to assist in predicting and evaluating risk.
- Recognition that other biomarkers such as apolipoprotein B, estimated glomerular filtration rate (eGFR); creatinine; lipoprotein (a), or Lp(a); and microalbumin warrant further study and may be considered for inclusion in future guidelines. 🍁

Studies have shown that coronary artery disease (CAD) is inversely related to LDLC particle number and size. The nuclear magnetic resonance (NMR) lipid profile uses NMR imaging spectroscopy to determine LDLC particle number and size in addition to measurement of the traditional lipid markers.

HDLC levels less than 40 mg/dL in men and women represent a coronary risk factor. There is an inverse relationship between HDLC and risk of CAD (i.e., lower HDLC levels represent a higher risk of CAD). Levels of LDLC in terms of risk for CAD are directly proportional to risk and vary by age group. The LDLC can be estimated using the Friedewald formula:

$$LDLC = (\text{Total Cholesterol}) - (HDLC) - (VLDLC)$$

Very-low-density lipoprotein cholesterol (VLDLC) is estimated by dividing the triglycerides (conventional units) by 5. Triglycerides in SI units would be divided by 2.18 to estimate VLDLC. It is important to note that the formula is valid only if the triglycerides are less than 400 mg/dL or 4.52 mmol/L.

This procedure is contraindicated for: N/A

INDICATIONS

- Determine the risk of CVD.
- Evaluate the response to dietary and drug therapy for hypercholesterolemia.
- Investigate hypercholesterolemia in light of family history of CVD.

POTENTIAL MEDICAL DIAGNOSIS

Although the exact pathophysiology is unknown, cholesterol is required for many functions at the cellular and organ levels. Elevations of cholesterol are associated with conditions caused by an inherited defect in lipoprotein metabolism, liver disease, kidney disease, or a disorder of the endocrine system. Decreases in cholesterol levels are associated with conditions caused by enzyme deficiencies, malnutrition, malabsorption, liver disease, and sudden increased utilization.

HDLC increased in

- Alcoholism
- Biliary cirrhosis
- Chronic hepatitis
- Exercise
- Familial hyper-α-lipoproteinemia

HDLC decreased in

- Abetalipoproteinemia
- Cholestasis
- Chronic kidney disease
- Fish-eye disease
- Genetic predisposition or enzyme/cofactor deficiency
- Hepatocellular disorders
- Hypertriglyceridemia
- Metabolic syndrome
- Nephrotic syndrome
- Obesity
- Premature CAD
- Sedentary lifestyle
- Smoking
- Tangier's disease
- Uncontrolled diabetes

LDLC increased in

- Anorexia nervosa
- Chronic kidney disease
- Corneal arcus
- Cushing's syndrome
- Diabetes
- Diet high in cholesterol and saturated fat
- Dysglobulinemias
- Hepatic disease
- Hepatic obstruction
- Hyperlipoproteinemia types IIA and IIB
- Hypothyroidism
- Metabolic syndrome
- Nephrotic syndrome
- Porphyria
- Pregnancy
- Premature CAD
- Tendon and tuberous xanthomas

LDLC decreased in

- Acute stress (severe burns, illness)
- Chronic anemias
- Chronic pulmonary disease
- Genetic predisposition or enzyme/cofactor deficiency
- Hyperthyroidism
- Hypolipoproteinemia and abetalipoproteinemia
- Inflammatory joint disease
- Myeloma
- Reye's syndrome
- Severe hepatocellular destruction or disease
- Tangier disease

CRITICAL FINDINGS: N/A

INTERFERING FACTORS

- Drugs and other substances that may increase HDLC levels include albuterol, anticonvulsants, cholestyramine, cimetidine, clofibrate and other fibric acid derivatives, estrogens, ethanol (moderate use), lovastatin, niacin, oral contraceptives, pindolol, pravastatin, prazosin hydrochloride, and simvastatin.
- Drugs and other substances that may decrease HDLC levels include acebutolol, atenolol, danazol, diuretics, etretinate, interferon, isotretinoin, linseed oil, metoprolol, neomycin, nonselective β-adrenergic blocking drugs, probucol, progesterone, steroids, and thiazides.
- Drugs and other substances that may increase LDLC levels include androgens, catecholamines, chenodiol, cyclosporine, danazol, diuretics, etretinate, glucogenic corticosteroids, and progestins.
- Drugs and other substances that may decrease LDLC levels include aminosalicylic acid, cholestyramine, colestipol estrogens, fibric acid derivatives, interferon, lovastatin, neomycin, niacin, pravastatin, prazosin, probucol, simvastatin, terazosin, and thyroxine.
- Some of the drugs used to lower total cholesterol and LDLC or increase HDLC may cause liver damage.
- Grossly elevated triglyceride levels invalidate the Friedewald formula for mathematical estimation of LDLC; if the triglyceride level is greater than 400 mg/dL (SI: 4.52 mmol/L), the formula should not be used.
- Fasting before specimen collection is highly recommended. Ideally, the patient should be on a stable diet for 3 wk and fast for 12 hr before specimen collection.
- Failure to follow dietary restrictions before the procedure may cause the procedure to be canceled or repeated.

NURSING IMPLICATIONS AND PROCEDURE

PRETEST:

- Positively identify the patient using at least two person-specific identifiers before services, treatments, or procedures are performed.
- ***Patient Teaching:*** Inform the patient this test can assist with evaluation of cholesterol level.
- Obtain a history of the patient's health concerns, symptoms, surgical procedures, and results of previously performed laboratory and diagnostic studies. Include a list of known allergens, especially allergies or sensitivities to latex. The presence of other risk factors, such as family history of heart disease, smoking, obesity, diet, lack of physical activity, hypertension, diabetes, previous myocardial infarction (MI), and previous vascular disease, should be investigated. Knowledge of genetics assists the nurse in identifying patients and family members who may benefit from additional education, risk assessment, and counseling. Genetics is the study and identification of genes, genetic mutations, and inheritance. For example, genetics provides some insight into the likelihood of inheriting a trait such as blue eyes or a medical condition such as CAD. Genomic studies evaluate the interaction of groups of genes. The combined activity or combined expression of groups of genes allows assumptions or predictions to be made. As an example, genomic studies measure the levels of activity in multiple genes to predict how they, along with environmental and lifestyle decisions, influence the development of type 2 diabetes, CAD, MI, or ischemic stroke.
- Obtain a list of the patient's current medications, including over-the-counter medications and dietary

supplements (see Effects of Natural Products on Laboratory Values online at Davis*Plus*).

- Review the procedure with the patient. Inform the patient that specimen collection takes approximately 5 to 10 min. Address concerns about pain and explain that there may be some discomfort during the venipuncture.
- ***Sensitivity to social and cultural issues,*** as well as concern for modesty, is important in providing psychological support before, during, and after the procedure.
- Instruct the patient to fast for 12 hr before specimen collection. Protocols may vary among facilities.
- Confirm with the requesting HCP that the patient should withhold medications known to influence test results, and instruct the patient accordingly.
- Note that there are no fluid restrictions unless by medical direction.

INTRATEST:

- Ensure that the patient has complied with dietary and medication restrictions as well as other pretesting preparations prior to the study, as instructed.
- Avoid the use of equipment containing latex if the patient has a history of allergic reaction to latex.
- Instruct the patient to cooperate fully and to follow directions. Direct the patient to breathe normally and to avoid unnecessary movement.
- Observe standard precautions, and follow the general guidelines in Patient Preparation and Specimen Collection online at Davis*Plus*. Positively identify the patient, and label the appropriate specimen container with the corresponding patient demographics, initials of the person collecting the specimen, date, and time of collection. Perform a venipuncture.
- Remove the needle and apply direct pressure with dry gauze to stop bleeding. Observe/assess venipuncture site for bleeding or hematoma formation and secure gauze with adhesive bandage.
- Promptly transport the specimen to the laboratory for processing and analysis.

POST-TEST:

- Inform the patient that a report of the results will be made available to the requesting HCP, who will discuss the results with the patient.
- Instruct the patient to resume usual diet, fluids, and medications, as directed by the HCP.
- ***Nutritional Considerations:*** Decreased HDLC level and increased LDLC level may be associated with CAD. Nutritional therapy is recommended for the patient identified to be at risk for developing CAD or for individuals who have specific risk factors and/or existing medical conditions (e.g., elevated LDL cholesterol levels, other lipid disorders, type 1 diabetes, type 2 diabetes, insulin resistance, or metabolic syndrome). Other changeable risk factors warranting patient education include strategies to encourage patients, especially those who are overweight and with high blood pressure, to safely decrease sodium intake, achieve a normal weight, ensure regular participation in moderate aerobic physical activity three to four times per week, eliminate tobacco use, and adhere to a heart-healthy diet. If triglycerides also are elevated, the patient should be advised to eliminate or reduce alcohol. A variety of dietary patterns are beneficial for people with CAD, and there are many meal-planning approaches with nutritional goals endorsed by the American Diabetes Association (ADA). The Guideline on Lifestyle Management to Reduce Cardiovascular Risk published by the ACC and AHA in conjunction with the NHLBI recommends a Mediterranean-style diet rather than a low-fat diet. The guideline emphasizes inclusion of vegetables, whole grains, fruits, low-fat dairy, nuts, legumes, and nontropical vegetable oils (e.g., olive, canola, peanut, sunflower, flaxseed) along with fish and lean poultry. 🍁 The DASH diet makes additional recommendations for the reduction of dietary sodium. Both dietary styles emphasize a reduction in consumption of red meats,

which are high in saturated fats and cholesterol, and other foods containing sugar, saturated fats, trans fats, and sodium. The ADA also includes a vegetarian diet as well as other potential weight loss diets such as Weight Watchers. 🍁 The nutritional needs of each patient need to be determined individually (especially during pregnancy) with the appropriate HCPs, particularly professionals educated in nutrition.

- ***Sensitivity to social and cultural issues:*** Numerous studies point to the prevalence of excess body weight in American children and adolescents. Experts estimate that obesity is present in 25% of the population ages 6 to 11 yr. The medical, social, and emotional consequences of excess body weight are significant. Special attention should be given to instructing the pediatric patient and caregiver regarding health risks and weight control education. 🍁
- Recognize anxiety related to test results, and be supportive of fear of shortened life expectancy. Discuss the implications of abnormal test results on the patient's lifestyle. Provide teaching and information regarding the clinical implications of the test results, as appropriate. Educate the patient regarding access to counseling services. Provide contact information, if desired, for the AHA (www.americanheart.org), NHLBI (www.nhlbi.nih.gov), Institute of Medicine of the National Academies (www.iom.edu), and the USDA's resource for nutrition (www.choosemyplate.gov). 🍁
- Reinforce information given by the patient's HCP regarding further testing, treatment, or referral to another HCP. Answer any questions or address any concerns voiced by the patient or family.
- Depending on the results of this procedure, additional testing may be performed to evaluate or monitor progression of the disease process and determine the need for a change in therapy. Evaluate test results in relation to the patient's symptoms and other tests performed.

RELATED STUDIES:

- Related tests include antidysrhythmic drugs, apolipoprotein A and B, ANP, blood gases, BNP, calcium, cholesterol total, CT cardiac scoring, CRP, CK and isoenzymes, echocardiography, genetic testing, glucose, glycated hemoglobin, Holter monitor, homocysteine, ketones, LDH and isoenzymes, lipoprotein electrophoresis, magnesium, MRI chest, MI scan, myocardial perfusion heart scan, myoglobin, PET heart, potassium, triglycerides, and troponin.
- Refer to the Cardiovascular System table online at Davis*Plus* for related tests by body system.

Cholesterol, Total

SYNONYM/ACRONYM: N/A

COMMON USE: To assess and monitor risk for coronary artery disease.

SPECIMEN: Serum collected in a gold-, red-, or red/gray-top tube. Plasma collected in a green-top (heparin) tube is also acceptable. It is important to use the same tube type when serial specimen collections are anticipated for consistency in testing.

NORMAL FINDINGS: (Method: Spectrophotometry)

Risk	Conventional Units	SI Units (Conventional Units × 0.0259)
Children and adolescents (less than 20 yr)		
Desirable	Less than 170 mg/dL	Less than 4.4 mmol/L
Borderline	170–199 mg/dL	4.4–5.2 mmol/L
High	Greater than 200 mg/dL	Greater than 5.2 mmol/L
Adults and older adults		
Desirable	Less than 200 mg/dL	Less than 5.2 mmol/L
Borderline	200–239 mg/dL	5.2–6.2 mmol/L
High	Greater than 240 mg/dL	Greater than 6.2 mmol/L

Plasma values may be 10% lower than serum values.

DESCRIPTION: Cholesterol is a lipid needed to form cell membranes, bile salts, adrenal corticosteroid hormones, and other hormones such as estrogen and the androgens. Cholesterol is obtained from the diet and also synthesized in the body, mainly by the liver and intestinal mucosa. Very low cholesterol values, as are sometimes seen in critically ill patients, can be as life-threatening as very high levels. Maintaining cholesterol levels less than 200 mg/dL (SI: Less than 5.2 mmol/L) significantly reduces the risk of coronary heart disease. Beyond the total cholesterol and high-density lipoprotein cholesterol (HDLC) values, other important risk factors must be considered. Many myocardial infarctions occur even in patients whose cholesterol levels are considered to be within acceptable limits or who are in a moderate-risk category. The combination of risk factors and lipid values helps identify individuals at risk so that appropriate interventions can be taken. If the cholesterol level is greater than 200 mg/dL (SI: Less than 5.2 mmol/L), repeat testing after a 12- to 24-hr fast is recommended.

Guidelines for the prevention of cardiovascular disease (CVD) have been developed by the American College of Cardiology (ACC) and the American Heart Association (AHA) in conjunction with members of the National Heart, Lung, and Blood Institute's (NHLBI) ATP intravenous Expert Panel. The updated, evidence-based guidelines redefine the condition of concern as *atherosclerotic cardiovascular disease (ASCVD)* and expand ASCVD to include CVD, stroke, and peripheral arterial disease. Some of the important highlights include the following:

- Movement away from the use of LDL cholesterol targets in determining treatment with statins. Recommendations that focus on selecting (a) the patients who fall into four groups most likely to benefit from statin therapy and (b) the level of statin intensity most likely to affect or reduce development of ASCVD.
- Development of a new 10-yr risk assessment tool based on findings from a large, diverse population. Evidence-based risk factors include age, sex, ethnicity, total cholesterol, HDLC, blood pressure,

blood-pressure treatment status, diabetes, and current use of tobacco products.
- Recommendations for aspects of lifestyle that would encourage prevention of ASCVD to include adherence to a Mediterranean-style or DASH (Dietary Approaches to Stop Hypertension)-style diet; dietary restriction of saturated fats, trans fats, sugar, and sodium; and regular participation in aerobic exercise. The guidelines contain reductions in body mass index (BMI) cutoffs for men and women designed to promote discussions between health-care providers (HCPs) and their patients regarding the benefits of maintaining a healthy weight.
- Recognition that additional biological markers, such as family history, high-sensitivity C-reactive protein, ankle-brachial index (ABI), and coronary artery calcium score, may be selectively used with the assessment tool to assist in predicting and evaluating risk.
- Recognition that other biomarkers such as apolipoprotein B, estimated glomerular filtration rate (eGFR), creatinine, lipoprotein (a) or Lp(a), and microalbumin warrant further study and may be considered for inclusion in future guidelines. 🍁

This procedure is contraindicated for: N/A

INDICATIONS

- Assist in determining risk of CVD.
- Assist in the diagnosis of nephrotic syndrome, hepatic disease, pancreatitis, and thyroid disorders.
- Evaluate the response to dietary and drug therapy for hypercholesterolemia.
- Investigate hypercholesterolemia in light of family history of CVD.

POTENTIAL MEDICAL DIAGNOSIS

Increased in:

Although the exact pathophysiology is unknown, cholesterol is required for many functions at the cellular and organ level. Elevations of cholesterol are associated with conditions caused by an inherited defect in lipoprotein metabolism, liver disease, kidney disease, or a disorder of the endocrine system.

- Acute intermittent porphyria
- Alcoholism
- Anorexia nervosa
- Cholestasis
- Chronic kidney disease
- Diabetes (with poor control)
- Diets high in cholesterol and fats
- Familial hyperlipoproteinemia
- Glomerulonephritis
- Glycogen storage disease (von Gierke's disease)
- Gout
- Hypothyroidism (primary)
- Ischemic heart disease
- Metabolic syndrome
- Nephrotic syndrome
- Obesity
- Pancreatic and prostatic malignancy
- Pregnancy
- Werner's syndrome

Decreased in:

Although the exact pathophysiology is unknown, cholesterol is required for many functions at the cellular and organ level. Decreases in cholesterol levels are associated with conditions caused by malnutrition, malabsorption, liver disease, and sudden increased utilization.

- Burns
- Chronic myelocytic leukemia
- Chronic obstructive pulmonary disease
- Hyperthyroidism

- Liver disease (severe)
- Malabsorption and malnutrition syndromes
- Myeloma
- Pernicious anemia
- Polycythemia vera
- Severe illness
- Sideroblastic anemias
- Tangier disease
- Thalassemia
- Waldenström's macroglobulinemia

CRITICAL FINDINGS: N/A

INTERFERING FACTORS

- Drugs and other substances that may increase cholesterol levels include amiodarone, androgens, β-blockers, calcitriol, cortisone, cyclosporine, danazol, diclofenac, disulfiram, glucogenic corticosteroids, ibuprofen, isotretinoin, levodopa, methyclothiazide, miconazole (owing to castor oil vehicle, not the drug), nafarelin, some oral contraceptives, phenobarbital, phenothiazines, prochlorperazine, sotalol, thiabendazole, thiouracil, tretinoin, and trifluoperazine.
- Drugs and other substances that may decrease cholesterol levels include acebutolol, amiloride, aminosalicylic acid, androsterone, ascorbic acid, asparaginase, atenolol, atorvastatin, beclobrate, bezafibrate, cerivastatin, cholestyramine, ciprofibrate, clofibrate, colestipol, doxazosin, enalapril, estrogens, fenofibrate, fluvastatin, gemfibrozil, haloperidol, hormone replacement therapy, hydralazine, hydrochlorothiazide, interferon, isoniazid, kanamycin, ketoconazole, lincomycin, lisinopril, lovastatin, metformin, neomycin, niacin, nicotinic acid, nifedipine, paromomycin, pravastatin, probucol, simvastatin, tamoxifen, terazosin, thyroxine, trazodone, triiodothyronine, ursodiol, valproic acid, and verapamil.
- Ingestion of alcohol 12 to 24 hr before the test can falsely elevate results.
- Ingestion of drugs that alter cholesterol levels within 12 hr of the test may give a false impression of cholesterol levels, unless the test is done to evaluate such effects.
- Positioning can affect results; lower levels are obtained if the specimen is from a patient who has been supine for 20 min.
- Failure to follow dietary restrictions before the procedure may cause the procedure to be canceled or repeated.

NURSING IMPLICATIONS AND PROCEDURE

POTENTIAL NURSING PROBLEMS:

Problem	Signs & Symptoms	Interventions
Pain ***(related to myocardial ischemia; myocardial infarction; pericarditis; coronary vasospasm;***	Reports of chest pain, new onset of angina, shortness of breath, pallor, weakness, diaphoresis, palpitations, nausea, vomiting,	Assess pain characteristics, squeezing pressure, location in substernal back, neck, or jaw; assess pain duration and onset (minimal exertion, sleep, or rest); identify pain modalities that have relieved pain in the past; monitor

(table continues on page 428)

C

Problem	Signs & Symptoms	Interventions
ventricular hypertrophy; embolism; epicardial artery inflammation)	epigastric pain or discomfort, increased blood pressure, increased heart rate	cardiac biomarkers (CK-MB, troponin, myoglobin); collaborate with ancillary departments to complete ordered echocardiography, exercise stress testing, pharmacological stress testing; administer prescribed pain medication; monitor and trend vital signs; administer prescribed oxygen; administer prescribed anticoagulants, antiplatelets, beta blockers, calcium channel blockers, angiotensin-converting enzyme (ACE) inhibitors, angiotensin II receptor blockers (ARBs), thrombolytic drugs
Cardiac output ***(related to increased preload; increased afterload; impaired cardiac contractility; cardiac muscle disease; altered cardiac conduction)***	Decreased peripheral pulses; decreased urinary output; cool, clammy skin; tachypnea; dyspnea; edema; altered level of consciousness; abnormal heart sounds; crackles in lungs; decreased activity tolerance; weight gain; fatigue; hypoxia	Assess peripheral pulses and capillary refill; monitor blood pressure and check for orthostatic changes; assess respiratory rate, breath sounds, and orthopnea; assess skin color and temperature; assess level of consciousness; monitor urinary output; use pulse oximetry to monitor oxygenation; monitor sodium and potassium levels; monitor B-type natriuretic peptide (BNP) levels; administer ordered ACE inhibitors, beta blockers, diuretics, aldosterone antagonists, and vasodilators; provide oxygen administration
Health management ***(related to failure to regulate diet; lack of exercise; alcohol use; smoking)***	Inability or failure to recognize or process information toward improving health and preventing illness with associated mental and physical effects	Encourage regular participation in weight-bearing exercise; assess diet, smoking, and alcohol use; teach the importance of adequate calcium intake with diet and supplements; refer to smoking cessation and alcohol treatment programs; collaborate with HCP for bone density evaluation

Problem	Signs & Symptoms	Interventions
Nutrition ***(related to excess caloric intake with large amounts of dietary sodium and fat; cultural lifestyle; overeating associated with anxiety, depression, compulsive disorder; genetics; inadequate or unhealthy food resources)***	Observable obesity; high-fat or sodium food selections; high BMI; high consumption of ethnic foods; sedentary lifestyle; dietary religious beliefs and food selections; binge eating; diet high in refined sugar; repetitive dieting and failure	Discuss ideal body weight and the purpose and relationship between ideal weight and caloric intake to support cardiac health; review ways to decrease intake of saturated fats and increase intake of polyunsaturated fats; discuss limiting cholesterol intake to less than 300 mg per day; discuss limiting the intake of refined processed sugar; teach limiting sodium intake to the HCP's recommended restriction; encourage intake of fresh fruits and vegetables, unprocessed carbohydrates, poultry, and grains

PRETEST:

- Positively identify the patient using at least two person-specific identifiers before services, treatments, or procedures are performed.
- *Patient Teaching:* Inform the patient this test can assist with evaluation of cholesterol level.
- Obtain a history of the patient's health concerns, symptoms, surgical procedures, and results of previously performed laboratory and diagnostic studies. Include a list of known allergens, especially allergies or sensitivities to latex. The presence of other risk factors, such as family history of heart disease, smoking, obesity, diet, lack of physical activity, hypertension, diabetes, previous myocardial infarction (MI), and previous vascular disease, should be investigated. Knowledge of genetics assists the nurse in identifying patients and family members who may benefit from additional education, risk assessment, and counseling. Genetics is the study and identification of genes, genetic mutations, and inheritance. For example, genetics provides some insight into the likelihood of inheriting a trait such as blue eyes or a medical condition such as CAD. Genomic studies evaluate the interaction of groups of genes. The combined activity or combined expression of groups of genes allows assumptions or predictions to be made. As an example, genomic studies measure the levels of activity in multiple genes to predict how they, along with environmental and lifestyle decisions, influence the development of type 2 diabetes, CAD, MI, or ischemic stroke.
- Obtain a list of the patient's current medications, including over-the-counter medications and dietary supplements (see Effects of Natural Products on Laboratory Values online at Davis*Plus*).
- Review the procedure with the patient. Inform the patient that specimen collection takes approximately 5 to 10 min. Address concerns about pain and explain that there may be some discomfort during the venipuncture.
- ***Sensitivity to social and cultural issues,*** as well as concern for modesty, is important in providing psychological support before, during, and after the procedure.

C

- Instruct the patient to withhold alcohol and drugs known to alter cholesterol levels for 12 to 24 hr before specimen collection, at the direction of the HCP.
- Note that there are no fluid or medication restrictions unless by medical direction.
- Instruct the patient to fast 6 to 12 hr before specimen collection; fasting is required if triglyceride measurements are included and recommended if cholesterol levels alone are measured for screening. Protocols may vary among facilities.

INTRATEST:

Potential Complications: N/A

- Ensure that the patient has complied with dietary restrictions and pretesting preparations; ensure that food has been restricted for at least 6 to 12 hr prior to the procedure if triglycerides are to be measured.
- Avoid the use of equipment containing latex if the patient has a history of allergic reaction to latex.
- Instruct the patient to cooperate fully and to follow directions. Direct the patient to breathe normally and to avoid unnecessary movement.
- Observe standard precautions, and follow the general guidelines in Patient Preparation and Specimen Collection online at Davis*Plus*. Positively identify the patient, and label the appropriate specimen container with the corresponding patient demographics, initials of the person collecting the specimen, date, and time of collection. Perform a venipuncture.
- Remove the needle and apply direct pressure with dry gauze to stop bleeding. Observe/assess venipuncture site for bleeding or hematoma formation and secure gauze with adhesive bandage.
- Promptly transport the specimen to the laboratory for processing and analysis.

POST-TEST:

- Inform the patient that a report of the results will be made available to the requesting HCP, who will discuss the results with the patient.
- Instruct the patient to resume usual diet as directed by the HCP.
- Secondary causes for increased cholesterol levels should be ruled out before therapy to decrease levels is initiated by use of drugs.
- ***Nutritional Considerations:*** Increases in total cholesterol levels may be associated with CAD. Nutritional therapy is recommended for the patient identified to be at risk for developing coronary artery disease (CAD) or for individuals who have specific risk factors and/or existing medical conditions (e.g., elevated LDL cholesterol levels, other lipid disorders, type 1 diabetes, type 2 diabetes, insulin resistance, or metabolic syndrome). Other changeable risk factors warranting patient education include strategies to encourage patients, especially those who are overweight and with high blood pressure, to safely decrease sodium intake, achieve a normal weight, ensure regular participation of moderate aerobic physical activity three to four times per week, eliminate tobacco use, and adhere to a heart-healthy diet. If triglycerides also are elevated, the patient should be advised to eliminate or reduce alcohol. A variety of dietary patterns are beneficial for people with CAD and there are many meal-planning approaches with nutritional goals endorsed by the American Diabetes Association (ADA). The Guideline on Lifestyle Management to Reduce Cardiovascular Risk published by the ACC and AHA in conjunction with the NHLBI recommends a Mediterranean-style diet rather than a low-fat diet. The guideline emphasizes inclusion of vegetables, whole grains, fruits, low-fat dairy, nuts, legumes, and nontropical vegetable oils (e.g., olive, canola, peanut, sunflower, flaxseed) along with fish and lean poultry. 🍁 The DASH diet makes additional recommendations for the reduction of dietary sodium. Both dietary styles emphasize a reduction in

consumption of red meats, which are high in saturated fats and cholesterol, and other foods containing sugar, saturated fats, trans fats, and sodium. The ADA also includes a vegetarian diet as well as other potential weight loss diets such as Weight Watchers. 🍁 The nutritional needs of each patient need to be determined individually (especially during pregnancy) with the appropriate HCPs, particularly professionals educated in nutrition.

- *Sensitivity to social and cultural issues,* Numerous studies point to the prevalence of excess body weight in American children and adolescents. Experts estimate that obesity is present in 25% of the population ages 6 to 11 yr. The medical, social, and emotional consequences of excess body weight are significant. Special attention should be given to instructing the pediatric patient and caregiver regarding health risks and weight control education. 🍁
- Recognize anxiety related to test results, and be supportive of fear of shortened life expectancy.
- Depending on the results of this procedure, additional testing may be performed to evaluate or monitor progression of the disease process and determine the need for a change in therapy. Evaluate test results in relation to the patient's symptoms and other tests performed.

Patient Education:

- Discuss the implications of abnormal test results on the patient's lifestyle.
- Provide teaching and information regarding the clinical implications of the test results, as appropriate.
- Educate the patient regarding access to counseling services.
- Provide contact information, if desired, for the AHA (www.americanheart.org), NHLBI (www.nhlbi.nih.gov), Institute of Medicine of the National Academies (www.iom.edu) and the USDA's resource for nutrition (www.choosemyplate.gov). 🍁
- Reinforce information given by the patient's HCP regarding further testing, treatment, or referral to another HCP.
- Answer any questions or address any concerns voiced by the patient or family.
- Explain to the patient and the family the anatomy and pathophysiology of the heart and coronary arteries.
- Explain to the patient and the family the risk factors for CAD.

Expected Patient Outcomes:

Understanding

- The patient and family differentiate between the signs and symptoms of MI and angina.
- The patient and family describe the signs and symptoms of heart attack.

Ability

- The patient and family demonstrate readiness to learn and identify their learning preferences.
- The patient and family demonstrate making food selections that are low in saturated fats and high in polyunsaturated fats.

Response

- The patient and family display an emotional response to the cardiac event that is appropriate to the circumstances.
- The patient and family comply with recommended lifestyle alterations and involvement in cardiac rehabilitation.

RELATED STUDIES:

- Related tests include antidysrhythmic drugs, apolipoprotein A and B, ANP, blood gases, BNP, calcium, cholesterol (HDL and LDL), CT cardiac scoring, CRP, CK and isoenzymes, echocardiography, genetic testing, glucose, glycated hemoglobin, Holter monitor, homocysteine, ketones, LDH and isoenzymes, lipoprotein electrophoresis, MRI chest, magnesium, MI scan, myocardial perfusion heart scan, myoglobin, PET heart, potassium, triglycerides, and troponin.
- Refer to the Cardiovascular, Gastrointestinal, and Hepatobiliary systems tables online at Davis*Plus* for related tests by body system.

Chromosome Analysis, Blood

C

SYNONYM/ACRONYM: N/A

COMMON USE: To test for suspected chromosomal disorders that result in birth defects such as Down syndrome.

SPECIMEN: Whole blood collected in a green-top (sodium heparin) tube.

NORMAL FINDINGS: (Method: Tissue culture and microscopic analysis) No chromosomal abnormalities identified.

DESCRIPTION: Cytogenetics is a specialization within the area of genetics that includes chromosome analysis or karyotyping. Chromosome analysis or karyotyping involves comparison of test samples against normal chromosome patterns of number and structure. A normal karyotype consists of 22 pairs of autosomal chromosomes and one pair of sex chromosomes, XX for female and XY for male. Variations in number or structure can be congenital or acquired. Variations can range from a small, single-gene mutation to abnormalities in an entire chromosome or set of chromosomes due to duplication, deletion, substitution, translocation, or other rearrangement. Molecular probe techniques are used to detect smaller, more subtle changes in chromosomes. Cells are incubated in culture media to increase the number of cells available for study and to allow for hybridization of the cellular DNA with fluorescent DNA probes in a technique called fluorescence in situ hybridization (FISH). The probes are designed to target areas of the chromosome known to correlate with genetic risk for a particular disease. When a suitable volume of hybridized sample is achieved, cell growth is chemically inhibited during the prophase and metaphase stages of mitosis (cell division), and cellular DNA is examined to detect fluorescence, which represents chromosomal abnormalities, in the targeted areas. Amniotic fluid, chorionic villus sampling, and cells from fetal tissue or products of conception can also be evaluated for chromosomal abnormalities.

Knowledge of genetics assists the nurse in identifying patients and family members who may benefit from additional education, risk assessment, and counseling. Genetics is the study and identification of genes, genetic mutations, and inheritance. For example, genetics provides some insight into the likelihood of inheriting a trait such as blue eyes or a medical condition such as Down syndrome. Down syndrome is an example of a chromosome disorder in which the cells have three copies of chromosome 21 (trisomy) instead of the normal two copies. Further information regarding inheritance of genes can be found in the study titled "Genetic Testing."

This procedure is contraindicated for

- Circumstances where the parents are not emotionally capable of understanding the test results and managing the ramifications of the test results.

INDICATIONS

- Evaluate conditions related to cryptorchidism, hypogonadism, primary amenorrhea, and infertility.
- Evaluate congenital anomaly, delayed development (physical or mental), intellectual disability, and ambiguous sexual organs.
- Investigate the carrier status of patients or relatives with known genetic abnormalities.
- Investigate the cause of still birth or multiple miscarriages.
- Investigate types of solid tumor or hematologic malignancies.
- Provide prenatal care or genetic counseling.

POTENTIAL MEDICAL DIAGNOSIS

The following tables list some common genetic defects.

Syndrome	Autosomal Chromosome Defect	Features
Angelman	Deletion 15q11–q13	Developmental delays (physical growth, communication, and motor skills); hyperactive behavior; overall happy demeanor with frequent laughter and hand-flapping actions; fascination with water
Beckwith-Wiedemann	Duplication 11p15	Macroglossia, omphalocele, earlobe creases
Bloom	Mutations of BLM, 15	Birth weight and length are below normal and stature remains below normal to adulthood; skin changes in response to sun exposure; increased risk of cancers which develop early in life; high-pitched voice; distinctive facial features (long, narrow face with a small jaw; large nose and ears)
Canavan	Mutations of ASPA, 17p13.3	Developmental delays that become obvious at 3 to 5 months of age; hypotonia that contributes to inability to roll over, sit upright, or swallow; macrocephaly; and intellectual disability
Cat's eye	Trisomy 2q11	Anal atresia, coloboma
Cri du chat	Deletion 5p	Catlike cry, microcephaly, hypertelorism, intellectual disability, retrognathia

(table continues on page 434)

C

Syndrome	Autosomal Chromosome Defect	Features
Cystic fibrosis	Mutations of CFTR, 7	Impaired transport of chloride affects the movement of water in and out of the cells lining the lungs and pancreas. The result is production of thick mucus that obstructs airways and prevents normal function of the affected organs; life-threatening, permanent lung damage
DiGeorge	Deletion 22q11.2	There is a wide variety in the type and severity of problems associated with this syndrome of impaired development of body systems, most commonly included: cardiac abnormalities or defects, poor immune system function (hypothymic or absent thymus), cleft palate, hypoparathyroidism (low calcium); behavioral disorders; distinctive facial features (long face with downturned mouth, asymmetric face when crying, microcephaly, hooded eye lids, malformed ears)
Down	Trisomy 21	Epicanthal folds, simian crease of palm, flat nasal bridge, intellectual disability, congenital heart disease
Edwards	Trisomy 18	Micrognathia, clenched third/fourth fingers with the fifth finger overlapping, rocker-bottom feet, intellectual disability, congenital heart disease
Gaucher's	Mutations of GBA, 1	Hepatomegaly and splenomegaly related to accumulation of lipids; anemia; thrombocytopenia; bone disease (bone pain, fractures, and arthritis)
Maple Syrup	Mutations of BCKDHA, BCKDHB, DBT, and DLD, 19	Developmental delays; poor feeding; lethargy; distinctive maple syrup odor in urine
Miller-Dieker	Deletion 17	Lissencephaly (incomplete or absent development of the folds of the cerebrum); microcephaly; developmental delays, especially in growth; intellectual disability with seizures; difficulty feeding and failure to thrive; cardiac malformations

Syndrome	Autosomal Chromosome Defect	Features
Niemann-Pick	Chromosome 14q24.3 (type C2), 18q11.2 (type C1), 11p15.4–p15.1 (types A & B)	Both types demonstrate symptoms that reflect abnormalities in liver and lung function; blood tests show hyperlipidemia (cholesterol and other fats) and thrombocytopenia
Pallister-Killian	Trisomy 12p	Psychomotor delay, sparse anterior scalp hair, micrognathia, hypotonia
Patau	Trisomy 13	Microcephaly, cleft palate or lip, polydactyly, intellectual disability, congenital heart disease
Prader-Willi	Deletion 15q11–q13	Delayed development; distinctive facial features (narrow forehead, almond-shaped eyes, triangular-shaped mouth, diminished stature with small hands and feet); hypotonia; childhood development of an insatiable appetite, hyperphagia, and obesity; mild to moderate intellectual disability; behavioral problems (outbursts of anger and compulsive behavior such as picking at the skin)
Smith-Magenis	Deletion 17p11.2	The major features of this condition include mild to moderate intellectual disability, delayed speech and language skills, distinctive facial features, sleep disturbances, and behavioral problems
Tay-Sachs	Mutations of HEXA, 15q24.1	Normal development until age 3 to 6 mo when development slows and hypotonia affects motor skills such as ability to turn over, sit upright, and crawl; exaggerated startle reaction to loud noises; seizures; eventual loss of vision (cherry red spot upon eye exam is characteristic) and hearing; intellectual disability
Warkam	Mosaic trisomy 8	Malformed ears, bulbous nose, deep palm creases, absent or hypoplastic patellae
Wolf-Hirschhorn	Deletion 4p16.3	Microcephaly, growth retardation, intellectual disability, carp mouth

Syndrome	Sex-Chromosome Defect	Features
Fragile X	Xq27.3	Intellectual disability; autism and autism spectrum disorders
XYY	47,XYY	Tall, increased risk of behavior problems
Klinefelter	47,XXY	Hypogonadism, infertility, underdeveloped secondary sex characteristics, learning disabilities
Rett	Mutations of Xq28	Severe and progressive developmental problems related to brain functions such as speech, motor and intelligence begin after 6 to 18 mo of normal growth; brain disorder almost exclusively affecting females; slower than normal physical growth; microcephaly; meaningful use of hands is lost in early childhood and replaced by repetitive random hand motions such as clapping or wringing.
Triple X	47,XXX	Increased risk of infertility and learning disabilities
Ullrich-Turner	45,X	Short, gonadal dysgenesis, webbed neck, low posterior hairline, renal and cardiovascular abnormalities

CRITICAL FINDINGS: N/A

INTERFERING FACTORS: N/A

NURSING IMPLICATIONS AND PROCEDURE

PRETEST:

- Positively identify the patient using at least two person-specific identifiers before services, treatments, or procedures are performed.
- ***Patient Teaching:*** Inform the patient this test can assist in identification of potential birth defects.
- Obtain a history of the patient's health concerns (especially family history of known or suspected genetic disorders), symptoms, surgical procedures, and results of previously performed laboratory and diagnostic studies. Include a list of known allergens, especially allergies or sensitivities to latex.
- Obtain a list of the patient's current medications, including over-the-counter medications and dietary supplements (see Effects of Natural Products on Laboratory Values online at Davis*Plus*).
- Review the procedure with the patient. Inform the patient that specimen collection takes approximately 5 to 10 min. Address concerns about pain and explain that there may be some discomfort during the venipuncture.
- ***Sensitivity to social and cultural issues,*** as well as concern for modesty, is important in providing psychological support before, during, and after the procedure.
- Note that there are no food, fluid, or medication restrictions unless by medical direction.

INTRATEST:

Potential Complications: N/A

- Avoid the use of equipment containing latex if the patient has a history of allergic reaction to latex.
- Instruct the patient to cooperate fully and to follow directions. Direct the patient to breathe normally and to avoid unnecessary movement.
- Observe standard precautions, and follow the general guidelines in Patient Preparation and Specimen Collection online at Davis*Plus*. Positively identify the patient, and label the appropriate specimen container with the corresponding patient demographics, initials of the person collecting the specimen, date, and time of collection. Perform a venipuncture.
- Remove the needle and apply direct pressure with dry gauze to stop bleeding. Observe/assess venipuncture site for bleeding or hematoma formation and secure gauze with adhesive bandage.
- Promptly transport the specimen to the laboratory for processing and analysis.

POST-TEST:

- Inform the patient that a report of the results will be made available to the requesting health-care provider (HCP), who will discuss the results with the patient.
- Recognize anxiety related to test results, and be supportive of the sensitive nature of the testing. Discuss the implications of abnormal test results on the patient's lifestyle. Provide teaching and information regarding the clinical implications of the test results, as appropriate. Educate the patient regarding access to counseling services.
- ***Social and Cultural Considerations:*** Encourage the family to seek counseling if they are contemplating pregnancy termination or to seek genetic counseling if a chromosomal abnormality is determined. Decisions regarding elective abortion should occur in the presence of both parents. Provide a nonjudgmental, nonthreatening atmosphere for discussing the risks and difficulties of delivering and raising a developmentally challenged infant, as well as exploring other options (termination of pregnancy or adoption). It is also important to discuss feelings the mother and father may experience (e.g., guilt, depression, anger) if fetal abnormalities are detected. Educate the patient and family regarding access to counseling services, as appropriate.
- Reinforce information given by the patient's HCP regarding further testing, treatment, or referral to another HCP. Answer any questions or address any concerns voiced by the patient or family.
- Depending on the results of this procedure, additional testing may be performed to evaluate or monitor changes in health status and determine the need for a change in therapy. Evaluate test results in relation to the patient's symptoms and other tests performed.

RELATED STUDIES:

- Related tests include α_1-fetoprotein, amniotic fluid analysis, biopsy chorionic villus, genetic testing, newborn screening, and US biophysical profile obstetric.
- Refer to the Reproductive System table online at Davis*Plus* for related tests by body system.

Clot Retraction

SYNONYM/ACRONYM: N/A

COMMON USE: To assist in the diagnosis of bleeding disorders.

Access Canadian content on Fast Find: Lab and Dx at davispl.us/vanleeuwen7

SPECIMEN: Whole blood collected in a full red-top tube.

NORMAL FINDINGS: (Method: Macroscopic observation of sample) A normal clot, gently separated from the side of the test tube and incubated at 37°C, shrinks to about half of its original size within 1 hr. The result is a firm, cylindrical fibrin clot that contains red blood cells and is sharply demarcated from the clear serum. Complete clot retraction can take 6 to 24 hr.

C

POTENTIAL MEDICAL DIAGNOSIS

Increased in:

- Anemia (severe) ***(related to inadequate numbers of red blood cells (RBCs) that quickly produce a clot)***
- Hypofibrinogenemia, dysfibrinogenemia, disseminated intravascular coagulation ***(evidenced by rapid formation of a small, loosely formed clot; absence of functional fibrinogen reduces fibrinolysis)***
- Medications like aspirin ***(related to effect of acetylsalicylic acid as a potentiator of platelet aggregation)***

Decreased in:

- Glanzmann's thrombasthenia ***(related to autosomal recessive abnormality of platelet glycoprotein IIb–IIIa required for platelet aggregation)***
- Polycythemia ***(related to excessive numbers of RBCs that physically limit the extent to which the clot can retract)***
- Thrombocytopenia ***(related to inadequate numbers of platelets to produce a well-formed clot)***
- von Willebrand disease ***(related to deficiency of von Willebrand factor required for platelet aggregation)***
- Waldenström's macroglobulinemia ***(related to excessive production of paraproteins that physically obstruct platelet aggregation)***

CRITICAL FINDINGS: N/A

Find and print out the full study on Fast Find at davispl.us/vanleeuwen7.

Coagulation Factors

SYNONYM/ACRONYM: See table.

COMMON USE: To detect factor deficiencies and related coagulopathies such as found in disseminated intravascular coagulation (DIC).

SPECIMEN: Whole blood collected in a completely filled blue-top (3.2% sodium citrate) tube. If the patient's hematocrit exceeds 55%, the volume of citrate in the collection tube must be adjusted.

NORMAL FINDINGS: (Method: Photo-optical clot detection) Activity from 50% to 150%.

	Preferred Name	Synonym	Role in Modern Coagulation Cascade Model	Coagulation Test Responses in the Presence of Factor Deficiency
Factor I	Fibrinogen	—	Assists in the formation of the fibrin clot	PT prolonged, aPTT prolonged
Factor II	Prothrombin	Prethrombin	Assists factor Xa in formation of trace thrombin in the initiation phase and assists factors VIIIa, IXa, Xa, and Va to form thrombin in the propagation phase of hemostasis	PT prolonged, aPTT prolonged
Tissue factor (formerly known as factor III)	Tissue factor	Tissue thromboplastin	Assists factor VII and Ca^{2+} in the activation of factors IX and X during the initiation phase of hemostasis	PT prolonged, aPTT prolonged
Calcium (formerly known as factor intravenous)	Calcium	Ca^{2+}	Essential to the activation of multiple clotting factors	N/A
Factor V	Proaccelerin	Labile factor, accelerator globulin (AcG)	Assists factors VIIIa, IXa, Xa, and II in the formation of thrombin during the amplification and propagation phases of hemostasis	PT prolonged, aPTT prolonged
Factor VII	Proconvertin	Stabile factor, serum prothrombin conversion accelerator, autoprothrombin I	Assists tissue factor and Ca^{2+} in the activation of factors IX and X	PT prolonged, aPTT normal
Factor VIII	Antihemophilic factor (AHF)	Antihemophilic globulin (AHG), antihemophilic factor A, platelet cofactor 1	Activated by trace thrombin during the initiation phase of hemostasis to amplify formation of additional thrombin	PT normal, aPTT prolonged

(table continues on page 440)

C

C

	Preferred Name	Synonym	Role in Modern Coagulation Cascade Model	Coagulation Test Responses in the Presence of Factor Deficiency
Factor IX	Plasma thromboplastin component (PTC)	Christmas factor, antihemophilic factor B, platelet cofactor 2	Assists factors Va and VIIIa in the amplification phase and factors VIIIa, Xa, Va, and II to form thrombin in the propagation phase	PT normal, aPTT prolonged
Factor X	Stuart-Prower factor	Autoprothrombin III, thrombokinase	Assists with formation of trace thrombin in the initiation phase and acts with factors VIIIa, IXa, Va, and II to form thrombin in the propagation phase	PT prolonged, aPTT prolonged
Factor XI	Plasma thromboplastin antecedent (PTA)	Antihemophilic factor C	Activated by thrombin produced in the extrinsic pathway to enhance production of additional thrombin inside the fibrin clot via the intrinsic pathway; this factor also participates in slowing down the process of fibrinolysis	PT normal, aPTT prolonged
Factor XII	Hageman factor	Glass factor, contact factor	Contact activator of the kinin system (e.g., prekallikrein, and high-molecular-weight kininogen)	PT normal, aPTT prolonged
Factor XIII	Fibrin-stabilizing factor (FSF)	Laki-Lorand factor (LLF), fibrinase, plasma transglutaminase	Activated by thrombin and assists in formation of bonds between fibrin strands to complete secondary hemostasis	PT normal, aPTT normal
von Willebrand factor	von Willebrand factor	vWF	Assists in platelet adhesion and thrombus formation	Ristocetin cofactor decreased

DESCRIPTION: Hemostasis involves three components: blood vessel walls, platelets, and plasma coagulation proteins. Primary hemostasis has three major stages involving platelet adhesion, platelet activation, and platelet aggregation. Platelet adhesion is initiated by exposure of the endothelium as a result of damage to blood vessels. Exposed tissue factor–bearing cells trigger the simultaneous binding of von Willebrand factor to exposed collagen and circulating platelets. Activated platelets release a number of procoagulant factors, including thromboxane, a very potent platelet activator, from storage granules. These factors enter the circulation and activate other platelets, and the cycle continues. The activated platelets aggregate at the site of vessel injury, and at this stage of hemostasis, the glycoprotein IIb/IIIa receptors on the activated platelets bind fibrinogen, causing the platelets to stick together and form a plug. There is a balance in health between the prothrombotic or clot formation process and the antithrombotic or clot disintegration process. Simultaneously, the coagulation process or secondary hemostasis occurs. In secondary hemostasis, the coagulation proteins respond to blood vessel injury in an overlapping chain of events. The contact activation and tissue factor pathways (also known respectively as the intrinsic and extrinsic pathways) of secondary hemostasis are a series of reactions involving the substrate protein fibrinogen, the coagulation factors (also known as *enzyme precursors* or *zymogens*), nonenzymatic cofactors (Ca^{2+}), and phospholipids. The factors were assigned Roman numerals in the order of their discovery, not their place in the coagulation sequence. Factor VI was originally thought to be a separate clotting factor. It was subsequently proved to be the same as a modified form of factor Va, and therefore, the number is no longer used.

The antithrombotic process includes tissue factor pathway inhibitor (TFPI), antithrombin, protein C, and fibrinolysis.

The coagulation factors are formed in the liver. They can be divided into three groups based on their common properties:

1. The contact group is activated in vitro by a surface such as glass and is activated in vivo by collagen. The contact group includes factor XI, factor XII, prekallikrein, and high-molecular-weight kininogen.
2. The prothrombin or vitamin K–dependent group includes factors II, VII, IX, and X.
3. The fibrinogen group includes factors I, V, VIII, and XIII. They are the most labile of the factors and are consumed during the coagulation process. The factors listed in the table are the ones most commonly measured.

For many years it was believed that the intrinsic and extrinsic pathways operated equally, in parallel. A more modern concept of the coagulation process has replaced the traditional model (formerly called the *coagulation cascade*) and is presented on the next page. The cellular-based model includes four overlapping phases in the formation of thrombin: initiation, amplification, propagation, and termination. It is now known that the tissue factor pathway is the primary pathway for the initiation of blood coagulation. Tissue factor (TF)–bearing cells (e.g., endothelial cells, smooth muscle cells, monocytes) can be induced to express TF and are the primary initiators of the coagulation cascade either by contact activation or trauma. The contact activation pathway is more related to inflammation, and although it plays an important role in the body's reaction to damaged endothelial surfaces, a deficiency in factor XII does not result in development of a bleeding disorder, which demonstrates the minor role of the intrinsic pathway in the process of blood coagulation. Substances such as endotoxins, tumor necrosis factor alpha, and lipoproteins can also stimulate expression of TF. TF, in combination with factor VII and calcium, forms a complex that then activates factors IX and X in the initiation phase. Activated factor X in the presence of factor II (prothrombin) leads to the formation of thrombin. TFPI quickly inactivates this stage of the pathway so that limited or trace amounts of thrombin are produced, which results in the activation of factors VIII and V. Activated factor IX, assisted by activated factors V and VIII, initiate amplification and propagation of thrombin in the cascade. Thrombin activates factor XIII and begins converting fibrinogen into fibrin monomers, which spontaneously polymerize and then become cross-linked into a stable clot by activated factor XIII.

Qualitative and quantitative factor deficiencies can affect the function of the coagulation pathways. Factor V and factor II (prothrombin) mutations are examples of qualitative deficiencies and are the most common inherited predisposing factors for blood clots. Hemophilia A is an inherited deficiency of factor VIII and occurs at a prevalence of about 1 in 5,000 to 10,000 male births. Hemophilia B is an inherited deficiency of factor IX and occurs at a prevalence of about 1 in about 20,000 to 34,000 male births. Genetic testing is available for inherited mutations associated with inherited coagulopathies. The tests are performed on samples of whole blood. Counseling and informed written consent are generally required for genetic testing.

Knowledge of genetics assists the nurse in identifying patients and family members who may benefit from additional education, risk assessment, and counseling. Genetics is the study and identification of genes, genetic mutations, and inheritance. For example, genetics provides some insight into the likelihood of inheriting a trait such as blue eyes or a medical condition such as hemophilia. Some conditions are the result of mutations involving a single gene, whereas other conditions may involve multiple genes and/or multiple chromosomes. Hemophilia is an example of a recessive sex-linked genetic disorder passed from a mother to male children. The factor V Leiden mutation in the F5 gene is an inherited autosomal genetic disorder that results in thrombophilia and the development of blood clots. Severity of the disorder depends on whether a single F5 mutation is inherited from one parent or two mutations are inherited, one from each parent. The risk of forming abnormal blood clots is also increased in people who have multiple mutations in the F5 gene or mutations in a different gene that also codes for products involved in the coagulation process, including factor V Leiden. Genomic studies evaluate the interaction of groups of genes. The combined activity or combined expression of groups of genes allows assumptions or predictions to be made. As an example, genomic studies measure the levels of activity in multiple genes to predict how they and other factors influence the prolonged development of abnormal blood clots. Other factors that may contribute to the development of blood clots in people with the factor V Leiden mutation include obesity, tissue injury (e.g., from surgery or trauma), smoking, pregnancy, exposure to hormones (e.g., oral contraceptives or hormone replacement therapy), and advancing age. Further information regarding inheritance of genes can be found in the study titled "Genetic Testing."

The PT/INR measures the function of the tissue factor pathway of coagulation and is used to monitor patients receiving warfarin or coumarin-derivative anticoagulant therapy. The aPTT measures the function of the contact activation pathway of coagulation and is used to monitor patients receiving heparin anticoagulant therapy.

This procedure is contraindicated for: N/A

INDICATIONS

- Identify the presence of inherited bleeding disorders.
- Identify the presence of qualitative or quantitative factor deficiency.

POTENTIAL MEDICAL DIAGNOSIS

Increased in: N/A

Decreased in:

- Congenital deficiency
- DIC ***(related to consumption of factors as part of the coagulation cascade)***
- Liver disease ***(related to inability of damaged liver to synthesize coagulation factors)***

CRITICAL FINDINGS:

Fibrinogen: Less than 80 mg/dL (SI: Less than 2.4 micromol/L).

Note and immediately report to the requesting health-care provider (HCP) any critical findings and related symptoms. A listing of these findings varies among facilities. Timely notification of a critical finding for laboratory or diagnostic studies is a role expectation of the professional nurse. The notification processes vary among facilities. Upon receipt of the critical finding, the information should be read back to the caller to verify accuracy.

Signs and symptoms of microvascular thrombosis include cyanosis, ischemic tissue necrosis, hemorrhagic necrosis, tachypnea, dyspnea, pulmonary emboli, venous distention, abdominal pain, and oliguria. Possible interventions include identification and treatment of the underlying cause, support through administration of required blood products (cryoprecipitate or fresh frozen plasma), and administration of heparin. Cryoprecipitate may be a more effective product than fresh frozen plasma in cases where the fibrinogen level is less than 100 mg/dL (SI: 2.94 micromol/L), the minimum level required for adequate hemostasis, because it delivers a concentrated amount of fibrinogen without as much plasma volume.

Coagulation Process

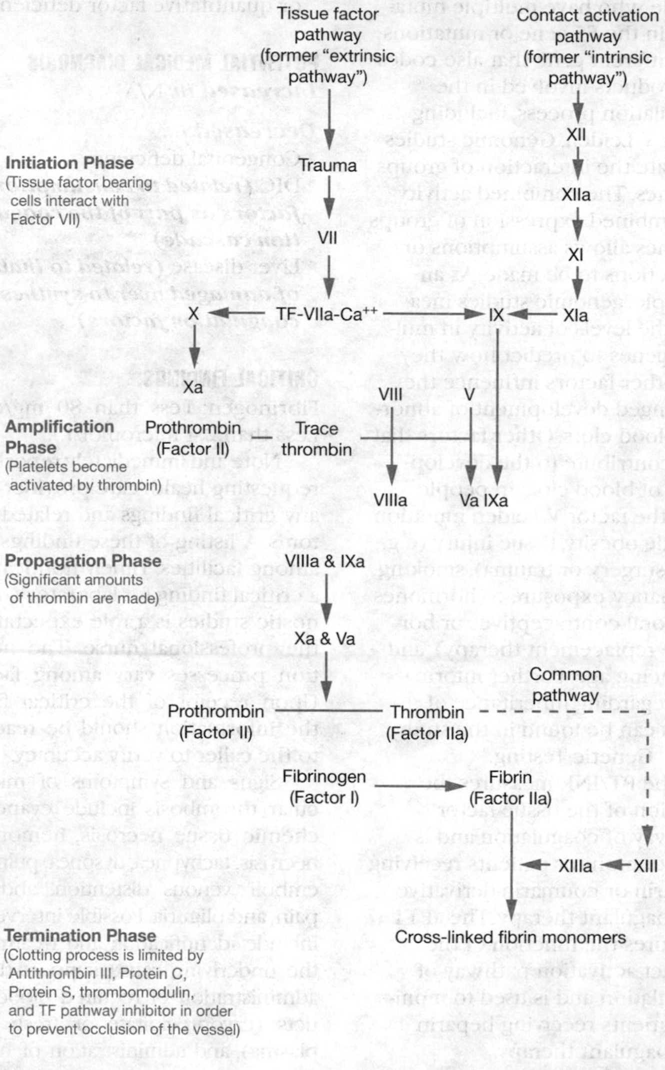

INTERFERING FACTORS

- Drugs and other substances that may decrease factor II levels include warfarin.
- Drugs and other substances that may increase factor V, VII, and X levels include anabolic steroids and oral contraceptives.
- Drugs and other substances that may decrease factor V levels include streptokinase.
- Drugs and other substances that may decrease factor VII levels include acetylsalicylic acid, asparaginase, cefamandole, ceftriaxone, dextran, dicumarol,

gemfibrozil, oral contraceptives, and warfarin.

- Drugs and other substances that may increase factor VIII levels include chlormadinone.
- Drugs and other substances that may decrease factor VIII levels include asparaginase.
- Drugs and other substances that may increase factor IX levels include chlormadinone and oral contraceptives.
- Drugs and other substances that may decrease factor IX levels include asparaginase and warfarin.
- Drugs that may decrease factor X levels include chlormadinone, dicumarol, oral contraceptives, and warfarin.
- Drugs that may decrease factor XI levels include asparaginase and captopril.
- Drugs that may decrease factor XII levels include captopril.
- Test results of patients on anticoagulant therapy are unreliable.
- Placement of tourniquet for longer than 1 min can result in venous stasis and changes in the concentration of plasma proteins to be measured. Platelet activation may also occur under these conditions, causing erroneous results.
- Vascular injury during phlebotomy can activate platelets and coagulation factors, causing erroneous results.
- Hemolyzed specimens must be rejected because hemolysis is an indication of platelet and coagulation factor activation.
- Icteric or lipemic specimens interfere with optical testing methods, producing erroneous results.
- Incompletely filled collection tubes, specimens contaminated with heparin, clotted specimens, or unprocessed specimens not delivered to the laboratory within 1 to 2 hr of collection should be rejected.

C

NURSING IMPLICATIONS AND PROCEDURE

POTENTIAL NURSING PROBLEMS:

Problem	Signs & Symptoms	Interventions
Bleeding ***(related to alerted clotting factors secondary to heparin use or depleted clotting factors)***	Altered level of consciousness; hypotension; increased heart rate; decreased Hgb and Hct; capillary refill greater than 3 sec; cool extremities	Increase frequency of vital sign assessment with variances in results; monitor for vital sign trends; administer blood or blood products as ordered; administer stool softeners as needed; monitor stool for blood; encourage intake of foods rich in vitamin K; monitor and trend Hgb/Hct; assess skin for petechiae, purpura, hematoma; monitor for blood in emesis, or sputum; institute bleeding precautions (prevent unnecessary venipuncture;

(table continues on page 446)

Problem	Signs & Symptoms	Interventions
		avoid intramuscular injections; prevent trauma; be gentle with oral care, suctioning; avoid use of a sharp razor); administer prescribed medications (recombinant human activated protein C; epsilon aminocaproic acid)
Gas exchange ***(related to deficient oxygen capacity of the blood)***	Irregular breathing pattern, use of accessory muscles; altered chest excursion; adventitious breath sounds (crackles, rhonchi, wheezes, diminished breath sounds); copious secretions; signs of hypoxia; altered blood gas results; confusion; lethargy; cyanosis	Monitor respiratory rate and effort based on assessment of patient condition; assess lung sounds frequently; monitor for secretions, bloody sputum; suction as necessary; use pulse oximetry to monitor oxygen saturation; collaborate with HCP to administer oxygen as needed; elevate the head of the bed 30 degrees or higher; monitor intravenous fluids and avoid aggressive fluid resuscitation; assess level of consciousness; anticipate the need for possible intubation
Tissue perfusion ***(related to compromised clotting factor; blood loss; deficient oxygen-carrying capacity of the blood)***	Hypotension; dizziness; cool extremities; capillary refill greater than 3 sec; weak pedal pulses; altered level of consciousness	Monitor blood pressure; assess for dizziness; check skin temperature for warmth; assess capillary refill; assess pedal pulses; monitor level of consciousness; administer prescribed vasodilators and inotropic drugs; use oxygen as required
Confusion ***(related to an alteration in the oxygen-carrying capacity of the blood; blood loss; compromised clotting factor)***	Disorganized thinking, restless, irritable, altered concentration and attention span, changeable mental function over the day, hallucinations; altered attention span; inability to follow directions; disorientation to person, place, time, and purpose; inappropriate affect	Treat the medical condition; correlate confusion with the need to reverse altered electrolytes; evaluate medications; prevent falls and injury through appropriate use of postural support, bed alarm, or restraints; consider pharmacological interventions; record accurate intake and output to assess fluid status; administer blood or blood products; monitor and trend Hgb/Hct

PRETEST:

- Positively identify the patient using at least two person-specific identifiers before providing care, treatment, or services.
- *Patient Teaching:* Inform the patient this test can assist in evaluating the effectiveness of blood clotting and identify deficiencies in blood factor levels.
- Obtain a history of the patient's health concerns, symptoms, surgical procedures, and results of previously performed laboratory and diagnostic studies. Include a list of known allergens, especially allergies or sensitivities to latex.
- Obtain a list of the patient's current medications, including over-the-counter medications, dietary supplements, anticoagulants, aspirin and other salicylates (see Effects of Natural Products on Laboratory Values online at Davis*Plus*). Such products should be discontinued by medical direction for the appropriate number of days prior to a surgical procedure. Note the last time and dose of medication taken.
- Review the procedure with the patient. Inform the patient that specimen collection takes approximately 5 to 10 min. Address concerns about pain and explain that there may be some discomfort during the venipuncture.
- ***Sensitivity to social and cultural issues,*** as well as concern for modesty, is important in providing psychological support before, during, and after the procedure.
- Note that there are no food, fluid, or medication restrictions unless by medical direction.

INTRATEST:

Potential Complications: N/A

- Avoid the use of equipment containing latex if the patient has a history of allergic reaction to latex.
- Instruct the patient to cooperate fully and to follow directions. Direct the patient to breathe normally and to avoid unnecessary movement.
- Observe standard precautions, and follow the general guidelines in Patient Preparation and Specimen Collection online at Davis*Plus*. Positively identify the patient, and label the appropriate specimen container with the corresponding patient demographics, initials of the person collecting the specimen, date, and time of collection. Perform a venipuncture. When multiple specimens are drawn, the blue-top tube should be collected after sterile (i.e., blood culture) tubes. Otherwise, when using a standard vacutainer system, the blue top is the first tube collected. When a butterfly is used and due to the added tubing, an extra red-top tube should be collected before the blue-top tube to ensure complete filling of the blue top tube.
- Remove the needle and apply direct pressure with dry gauze to stop bleeding. Observe/assess venipuncture site for bleeding or hematoma formation and secure gauze with adhesive bandage.
- Promptly transport the specimen to the laboratory for processing and analysis. The recommendation for processed and unprocessed samples stored in unopened tubes is that testing should be completed within 1 to 4 hr of collection.

POST-TEST:

- Inform the patient that a report of the results will be made available to the requesting HCP, who will discuss the results with the patient.
- Depending on the results of this procedure, additional testing may be performed to evaluate or monitor progression of the disease process and determine the need for a change in therapy. Evaluate test results in relation to the patient's symptoms and other tests performed.

Patient Education:

- Instruct the patient to report immediately any signs of unusual bleeding or bruising.
- Inform the patient with decreased factor levels of the importance of taking precautions against bruising and bleeding.

C

- Reinforce information given by the patient's HCP regarding further testing, treatment, or referral to another HCP.
- Answer any questions or address any concerns voiced by the patient or family.

Expected Patient Outcomes:

Understanding

- The patient and family state bleeding precautions that include the use of a soft bristle toothbrush, use of an electric razor, avoidance of constipation, avoidance of acetylsalicylic acid and similar products, and avoidance of intramuscular injections.
- The patient and family state the importance of monitoring stool, sputum, and urine for blood.

Ability

- The patient demonstrates proficiency in self-administering prescribed medications.
- The patient and family demonstrate proficiency in adequately elevating the head of the bed to facilitate adequate gas exchange.

Response

- The patient complies with the recommendation to refrain from risky behavior that could result in trauma and bleeding.
- The patient and family comply with the recommendation to report any new bleeding to the HCP.

RELATED STUDIES:

- Related tests include aPTT, ALT, ALP, AT-IIII, AST, clot retraction, CBC platelet count, copper, fibrinogen, FDP, plasminogen, procalcitonin, protein C, protein S, PT/INR, and vitamin K.
- Refer to the Hematopoietic and Hepatobiliary systems tables online at Davis*Plus* for related tests by body system.

Cold Agglutinin Titer

SYNONYM/ACRONYM: Mycoplasma serology.

COMMON USE: To identify and confirm the presence of viral infections such as found in atypical pneumonia.

SPECIMEN: Serum collected in a red-top tube. The tube must be placed in a water bath or heat block at 37°C for 1 hr and allowed to clot before the serum is separated from the red blood cells (RBCs).

NORMAL FINDINGS: (Method: Patient serum containing autoantibodies titered against type O RBCs at 2°C to 8°C. Type O cells are used because they have no antigens on the cell membrane surface. Agglutination with patient sera would not occur because of reaction between RBC blood type antigens and patient blood type antibodies.) Negative: Single titer less than 1:32 or less than a four-fold increase in titer over serial samples. High titers may appear spontaneously in older adult patients and persist for many years.

POTENTIAL MEDICAL DIAGNOSIS

Increased in:

Mycoplasma *infection stimulates production of antibodies against specific RBC antigens in affected individuals.*

- Cirrhosis
- Gangrene
- Hemolytic anemia
- Infectious diseases (e.g., staphylococcemia, influenza, tuberculosis)

- Infectious mononucleosis
- Malaria
- *M. pneumoniae* (primary atypical pneumonia)
- Multiple myeloma
- Pulmonary embolism
- Raynaud's disease (severe)
- Systemic lupus erythematosus
- Trypanosomiasis

Decreased in: N/A

CRITICAL FINDINGS: N/A

Find and print out the full study on Fast Find at davispl.us/vanleeuwen7.

C

Collagen Cross-Linked N-Telopeptide

SYNONYM/ACRONYM: NT_x.

COMMON USE: To evaluate the effectiveness of treatment for osteoporosis.

SPECIMEN: Urine from a random specimen collected in a clean plastic container.

NORMAL FINDINGS: (Method: Immunoassay)

Adult male 18–29 yr	Less than 100 mmol bone collagen equivalents (BCE)/mmol creatinine
Adult male 30–59 yr	Less than 65 mmol BCE/mmol creatinine
Adult female (premenopausal)	Less than 65 mmol BCE/mmol creatinine

DESCRIPTION: Osteoporosis is the most common bone disease in the West. It is often called the "silent disease" because bone loss occurs without symptoms. The formation and maintenance of bone mass is dependent on a combination of factors that include genetics, nutrition, exercise, and hormone function. Normally, the rate of bone formation is equal to the rate of bone resorption. After midlife, the rate of bone loss begins to increase. Osteoporosis is more commonly identified in women than in men. Other risk factors include thin, small-framed body structure; family history of osteoporosis; diet low in calcium; white or Asian ancestry; excessive use of alcohol; cigarette smoking; sedentary lifestyle; long-term use of corticosteroids, thyroid replacement medications, or antiepileptics; history of bulimia, anorexia nervosa, chronic liver disease, or malabsorption disorders; and postmenopausal state. Knowledge of genetics assists the nurse in identifying patients and family members who may benefit from additional education, risk assessment, and counseling. Genetics is the study and identification of genes, genetic mutations, and inheritance. Genomic studies evaluate the interaction of groups

C

of genes. The combined activity or combined expression of groups of genes allows assumptions or predictions to be made. As an example, genomic studies measure the levels of activity in multiple genes to predict how they, along with environmental and lifestyle decisions, influence the development of type 2 diabetes, coronary artery disease, reduction in bone mass, or ischemic stroke. Further information regarding inheritance of genes can be found in the study titled "Genetic Testing."

Osteoporosis is a major consequence of menopause in women owing to the decline of estrogen production. Osteoporosis is rare in premenopausal women. Estrogen replacement therapy (after menopause) is one strategy that has been commonly employed to prevent osteoporosis, although its exact protective mechanism is unknown. Results of some recently published studies indicate that there may be significant adverse effects to estrogen replacement therapy; more research is needed to understand the long-term effects (positive and negative) of this therapy. Other treatments include raloxifene 🍁 (selectively modulates estrogen receptors), calcitonin (interacts directly with osteoclasts), and bisphosphates (inhibit osteoclast-mediated bone resorption).

A noninvasive test to detect the presence of collagen cross-linked N-telopeptide (NT_x) is used to follow the progress of patients who have begun treatment for osteoporosis. NT_x is formed when collagenase acts on bone. Small NT_x fragments are excreted in the urine after bone resorption. A desirable response, 2 to 3 mo after therapy is initiated, is a 30% reduction in NT_x and a reduction of 50% below baseline by 12 mo.

This procedure is contraindicated for: N/A

INDICATIONS

- Assist in the evaluation of osteoporosis.
- Assist in the management and treatment of osteoporosis.
- Monitor effects of estrogen replacement therapy.

POTENTIAL MEDICAL DIAGNOSIS

Increased in:

Conditions that reflect increased bone resorption are associated with increased levels of N-telopeptide in the urine.

- Alcoholism ***(related to inadequate nutrition)***
- Chronic immobilization
- Chronic treatment with anticonvulsants, corticosteroids, gonadotropin releasing hormone agonists, heparin, or thyroid hormone
- Conditions that include hypercortisolism, hyperparathyroidism, hyperthyroidism, and hypogonadism
- Gastrointestinal disease ***(related to inadequate dietary intake or absorption of minerals required for bone formation and maintenance)***
- Growth disorders (acromegaly, growth hormone deficiency, osteogenesis imperfecta)
- Hyperparathyroidism ***(related to imbalance in calcium and phosphorus that affects the rate of bone resorption)***
- Multiple myeloma and metastatic tumors

- Osteomalacia ***(related to defective bone mineralization)***
- Osteoporosis
- Paget's disease
- Postmenopausal women ***(related to estrogen deficiency)***
- Recent fracture
- Renal insufficiency ***(related to excessive loss through renal dysfunction)***
- Rheumatoid arthritis and other connective tissue diseases ***(related to inadequate diet due to loss of appetite)***

Decreased in:

- Effective therapy for osteoporosis

CRITICAL FINDINGS: N/A

INTERFERING FACTORS

- NT_x levels are affected by urinary excretion, and values may be influenced by the presence of kidney disease.

C

NURSING IMPLICATIONS AND PROCEDURE

POTENTIAL NURSING PROBLEMS:

Problem	Signs & Symptoms	Interventions
Health maintenance ***(related to failure to regulate diet; lack of exercise; alcohol use; smoking)***	Inability or failure to recognize or process information toward improving health and preventing illness with associated mental and physical effects	Encourage regular participation in weight-bearing exercise; assess diet, smoking, and alcohol use; teach the importance of adequate calcium intake with diet and supplements; refer to smoking cessation and alcohol treatment programs; collaborate with health-care provider (HCP) for bone density evaluation
Socialization ***(related to altered body image and associated change in physical appearance)***	Expresses concern about changes in appearance related to kyphosis or lordosis; isolates self at home and refuses to participate in usual social or familial activities; expresses discomfort with social situations; fear of falling	Encourage continuation of activities inclusive of those with whom there is an established friend or family relationship; encourage participation in a community support group; encourage realistic view of physical appearance; acknowledge patient's perception of changed image and the impact on his or her life

(table continues on page 452)

Problem	Signs & Symptoms	Interventions
Self-care ***(related to loss of bone mass and physical deformity; pain; and limited range of motion)***	Difficulty fastening clothing; difficulty performing personal hygiene; inability to maintain appropriate appearance; difficulty with independent mobility	Reinforce self-care techniques as taught by occupational therapy; ensure the patient has adequate time to perform self-care; encourage use of assistive devices to maintain independence; ask if there is any interference with lifestyle activities
Fall risk ***(related to altered mobility associated with loss of bone mass)***	Postural instability; jerky movement; uncoordinated movement; slow, unsteady movement	Teach about fall precautions; assess home environment for fall risk; evaluate medications for contributory cause related to recent falls; encourage physical therapy to facilitate moderate exercise; teach that low, comfortable walking shoes can promote safe ambulation and decrease fall risk

PRETEST:

- Positively identify the patient using at least two person-specific identifiers before services, treatments, or procedures are performed.
- *Patient Teaching:* Inform the patient this test can assist in diagnosing osteoporosis and evaluating the effectiveness of therapy.
- Obtain a history of the patient's health concerns, symptoms, surgical procedures, and results of previously performed laboratory and diagnostic studies. Include a list of known allergens, especially allergies or sensitivities to latex.
- Obtain a list of the patient's current medications, including over-the-counter medications and dietary supplements (see Effects of Natural Products on Laboratory Values online at Davis*Plus*).
- Review the procedure with the patient. Inform the patient that specimen collection takes approximately 5 to 10 min. Address concerns about pain and explain that there should be no discomfort during the procedure.
- *Sensitivity to social and cultural issues,* as well as concern for modesty, is important in providing psychological support before, during, and after the procedure.
- Note that there are no food, fluid, or medication restrictions unless by medical direction.

INTRATEST:

Potential Complications: N/A

- Instruct the patient to cooperate fully and to follow directions.
- Observe standard precautions, and follow the general guidelines

in Patient Preparation and Specimen Collection online at Davis*Plus*. Positively identify the patient, and label the appropriate specimen container with the corresponding patient demographics, initials of the person collecting the specimen, date, and time of collection.

- Instruct the patient to collect a second-void morning specimen as follows: (1) void and then drink a glass of water; (2) wait 30 min, and then try to void again.
- Promptly transport the specimen to the laboratory for processing and analysis.

POST-TEST:

- Inform the patient that a report of the results will be made available to the requesting HCP, who will discuss the results with the patient.
- ***Nutritional Considerations:*** Increased NT_x levels may be associated with osteoporosis. Nutritional therapy may be indicated for patients identified as being at high risk for developing osteoporosis. Educate the patient about the National Osteoporosis Foundation's guidelines regarding a regular regimen of weight-bearing exercises, limited alcohol intake, avoidance of tobacco products, and adequate dietary intake of vitamin D and calcium. Dietary calcium can be obtained from animal or plant sources. Almonds (milk, nuts), beet greens, broccoli, cheese, clams, kale, legumes, milk and milk products, oysters, rhubarb, salmon (canned), sardines (canned), spinach, tofu, yogurt, and calcium fortified foods such as orange juice are high in calcium. Milk and milk products also contain vitamin D and lactose, which assist calcium absorption.
- Recognize anxiety related to test results, and be supportive of impaired activity related to lack of muscular control, perceived loss of independence, and fear of shortened life expectancy.
- Depending on the results of this procedure, additional testing may be performed to evaluate or monitor progression of the disease process and determine the need for a change in therapy. Evaluate test results in relation to the patient's symptoms and other tests performed.

Patient Education:

- Instruct the patient to resume usual diet, fluids, medications, and activity, as directed by the HCP.
- Discuss the implications of abnormal test results on the patient's lifestyle.
- Provide teaching and information regarding the clinical implications of the test results, as appropriate.
- Educate the patient regarding access to counseling services. Provide contact information, if desired, for the National Osteoporosis Foundation (www.nof.org), Institute of Medicine of the National Academies (www.iom.edu), or American College of Rheumatology (www.rheumatology.org).
- Reinforce information given by the patient's HCP regarding further testing, treatment, or referral to another HCP.
- Answer any questions or address any concerns voiced by the patient or family.
- Discuss with the patient the effect of alcohol consumption on nutritional status and calcium intake.

Expected Patient Outcomes:

Understanding

- The patient and family identify the importance of adhering to the recommended therapeutic regime to maintain health.
- The patient and family describe the importance of early intervention on preserving bone density and reducing future risk of falls and fractures.

Ability

- The patient proficiently demonstrates the proper use of assistive devices to support mobility and increase activity.
- The patient independently demonstrates weight-bearing exercises designed to promote bone growth.

Response

- The patient discusses perceived change in physical appearance with a positive attitude.

- The patient and family select positive changes in lifestyle that can preserve bone health.

RELATED STUDIES:

- Related tests include ALP, BMD, calcitonin, calcium, creatinine, creatinine clearance, genetic testing, osteocalcin, PTH, phosphorus, radiography bone, and vitamin D.
- Refer to the Musculoskeletal System table online at Davis*Plus* for related tests by body system.

C

Colonoscopy

SYNONYM/ACRONYM: Full colonoscopy, lower endoscopy, lower panendoscopy.

COMMON USE: To visualize and assess the lower colon for tumor, cancer, and infection.

AREA OF APPLICATION: Colon.

DESCRIPTION: Colonoscopy, a radiological examination of the colon, follows instillation of barium (single contrast study) using a rectal tube inserted into the rectum. The patient retains the contrast while a series of images are obtained, recorded, and available for viewing. Visualization can be improved by draining the barium and using air contrast (double contrast study); some of the barium remains on the surface of the colon wall, allowing for greater detail in the images. A combination of x-ray and fluoroscopic techniques are used to allow inspection of the mucosa of the entire colon, ileocecal valve, and terminal ileum using a flexible fiberoptic colonoscope inserted through the anus and advanced to the terminal ileum. The colonoscope, a multichannel instrument, allows viewing of the gastrointestinal (GI) tract lining, insufflation of air, aspiration of fluid, collection of tissue biopsy samples, and passage of a laser beam for obliteration of tissue and control of bleeding. Mucosal surfaces of the lower GI tract are examined for ulcerations, polyps, chronic diarrhea, hemorrhagic sites, neoplasms, and strictures. During the procedure, tissue samples may be obtained for cytology, and some therapeutic procedures may be performed, such as excision of small tumors or polyps, coagulation of bleeding sites, and removal of foreign bodies. Computed tomography (CT) colonoscopy may be indicated for patients who have diseases rendering them unable to undergo conventional colonoscopy (e.g., bleeding disorders, lung or heart disease) and for patients who are unable to undergo the sedation required for traditional colonoscopy.

This procedure is contraindicated for

- Patients with bleeding disorders or cardiac conditions.
- Patients with bowel perforation, acute peritonitis, acute colitis, ischemic bowel necrosis, toxic colitis, recent bowel surgery, advanced pregnancy, severe cardiac or pulmonary disease, recent myocardial infarction, known or

suspected pulmonary embolus, and large abdominal aortic or iliac aneurysm.

Patients who have had a colon anastomosis within the past 14 to 21 days, ***because an anastomosis may break down with gas insufflation.***

INDICATIONS

- Assess GI function in a patient with a personal or family history of colon cancer, polyps, or ulcerative colitis.
- Confirm diagnosis of colon cancer and inflammatory bowel disease.
- Detect Hirschsprung's disease and determine the areas affected by the disease.
- Determine cause of lower GI disorders, especially when barium enema and proctosigmoidoscopy are inconclusive.
- Determine source of rectal bleeding and perform hemostasis by coagulation.
- Evaluate postsurgical status of colon resection.
- Evaluate stools that show a positive occult blood test, lower GI bleeding, or change in bowel habits.
- Follow up on previously diagnosed and treated colon cancer.
- Investigate iron-deficiency anemia of unknown origin.
- Reduce volvulus and intussusception in children.
- Remove colon polyps.
- Remove foreign bodies and sclerosing strictures by laser.

POTENTIAL MEDICAL DIAGNOSIS

Normal findings

- Normal intestinal mucosa with no abnormalities of structure, function, or mucosal surface in the colon or terminal ileum

Abnormal findings related to

- Benign lesions
- Bleeding sites
- Bowel distention
- Bowel infection or inflammation
- Colitis
- Colon cancer
- Crohn's disease
- Diverticula
- Foreign bodies
- Hemorrhoids
- Polyps
- Proctitis
- Tumors
- Vascular abnormalities

CRITICAL FINDINGS: N/A

INTERFERING FACTORS

Factors that may alter the results of the study

- Gas or feces in the GI tract resulting from inadequate cleansing or failure to restrict food intake before the study.
- Retained barium from a previous radiological procedure.
- Metallic objects (e.g., jewelry, body rings) within the examination field, which may inhibit organ visualization and cause unclear images.
- Inability of the patient to cooperate or remain still during the procedure because of age, significant pain, or mental status.
- Severe lower GI bleeding or the presence of feces, barium, blood, or blood clots, which can interfere with visualization.
- Spasm of the colon, which can mimic the radiographic signs of cancer. (*Note:* The use of intravenous (IV) glucagon minimizes spasm.)
- Inability of the patient to tolerate introduction of or retention of barium, air, or both in the bowel.

Other considerations

- The procedure may be terminated if chest pain or severe cardiac dysrhythmias occur.
- Failure to follow dietary restrictions and other pretesting preparations may cause the procedure to be canceled or repeated.

- **The procedure may be canceled if the patient's weight exceeds the safety limit for the equipment.**
- **Bowel preparations that include laxatives or enemas should be avoided in pregnant patients or patients with inflammatory bowel disease unless specifically directed by a health-care provider (HCP).**

C

NURSING IMPLICATIONS AND PROCEDURE

PRETEST:

- Positively identify the patient using at least two person-specific identifiers before services, treatments, or procedures are performed.
- *Patient Teaching:* Inform the patient this procedure can assist in assessing the colon for disease.
- Obtain a history of the patient's health concerns, symptoms, surgical procedures, and results of previously performed laboratory and diagnostic studies. Include a list of known allergens, especially allergies or sensitivities to latex, anesthetics, or sedatives.
- Note any recent procedures that can interfere with test results, including examinations using barium- or iodine-based contrast medium. Ensure that barium studies were performed more than 4 days before the CT scan.
- Ensure that this procedure is performed before an upper GI study or barium swallow.
- Record the date of the last menstrual period and determine the possibility of pregnancy in perimenopausal women.
- Obtain a list of the patient's current medications, including over-the-counter medications, dietary supplements, anticoagulants, aspirin and other salicylates (see Effects of Natural Products on Laboratory Values online at Davis*Plus*). Such products should be discontinued by medical direction for the appropriate number of days prior to a surgical procedure. Note the last time and dose of medication taken.
- Note intake of oral iron preparations within 1 wk before the procedure because these cause black, sticky feces that are difficult to remove with bowel preparation.
- Review the procedure with the patient. Address concerns about pain and explain that some pain may be experienced during the test, and there may be moments of discomfort. Inform the patient that the procedure is performed in a GI laboratory, by an HCP, with support staff, and takes approximately 30 to 60 min.
- ***Sensitivity to social and cultural issues,*** as well as concern for modesty, is important in providing psychological support before, during, and after the procedure.
- Explain that an IV line may be inserted to allow infusion of fluids such as saline, anesthetics, sedatives, or emergency medications.
- Inform the patient that it is important that the bowel be cleaned thoroughly so that the HCP can visualize the colon. Inform the patient that a laxative and cleansing enema may be needed the day before the procedure, with cleansing enemas on the morning of the procedure, depending on the institution's policy.
- Instruct the patient to remove all external metallic objects from the area to be examined.
- Instruct the patient to eat a low-residue diet for several days before the procedure and to consume only clear liquids the evening before the test.
- Instruct the patient that to reduce the risk of aspiration related to nausea and vomiting, solid food and milk or milk products are restricted for at least 6 hr, and clear liquids are restricted for at least 2 hr prior to general anesthesia, regional anesthesia, or sedation/analgesia (monitored anesthesia). The American Society of Anesthesiologists has fasting guidelines for risk levels according to patient status. More information can be located at www.asahq.org. 🍁 Patients on beta blockers before the surgical procedure

should be instructed to take their medication as ordered during the perioperative period. Protocols may vary among facilities.
- *Make sure a written and informed consent has been signed prior to the procedure and before administering any medications.*

INTRATEST:

Potential Complications:

Complications of the procedure may include bleeding and cardiac dysrhythmias.
- Observe standard precautions, and follow the general guidelines in Patient Preparation and Specimen Collection online at Davis*Plus*. Positively identify the patient, and label the appropriate specimen container with the corresponding patient demographics, initials of the person collecting the specimen, date, and time of collection.
- Ensure that the patient has complied with dietary, fluid and medication restrictions, and pretesting preparations prior to the study, as instructed.
- Ensure that ordered laxatives were administered late in the afternoon of the day before the procedure.
- Assess for completion of bowel preparation according to the institution's procedure.
- Instruct the patient to remove all external metallic objects from the area to be examined.
- Avoid the use of equipment containing latex if the patient has a history of allergic reaction to latex.
- Have emergency equipment readily available.
- Instruct the patient to void prior to the procedure and to change into the gown, robe, and foot coverings provided.
- Instruct the patient to cooperate fully and to follow directions. Instruct the patient to remain still throughout the procedure because movement produces unreliable results.
- Obtain and record baseline vital signs.
- Establish an IV fluid line for the injection of saline, sedatives, or emergency medications.
- Administer medications, as ordered, to reduce discomfort and to promote relaxation and sedation.
- Place the patient on an examination table in the left lateral decubitus position and drape with the buttocks exposed.
- The HCP performs a visual inspection of the perianal area and a digital rectal examination.
- Instruct the patient to bear down as if having a bowel movement as the fiberoptic tube is inserted through the rectum.
- The scope is advanced through the sigmoid. The patient's position is changed to supine to facilitate passage into the transverse colon. Air is insufflated through the tube during passage to aid in visualization.
- Instruct the patient to take deep breaths to aid in movement of the scope downward through the ascending colon to the cecum and into the terminal portion of the ileum.
- Air is insufflated to distend the GI tract, as needed. Biopsies, cultures, or any endoscopic surgery is performed.
- Foreign bodies or polyps are removed and placed in appropriate specimen containers, labelled, and sent to the laboratory.
- Photographs are obtained for future reference.
- At the end of the procedure, excess air and secretions are aspirated through the scope, and the colonoscope is removed.

POST-TEST:

- Inform the patient that a report of the results will be made available to the requesting HCP, who will discuss the results with the patient.
- Monitor the patient for signs of respiratory depression.
- Monitor vital signs and neurological status every 15 min for 1 hr, then every 2 hr for 4 hr, or as ordered. Take temperature every 4 hr for 24 hr.

Monitor intake and output at least every 8 hr. Compare with baseline values. Notify the HCP if temperature is elevated. Protocols may vary among facilities.

- Observe the patient until the effects of the sedation have worn off.
- Instruct the patient to resume usual diet, fluids, medications, and activity, as directed by the HCP.
- Monitor for any rectal bleeding. Instruct the patient to expect slight rectal bleeding for 2 days after removal of polyps or biopsy specimens but that an increasing amount of bleeding or sustained bleeding should be reported to the HCP immediately.
- Instruct the patient to immediately report symptoms such as fast heart rate, difficulty breathing, skin rash, itching, chest pain, persistent right shoulder pain, or abdominal pain. Immediately report symptoms to the appropriate HCP.
- Inform the patient that belching, bloating, or flatulence is the result of air insufflation.
- Encourage the patient to drink several glasses of water to help replace fluids lost during the preparation for the test.
- Carefully monitor the patient for fatigue and fluid and electrolyte imbalance.
- Recognize anxiety related to test results. Discuss the implications of abnormal test results on the patient's lifestyle. Provide teaching and information regarding the clinical implications of the test results, as appropriate.
- Reinforce information given by the patient's HCP regarding further testing, treatment, or referral to another HCP. Decisions regarding the need for and frequency of occult blood testing, colonoscopy, or other cancer screening procedures should be made after consultation between the patient and HCP. The American Cancer Society recommends regular screening for colon cancer, beginning at age 50 yr for individuals without identified risk factors and sooner for those with identified risk factors. Its recommendations for frequency of screening are as follows: annually for occult blood testing (fecal occult blood testing or fecal immunochemical testing); or every 5 yr for flexible sigmoidoscopy, double contrast barium enema, or CT colonography; or every 10 yr for colonoscopy; or every 3 yr for stool DNA testing. 🍁 Abnormal findings should be followed up by colonoscopy. There are advantages and disadvantages to the screening tests that are available today. Methods to use DNA testing of stool are being investigated and are designed to identify abnormal changes in DNA from the cells in the lining of the colon that are normally shed and excreted in stool. The DNA tests under development use multiple markers to identify colon cancers that demonstrate different, abnormal DNA changes. Unlike some of the current screening methods, the DNA tests would be able to detect precancerous polyps. The most current guidelines for colon cancer screening of the general population as well as of individuals with increased risk are available from the American Cancer Society (www.cancer.org), U.S. Preventive Services Task Force (www.uspreventiveservicestaskforce.org), and American College of Gastroenterology (www.gi.org). 🍁
- Depending on the results of this procedure, additional testing may be needed to evaluate or monitor progression of the disease process and determine the need for a change in therapy. Evaluate test results in relation to the patient's symptoms and other tests performed.

RELATED STUDIES:

- Related tests include barium enema, biopsy intestinal, capsule endoscopy, carcinoembryonic and cancer antigens, CT abdomen, CT colonoscopy, fecal analysis, KUB, MRI abdomen, and proctosigmoidoscopy.
- Refer to the Gastrointestinal System table online at Davis*Plus* for related tests by body system.

C

Color Perception Test

SYNONYM/ACRONYM: Color blindness test, Ishihara color perception test, Ishihara pseudoisochromatic plate test.

COMMON USE: To assist in the diagnosis of color blindness.

AREA OF APPLICATION: Eyes.

POTENTIAL MEDICAL DIAGNOSIS

Normal findings

- Normal visual color discrimination; no difficulty in identification of color combinations

Abnormal findings related to

- Identification of some but not all colors

CRITICAL FINDINGS: N/A

Find and print out the full study on Fast Find at davispl.us/vanleeuwen7.

Colposcopy

SYNONYM/ACRONYM: Cervical biopsy, endometrial biopsy.

COMMON USE: To visualize and assess the cervix and vagina related to suspected cancer or other disease.

AREA OF APPLICATION: Vagina and cervix.

POTENTIAL MEDICAL DIAGNOSIS

Normal findings

- Normal appearance of the vagina and cervix
- No abnormal cells or tissues

Abnormal findings related to

- Atrophic changes
- Cervical erosion
- Cervical intraepithelial neoplasia
- Infection
- Inflammation
- Invasive carcinoma
- Leukoplakia
- Papilloma, including condyloma

CRITICAL FINDINGS: N/A

Find and print out the full study on Fast Find at davispl.us/vanleeuwen7.

Complement C3 and Complement C4

SYNONYM/ACRONYM: C3 and C4.

COMMON USE: To assist in the diagnosis of immunological diseases, such as rheumatoid arthritis, and systemic lupus erythematosus (SLE), in which complement is consumed at an increased rate, or to detect inborn deficiency.

SPECIMEN: Serum collected in a red- or red/gray-top tube. Place separated serum into a standard transport tube within 2 hr of collection.

NORMAL FINDINGS: (Method: Immunoturbidimetric)

C3

Age	Conventional Units	SI Units (Conventional Units × 0.01)
Newborn	57–116 mg/dL	0.57–1.16 g/L
6 mo–adult	74–166 mg/dL	0.74–1.66 g/L
Adult	83–177 mg/dL	0.83–1.77 g/L

C4

Age	Conventional Units	SI Units (Conventional Units × 0.01)
Newborn	10–31 mg/dL	0.1–0.31 g/L
6 mo–6 yr	15–52 mg/dL	0.15–0.52 g/L
7–12 yr	19–40 mg/dL	0.19–0.4 g/L
13–15 yr	19–57 mg/dL	0.19–0.57 g/L
16–18 yr	19–42 mg/dL	0.19–0.42 g/L
Adult	12–36 mg/dL	0.12–0.36 g/L

DESCRIPTION: Complement is a system of 25 to 30 distinct cell membrane and plasma proteins, numbered C1 through C9. Once activated, the proteins interact with each other in a specific sequence called the complement cascade. The classical pathway is triggered by antigen-antibody complexes and includes participation of all complement proteins C1 through C9. The alternate pathway occurs when C3, C5, and C9 are activated without participation of C1, C2, and C4 or the presence of antigen-antibody complexes. Complement proteins act as enzymes that aid in the immunological and inflammatory response. The complement system is an important mechanism for the destruction and removal of foreign materials. Serum complement levels are used to detect autoimmune diseases. C3 and C4 are the most frequently assayed complement proteins, along with total complement.

Circulating C3 is synthesized in the liver and comprises 70% of the complement system, but cells in other tissues can also produce C3. C3 is an essential activating protein in the classic and alternate complement cascades. It is decreased in patients with immunological diseases, in whom it is consumed at an increased rate. C4 is produced primarily in the liver but can also be produced by monocytes, fibroblasts, and macrophages. C4 participates in the classic complement pathway.

This procedure is contraindicated for: N/A

INDICATIONS

- Detect genetic deficiencies.
- Evaluate immunological diseases.

POTENTIAL MEDICAL DIAGNOSIS

Normal C4 and decreased C3	Acute glomerulonephritis, membranous glomerulonephritis, immune complex diseases, SLE, C3 deficiency
Decreased C4 and normal C3	Immune complex diseases, cryoglobulinemia, C4 deficiency, hereditary angioedema
Decreased C4 and decreased C3	Immune complex diseases

Increased in:

Response to sudden increased demand

- C3 and C4
  Acute-phase reactions
- C3
  Amyloldosis
  Cancer
  Diabetes
  Myocardial infarction
  Pneumococcal pneumonia
  Pregnancy
  Rheumatic disease
  Thyroiditis
  Viral hepatitis
- C4
  Certain malignancies

Decreased in:

Related to overconsumption during immune response

- C3 and C4
  Hereditary deficiency ***(insufficient production)***
  Liver disease ***(insufficient production related to damaged liver cells)***
  SLE
- C3
  Chronic infection (bacterial, parasitic, viral)
  Post–membranoproliferative glomerulonephritis
  Post–streptococcal infection
  Rheumatic arthritis
- C4
  Angioedema ***(hereditary and acquired)***
  Autoimmune hemolytic anemia
  Autoimmune thyroiditis
  Cryoglobulinemia
  Glomerulonephritis
  Juvenile dermatomyositis
  Meningitis (bacterial, viral)
  Pneumonia
  Streptococcal or staphylococcal sepsis

CRITICAL FINDINGS: N/A

INTERFERING FACTORS

- **Drugs and other substances that may increase C3 levels include cimetidine and cyclophosphamide.**
- **Drugs and other substances that may decrease C3 levels include danazol, methyldopa, and phenytoin.**
- **Drugs and other substances that may increase C4 levels include cimetidine, cyclophosphamide, and danazol.**
- **Drugs and other substances that may decrease C4 levels include dextran and penicillamine.**

NURSING IMPLICATIONS AND PROCEDURE

PRETEST:

- Positively identify the patient using at least two person-specific identifiers before services, treatments, or procedures are performed.
- ***Patient Teaching:*** Inform the patient this test can assist in diagnosing diseases of the immune system.
- Obtain a history of the patient's health concerns, symptoms, surgical procedures, and results of previously performed laboratory and diagnostic studies. Include a list of known allergens, especially allergies or sensitivities to latex.
- Obtain a list of the patient's current medications, including over-the-counter medications and dietary supplements (see Effects of Natural Products on Laboratory Values online at Davis*Plus*).

- Review the procedure with the patient. Inform the patient that specimen collection takes approximately 5 to 10 min. Address concerns about pain and explain that there may be some discomfort during the venipuncture.
- *Sensitivity to social and cultural issues,* as well as concern for modesty, is important in providing psychological support before, during, and after the procedure.
- Note that there are no food, fluid, or medication restrictions unless by medical direction.

INTRATEST:

Potential Complications: N/A

- Avoid the use of equipment containing latex if the patient has a history of allergic reaction to latex.
- Instruct the patient to cooperate fully and to follow directions. Direct the patient to breathe normally and to avoid unnecessary movement.
- Observe standard precautions, and follow the general guidelines in Patient Preparation and Specimen Collection online at Davis*Plus*. Positively identify the patient, and label the appropriate specimen container with the corresponding patient demographics, initials of the person collecting the specimen, date, and time of collection. Perform a venipuncture.
- Remove the needle and apply direct pressure with dry gauze to stop bleeding. Observe/assess venipuncture site for bleeding or hematoma formation and secure gauze with adhesive bandage.
- Promptly transport the specimen to the laboratory for processing and analysis.

POST-TEST:

- Inform the patient that a report of the results will be made available to the requesting health-care provider (HCP), who will discuss the results with the patient.
- Reinforce information given by the patient's HCP regarding further testing, treatment, or referral to another HCP. Answer any questions or address any concerns voiced by the patient or family.
- Depending on the results of this procedure, additional testing may be performed to evaluate or monitor progression of the disease process and determine the need for a change in therapy. Evaluate test results in relation to the patient's symptoms and other tests performed.

RELATED STUDIES:

- Related tests include anticardiolipin antibody, ANA, complement total, cryoglobulin, and ESR.
- Refer to the Immune System table online at Davis*Plus* for related tests by body system.

Complement, Total

SYNONYM/ACRONYM: Total hemolytic complement, CH_{50}, CH_{100}.

COMMON USE: To evaluate immune diseases related to complement activity and follow up on a patient's response to therapy such as treatment for systemic lupus erythematosus (SLE).

SPECIMEN: Serum collected in a red-top tube.

NORMAL FINDINGS: (Method: Quantitative hemolysis)

Conventional Units	SI Units (Conventional Units × 1)
25–110 CH_{50} units/mL	25–110 CH_{50} kilo units/L

Access Canadian content on Fast Find: Lab and Dx at davispl.us/vanleeuwen7

POTENTIAL MEDICAL DIAGNOSIS

Increased in:

- Acute-phase immune response ***(related to sudden response to increased demand)***

Decreased in:

- Autoimmune diseases ***(related to continuous demand)***
- Autoimmune hemolytic anemia ***(related to consumption during hemolytic process)***
- Burns ***(related to increased consumption from initiation of complement cascade)***
- Cryoglobulinemia ***(related to increased consumption)***
- Hereditary deficiency ***(related to insufficient production)***
- Infections ***(bacterial, parasitic, viral; related to increased consumption during immune response)***
- Liver disease ***(related to decreased production by damaged liver cells)***
- Malignancy ***(related to consumption during cellular immune response)***
- Membranous glomerulonephritis ***(related to consumption during cellular immune response)***
- Rheumatoid arthritis ***(related to consumption during immune response)***
- SLE ***(related to consumption during immune response)***
- Trauma ***(related to consumption during immune response)***
- Vasculitis ***(related to consumption during cellular immune response)***

CRITICAL FINDINGS: N/A

Find and print out the full study on Fast Find at davispl.us/vanleeuwen7.

Complete Blood Count

SYNONYM/ACRONYM: CBC.

COMMON USE: To evaluate numerous conditions involving red blood cells, white blood cells, and platelets. This test is also used to indicate inflammation, infection, and response to chemotherapy.

SPECIMEN: Whole blood from one full lavender-top (EDTA) tube or Microtainer. Whole blood from a green-top (lithium or sodium heparin) tube may be submitted, but the following automated values may not be reported: white blood cell (WBC) count, WBC differential, platelet count, immature platelet fraction (IPF), and mean platelet volume.

NORMAL FINDINGS: (Method: Automated, computerized, multichannel analyzers. Many of these analyzers are capable of determining a five- or six-part WBC differential.) This battery of tests includes hemoglobin, hematocrit, red blood cell (RBC) count, RBC morphology, RBC indices, RBC distribution width index (RDWCV and RDWSD), platelet count, platelet size, IPF, WBC count, and WBC differential. The six-part automated WBC differential identifies and enumerates neutrophils, lymphocytes, monocytes, eosinophils, basophils, and immature granulocytes (IG), where IG represents the combined enumeration of promyelocytes, metamyelocytes, and myelocytes as both an absolute number and a percentage. The five-part WBC differential includes all but the IG parameters.

Hemoglobin

Age	Conventional Units	SI Units (Conventional Units × 10)
Cord blood	13.5–20.7 g/dL	135–207 g/L
0–1 wk	15.2–23.6 g/dL	152–236 g/L
2–3 wk	13.3–18.7 g/dL	133–187 g/L
1–2 mo	10.7–18 g/dL	107–180 g/L
3–6 mo	11.7–16.3 g/dL	117–163 g/L
7 mo–1 yr	10.3–14.3 g/dL	103–143 g/L
2–6 yr	10–13.3 g/dL	100–133 g/L
7–15 yr	10.7–14 g/dL	107–140 g/L
16–18 yr	11–15 g/dL	110–150 g/L
Adult		
Male	14–17.3 g/dL	140–173 g/L
Female	11.7–15.5 g/dL	117–155 g/L
Pregnant Female		
1st Trimester	11.6–13.9 g/dL	116–139 g/L
2nd and 3rd Trimester	9.5–11 g/dL	95–110 g/L

Values are slightly lower in older adults.
Reference range values may vary between laboratories.
Note: See "Complete Blood Count, Hemoglobin" study for more detailed information.

Hematocrit

Age	Conventional Units (%)	SI Units (Conventional Units × 0.01) (Volume Fraction)
Cord blood	42–62	0.42–0.62
0–1 wk	46–68	0.46–0.68
2–3 wk	41–56	0.41–0.56
1–2 mo	39–59	0.39–0.59
3–6 mo	35–49	0.35–0.49
7 mo–1 yr	31–43	0.31–0.43
2–6 yr	30–40	0.3–0.4
7–15 yr	32–42	0.32–0.42
16–18 yr	33–45	0.33–0.45
Adult		
Male	42–52	0.42–0.52
Female	36–48	0.36–0.48
Pregnant Female		
1st Trimester	35–42	0.35–0.42
2nd and 3rd Trimester	28–33	0.28–0.33

Values are slightly lower in older adults.
Reference range values may vary between laboratories.
Note: See "Complete Blood Count, Hematocrit" study for more detailed information.

C

White Blood Cell Count and Differential

Age	Conventional Units WBC × 10^3/microL	Neutrophils	Lymphocytes	Monocytes	Eosinophils	Basophils
		(Absolute) and %	(Absolute) and %	(Absolute) and %	(Absolute) and %	(Absolute) and %
Birth	9.1–30.1	(5.5–18.3) 24%–58%	(2.8–9.3) 26%–56%	(0.5–1.7) 7%–13%	(0.02–0.7) 0%–8%	(0.1–0.2) 0%–2.5%
1–23 mo	6.1–17.5	(1.9–5.4) 21%–67%	(3.7–10.7) 20%–64%	(0.3–0.8) 4%–11%	(0.2–0.5) 0%–3.3%	(0–0.1) 0%–1%
2–10 yr	4.5–13.5	(2.4–7.3) 30%–77%	(1.7–5.1) 14%–50%	(0.2–0.6) 4%–9%	(0.1–0.3) 0%–5.8%	(0–0.1) 0%–1%
11 yr–older adult	4.5–11.1	(2.7–6.5) 40%–75%	(1.5–3.7) 12%–44%	(0.2–0.4) 4%–9%	(0.05–0.5) 0%–5.5%	(0–0.1) 0%–1%

*SI Units (Conventional Units × 1 or WBC × 10^9/L).
Note: See "Complete Blood Count, WBC Count and Differential" study for more detailed information.

White Blood Cell Count and Differential

Age	Immature Granulocytes (Absolute) (10^3/microL)	Immature Granulocyte Fraction (IGF) (%)
Birth–9 yr	0–0.03	0%–0.4%
10 yr–older adult	0–0.09	0%–0.9%

C

Red Blood Cell Count

Age	Conventional Units (10^6 cells/microL)	SI Units (10^{12} cells/L) (Conventional Units × 1)
Cord blood	3.61–5.81	3.61–5.81
0–1 wk	4.51–6.01	4.51–6.01
2–3 wk	3.99–6.11	3.99–6.11
1–2 mo	3.71–6.11	3.71–6.11
3–6 mo	3.81–5.61	3.81–5.61
7 mo–1 yr	3.81–5.21	3.81–5.21
2–6 yr	3.91–5.31	3.91–5.31
7–15 yr	3.99–5.21	3.99–5.21
16–18 yr	4.21–5.41	4.21–5.41
Adult		
Male	4.21–5.81	4.21–5.81
Female	3.61–5.11	3.61–5.11

Values are decreased in pregnancy related to the dilutional effects of increased fluid volume and potential nutritional deficiency related to decreased intake, nausea, and/or vomiting. Values are slightly lower in older adults associated with potential nutritional deficiency. Values are slightly lower in older adults.

Note: See "Complete Blood Count, RBC Count" study for more detailed information.

Red Blood Cell Indices

Age	MCV (fl)	MCH (pg/cell)	MCHC (g/dL)	RDWCV	RDWSD
Cord blood	107–119	35–39	31–35	14.9–18.7	51–66
0–1 wk	104–116	29–45	24–36	14.9–18.7	51–66
2–3 wk	95–117	26–38	26–34	14.9–18.7	51–66
1–2 mo	81–125	25–37	26–34	14.9–18.7	44–55
3–11 mo	78–110	22–34	26–34	14.9–18.7	35–46
1–5 yr	74–94	24–32	30–34	11.6–14.8	35–42
6–8 yr	73–93	24–32	32–36	11.6–14.8	35–42
9–14 yr	74–94	25–33	32–36	11.6–14.8	37–44
15 yr–adult					
Male	77–97	26–34	32–36	11.6–14.8	38–48
Female	78–98	26–34	32–36	11.6–14.8	38–48
Older adult					
Male	79–103	27–35	32–36	11.6–14.8	38–48
Female	78–102	27–35	32–36	11.6–14.8	38–48

MCH = mean corpuscular hemoglobin; MCHC = mean corpuscular hemoglobin concentration; MCV = mean corpuscular volume; RDWCV = coefficient of variation in RBC distribution width index;
RDWSD = standard deviation in RBC distribution width index.

Note: See "Complete Blood Count, RBC Indices" study for more detailed information.

Red Blood Cell Morphology

Morphology	Within Normal Limits	1+	2+	3+	4+
Size					
Anisocytosis	0–5	5–10	10–20	20–50	Greater than 50
Macrocytes	0–5	5–10	10–20	20–50	Greater than 50
Microcytes	0–5	5–10	10–20	20–50	Greater than 50
Shape					
Poikilocytes	0–2	3–10	10–20	20–50	Greater than 50
Burr cells	0–2	3–10	10–20	20–50	Greater than 50
Acanthocytes	Less than 1	2–5	5–10	10–20	Greater than 20
Schistocytes	Less than 1	2–5	5–10	10–20	Greater than 20
Dacryocytes (teardrop cells)	0–2	2–5	5–10	10–20	Greater than 20
Codocytes (target cells)	0–2	2–10	10–20	20–50	Greater than 50
Spherocytes	0–2	2–10	10–20	20–50	Greater than 50
Ovalocytes	0–2	2–10	10–20	20–50	Greater than 50
Stomatocytes	0–2	2–10	10–20	20–50	Greater than 50
Drepanocytes (sickle cells)	Absent	Reported as present or absent			
Helmet cells	Absent	Reported as present or absent			
Agglutination	Absent	Reported as present or absent			
Rouleaux	Absent	Reported as present or absent			
Hemoglobin Content					
Hypochromia	0–2	3–10	10–50	50–75	Greater than 75
Polychromasia					
Adult	Less than 1	2–5	5–10	10–20	Greater than 20
Newborn	1–6	7–15	15–20	20–50	Greater than 50

Note: See "Complete Blood Count, RBC Morphology and Inclusions" study for more detailed information.

C

Red Blood Cell Inclusions

Inclusions	Within Normal Limits	1+	2+	3+	4+
Cabot's rings	Absent	Reported as present or absent			
Basophilic stippling	0–1	1–5	5–10	10–20	Greater than 20
Howell-Jolly bodies	Absent	1–2	3–5	5–10	Greater than 10
Heinz bodies	Absent	Reported as present or absent			
Hemoglobin C crystals	Absent	Reported as present or absent			
Pappenheimer bodies	Absent	Reported as present or absent			
Intracellular parasites (e.g., *Plasmodium, Babesia*, trypanosomes)	Absent	Reported as present or absent			

Note: See "Complete Blood Count, RBC Morphology and Inclusions" study for more detailed information.

Platelet Count

Age	Conventional Units	SI Units (Conventional Units × 1)	MPV (fl)	IPF (%)
Birth	150–450 × 10^3/microL	150–450 × 10^9/L	7.1–10.2	1.1–7.1
Child/Adult/ Older adult	140–400 × 10^3/microL	140–400 × 10^9/L	7.1–10.2	1.1–7.1

Note: See "Complete Blood Count, Platelet Count" study for more detailed information. Platelet counts may decrease slightly with age.

DESCRIPTION: A CBC is a group of tests used for basic screening purposes. It is probably the most widely ordered laboratory test. Results provide the enumeration of the cellular elements of the blood, measurement of RBC indices, and determination of cell morphology by automation and evaluation of stained smears. The results can provide valuable diagnostic information regarding the overall health of the patient and the patient's response to disease and treatment. Detailed information is found in studies titled "Complete Blood Count, Hemoglobin," "Complete Blood Count, Hematocrit," "Complete Blood Count, RBC Indices," "Complete

Blood Count, RBC Morphology and Inclusions," "Complete Blood Count, RBC Count," "Complete Blood Count, Platelet Count," and "Complete Blood Count, WBC Count and Cell Differential."

This procedure is contraindicated for: N/A

INDICATIONS

- Detect hematological disorder, neoplasm, leukemia, or immunological abnormality.
- Determine the presence of hereditary hematological abnormality.
- Evaluate known or suspected anemia and related treatment.
- Monitor blood loss and response to blood replacement.
- Monitor the effects of physical or emotional stress.
- Monitor fluid imbalances or treatment for fluid imbalances.
- Monitor hematological status during pregnancy.
- Monitor progression of nonhematological disorders, such as chronic obstructive pulmonary disease, malabsorption syndromes, cancer, and kidney disease.
- Monitor response to chemotherapy and evaluate undesired reactions to drugs that may cause blood dyscrasias.
- Provide screening as part of a general physical examination, especially on admission to a health-care facility or before surgery.

POTENTIAL MEDICAL DIAGNOSIS

- See studies titled "Complete Blood Count, Hemoglobin," "Complete Blood Count, Hematocrit," "Complete Blood Count, RBC Indices," "Complete Blood Count, RBC Morphology and Inclusions," "Complete Blood Count, RBC Count," "Complete Blood Count, Platelet Count," and "Complete Blood Count, WBC Count and Differential."

Increased in:

- See above-listed studies.

Decreased in:

- See above-listed studies.

CRITICAL FINDINGS:

Hemoglobin

Adults & children

- Less than 6.6 g/dL (SI: Less than 66 mmol/L)
- Greater than 20 g/dL (SI: Greater than 200 mmol/L)

Newborns

- Less than 9.5 g/dL (SI: Less than 95 mmol/L)
- Greater than 22.3 g/dL (SI: Greater than 223 mmol/L)

Hematocrit

Adults & children

- Less than 19.8% (SI: Less than 0.2 volume fraction)
- Greater than 60% (SI: Greater than 0.6 volume fraction)

Newborns

- Less than 28.5% (SI: Less than 0.28 volume fraction)
- Greater than 66.9% (SI: Greater than 0.67 volume fraction)

WBC Count (on Admission)

- Less than 2×10^3/microL (SI: Less than 2×10^9/L)
- Absolute neutrophil count of less than 0.5×10^3/microL (SI: Less than 0.5×10^9/L)
- Greater than 30×10^3/microL (SI: Greater than 30×10^9/L)

Platelet Count

- Less than 30×10^3/microL (SI: Less than 30×10^9/L)
- Greater than $1{,}000 \times 10^3$/microL (SI: Greater than $1{,}000 \times 10^9$/L)

Consideration may be given to verifying the critical findings before action is taken. Policies vary among facilities and may include requesting immediate recollection and retesting by the laboratory or retesting using a rapid point-of-care instrument at the bedside, if available.

C

Note and immediately report to the requesting health-care provider (HCP) any critical findings and related symptoms. A listing of these findings varies among facilities. Timely notification of a critical finding for laboratory or diagnostic studies is a role expectation of the professional nurse. The notification processes vary among facilities. Upon receipt of the critical finding, the information should be read back to the caller to verify accuracy.

The presence of abnormal cells, other morphological characteristics, or cellular inclusions may signify a potentially life-threatening or serious health condition and should be investigated. Examples are the presence of sickle cells, moderate numbers of spherocytes, marked schistocytosis, oval macrocytes, basophilic stippling, eosinophil count greater than 10%, monocytosis greater than 15%, nucleated RBCs (if patient is not an infant), malarial organisms, hypersegmented neutrophils, agranular neutrophils, blasts or other immature cells, Auer rods, Döhle bodies, marked toxic granulation, or plasma cells.

INTERFERING FACTORS

- Failure to fill the tube sufficiently (less than three-fourths full) may yield inadequate sample volume for automated analyzers and may be a reason for specimen rejection.
- Hemolyzed or clotted specimens should be rejected for analysis.
- Elevated serum glucose or sodium levels may produce elevated mean corpuscular volume values because of swelling of erythrocytes.
- Recent transfusion history should be considered when evaluating the CBC.

NURSING IMPLICATIONS AND PROCEDURE

PRETEST:

- Positively identify the patient using at least two person-specific identifiers before services, treatments, or procedures are performed.
- ***Patient Teaching:*** Inform the patient this test can assist in evaluating general health and the body's response to illness.
- Obtain a history of the patient's health concerns, including a list of known allergens, especially allergies or sensitivities to latex.
- Obtain a history of the patient's gastrointestinal, hematopoietic, immune, and respiratory systems as well as results of previously performed laboratory tests and diagnostic and surgical procedures.
- Obtain a list of the patient's current medications, including over-the-counter medications, dietary supplements, anticoagulants, aspirin and other salicylates (see Effects of Natural Products on Laboratory Values online at Davis*Plus*). Such products should be discontinued by medical direction for the appropriate number of days prior to a surgical procedure. Note the last time and dose of medication taken.
- Review the procedure with the patient. Inform the patient that specimen collection takes approximately 5 to 10 min. Address concerns about pain and explain that there may be some discomfort during the venipuncture.
- ***Sensitivity to social and cultural issues,*** as well as concern for modesty, is important in providing psychological support before, during, and after the procedure.
- Note that there are no food, fluid, or medication restrictions unless by medical direction.

INTRATEST:

Potential Complications: N/A

- Avoid the use of equipment containing latex if the patient has a history of allergic reaction to latex.
- Instruct the patient to cooperate fully and to follow directions. Direct the patient to breathe normally and to avoid unnecessary movement.
- Observe standard precautions, and follow the general guidelines in Patient Preparation and Specimen Collection online at Davis*Plus*. Positively identify the patient, and label the appropriate specimen container with the corresponding patient demographics, initials of the person collecting the specimen, date, and time of collection. Perform a venipuncture. An EDTA Microtainer sample may be obtained from infants, children, and adults for whom venipuncture may not be feasible. The specimen should be analyzed within 24 hr when stored at room temperature or within 48 hr if stored at refrigerated temperature. If it is anticipated the specimen will not be analyzed within 24 hr, two blood smears should be made immediately after the venipuncture and submitted with the blood sample. Smears made from specimens older than 24 hr may contain an unacceptable number of misleading artifactual abnormalities of the RBCs, such as echinocytes and spherocytes, as well as necrobiotic white blood cells.
- Remove the needle and apply direct pressure with dry gauze to stop bleeding. Observe/assess venipuncture site for bleeding or hematoma formation and secure gauze with adhesive bandage.
- Promptly transport the specimen to the laboratory for processing and analysis.

POST-TEST:

- Inform the patient that a report of the results will be made available to the requesting HCP, who will discuss the results with the patient.
- *Nutritional Considerations:* Instruct patients to consume a variety of foods within the basic food groups, maintain a healthy weight, be physically active, limit salt intake, limit alcohol intake, and avoid use of tobacco.
- Reinforce information given by the patient's HCP regarding further testing, treatment, or referral to another HCP. Answer any questions or address any concerns voiced by the patient or family.
- Depending on the results of this procedure, additional testing may be performed to evaluate or monitor progression of the disease process and determine the need for a change in therapy. Evaluate test results in relation to the patient's symptoms and other tests performed.

RELATED STUDIES:

- Related tests include alveolar arterial ratio, biopsy bone marrow, blood gases, blood groups and antibodies, erythropoietin, ferritin, CBC hematocrit, CBC hemoglobin, CBC platelet count, CBC RBC count, CBC RBC indices, CBC RBC morphology, CBC WBC count and cell differential, iron/TIBC, lead, pulse oximetry, and reticulocyte count.
- Refer to the Gastrointestinal, Hematopoietic, Immune, and Respiratory systems tables online at Davis*Plus* for related tests by body system.

Complete Blood Count, Hematocrit

SYNONYM/ACRONYM: Packed cell volume (PCV), Hct.

COMMON USE: To evaluate anemia, polycythemia, and hydration status and to monitor therapy.

SPECIMEN: Whole blood from one full lavender-top (EDTA) tube, Microtainer, or capillary. Whole blood from a green-top (lithium or sodium heparin) tube may also be submitted.

NORMAL FINDINGS: (Method: Automated, computerized, multichannel analyzers)

Age	Conventional Units (%)	SI Units (Conventional Units × 0.01) (Volume Fraction)
Cord blood	42–62	0.42–0.62
0–1 wk	46–68	0.46–0.68
2–3 wk	41–56	0.41–0.56
1–2 mo	39–59	0.39–0.59
3–6 mo	35–49	0.35–0.49
7 mo–1 yr	31–43	0.31–0.43
2–6 yr	30–40	0.3–0.4
7–15 yr	32–42	0.32–0.42
16–18 yr	33–45	0.33–0.45
Adult		
Male	42–52	0.42–0.52
Female	36–48	0.36–0.48
Pregnant Female		
1st Trimester	35–42	0.35–0.42
2nd and 3rd Trimester	28–33	0.28–0.33

Values are slightly lower in older adults.
Reference range values may vary between laboratories.

DESCRIPTION: Blood consists of a liquid plasma portion and a solid cellular portion. The solid portion is comprised of red blood cells (RBCs), white blood cells (WBCs), and platelets. It is important to be able to assess whether there is a sufficient number of circulating RBCs to transport the required amount of oxygen throughout the body. The hematocrit (Hct) is a mathematical expression of the number of RBCs, or packed cell volume, expressed as a percentage of whole blood. For example, a packed cell volume, or Hct of 45% means that a 100-mL sample of blood contains 45 mL of packed RBCs, which would reflect an acceptable level of RBCs for a patient of any given age. The Hct depends primarily on the number of RBCs, however the average size of the RBCs influences Hct. Conditions that cause RBC size to be increased (e.g., swelling of the RBC due to change in osmotic pressure related to elevated sodium levels) may increase the Hct while conditions that result in smaller than normal RBCs (e.g., microcytosis related to iron deficiency anemia) may decrease the Hct. Hct can be estimated directly by centrifuging a sample of whole blood for a specific time period. As the blood spins it is separated into fractions. The RBC fraction is read against a scale. Most often the Hct is measured indirectly, by multiplying the RBC count and mean cell volume (MCV), using an automated cell counter. Hct can also be estimated by multiplying the hemoglobin (Hgb) by three.

The Hct level is part of the complete blood count (CBC). Frequently, Hct and Hgb measures are requested together as an H&H. H&H levels parallel each other and are the best determinant of the degree of anemia or polycythemia. *Polycythemia* is a term used in conjunction with conditions resulting from an abnormal increase in Hgb, Hct, and RBC counts. *Anemia* is a term associated with conditions resulting from an abnormal decrease in Hgb, Hct, and RBC counts. Results of the Hgb, Hct, and RBC counts should be evaluated simultaneously because the same underlying conditions affect this triad of tests similarly. The RBC count multiplied by 3 should approximate the Hgb concentration. The Hct should be within 3 times the Hgb if the RBC population is normal in size and shape. The Hct plus 6 should approximate the first two figures of the RBC count within 3 (e.g., Hct is 40%; therefore, 40 + 6 = 46, and the RBC count should be 4.6 or in the range of 4.3 to 4.9). There are some ethnic variations in H&H values. After the first decade of life, the mean Hgb in African Americans is 0.5 to 1 g lower than in individuals of European descent.

This procedure is contraindicated for: N/A

INDICATIONS

- Detect hematological disorder, neoplasm, or immunological abnormality.
- Determine the presence of hereditary hematological abnormality.
- Evaluate known or suspected anemia and related treatment, in combination with Hgb.
- Monitor blood loss and response to blood replacement, in combination with Hgb.
- Monitor the effects of physical or emotional stress on the patient.
- Monitor fluid imbalances or their treatment.
- Monitor hematological status during pregnancy, in combination with Hgb.
- Monitor the progression of nonhematological disorders such as chronic obstructive pulmonary disease, malabsorption syndromes, cancer, and renal disease.
- Monitor response to drugs or chemotherapy, and evaluate undesired reactions to drugs that may cause blood dyscrasias.
- Provide screening as part of a CBC in a general physical examination, especially upon admission to a health-care facility or before surgery.

POTENTIAL MEDICAL DIAGNOSIS

Increased in:

- Burns ***(related to dehydration; total blood volume is decreased, but RBC count remains the same)***
- Chronic obstructive pulmonary disease ***(related to chronic hypoxia that stimulates production of RBC and a corresponding increase in Hct)***
- Dehydration ***(total blood volume is decreased, but RBC count remains the same)***
- Erythrocytosis ***(total blood volume remains the same, but RBC count is increased)***
- Heart failure ***(when the underlying cause is anemia, the body responds by increasing production of RBCs with a corresponding increase in Hct)***

- Hemoconcentration ***(same effect as seen in dehydration)***
- High altitudes ***(related to hypoxia that stimulates production of RBC and therefore increases Hct)***
- Polycythemia ***(abnormal bone marrow response resulting in overproduction of RBC)***
- Shock

C

Decreased in:

- Anemia ***(overall decrease in RBC and corresponding decrease in Hct)***
- Blood loss (acute and chronic) ***(overall decrease in RBC and corresponding decrease in Hct)***
- Bone marrow hyperplasia ***(bone marrow failure that results in decreased RBC production)***
- Carcinoma ***(anemia is often associated with chronic disease)***
- Chronic disease ***(anemia is often associated with chronic disease)***
- Chronic kidney disease ***(related to decreased levels of erythropoietin, which stimulates production of RBCs)***
- Cirrhosis ***(related to accumulation of fluid)***
- Fluid retention ***(dilutional effect of increased blood volume while RBC count remains stable)***
- Hemoglobinopathies ***(reduced RBC survival with corresponding decrease in Hgb)***
- Hemolytic disorders (e.g., hemolytic anemias, prosthetic valves) ***(reduced RBC survival with corresponding decrease in Hct)***
- Hemorrhage (acute and chronic) ***(related to loss of RBC that exceeds rate of production)***
- Hodgkin's disease ***(bone marrow failure that results in decreased RBC production)***
- Incompatible blood transfusion ***(reduced RBC survival with corresponding decrease in Hgb)***
- Intravenous (IV) overload ***(dilutional effect)***
- Fluid retention ***(dilutional effect of increased blood volume while RBC count remains stable)***
- Leukemia ***(bone marrow failure that results in decreased RBC production)***
- Lymphomas ***(bone marrow failure that results in decreased RBC production)***
- Nutritional deficit ***(anemia related to dietary deficiency in iron, vitamins, folate needed to produce sufficient RBC; decreased RBC count with corresponding decrease in Hct)***
- Pregnancy ***(related to anemia)***
- Splenomegaly ***(total blood volume remains the same, but spleen retains RBCs and Hct reflects decreased RBC count)***

CRITICAL FINDINGS:

Adults & children

- Less than 19.8% (SI: Less than 0.2 volume fraction)
- Greater than 60% (SI: Greater than 0.6 volume fraction)

Newborns

- Less than 28.5% (SI: Less than 0.28 volume fraction)
- Greater than 66.9% (SI: Greater than 0.67 volume fraction)

Note and immediately report to the requesting health-care provider (HCP) any critical findings and related symptoms. A listing of these findings varies among facilities. Timely notification of a critical finding for laboratory or diagnostic studies is a role expectation of the professional nurse. The notification processes vary among facilities. Upon receipt of the critical finding, the information should be read back to the caller to verify accuracy.

Consideration may be given to verifying the critical findings before action is taken. Policies vary among facilities and may include requesting immediate recollection and retesting by the laboratory.

Low Hct leads to anemia. Anemia can be caused by blood loss, decreased blood cell production, increased blood cell destruction, and hemodilution. Causes of blood loss include menstrual excess or frequency, gastrointestinal bleeding, inflammatory bowel disease, and hematuria. Decreased blood cell production can be caused by folic acid deficiency, vitamin B_{12} deficiency, iron deficiency, and chronic disease. Increased blood cell destruction can be caused by a hemolytic reaction, chemical reaction, medication reaction, and sickle cell disease. Hemodilution can be caused by heart failure, chronic kidney disease, polydipsia, and overhydration. Symptoms of anemia (due to these causes) include anxiety, dyspnea, edema, hypertension, hypotension, hypoxia, jugular venous distention, fatigue, pallor, rales, restlessness, and weakness. Treatment of anemia depends on the cause.

High Hct leads to polycythemia. Polycythemia can be caused by dehydration, decreased oxygen levels in the body, and an overproduction of RBCs by the bone marrow. Dehydration from diuretic use, vomiting, diarrhea, excessive sweating, severe burns, or decreased fluid intake decreases the plasma component of whole blood, thereby increasing the ratio of RBCs to plasma, and leads to a higher than normal Hct. Causes of decreased oxygen include smoking, exposure to carbon monoxide, high altitude, and chronic lung disease, which leads to a mild hemoconcentration of blood in the body to carry more oxygen to the body's tissues. An overproduction of RBCs by the bone marrow leads to polycythemia vera, which is a rare chronic myeloproliferative disorder that leads to a severe hemoconcentration of blood. Severe hemoconcentration can lead to thrombosis (spontaneous blood clotting). Symptoms of hemoconcentration include decreased pulse pressure and volume, loss of skin turgor, dry mucous membranes, headaches, hepatomegaly, low central venous pressure, orthostatic hypotension, pruritus (especially after a hot bath), splenomegaly, tachycardia, thirst, tinnitus, vertigo, and weakness. Treatment of polycythemia depends on the cause. Possible interventions for hemoconcentration due to dehydration include IV fluids and discontinuance of diuretics if they are believed to be contributing to critically elevated Hct. Polycythemia due to decreased oxygen states can be treated by removal of the offending substance, such as smoke or carbon monoxide. Treatment includes oxygen therapy in cases of smoke inhalation, carbon monoxide poisoning, and desaturating chronic lung disease. Symptoms of polycythemic overload crisis include signs of thrombosis, pain and redness in the extremities, facial flushing, and irritability. Possible interventions for hemoconcentration due to polycythemia include therapeutic phlebotomy and IV fluids.

INTERFERING FACTORS

- Drugs and other substances that may cause a decrease in Hct include those that induce hemolysis due to drug sensitivity or enzyme deficiency and those that result in anemia (see study titled "Complete Blood Count, RBC Count").
- Some drugs and other substances may also affect Hct values by increasing the RBC count (see study titled "Complete Blood Count, RBC Count").
- The results of RBC counts may vary depending on the patient's

position: Hct can decrease when the patient is recumbent as a result of hemodilution and can increase when the patient rises as a result of hemoconcentration.

- Leaving the tourniquet in place for longer than 60 sec can falsely increase Hct levels by 2% to 5%.
- Traumatic venipuncture and hemolysis may result in falsely decreased Hct values.
- Failure to fill the tube sufficiently (i.e., tube less than three-quarters full) may yield inadequate sample volume for automated analyzers and may be a reason for specimen rejection.
- Clotted or hemolyzed specimens must be rejected for analysis.
- The results of a CBC should be carefully evaluated during transfusion or acute blood loss because the body is not in a state of homeostasis and values may be misleading. Considerations for draw times after transfusion include the type of product, the amount of product transfused, and the patient's clinical situation. Generally, specimens collected an hour after transfusion will provide an acceptable reflection of the effects of the transfused product. Measurements taken during a massive transfusion are an exception, providing essential guidance for therapeutic decisions during critical care.
- Abnormalities in the RBC size (macrocytes, microcytes) or shape (spherocytes, sickle cells) may alter Hct values, as in diseases and conditions including sickle cell anemia, hereditary spherocytosis, and iron deficiency.
- Elevated blood glucose or serum sodium levels may produce elevated Hct levels because of swelling of the erythrocytes.

NURSING IMPLICATIONS AND PROCEDURE

PRETEST:

- Positively identify the patient using at least two person-specific identifiers before services, treatments, or procedures are performed.
- ***Patient Teaching:*** Inform the patient this test can assist in evaluating the body's blood cell volume status.
- Obtain a history of the patient's health concerns, symptoms, surgical procedures, and results of previously performed laboratory and diagnostic studies. Include a list of known allergens, especially allergies or sensitivities to latex.
- Note any recent procedures that can interfere with test results.
- Obtain a list of the patient's current medications, including over-the-counter medications and dietary supplements (see Effects of Natural Products on Laboratory Values online at Davis*Plus*).
- Review the procedure with the patient. Inform the patient that specimen collection takes approximately 5 to 10 min. Address concerns about pain and explain that there may be some discomfort during the venipuncture.
- ***Sensitivity to social and cultural issues,*** as well as concern for modesty, is important in providing psychological support before, during, and after the procedure.
- Note that there are no food, fluid, or medication restrictions unless by medical direction.

INTRATEST:

Potential Complications: N/A

- Avoid the use of equipment containing latex if the patient has a history of allergic reaction to latex.
- Instruct the patient to cooperate fully and to follow directions. Direct the patient to breathe normally and to avoid unnecessary movement.
- Observe standard precautions, and follow the general guidelines

in Patient Preparation and Specimen Collection online at DavisPlus. Positively identify the patient, and label the appropriate tubes with the corresponding patient demographics, date, and time of collection. Perform a venipuncture; collect the specimen in a 5-mL lavender-top (EDTA) tube. An EDTA Microtainer sample may be obtained from infants, children, and adults for whom venipuncture may not be feasible. The specimen should be mixed gently by inverting the tube 10 times. The specimen should be analyzed within 24 hr when stored at room temperature or within 48 hr if stored at refrigerated temperature. If it is anticipated the specimen will not be analyzed within 24 hr, two blood smears should be made immediately after the venipuncture and submitted with the blood sample. Smears made from specimens older than 24 hr may contain an unacceptable number of misleading artifactual abnormalities of the RBCs, such as echinocytes and spherocytes, as well as necrobiotic white blood cells.

- Remove the needle and apply direct pressure with dry gauze to stop bleeding. Observe/assess venipuncture site for bleeding or hematoma formation and secure gauze with adhesive bandage.
- Promptly transport the specimen to the laboratory for processing and analysis.

POST-TEST:

- Inform the patient that a report of the results will be made available to the requesting HCP, who will discuss the results with the patient.
- ***Nutritional Considerations:*** Nutritional therapy may be indicated for patients with increased Hct if iron levels are also elevated. Educate the patient with abnormally elevated iron values, as appropriate, on the importance of reading food labels. Patients with hemochromatosis or acute pernicious anemia should be educated to avoid foods rich in iron. Iron absorption is affected by numerous factors that may enhance or decrease absorption regardless of the original content of the iron-containing dietary source (see study titled "Iron"). Iron levels in foods can be increased if foods are cooked in cookware containing iron. Consumption of large amounts of alcohol damages the intestine and allows increased absorption of iron. A high intake of calcium and ascorbic acid also increases iron absorption. Iron absorption after a meal is also increased by factors in meat, fish, and poultry.
- ***Nutritional Considerations:*** Nutritional therapy may be indicated for patients with decreased Hct. Iron deficiency is the most common nutrient deficiency in the United States. Patients at risk (e.g., children, pregnant women, women of childbearing age, and low-income populations) should be instructed to include in their diet foods that are high in iron, such as meats (especially liver), eggs, grains, green leafy vegetables, and multivitamins with iron. Educate the patient with abnormally elevated iron values, as appropriate, on the importance of reading food labels. Iron absorption is decreased by the absence (gastric resection) or diminished presence (use of antacids) of gastric acid.
- Reinforce information given by the patient's HCP regarding further testing, treatment, or referral to another HCP. Answer any questions or address any concerns voiced by the patient or family. Educate the patient regarding access to nutritional counseling services. Provide contact information, if desired, for the Institute of Medicine of the National Academies (www.iom.edu) or the USDA's resource for nutrition (www.choosemyplate.gov). 🍁
- Depending on the results of this procedure, additional testing may be performed to evaluate or monitor progression of the disease process and determine the need for a change in therapy. Evaluate test results in relation to the patient's symptoms and other tests performed.

RELATED STUDIES:

- Related tests include biopsy bone marrow, CBC, CBC hemoglobin, CBC RBC indices, CBC RBC morphology, erythropoietin, ferritin, iron/TIBC, and reticulocyte count.
- Refer to the Cardiovascular, Gastrointestinal, Hematopoietic, Hepatobiliary, Immune, and Respiratory systems tables online at Davis*Plus* for related tests by body system.

Complete Blood Count, Hemoglobin

SYNONYM/ACRONYM: Hgb.

COMMON USE: To evaluate anemia, polycythemia, hydration status, and monitor therapy such as transfusion.

SPECIMEN: Whole blood from one full lavender-top (EDTA) tube, Microtainer, or capillary. Whole blood from a green-top (lithium or sodium heparin) tube may also be submitted.

NORMAL FINDINGS: (Method: Spectrophotometry)

Age	Conventional Units	SI Units (Conventional Units × 10)
Cord blood	13.5–20.7 g/dL	135–207 g/L
0–1 wk	15.2–23.6 g/dL	152–236 g/L
2–3 wk	13.3–18.7 g/dL	133–187 g/L
1–2 mo	10.7–18 g/dL	107–180 g/L
3–6 mo	11.7–16.3 g/dL	117–163 g/L
7 mo–1 yr	10.3–14.3 g/dL	103–143 g/L
2–6 yr	10–13.3 g/dL	100–133 g/L
7–15 yr	10.7–14 g/dL	107–140 g/L
16–18 yr	11–15 g/dL	110–150 g/L
Adult		
Male	14–17.3 g/dL	140–173 g/L
Female	11.7–15.5 g/dL	117–155 g/L
Pregnant Female		
1st Trimester	11.6–13.9 g/dL	116–139 g/L
2nd and 3rd Trimester	9.5–11 g/dL	95–110 g/L

Values are slightly lower in older adults.
Reference range values may vary between laboratories.

DESCRIPTION: Hemoglobin (Hgb) is the main intracellular protein of erythrocytes. It carries oxygen (O_2) to and removes carbon dioxide (CO_2) from red blood cells (RBCs). It also serves as a buffer to maintain acid-base balance in the extracellular fluid. Each Hgb molecule consists of heme and globulin. Copper is a cofactor necessary for the enzymatic incorporation of iron molecules into heme. Heme contains iron and porphyrin molecules that have a high affinity for O_2. The affinity of Hgb molecules for O_2 is influenced by 2,3-diphosphoglycerate (2,3-DPG), a substance produced by anaerobic glycolysis to generate energy for the RBCs. When Hgb binds with 2,3-DPG, O_2 affinity decreases. The ability of Hgb to bind and release O_2 can be graphically represented by an oxyhemoglobin dissociation curve. The term *shift to the left* describes an increase in the affinity of Hgb for O_2. Conditions that can cause this leftward shift include decreased body temperature, decreased 2,3-DPG, decreased CO_2 concentration, and increased pH. Conversely, a *shift to the right* represents a decrease in the affinity of Hgb for O_2. Conditions that can cause a rightward shift include increased body temperature, increased 2,3-DPG levels, increased CO_2 concentration, and decreased pH.

Hgb levels are a direct reflection of the O_2-combining capacity of the blood. It is the combination of heme and O_2 that gives blood its characteristic red color. RBC counts parallel the O_2-combining capacity of Hgb, but because some RBCs contain more Hgb than others, the relationship is not directly proportional. As CO_2 diffuses into RBCs, an enzyme called carbonic anhydrase converts the CO_2 into bicarbonate and hydrogen ions. Hgb that is not bound to O_2 combines with the free hydrogen ions, increasing pH. As this binding is occurring, bicarbonate is leaving the RBC in exchange for chloride ions. (For additional information about the relationship between the respiratory and renal components of this buffer system, see study titled "Blood Gases.")

Hgb is included in the complete blood count (CBC). Frequently, Hct and Hgb measures are requested together as an H&H. H&H levels parallel each other and are frequently used to evaluate anemia. *Polycythemia* is a condition resulting from an abnormal increase in Hgb, Hct, and RBC count. *Anemia* is a condition resulting from an abnormal decrease in Hgb, Hct, and RBC count. Results of the Hgb, Hct, and RBC count should be evaluated simultaneously because the same underlying conditions affect this triad of tests similarly. The RBC count multiplied by 3 should approximate the Hgb concentration. The Hct should be within three times the Hgb if the RBC population is normal in size and shape. The Hct plus 6 should approximate the first two figures of the RBC count within 3 (e.g., Hct is 40%; therefore, 40 + 6 = 46, and the RBC count should be 4.6 or in the range of 4.3 to 4.9). There are some ethnic variations in H&H values. After the first decade of life, the mean Hgb in African Americans is 0.5 to 1 g lower than in individuals of European descent.

This procedure is contraindicated for: N/A

INDICATIONS

- Detect hematological disorder, neoplasm, or immunological abnormality.
- Determine the presence of hereditary hematological abnormality.
- Evaluate known or suspected anemia and related treatment, in combination with Hct.

C

C

- Monitor blood loss and response to blood replacement, in combination with Hct.
- Monitor the effects of physical or emotional stress on the patient.
- Monitor fluid imbalances or their treatment.
- Monitor hematological status during pregnancy, in combination with Hct.
- Monitor the progression of nonhematological disorders, such as chronic obstructive pulmonary disease (COPD), malabsorption syndromes, cancer, and kidney disease.
- Monitor response to drugs or chemotherapy and evaluate undesired reactions to drugs that may cause blood dyscrasias.
- Provide screening as part of a CBC in a general physical examination, especially upon admission to a health-care facility or before surgery.

POTENTIAL MEDICAL DIAGNOSIS

Increased in:

- Burns ***(related to dehydration; total blood volume is decreased, but RBC count remains the same)***
- COPD ***(related to chronic hypoxia that stimulates production of RBCs and a corresponding increase in Hgb)***
- Dehydration ***(total blood volume is decreased, but RBC count remains the same)***
- Erythrocytosis ***(total blood volume remains the same, but RBC count is increased)***
- Heart failure ***(when the underlying cause is anemia, the body responds by increasing production of RBCs with a corresponding increase in Hct)***
- Hemoconcentration ***(same effect as seen in dehydration)***
- High altitudes ***(related to hypoxia that stimulates production of RBCs and therefore increases Hgb)***
- Polycythemia vera ***(abnormal bone marrow response resulting in overproduction of RBCs)***
- Shock

Decreased in:

- Anemias ***(overall decrease in RBCs and corresponding decrease in Hgb)***
- Blood loss (acute and chronic) ***(overall decrease in RBC and corresponding decrease in Hct)***
- Bone marrow hyperplasia ***(bone marrow failure that results in decreased RBC production)***
- Carcinoma ***(anemia is often associated with chronic disease)***
- Chronic disease ***(anemia is often associated with chronic disease)***
- Chronic kidney disease ***(related to decreased levels of erythropoietin, which stimulates production of RBCs)***
- Cirrhosis ***(related to accumulation of fluid)***
- Fluid retention ***(dilutional effect of increased blood volume while RBC count remains stable)***
- Hemoglobinopathies ***(reduced RBC survival with corresponding decrease in Hgb)***
- Hemolytic disorders (e.g., hemolytic anemias, prosthetic valves) ***(reduced RBC survival with corresponding decrease in Hct)***
- Hemorrhage (acute and chronic) ***(overall decrease in RBCs and corresponding decrease in Hgb)***
- Hodgkin's disease ***(bone marrow failure that results in decreased RBC production)***
- Incompatible blood transfusion ***(reduced RBC survival with corresponding decrease in Hgb)***
- Intravenous (IV) overload ***(dilutional effect)***
- Leukemia ***(bone marrow failure that results in decreased RBC production)***

- Lymphomas ***(bone marrow failure that results in decreased RBC production)***
- Nutritional deficit ***(anemia related to dietary deficiency in iron, vitamins, folate needed to produce sufficient RBCs; decreased RBC count with corresponding decrease in Hgb)***
- Pregnancy ***(related to anemia)***
- Splenomegaly ***(total blood volume remains the same, but spleen retains RBCs and Hgb reflects decreased RBC count)***

CRITICAL FINDINGS:

Adults & children

- Less than 6.6 g/dL (SI: Less than 66 mmol/L)
- Greater than 20 g/dL (SI: Greater than 200 mmol/L)

Newborns

- Less than 9.5 g/dL (SI: Less than 95 mmol/L)
- Greater than 22.3 g/dL (SI: Greater than 223 mmol/L)

Note and immediately report to the requesting health-care provider (HCP) any critical findings and related symptoms. A listing of these findings varies among facilities. Timely notification of a critical finding for laboratory or diagnostic studies is a role expectation of the professional nurse. The notification processes vary among facilities. Upon receipt of the critical finding, the information should be read back to the caller to verify accuracy.

Consideration may be given to verifying the critical findings before action is taken. Policies vary among facilities and may include requesting immediate recollection and retesting by the laboratory.

Low Hgb leads to anemia. Anemia can be caused by blood loss, decreased blood cell production, increased blood cell destruction, and hemodilution. Causes of blood loss include menstrual excess or frequency, gastrointestinal bleeding, inflammatory bowel disease, and hematuria. Decreased blood cell production can be caused by folic acid deficiency, vitamin B_{12} deficiency, iron deficiency, and chronic disease. Increased blood cell destruction can be caused by a hemolytic reaction, chemical reaction, medication reaction, and sickle cell disease. Hemodilution can be caused by heart failure, chronic kidney disease, polydipsia, and overhydration. Symptoms of anemia (due to these causes) include anxiety, dyspnea, edema, fatigue, hypertension, hypotension, hypoxia, jugular venous distention, pallor, rales, restlessness, and weakness. Treatment of anemia depends on the cause.

High Hgb leads to polycythemia. Polycythemia can be caused by dehydration, decreased oxygen levels in the body, and an overproduction of RBCs by the bone marrow. Dehydration from diuretic use, vomiting, diarrhea, excessive sweating, severe burns, or decreased fluid intake decreases the plasma component of whole blood, thereby increasing the ratio of RBCs to plasma, and leads to a higher than normal Hgb. Causes of decreased oxygen include smoking, exposure to carbon monoxide, high altitude, and chronic lung disease, which leads to a mild hemoconcentration of blood in the body to carry more oxygen to the body's tissues. An overproduction of RBCs by the bone marrow leads to polycythemia vera, which is a rare chronic myeloproliferative disorder that leads to a severe hemoconcentration of blood. Severe hemoconcentration can lead to thrombosis (spontaneous blood clotting). Symptoms of hemoconcentration include decreased pulse pressure and volume,

C

loss of skin turgor, dry mucous membranes, headaches, hepatomegaly, low central venous pressure, orthostatic hypotension, pruritus (especially after a hot bath), splenomegaly, tachycardia, thirst, tinnitus, vertigo, and weakness. Treatment of polycythemia depends on the cause. Possible interventions for hemoconcentration due to dehydration include IV fluids and discontinuance of diuretics if they are believed to be contributing to critically elevated Hgb. Polycythemia due to decreased oxygen states can be treated by removal of the offending substance, such as smoke or carbon monoxide. Treatment includes oxygen therapy in cases of smoke inhalation, carbon monoxide poisoning, and desaturating chronic lung disease. Symptoms of polycythemic overload crisis include signs of thrombosis, pain and redness in extremities, facial flushing, and irritability. Possible interventions for hemoconcentration due to polycythemia include therapeutic phlebotomy and IV fluids.

C

INTERFERING FACTORS

- Drugs and other substances that may cause a decrease in Hgb include those that induce hemolysis due to drug sensitivity or enzyme deficiency and those that result in anemia (see study titled "Complete Blood Count, RBC Count").
- Some drugs and other substances may also affect Hgb values by increasing the RBC count (see study titled "Complete Blood Count, RBC Count").
- The results of RBC counts may vary depending on the patient's position: Hgb can decrease when the patient is recumbent as a result of hemodilution and can increase when the patient rises as a result of hemoconcentration.
- Use of the nutraceutical liver extract is strongly contraindicated in iron-storage disorders, such as hemochromatosis, because it is rich in heme (the iron-containing pigment in Hgb).
- A severe copper deficiency may result in decreased Hgb levels.
- Cold agglutinins may falsely increase the mean corpuscular Hgb concentration (MCHC) and decrease the RBC count, affecting Hgb values. This can be corrected by warming the blood or replacing the plasma with warmed saline and repeating the analysis.
- Leaving the tourniquet in place for longer than 60 sec can falsely increase Hgb levels by 2% to 5%.
- Failure to fill the tube sufficiently (i.e., tube less than three-quarters full) may yield inadequate sample volume for automated analyzers and may be a reason for specimen rejection.
- Clotted or hemolyzed specimens must be rejected for analysis.
- Care should be taken in evaluating the Hgb during the first few hours after transfusion or acute blood loss because the value may appear to be normal and may not be a reliable indicator of anemia or therapeutic response to treatment.
- Abnormalities in the RBC size (macrocytes, microcytes) or shape (spherocytes, sickle cells) may alter Hgb values, as in diseases and conditions including sickle cell anemia, hereditary spherocytosis, and iron deficiency.
- Lipemia will falsely increase the Hgb measurement, also affecting the mean corpuscular volume (MCV) and MCHC. This can be corrected by replacing the plasma with saline, repeating the measurement, and manually correcting the Hgb, MCH, and MCHC using specific mathematical formulas.

C

NURSING IMPLICATIONS AND PROCEDURE

POTENTIAL NURSING PROBLEMS:

Problem	Signs & Symptoms	Interventions
Fatigue ***(related to decreased oxygenation associated with a decreased number of RBCs)***	Verbalization of fatigue; altered ability to perform activities of daily living due to lack of energy; shortness of breath with exertion; increasingly frequent rest periods; presence of fatigue after sleep; inability to adhere to daily routine; altered level of concentration; reports of tiredness	Monitor and trend CBC, Hgb, Hct; monitor for shortness of breath; use oxygen administration and pulse oximetry as appropriate; assess ability to perform self-care; assess nutritional intake; encourage frequent rest periods; teach techniques for conserving energy expenditure; administer blood and blood products as ordered; monitor urine, stool, and sputum for bleeding; assess for medical or psychological factors contributing to fatigue; prioritize and bundle activities to conserve energy and decrease fatigue; administer prescribed erythropoietin
Bleeding ***(related to malfunction of bone marrow)***	Altered level of consciousness; hypotension; increased heart rate; decreased Hgb and Hct; capillary refill greater than 3 sec; cool extremities	Monitor and trend platelet count; increase frequency of vital sign assessment with variances in results; monitor for vital sign trends; administer blood or blood products as ordered; administer stool softeners as needed; monitor and assess stool, urine, sputum, gums, and nose for blood; coordinate laboratory draws to decrease frequency of venipuncture; institute bleeding precautions (avoid intramuscular injections, prevent trauma, be gentle with oral care and suctioning, avoid use of a sharp razor); administer prescribed medications; assess diet for iron-rich foods and foods with vitamin K

(table continues on page 484)

C

Problem	Signs & Symptoms	Interventions
Activity ***(related to decreased oxygen-carrying capacity of the blood secondary to anemia; decreased number of RBCs)***	Weakness; fatigue; shortness of breath with activity; dizziness; palpitations; headache; verbalization of difficulty with activity tolerance	Assess for fall risk and implement strategies commensurate with level of risk; administer prescribed oxygen; use pulse oximetry; administer blood and blood products as ordered; monitor for transfusion reaction; coordinate episodes of activity with rest periods; increase activity gradually as anemia resolves
Knowledge ***(related to lack of resources; unfamiliarity with disease process; complexity of disease process and treatment; new disease process)***	Asks multiple questions; asks too few questions; inaccurate verbalization of information; noncompliance or inaccurate treatment choices	Assess understanding of anemia; assess understanding of iron deficiency; assess current level of knowledge regarding disease process; explain the functions of RBCs within the body in relation to overall health; examine dietary selections; teach how to choose foods that will support RBC formation; teach about the importance of taking prescribed iron or folic acid

PRETEST:

- Positively identify the patient using at least two person-specific identifiers before services, treatments, or procedures are performed.
- ***Patient Teaching:*** Inform the patient this test can assist in evaluating the amount of hemoglobin in the blood to assist in diagnosis and monitor therapy.
- Obtain a history of the patient's health concerns, symptoms, surgical procedures, and results of previously performed laboratory and diagnostic studies. Include a list of known allergens, especially allergies or sensitivities to latex.
- Note any recent procedures that can interfere with test results.
- Obtain a list of the patient's current medications, including over-the-counter medications and dietary supplements (see Effects of Natural Products on Laboratory Values online at Davis*Plus*).
- Review the procedure with the patient. Inform the patient that specimen collection takes approximately 5 to 10 min. Address concerns about pain and explain that there may be some discomfort during the venipuncture.
- ***Sensitivity to social and cultural issues,*** as well as concern for modesty, is important in providing psychological support before, during, and after the procedure.
- Note that there are no food, fluid, or medication restrictions unless by medical direction.

INTRATEST:

Potential Complications: N/A

- Avoid the use of equipment containing latex if the patient has a history of allergic reaction to latex.
- Instruct the patient to cooperate fully and to follow directions. Direct the

patient to breathe normally and to avoid unnecessary movement.

- Observe standard precautions, and follow the general guidelines in Patient Preparation and Specimen Collection online at Davis*Plus*. Positively identify the patient, and label the appropriate tubes with the corresponding patient demographics, date, and time of collection. Perform a venipuncture; collect the specimen in a 5-mL lavender-top (EDTA) tube. An EDTA Microtainer sample may be obtained from infants, children, and adults for whom venipuncture may not be feasible. The specimen should be mixed gently by inverting the tube 10 times. The specimen should be analyzed within 24 hr when stored at room temperature or within 48 hr if stored at refrigerated temperature. If it is anticipated the specimen will not be analyzed within 24 hr, two blood smears should be made immediately after the venipuncture and submitted with the blood sample. Smears made from specimens older than 24 hr may contain an unacceptable number of misleading artifactual abnormalities of the RBCs, such as echinocytes and spherocytes, as well as necrobiotic white blood cells.
- Remove the needle and apply direct pressure with dry gauze to stop bleeding. Observe/assess venipuncture site for bleeding or hematoma formation and secure gauze with adhesive bandage.
- Promptly transport the specimen to the laboratory for processing and analysis.

POST-TEST:

- Inform the patient that a report of the results will be made available to the requesting HCP, who will discuss the results with the patient.
- The results of a CBC should be carefully evaluated during transfusion or acute blood loss because the body is not in a state of homeostasis and values may be misleading. Considerations for draw times after transfusion include the type of product, the amount of product transfused, and the patient's clinical situation. Generally, specimens collected an hour after transfusion will provide an acceptable reflection of the effects of the transfused product. Measurements taken during a massive transfusion are an exception, providing essential guidance for therapeutic decisions during critical care.
- Recognize anxiety related to test results, and assess the color of the patient's skin as pallor is an indication of poor tissue perfusion. Inform the patient, as appropriate, that oxygen or blood product transfusion may be necessary to alleviate some of the symptoms the patient is experiencing due to the effects of the anemia. Frequently assess vital signs and explain to the patient that elevating the head of the bed may reduce difficulty in breathing. Educate the patient regarding access to nutritional counseling services.
- ***Nutritional Considerations:*** Nutritional therapy may be indicated for patients with increased Hgb if iron levels are also elevated. Educate the patient with abnormally elevated iron values, as appropriate, on the importance of reading food labels. Patients with hemochromatosis or acute pernicious anemia should be educated to avoid foods rich in iron. Iron absorption is affected by numerous factors that may enhance or decrease absorption regardless of the original content of the iron-containing dietary source (see study titled "Iron"). Iron levels in foods can be increased if foods are cooked in cookware containing iron. Consumption of large amounts of alcohol damages the intestine and allows increased absorption of iron. A high intake of calcium and ascorbic acid also increases iron absorption. Iron absorption after a meal is also increased by factors in meat, fish, and poultry.
- ***Nutritional Considerations:*** Nutritional therapy may be indicated for patients with decreased Hgb, which may indicate corresponding iron deficiency. Iron deficiency is the most common nutrient deficiency in the United States. Patients at risk (e.g., children,

pregnant women, women of childbearing age, and low-income populations) should be instructed to include in their diet foods that are high in iron, such as meats (especially liver), eggs, grains, green leafy vegetables, and multivitamins with iron. Instruct these patients in the administration of iron supplements, including adverse effects, as appropriate. The Hgb level should increase by about 1 g/dL (SI: 10 g/L) after 3 to 4 wk of oral iron supplementation. Educate the patient with abnormally decreased Hgb values, as appropriate, about the importance of reading food labels and of dietary inclusion of iron-rich foods. Iron absorption is affected by numerous factors that may enhance or decrease absorption regardless of the original content of the iron-containing dietary source. Iron absorption is decreased by the absence (gastric resection) or diminished presence (use of antacids) of gastric acid.

- Depending on the results of this procedure, additional testing may be performed to evaluate or monitor progression of the disease process and determine the need for a change in therapy. Evaluate test results in relation to the patient's symptoms and other tests performed.

Patient Education:

- Reinforce information given by the patient's HCP regarding further testing, treatment, or referral to another HCP.
- Answer any questions or address any concerns voiced by the patient or family.
- Educate the patient regarding access to nutritional counseling services. Provide contact information, if desired, for the Institute of Medicine of the National Academies (www.iom.edu) or the USDA's resource for nutrition (www.choosemyplate.gov). 🍁

Expected Patient Outcomes:

Understanding

- The patient and family state that activity tolerance will increase as anemia resolves.
- The patient and family state that erythropoietin replacement therapy will be needed until anemia resolves.

Ability

- The patient demonstrates proficiency in the self-administration of erythropoietin.
- The patient demonstrates proficiency in the self-administration of iron or folic acid supplements.

Response

- The patient and family discuss the risks and benefits associated with blood transfusion.
- The patient complies with the request to include dietary foods high in iron.

RELATED STUDIES:

- Related tests include biopsy bone marrow, biopsy lymph node, biopsy kidney, blood groups and antibodies, CBC, CBC hematocrit, Coombs' antiglobulin, CT thoracic, erythropoietin, fecal analysis (occult blood), ferritin, gallium scan, haptoglobin, hemoglobin electrophoresis, iron/TIBC, lymphangiogram, Meckel's diverticulum scan, reticulocyte count, and sickle cell screen.
- Refer to the Cardiovascular, Gastrointestinal, Hematopoietic, Hepatobiliary, Immune, and Respiratory systems tables online at Davis*Plus* for related tests by body system.

Complete Blood Count, Platelet Count

SYNONYM/ACRONYM: Thrombocytes.

COMMON USE: To assist in diagnosing and evaluating treatment for blood disorders such as thrombocytosis and thrombocytopenia and to evaluate preprocedure or preoperative coagulation status.

SPECIMEN: Whole blood from one full lavender-top (EDTA) tube.

NORMAL FINDINGS: (Method: Automated, computerized, multichannel analyzers)

Age	Platelet Count*	SI Units (Conventional Units × 1)	MPV (fL)	IPF (%)
Birth	150–450 × 10^3/microL	150–450 × 10^9/L	7.1–10.2	1.1–7.1
Child/Adult/ Older adult	140–400 × 10^3/microL	140–400 × 10^9/L	7.1–10.2	1.1–7.1

Note: Platelet counts may decrease slightly with age.
*Conventional units.
MPV = mean platelet volume.

DESCRIPTION: *Platelets* are non-nucleated, cytoplasmic, round or oval disks formed by budding off of large, multinucleated cells (megakaryocytes). Platelets have an essential function in coagulation, hemostasis, and blood thrombus formation. Activated platelets release a number of procoagulant factors, including thromboxane, a very potent platelet activator, from storage granules. These factors enter the circulation and activate other platelets and the cycle continues. The activated platelets aggregate at the site of vessel injury, and at this stage of hemostasis the glycoprotein IIb/IIIa receptors on the activated platelets bind fibrinogen, causing the platelets to stick together and form a plug. Coagulation must be localized to the site of vessel wall injury, or the growing platelet plug would eventually occlude the affected vessel. The fibrinolytic system, under normal circumstances, begins to work, once fibrin begins to form, to ensure coagulation is limited to the appropriate site. *Thrombocytosis* is an increase in platelet count. In reactive thrombocytosis, the increase is transient and short-lived, and it usually does not pose a health risk. One exception may be reactive thrombocytosis occurring after coronary bypass surgery. This circumstance has been identified as an important risk factor for postoperative infarction and thrombosis. The term *thrombocythemia* describes platelet increases associated with chronic myeloproliferative disorders; *thrombocytopenia* describes platelet counts of less than 140 × 10^3/microL 🍁. Decreased platelet counts occur whenever the body's need for platelets exceeds the rate of platelet production; this circumstance will arise if production rate decreases or platelet loss increases. The severity of bleeding is related to platelet count as well as platelet function. Platelet counts can be within normal limits, but the patient may exhibit signs of internal bleeding; this circumstance usually indicates an anomaly in platelet function. Abnormal findings by automated cell counters may indicate the need to review a smear of peripheral blood for platelet estimate. Abnormally large or giant platelets may result in underestimation of automated counts by 30% to 50%. A large discrepancy between the automated count and the estimate requires that a manual count be performed. Platelet clumping may result in the underestimation of the platelet count. Clumping may be detected by the automated cell counter or upon microscopic review of a blood smear. A citrated platelet count, performed on a specimen collected in a blue-top tube, can be performed to obtain an accurate platelet count from patients who demonstrate platelet clumping in EDTA-preserved samples.

C

Thrombopoiesis or platelet production is reflected by the measurement of the immature platelet fraction (IPF). This parameter can be correlated to the total platelet count in the investigation of platelet disorders. A low platelet count with a low IPF can indicate a disorder of platelet production (e.g., drug toxicity, aplastic anemia or bone marrow failure of another cause), whereas a low platelet count with an increased IPF might indicate platelet destruction or abnormally high platelet consumption (e.g., mechanical destruction, disseminated intravascular coagulation, idiopathic thrombocytopenic purpura [ITP], thrombotic thrombocytopenic purpura).

Platelet size, reflected by mean platelet volume (MPV), and cellular age are inversely related; that is, younger platelets tend to be larger. An increase in MPV indicates an increase in platelet turnover. Therefore, in a healthy patient, the platelet count and MPV have an inverse relationship. Abnormal platelet size may also indicate the presence of a disorder. MPV and platelet distribution width are both increased in ITP. MPV is also increased in May-Hegglin anomaly, Bernard-Soulier syndrome, myeloproliferative disorders, hyperthyroidism, and pre-eclampsia. MPV is decreased in Wiskott-Aldrich syndrome, septic thrombocytopenia, and hypersplenism.

Platelets have receptor sites that are essential for normal platelet function and activation. Drugs such as clopidogrel, abciximab (ReoPro), eptifibatide (Integrilin), and tirofiban block these receptor sites and inhibit platelet function. Aspirin also can affect platelet function by the irreversible inactivation of a crucial cyclooxygenase enzyme. Medications like clopidogrel (Plavix) and aspirin are prescribed to prevent heart attack, stroke, and blockage of coronary stents. Studies have confirmed that up to 30% of patients receiving these medications may be nonresponsive. There are several commercial test systems that can assess aspects of platelet function in addition to platelet count and size. Platelet adhesion, platelet aggregation, or bleeding time studies provide measurable responses that represent the time it might take for platelet closure to occur after a vascular injury. Platelet function testing helps ensure alternative or additional platelet therapy is instituted, if necessary. The test results can also be used preoperatively to determine whether antiplatelet medications have been sufficiently cleared from the patient's circulation such that surgery can safely be performed without risk of excessive bleeding. Thromboxane A2 is a potent stimulator of platelet activation. 11-D B2 is the stable, inactive product of thromboxane A2 metabolism, released by activated platelets. Urine levels of

11-dehydrothromboxane B2 can be used to monitor response to aspirin therapy.

The metabolism of many commonly prescribed medications is driven by the cytochrome P450 (CYP450) family of enzymes. Genetic variants can alter enzymatic activity that results in a spectrum of effects ranging from the total absence of drug metabolism to ultrafast metabolism. Impaired drug metabolism can prevent the intended therapeutic effect or even lead to serious adverse drug reactions. Poor metabolizers are at increased risk for drug-induced adverse effects due to accumulation of drug in the blood, while ultra-rapid metabolizers require a higher than normal dosage because the drug is metabolized over a shorter duration than intended. Other genetic phenotypes used to report CYP450 results are intermediate metabolizer and extensive metabolizer. CYP2C19 is a gene in the CYP450 family that metabolizes drugs such as clopidogrel (Plavix). Genetic testing can be performed on blood samples submitted to a laboratory. Testing for the most common genetic variants of CYP2C19 is used to predict altered enzyme activity and anticipate the most effective therapeutic plan. The test method commonly used is polymerase chain reaction. Counseling and informed written consent are generally required for genetic testing.

Knowledge of genetics assists the nurse in identifying patients and family members who may benefit from additional education, risk assessment, and counseling. Genetics is the study and identification of genes, genetic mutations, and inheritance. For example, genetics provides some insight into the likelihood of inheriting a trait such as blue eyes or a tendency to abnormally metabolize drugs. Some conditions are the result of mutations involving a single gene, whereas other conditions may involve multiple genes and/or multiple chromosomes. Further information regarding inheritance of genes can be found in the study titled "Genetic Testing."

This procedure is contraindicated for: N/A

INDICATIONS

- Confirm an elevated platelet count (thrombocytosis), which can cause increased clotting.
- Confirm a low platelet count (thrombocytopenia), which can be associated with bleeding.
- Identify the possible cause of abnormal bleeding, such as epistaxis, hematoma, gingival bleeding, hematuria, and menorrhagia.
- Provide screening as part of a complete blood count (CBC) in a general physical examination, especially upon admission to a health-care facility or before surgery.

POTENTIAL MEDICAL DIAGNOSIS

Increased in:

Conditions that involve inflammation activate and increase the number of circulating platelets:

- Acute infections
- After exercise (transient)
- Anemias (posthemorrhagic, hemolytic, iron deficiency) ***(bone marrow response to anemia; platelet formation is unaffected by iron deficiency)***
- Cirrhosis
- Essential thrombocythemia
- Leukemias (chronic)

- Malignancies (carcinoma, Hodgkin's, lymphomas)
- Pancreatitis (chronic)
- Polycythemia vera ***(hyperplastic bone marrow response in all cell lines)***
- Rebound recovery from thrombocytopenia ***(initial response)***
- Rheumatic fever (acute)
- Rheumatoid arthritis
- Splenectomy (2 mo postprocedure) ***(normal function of the spleen is to cull aging cells from the blood; without the spleen, the count increases)***
- Surgery (2 wk postprocedure)
- Trauma
- Tuberculosis
- Ulcerative colitis

Decreased in:

Decreased in (as a result of megakaryocytic hypoproliferation)
- Alcohol toxicity
- Aplastic anemia
- Congenital abnormalities (Fanconi's syndrome, May-Hegglin anomaly, Bernard-Soulier syndrome, Wiskott-Aldrich syndrome, Gaucher's disease, Chédiak-Higashi syndrome)
- Drug toxicity
- Prolonged hypoxia

Decreased in (as a result of ineffective thrombopoiesis)
- Ethanol misuse without malnutrition
- Iron-deficiency anemia
- Megaloblastic anemia (B_{12}/folate deficiency)
- Paroxysmal nocturnal hemoglobinuria
- Thrombopoietin deficiency
- Viral infection

Decreased in (as a result of bone marrow replacement)
- Lymphoma
- Granulomatous infections
- Metastatic carcinoma
- Myelofibrosis

Increased in:

Increased destruction in (as a result of increased loss/consumption)
- Contact with foreign surfaces (dialysis membranes, artificial organs, grafts, prosthetic devices)
- Disseminated intravascular coagulation
- Extensive transfusion
- HELLP syndrome of pregnancy (hemolysis, elevated liver enzymes, low platelet count)
- Severe hemorrhage
- Thrombotic thrombocytopenic purpura
- Uremia

Increased destruction in (as a result of immune reaction)
- Antibody/human leukocyte antigen reactions
- Hemolytic disease of the newborn ***(target is platelets instead of RBCs)***
- Idiopathic thrombocytopenic purpura
- Refractory reaction to platelet transfusion

Increased destruction in (as a result of immune reaction secondary to infection)
- Bacterial infections
- Burns
- Congenital infections (cytomegalovirus, herpes, syphilis, toxoplasmosis)
- Histoplasmosis
- Malaria
- Rocky Mountain spotted fever

Increased destruction in (as a result of other causes)
- Radiation
- Splenomegaly caused by liver disease

CRITICAL FINDINGS:

- Less than 30×10^3/microL (SI: Less than 30×10^9/L)
- Greater than $1{,}000 \times 10^3$/microL (SI: Greater than $1{,}000 \times 10^9$/L)

Note and immediately report to the requesting health-care provider (HCP) any critical findings and related symptoms. A listing of these findings varies among facilities. Timely notification of a critical finding for laboratory or diagnostic studies is a role expectation of the professional nurse. The notification processes vary among facilities. Upon receipt of the critical finding, the information should be read back to the caller to verify accuracy.

Consideration may be given to verifying the critical findings before action is taken. Policies vary among facilities and may include requesting immediate recollection and retesting by the laboratory.

Critically low platelet counts can lead to brain bleeds or gastrointestinal hemorrhage, which can be fatal. Some signs and symptoms of decreased platelet count include spontaneous nose bleeds or bleeding from the gums, bruising easily, prolonged bleeding from minor cuts and scrapes, or bloody stool. Possible interventions for decreased platelet count may include transfusion of platelets or changes in anticoagulant therapy.

INTERFERING FACTORS

- Drugs and other substances that may decrease platelet counts include acetophenazine, amphotericin B, antazoline, anticonvulsants, antimony compounds, arsenicals, azathioprine, barbiturates, benzene, busulfan, butaperazine, chlordane, chlorophenothane, dactinomycin, dextromethorphan, diethylstilbestrol, ethoxzolamide, floxuridine, hydantoin derivatives, hydroxychloroquine, iproniazid, mechlorethamine, mefenamic acid, miconazole, mitomycin, nitrofurantoin, novobiocin, nystatin, phenolphthalein, phenothiazine, pipamazine, plicamycin, procarbazine, pyrazolones, streptomycin, sulfonamides, tetracycline, thiabendazole, thiouracil, tolazamide, tolazoline, tolbutamide, trifluoperazine, and urethane.
- Drugs and other substances that may increase platelet counts include glucocorticoids.
- X-ray therapy may also decrease platelet counts.
- The results of blood counts may vary depending on the patient's position. Platelet counts can decrease when the patient is recumbent, as a result of hemodilution, and can increase when the patient rises, as a result of hemoconcentration.
- Platelet counts normally increase under a variety of stressors, such as high altitudes or strenuous exercise.
- Platelet counts are normally decreased before menstruation and during pregnancy.
- Leaving the tourniquet in place for longer than 60 sec can affect the results.
- Traumatic venipunctures may lead to erroneous results as a result of activation of the coagulation sequence.
- Failure to fill the tube sufficiently (i.e., tube less than three-quarters full) may yield inadequate sample volume for automated analyzers and may be a reason for specimen rejection.
- Hemolysis or clotted specimens are reasons for rejection.
- CBC should be carefully evaluated after transfusion or acute blood loss because the value may appear to be normal.

C

NURSING IMPLICATIONS AND PROCEDURE

POTENTIAL NURSING PROBLEMS:

Problem	Signs & Symptoms	Interventions
Protection ***(related to decreased platelet count; bleeding risk)***	Ease of bruising; blood in urine, stool, sputum, nosebleed, bleeding gums; presence of hematoma or petechiae; headache; vision changes	Assess for bruising, petechiae, hematoma; monitor and trend platelet count; administer blood or blood products, platelets; administer stool softeners; administer prescribed corticosteroids; increase frequency of vital sign assessment with variances in results; monitor for vital sign trends; assess stool, urine, sputum, gums, nose, for blood; coordinate laboratory draws to decrease frequency of venipuncture; institute bleeding precautions avoid intramuscular (IM) injections, prevent trauma, be gentle with oral care and suctioning avoid use of a sharp razor; administer prescribed medications (intravenous (IV) immunoglobulin, recombinant interleukin, Rh(D) immune globulin RhoGAM IM or Rhophylac IM or IV 🍁)
Tissue perfusion (cerebral, peripheral, renal) ***(related to altered blood flow associated with platelet clumping)***	Confusion; altered mental status; headaches; dizziness; visual disturbances; hypotension; cool extremities; capillary refill greater than 3 sec; weak pedal pulses; altered level of consciousness; decreased urine output	Monitor blood pressure; assess for dizziness; check skin temperature for warmth; assess capillary refill; assess pedal pulses; monitor level of consciousness; monitor urine output to be in excess of 30 mL/hr; ensure adequate fluid intake or administer IV fluids as ordered
Pain ***(related to joint disturbances associated with bleeding; bleeding into the tissues)***	Expression of pain, facial grimace, moaning, crying; report of pain	Assess level of pain and identify pain characteristics (what makes it better or worse); use a foot cradle to keep pressure off of legs; support joints with pillows; use socks to keep

🍁 Access Canadian content on Fast Find: Lab and Dx at davispl.us/vanleeuwen7

Problem	Signs & Symptoms	Interventions
		feet warm; administer prescribed analgesics; assess effectiveness of analgesics and collaborate with HCP to provide adequate pain management
Confusion ***(related to decreased tissue perfusion secondary to platelet clumping and altered blood flow)***	Disorganized thinking, restless, irritable, altered concentration and attention span, changeable mental function over the day, hallucinations; altered attention span; inability to follow directions; disoriented to person, place, time, and purpose; inappropriate affect	Treat the medical condition; monitor and trend platelet count; evaluate medications; prevent falls and injury through appropriate use of postural support, bed alarm, or restraints; administer prescribed medications (IV immunoglobulin, recombinant interleukin, Rh(D) immune globulin RhoGAM IM or Rhophylac IM or IV)

PRETEST:

- Positively identify the patient using at least two person-specific identifiers before services, treatments, or procedures are performed.
- ***Patient Teaching:*** Inform the patient this test can assist in diagnosing, evaluating, and monitoring bleeding disorders.
- Obtain a history of the patient's health concerns, symptoms, surgical procedures, and results of previously performed laboratory and diagnostic studies. Include a list of known allergens, especially allergies or sensitivities to latex.
- Note any recent procedures that can interfere with test results.
- Obtain a list of the patient's current medications, including over-the-counter medications, dietary supplements, anticoagulants, aspirin and other salicylates (see Effects of Natural Products on Laboratory Values online at Davis*Plus*). Such products should be discontinued by medical direction for the appropriate number of days prior to a surgical procedure. Note the last time and dose of medication taken.
- Review the procedure with the patient. Inform the patient that specimen collection takes approximately 5 to 10 min. Address concerns about pain and explain that there may be some discomfort during the venipuncture.
- ***Sensitivity to social and cultural issues,*** as well as concern for modesty, is important in providing psychological support before, during, and after the procedure.
- Note that there are no food, fluid, or medication restrictions unless by medical direction.

INTRATEST:

Potential Complications: N/A

- Avoid the use of equipment containing latex if the patient has a history of allergic reaction to latex.
- Instruct the patient to cooperate fully and to follow directions. Direct the patient to breathe normally and to avoid unnecessary movement.
- Observe standard precautions, and follow the general guidelines in Patient Preparation and Specimen Collection online at Davis*Plus*.

Positively identify the patient, and label the appropriate specimen container with the corresponding patient demographics, initials of the person collecting the specimen, date, and time of collection. Perform a venipuncture. The specimen should be mixed gently by inverting the tube 10 times. The specimen should be analyzed within 24 hr when stored at room temperature or within 48 hr if stored at refrigerated temperature. If it is anticipated the specimen will not be analyzed within 24 hr, two blood smears should be made immediately after the venipuncture and submitted with the blood sample.

- Remove the needle and apply direct pressure with dry gauze to stop bleeding. Observe/assess venipuncture site for bleeding or hematoma formation and secure gauze with adhesive bandage.
- Promptly transport the specimen to the laboratory for processing and analysis.

POST-TEST:

- Inform the patient that a report of the results will be made available to the requesting HCP, who will discuss the results with the patient.
- The results of a CBC should be carefully evaluated during transfusion or acute blood loss because the body is not in a state of homeostasis and values may be misleading. Considerations for draw times after transfusion include the type of product, the amount of product transfused, and the patient's clinical situation. Generally, specimens collected an hour after transfusion will provide an acceptable reflection of the effects of the transfused product. Measurements taken during a massive transfusion are an exception, providing essential guidance for therapeutic decisions during critical care.
- ***Nutritional Considerations:*** Instruct patients to consume a variety of foods within the basic food groups, maintain a healthy weight, be physically active, limit salt intake, limit alcohol intake, and avoid the use of tobacco.
- Recognize anxiety related to test results. Discuss the implications of abnormal test results on the patient's lifestyle. Provide teaching and information regarding the clinical implications of the test results, as appropriate.
- Depending on the results of this procedure, additional testing may be performed to evaluate or monitor progression of the disease process and determine the need for a change in therapy. Evaluate test results in relation to the patient's symptoms and other tests performed.

Patient Education:

- Instruct the patient to report bleeding from any areas of the skin or mucous membranes.
- Inform the patient of the importance of periodic laboratory testing if he or she is taking an anticoagulant.
- Reinforce information given by the patient's HCP regarding further testing, treatment, or referral to another HCP.
- Answer any questions or address any concerns voiced by the patient or family.

Expected Patient Outcomes:

Understanding

- The patient states the importance of taking a stool softener to prevent straining while having a bowel movement.
- The patient and family state the importance of taking precautions against bruising and bleeding, including the use of a soft bristle toothbrush, use of an electric razor, avoidance of constipation, avoidance of acetylsalicylic acid and similar products, and avoidance of intramuscular injections

Ability

- The patient and family identify symptoms of bleeding that should be reported to the HCP.
- The patient identifies pain management therapy that provides the best pain relief.

Response

- The patient complies with the request to refrain from participating in at-risk activities that could cause trauma and bleeding.
- The patient complies with the request to take stool softeners to prevent constipation and bleeding.

RELATED STUDIES:

- Related tests include antidysrhythmic drugs (quinidine), biopsy bone marrow, bleeding time, blood groups and antibodies, clot retraction, coagulation factors, CBC, CBC RBC morphology and inclusions, CBC WBC count and differential, CT angiography, CT brain, FDP, fibrinogen, genetic testing, PTT, platelet antibodies, procalcitonin, PT/INR, and US pelvis.
- Refer to the Hematopoietic and Immune systems tables online at Davis*Plus* for related tests by body system.

C

Complete Blood Count, RBC Count

SYNONYM/ACRONYM: RBC.

COMMON USE: To evaluate the number of circulating red cells in the blood toward diagnosing disease and monitoring therapeutic treatment. Variations in the number of cells is most often seen in anemias, cancer, and hemorrhage.

SPECIMEN: Whole blood collected in a lavender-top (EDTA) tube.

NORMAL FINDINGS: (Method: Automated, computerized, multichannel analyzers)

Age	Conventional Units (10^6 cells/microL)	SI Units (10^{12} cells/L) (Conventional Units × 1)
Cord blood	3.61–5.81	3.61–5.81
0–1 wk	4.51–6.01	4.51–6.01
2–3 wk	3.99–6.11	3.99–6.11
1–2 mo	3.71–6.11	3.71–6.11
3–6 mo	3.81–5.61	3.81–5.61
7 mo–1 yr	3.81–5.21	3.81–5.21
2–6 yr	3.91–5.31	3.91–5.31
7–15 yr	3.99–5.21	3.99–5.21
16–18 yr	4.21–5.41	4.21–5.41
Adult		
Male	4.21–5.81	4.21–5.81
Female	3.61–5.11	3.61–5.11

Values are decreased in pregnancy related to the dilutional effects of increased fluid volume and potential nutritional deficiency related to decreased intake, nausea, and/or vomiting. Values are slightly lower in older adults associated with potential nutritional deficiency. Values are slightly lower in older adults.

DESCRIPTION: The red blood cell (RBC) count is a component of the CBC. It determines the number of RBCs per cubic millimeter of whole blood. The main role of RBCs, which contain the pigmented protein hemoglobin (Hgb), is the transport and exchange of oxygen to the tissues. Some carbon dioxide is returned from the tissues to the lungs by RBCs. RBC production in healthy adults takes place in the bone marrow of the vertebrae, pelvis, ribs, sternum, skull, and proximal ends of the femur and humerus. Production of RBCs is regulated by a hormone called erythropoietin which is produced and secreted by the kidneys. Normal RBC development and function are dependent on adequate levels of vitamin B_{12}, folic acid, vitamin E, and iron. The average life span of normal RBCs is 120 days. Old or damaged RBCs are removed from circulation by the spleen. The liver is responsible for the breakdown of hemoglobin and other cellular contents released from destroyed RBCs. *Polycythemia* is a condition resulting from an abnormal increase in Hgb, hematocrit (Hct), and RBC count. *Anemia* is a condition resulting from an abnormal decrease in Hgb, Hct, and RBC count. Results of the Hgb, Hct, and RBC count should be evaluated simultaneously because the same underlying conditions affect this triad of tests similarly. The RBC count multiplied by 3 should approximate the Hgb concentration. The Hct should be within three times the Hgb if the RBC population is normal in size and shape. The Hct plus 6 should approximate the first two figures of the RBC count within 3 (e.g., Hct is 40%; therefore 40 + 6 = 46, and the RBC count should be 4.6 or in the range 4.3 to 4.9). (See "Complete Blood Count, Hematocrit," "Complete Blood Count, Hemoglobin," and "Complete Blood Count, RBC Indices.")

This procedure is contraindicated for: N/A

INDICATIONS

- Detect a hematological disorder involving RBC destruction (e.g., hemolytic anemia).
- Determine the presence of hereditary hematological abnormality.
- Monitor the effects of acute or chronic blood loss.
- Monitor the effects of physical or emotional stress on the patient.
- Monitor patients with disorders associated with elevated erythrocyte counts (e.g., polycythemia vera, chronic obstructive pulmonary disease [COPD]).
- Monitor the progression of nonhematological disorders associated with elevated erythrocyte counts, such as COPD, liver disease, hypothyroidism, adrenal dysfunction, bone marrow failure, malabsorption syndromes, cancer, and chronic kidney disease.
- Monitor the response to drugs or chemotherapy and evaluate undesired reactions to drugs that may cause blood dyscrasias.
- Provide screening as part of a CBC in a general physical examination, especially upon admission to a health-care facility or before surgery.

POTENTIAL MEDICAL DIAGNOSIS

Increased in:

- Anxiety or stress ***(related to physiological response)***
- Bone marrow failure ***(initial response is stimulation of RBC production)***
- COPD with hypoxia and secondary polycythemia ***(related to chronic hypoxia that stimulates production of RBCs and a corresponding increase in RBCs)***

- Dehydration with hemoconcentration ***(related to decrease in total blood volume relative to unchanged RBC count)***
- Erythremic erythrocytosis ***(related to unchanged total blood volume relative to increase in RBC count)***
- High altitude ***(related to hypoxia that stimulates production of RBCs)***
- Polycythemia vera ***(related to abnormal bone marrow response resulting in overproduction of RBCs)***

Decreased in:

- Chemotherapy ***(related to reduced RBC survival)***
- Chronic inflammatory diseases ***(related to anemia of chronic disease)***
- Chronic kidney disease ***(related to decreased production of erythropoietin)***
- Hemoglobinopathy ***(related to reduced RBC survival)***
- Hemolytic anemia ***(related to reduced RBC survival)***
- Hemorrhage ***(related to overall decrease in RBC count)***
- Hodgkin's disease ***(evidenced by bone marrow failure that results in decreased RBC production)***
- Leukemia ***(evidenced by bone marrow failure that results in decreased RBC production)***
- Multiple myeloma ***(evidenced by bone marrow failure that results in decreased RBC production)***
- Nutritional deficit ***(related to deficiency of iron or vitamins required for RBC production and/or maturation)***
- Overhydration ***(related to increase in blood volume relative to unchanged RBC count)***
- Pregnancy ***(related to anemia; normal dilutional effect)***
- Subacute endocarditis

CRITICAL FINDINGS:

The presence of abnormal cells, other morphological characteristics, or cellular inclusions may signify a potentially life-threatening or serious health condition and should be investigated. Examples are the presence of sickle cells, moderate numbers of spherocytes, marked schistocytosis, oval macrocytes, basophilic stippling, nucleated RBCs (if the patient is not an infant), or malarial organisms.

Note and immediately report to the requesting health-care provider (HCP) any critical findings and related symptoms. A listing of these findings varies among facilities. Timely notification of a critical finding for laboratory or diagnostic studies is a role expectation of the professional nurse. The notification processes vary among facilities. Upon receipt of the critical finding, the information should be read back to the caller to verify accuracy.

Consideration may be given to verifying the critical findings before action is taken. Policies vary among facilities and may include requesting immediate recollection and retesting by the laboratory or retesting using a rapid Point of Care instrument at the bedside, if available.

Low RBC count leads to anemia. Anemia can be caused by blood loss, decreased blood cell production, increased blood cell destruction, or hemodilution. Causes of blood loss include menstrual excess or frequency, gastrointestinal bleeding, inflammatory bowel disease, or hematuria. Decreased blood cell production can be caused by folic acid deficiency, vitamin B_{12} deficiency, iron deficiency, or chronic disease. Increased blood cell destruction can be caused by a hemolytic reaction, chemical reaction, medication reaction, or sickle cell disease. Hemodilution can be caused by heart failure, chronic kidney disease, polydipsia, or overhydration. Symptoms of anemia (due to these causes) include anxiety, dyspnea, edema, hypertension, hypotension, hypoxia, jugular venous distention, fatigue, pallor, rales, restlessness, and weakness. Treatment of anemia depends on the cause.

High RBC count leads to polycythemia. Polycythemia can be caused by dehydration, decreased oxygen levels in the body, and an overproduction of RBCs by the bone marrow. Dehydration by diuretic use, vomiting, diarrhea, excessive sweating, severe burns, or decreased fluid intake decreases the plasma component of whole blood, thereby increasing the ratio of RBCs to plasma, and leads to a higher than normal Hct. Causes of decreased oxygen include smoking, exposure to carbon monoxide, high altitude, and chronic lung disease, which leads to a mild hemoconcentration of blood in the body to carry more oxygen to the body's tissues. An overproduction of RBCs by the bone marrow leads to polycythemia vera, which is a rare chronic myeloproliferative disorder that leads to a severe hemoconcentration of blood. Severe hemoconcentration can lead to thrombosis (spontaneous blood clotting). Symptoms of hemoconcentration include decreased pulse pressure and volume, loss of skin turgor, dry mucous membranes, headaches, hepatomegaly, low central venous pressure, orthostatic hypotension, pruritus (especially after a hot bath), splenomegaly, tachycardia, thirst, tinnitus, vertigo, and weakness. Treatment of polycythemia depends on the cause. Possible interventions for hemoconcentration due to dehydration include intravenous (IV) fluids and discontinuance of diuretics if they are believed to be contributing to critically elevated Hct. Polycythemia due to decreased oxygen states can be treated by removal of the offending substance, such as smoke or carbon monoxide. Treatment includes oxygen therapy in cases of smoke inhalation, carbon monoxide poisoning, and desaturating chronic lung disease. Symptoms of polycythemic overload crisis include signs of thrombosis, pain and redness in extremities, facial flushing, and irritability. Possible interventions for hemoconcentration due to polycythemia include therapeutic phlebotomy and IV fluids.

INTERFERING FACTORS

- Drugs and other substances that may decrease RBC count by causing hemolysis resulting from drug sensitivity or enzyme deficiency include acetaminophen, aminosalicylic acid, amphetamine, anticonvulsants, antipyrine, arsenicals, benzene, busulfan, carbenicillin, cephalothin, chemotherapy drugs, chlorate, chloroquine, chlorothiazide, chlorpromazine, colchicine, diphenhydramine, dipyrone, glucosulfone, gold, indomethacin, nalidixic acid, neomycin, nitrofurantoin, penicillin, phenacemide, phenazopyridine, and phenothiazine.
- Drugs and other substances that may decrease RBC count by causing anemia include miconazole, penicillamine, phenylhydrazine, primaquine, probenecid, pyrazolones, pyrimethamine, quinines, streptomycin, sulfamethizole, sulfamethoxypyridazine, sulfisoxazole, suramin, thioridazine, tolbutamide, trimethadione, and tripelennamine.
- Drugs that may decrease RBC count by causing bone marrow suppression include floxuridineand phenylbutazone.
- Drugs and vitamins that may increase the RBC count include amphotericin B, erythropoietin, glucocorticosteroids, pilocarpine, and vitamin B_{12}.
- Use of the nutraceutical liver extract is strongly contraindicated

in patients with iron-storage disorders such as hemochromatosis because it is rich in heme (the iron-containing pigment in Hgb).

- Hemodilution (e.g., excessive administration of IV fluids, normal pregnancy) in the presence of a normal number of RBCs may lead to false decreases in RBC count.
- Cold agglutinins may falsely increase the mean corpuscular volume and decrease the RBC count. This can be corrected by warming the blood or diluting the sample with warmed saline and repeating the analysis.
- Excessive exercise, anxiety, pain, and dehydration may cause false elevations in RBC count.
- The results of a CBC should be carefully evaluated during transfusion or acute blood loss because the body is not in a state of homeostasis and values may be misleading. Considerations for draw times after transfusion include the type of product, the amount of product transfused, and the patient's clinical situation. Generally, specimens collected an hour after transfusion will provide an acceptable reflection of the effects of the transfused product. Measurements taken during a massive transfusion are an exception, providing essential guidance for therapeutic decisions during critical care.
- RBC counts can vary depending on the patient's position, decreasing when the patient is recumbent as a result of hemodilution and increasing when the patient rises as a result of hemoconcentration.
- Venous stasis can falsely elevate RBC counts; therefore, the tourniquet should not be left on the arm for longer than 60 sec.
- Failure to fill the tube sufficiently (i.e., tube less than three-quarters full) may yield inadequate sample volume for automated analyzers and may be a reason for specimen rejection.
- Hemolyzed or clotted specimens must be rejected for analysis.

NURSING IMPLICATIONS AND PROCEDURE

C

PRETEST:

- Positively identify the patient using at least two person-specific identifiers before services, treatments, or procedures are performed.
- ***Patient Teaching:*** Inform the patient this test can assist in assessing for anemia and disorders affecting the number of circulating RBCs.
- Obtain a history of the patient's health concerns, symptoms, surgical procedures, and results of previously performed laboratory and diagnostic studies. Include a list of known allergens, especially allergies or sensitivities to latex.
- Note any recent procedures that can interfere with test results.
- Obtain a list of the patient's current medications, including over-the-counter medications and dietary supplements (see Effects of Natural Products on Laboratory Values online at Davis*Plus*).
- Review the procedure with the patient. Inform the patient that specimen collection takes approximately 5 to 10 min. Address concerns about pain and explain that there may be some discomfort during the venipuncture.
- ***Sensitivity to social and cultural issues,*** as well as concern for modesty, is important in providing psychological support before, during, and after the procedure.
- Note that there are no food, fluid, or medication restrictions unless by medical direction.

INTRATEST:

Potential Complications: N/A

- Avoid the use of equipment containing latex if the patient has a history of allergic reaction to latex.

C

- Instruct the patient to cooperate fully and to follow directions. Direct the patient to breathe normally and to avoid unnecessary movement.
- Observe standard precautions, and follow the general guidelines in Patient Preparation and Specimen Collection online at Davis*Plus*. Positively identify the patient, and label the appropriate specimen container with the corresponding patient demographics, initials of the person collecting the specimen, date, and time of collection. Perform a venipuncture. An EDTA Microtainer sample may be obtained from infants, children, and adults for whom venipuncture may not be feasible. The specimen should be mixed gently by inverting the tube 10 times. The specimen should be analyzed within 24 hr when stored at room temperature or within 48 hr if stored at refrigerated temperature. If it is anticipated the specimen will not be analyzed within 24 hr, two blood smears should be made immediately after the venipuncture and submitted with the blood sample. Smears made from specimens older than 24 hr will contain an unacceptable number of misleading artifactual abnormalities of the RBCs, such as echinocytes and spherocytes, as well as necrobiotic WBCs.
- Remove the needle and apply direct pressure with dry gauze to stop bleeding. Observe/assess venipuncture site for bleeding or hematoma formation and secure gauze with adhesive bandage.
- Promptly transport the specimen to the laboratory for processing and analysis.

POST-TEST:

- Inform the patient that a report of the results will be made available to the requesting HCP, who will discuss the results with the patient.
- ***Nutritional Considerations:*** Nutritional therapy may be indicated for patients with decreased RBC count. Iron deficiency is the most common nutrient deficiency in the United States. Patients at risk (e.g., children, pregnant women and women of childbearing age, low-income populations) should be instructed to include foods that are high in iron in their diet, such as meats (especially liver), eggs, grains, green leafy vegetables, and multivitamins with iron. Iron absorption is affected by numerous factors (see study titled "Iron").
- ***Nutritional Considerations:*** Patients at risk for vitamin B_{12} or folate deficiency include those with the following conditions: malnourishment (inadequate intake), pregnancy (increased need), infancy, malabsorption syndromes (inadequate absorption/increased metabolic rate), infections, cancer, hyperthyroidism, serious burns, excessive blood loss, and gastrointestinal damage. Instruct the patient with vitamin B_{12} deficiency, as appropriate, in the use of vitamin supplements. Inform the patient, as appropriate, that the best dietary sources of vitamin B_{12} are meats, milk, cheese, eggs, and fortified soy milk products. Instruct the folate-deficient patient (especially pregnant women), as appropriate, to eat foods rich in folate, such as meats (especially liver), salmon, eggs, beets, asparagus, green leafy vegetables such as spinach, cabbage, oranges, broccoli, sweet potatoes, kidney beans, and whole wheat.
- ***Nutritional Considerations:*** A diet deficient in vitamin E puts the patient at risk for increased RBC destruction, which could lead to anemia. Nutritional therapy may be indicated for these patients. Educate the patient with a vitamin E deficiency, if appropriate, that the main dietary sources of vitamin E are vegetable oils including olive oil, whole grains, wheat germ, nuts, milk, eggs, meats, fish, and green leafy vegetables. Vitamin E is fairly stable at most cooking temperatures (except frying) and when exposed to acidic foods. Supplemental vitamin E may also be taken, but the danger of toxicity should be explained to the patient. Very large supplemental doses, in excess of 600 mg of vitamin E over a period of 1 yr, may result in excess

bleeding. Vitamin E is heat stable but is very negatively affected by light.

- Reinforce information given by the patient's HCP regarding further testing, treatment, or referral to another HCP. Answer any questions or address any concerns voiced by the patient or family. Educate the patient regarding access to nutritional counseling services. Provide contact information, if desired, for the Institute of Medicine of the National Academies (www.iom.edu) or the USDA's resource for nutrition (www.choosemyplate.gov). 🍁
- Depending on the results of this procedure, additional testing may be performed to evaluate or monitor progression of the disease process and determine the need for a change in therapy. Evaluate test results in relation to the patient's symptoms and other tests performed.

RELATED STUDIES:

- Related tests include biopsy bone marrow, biopsy kidney, blood groups and antibodies, CBC, CBC hematocrit, CBC hemoglobin, CBC RBC morphology and inclusions, Coombs' antiglobulin, erythropoietin, fecal analysis, ferritin, folate, gallium scan, haptoglobin, iron/TIBC, lymphangiogram, Meckel's diverticulum scan, reticulocyte count, and vitamin B_{12}.
- Refer to the Cardiovascular, Gastrointestinal, Genitourinary, Hematopoietic, Hepatobiliary, Immune, and Respiratory systems tables online at Davis*Plus* for related tests by body system.

Complete Blood Count, RBC Indices

SYNONYM/ACRONYM: Mean corpuscular hemoglobin (MCH), mean corpuscular volume (MCV), mean corpuscular hemoglobin concentration (MCHC), red blood cell distribution width (RDW).

COMMON USE: To evaluate cell size, shape, weight, and hemoglobin (Hgb) concentration. Used to diagnose and monitor therapy for diagnoses such as iron-deficiency anemia.

SPECIMEN: Whole blood collected in a lavender-top (EDTA) tube.

NORMAL FINDINGS: (Method: Automated, computerized, multichannel analyzers)

Age	MCV (fL)	MCH (pg/cell)	MCHC (g/dL)	RDWCV	RDWSD
Cord blood	107–119	35–39	31–35	14.9–18.7	51–66
0–1 wk	104–116	29–45	24–36	14.9–18.7	51–66
2–3 wk	95–117	26–38	26–34	14.9–18.7	51–66
1–2 mo	81–125	25–37	26–34	14.9–18.7	44–55
3–11 mo	78–110	22–34	26–34	14.9–18.7	35–46
1–5 yr	74–94	24–32	30–34	11.6–14.8	35–42
6–8 yr	73–93	24–32	32–36	11.6–14.8	35–42
9–14 yr	74–94	25–33	32–36	11.6–14.8	37–44
15 yr–adult					
Male	77–97	26–34	32–36	11.6–14.8	38–48
Female	78–98	26–34	32–36	11.6–14.8	38–48

(table continues on page 502)

Age	MCV (fL)	MCH (pg/cell)	MCHC (g/dL)	RDWCV	RDWSD
Older adult					
Male	79–103	27–35	32–36	11.6–14.8	38–48
Female	78–102	27–35	32–36	11.6–14.8	38–48

MCV = mean corpuscular volume; MCH = mean corpuscular hemoglobin; MCHC = mean corpuscular hemoglobin concentration; RDWCV = coefficient of variation in red blood cell distribution width; RDWSD = standard deviation in RBC distribution width.

DESCRIPTION: Red blood cell (RBC) indices provide information about RBC size and Hgb content. The indices are derived from mathematical relationships between the RBC count, Hgb level, and hematocrit (Hct) percentage. RBC indices are frequently used to assist in the classification of anemias. The MCV reflects the average size of circulating RBCs and classifies size as normocytic, microcytic (smaller than normal), and macrocytic (larger than normal). MCV is determined by dividing the Hct by the total RBC. The RDW is a measurement of cell size distribution. Many of the commonly used automated cell counters report the more sophisticated statistical indices, the coefficient of variation in red blood cell distribution width (RDWCV) and the standard deviation in RBC distribution width (RDWSD) instead of RDW. The RDWCV is an indication of variation in cell size over the circulating RBC population. The RDWSD is also an indicator of variation in RBC size, is not affected by the MCV as with the RDWCV index, and is a more accurate measurement of the degree of variation in cell size. Review of peripheral smears is used to corroborate findings from automated instruments. Excessive variations in cell size are graded from 1+ to 4+, with 4+ indicating the most severe degree of anisocytosis, or variation in cell size. MCH, or average amount of Hgb in RBCs, and MCHC, or average amount of Hgb per volume of RBCs, are used to measure Hgb content. Microscopic review of the peripheral smear can also be used to visually confirm automated values. Terms used to describe the Hgb content of RBCs are *normochromic, hypochromic,* and *hyperchromic.* The findings are also visually graded from 1+ to 4+. The MCH is determined by dividing the total Hgb by the RBC count. MCHC is determined by dividing total Hgb by Hct. (See "Complete Blood Count, Hemoglobin," "Complete Blood Count, Hematocrit," "Complete Blood Count, RBC Count," and "Complete Blood Count, RBC Morphology and Inclusions.")

This procedure is contraindicated for: N/A

INDICATIONS

- Assist in the diagnosis of anemia.
- Detect a hematological disorder, neoplasm, or immunological abnormality.
- Determine the presence of a hereditary hematological abnormality.
- Monitor the effects of physical or emotional stress.
- Monitor the progression of nonhematological disorders such as chronic obstructive pulmonary

disease, malabsorption syndromes, cancer, and chronic kidney disease.
- Monitor the response to drugs or chemotherapy, and evaluate undesired reactions to drugs that may cause blood dyscrasias.
- Provide screening as part of a complete blood count (CBC) in a general physical examination, especially upon admission to a healthcare facility or before surgery.

POTENTIAL MEDICAL DIAGNOSIS

Increased in:

MCV
- Alcoholism ***(vitamin deficiency related to malnutrition)***
- Antimetabolite therapy ***(the therapy inhibits vitamin B_{12} and folate)***
- Liver disease ***(complex effect on RBCs that includes malnutrition, alterations in RBC shape and size, effects of chronic disease)***
- Pernicious anemia (vitamin B_{12}/folate anemia)

MCH
- Macrocytic anemias ***(related to increased Hgb or cell size)***

MCHC
- Spherocytosis ***(artifact in measurement caused by abnormal cell shape)***

RDW
- Anemias with heterogeneous cell size as a result of hemoglobinopathy, hemolytic anemia, anemia following acute blood loss, iron-deficiency anemia, vitamin- and folate-deficiency anemia ***(related to a mixture of cell sizes as the bone marrow responds to the anemia and/or to a mixture of cell shapes due to cell fragmentation as a result of the disease)***

Decreased in:

MCV
- Iron-deficiency anemia ***(related to low Hgb)***
- Thalassemias ***(related to low Hgb)***

MCH
- Hypochromic anemias ***(related to low Hgb)***
- Microcytic anemias ***(related to low Hgb)***

MCHC
- Iron-deficiency anemia ***(the amount of Hgb in the RBC is small relative to RBC size)***

RDW: N/A

CRITICAL FINDINGS: N/A

INTERFERING FACTORS

- Drugs and other substances that may decrease the MCHC include styrene (occupational exposure).
- Drugs and other substances that may decrease the MCV include nitrofurantoin.
- Drugs and other substances that may increase the MCV include colchicine, pentamidine, pyrimethamine, and triamterene.
- Drugs and other substances that may increase the MCH and MCHC include oral contraceptives (long-term use).
- Diseases that cause agglutination of RBCs will alter test results.
- Cold agglutinins may falsely increase the MCV and decrease the RBC count. This can be corrected by warming the blood or diluting the sample with warmed saline and then correcting the RBC count mathematically.
- RBC counts can vary depending on the patient's position, decreasing when the patient is

recumbent as a result of hemodilution and increasing when the patient rises as a result of hemoconcentration.

- The results of a CBC should be carefully evaluated during transfusion or acute blood loss because the body is not in a state of homeostasis and values may be misleading. Considerations for draw times after transfusion include the type of product, the amount of product transfused, and the patient's clinical situation. Generally, specimens collected an hour after transfusion will provide an acceptable reflection of the effects of the transfused product. Measurements taken during a massive transfusion are an exception, providing essential guidance for therapeutic decisions during critical care.
- Venous stasis can falsely elevate RBC counts; therefore, the tourniquet should not be left on the arm for longer than 60 sec.
- Failure to fill the tube sufficiently (i.e., tube less than three-quarters full) may yield inadequate sample volume for automated analyzers and may be a reason for specimen rejection.
- Hemolyzed or clotted specimens should be rejected.
- Lipemia will falsely increase the hemoglobin measurement, also affecting the MCV and MCH.

NURSING IMPLICATIONS AND PROCEDURE

PRETEST:

- Positively identify the patient using at least two person-specific identifiers before services, treatments, or procedures are performed.
- *Patient Teaching:* Inform the patient this test can assist in assessing RBC shape and size.
- Obtain a history of the patient's health concerns, symptoms, surgical procedures, and results of previously performed laboratory and diagnostic studies. Include a list of known allergens, especially allergies or sensitivities to latex.
- Note any recent procedures that can interfere with test results.
- Obtain a list of the patient's current medications, including over-the-counter medications and dietary supplements (see Effects of Natural Products on Laboratory Values online at Davis*Plus*).
- Review the procedure with the patient. Inform the patient that specimen collection takes approximately 5 to 10 min. Address concerns about pain and explain that there may be some discomfort during the venipuncture.
- *Sensitivity to social and cultural issues,* as well as concern for modesty, is important in providing psychological support before, during, and after the procedure.
- Note that there are no food, fluid, or medication restrictions unless by medical direction.

INTRATEST:

Potential Complications: N/A

- Avoid the use of equipment containing latex if the patient has a history of allergic reaction to latex.
- Instruct the patient to cooperate fully and to follow directions. Direct the patient to breathe normally and to avoid unnecessary movement.
- Observe standard precautions, and follow the general guidelines in Patient Preparation and Specimen Collection online at Davis*Plus*. Positively identify the patient, and label the appropriate specimen container with the corresponding patient demographics, initials of the person collecting the specimen, date, and time of collection. Perform a venipuncture. An EDTA Microtainer sample may be obtained from infants, children, and adults for whom venipuncture may not be feasible. The specimen should

be mixed gently by inverting the tube 10 times. The specimen should be analyzed within 24 hr when stored at room temperature or within 48 hr if stored at refrigerated temperature. If it is anticipated the specimen will not be analyzed within 24 hr, two blood smears should be made immediately after the venipuncture and submitted with the blood sample. Smears made from specimens older than 24 hr may contain an unacceptable number of misleading artifactual abnormalities of the RBCs, such as echinocytes and spherocytes, as well as necrobiotic white blood cells.

- Remove the needle and apply direct pressure with dry gauze to stop bleeding. Observe/assess venipuncture site for bleeding or hematoma formation and secure gauze with adhesive bandage.
- Promptly transport the specimen to the laboratory for processing and analysis.

POST-TEST:

- Inform the patient that a report of the results will be made available to the requesting health care provider (HCP), who will discuss the results with the patient.
- Reinforce information given by the patient's HCP regarding further testing, treatment, or referral to another HCP. Answer any questions or address any concerns voiced by the patient or family.
- Depending on the results of this procedure, additional testing may be performed to evaluate or monitor progression of the disease process and determine the need for a change in therapy. Evaluate test results in relation to the patient's symptoms and other tests performed.

RELATED STUDIES:

- Related tests include biopsy bone marrow, CBC, CBC hematocrit, CBC hemoglobin, CBC RBC count, CBC RBC morphology and inclusions, CBC WBC count and differential, erythropoietin, ferritin, folate, Hgb electrophoresis, iron/TIBC, lead, reticulocyte count, sickle cell screen, and vitamin B_{12}.
- Refer to the Gastrointestinal, Hematopoietic, Immune, and Respiratory systems tables online at Davis*Plus* for related tests by body system.

Complete Blood Count, RBC Morphology and Inclusions

SYNONYM/ACRONYM: N/A

COMMON USE: To make a visual evaluation of the red blood cell (RBC) shape and/or size as a confirmation in assisting to diagnose and monitor disease progression.

SPECIMEN: Whole blood from one full lavender-top (EDTA) tube or Wright's-stained, thin-film peripheral blood smear. The laboratory should be consulted as to the necessity of thick-film smears for the evaluation of malarial inclusions.

NORMAL FINDINGS: (Method: Microscopic, manual review of stained blood smear)

C

RBC Morphology	Within Normal Limits	1+	2+	3+	4+
Size					
Anisocytosis	0–5	5–10	10–20	20–50	Greater than 50
Macrocytes	0–5	5–10	10–20	20–50	Greater than 50
Microcytes	0–5	5–10	10–20	20–50	Greater than 50
Shape					
Poikilocytes	0–2	3–10	10–20	20–50	Greater than 50
Burr cells	0–2	3–10	10–20	20–50	Greater than 50
Acanthocytes	Less than 1	2–5	5–10	10–20	Greater than 20
Schistocytes	Less than 1	2–5	5–10	10–20	Greater than 20
Dacryocytes (teardrop cells)	0–2	2–5	5–10	10–20	Greater than 20
Codocytes (target cells)	0–2	2–10	10–20	20–50	Greater than 50
Spherocytes	0–2	2–10	10–20	20–50	Greater than 50
Ovalocytes	0–2	2–10	10–20	20–50	Greater than 50
Stomatocytes	0–2	2–10	10–20	20–50	Greater than 50
Drepanocytes (sickle cells)	Absent	Reported as present or absent			
Helmet cells	Absent	Reported as present or absent			
Agglutination	Absent	Reported as present or absent			
Rouleaux	Absent	Reported as present or absent			
Hemoglobin (Hgb) Content					
Hypochromia	0–2	3–10	10–50	50–75	Greater than 75
Polychromasia					
Adult	Less than 1	2–5	5–10	10–20	Greater than 20
Newborn	1–6	7–15	15–20	20–50	Greater than 50
Inclusions					
Cabot rings	Absent	Reported as present or absent			
Basophilic stippling	0–1	1–5	5–10	10–20	Greater than 20
Howell-Jolly bodies	Absent	1–2	3–5	5–10	Greater than 10

RBC Morphology	Within Normal Limits	1+	2+	3+	4+
Heinz bodies	Absent	Reported as present or absent			
Hgb C crystals	Absent	Reported as present or absent			
Pappenheimer bodies	Absent	Reported as present or absent			
Intracellular parasites (e.g., *Plasmodium, Babesia, Trypanosoma*)	Absent	Reported as present or absent			

DESCRIPTION: The decision to manually review a peripheral blood smear for abnormalities in RBC shape or size is made on the basis of criteria established by the reporting laboratory. Cues in the results of the complete blood count (CBC) will point to specific abnormalities that can be confirmed visually by microscopic review of the sample on a stained blood smear.

This procedure is contraindicated for: N/A

INDICATIONS

- Assist in the diagnosis of anemia.
- Detect a hematological disorder, neoplasm, or immunological abnormality.
- Determine the presence of a hereditary hematological abnormality.
- Monitor the effects of physical or emotional stress on the patient.
- Monitor the progression of nonhematological disorders, such as chronic obstructive pulmonary disease, malabsorption syndromes, cancer, and renal disease.
- Monitor the response to drugs or chemotherapy, and evaluate undesired reactions to drugs that may cause blood dyscrasias.
- Provide screening as part of a CBC in a general physical examination, especially upon admission to a health-care facility or before surgery.

POTENTIAL MEDICAL DIAGNOSIS

RBC Size

Increased in:

Cell Size

- Alcoholism
- Aplastic anemia
- Chemotherapy
- Chronic hemolytic anemia
- Grossly elevated glucose (hyperosmotic)
- Hemolytic disease of the newborn
- Hypothyroidism
- Leukemia
- Lymphoma
- Metastatic carcinoma

- Myelofibrosis
- Myeloma
- Refractory anemia
- Sideroblastic anemia
- Vitamin B_{12}/folate deficiency ***(related to impaired DNA synthesis and delayed cell division, which permits the cells to grow for a longer period than normal)***

C

Decreased in:

Cell Size

- Hemoglobin (Hgb) C disease
- Hemolytic anemias
- Hereditary spherocytosis
- Inflammation
- Iron-deficiency anemia
- Thalassemias

RBC Shape

Variations in cell shape are the result of hereditary conditions such as elliptocytosis, sickle cell anemia, spherocytosis, thalassemias, or hemoglobinopathies (e.g., hemoglobin C disease). Irregularities in cell shape can also result from acquired conditions, such as physical/mechanical cellular trauma, exposure to chemicals, or reactions to medications.

- Acquired spherocytosis can result from Heinz body hemolytic anemia, microangiopathic hemolytic anemia, secondary isoimmunohemolytic anemia, and transfusion of old banked blood.
- Acanthocytes are associated with acquired conditions such as alcoholic cirrhosis with hemolytic anemia, disorders of lipid metabolism, hepatitis of newborns, malabsorptive diseases, metastatic liver disease, the postsplenectomy period, and pyruvate kinase deficiency.
- Burr cells are commonly seen in acquired renal insufficiency, burns, cardiac valve disease, disseminated intravascular coagulation (DIC), hypertension, IV fibrin deposition, metastatic malignancy, normal neonatal period, and uremia.
- Codocytes are seen in hemoglobinopathies, iron-deficiency anemia, obstructive liver disease, and the postsplenectomy period.
- Dacryocytes are most commonly associated with metastases to the bone marrow, myelofibrosis, myeloid metaplasia, pernicious anemia, and tuberculosis.
- Schistocytes are seen in burns, cardiac valve disease, DIC, glomerulonephritis, hemolytic anemia, microangiopathic hemolytic anemia, renal graft rejection, thrombotic thrombocytopenic purpura, uremia, and vasculitis.

RBC Hemoglobin Content

- RBCs with a normal Hgb level have a clear central pallor and are referred to as *normochromic.*
- Cells with low Hgb and lacking in central pallor are referred to as *hypochromic.* Hypochromia is associated with iron-deficiency anemia, thalassemias, and sideroblastic anemia.
- Cells with excessive Hgb levels are referred to as *hyperchromic* even though they technically lack a central pallor. Hyperchromia is usually associated with an elevated mean corpuscular Hgb concentration as well as hemolytic anemias.
- Cells referred to as *polychromic* are young erythrocytes that still contain ribonucleic acid (RNA). The RNA is picked up by the Wright's stain. Polychromasia is indicative of premature release of RBCs from bone marrow secondary to increased erythropoietin stimulation.

RBC Inclusions

RBC inclusions can result from certain types of anemia, abnormal Hgb precipitation, or parasitic infection.

- Cabot rings may be seen in megaloblastic and other anemias, lead poisoning, and conditions in which RBCs are destroyed before they are released from bone marrow.
- Basophilic stippling is seen whenever there is altered Hgb synthesis, as in thalassemias, megaloblastic anemias, alcoholism, and lead or arsenic intoxication.
- Howell-Jolly bodies are seen in sickle cell anemia, other hemolytic anemias, megaloblastic anemia, congenital absence of the spleen, and the postsplenectomy period.
- Pappenheimer bodies may be seen in cases of sideroblastic anemia, thalassemias, refractory anemia, dyserythropoietic anemias, hemosiderosis, and hemochromatosis.
- Heinz bodies are most often seen in the blood of patients who have ingested drugs known to induce the formation of these inclusion bodies. They are also seen in patients with hereditary glucose-6-phosphate dehydrogenase (G6PD) deficiency.
- Hgb C crystals can often be identified in stained peripheral smears of patients with hereditary hemoglobin C disease.
- Parasites such as *Plasmodium* (transmitted by mosquitoes and causing malaria) and *Babesia* (transmitted by ticks), known to invade human RBCs, can be visualized with Wright's stain and other special stains of the peripheral blood.

CRITICAL FINDINGS:

The presence of sickle cells or parasitic inclusions should be brought to the immediate attention of the requesting health-care provider (HCP).

Note and immediately report to the requesting HCP any critical findings and related symptoms. A listing of these findings varies among facilities. Timely notification of a critical finding for laboratory or diagnostic studies is a role expectation of the professional nurse. The notification processes vary among facilities. Upon receipt of the critical finding, the information should be read back to the caller to verify accuracy.

INTERFERING FACTORS

- Drugs and other substances that may increase Heinz body formation as an initial precursor to significant hemolysis include acetanilid, acetylsalicylic acid, antimalarials, antipyretics, furazolidone, methylene blue, naphthalene, and nitrofurans.
- The results of a CBC should be carefully evaluated during transfusion or acute blood loss because the body is not in a state of homeostasis and values may be misleading. Considerations for draw times after transfusion include the type of product, the amount of product transfused, and the patient's clinical situation. Generally, specimens collected an hour after transfusion will provide an acceptable reflection of the effects of the transfused product. Measurements taken during a massive transfusion are an exception, providing essential guidance for therapeutic decisions during critical care.
- Leaving the tourniquet in place for longer than 60 sec can falsely affect the results.
- Morphology can be evaluated to some extent via indices; therefore, failure to fill the tube sufficiently (i.e., tube less than three-quarters full) may yield inadequate sample volume for automated analyzers and may be a reason for specimen rejection.
- Hemolyzed or clotted specimens should be rejected.

NURSING IMPLICATIONS AND PROCEDURE

C

PRETEST:

- Positively identify the patient using at least two person-specific identifiers before services, treatments, or procedures are performed.
- ***Patient Teaching:*** Inform the patient this test can assist in assessing red cell appearance.
- Obtain a history of the patient's health concerns, symptoms, surgical procedures, and results of previously performed laboratory and diagnostic studies. Include a list of known allergens, especially allergies or sensitivities to latex.
- Note any recent procedures that can interfere with test results.
- Obtain a list of the patient's current medications, including over-the-counter medications and dietary supplements (see Effects of Natural Products on Laboratory Values online at Davis*Plus*).
- Review the procedure with the patient. Inform the patient that specimen collection takes approximately 5 to 10 min. Address concerns about pain and explain that there may be some discomfort during the venipuncture.
- ***Sensitivity to social and cultural issues,*** as well as concern for modesty, is important in providing psychological support before, during, and after the procedure.
- Note that there are no food, fluid, or medication restrictions unless by medical direction.

INTRATEST:

Potential Complications: N/A

- Avoid the use of equipment containing latex if the patient has a history of allergic reaction to latex.
- Instruct the patient to cooperate fully and to follow directions. Direct the patient to breathe normally and to avoid unnecessary movement.
- Observe standard precautions, and follow the general guidelines in Patient Preparation and Specimen Collection online at Davis*Plus*. Positively identify the patient, and label the appropriate specimen container with the corresponding patient demographics, initials of the person collecting the specimen, date, and time of collection. Perform a venipuncture. An EDTA Microtainer sample may be obtained from infants, children, and adults for whom venipuncture may not be feasible. The specimen should be mixed gently by inverting the tube 10 times. The specimen should be analyzed within 6 hr when stored at room temperature or within 24 hr if stored at refrigerated temperature. if it is anticipated the specimen will not be analyzed within 4 to 6 hr, two blood smears should be made immediately after the venipuncture and submitted with the blood sample. Smears made from specimens older than 6 hr will contain an unacceptable number of misleading artifactual abnormalities of the RBCs, such as echinocytes and spherocytes, as well as necrobiotic white blood cells.
- Remove the needle and apply direct pressure with dry gauze to stop bleeding. Observe/assess venipuncture site for bleeding or hematoma formation and secure gauze with adhesive bandage.
- Promptly transport the specimen to the laboratory for processing and analysis.

POST-TEST:

- Inform the patient that a report of the results will be made available to the requesting HCP, who will discuss the results with the patient.
- ***Nutritional Considerations:*** Instruct patients to consume a variety of foods within the basic food groups, maintain a healthy weight, be physically active, limit salt intake, limit alcohol intake, and avoid the use of tobacco.
- Reinforce information given by the patient's HCP regarding further testing, treatment, or referral to another HCP. Answer any questions or address any concerns voiced by the patient or family.

- Depending on the results of this procedure, additional testing may be performed to evaluate or monitor progression of the disease process and determine the need for a change in therapy. Evaluate test results in relation to the patient's symptoms and other tests performed.

RELATED STUDIES:

- Related tests include biopsy bone marrow, CBC, CBC hematocrit, CBC hemoglobin, CBC platelet count, CBC RBC count, CBC RBC indices, CBC WBC count with differential, δ-aminolevulinic acid, erythropoietin, ferritin, G6PD, hemoglobin electrophoresis, iron/TIBC, lead, and reticulocyte count.
- Refer to the Gastrointestinal, Hematopoietic, Hepatobiliary, Immune, and Respiratory systems tables online at Davis*Plus* for related tests by body system.

C

Complete Blood Count, WBC Count and Differential

SYNONYM/ACRONYM: WBC with diff, leukocyte count, white cell count.

COMMON USE: To evaluate viral and bacterial infections and to assist in diagnosing and monitoring leukemic disorders.

SPECIMEN: Whole blood from one full lavender-top (EDTA) tube.

NORMAL FINDINGS: (Method: Automated, computerized, multichannel analyzers. Many analyzers can determine a five- or six-part WBC differential. The six-part automated white blood cell [WBC] differential identifies and enumerates neutrophils, lymphocytes, monocytes, eosinophils, basophils, and immature granulocytes [IG], where IG represents the combined enumeration of promyelocytes, metamyelocytes, and myelocytes as both an absolute number and a percentage. The five-part WBC differential includes all but the immature granulocyte parameters.)

C

WBC Count and Differential

Age	Conventional Units WBC × 10^3/microL	Neutrophils (Absolute) and %	Lymphocytes (Absolute) and %	Monocytes (Absolute) and %	Eosinophils (Absolute) and %	Basophils (Absolute) and %
Birth	9.1–30.1	(5.5–18.3) 24%–58%	(2.8–9.3) 26%–56%	(0.5–1.7) 7%–13%	(0.02–0.7) 0%–8%	(0.1–0.2) 0%–2.5%
1–23 mo	6.1–17.5	(1.9–5.4) 21%–67%	(3.7–10.7) 20%–64%	(0.3–0.8) 4%–11%	(0.2–0.5) 0%–3.3%	(0–0.1) 0%–1%
2–10 yr	4.5–13.5	(2.4–7.3) 30%–77%	(1.7–5.1) 14%–50%	(0.2–0.6) 4%–9%	(0.1–0.3) 0%–5.8%	(0–0.1) 0%–1%
11 yr–older adult	4.5–11.1	(2.7–6.5) 40%–75%	(1.5–3.7) 12%–44%	(0.2–0.4) 4%–9%	(0.05–0.5) 0%–5.5%	(0–0.1) 0%–1%

*SI Units (conventional units × 1 or WBC count × 10^9/L).

WBC Count and Differential

Age	Immature Granulocytes (Absolute) (10^3/microL)	Immature Granulocyte Fraction (IGF) (%)
Birth–9 yr	0–0.03	0%–0.4%
10 yr–older adult	0–0.09	0%–0.9%

DESCRIPTION: WBCs constitute the body's primary defense system against foreign organisms, tissues, and other substances. The life span of a normal WBC is 13 to 20 days. Old WBCs are destroyed by the lymphatic system and excreted in the feces. Reference values for WBC counts vary significantly with age. WBC counts vary diurnally, with counts being lowest in the morning and highest in the late afternoon. Other variables such as stress and high levels of activity or physical exercise can trigger transient increases of 2×10^3/microL to 5×10^3/microL. The main WBC types are neutrophils (band and segmented neutrophils), eosinophils, basophils, monocytes, and lymphocytes. WBCs are produced in the bone marrow. B-cell lymphocytes remain in the bone marrow to mature. T-cell lymphocytes migrate to and mature in the thymus. The WBC count can be performed alone with the differential cell count or as part of the complete blood count (CBC). The WBC differential can be performed by an automated instrument or manually on a slide prepared from a stained peripheral blood sample. Automated instruments provide excellent, reliable information, but the accuracy of the WBC count can be affected by the presence of circulating nucleated red blood cells (RBCs), clumped platelets, fibrin strands, cold agglutinins, cryoglobulins, intracellular parasitic organisms, or other significant blood cell inclusions and may not be identified in the interpretation of an automated blood count. The decision to report a manual or automated differential is based on specific criteria established by the laboratory. The criteria are designed to identify findings that warrant further investigation or confirmation by manual review. An increased WBC count is termed *leukocytosis,* and a decreased WBC count is termed *leukopenia.* A total WBC count indicates the degree of response to a pathological process, but a more complete evaluation for specific diagnoses for any one disorder is provided by the differential count. The WBCs in the count and differential are reported as an ***absolute value*** and as a percentage. The relative percentages of cell types are arrived at by basing the enumeration of each cell type on a 100-cell count. The absolute value is obtained by multiplying the relative percentage value of each cell type by the total WBC count. For example, on a CBC report, with a total WBC of 9×10^3/microL ✱ and WBC differential with 92% segmented neutrophils, 1% band neutrophils, 5% lymphocytes, and 1% monocytes the absolute values are calculated as follows: $92/100 \times 9 = 8.3$ segs, $1/100 \times 9 = 0.09$ bands, $5/100 \times 9 = 0.45$ lymphs, $1/100 \times 9 = 0.1$ monos for a total of 9 WBC count. The absolute neutrophil count (ANC) for this patient would be 9 × (0.92 + 0.01) = 8.4.

The ANC reflects the number of segmented and band type neutrophils in the total WBC count. It is used as an indicator of immune status because it reflects the type and number of WBC available to rapidly respond to an infection. Neutropenia is a decrease below normal in the number of neutrophils. ANC = Total WBC × [(Segs/100) + (Bands/100)] or total WBC × (% Segs + % Bands). The normal value varies with age but in general mild neutropenia is less than 1.5, moderate neutropenia is between 0.5 and 1, and severe neutropenia is less than 0.5. The ANC is helpful when managing patients receiving chemotherapy. It can drive decisions to place a hospitalized patient in isolation in order to protect them from exposure to infectious agents. When the patient is aware of their ANC they can also make informed decisions in taking actions to avoid exposure to crowds, avoid touching things in public places that may carry germs, or avoiding friends and family who may be sick.

Acute leukocytosis is initially accompanied by changes in the WBC count population, followed by changes within the individual WBCs. Leukocytosis usually occurs by way of increase in a single WBC family rather than a proportional increase in all cell types. Toxic granulation and vacuolation are commonly seen in leukocytosis accompanied by a *shift to the left,* or increase in the percentage of immature neutrophils to mature segmented neutrophils. An increased number or percentage of immature granulocytes, reflected by a shift to the left, represents production of WBCs and is useful as an indicator of infection. Immature neutrophils are called bands and can represent 3% to 5% of total circulating neutrophils in healthy individuals. *Bandemia* is defined by the presence of greater than 6% to 10% band neutrophils in the total neutrophil cell population. These changes in the white cell population are most commonly associated with an infectious process, usually bacterial, but they can occur in healthy individuals who are under stress (in response to epinephrine production), such as women in childbirth and very young infants. The WBC count and differential of a woman in labor or of an actively crying infant may show an overall increase in WBCs with a shift to the left. Before initiating any kind of intervention, it is important to determine whether an increased WBC count is the result of a normal condition involving physiological stress or a pathological process. The use of multiple specimen types may confuse the interpretation of results in infants. Multiple samples from the same collection site (i.e., capillary versus venous) may be necessary to obtain an accurate assessment of the WBC picture in these young patients.

Neutrophils are normally found as the predominant WBC type in the circulating blood. Also called *polymorphonuclear cells,* they are the body's first line of defense through the process of phagocytosis. They also contain enzymes and pyogenes, which combat foreign invaders.

Lymphocytes are agranular, mononuclear blood cells that are

smaller than granulocytes. They are found in the next highest percentage in normal circulation. Lymphocytes are classified as B cells and T cells. Both types are formed in the bone marrow, but B cells mature in the bone marrow and T cells mature in the thymus. Lymphocytes play a major role in the body's natural defense system. B cells differentiate into immunoglobulin-synthesizing plasma cells. T cells function as cellular mediators of immunity and comprise helper/inducer (CD4) lymphocytes, delayed hypersensitivity lymphocytes, cytotoxic (CD8 or CD4) lymphocytes, and suppressor (CD8) lymphocytes.

Monocytes are mononuclear cells similar to lymphocytes, but they are related more closely to granulocytes in terms of their function. They are formed in the bone marrow from the same cells as those that produce neutrophils. The major function of monocytes is phagocytosis. Monocytes stay in the peripheral blood for about 70 hr, after which they migrate into the tissues and become macrophages.

The function of eosinophils is phagocytosis of antigen-antibody complexes. They become active in the later stages of inflammation. Eosinophils respond to allergic and parasitic diseases: They have granules that contain histamine used to kill foreign cells in the body and proteolytic enzymes that damage parasitic worms (see study titled "Eosinophil Count").

Basophils are found in small numbers in the circulating blood. They have a phagocytic function and, similar to eosinophils, contain numerous specific granules. Basophilic granules contain heparin, histamines, and serotonin. Basophils may also be found in tissue and as such are classified as mast cells. Basophilia is noted in conditions such as leukemia, Hodgkin's disease, polycythemia vera, ulcerative colitis, nephrosis, and chronic hypersensitivity states.

This procedure is contraindicated for: N/A

INDICATIONS

- Assist in confirming suspected bone marrow depression.
- Assist in determining the cause of an elevated WBC count (e.g., infection, inflammatory process).
- Detect hematological disorder, neoplasm, or immunological abnormality.
- Determine the presence of a hereditary hematological abnormality.
- Monitor the effects of physical or emotional stress.
- Monitor the progression of nonhematological disorders, such as chronic obstructive pulmonary disease, malabsorption syndromes, cancer, and kidney disease.
- Monitor the response to drugs or chemotherapy and evaluate undesired reactions to drugs that may cause blood dyscrasias.
- Provide screening as part of a CBC in a general physical examination, especially on admission to a healthcare facility or before surgery.

POTENTIAL MEDICAL DIAGNOSIS

Increased in:

Leukocytosis

- Normal physiological and environmental conditions:

  Early infancy ***(increases are believed to be related to the physiological stress of birth and metabolic demands of rapid development)***

  Emotional stress ***(related to secretion of epinephrine)***

Exposure to extreme heat or cold ***(related to physiological stress)***
Pregnancy and labor ***(WBC counts may be modestly elevated due to increased neutrophils into the third trimester and during labor, returning to normal within a week postpartum)***
Strenuous exercise ***(related to epinephrine secretion; increases are short in duration, minutes to hours)***
Ultraviolet light ***(related to physiological stress and possible inflammatory response)***

- Pathological conditions:

Acute hemolysis, especially due to splenectomy or transfusion reactions ***(related to leukocyte response to remove lysed RBC fragments)***
All types of infections ***(related to an inflammatory or infectious response)***
Anemias ***(bone marrow disorders affecting RBC production may result in elevated WBC count)***
Appendicitis
Collagen disorders ***(related to an inflammatory or infectious response)***
Cushing's disease ***(related to overproduction of cortisol, a corticosteroid, which stimulates WBC production)***
Inflammatory disorders ***(related to an inflammatory or infectious response)***
Leukemias and other malignancies ***(related to bone marrow disorders that result in abnormal WBC production)***
Parasitic infestations ***(related to an inflammatory or infectious response)***
Polycythemia vera ***(myeloproliferative bone marrow disorder causing an increase in all cell lines)***

Decreased in:

Leukopenia

- Normal physiological conditions

Diurnal rhythms (lowest in the morning)

- Pathological conditions

Alcoholism ***(related to WBC changes associated with nutritional deficiencies of vitamin B_{12} or folate)***
Anemias ***(related to WBC changes associated with nutritional deficiencies of vitamin B_{12} or folate, especially in megaloblastic anemias)***
Bone marrow depression ***(related to decreased production)***
Malaria ***(related to hypersplenism)***
Malnutrition ***(related to WBC changes associated with nutritional deficiencies of vitamin B_{12} or folate)***
Radiation ***(related to physical cell destruction due to toxic effects of radiation)***
Rheumatoid arthritis ***(related to adverse effect of medications used to treat the condition)***
Systemic lupus erythematosus (SLE) and other autoimmune disorders ***(related to adverse effect of drugs used to treat the condition)***
Toxic and antineoplastic drugs ***(related to bone marrow suppression)***
Very low birth weight neonates ***(related to bone marrow activity being diverted to develop RBCs in response to hypoxia)***
Viral infections ***(leukopenia, lymphocytopenia, and abnormal lymphocytes may be present in the early stages of viral infections)***

Neutrophils Increased (Neutrophilia)

- Acute hemolysis
- Acute hemorrhage
- Extremes in temperature
- Infectious diseases
- Inflammatory conditions (rheumatic fever, gout, rheumatoid arthritis, vasculitis, myositis)
- Malignancies
- Metabolic disorders (uremia, eclampsia, diabetic ketoacidosis, thyroid storm, Cushing's syndrome)
- Myelocytic leukemia
- Physiological stress (e.g., allergies, asthma, exercise, childbirth, surgery)
- Tissue necrosis (burns, crushing injuries, abscesses, myocardial infarction)
- Tissue poisoning with toxins and venoms

Neutrophils Decreased (Neutropenia)
- Acromegaly
- Addison's disease
- Anaphylaxis
- Anorexia nervosa, starvation, malnutrition
- Bone marrow depression (viruses, toxic chemicals, overwhelming infection, radiation, Gaucher's disease)
- Disseminated SLE
- Thyrotoxicosis
- Viral infection (mononucleosis, hepatitis, influenza)
- Vitamin B_{12} or folate deficiency

Lymphocytes Increased (Lymphocytosis)
- Addison's disease
- Felty's syndrome
- Infections (viral, e.g., cytomegalovirus, hepatitis, HIV, infectious mononucleosis, rubella, varicella; or bacterial, e.g., tuberculosis, whooping cough)
- Lymphocytic leukemia
- Lymphomas
- Lymphosarcoma
- Myeloma
- Rickets
- Thyrotoxicosis
- Ulcerative colitis
- Waldenström's macroglobulinemia

Lymphocytes Decreased (Lymphopenia)
- Antineoplastic drugs
- Aplastic anemia
- Bone marrow failure
- Burns
- Gaucher's disease
- Hemolytic disease of the newborn
- High doses of adrenocorticosteroids
- Hodgkin's disease
- Hypersplenism
- Immunodeficiency diseases
- Infections
- Malnutrition
- Pernicious anemia
- Pneumonia
- Radiation
- Rheumatic fever
- Septicemia
- Thrombocytopenic purpura
- Toxic chemical exposure
- Transfusion reaction

Monocytes Increased (Monocytosis)
- Carcinomas
- Cirrhosis
- Collagen diseases
- Gaucher's disease
- Hemolytic anemias
- Hodgkin's disease
- Infections
- Lymphomas
- Monocytic leukemia
- Polycythemia vera
- Radiation
- Sarcoidosis
- SLE
- Thrombocytopenic purpura
- Ulcerative colitis

CRITICAL FINDINGS:
- Total WBC count of less than 2×10^3/microL (SI: Less than 2×10^9/L)
- Absolute neutrophil count of less than 0.5×10^3/microL (SI: Less than 0.5×10^9/L)
- Total WBC count of greater than 30×10^3/microL (SI: Greater than 30×10^9/L)

Note and immediately report to the requesting health-care provider (HCP) any critical findings and related symptoms. A listing of these findings varies among facilities. Timely notification of a critical finding for laboratory or diagnostic studies is a role expectation of the professional nurse. The notification processes vary among facilities. Upon receipt of the critical finding, the information should be read back to the caller to verify accuracy.

C

Consideration may be given to verifying the critical findings before action is taken. Policies vary among facilities and may include requesting immediate recollection and retesting by the laboratory.

The presence of abnormal cells, other morphological characteristics, or cellular inclusions may signify a potentially life-threatening or serious health condition and should be investigated. Examples are hypersegmented neutrophils, agranular neutrophils, blasts or other immature cells, Auer rods, Döhle bodies, marked toxic granulation, or plasma cells.

C

INTERFERING FACTORS

- Drugs and other substances that may decrease the overall WBC count include acetylsalicylic acid, aminosalicylic acid, ampicillin, amsacrine, antazoline, anticonvulsants, antineoplastic drugs (therapeutic intent), antipyrine, barbiturates, busulfan, carmustine, chlorambucil, chloramphenicol, chlordane, chlorophenothane, chlorpromazine, chlorthalidone, cisplatin, colchicine, colistimethate, cycloheximide, cyclophosphamide, cytarabine, dacarbazine, dactinomycin, diazepam, diethylpropion, digitalis, dipyridamole, dipyrone, fumagillin, glaucarubin, glucosulfone, hexachlorobenzene, hydroxychloroquine, iothiouracil, iproniazid, lincomycin, local anesthetics, mefenamic acid, meprobamate, mercaptopurine, methotrexate, methylpromazine, mitomycin, paramethadione, parathion, penicillin, phenacemide, phenothiazine, pipamazine, prednisone (by Coulter S method), primaquine, procainamide, procarbazine, prochlorperazine, promethazine, pyrazolones, pyrimethamine, quinacrine, quinines, radioactive compounds, razoxane, ristocetin, sulfa drugs, tamoxifen, tetracycline, thenalidine, thioridazine, tolazamide, tolazoline, tolbutamide, trimethadione, and urethane.
- A significant decrease in basophil count occurs rapidly after intravenous (IV) injection of propanidid and thiopental.
- A significant decrease in lymphocyte count occurs rapidly after administration of corticotropin, mechlorethamine, methysergide, and x-ray therapy; and after megadoses of niacin, pyridoxine, and thiamine. 🍁
- Drugs and other substances that may increase the overall WBC count include amphetamine, amphotericin B, chloramphenicol, chloroform (normal response to anesthesia), colchicine (leukocytosis follows leukopenia), corticotropin, erythromycin, ether (normal response to anesthesia), isoflurane (normal response to anesthesia), niacinamide, phenylbutazone, prednisone, and quinine.
- Drug allergies may have a significant effect on eosinophil count and may affect the overall WBC count. Refer to the study titled "Eosinophil Count" for a detailed listing of interfering drugs.
- The WBC count may vary depending on the patient's position, decreasing when the patient is recumbent owing to hemodilution and increasing when the patient rises owing to hemoconcentration.
- Venous stasis can falsely elevate results; the tourniquet should not be left on the arm for longer than 60 sec.
- Failure to fill the tube sufficiently (i.e., tube less than three-quarters full) may yield inadequate sample volume for automated analyzers and may be reason for specimen rejection.

- Hemolyzed or clotted specimens should be rejected for analysis.
- The presence of nucleated red blood cells or giant or clumped platelets affects the automated WBC, requiring a manual correction of the WBC count.
- Care should be taken in evaluating the CBC during the first few hours after transfusion.
- Patients with cold agglutinins or monoclonal gammopathies may have a falsely decreased WBC count as a result of cell clumping.

C

NURSING IMPLICATIONS AND PROCEDURE

POTENTIAL NURSING PROBLEMS:

Problem	Signs & Symptoms	Interventions
Infection ***(related to metabolic or endocrine dysfunction; chronic debilitating illness; cirrhosis; trauma; vectors; decreased tissue perfusion; presence of gram-positive or gram-negative organisms)***	Temperature; increased heart rate; increased blood pressure; shaking; chills; mottled skin; lethargy; fatigue; swelling; edema; pain; localized pressure; diaphoresis; night sweats; confusion; vomiting; nausea; headache	Promote good hygiene; assist with hygiene as needed; administer prescribed antibiotics, antipyretics; provide cooling measures; administer prescribed IV fluids; monitor vital signs and trend temperatures; encourage oral fluids; adhere to standard or universal precautions; isolate as appropriate; obtain cultures as ordered; encourage use of lightweight clothing and bedding; monitor and trend indicators of infection (WBC, C-reactive protein [CRP])
Fluid volume ***(related to metabolic imbalances associated with disease process; insensible fluid loss; excessive diaphoresis)***	**Deficient:** Decreased urinary output, fatigue, sunken eyes, dark urine, decreased blood pressure, increased heart rate, and altered mental status	Record daily weight and monitor trends; record accurate intake and output; collaborate with HCP with administration of IV fluids to support hydration; monitor laboratory values that reflect alterations in fluid status (potassium, blood urea nitrogen, creatinine, calcium, hemoglobin, and hematocrit); manage underlying cause of fluid alteration; monitor urine characteristics and respiratory status; establish baseline assessment data; collaborate with HCP to adjust oral and IV fluids to provide optimal hydration status; administer replacement electrolytes as ordered

(table continues on page 520)

Problem	Signs & Symptoms	Interventions
Fever ***(related to increased basal metabolic rate; infection)***	Elevated temperature; flushed, warm skin; diaphoresis; skin warm to touch; tachycardia; tachypnea; seizures; convulsions	Assess the patient's temperature frequently; monitor for emotional labile events that could precipitate a thyroid storm or crisis and precipitate an elevation in temperature; ensure the patient's immediate environment remains cool; encourage the use of light bedding and lightweight clothing to prevent overheating; increase fluid intake to offset insensible fluid loss; encourage bathing with tepid water for comfort and promotion of cooling; administer prescribed antithyroid therapy
Health management ***(related to failure to regulate diet; lack of exercise; alcohol use; smoking; complexity of health-care system; complexity of therapeutic management; altered metabolic process; knowledge deficit; conflicted decision making; cultural family health patterns; barriers to healthy decisions; mistrust of HCP)***	Inability or failure to recognize or process information toward improving health and preventing illness with associated mental and physical effects; ineffective health choices; increasing symptoms of illness; verbalizes that therapeutic regime is too difficult; patient and family do not support HCP's suggestions for health improvement; refusal to follow recommended therapeutic regime	Ensure regular participation in weight-bearing exercise; assess diet, smoking, and alcohol use; teach the importance of adequate calcium intake with diet and supplements; refer to smoking cessation and alcohol treatment programs; teach the signs and symptoms of infection; assess family or cultural factors that impact the success of the therapeutic regime; assess the patient's self-assessment of his or her health status; include the patient and family in designing the plan of care; tailor the plan of care to the patient's lifestyle; collaborate with the patient and family to develop a system of managing own health; focus on behaviors that will make the biggest positive impact on improved health

PRETEST:

- Positively identify the patient using at least two person-specific identifiers before services, treatments, or procedures are performed.
- *Patient Teaching:* Inform the patient this test can assist in assessing for infection or monitoring leukemia.
- Obtain a history of the patient's health concerns, symptoms, surgical procedures, and results of previously performed laboratory and diagnostic studies. Include a list of known allergens, especially allergies or sensitivities to latex.
- Note any recent procedures that can interfere with test results.
- Obtain a list of the patient's current medications, including over-the-counter medications and dietary supplements (see Effects of Natural Products on Laboratory Values online at Davis*Plus*).
- Review the procedure with the patient. Inform the patient that specimen collection takes approximately 5 to 10 min. Address concerns about pain and explain that there may be some discomfort during the venipuncture.
- *Sensitivity to social and cultural issues,* as well as concern for modesty, is important in providing psychological support before, during, and after the procedure.
- Note that there are no food, fluid, or medication restrictions unless by medical direction.

INTRATEST:

Potential Complications: N/A

- Avoid the use of equipment containing latex if the patient has a history of allergic reaction to latex.
- Instruct the patient to cooperate fully and to follow directions. Direct the patient to breathe normally and to avoid unnecessary movement.
- Observe standard precautions, and follow the general guidelines in Patient Preparation and Specimen Collection online at Davis*Plus*. Positively identify the patient, and label the appropriate specimen container with the corresponding patient demographics, initials of the person collecting the specimen, date, and time of collection. Perform a venipuncture. The specimen should be mixed gently by inverting the tube 10 times. The specimen should be analyzed within 24 hr when stored at room temperature or within 48 hr if stored at refrigerated temperature. If it is anticipated the specimen will not be analyzed within 24 hr, two blood smears should be made immediately after the venipuncture and submitted with the blood sample. Smears made from specimens older than 24 hr may contain an unacceptable number of misleading artifactual abnormalities of the RBCs, such as echinocytes and spherocytes, as well as necrobiotic white blood cells.
- Remove the needle and apply direct pressure with dry gauze to stop bleeding. Observe/assess venipuncture site for bleeding or hematoma formation and secure gauze with adhesive bandage.
- Promptly transport the specimen to the laboratory for processing and analysis.

POST-TEST:

- Inform the patient that a report of the results will be made available to the requesting HCP, who will discuss the results with the patient.
- *Nutritional Considerations:* Infection, fever, sepsis, and trauma can result in an impaired nutritional status. Malnutrition can occur for many reasons, including fatigue, lack of appetite, and gastrointestinal distress.
- *Nutritional Considerations:* Adequate intake of vitamins A and C, and zinc are also important for regenerating body stores depleted by the effort exerted in fighting infections. Educate the patient or caregiver regarding the importance of following the prescribed diet.
- *Nutritional Considerations:* Educate the patient with vitamin A deficiency, as appropriate, that the main dietary

C

source of vitamin A comes from carotene, a yellow pigment noticeable in most fruits and vegetables, especially carrots, sweet potatoes, squash, apricots, and cantaloupe. It is also present in spinach, collards, broccoli, and cabbage. This vitamin is fairly stable at most cooking temperatures, but it is destroyed easily by light and oxidation.

C

Vitamin C

- *Nutritional Considerations:* Educate the patient with vitamin C deficiency, as appropriate, that citrus fruits are excellent dietary sources of vitamin C. Other good sources are green and red peppers, tomatoes, white potatoes, cabbage, broccoli, chard, kale, turnip greens, asparagus, berries, melons, pineapple, and guava. Vitamin C is destroyed by exposure to air, light, heat, or alkalis. Boiling water before cooking eliminates dissolved oxygen that destroys vitamin C in the process of boiling. Vegetables should be crisp and cooked as quickly as possible.
- *Nutritional Considerations:* Topical or oral supplementation may be ordered for patients with zinc deficiency. Dietary sources high in zinc include shellfish, red meat, wheat germ, nuts, and processed foods such as canned pork and beans and canned chili. Patients should be informed that phytates (from whole grains, coffee, cocoa, or tea) bind zinc and prevent it from being absorbed. Decreases in zinc also can be induced by increased intake of iron, copper, or manganese. Vitamin and mineral supplements with a greater than 3:1 iron/zinc ratio inhibit zinc absorption.
- Recognize anxiety related to test results, and be supportive of fear of shortened life expectancy.
- Depending on the results of this procedure, additional testing may be performed to evaluate or monitor progression of the disease process and determine the need for a change in therapy. Evaluate test results in relation to the patient's symptoms and other tests performed.

Patient Education:

- Discuss the implications of abnormal test results on the patient's lifestyle.
- Provide teaching and information regarding the clinical implications of the test results, as appropriate.
- Educate the patient regarding access to counseling services.
- Provide contact information, if desired, for the Institute of Medicine of the National Academies (www.iom.edu) or the USDA's resource for nutrition (www.choosemyplate.gov). 🍁 Additional resources are available through the National Cancer Institute (www.nci.nih.org) or American Cancer Society (www.cancer.org). 🍁
- Reinforce information given by the patient's HCP regarding further testing, treatment, or referral to another HCP.
- Answer any questions or address any concerns voiced by the patient or family.

Expected Patient Outcomes:

Understanding

- The patient and family state the signs and symptoms of infection.
- The patient and family state the importance of compliance with follow-up laboratory tests to manage disease process.

Ability

- The patient demonstrates proficiency in taking prescribed antibiotics.
- The patient and family demonstrate proficiency in taking and recording temperature.

Response

- The patient and family comply with the request to make lifestyle alterations that will decrease infection risk.
- The patient complies with the request to increase fluid intake to offset fluid loss and prevent dehydration.

RELATED STUDIES:

- Related tests include albumin, antibody anti–neutrophilic cytoplasmic biopsy bone marrow, biopsy lymph node, CBC, CBC RBC count, CBC RBC indices, CBC RBC morphology, culture bacterial (see individually listed culture studies), culture fungal, culture viral, eosinophil count, ESR, fecal analysis, Gram stain, infectious mononucleosis, LAP, procalcitonin, UA, US abdomen, and WBC scan.

- Refer to the Hematopoietic, Immune, and Respiratory systems tables online at Davis*Plus* for related tests by body system.

Computed Tomography, Abdomen

C

SYNONYM/ACRONYM: Computed axial tomography (CAT), computed transaxial tomography (CTT), abdominal CT, helical/spiral CT.

COMMON USE: To visualize and assess abdominal structures and to assist in diagnosing tumors, cancer, bleeding, and abscess. Used as an evaluation tool for surgical, radiation, and medical therapeutic interventions.

AREA OF APPLICATION: Abdomen.

DESCRIPTION: Abdominal computed tomography (CT) is a noninvasive procedure used to enhance certain anatomic views of the abdominal structures. It becomes invasive when contrast medium is used. During the procedure, the patient lies on a motorized table. The table is moved in and out of a circular opening in a doughnut-like device called a *gantry,* which houses the x-ray tube and associated electronics. A beam of x-rays irradiates the patient as the table moves in and out of the scanner in a series of phases. The x-rays penetrate liquids and solids of different densities by varying degrees. Multiple detectors rotate around the patient to collect numeric data associated with the density coefficients assigned to each degree of tissue density. The imaging system's computer converts the numeric data obtained from the scanner into digital images. Air appears black; bone appears white; and body fluids, fat, and soft tissue structures are represented in various shades between black and white. The cross-sectional views, or *slices,* of the liver, biliary tract, gallbladder, pancreas, kidneys, adrenal glands, spleen, intestines, and associated vascular system can be reviewed individually or as a three-dimensional image to allow differentiations of solid, cystic, inflammatory, or vascular lesions as well as identification of suspected hematomas and aneurysms. The scan may be repeated after administration of contrast medium given orally, by intravenous (IV) injection, or rectally. Contrast is used to differentiate, enhance, or "light up" areas of interest depending on the type of study to be performed, type of contrast medium to be used, and method of administration. The medium works by creating a contrast between areas of interest based on density; penetration of the x-rays is weaker in areas where the contrast medium is detected by the scanner, showing the blood vessels, organs, and tissue as whitish areas that either outline the area of interest or completely fill it. Oral ingestion of contrast medium can be used

C

for opacification to distinguish the bowel, adjacent abdominal organs, other types of tissue, and blood vessels as the medium moves through the digestive tract. IV injection of contrast medium is used for evaluation of blood flow through vessels and greater enhancement of tissue density and organ visualization. In some cases, scans may be repeated after multiple types of contrast are administered. Multislice or multidetector CT scanners continuously collect images in a helical or spiral fashion instead of a series of individual images, as with standard scanners. Helical CT can collect many images over a short period of time (seconds), is sensitive in identifying small abnormalities, and produces high-quality images. Positron emission tomography (PET) and single-photon emission tomography (SPECT) are types of nuclear medicine studies that offer insights into functionality such as movement of blood flow or uptake and distribution of metabolites into tumors. PET/CT and SPECT/CT are imaging applications that superimpose PET or SPECT and CT findings. The images are collected and produced by a single gantry system. The co-registered or image fusion of PET/CT or SPECT/CT findings can provide a detailed combination of anatomical and functional images. Images can be recorded on photographic or x-ray film or stored in digital format as digitized computer data. The CT scan can be used to guide biopsy needles into areas of suspected tumors to obtain tissue for laboratory analysis and to guide placement of catheters for drainage of cysts or abscesses. Tumor staging and progression, before and after therapy, and effectiveness of medical interventions may be monitored by PET/CT or SPECT/CT scanning. The images can be reevaluated and manipulated for further, detailed examination without having to repeat the procedure.

This procedure is contraindicated for

- Patients who are pregnant or suspected of being pregnant, unless the potential benefits of a procedure using radiation far outweigh the risk of radiation exposure to the fetus and mother.
- Patients who are claustrophobic.
- Patients with conditions associated with adverse reactions to contrast medium (e.g., asthma, food allergies, or allergy to contrast medium).

  Although patients are asked specifically if they have a known allergy to iodine or shellfish, it has been well established that the reaction is not to iodine, in fact an actual iodine allergy would be problematic because iodine is required for the production of thyroid hormones. In the case of shellfish the reaction is to a muscle protein called tropomyosin; in the case of iodinated contrast medium the reaction is to the noniodinated part of the contrast molecule. Patients with a known hypersensitivity to the medium may benefit from premedication with corticosteroids and diphenhydramine; the use of nonionic contrast or an alternative noncontrast imaging study, if available, may be considered for patients who have severe asthma or who have experienced moderate to severe reactions to ionic contrast medium.
- Patients with conditions associated with preexisting renal insufficiency (e.g., chronic kidney disease, single kidney transplant, nephrectomy,

diabetes, multiple myeloma, treatment with aminoglycosides and NSAIDs) ***because iodinated contrast is nephrotoxic.***

Patients who are chronically dehydrated before the test, especially older adults and patients whose health is already compromised, ***because of their risk of contrast-induced acute kidney injury.***

Patients with pheochromocytoma ***because iodinated contrast may cause a hypertensive crisis.***

Patients with bleeding disorders or receiving anticoagulant therapy ***because the puncture site may not stop bleeding.***

INDICATIONS

- Assist in differentiating between benign and malignant tumors.
- Detect aortic aneurysms.
- Detect tumor extension of masses and metastasis into the abdominal area.
- Differentiate aortic aneurysms from tumors near the aorta.
- Differentiate between infectious and inflammatory processes.
- Evaluate cysts, masses, abscesses, renal calculi, gastrointestinal (GI) bleeding and obstruction, and trauma.
- Evaluate retroperitoneal lymph nodes.
- Monitor and evaluate the effectiveness of medical, radiation, or surgical therapies.

POTENTIAL MEDICAL DIAGNOSIS

Normal findings

- Normal size, position, and shape of abdominal organs and vascular system

Abnormal findings related to

Identification of abnormal findings is assisted by comparison of parameters such as size, shape, symmetry, density, and location. For example, areas of altered density in either an expected or unexpected location may indicate enlargement of an organ or the presence of blood or other fluids, tumors, or cysts. Comparison by type of abnormal findings may also assist in evaluating areas of altered density. For example, well-defined round or oval areas, smaller in size and having lower density than a primary tumor, may indicate a cyst.

- Abdominal abscess
- Abdominal aortic aneurysm
- Abnormal accumulations of blood, fat, or body fluid
- Adrenal tumor or hyperplasia
- Appendicitis
- Bowel obstruction
- Bowel perforation
- Cirrhosis
- Dilation of the common hepatic duct, common bile duct, or gallbladder
- Diverticulitis or irritable bowel
- Gallstones
- GI bleeding
- Hematomas
- Hemoperitoneum
- Hepatic cysts or abscesses
- Infarction (e.g., intestinal, omental)
- Infection
- Pancreatic pseudocyst
- Primary and metastatic neoplasms in bone, organs, glands, ducts, or ligaments
- Renal calculi
- Splenic laceration
- Trauma

CRITICAL FINDINGS:

- Abscess
- Acute GI bleed
- Aortic aneurysm
- Appendicitis
- Aortic dissection
- Bowel perforation
- Bowel obstruction
- Mesenteric torsion
- Tumor with significant mass effect

- Visceral injury; significant solid organ laceration

Note and immediately report to the requesting health-care provider (HCP) any critical findings and related symptoms. A listing of these findings varies among facilities. Timely notification of a critical finding for laboratory or diagnostic studies is a role expectation of the professional nurse. The notification processes vary among facilities. Upon receipt of the critical finding, the information should be read back to the caller to verify accuracy.

C

INTERFERING FACTORS

Factors that may alter the results of the study

- Gas or feces in the GI tract resulting from inadequate cleansing or failure to restrict food intake before the study.
- Retained barium from a previous radiological procedure.
- Metallic objects within the examination field (e.g., jewelry, body rings), which may inhibit organ visualization and cause unclear images.
- Patients who are extremely obese may require more radiation to obtain a clear image.
- Patients with extreme claustrophobia unless sedation is given before the study.
- Inability of the patient to cooperate or remain still during the procedure because of age, significant pain, or mental status.

Other considerations

- The procedure may be terminated if chest pain or severe cardiac dysrhythmias occur.
- Failure to follow dietary restrictions and other pretesting preparations may cause the procedure to be canceled or repeated.
- The procedure may be canceled if the patient's weight exceeds the safety limit for the equipment.

NURSING IMPLICATIONS AND PROCEDURE

See Potential Nursing Problems on Fast Find at davispl.us/vanleeuwen7

PRETEST:

- Positively identify the patient using at least two person-specific identifiers before services, treatments, or procedures are performed.
- ***Patient Teaching:*** Inform the patient this procedure can assist in assessing the abdominal organs.
- Obtain a history of the patient's health concerns, symptoms, surgical procedures, and results of previously performed laboratory and diagnostic studies. Include a list of known allergens, especially allergies or sensitivities to latex, anesthetics, sedatives, or contrast medium. Ensure results of coagulation testing are obtained and recorded prior to the procedure; a creatinine level is also needed before contrast medium is to be used.
- Note any recent procedures that can interfere with test results, including examinations using barium- or iodine-based contrast medium. Ensure that barium studies were performed more than 4 days before the CT scan.
- Record the date of the last menstrual period and determine the possibility of pregnancy in perimenopausal women.
- Obtain a list of the patient's current medications, including over-the-counter medications, anticoagulants, aspirin and other salicylates, and dietary supplements (see Effects of Natural Products on Laboratory Values online at Davis*Plus*). Such products should be discontinued by medical direction for the appropriate number of days prior to a surgical procedure. Note the last time and dose of medication taken.
- If iodinated contrast medium is scheduled to be used in patients receiving metformin (Glucophage) for type 2 diabetes, the drug should be discontinued on the day of the test and continue to be withheld for 48 hr

after the test. Iodinated contrast can temporarily impair kidney function, and failure to withhold metformin may indirectly result in drug-induced lactic acidosis, a dangerous and sometimes fatal adverse effect of metformin ***related to renal impairment that does not support sufficient excretion of metformin.***

- Review the procedure with the patient. Explain the purpose of the test and how the procedure is performed. Address concerns about pain and explain that there may be moments of discomfort and some pain experienced during the test. Inform the patient that the procedure is performed in a radiology suite, usually by an HCP, and takes approximately 15 to 30 min depending on factors such as the type of study ordered, whether contrast will be used, and the type of contrast used.
- *Sensitivity to social and cultural issues,* as well as concern for modesty, is important in providing psychological support before, during, and after the procedure.
- Explain that an IV line may be inserted to allow infusion of fluids such as saline, anesthetics, contrast medium, or sedatives.
- Inform the patient that he or she may experience nausea, a feeling of warmth, a salty or metallic taste, or a transient headache after injection of contrast medium, if given.
- Advise the patient that he or she may be requested to drink approximately 450 mL of a dilute barium solution (approximately 1% barium) or a water-soluble oral contrast; the oral contrast is given within a specified time period prior to the study. Oral contrast is administered to distinguish GI organs from the other abdominal organs and to enhance other areas of interest.
- Instruct the patient to remove all external metallic objects from the area to be examined.
- Inform the patient, as appropriate, that CT studies performed without contrast usually do not require the patient to fast before the procedure. Instruct the patient, if required, to fast and restrict fluids for the specified time period prior to the procedure; fasting may be ordered as a precaution against aspiration related to nausea and vomiting during the administration of contrast. Also instruct the patient to avoid taking anticoagulant medication or to reduce dosage as ordered prior to the procedure due to increased risk of bleeding at the IV insertion site. Protocols may vary among facilities.
- *Make sure a written and informed consent has been signed prior to the procedure and before administering any medications.*

INTRATEST:

Potential Complications:

Injection of the contrast through IV tubing into a blood vessel is an invasive procedure. Complications are rare but do include risk for allergic reaction ***related to contrast reaction,*** cardiac dysrhythmias, hematoma ***related to blood leakage into the tissue following insertion of the IV needle,*** or infection ***that might occur if bacteria from the skin surface is introduced at the IV needle insertion site.***

- Observe standard precautions, and follow the general guidelines in Patient Preparation and Specimen Collection online at Davis*Plus*. Positively identify the patient.
- Ensure the patient has complied with dietary, fluids, medication restrictions and other pretesting instructions, as required, prior to the procedure.
- Ensure the patient has removed all external metallic objects from the area to be examined.
- Administer ordered prophylactic steroids or antihistamines before the procedure if the patient has a history of allergic reactions to any substance or drug.
- Avoid the use of equipment containing latex if the patient has a history of allergic reaction to latex.
- Have emergency equipment readily available.

C

- Instruct the patient to void prior to the procedure and to change into the gown, robe, and foot coverings provided.
- Instruct the patient to cooperate fully and to follow directions. Instruct the patient to remain still throughout the procedure because movement produces unreliable results.
- Record baseline vital signs, and continue to monitor throughout the procedure. Protocols may vary among facilities.
- Establish an IV fluid line for the injection of contrast, emergency drugs, and sedatives.
- Administer an antianxiety drug, as ordered, if the patient has claustrophobia. Administer a sedative to a child or to an adult who is uncooperative, as ordered.
- Place the patient in the supine position on an examination table.
- If IV contrast media is used, during and after injection a rapid series of images is taken.
- Instruct the patient to inhale deeply and hold his or her breath while the images are taken, and then to exhale after the images are taken.
- Instruct the patient to take slow, deep breaths if nausea occurs during the procedure.
- Monitor the patient for complications related to the procedure (e.g., allergic reaction, anaphylaxis, bronchospasm) if contrast is used.
- The needle is removed, and a pressure dressing is applied over the puncture site.
- Observe/assess the needle site for bleeding, inflammation, or hematoma formation.

POST-TEST:

- Inform the patient that a report of the results will be made available to the requesting HCP, who will discuss the results with the patient.
- Instruct the patient to resume usual diet, fluids, medications, and activity, as directed by the HCP. Kidney function should be assessed before metformin is resumed, if contrast was used.
- Monitor vital signs and neurological status every 15 min for 1 hr, then every 2 hr for 4 hr, and then as ordered by the HCP. Monitor temperature every 4 hr for 24 hr. Monitor intake and output at least every 8 hr. Compare with baseline values. Notify the HCP if temperature is elevated. Protocols may vary among facilities.
- If contrast was used, observe for delayed allergic reactions, such as rash, urticaria, tachycardia, hyperpnea, hypertension, palpitations, nausea, or vomiting. Antihistamines may be ordered and given to alleviate symptoms of allergic reaction.
- Instruct the patient to immediately report symptoms such as fast heart rate, difficulty breathing, skin rash, itching, chest pain, persistent right shoulder pain, or abdominal pain. Immediately report symptoms to the appropriate HCP.
- Observe/assess the needle insertion site for bleeding, inflammation, or hematoma formation.
- Instruct the patient in the care and assessment of the site.
- Instruct the patient to apply cold compresses to the insertion site as needed, to reduce discomfort or edema.
- Instruct the patient to increase fluid intake to help eliminate the contrast medium, if used.
- Inform the patient that diarrhea may occur after ingestion of oral contrast medium.
- Recognize anxiety related to test results. Discuss the implications of abnormal test results on the patient's lifestyle. Provide teaching and information regarding the clinical implications of the test results, as appropriate.
- Reinforce information given by the patient's HCP regarding further testing, treatment, or referral to another HCP. Answer any questions or address any concerns voiced by the patient or family.
- Depending on the results of this procedure, additional testing may be needed to evaluate or monitor progression of the disease process

and determine the need for a change in therapy. Evaluate test results in relation to the patient's symptoms and other tests performed.

Patient Education:

- Teach the patient the importance of managing hypertension to decrease bleeding risk.
- Teach the signs and symptoms of transfusion reaction.

Expected Patient Outcomes:

Understanding

- The patient and family discuss the medical versus surgical options for aneurysm management.
- The patient and family discuss the risks and benefits of blood transfusion and the types of transfusion available.

Ability

- The patient and family successfully create a quiet environment.
- The patient successfully demonstrates how to take own blood pressure using an approved medical device.

Response

- The patient and family agree to vigilant follow-up care to monitor the size of the aneurysm.
- The patient agrees to blood replacement therapy.

RELATED STUDIES:

- Related tests include ACTH and challenge tests, amylase, angiography abdomen, biopsy intestinal, BUN, calculus kidney stone panel, CBC, CBC hematocrit, CBC hemoglobin, cortisol and challenge tests, creatinine, cystoscopy, hepatobiliary scan, IVP, KUB studies, MRI abdomen, peritoneal fluid analysis, PT/INR, renogram, US abdomen, and US pelvis.
- Refer to the Gastrointestinal and Hepatobiliary systems tables online at Davis*Plus* for related tests by body system.

Computed Tomography, Angiography

SYNONYM/ACRONYM: Computed axial tomography (CAT) angiography, CTA.

COMMON USE: To visualize and assess the vascular structure to assist in the diagnosis of aneurysm, embolism, or stenosis.

AREA OF APPLICATION: Vessels.

DESCRIPTION: Computed tomography angiography (CTA) is a noninvasive procedure that enhances certain anatomic views of vascular structures. It becomes invasive when contrast medium is used. This procedure complements traditional angiography and allows reconstruction of the images in different planes and removal of surrounding structures, leaving only the vessels to be studied. During the procedure, the patient lies on a motorized table. The table is moved in and out of a circular opening in a doughnut-like device called a *gantry,* which houses the x-ray tube and associated electronics. A beam of x-rays irradiates the patient as the table moves in and out of the scanner in a series of phases. The x-rays penetrate liquids and solids of different densities by varying degrees. Multiple detectors rotate around the patient to collect numeric data associated with the density coefficients assigned to each degree of tissue density. The imaging system's computer

C

converts the numeric data obtained from the scanner into digital images. Air appears black; bone appears white; and body fluids, fat, and soft tissue structures are represented in various shades between black and white. The cross-sectional views, or *slices,* of the vascular system that supports major organs (brain, heart, lungs, kidneys) and anatomical areas such as the head, neck, arms, and legs can be reviewed individually or as a three-dimensional image to allow differentiations of solid, cystic, or vascular obstructions as well as identification of suspected hematomas and aneurysms. The scan may be repeated after intravenous (IV) administration of contrast medium. Contrast is used to differentiate, enhance, or "light up" areas of interest depending on the type of study to be performed, type of contrast medium to be used, and method of administration. The medium works by creating a contrast between areas of interest based on density; penetration of the x-rays is weaker in areas where the contrast medium is detected by the scanner, showing the blood vessels, organs, and tissue as whitish areas that either outline the area of interest or completely fill it. These images are helpful when vessels are heavily calcified, and the images give the most precise information regarding the true extent of stenosis. They can also evaluate intracerebral aneurysms. Small ulcerations and plaque irregularity are readily seen with CTA; the degree of stenosis can be closely estimated with CTA because of the increased number of imaging planes. Multislice or multidetector CT scanners continuously collect images in a helical or spiral fashion instead of a series of individual images, as with standard scanners. Helical CT can collect many images over a short period of time (seconds), is sensitive in identifying small abnormalities, and produces high-quality images. Images can be recorded on photographic or x-ray film or stored in digital format as digitized computer data. The CT scan can be used to guide biopsy needles into areas of suspected tumors to obtain tissue for laboratory analysis and to guide placement of catheters for angioplasty or biopsy. Tumor staging and progression, before and after therapy, and effectiveness of medical interventions may be monitored by CT scanning. The images can be reevaluated and manipulated for further, detailed examination without having to repeat the procedure.

This procedure is contraindicated for

- Patients who are pregnant or suspected of being pregnant, unless the potential benefits of a procedure using radiation far outweigh the risk of radiation exposure to the fetus and mother.
- Patients who are claustrophobic.
- Patients with conditions associated with adverse reactions to contrast medium (e.g., asthma, food allergies, or allergy to contrast medium).

Although patients are asked specifically if they have a known allergy to iodine or shellfish, it has been well established that the reaction is not to iodine; an actual iodine allergy would be problematic because iodine is required for the production of thyroid hormones.

In the case of shellfish, the reaction is to a muscle protein called tropomyosin; in the case of iodinated contrast medium, the reaction is to the noniodinated part of the contrast molecule. Patients with a known hypersensitivity to the medium may benefit from premedication with corticosteroids and diphenhydramine; the use of nonionic contrast or an alternative noncontrast imaging study, if available, may be considered for patients who have severe asthma or who have experienced moderate to severe reactions to ionic contrast medium.

Patients with conditions associated with preexisting renal insufficiency (e.g., chronic kidney disease, single kidney transplant, nephrectomy, diabetes, multiple myeloma, treatment with aminoglycosides and NSAIDs) ***because iodinated contrast is nephrotoxic.***

Patients who are chronically dehydrated before the test, especially older adults and patients whose health is already compromised, ***because of their risk of contrast-induced acute kidney injury.***

Patients with pheochromocytoma ***because iodinated contrast may cause a hypertensive crisis.***

Patients with bleeding disorders or receiving anticoagulant therapy ***because the puncture site may not stop bleeding.***

INDICATIONS

- Detect aneurysms.
- Detect embolism or other occlusions.
- Detect fistula.
- Detect stenosis.
- Detect peripheral arterial disease (PAD).
- Differentiate aortic aneurysms from tumors near the aorta.
- Differentiate between vascular and nonvascular tumors.
- Evaluate atherosclerosis.
- Evaluate hemorrhage or trauma.
- Monitor and evaluate the effectiveness of medical or surgical therapies.

POTENTIAL MEDICAL DIAGNOSIS

Normal findings

- Normal size, position, and shape of vascular structures

Abnormal findings related to

Identification of abnormal findings is assisted by comparison of parameters such as size, shape, symmetry, density, and location. For example, areas of altered density in either an expected or unexpected location may indicate enlargement of an organ or the presence of blood or other fluids, tumors, or cysts. Comparison by type of abnormal findings may also assist in evaluating areas of altered density. For example, well-defined round or oval areas, smaller in size and having lower density than a primary tumor, may indicate a cyst; unusual vascularity may indicate the site of a tumor; vessels that demonstrate narrowing may indicate areas of decreased blood flow.

- Aortic aneurysm
- Cysts or abscesses
- Dissected aorta
- Emboli
- Hemorrhage
- Occlusion
- PAD
- Pericarditis
- Shunting
- Stenosis
- Tumor

CRITICAL FINDINGS:

- Brain or spinal cord ischemia
- Emboli
- Hemorrhage
- Leaking aortic aneurysm
- Occlusion
- Tumor with significant mass effect

C

Note and immediately report to the requesting health-care provider (HCP) any critical findings and related symptoms. A listing of these findings varies among facilities. Timely notification of a critical finding for laboratory or diagnostic studies is a role expectation of the professional nurse. The notification processes vary among facilities. Upon receipt of the critical finding, the information should be read back to the caller to verify accuracy.

INTERFERING FACTORS

Factors that may alter the results of the study

- Gas or feces in the gastrointestinal tract resulting from inadequate cleansing or failure to restrict food intake before the study.
- Retained barium from a previous radiological procedure.
- Metallic objects within the examination field (e.g., jewelry, body rings), which may inhibit organ visualization and cause unclear images.
- Patients who are extremely obese may require more radiation to obtain a clear image.
- Patients with extreme claustrophobia unless sedation is given before the study.
- Patients who are unable to cooperate or remain still during the procedure because of age, significant pain, or mental status.

Other considerations

- The procedure may be terminated if chest pain or severe cardiac dysrhythmias occur.
- Failure to follow dietary restrictions and other pretesting preparations may cause the procedure to be canceled or repeated.
- The procedure may be canceled if the patient's weight exceeds the safety limit for the equipment.

NURSING IMPLICATIONS AND PROCEDURE

See Potential Nursing Problems on Fast Find at davispl.us/vanleeuwen7

PRETEST:

- Positively identify the patient using at least two person-specific identifiers before services, treatments, or procedures are performed.
- ***Patient Teaching:*** Inform the patient this procedure can assist in assessing the cardiovascular system.
- Obtain a history of the patient's health concerns, symptoms, surgical procedures, and results of previously performed laboratory and diagnostic studies. Include a list of known allergens, especially allergies or sensitivities to latex, anesthetics, contrast medium, or sedatives. Ensure results of coagulation testing are obtained and recorded prior to the procedure; a creatinine level is also needed before contrast medium is to be used.The presence of other risk factors, such as family history of heart disease, smoking, obesity, diet, lack of physical activity, hypertension, diabetes, previous myocardial infarction (MI), and previous vascular disease, should be investigated. Knowledge of genetics assists the nurse in identifying patients and family members who may benefit from additional education, risk assessment, and counseling. Genetics is the study and identification of genes, genetic mutations, and inheritance. For example, genetics provides some insight into the likelihood of inheriting a trait such as blue eyes or a medical condition such as coronary artery disease (CAD). Genomic studies evaluate the interaction of groups of genes. The combined activity or combined expression of groups of genes allows assumptions or predictions to be made. As an example, genomic studies measure the levels of activity in multiple genes to predict how they, along with environmental and lifestyle decisions, influence the development

of type 2 diabetes, CAD, MI, or ischemic stroke. Further information regarding inheritance of genes can be found in the study titled "Genetic Testing."

- Note any recent procedures that can interfere with test results, including examinations using barium- or iodine-based contrast medium. Ensure that barium studies were performed more than 4 days before the CT scan.
- Record the date of the last menstrual period and determine the possibility of pregnancy in perimenopausal women.
- Obtain a list of the patient's current medications, including over-the-counter medications, anticoagulants, aspirin and other salicylates, and dietary supplements (see Effects of Natural Products on Laboratory Values online at Davis*Plus*). Such products should be discontinued by medical direction for the appropriate number of days prior to a surgical procedure. Note the last time and dose of medication taken.
- If iodinated contrast medium is scheduled to be used in patients receiving metformin (Glucophage) for type 2 diabetes, the drug should be discontinued on the day of the test and continue to be withheld for 48 hr after the test. Iodinated contrast can temporarily impair kidney function, and failure to withhold metformin may indirectly result in drug-induced lactic acidosis, a dangerous and sometimes fatal adverse effect of metformin ***related to renal impairment that does not support sufficient excretion of metformin.***
- Review the procedure with the patient. Address concerns about pain and explain that there may be moments of discomfort and some pain experienced during the test. Inform the patient that the procedure is usually performed in a radiology suite by an HCP specializing in this procedure, with support staff, and takes approximately 15 to 30 min depending on factors such as the type of study ordered, whether contrast is used, and the type of contrast used.
- *Sensitivity to social and cultural issues,* as well as concern for modesty, important in providing psychological support before, during, and after the procedure.
- Explain that an IV line may be inserted to allow infusion of fluids such as saline, anesthetics, contrast medium, or sedatives.
- Inform the patient that a burning and flushing sensation may be felt throughout the body during injection of the contrast medium. After injection of the contrast medium, the patient may experience an urge to cough, flushing, nausea, or a salty or metallic taste.
- Instruct the patient to remove all external metallic objects from the area to be examined.
- Inform the patient, as appropriate, that CT studies performed without contrast usually do not require the patient to fast before the procedure. Instruct the patient, if required, to fast and restrict fluids for the specified time period prior to the procedure; fasting may be ordered as a precaution against aspiration related to nausea and vomiting during the administration of contrast. Also instruct the patient to avoid taking anticoagulant medication or to reduce dosage as ordered prior to the procedure due to increased risk of bleeding at the IV insertion site. Protocols may vary among facilities.
- *Make sure a written and informed consent has been signed prior to the procedure and before administering any medications.*

INTRATEST:

Potential Complications:

Injection of the contrast through IV tubing into a blood vessel is an invasive procedure. Complications are rare but do include risk for allergic reaction ***related to contrast reaction,*** cardiac dysrhythmias, hematoma ***related to blood leakage into the tissue following insertion of the IV needle,*** or infection ***that might occur if bacteria from the skin surface is introduced at the IV needle insertion site.***

C

- Observe standard precautions, and follow the general guidelines in Patient Preparation and Specimen Collection online at Davis*Plus*. Positively identify the patient.
- Ensure the patient has complied with-dietary, fluids, medication restrictions, and other pretesting preparations prior to the study, as instructed.
- Ensure that the patient has removed all external metallic objects from the area to be examined.
- Administer ordered prophylactic steroids or antihistamines before the procedure if the patient has a history of allergic reactions to any substance or drug.
- Avoid the use of equipment containing latex if the patient has a history of allergic reaction to latex.
- Have emergency equipment readily available.
- Instruct the patient to void prior to the procedure and to change into the gown, robe, and foot coverings provided.
- Instruct the patient to cooperate fully and to follow directions. Instruct the patient to remain still throughout the procedure because movement produces unreliable results.
- Establish an IV fluid line for the injection of contrast, emergency drugs, and sedatives.
- Administer an antianxiety drug, as ordered, if the patient has claustrophobia. Administer a sedative to a child or to an adult who is uncooperative, as ordered.
- Place the patient in the supine position on an examination table.
- If IV contrast media is used, a rapid series of images is taken during and after the filling of the vessels to be examined. Delayed images may be taken to examine the vessels after a time and to monitor the venous phase of the procedure.
- Ask the patient to inhale deeply and hold his or her breath while the images are taken, and then to exhale after the images are taken.
- Instruct the patient to take slow, deep breaths if nausea occurs during the procedure. Monitor and administer an antiemetic drug if ordered. Ready an emesis basin for use.
- Monitor the patient for complications related to the procedure (e.g., allergic reaction, anaphylaxis, bronchospasm).
- The needle is removed and a pressure dressing is applied over the puncture site.
- Observe/assess the needle site for bleeding, inflammation, or hematoma formation.

POST-TEST:

- Inform the patient that a report of the results will be made available to the requesting HCP, who will discuss the results with the patient.
- Instruct the patient to resume pretesting diet, as directed by the HCP. Assess the patient's ability to swallow before allowing the patient to attempt liquids or solid foods. Kidney function should be assessed before metformin is resumed.
- Monitor vital signs and neurological status every 15 min for 1 hr, then every 2 hr for 4 hr, and then as ordered by the HCP. Monitor temperature every 4 hr for 24 hr. Monitor intake and output at least every 8 hr. Compare with baseline values. Notify the HCP if temperature is elevated. Protocols may vary among facilities.
- If contrast was used, observe for delayed allergic reactions, such as rash, urticaria, tachycardia, hyperpnea, hypertension, palpitations, nausea, or vomiting. Antihistamines may be ordered and given to alleviate symptoms of allergic reaction.
- Instruct the patient to immediately report symptoms such as fast heart rate, difficulty breathing, skin rash, itching, chest pain, persistent right shoulder pain, or abdominal pain. Immediately report symptoms to the appropriate HCP.
- Assess extremities for signs of ischemia or absence of distal pulse caused by a catheter-induced thrombus.
- Observe/assess the needle insertion site for bleeding, inflammation, or hematoma formation.

- Instruct the patient to apply cold compresses to the insertion site as needed, to reduce discomfort or edema.
- Instruct the patient to increase fluid intake to help eliminate the contrast medium, if used.
- Instruct the patient to maintain bed rest for 4 to 6 hr after the procedure.
- ***Nutritional Considerations:*** Abnormal findings may be associated with cardiovascular disease. Nutritional therapy is recommended for the patient identified to be at risk for developing CAD or for individuals who have specific risk factors and/or existing medical conditions (e.g., elevated LDL cholesterol levels, other lipid disorders, type 1 diabetes, type 2 diabetes, insulin resistance, or metabolic syndrome). Other changeable risk factors warranting patient education include strategies to encourage patients, especially those who are overweight and with high blood pressure, to safely decrease sodium intake, achieve a normal weight, ensure regular participation in moderate aerobic physical activity three to four times per week, eliminate tobacco use, and adhere to a heart-healthy diet. If triglycerides also are elevated, the patient should be advised to eliminate or reduce alcohol. A variety of dietary patterns are beneficial for people with CAD, and there are many meal-planning approaches with nutritional goals endorsed by the American Diabetes Association (ADA). The Guideline on Lifestyle Management to Reduce Cardiovascular Risk published by the American College of Cardiology (ACC) and the American Heart Association (AHA) in conjunction with the National Heart, Lung, and Blood Institute (NHLBI) recommends a Mediterranean-style diet rather than a low-fat diet. The guideline emphasizes inclusion of vegetables, whole grains, fruits, low-fat dairy, nuts, legumes, and nontropical vegetable oils (e.g., olive, canola, peanut, sunflower, flaxseed) along with fish and lean poultry. 🍁 A similar dietary pattern known as the Dietary Approaches to Stop Hypertension (DASH) diet makes additional recommendations for the reduction of dietary sodium. Both dietary styles emphasize a reduction in consumption of red meats, which are high in saturated fats and cholesterol, and other foods containing sugar, saturated fats, trans fats, and sodium. The ADA also includes a vegetarian diet as well as other potential weight loss diets such as Weight Watchers. 🍁 The nutritional needs of each patient need to be determined individually (especially during pregnancy) with the appropriate HCPs, particularly professionals educated in nutrition.
- ***Sensitivity to social and cultural issues:*** Numerous studies point to the prevalence of excess body weight in American children and adolescents. Experts estimate that obesity is present in 25% of the population ages 6 to 11 yr. The medical, social, and emotional consequences of excess body weight are significant. Special attention should be given to instructing the pediatric patient and caregiver regarding health risks and weight control education. 🍁
- Recognize anxiety related to test results, and be supportive of fear of shortened life expectancy. Discuss the implications of abnormal test results on the patient's lifestyle. Provide teaching and information regarding the clinical implications of the test results, as appropriate. Educate the patient regarding access to counseling services. Provide contact information, if desired, for the American Heart Association (www.americanheart.org), NHLBI (www.nhlbi.nih.gov), Institute of Medicine of the National Academies (www.iom.edu), or the USDA's resource for nutrition (www.choosemyplate.gov). 🍁
- Recognize anxiety related to test results. Discuss the implications of abnormal test results on the patient's lifestyle. Provide teaching and information regarding the clinical implications of the test results, as appropriate.

- Reinforce information given by the patient's HCP regarding further testing, treatment, or referral to another HCP. Answer any questions or address any concerns voiced by the patient or family.
- Instruct the patient in the use of any ordered medications. Explain the importance of adhering to the therapy regimen. As appropriate, instruct the patient in significant adverse effects associated with the prescribed medication. Encourage him or her to review corresponding literature provided by a pharmacist.
- Depending on the results of this procedure, additional testing may be needed to evaluate or monitor progression of the disease process and determine the need for a change in therapy. Evaluate test results in relation to the patient's symptoms and other tests performed.

Patient Education:

- Teach the patient the importance of managing hypertension to decrease bleeding risk.
- Teach the signs and symptoms of transfusion reaction.

Expected Patient Outcomes:

Understanding

- The patient and family discuss the medical versus surgical options for aneurysm management.
- The patient and family discuss the risks and benefits of blood transfusion and the types of transfusion available.

Ability

- The patient and family successfully create a quiet environment.
- The patient successfully demonstrates how to take own blood pressure using an approved medical device.

Response

- The patient and family agree to vigilant follow-up care to monitor the size of the aneurysm.
- The patient agrees to blood replacement therapy.

RELATED STUDIES:

- Related tests include angiography of the specific area (abdomen, adrenal, carotid, coronary, pulmonary, renal), blood pool imaging, BUN, chest x-ray, colonoscopy, CBC, CBC hematocrit, CBC hemoglobin, CT of the specific area (abdomen, biliary/liver, brain, pituitary, renal, spine, spleen, thoracic), creatinine echocardiography, echocardiography transesophageal, fluorescein angiography, fundoscopy with or without photography, genetic testing, MRA, MRI of the specific area (abdomen, brain, chest, pituitary), MRI venography, MI scan, plethysmography, PET (brain, heart), proctosigmoidoscopy, PT/INR, US carotid, and US venous Doppler extremity.
- Refer to the Cardiovascular System table online at Davis*Plus* for related tests by body system.

Computed Tomography, Biliary Tract and Liver

SYNONYM/ACRONYM: Computed axial tomography (CAT), computed transaxial tomography (CTT), abdominal CT, helical/spiral CT.

COMMON USE: To visualize and assess the structure of the liver and biliary tract toward the diagnosis of tumor, obstruction, bleeding, and infection. Used as an evaluation tool for surgical, radiation, and medical therapeutic interventions.

AREA OF APPLICATION: Liver, biliary tract, and adjacent structures.

DESCRIPTION: Computed tomography (CT) of the liver and biliary tract is a noninvasive procedure that enhances certain anatomic views of these structures. It becomes invasive with the use of contrast medium. During the procedure, the patient lies on a motorized table. The table is moved in and out of a circular opening in a doughnut-like device called a *gantry,* which houses the x-ray tube and associated electronics. A beam of x-rays irradiates the patient as the table moves in and out of the scanner in a series of phases. The x-rays penetrate liquids and solids of different densities by varying degrees. Multiple detectors rotate around the patient to collect numeric data associated with the density coefficients assigned to each degree of tissue density. The imaging system's computer converts the numeric data obtained from the scanner into digital images. Air appears black; bone appears white; and body fluids, fat, and soft tissue structures are represented in various shades between black and white. The cross-sectional views, or *slices,* of the liver, biliary tract, and associated vascular system can be reviewed individually or as a three-dimensional image to allow differentiations of solid, cystic, inflammatory, or vascular lesions as well as identification of suspected hematomas. The scan may be repeated after administration of contrast medium given orally or by intravenous (IV) injection. Contrast is used to differentiate, enhance, or "light up" areas of interest depending on the type of study to be performed, type of contrast medium to be used, and method of administration. The medium works by creating a contrast between areas of interest based on density; penetration of the x-rays is weaker in areas where the contrast medium is detected by the scanner, showing the blood vessels, organs, and tissue as whitish areas that either outline the area of interest or completely fill it. Oral ingestion of contrast medium can be used for opacification to distinguish the bowel, adjacent abdominal organs, other types of tissue, and blood vessels as the medium moves through the digestive tract. IV injection of contrast medium is used for evaluation of blood flow through vessels and greater enhancement of tissue density and organ visualization. In some cases, scans may be repeated after both types of contrast are administered. Multislice or multidetector CT scanners continuously collect images in a helical or spiral fashion instead of a series of individual images, as with standard scanners. Helical CT can collect many images over a short period of time (seconds), is sensitive in identifying small abnormalities, and produces high-quality images. Positron emission tomography (PET) and single-photon emission tomography (SPECT) are types of nuclear medicine studies that offer insights into functionality such as movement of blood flow or uptake and distribution of metabolites into tumors. PET/CT and SPECT/CT are imaging applications that superimpose PET or SPECT and CT findings. The images are collected and produced by a single gantry system. The co-registered or image fusion of PET/CT or SPECT/CT findings can provide a detailed combination of anatomical and functional images. Images can be recorded on photographic or x-ray film or stored in digital format as digitized computer data. The CT scan can be used to guide biopsy needles into areas of suspected tumors to obtain tissue for laboratory analysis and to guide placement of catheters for drainage of cysts or abscesses. Tumor staging and progression, before and after therapy, and effectiveness of medical interventions may be monitored by PET/CT or SPECT/CT scanning. The images can be reevaluated and manipulated for further, detailed examination without having to repeat the procedure.

This procedure is contraindicated for

- Patients who are pregnant or suspected of being pregnant, unless the potential benefits of a procedure using radiation far outweigh the risk of radiation exposure to the fetus and mother.
- Patients who are claustrophobic.
- Patients with conditions associated with adverse reactions to contrast medium (e.g., asthma, food allergies, or allergy to contrast medium).

Although patients are asked specifically if they have a known allergy to iodine or shellfish, it has been well established that the reaction is not to iodine; an actual iodine allergy would be problematic because iodine is required for the production of thyroid hormones. In the case of shellfish, the reaction is to a muscle protein called tropomyosin; in the case of iodinated contrast medium, the reaction is to the noniodinated part of the contrast molecule. Patients with a known hypersensitivity to the medium may benefit from premedication with corticosteroids and diphenhydramine; the use of nonionic contrast or an alternative noncontrast imaging study, if available, may be considered for patients who have severe asthma or who have experienced moderate to severe reactions to ionic contrast medium.

- Patients with conditions associated with preexisting renal insufficiency (e.g., chronic kidney disease, single kidney transplant, nephrectomy, diabetes, multiple myeloma, treatment with aminoglycosides and NSAIDs) ***because iodinated contrast is nephrotoxic.***
- Patients who are chronically dehydrated before the test, especially older adults and patients whose health is already compromised, ***because of their risk of contrast-induced acute kidney injury.***
- Patients with pheochromocytoma ***because iodinated contrast may cause a hypertensive crisis.***
- Patients with bleeding disorders or receiving anticoagulant therapy ***because the puncture site may not stop bleeding.***

INDICATIONS

- Assist in differentiating between benign and malignant tumors.
- Detect dilation or obstruction of the biliary ducts with or without calcification or gallstone
- Detect liver abnormalities, such as cirrhosis with ascites and fatty liver.
- Detect tumor extension of masses and metastasis into the hepatic area.
- Differentiate aortic aneurysms from tumors near the aorta.
- Differentiate between obstructive and nonobstructive jaundice.
- Differentiate infectious from inflammatory processes.
- Evaluate hepatic cysts, masses, abscesses, and hematomas, or hepatic trauma.

- Monitor and evaluate effectiveness of medical, radiation, or surgical therapies.

POTENTIAL MEDICAL DIAGNOSIS

Normal findings

- Normal size, position, and contour of the liver and biliary ducts

Abnormal findings related to

Identification of abnormal findings is assisted by comparison of parameters such as size, shape, symmetry, density, and location. For example, areas of altered density in either an expected or unexpected location may indicate enlargement of an organ or the presence of blood or other fluids, tumors, or cysts; a crescent-shaped area of abnormal density that alters the proximity of the liver to the Glisson's capsule may indicate a hematoma; areas of less than normal density may indicate hepatic lesions; and dilation of the associated ducts may indicate an obstruction. Comparison by type of abnormal findings may also assist in evaluating areas of altered density. For example, well-defined round or oval areas, smaller in size and having lower density than a primary tumor, may indicate a cyst.

- Dilation of the common hepatic duct, common bile duct, or gallbladder
- Gallstones
- Hematomas
- Hepatic cysts or abscesses
- Jaundice (obstructive or nonobstructive)
- Primary and metastatic neoplasms

CRITICAL FINDINGS: N/A

INTERFERING FACTORS

Factors that may alter the results of the study

- Gas or feces in the gastrointestinal (GI) tract resulting from inadequate cleansing or failure to restrict food intake before the study.
- Retained barium from a previous radiological procedure.
- Metallic objects (e.g., jewelry, body rings) within the examination field, which may inhibit organ visualization and cause unclear images.
- Patients who are extremely obese may require more radiation to obtain a clear image.
- Patients with extreme claustrophobia unless sedation is given before the study.
- Patients who are unable to cooperate or remain still during the procedure because of age, significant pain, or mental status.

Other considerations

- The procedure may be terminated if chest pain or severe cardiac dysrhythmias occur.
- Failure to follow dietary restrictions and other pretesting preparations may cause the procedure to be canceled or repeated.
- The procedure may be canceled if the patient's weight exceeds the safety limit for the equipment.

NURSING IMPLICATIONS AND PROCEDURE

See Potential Nursing Problems on Fast Find at davispl.us/vanleeuwen7

PRETEST:

- Positively identify the patient using at least two person-specific identifiers before services, treatments, or procedures are performed.
- *Patient Teaching:* Inform the patient this procedure can assist in assessing the liver, biliary tract, and surrounding structures.
- Obtain a history of the patient's health concerns, symptoms, surgical procedures, and results of previously performed laboratory and diagnostic studies. Include a list of

known allergens, especially allergies or sensitivities to latex, anesthetics, sedatives, or contrast medium. Ensure results of coagulation testing are obtained and recorded prior to the procedure; a creatinine level is also needed before contrast medium is to be used.

C

- Note any recent procedures that can interfere with test results, including examinations using barium- or iodine-based contrast medium. Ensure that barium studies were performed more than 4 days before the CT scan.
- Record the date of the last menstrual period and determine the possibility of pregnancy in perimenopausal women.
- Obtain a list of the patient's current medications, including over-the-counter medications, anticoagulants, aspirin and other salicylates, and dietary supplements (see Effects of Natural Products on Laboratory Values online at Davis*Plus*). Such products should be discontinued by medical direction for the appropriate number of days prior to a surgical procedure. Note the last time and dose of medication taken.
- If iodinated contrast medium is scheduled to be used in patients receiving metformin (Glucophage) for type 2 diabetes, the drug should be discontinued on the day of the test and continue to be withheld for 48 hr after the test. Iodinated contrast can temporarily impair kidney function, and failure to withhold metformin may indirectly result in drug-induced lactic acidosis, a dangerous and sometimes fatal adverse effect of metformin ***related to renal impairment that does not support sufficient excretion of metformin.***
- Review the procedure with the patient. Address concerns about pain and explain that there may be moments of discomfort and some pain experienced during the test. Inform the patient the procedure is usually performed in a radiology suite by a health-care provider (HCP) specializing in this procedure, with support staff, and takes approximately 15 to 30 min depending on factors such as the type of study ordered, whether contrast will be used, and the type of contrast used.
- ***Sensitivity to social and cultural issues,*** as well as concern for modesty, is important in providing psychological support before, during, and after the procedure.
- Explain that an IV line may be inserted to allow infusion of fluids such as saline, anesthetics, contrast medium, or sedatives.
- Inform the patient that he or she may experience nausea, a feeling of warmth, a salty or metallic taste, or a transient headache after injection of contrast medium, if given.
- Advise the patient that he or she may be requested to drink approximately 450 mL of a dilute barium solution (approximately 1% barium) or a water-soluble oral contrast; the oral contrast is given within a specified time period prior to the study. Oral contrast is administered to distinguish GI organs from the other abdominal organs and to enhance other areas of interest.
- Instruct the patient to remove all external metallic objects from the area to be examined.
- Inform the patient, as appropriate, that CT studies performed without contrast usually do not require the patient to fast before the procedure. Instruct the patient, if required, to fast and restrict fluids for the specified time period prior to the procedure; fasting may be ordered as a precaution against aspiration related to nausea and vomiting during the administration of contrast. Also instruct the patient to avoid taking anticoagulant medication or to reduce dosage as ordered prior to the procedure due to increased risk of bleeding at the IV insertion site. Protocols may vary among facilities.
- *Make sure a written and informed consent has been signed prior to the procedure and before administering any medications.*

INTRATEST:

Potential Complications:

Injection of the contrast through IV tubing into a blood vessel is an invasive procedure. Complications are rare but do include risk for allergic reaction ***related to contrast reaction***, cardiac dysrhythmias, hematoma ***related to blood leakage into the tissue following insertion of the IV needle***, or infection ***that might occur if bacteria from the skin surface is introduced at the IV needle insertion site.***

- Observe standard precautions, and follow the general guidelines in Patient Preparation and Specimen Collection online at Davis*Plus*. Positively identify the patient.
- Ensure the patient has complied with dietary, fluids, medication restrictions, and other pretesting preparations prior to the study, as instructed.
- Ensure the patient has removed all external metallic objects from the area to be examined.
- Administer ordered prophylactic steroids or antihistamines before the procedure if the patient has a history of allergic reactions to any substance or drug.
- Avoid the use of equipment containing latex if the patient has a history of allergic reaction to latex.
- Have emergency equipment readily available.
- Instruct the patient to void prior to the procedure and to change into the gown, robe, and foot coverings provided.
- Instruct the patient to cooperate fully and to follow directions. Instruct the patient to remain still throughout the procedure because movement produces unreliable results.
- Record baseline vital signs, and continue to monitor throughout the procedure. Protocols may vary among facilities.
- Establish an IV fluid line for the injection of contrast medium, emergency drugs, and sedatives.
- Administer an antianxiety drug, as ordered, if the patient has claustrophobia. Administer a sedative to a child or to an adult who is uncooperative, as ordered.
- Place the patient in the supine position on an examination table.
- If IV contrast medium is used, a rapid series of images is taken during and after injection.
- Instruct the patient to inhale deeply and hold his or her breath while the images are taken, and then to exhale after the images are taken.
- Instruct the patient to take slow, deep breaths if nausea occurs during the procedure.
- Monitor the patient for complications related to the procedure (e.g., allergic reaction, anaphylaxis, bronchospasm) if contrast is used.
- The needle is removed, and a pressure dressing is applied over the puncture site.
- Observe/assess the needle site for bleeding, inflammation, or hematoma formation.

POST-TEST:

- Inform the patient that a report of the results will be made available to the requesting HCP, who will discuss the results with the patient.
- Instruct the patient to resume usual diet, fluids, medications, and activity, as directed by the HCP. Kidney function should be assessed before metformin is resumed, if contrast was used.
- Monitor vital signs and neurological status every 15 min for 1 hr, then every 2 hr for 4 hr, and then as ordered by the HCP. Monitor temperature every 4 hr for 24 hr. Monitor intake and output at least every 8 hr. Compare with baseline values. Notify the HCP if temperature is elevated. Protocols may vary among facilities.
- If contrast was used, observe for delayed allergic reactions, such as rash, urticaria, tachycardia, hyperpnea, hypertension, palpitations, nausea, or vomiting. Antihistamines may be ordered and given to alleviate symptoms of allergic reaction.
- Instruct the patient to immediately report symptoms such as fast heart

C

rate, difficulty breathing, skin rash, itching, chest pain, persistent right shoulder pain, or abdominal pain. Immediately report symptoms to the appropriate HCP.

- Observe/assess the needle insertion site for bleeding, inflammation, or hematoma formation.
- Instruct the patient in the care and assessment of the site.
- Instruct the patient to apply cold compresses to the insertion site as needed, to reduce discomfort or edema.
- Instruct the patient to increase fluid intake to help eliminate the contrast medium, if used.
- Inform the patient that diarrhea may occur after ingestion of oral contrast media.
- Recognize anxiety related to test results. Discuss the implications of abnormal test results on the patient's lifestyle. Provide teaching and information regarding the clinical implications of the test results, as appropriate.
- Reinforce information given by the patient's HCP regarding further testing, treatment, or referral to another HCP. Answer any questions or address any concerns voiced by the patient or family.
- Depending on the results of this procedure, additional testing may be needed to evaluate or monitor progression of the disease process and determine the need for a change in therapy. Evaluate test results in relation to the patient's symptoms and other tests performed.

Patient Education:

- Teach the patient to avoid fatty foods in his or her diet.
- Teach the patient to increase oral fluids to decrease dehydration.

Expected Patient Outcomes:

Understanding

- The patient and family identify fatty foods that should be omitted from the diet to prevent pain and distress.
- The patient and family successfully repeat information provided by the nurse related to disease process.

Ability

- The patient and family demonstrate the correct method of measuring and documenting intake and output.
- The patient and family create a quiet environment that will assist in their own learning.

Response

- The patient agrees to use alternative pain interventions to control pain.
- The patient and family agree to make lifestyle changes that will promote a healthy gallbladder.

RELATED STUDIES:

- Related tests include ALT, AST, bilirubin, biopsy liver, BUN, CBC, CBC hematocrit, CBC hemoglobin, creatinine, GGT, hepatobiliary scan, KUB, liver and spleen scan, MRI abdomen, PT/INR, and US liver.
- Refer to the Hepatobiliary System table online at Davis*Plus* for related tests by body system.

Computed Tomography, Brain and Head

SYNONYM/ACRONYM: Computed axial tomography (CAT) of the head, computed transaxial tomography (CTT) of the head, brain CT, helical/spiral CT.

COMMON USE: To visualize and assess the brain to assist in diagnosing tumor, bleeding, infarct, infection, structural changes, and edema. Also valuable in evaluation of medical, radiation, and surgical interventions.

AREA OF APPLICATION: Brain.

DESCRIPTION: Computed tomography (CT) of the brain and head is a noninvasive procedure used to assist in diagnosing abnormalities of the head, neck, brain, orbits, sinuses, mastoids, auditory canals of the inner ear, cerebrospinal fluid, and blood circulation. It becomes invasive if contrast medium is used. During the procedure, the patient lies on a motorized table. The table is moved in and out of a circular opening in a doughnut-like device called a *gantry,* which houses the x-ray tube and associated electronics. A beam of x-rays irradiates the patient as the table moves in and out of the scanner in a series of phases. The x-rays penetrate liquids and solids of different densities by varying degrees. Multiple detectors rotate around the patient to collect numeric data associated with the density coefficients assigned to each degree of tissue density. The imaging system's computer converts the numeric data obtained from the scanner into digital images. Air appears black; bone appears white; and body fluids, fat, and soft tissue structures are represented in various shades between black and white. The cross-sectional views, or *slices,* of the head, brain, neck, thyroid gland, and associated vascular system can be reviewed individually or as a three-dimensional image to allow differentiations of solid, cystic, inflammatory, or vascular lesions as well as identification of suspected aneurysms, intracranial bleeds, and subdural or epidural hematomas. The scan may be repeated after administration of contrast medium given by intravenous injection. Contrast is used to differentiate, enhance, or "light up" areas of interest depending on the type of study to be performed, type of contrast medium to be used, and method of administration. The medium works by creating a contrast between areas of interest based on density; penetration of the x-rays is weaker in areas where the contrast medium is detected by the scanner, showing the blood vessels, organs, and tissue as whitish areas that either outline the area of interest or completely fill it. IV injection of contrast medium is used for evaluation of blood flow through vessels and greater enhancement of tissue density and organ visualization. Multislice or multidetector CT scanners continuously collect images in a helical or spiral fashion instead of a series of individual images, as with standard scanners. Helical CT can collect many images over a short period of time (seconds), is sensitive in identifying small abnormalities, and produces high-quality images. Positron emission tomography (PET) and single-photon emission tomography (SPECT) are types of nuclear medicine studies that offer insights into functionality such as movement of blood flow or uptake and distribution of metabolites into tumors. PET/CT and SPECT/CT are imaging applications that superimpose PET or SPECT and CT findings. The images are collected and produced by a single gantry system. The co-registered or image fusion of PET/CT or SPECT/CT findings can provide a detailed combination of anatomical and functional images. Images can be recorded on photographic or x-ray film or stored in digital format as

C

digitized computer data. The CT scan can be used to guide biopsy needles into areas of suspected tumors to obtain tissue for laboratory analysis and to guide placement of catheters for drainage of cysts or abscesses. Tumor staging and progression, before and after therapy, and effectiveness of medical interventions may be monitored by PET/CT, SPECT/CT, or PET scanning. The images can be reevaluated and manipulated for further, detailed examination without having to repeat the procedure. Xenon-enhanced CT scanning is an imaging method used to assess cerebral blood flow. Xenon-133 is an odorless, colorless, radioactive gas that can be either inhaled or injected. The isotope moves rapidly through the blood into the brain. The diffused gas demonstrates how much blood goes to each area of the brain. Sensitivity of stroke detection in the acute phase is increased by using Xenon.

This procedure is contraindicated for

- Patients who are pregnant or suspected of being pregnant, unless the potential benefits of a procedure using radiation far outweigh the risk of radiation exposure to the fetus and mother.
- Patients who are claustrophobic.
- Patients with conditions associated with adverse reactions to contrast medium (e.g., asthma, food allergies, or allergy to contrast medium).

Although patients are asked specifically if they have a known allergy to iodine or shellfish, it has been well established that the reaction is not to iodine; an actual iodine allergy would be problematic because iodine is required for the production of thyroid hormones. In the case of shellfish, the reaction is to a muscle protein called tropomyosin; in the case of iodinated contrast medium, the reaction is to the noniodinated part of the contrast molecule. Patients with a known hypersensitivity to the medium may benefit from premedication with corticosteroids and diphenhydramine; the use of nonionic contrast or an alternative noncontrast imaging study, if available, may be considered for patients who have severe asthma or who have experienced moderate to severe reactions to ionic contrast medium.

- Patients with conditions associated with preexisting renal insufficiency (e.g., chronic kidney disease, single kidney transplant, nephrectomy, diabetes, multiple myeloma, treatment with aminoglycosides and NSAIDs) ***because iodinated contrast is nephrotoxic.***
- Patients who are chronically dehydrated before the test, especially older adults and patients whose health is already compromised, ***because of their risk of contrast-induced acute kidney injury.***
- Patients with pheochromocytoma ***because iodinated contrast may cause a hypertensive crisis.***
- Patients with bleeding disorders or receiving anticoagulant therapy ***because the puncture site may not stop bleeding.***

INDICATIONS

- Detect brain infection, abscess, or necrosis, as evidenced by decreased density on the image.
- Detect ventricular enlargement or displacement by increased cerebrospinal fluid.
- Determine benign and cancerous tumors and cyst formation, as evidenced by changes in tissue densities.

- Determine cause of increased intracranial pressure.
- Determine presence and type of hemorrhage in infants and children experiencing signs and symptoms of intracranial trauma or congenital conditions such as hydrocephalus and arteriovenous malformations (AVMs).
- Determine presence of multiple sclerosis, as evidenced by sclerotic plaques.
- Determine lesion size and location causing infarct or hemorrhage.
- Differentiate hematoma location after trauma (e.g., subdural, epidural, cerebral) and determine extent of edema, as evidenced by higher blood densities.
- Differentiate between cerebral infarction and hemorrhage.
- Evaluate abnormalities of the middle ear ossicles, auditory nerve, and optic nerve.
- Evaluate for thyroid cancer.
- Monitor and evaluate the effectiveness of medical, radiation, or surgical therapies.

POTENTIAL MEDICAL DIAGNOSIS

Normal findings

- Normal size, position, and shape of intracranial, head, and neck structures and associated vascular system

Abnormal findings related to

Identification of abnormal findings is assisted by comparison of parameters such as size, shape, symmetry, density, and location. For example, areas of altered density in either an expected or unexpected location may indicate abnormal anatomical enlargement or the presence of blood or other fluids, tumors, or cysts. Comparison by type of abnormal findings may also assist in evaluating areas of altered density. For example, well-defined round or oval areas, smaller in size and having lower density than a primary tumor, may indicate a cyst.

- Abscess
- Alzheimer's disease
- Aneurysm
- AVMs
- Cerebral atrophy
- Cerebral edema
- Cerebral infarction
- Congenital abnormalities
- Craniopharyngioma
- Cysts
- Foreign body
- Hematomas (e.g., epidural, subdural, intracerebral)
- Hemorrhage
- Hydrocephaly
- Increased intracranial pressure or trauma
- Infarction
- Infection
- Pheochromocytoma
- Sclerotic plaques suggesting multiple sclerosis
- Sinusitis
- Trauma
- Tumor
- Ventricular or tissue displacement or enlargement

CRITICAL FINDINGS:

- Abscess
- Acute hemorrhage
- Aneurysm
- Infarction
- Infection
- Tumor with significant mass effect

Note and immediately report to the requesting health-care provider (HCP) any critical findings and related symptoms. A listing of these findings varies among facilities. Timely notification of a critical finding for laboratory or diagnostic studies is a role expectation of the professional nurse. The notification processes vary among facilities. Upon receipt of the critical finding, the information should be read back to the caller to verify accuracy.

INTERFERING FACTORS

Factors that may alter the results of the study

- **Metallic objects (e.g., jewelry, dentures, body rings) within the examination field, which may inhibit organ visualization and cause unclear images.**
- **Patients who are extremely obese may require more radiation to obtain a clear image.**
- **Patients with extreme claustrophobia unless sedation is given before the study.**
- **Patient who are unable to cooperate or remain still during the procedure because of age, significant pain, or mental status.**

Other considerations

- **The procedure may be terminated if chest pain or severe cardiac dysrhythmias occur.**
- **Failure to follow dietary restrictions and other pretesting preparations may cause the procedure to be canceled or repeated.**
- **The procedure may be canceled if the patient's weight exceeds the safety limit for the equipment.**

NURSING IMPLICATIONS AND PROCEDURE

See Potential Nursing Problems on Fast Find at davispl.us/vanleeuwen7

PRETEST:

- Positively identify the patient using at least two person-specific identifiers before services, treatments, or procedures are performed.
- *Patient Teaching:* Inform the patient this procedure can assist in assessing the brain, neck, and head.
- Obtain a history of the patient's health concerns, symptoms, surgical procedures, and results of previously performed laboratory and diagnostic studies. Include a list of known allergens, especially allergies or sensitivities to latex, anesthetics, sedatives, or contrast medium. Ensure results of coagulation testing are obtained and recorded prior to the procedure; a creatinine level is also needed before contrast medium is to be used.
- Note any recent procedures that can interfere with test results, including examinations using barium- or iodine-based contrast medium. Ensure that barium studies were performed more than 4 days before the CT scan.
- Record the date of the last menstrual period and determine the possibility of pregnancy in perimenopausal women.
- Obtain a list of the patient's current medications, including over-the-counter medications, anticoagulants, aspirin and other salicylates, and dietary supplements (see Effects of Natural Products on Laboratory Values online at Davis*Plus*). Such products should be discontinued by medical direction for the appropriate number of days prior to a surgical procedure. Note the last time and dose of medication taken.
- If iodinated contrast medium is scheduled to be used in patients receiving metformin (Glucophage) for type 2 diabetes, the drug should be discontinued on the day of the test and continue to be withheld for 48 hr after the test. Iodinated contrast can temporarily impair kidney function, and failure to withhold metformin may indirectly result in drug-induced lactic acidosis, a dangerous and sometimes fatal adverse effect of metformin ***related to renal impairment that does not support sufficient excretion of metformin.***
- Review the procedure with the patient. Address concerns about pain and explain that there may be moments of discomfort and some pain experienced during the test. Inform the patient the procedure is usually performed in a radiology suite by an HCP specializing in this procedure, with support staff, and takes approximately 15 to 30 min.
- *Sensitivity to social and cultural issues,* as well as concern for modesty, is important in providing psychological

support before, during, and after the procedure.

- Explain that an IV line may be inserted to allow infusion of fluids such as saline, anesthetics, contrast medium, dye, or sedatives.
- Inform the patient that he or she may experience nausea, a feeling of warmth, a salty or metallic taste, or a transient headache after injection of contrast medium.
- Instruct the patient to remove dentures and all external metallic objects from the area to be examined.
- Inform the patient, as appropriate, that CT studies performed without contrast usually do not require the patient to fast before the procedure. Instruct the patient, if required, to fast and restrict fluids for the specified time period prior to the procedure; fasting may be ordered as a precaution against aspiration related to nausea and vomiting during the administration of contrast. Also instruct the patient to avoid taking anticoagulant medication or to reduce dosage as ordered prior to the procedure due to increased risk of bleeding at the IV insertion site. Protocols may vary among facilities.
- *Make sure a written and informed consent has been signed prior to the procedure and before administering any medications.*

INTRATEST:

Potential Complications:

Injection of the contrast through IV tubing into a blood vessel is an invasive procedure. Complications are rare but do include risk for allergic reaction ***related to contrast reaction,*** cardiac dysrhythmias, hematoma ***related to blood leakage into the tissue following insertion of the IV needle,*** or infection ***that might occur if bacteria from the skin surface is introduced at the IV needle insertion site.***

- Observe standard precautions, and follow the general guidelines in Patient Preparation and Specimen Collection online at Davis*Plus*. Positively identify the patient.
- Ensure the patient has complied with dietary, fluids, medication restrictions, and other pretesting preparations prior to the study, as instructed.
- Ensure the patient has removed dentures and all external metallic objects from the area to be examined prior to the procedure.
- Administer ordered prophylactic steroids or antihistamines before the procedure if the patient has a history of allergic reactions to any substance or drug.
- Avoid the use of equipment containing latex if the patient has a history of allergic reaction to latex.
- Have emergency equipment readily available.
- Instruct the patient to cooperate fully and to follow directions. Instruct the patient to remain still throughout the procedure because movement produces unreliable results.
- Record baseline vital signs, and continue to monitor throughout the procedure. Protocols may vary among facilities.
- Establish an IV fluid line for the injection of contrast medium, emergency drugs, and sedatives.
- Administer an antianxiety drug, as ordered, if the patient has claustrophobia. Administer a sedative to a child or to an adult who is uncooperative, as ordered.
- Place the patient in the supine position on an examination table.
- If contrast media is used, a rapid series of images is taken during and after injection.
- Instruct the patient to inhale deeply and hold his or her breath while the images are taken, and then to exhale after the images are taken.
- Instruct the patient to take slow, deep breaths if nausea occurs during the procedure.
- Monitor the patient for complications related to the procedure (e.g., allergic reaction, anaphylaxis, bronchospasm) if contrast is used.
- The needle is removed, and a pressure dressing is applied over the puncture site.

- Observe/assess the needle insertion site for bleeding, inflammation, or hematoma formation.

POST-TEST:

- Inform the patient that a report of the results will be made available to the requesting HCP, who will discuss the results with the patient.
- Instruct the patient to resume medications and activity, as directed by the HCP. Kidney function should be assessed before metformin is resumed if contrast was used.
- Monitor vital signs and neurological status every 15 min for 1 hr, then every 2 hr for 4 hr, and then as ordered by the HCP. Monitor temperature every 4 hr for 24 hr. Monitor intake and output at least every 8 hr. Compare with baseline values. Notify the HCP if temperature is elevated. Protocols may vary among facilities.
- If contrast was used, observe for delayed allergic reactions, such as rash, urticaria, tachycardia, hyperpnea, hypertension, palpitations, nausea, or vomiting. Antihistamines may be ordered and given to alleviate symptoms of allergic reaction.
- Instruct the patient to immediately report symptoms such as fast heart rate, difficulty breathing, skin rash, itching, chest pain, persistent right shoulder pain, or abdominal pain. Immediately report symptoms to the appropriate HCP.
- Observe/assess the needle insertion site for bleeding, inflammation, or hematoma formation.
- Instruct the patient in the care and assessment of the site.
- Instruct the patient to apply cold compresses to the puncture site as needed, to reduce discomfort or edema.
- Instruct the patient to increase fluid intake to help eliminate the contrast medium, if used.
- Recognize anxiety related to test results. Discuss the implications of abnormal test results on the patient's lifestyle. Provide teaching and information regarding the clinical implications of the test results, as appropriate.
- Reinforce information given by the patient's HCP regarding further testing, treatment, or referral to another HCP. Answer any questions or address any concerns voiced by the patient or family.
- Depending on the results of this procedure, additional testing may be needed to evaluate or monitor progression of the disease process and determine the need for a change in therapy. Evaluate test results in relation to the patient's symptoms and other tests performed.

Patient Education:

- Teach the patient, parent, or significant other reportable symptoms related to bleeding due to medication use.
- Teach the patient, parent, or significant other bleeding precautions that should be used with specific medications.

Expected Patient Outcomes:

Understanding

- The patient and family state the importance of refraining from risky activity that would result in trauma and bleeding.
- The patient and family state the importance of frequent positioning to decrease risk of pressure ulcer development.

Ability

- The patient successfully demonstrates range-of-motion technique.
- The patient successfully demonstrates the use of assistive devices.

Response

- The patient and family agree to follow-up laboratory studies to manage medications to prevent stroke.
- The patient agrees to call for assistance when getting out of bed to decrease fall risk.

RELATED STUDIES:

- Related tests include angiography carotid, audiometry hearing loss, BUN, CSF analysis, CBC, CBC hematocrit, CBC hemoglobin, CT angiography, creatinine, EEG, EMG, evoked brain potentials, MR angiography, MRI brain, nerve fiber analysis, otoscopy, PET brain, PT/INR, spondee speech reception threshold, and tuning fork tests.

Refer to the Musculoskeletal System table online at Davis*Plus* for related tests by body system.

Computed Tomography, Cardiac Scoring

C

SYNONYM/ACRONYM: Computed axial tomography (CAT), computed transaxial tomography (CTT), heart vessel calcium CT, helical/spiral CT, cardiac plaque CT.

COMMON USE: To visualize and assess coronary artery status related to plaque buildup, associated with coronary artery disease and heart failure. Used as an evaluation tool for surgical, radiation, and medical therapeutic interventions.

AREA OF APPLICATION: Heart.

DESCRIPTION: Cardiac scoring computed tomography (CT) is a noninvasive procedure used to enhance certain anatomic views of the heart for quantifying coronary artery calcium content. Coronary artery disease (CAD) occurs when the arteries that carry blood and oxygen to the heart muscle become clogged or built up with plaque. Plaque buildup slows the flow of blood to the heart muscle, causing ischemia and increasing the risk of heart failure. During the procedure, the patient lies on a motorized table. The table is moved in and out of a circular opening in a doughnut-like device called a *gantry,* which houses the x-ray tube and associated electronics. A beam of x-rays irradiates the patient as the table moves in and out of the scanner in a series of phases. The x-rays penetrate liquids and solids of different densities by varying degrees. Multiple detectors rotate around the patient to collect numeric data associated with the density coefficients assigned to each degree of tissue density. The imaging system's computer converts the numeric data obtained from the scanner into digital images. Air appears black; bone appears white; and body fluids, fat, plaque, and soft tissue structures are represented in various shades between black and white. The cross-sectional views, or *slices,* of the arteries demonstrate the location and degree of plaque accumulation (calcium score) and can be reviewed individually or as a three-dimensional image. Images can be recorded on photographic or x-ray film or stored in digital format as digitized computer data. The images can be reevaluated and manipulated for further, detailed examination without having to repeat the procedure. The Agatston score is the most frequently used scale to quantitate the amount of calcium in atherosclerotic plaque. The score is graded in levels from 0 to greater than 400, where a score of 0 is associated with a finding of no evidence of CAD, and a score of greater than 400 is associated with a finding of extensive evidence of CAD. Levels of 1–10, 11–100, and 101–400 respectively define minimal, mild, and moderate evidence of CAD.

This procedure is contraindicated for

Patients who are pregnant or suspected of being pregnant, unless the potential benefits of a procedure using radiation far outweigh the risk of radiation exposure to the fetus and mother.

Patients who are claustrophobic.

INDICATIONS

- Detect and quantify coronary artery calcium content
  - CAD is the leading cause of death in most industrialized nations.
  - Estimation of 10-year cardiovascular risk using a scoring system such as the gender-specific Framingham risk score is a more powerful predictor of CAD than cholesterol screening.
  - Of all myocardial infarctions (MIs), 45% occur in people younger than age 65.
  - Of women who have had MIs, 44% will die within 1 yr after the attack.
  - Women are more likely to die of heart disease than of breast cancer.
- Family history of heart disease
- Screening for coronary artery calcium in patients with
  - Diabetes
  - High blood pressure
  - High cholesterol
  - High-stress lifestyle
  - Overweight by 20% or more
  - Personal history of smoking
  - Sedentary lifestyle
- Screening for coronary artery plaque in patients with chest pain of unknown cause

POTENTIAL MEDICAL DIAGNOSIS

Normal findings

- If the Agatston score is 100 or less, the probability of having significant CAD is minimal or is unlikely to be causing a narrowing at the time of the examination.

Abnormal findings related to

Calcified plaque in the coronary arteries is similar in composition to bone and if present will appear as areas of whiteness depending on the amount of accumulated calcification.

- If the Agatston score is between 100 and 400, a significant amount of calcified plaque was found in the coronary arteries. There is an increased risk of a future MI, and a medical assessment of cardiac risk factors needs to be done. Additional testing may be needed.
- If the Agatston score is greater than 400, the procedure has detected extensive calcified plaque in the coronary arteries, which may have caused a critical narrowing of the vessels. A full medical assessment is needed as soon as possible. Further testing may be needed, and treatment may be needed to reduce the risk of MI.

CRITICAL FINDINGS: N/A

INTERFERING FACTORS

Factors that may alter the results of the study

- Retained barium or radiological contrast from a previous radiological procedure.
- Metallic objects (e.g., jewelry, body rings) within the examination field, which may inhibit organ visualization and cause unclear images.
- Improper adjustment of the radiographic equipment to accommodate obese or thin patients, which can cause overexposure or underexposure and a poor-quality study.
- Patients with extreme claustrophobia unless sedation is given before the study.
- Inability of the patient to cooperate or remain still during the procedure because of age, significant pain, or mental status.

Other considerations

- **The procedure may be terminated if chest pain or severe cardiac dysrhythmias occur.**

NURSING IMPLICATIONS AND PROCEDURE

PRETEST:

- Positively identify the patient using at least two person-specific identifiers before services, treatments, or procedures are performed.
- ***Patient Teaching:*** Inform the patient this procedure can assist in assessing the coronary arteries for the presence of plaque.
- Obtain a history of the patient's health concerns, symptoms, surgical procedures, and results of previously performed laboratory and diagnostic studies. Include a list of known allergens, especially allergies or sensitivities to latex, anesthetics, or sedatives. The presence of other risk factors, such as family history of heart disease, smoking, obesity, diet, lack of physical activity, hypertension, diabetes, previous myocardial infarction, and previous vascular disease, should be investigated. Knowledge of genetics assists the nurse in identifying patients and family members who may benefit from additional education, risk assessment, and counseling. Genetics is the study and identification of genes, genetic mutations, and inheritance. For example, genetics provides some insight into the likelihood of inheriting a trait such as blue eyes or a medical condition such as CAD. Genomic studies evaluate the interaction of groups of genes. The combined activity or combined expression of groups of genes allows assumptions or predictions to be made. As an example, genomic studies measure the levels of activity in multiple genes to predict how they, along with environmental and lifestyle decisions, influence the development of type 2 diabetes, CAD, MI, or ischemic stroke. Further information regarding inheritance of genes can be found in the study titled "Genetic Testing."
- Note any recent procedures that can interfere with test results, including examinations using barium- or iodine-based contrast medium. Ensure that barium studies were performed more than 4 days before the CT scan.
- Record the date of the last menstrual period and determine the possibility of pregnancy in perimenopausal women.
- Obtain a list of the patient's current medications, including over-the-counter medications, anticoagulants, aspirin and other salicylates, and dietary supplements (see Effects of Natural Products on Laboratory Values online at Davis*Plus*). Such products should be discontinued by medical direction for the appropriate number of days prior to a surgical procedure. Note the last time and dose of medication taken.
- Review the procedure with the patient. Address concerns about pain and explain that there may be moments of discomfort and some pain experienced during the test. Inform the patient the procedure is usually performed in a radiology suite by a health-care provider (HCP) specializing in this procedure, with support staff, and takes approximately 10 to 15 min.
- ***Sensitivity to social and cultural issues,*** as well as concern for modesty, is important in providing psychological support before, during, and after the procedure.
- Explain that an intravenous (IV) line may be inserted to allow infusion of fluids such as saline, anesthetics, or sedatives.
- Note that there are no medication restrictions unless by medical direction. Instruct the patient to abstain from caffeine and tobacco products for 4 hr prior to the study. Protocols may vary among facilities.
- Instruct the patient to remove all external metallic objects from the area to be examined.

C

INTRATEST:

Potential Complications:

Establishing an IV line is an invasive procedure. Complications are rare but do include risk for hematoma ***related to blood leakage into the tissue following insertion of the IV needle*** or infection ***that might occur if bacteria from the skin surface is introduced at the IV needle insertion site.***

- Observe standard precautions, and follow the general guidelines in Patient Preparation and Specimen Collection online at Davis*Plus*. Positively identify the patient.
- Ensure the patient has complied with pretesting preparations prior to the study, as instructed.
- Ensure that the patient has removed all external metallic objects from the area to be examined.
- Administer ordered prophylactic steroids or antihistamines before the procedure if the patient has a history of allergic reactions to any substance or drug.
- Have emergency equipment readily available.
- Instruct the patient to void prior to the procedure and to change into the gown, robe, and foot coverings provided.
- Instruct the patient to cooperate fully and to follow directions. Instruct the patient to remain still throughout the procedure because movement produces unreliable results.
- Place ECG electrodes to the appropriate locations on the patient's chest. The CT scanner will be synchronized with the patient's heart rate in order to record images when the heart is at rest.
- Record baseline vital signs, and continue to monitor throughout the procedure. Protocols may vary among facilities.
- Establish an IV fluid line for the injection of emergency drugs and sedatives.
- Administer an antianxiety drug, as ordered, if the patient has claustrophobia. Administer a sedative to a child or to an adult who is uncooperative, as ordered.
- Place the patient in the supine position on an examination table. A rapid series of images is taken of the vessels to be examined.
- Instruct the patient to inhale deeply and hold his or her breath while the images are taken, and then to exhale after the images are taken.
- Instruct the patient to take slow, deep breaths if nausea occurs during the procedure.
- The IV needle is removed, and a pressure dressing is applied over the puncture site.
- Observe/assess the needle site for bleeding, inflammation, or hematoma formation.

POST-TEST:

- Inform the patient that a report of the results will be made available to the requesting HCP, who will discuss the results with the patient.
- When the procedure is complete, remove the electrodes and clean the skin where the electrode was applied.
- Instruct the patient to resume usual diet, fluids, medications, and activity, as directed by the HCP.
- Instruct the patient in the care and assessment of the IV site.
- Instruct the patient to apply cold compresses to the insertion site as needed, to reduce discomfort or edema.
- Recognize anxiety related to test results. Discuss the implications of abnormal test results on the patient's lifestyle. Provide teaching and information regarding the clinical implications of the test results, as appropriate.
- ***Nutritional Considerations:*** Abnormal findings may be associated with cardiovascular disease. Nutritional therapy is recommended for the patient identified to be at risk for developing CAD or for individuals who have specific risk factors and/or existing medical conditions (e.g., elevated LDL cholesterol levels, other lipid disorders, type 1 diabetes,

type 2 diabetes, insulin resistance, or metabolic syndrome). Other changeable risk factors warranting patient education include strategies to encourage patients, especially those who are overweight and with high blood pressure, to safely decrease sodium intake, achieve a normal weight, ensure regular participation in moderate aerobic physical activity three to four times per week, eliminate tobacco use, and adhere to a heart-healthy diet. If triglycerides also are elevated, the patient should be advised to eliminate or reduce alcohol. A variety of dietary patterns are beneficial for people with CAD, and there are many meal-planning approaches with nutritional goals endorsed by the American Diabetes Association (ADA). The Guideline on Lifestyle Management to Reduce Cardiovascular Risk published by the American College of Cardiology (ACC) and the American Heart Association (AHA) in conjunction with the National Heart, Lung, and Blood Institute (NHLBI) recommends a Mediterranean-style diet rather than a low-fat diet. The guideline emphasizes inclusion of vegetables, whole grains, fruits, low-fat dairy, nuts, legumes, and nontropical vegetable oils (e.g., olive, canola, peanut, sunflower, flaxseed) along with fish and lean poultry. 🍁 A similar dietary pattern known as the Dietary Approaches to Stop Hypertension (DASH) diet makes additional recommendations for the reduction of dietary sodium. Both dietary styles emphasize a reduction in consumption of red meats, which are high in saturated fats and cholesterol, and other foods containing sugar, saturated fats, trans fats, and sodium. The ADA also includes a vegetarian diet as well as other potential weight loss diets such as Weight Watchers. 🍁 The nutritional needs of each patient need to be determined individually (especially during pregnancy) with the appropriate HCPs, particularly professionals educated in nutrition.

- Recognize anxiety related to test results, and be supportive of fear of shortened life expectancy. Discuss the implications of abnormal test results on the patient's lifestyle. Provide teaching and information regarding the clinical implications of the test results, as appropriate. Educate the patient regarding access to counseling services. Provide contact information, if desired, for the American Heart Association (www.americanheart.org), NHLBI (www.nhlbi.nih.gov), Institute of Medicine of the National Academies (www.iom.edu), or the USDA's resource for nutrition (www.choosemyplate.gov). 🍁
- Reinforce information given by the patient's HCP regarding further testing, treatment, or referral to another HCP. Answer any questions or address any concerns voiced by the patient or family.
- Depending on the results of this procedure, additional testing may be needed to evaluate or monitor progression of the disease process and determine the need for a change in therapy. Evaluate test results in relation to the patient's symptoms and other tests performed.

RELATED STUDIES:

- Related tests include antidysrhythmic drugs, apolipoprotein A and B, AST, atrial natriuretic peptide, BNP, BUN, calcium, chest x-ray, cholesterol (total, HDL, LDL), CRP, CBC, CBC hematocrit, CBC hemoglobin, coronary angiography, CT thorax, CK and isoenzymes, creatinine echocardiography, echocardiography transesophageal ECG, genetic testing, glucose, glycated hemoglobin, Holter monitor, homocysteine, ketones, LDH and isoenzymes, lipoprotein electrophoresis, lung scan, magnesium, MRI chest, MI scan, myocardial perfusion heart scan, myoglobin, PET heart, potassium, PT/INR, triglycerides, and troponin.
- Refer to the Cardiovascular System table online at Davis*Plus* for related tests by body system.

Computed Tomography, Colonoscopy

SYNONYM/ACRONYM: Computed axial tomography (CAT), computed transaxial tomography (CTT), CT colonography, CT virtual colonoscopy.

COMMON USE: To visualize and assess the rectum and colon related to identification and evaluation of large polyps, lesions, and tumors. Also used to assess the effectiveness of therapeutic interventions such as surgery and primarily used for patients who cannot tolerate conventional colonoscopy.

AREA OF APPLICATION: Colon.

DESCRIPTION: Computed tomography (CT) colonoscopy is a noninvasive technique that involves examining the colon by taking multiple CT scans of the patient's colon and rectum and using computer software to create three-dimensional images. It becomes invasive when contrast medium is used. During the procedure, the patient lies on a motorized table. The table is moved in and out of a circular opening in a doughnut-like device called a *gantry,* which houses the x-ray tube and associated electronics. A beam of x-rays irradiates the patient as the table moves in and out of the scanner in a series of phases. The x-rays penetrate liquids and solids of different densities by varying degrees. Multiple detectors rotate around the patient to collect numeric data associated with the density coefficients assigned to each degree of tissue density. The imaging system's computer converts the numeric data obtained from the scanner into digital images. Air appears black; bone appears white; and body fluids, fat, and soft tissue structures are represented in various shades between black and white. The cross-sectional views, or *slices,* of the colon can be reviewed individually or as a three-dimensional image to allow differentiations of solid, cystic, inflammatory, or vascular lesions. The scan may be repeated after administration of contrast medium given orally, by intravenous (IV) injection, or rectally. Contrast is used to differentiate, enhance, or "light up" areas of interest depending on the type of study to be performed, type of contrast medium to be used, and method of administration. The medium works by creating a contrast between areas of interest based on density; penetration of the x-rays is weaker in areas where the contrast medium is detected by the scanner, showing the blood vessels, organs, and tissue as whitish areas that either outline the area of interest or completely fill it. Oral ingestion of contrast medium can be used for opacification to distinguish the bowel, adjacent abdominal organs, other types of tissue, and blood vessels as the medium moves through the digestive tract. An IV injection of contrast medium is used for evaluation of blood flow through vessels and greater enhancement of tissue density and organ visualization. In some cases, scans may be repeated after multiple types of contrast are administered. Multislice or multidetector CT scanners continuously collect images in a helical or spiral fashion instead of a series of individual images, as with standard scanners. Helical CT can collect many images over a short period of time (seconds), is sensitive in identifying small abnormalities, and produces high-quality images. PET/CT is an imaging application that superimposes PET and CT findings. The images are collected and produced by a single gantry system. The co-registered or image fusion PET/CT findings can provide a detailed combination of anatomical and functional images. Images can be recorded on photographic or x-ray film or stored in digital format as digitized computer data. The procedure is used primarily to detect polyps, which are growths of tissue in the colon or rectum. Some types of polyps increase the risk of colon cancer, especially if they are large or if a patient has several polyps. Compared to conventional colonoscopy, CT colonoscopy is less effective in detecting polyps smaller than 5 mm, more effective when the polyps are between 5 and 9.9 mm, and most effective when the polyps are 10 mm or larger. This test may be valuable for patients who have diseases rendering them unable to undergo conventional colonoscopy (e.g., bleeding disorders, lung or heart disease) and for patients who are unable to undergo the sedation required for traditional colonoscopy. The procedure is less invasive than conventional colonoscopy, with little risk of complications and no recovery time. CT colonoscopy can be done as an outpatient procedure, and the patient may return to work or usual activities the same day. The CT scan can be used to guide biopsy needles into areas of suspected tumors to obtain tissue for laboratory analysis and to guide placement of catheters for drainage of abscesses. Tumor staging and progression, before and after therapy, and effectiveness of medical interventions may be monitored by CT scanning. The images can be reevaluated and manipulated for further, detailed examination without having to repeat the procedure.

CT colonoscopy and conventional colonoscopy require the bowel to be cleansed before the examination. The screening procedure requires no contrast medium injections, but if a suspicious area or abnormality is detected, a repeat series of images may be completed after IV contrast medium is given. These density measurements are sent to a computer that produces a digital analysis of the anatomy, enabling a health-care provider (HCP) to look at slices or thin sections of certain anatomic views of the colon and vascular system. A drawback of CT colonoscopy is that polyp removal and biopsies of tissue in the colon must be done using conventional colonoscopy. Therefore, if polyps are discovered during CT colonoscopy and biopsy becomes necessary, the patient must undergo bowel preparation a second time.

This procedure is contraindicated for

- Patients who are pregnant or suspected of being pregnant, unless the potential benefits of a procedure using radiation far outweigh the risk of radiation exposure to the fetus and mother.

- Patients who are claustrophobic.

- Patients with conditions associated with adverse reactions to contrast medium (e.g., asthma, food allergies, or allergy to contrast medium).

Although patients are asked specifically if they have a known allergy to iodine or shellfish, it has been well established that the reaction is not to iodine; an actual iodine allergy would be problematic because iodine is required for the production of thyroid hormones. In the case of shellfish, the reaction is to a muscle protein called tropomyosin; in the case of iodinated contrast medium, the reaction is to the noniodinated part of the contrast molecule. Patients with a known hypersensitivity to the medium may benefit from premedication with corticosteroids and diphenhydramine; the use of nonionic contrast or an alternative noncontrast imaging study, if available, may be considered for patients who have severe asthma or who have experienced moderate to severe reactions to ionic contrast medium.

- Patients with conditions associated with preexisting renal insufficiency (e.g., chronic kidney disease, single kidney transplant, nephrectomy, diabetes, multiple myeloma, treatment with aminoglycosides and NSAIDs) ***because iodinated contrast is nephrotoxic.***

- Patients who are chronically dehydrated before the test, especially older adults and patients whose health is already compromised, ***because of their risk of contrast-induced acute kidney injury.***

- Patients with pheochromocytoma ***because iodinated contrast may cause a hypertensive crisis.***

- Patients with bleeding disorders or receiving anticoagulant therapy ***because the puncture site may not stop bleeding.***

INDICATIONS

- Detect polyps in the colon.
- Evaluate the colon for metachronous lesions.
- Evaluate the colon in patients with obstructing rectosigmoid disease.
- Evaluate polyposis syndromes.
- Evaluate the site of resection for local recurrence of lesions.
- Examine the colon in patients with heart or lung disease, patients unable to be sedated, and patients unable to undergo colonoscopy.
- Failure to visualize the entire colon during conventional colonoscopy.
- Identify metastases.
- Investigate cause of positive occult blood test.
- Investigate further after an abnormal barium enema.
- Investigate further when flexible sigmoidoscopy is positive for polyps.

POTENTIAL MEDICAL DIAGNOSIS

Normal findings

- Normal colon and rectum, with no evidence of polyps or growths

Abnormal findings related to

Identification of abnormal findings is assisted by comparison of parameters such as size, shape, symmetry, density, and location. For example, areas of altered density in either an expected or unexpected location may indicate enlargement of an organ or the presence of blood or other fluids, tumors, or cysts. Comparison by type of abnormal findings may also assist in evaluating areas of altered density. For example, well-defined round or oval areas, smaller in size and having lower density than a primary tumor, may indicate a cyst.

- Abnormal endoluminal wall of the colon
- Extraluminal extension of primary cancer
- Mesenteric and retroperitoneal lymphadenopathy
- Metachronous lesions
- Metastases of cancer
- Polyps or growths in colon or rectum
- Tumor recurrence after surgery

CRITICAL FINDINGS: N/A

INTERFERING FACTORS

Factors that may alter the results of the study

- Gas or feces in the gastrointestinal tract resulting from inadequate cleansing or failure to restrict food intake before the study.
- Retained barium from a previous radiological procedure.
- Metallic objects (e.g., jewelry, body rings) within the examination field, which may inhibit organ visualization and cause unclear images.
- Patients who are extremely obese may require more radiation to obtain a clear image.
- Patients with extreme claustrophobia unless sedation is given before the study.
- Inability of the patient to cooperate or remain still during the procedure because of age, significant pain, or mental status.

Other considerations

- The procedure may be terminated if chest pain or severe cardiac dysrhythmias occur.
- Failure to follow dietary restrictions and other pretesting preparations may cause the procedure to be canceled or repeated.
- The procedure may be canceled if the patient's weight exceeds the safety limit for the equipment.

NURSING IMPLICATIONS AND PROCEDURE

PRETEST:

- Positively identify the patient using at least two person-specific identifiers before services, treatments, or procedures are performed.
- *Patient Teaching:* Inform the patient this procedure can assist in assessing the colon.
- Obtain a history of the patient's health concerns, symptoms, surgical procedures, and results of previously performed laboratory and diagnostic studies. Include a list of known allergens, especially allergies or sensitivities to latex, anesthetics, sedatives, or contrast medium. Ensure results of coagulation testing are obtained and recorded prior to the procedure; a creatinine level is also needed before contrast medium is to be used.
- Note any recent procedures that can interfere with test results, including examinations using barium- or iodine-based contrast medium. Ensure that barium studies were performed more than 4 days before the CT scan.
- Record the date of the last menstrual period and determine the possibility of pregnancy in perimenopausal women.
- Obtain a list of the patient's current medications, including over-the-counter medications, anticoagulants, aspirin and other salicylates, and dietary supplements (see Effects of Natural Products on Laboratory Values online at Davis*Plus*). Such products should be discontinued by medical direction for the appropriate number of days prior to a surgical procedure. Note the last time and dose of medication taken.
- If iodinated contrast medium is scheduled to be used in patients receiving metformin (Glucophage) for type 2 diabetes, the drug should be discontinued on the day of the test and continue to be withheld for 48 hr after the test. Iodinated contrast can temporarily impair kidney function,

and failure to withhold metformin may indirectly result in drug-induced lactic acidosis, a dangerous and sometimes fatal adverse effect of metformin ***related to renal impairment that does not support sufficient excretion of metformin.***

- Review the procedure with the patient. Address concerns about pain and explain that some pain may be experienced during the test, and there may be moments of discomfort. Inform the patient that the procedure is performed in a radiology department, usually by an HCP specializing in this procedure, with support staff, and takes approximately 15 to 30 min depending on factors such as the type of study ordered, whether contrast will be used, and the type of contrast used.
- *Sensitivity to social and cultural issues,* as well as concern for modesty, is important in providing psychological support before, during, and after the procedure.
- Explain that an IV line may be inserted to allow infusion of fluids such as saline, anesthetics, contrast medium, or sedatives.
- Inform the patient that it is important that the bowel be cleaned thoroughly so that the HCP can visualize the colon. Inform the patient that a laxative and cleansing enema may be needed the day before the procedure, with cleansing enemas on the morning of the procedure, depending on the institution's policy.
- Inform the patient that he or she may experience nausea, a feeling of warmth, a salty or metallic taste, or a transient headache after injection of contrast medium.
- Advise the patient that he or she may be requested to drink approximately 450 mL of a dilute barium solution (approximately 1% barium) or a water soluble oral contrast; the oral contrast is given within a specified time period prior to the study. Oral contrast is administered to distinguish GI organs from the other abdominal organs and to enhance other areas of interest.
- Instruct the patient to remove jewelry and other metallic objects from the area to be examined.
- Inform the patient, as appropriate, that CT studies performed without contrast usually do not require the patient to fast before the procedure. Instruct the patient, if required, to fast and restrict fluids for the specified time period prior to the procedure; fasting may be ordered as a precaution against aspiration related to nausea and vomiting during the administration of contrast. Also instruct the patient to avoid taking anticoagulant medication or to reduce dosage as ordered prior to the procedure due to increased risk of bleeding at the IV insertion site. Protocols may vary among facilities.
- *Make sure a written and informed consent has been signed prior to the procedure and before administering any medications.*

INTRATEST:

Potential Complications:

Injection of the contrast through IV tubing into a blood vessel is an invasive procedure. Complications are rare but do include risk for allergic reaction ***related to contrast reaction,*** cardiac dysrhythmias, hematoma ***related to blood leakage into the tissue following insertion of the IV needle,*** or infection ***that might occur if bacteria from the skin surface is introduced at the IV needle insertion site.***

- Observe standard precautions, and follow the general guidelines in Patient Preparation and Specimen Collection online at Davis*Plus*. Positively identify the patient.
- Ensure the patient has complied with dietary, fluids, medication restrictions, and other pretesting preparations prior to the study, as instructed.
- Ensure that the patient has removed all external metallic objects from the area to be examined prior to the procedure.
- Administer ordered prophylactic steroids or antihistamines before the

procedure if the patient has a history of allergic reactions to any substance or drug.

- Avoid the use of equipment containing latex if the patient has a history of allergic reaction to latex.
- Have emergency equipment readily available.
- Instruct the patient to void prior to the procedure and to change into the gown, robe, and foot coverings provided.
- Instruct the patient to cooperate fully and to follow directions. Instruct the patient to remain still throughout the procedure because movement produces unreliable results.
- Record baseline vital signs, and continue to monitor throughout the procedure. Protocols may vary among facilities.
- Establish an IV fluid line for the injection of contrast (if used), emergency drugs, and sedatives.
- Administer an antianxiety drug, as ordered, if the patient has claustrophobia. Administer a sedative to a child or to an adult who is uncooperative, as ordered.
- Place the patient in the supine position on an examination table.
- The colon is distended with room air or carbon dioxide by means of a rectal tube and balloon retention device to allow visualization of polyps or tumors that may be otherwise obscured in folds of the colon wall. Maximal colonic distention is guided by patient tolerance.
- If IV contrast is used, a rapid series of images is taken during and after injection.
- Instruct the patient to inhale deeply and hold his or her breath while the images are taken, and then to exhale after the images are taken.
- The sequence of images is repeated in the prone position.
- Instruct the patient to take slow, deep breaths if nausea occurs during the procedure.
- Monitor the patient for complications related to the procedure (e.g., allergic reaction, anaphylaxis, bronchospasm) if contrast is used.
- The needle is removed, and a pressure dressing is applied over the puncture site.
- Observe/assess the needle site for bleeding, inflammation, or hematoma formation.

POST-TEST:

- Inform the patient that a report of the results will be made available to the requesting HCP, who will discuss the results with the patient.
- Instruct the patient to resume usual diet, fluids, medications, and activity, as directed by the HCP. Kidney function should be assessed before metformin is resumed, if contrast was used.
- Monitor vital signs and neurological status every 15 min for 1 hr, then every 2 hr for 4 hr, and then as ordered by the HCP. Monitor temperature every 4 hr for 24 hr. Monitor intake and output at least every 8 hr. Compare with baseline values. Notify the HCP if temperature is elevated. Protocols may vary among facilities.
- If contrast was used, observe for delayed allergic reactions, such as rash, urticaria, tachycardia, hyperpnea, hypertension, palpitations, nausea, or vomiting. Antihistamines may be ordered and given to alleviate symptoms of allergic reaction.
- Instruct the patient to immediately report symptoms such as fast heart rate, difficulty breathing, skin rash, itching, chest pain, persistent right shoulder pain, or abdominal pain. Immediately report symptoms to the appropriate HCP.
- Observe/assess the needle/catheter insertion site for bleeding, inflammation, or hematoma formation.
- Instruct the patient in the care and assessment of the site.
- Instruct the patient to apply cold compresses to the puncture site as needed, to reduce discomfort or edema.
- Instruct the patient to increase fluid intake to help eliminate the contrast medium, if used.

C

- Inform the patient that diarrhea may occur after ingestion of oral contrast media.
- Recognize anxiety related to test results. Discuss the implications of abnormal test results on the patient's lifestyle. Provide teaching and information regarding the clinical implications of the test results, as appropriate.
- Reinforce information given by the patient's HCP regarding further testing, treatment, or referral to another HCP. Decisions regarding the need for and frequency of occult blood testing, colonoscopy, or other cancer-screening procedures should be made after consultation between the patient and HCP. The American Cancer Society (ACS) recommends regular screening for colon cancer, beginning at age 50 yr for individuals without identified risk factors. Its recommendations for frequency of screening are as follows: annually for occult blood testing (fecal occult blood testing or fecal immunochemical testing); every 5 yr for flexible sigmoidoscopy, double contrast barium enema, and CT colonography; and every 10 yr for colonoscopy. 🍁 There are both advantages and disadvantages to the screening tests that are available today. Methods to use DNA testing of stool are being investigated and awaiting FDA approval. The DNA test is designed to identify abnormal changes in DNA from the cells in the lining of the colon that are normally shed and excreted in stool. The DNA tests under development would use multiple markers to identify colon cancers with various, abnormal DNA changes and would be able to detect precancerous polyps. The most current guidelines for colon cancer screening of the general population as well as of individuals with increased risk are available from the ACS (www.cancer.org), U.S. Preventive Services Task Force (www.uspreventiveservicestaskforce.org), and the American College of Gastroenterology (www.gi.org). 🍁
- Depending on the results of this procedure, additional testing may be needed to evaluate or monitor progression of the disease process and determine the need for a change in therapy. Evaluate test results in relation to the patient's symptoms and other tests performed.

RELATED STUDIES:

- Related tests include barium enema, BUN, cancer antigens, capsule endoscopy, colonoscopy, CBC, CBC hematocrit, CBC hemoglobin, CT abdomen, creatinine, fecal analysis, KUB studies, MRI abdomen, PET pelvis, proctosigmoidoscopy, PT/INR, and US pelvis.
- Refer to the Gastrointestinal System table online at Davis*Plus* for related tests by body system.

Computed Tomography, Kidneys

SYNONYM/ACRONYM: Computed axial tomography (CAT), computed transaxial tomography (CTT), kidney CT, helical/spiral CT.

COMMON USE: To visualize and assess the kidney and surrounding structures to assist in diagnosing cancer, tumor, infection, and congenital anomalies. Used to evaluate the success of therapeutic medical, surgical, and radiation interventions.

AREA OF APPLICATION: Kidney.

DESCRIPTION: Kidney computed tomography (CT) is a noninvasive procedure used to enhance certain anatomic views of the renal structures. It becomes an invasive procedure when contrast medium is used. During the procedure, the patient lies on a motorized table. The table is moved in and out of a circular opening in a doughnut-like device called a *gantry,* which houses the x-ray tube and associated electronics. A beam of x-rays irradiates the patient as the table moves in and out of the scanner in a series of phases. The x-rays penetrate liquids and solids of different densities by varying degrees. Multiple detectors rotate around the patient to collect numeric data associated with the density coefficients assigned to each degree of tissue density. The imaging system's computer converts the numeric data obtained from the scanner into digital images. Air appears black; bone appears white; and body fluids, fat, and soft tissue structures are represented in various shades between black and white. The cross-sectional views, or *slices,* of the kidneys, bladder, ureters, and associated vascular system can be reviewed individually or as a three-dimensional image to allow differentiations of solid, cystic, inflammatory, or vascular lesions as well as identification of suspected hematomas and aneurysms. The scan may be repeated after administration of contrast medium given orally or by intravenous (IV) injection. Contrast is used to differentiate, enhance, or "light up" areas of interest depending on the type of study to be performed, type of contrast medium to be used, and method of administration. The medium works by creating a contrast between areas of interest based on density; penetration of the x-rays is weaker in areas where the contrast medium is detected by the scanner, showing the blood vessels, organs, and tissue as whitish areas that either outline the area of interest or completely fill it. IV injection of contrast medium is used for evaluation of blood flow through vessels and greater enhancement of tissue density and organ visualization. Multislice or multidetector CT scanners continuously collect images in a helical or spiral fashion instead of a series of individual images, as with standard scanners. Helical CT can collect many images over a short period of time (seconds), is sensitive in identifying small abnormalities, and produces high-quality images. Positron emission tomography–computed tomography (PET/CT) is an imaging application that superimposes PET and CT findings. The images are collected and produced by a single gantry system. The co-registered or image fusion PET/CT findings can provide a detailed combination of anatomical and functional images. Images can be recorded on photographic or x-ray film or stored in digital format as digitized computer data. The CT scan can be used to guide biopsy needles into areas of suspected tumors to obtain tissue for laboratory analysis and to guide placement of catheters for drainage of abscesses. Tumor staging and progression, before and after therapy, and effectiveness of medical interventions may be monitored by CT scanning. The images can be reevaluated and manipulated for further, detailed examination without having to repeat the procedure.

This procedure is contraindicated for

- Patients who are pregnant or suspected of being pregnant, unless the potential benefits of a procedure using radiation far outweigh the risk of radiation exposure to the fetus and mother.
- Patients who are claustrophobic.
- Patients with conditions associated with adverse reactions to contrast medium (e.g., asthma, food allergies, or allergy to contrast medium).

Although patients are asked specifically if they have a known allergy to iodine or shellfish, it has been well established that the reaction is not to iodine; an actual iodine allergy would be problematic because iodine is required for the production of thyroid hormones. In the case of shellfish, the reaction is to a muscle protein called tropomyosin; in the case of iodinated contrast medium, the reaction is to the noniodinated part of the contrast molecule. Patients with a known hypersensitivity to the medium may benefit from premedication with corticosteroids and diphenhydramine; the use of nonionic contrast or an alternative noncontrast imaging study, if available, may be considered for patients who have severe asthma or who have experienced moderate to severe reactions to ionic contrast medium.

- Patients with conditions associated with preexisting renal insufficiency (e.g., chronic kidney disease, single kidney transplant, nephrectomy, diabetes, multiple myeloma, treatment with aminoglycosides and NSAIDs) ***because iodinated contrast is nephrotoxic.***
- Patients who are chronically dehydrated before the test, especially older adults and patients whose health is already compromised, ***because of their risk of contrast-induced acute kidney injury.***
- Patients with pheochromocytoma ***because iodinated contrast may cause a hypertensive crisis.***
- Patients with bleeding disorders or receiving anticoagulant therapy ***because the puncture site may not stop bleeding.***

INDICATIONS

- Aid in the diagnosis of congenital anomalies, such as polycystic kidney disease, horseshoe kidney, absence of one kidney, or kidney displacement.
- Aid in the diagnosis of perirenal hematomas and abscesses and assist in localizing for drainage.
- Assist in differentiating between benign and malignant tumors.
- Assist in differentiating between an infectious and an inflammatory process.
- Detect aneurysms and vascular abnormalities.
- Detect bleeding or hyperplasia of the adrenal glands.
- Detect tumor extension of masses and metastasis into the renal area.
- Determine kidney size and location in relation to the bladder in posttransplant patients.
- Determine presence and type of adrenal tumor, such as benign adenoma, cancer, or pheochromocytoma.
- Evaluate abnormal fluid accumulation around the kidney.
- Evaluate cysts, masses, abscesses, renal calculi, obstruction, and trauma.
- Evaluate spread of a tumor or invasion of nearby retroperitoneal organs.

- Monitor and evaluate effectiveness of medical, radiation, or surgical therapies.

POTENTIAL MEDICAL DIAGNOSIS

Normal findings

- Normal size, position, and shape of kidneys and vascular system

Abnormal findings related to

Identification of abnormal findings is assisted by comparison of parameters such as size, shape, symmetry, density, and location. For example, areas of altered density in either an expected or unexpected location may indicate enlargement of an organ or the presence of blood or other fluids, tumors, or cysts. Comparison by type of abnormal findings may also assist in evaluating areas of altered density. For example, well-defined round or oval areas, smaller in size and having lower density than a primary tumor, may indicate a cyst.

- Adrenal tumor or hyperplasia
- Congenital anomalies, such as polycystic kidney disease, horseshoe kidney, absence of one kidney, or kidney displacement
- Dilation of the common hepatic duct, common bile duct, or gallbladder
- Renal artery aneurysm
- Renal calculi and ureteral obstruction
- Renal cell carcinoma
- Renal cysts or abscesses
- Renal laceration, fracture, tumor, and trauma
- Perirenal abscesses and hematomas
- Primary and metastatic neoplasms

CRITICAL FINDINGS: N/A

INTERFERING FACTORS

Factors that may alter the results of the study

- Gas or feces in the gastrointestinal (GI) tract resulting from inadequate cleansing or failure to restrict food intake before the study.
- Retained barium from a previous radiological procedure.
- Metallic objects (e.g., jewelry, body rings) within the examination field, which may inhibit organ visualization and cause unclear images.
- Patients who are extremely obese may require more radiation to obtain a clear image.
- Patients with extreme claustrophobia unless sedation is given before the study.
- Inability of the patient to cooperate or remain still during the procedure because of age, significant pain, or mental status.

Other considerations

- The procedure may be terminated if chest pain or severe cardiac dysrhythmias occur.
- Failure to follow dietary restrictions and other pretesting preparations may cause the procedure to be canceled or repeated.
- The procedure may be canceled if the patient's weight exceeds the safety limit for the equipment.

NURSING IMPLICATIONS AND PROCEDURE

See Potential Nursing Problems on Fast Find at davispl.us/vanleeuwen7

PRETEST:

- Positively identify the patient using at least two person-specific identifiers before services, treatments, or procedures are performed.
- *Patient Teaching:* Inform the patient this procedure can assist in assessing the kidney.
- Obtain a history of the patient's health concerns, symptoms, surgical procedures, and results of previously performed laboratory and diagnostic studies. Include a list of known allergens, especially allergies

or sensitivities to latex, anesthetics, sedatives, or contrast medium. Ensure results of coagulation testing are obtained and recorded prior to the procedure; a creatinine level is also needed before contrast medium is to be used.

- Note any recent procedures that can interfere with test results, including examinations using barium- or iodine-based contrast medium. Ensure that barium studies were performed more than 4 days before the CT scan.
- Record the date of the last menstrual period and determine the possibility of pregnancy in perimenopausal women.
- Obtain a list of the patient's current medications, including over-the-counter medications, anticoagulants, aspirin and other salicylates, and dietary supplements (see Effects of Natural Products on Laboratory Values online at Davis*Plus*). Such products should be discontinued by medical direction for the appropriate number of days prior to a surgical procedure. Note the last time and dose of medication taken.
- If iodinated contrast medium is scheduled to be used in patients receiving metformin (Glucophage) for type 2 diabetes, the drug should be discontinued on the day of the test and continue to be withheld for 48 hr after the test. Iodinated contrast can temporarily impair kidney function, and failure to withhold metformin may indirectly result in drug-induced lactic acidosis, a dangerous and sometimes fatal adverse effect of metformin ***related to renal impairment that does not support sufficient excretion of metformin.***
- Review the procedure with the patient. Address concerns about pain and explain that there may be moments of discomfort and some pain experienced during the test. Inform the patient the procedure is usually performed in a radiology suite by a health-care provider (HCP) specializing in this procedure, with support staff, and takes approximately 15 to 30 min depending on factors such as the type of study ordered, whether contrast will be used, and the type of contrast used.
- *Sensitivity to social and cultural issues,* as well as concern for modesty, is important in providing psychological support before, during, and after the procedure.
- Explain that an IV line may be inserted to allow infusion of fluids such as saline, anesthetics, contrast medium, or sedatives.
- Inform the patient that he or she may experience nausea, a feeling of warmth, a salty or metallic taste, or a transient headache after injection of contrast medium.
- Advise the patient that he or she may be requested to drink approximately 450 mL of a dilute barium solution (approximately 1% barium) or a water-soluble oral contrast; the oral contrast is given within a specified time period, usually 20 to 30 min prior to the study. Oral contrast is administered to distinguish GI organs from the other abdominal organs and to enhance other areas of interest.
- Instruct the patient to remove all external metallic objects from the area to be examined.
- Inform the patient, as appropriate, that CT studies performed without contrast usually do not require the patient to fast before the procedure. Instruct the patient, if required, to fast and restrict fluids for the specified time period prior to the procedure; fasting may be ordered as a precaution against aspiration related to nausea and vomiting during the administration of contrast. Also instruct the patient to avoid taking anticoagulant medication or to reduce dosage as ordered prior to the procedure due to increased risk of bleeding at the IV insertion site. Protocols may vary among facilities.
- *Make sure a written and informed consent has been signed prior to the procedure and before administering any medications.*

INTRATEST:

Potential Complications:
Injection of the contrast through IV tubing into a blood vessel is an invasive procedure. Complications are rare but do include risk for allergic reaction ***related to contrast reaction,*** cardiac dysrhythmias, hematoma ***related to blood leakage into the tissue following insertion of the IV needle,*** or infection ***that might occur if bacteria from the skin surface is introduced at the IV needle insertion site.***

- Observe standard precautions, and follow the general guidelines in Patient Preparation and Specimen Collection online at Davis*Plus*. Positively identify the patient.
- Ensure the patient has complied with dietary, fluids, medication restrictions, and other pretesting preparations prior to the study, as instructed.
- Ensure the patient has removed all external metallic objects from the area to be examined prior to the procedure.
- Administer ordered prophylactic steroids or antihistamines before the procedure if the patient has a history of allergic reactions to any substance or drug. Use nonionic contrast medium for the procedure.
- Avoid the use of equipment containing latex if the patient has a history of allergic reaction to latex.
- Have emergency equipment readily available.
- Instruct the patient to void prior to the procedure and to change into the gown, robe, and foot coverings provided.
- Instruct the patient to cooperate fully and to follow directions. Instruct the patient to remain still throughout the procedure because movement produces unreliable results.
- Record baseline vital signs, and continue to monitor throughout the procedure. Protocols may vary among facilities.
- Establish an IV fluid line for the injection of contrast, emergency drugs, and sedatives.
- Administer an antianxiety drug, as ordered, if the patient has claustrophobia. Administer a sedative to a child or to an adult who is uncooperative, as ordered.
- Place the patient in the supine position on an examination table.
- If IV contrast is used, a rapid series of images is taken during and after injection.
- Instruct the patient to inhale deeply and hold his or her breath while the images are taken, and then to exhale after the images are taken.
- Instruct the patient to take slow, deep breaths if nausea occurs during the procedure.
- Monitor the patient for complications related to the procedure (e.g., allergic reaction, anaphylaxis, bronchospasm) if contrast is used.
- The needle is removed, and a pressure dressing is applied over the puncture site.
- Observe/assess the needle site for bleeding, inflammation, or hematoma formation.

POST-TEST:

- Inform the patient that a report of the results will be made available to the requesting HCP, who will discuss the results with the patient.
- Instruct the patient to resume usual diet, fluids, medications, and activity, as directed by the HCP. Kidney function should be assessed before metformin is resumed, if contrast was used.
- Monitor vital signs and neurological status every 15 min for 1 hr, then every 2 hr for 4 hr, and then as ordered by the HCP. Monitor temperature every 4 hr for 24 hr. Monitor intake and output at least every 8 hr. Compare with baseline values. Notify the HCP if temperature is elevated. Protocols may vary among facilities.
- If contrast was used, observe for delayed allergic reactions, such as rash, urticaria, tachycardia, hyperpnea, hypertension, palpitations, nausea, or vomiting. Antihistamines may be ordered and given to alleviate symptoms of allergic reaction.

- Instruct the patient to immediately report symptoms such as fast heart rate, difficulty breathing, skin rash, itching, chest pain, persistent right shoulder pain, or abdominal pain. Immediately report symptoms to the appropriate HCP.
- Observe/assess the needle insertion site for bleeding, inflammation, or hematoma formation.
- Instruct the patient in the care and assessment of the site.
- Instruct the patient to apply cold compresses to the insertion site as needed, to reduce discomfort or edema.
- Instruct the patient to increase fluid intake to help eliminate the contrast medium, if used.
- Inform the patient that diarrhea may occur after ingestion of oral contrast medium.
- Recognize anxiety related to test results. Discuss the implications of abnormal test results on the patient's lifestyle. Provide teaching and information regarding the clinical implications of the test results, as appropriate.
- Reinforce information given by the patient's HCP regarding further testing, treatment, or referral to another HCP. Answer any questions or address any concerns voiced by the patient or family.
- Depending on the results of this procedure, additional testing may be needed to evaluate or monitor progression of the disease process and determine the need for a change in therapy. Evaluate test results in relation to the patient's symptoms and other tests performed.

Patient Education:

- Teach the patient diagnosed with stones to avoid foods that facilitate stone formation, such as tea, beer, chocolate, and tea.
- Teach the patient foods that can discourage stone formation, such as milk and milk products.

Expected Patient Outcomes:

Understanding

- The patient and family acknowledge the importance of increased oral intake to renal health.
- The patient and family acknowledge the importance of completing the prescribed antibiotic regime.

Ability

- The patient and family successfully demonstrate the ability to strain the urine.
- The patient and family successfully demonstrate how to measure and record intake an output.

Response

- The patient agrees to diet changes that will facilitate kidney health.
- The patient and family agree to HCPs recommended follow-up evaluations.

RELATED STUDIES:

- Related tests include ACTH, angiography adrenal, biopsy kidney, BUN, calculus/kidney stone panel, catecholamines, CBC, CBC hematocrit, CBC hemoglobin, creatinine, CT abdomen, homovanillic acid, IVP, KUB, MRI abdomen, PT/INR, US kidney, and VMA.
- Refer to the Genitourinary System table online at Davis*Plus* for related tests by body system.

Computed Tomography, Pancreas

SYNONYM/ACRONYM: Computed axial tomography (CAT), computed transaxial tomography (CTT), abdominal CT, helical/spiral CT.

COMMON USE: To visualize and assess the pancreas toward assisting in diagnosing tumors, masses, cancer, bleeding, infection, and abscess. Used as an evaluation tool for surgical, radiation, and medical therapeutic interventions.

AREA OF APPLICATION: Pancreas.

Access Canadian content on Fast Find: Lab and Dx at davispl.us/vanleeuwen7

DESCRIPTION: Computed tomography (CT) is a noninvasive procedure used to enhance certain anatomic views of the abdominal structures. It becomes an invasive procedure when contrast medium is used. CT of the pancreas aids in the diagnosis or evaluation of pancreatic cysts, pseudocysts, inflammation, tumors, masses, metastases, abscesses, and trauma. In all patients but the thinnest or most emaciated, the pancreas is surrounded by fat that clearly defines its margins. During the procedure, the patient lies on a motorized table. The table is moved in and out of a circular opening in a doughnut-like device called a *gantry,* which houses the x-ray tube and associated electronics. A beam of x-rays irradiates the patient as the table moves in and out of the scanner in a series of phases. The x-rays penetrate liquids and solids of different densities by varying degrees. Multiple detectors rotate around the patient to collect numeric data associated with the density coefficients assigned to each degree of tissue density. The imaging system's computer converts the numeric data obtained from the scanner into digital images. Air appears black; bone appears white; and body fluids, fat, and soft tissue structures are represented in various shades between black and white. The cross-sectional views, or *slices,* of the pancreas can be reviewed individually or as a three-dimensional image to allow differentiations of solid, cystic, inflammatory, or vascular lesions as well as identification of suspected areas of enlargement, atrophy, or obstructed ducts. The scan may be repeated after administration of contrast medium given orally, by intravenous (IV) injection, or rectally. Contrast is used to differentiate, enhance, or "light up" areas of interest depending on the type of study to be performed, type of contrast medium to be used, and method of administration. The medium works by creating a contrast between areas of interest based on density; penetration of the x-rays is weaker in areas where the contrast medium is detected by the scanner, showing the blood vessels, organs, and tissue as whitish areas that either outline the area of interest or completely fill it. Oral ingestion of contrast medium can be used for opacification to distinguish the bowel, adjacent abdominal organs, other types of tissue, and blood vessels as the medium moves through the digestive tract. IV injection of contrast medium is used for evaluation of blood flow through vessels and greater enhancement of tissue density and organ visualization. In some cases, scans may be repeated after multiple types of contrast are administered. Multislice or multidetector CT scanners continuously collect images in a helical or spiral fashion instead of a series of individual images as with standard scanners. Helical CT can collect many images over a short period of time (seconds), is sensitive in identifying small abnormalities, and produces high-quality images. Positron emission tomography–computed tomography (PET/CT) is an imaging application that superimposes PET and CT findings. The images are collected and produced by a single gantry system. The co-registered or image fusion PET/CT findings can provide a detailed combination of anatomical and functional images. Images can be recorded on photographic or x-ray film or stored in digital format as digitized computer data. The CT scan can be used to guide biopsy needles into areas of suspected tumors to obtain tissue for laboratory analysis and to guide placement of catheters for drainage of abscesses. Tumor staging and progression, before and after therapy, and effectiveness of medical interventions may be monitored by CT scanning. The images can be reevaluated and manipulated for further, detailed examination without having to repeat the procedure.

C

This procedure is contraindicated for

Patients who are pregnant or suspected of being pregnant, unless the potential benefits of a procedure using radiation far outweigh the risk of radiation exposure to the fetus and mother.

Patients who are claustrophobic.

Patients with conditions associated with adverse reactions to contrast medium (e.g., asthma, food allergies, or allergy to contrast medium).

Although patients are asked specifically if they have a known allergy to iodine or shellfish, it has been well established that the reaction is not to iodine; an actual iodine allergy would be problematic because iodine is required for the production of thyroid hormones. In the case of shellfish, the reaction is to a muscle protein called tropomyosin; in the case of iodinated contrast medium, the reaction is to the noniodinated part of the contrast molecule. Patients with a known hypersensitivity to the medium may benefit from premedication with corticosteroids and diphenhydramine; the use of nonionic contrast or an alternative noncontrast imaging study, if available, may be considered for patients who have severe asthma or who have experienced moderate to severe reactions to ionic contrast medium.

Patients with conditions associated with preexisting renal insufficiency (e.g., chronic kidney disease, single kidney transplant, nephrectomy, diabetes, multiple myeloma, treatment with aminoglycosides and NSAIDs) ***because iodinated contrast is nephrotoxic.***

Patients who are chronically dehydrated before the test, especially older adults and patients whose health is already compromised, ***because of their risk of contrast-induced acute kidney injury.***

Patients with pheochromocytoma ***because iodinated contrast may cause a hypertensive crisis.***

Patients with bleeding disorders or receiving anticoagulant therapy ***because the puncture site may not stop bleeding.***

INDICATIONS

- Detect dilation or obstruction of the pancreatic ducts.
- Differentiate between pancreatic disorders and disorders of the retroperitoneum.
- Evaluate benign or cancerous tumors or metastasis to the pancreas.
- Evaluate pancreatic abnormalities (e.g., bleeding, pancreatitis, pseudocyst, abscesses).
- Evaluate unexplained weight loss, jaundice, and epigastric pain.
- Monitor and evaluate effectiveness of medical or surgical therapies.

POTENTIAL MEDICAL DIAGNOSIS

Normal findings

- Normal size, position, and contour of the pancreas, which lies obliquely in the upper abdomen

Abnormal findings related to

Identification of abnormal findings is assisted by comparison of parameters such as size, shape, symmetry, density, and location. For example, areas of altered density in either an expected or unexpected location may indicate enlargement of an organ or the presence of blood or other fluids, tumors, or cysts. Comparison by type of abnormal findings may also assist in evaluating areas of altered density. For example, well-defined round or oval areas, smaller in size and having lower density than a primary tumor, may indicate a cyst.

- Acute or chronic pancreatitis
- Obstruction of the pancreatic ducts
- Pancreatic abscesses
- Pancreatic carcinoma
- Pancreatic pseudocyst
- Pancreatic tumor

CRITICAL FINDINGS: N/A

INTERFERING FACTORS

Factors that may alter the results of the study

- Gas or feces in the gastrointestinal (GI) tract resulting from inadequate cleansing or failure to restrict food intake before the study.
- Retained barium from a previous radiological procedure.
- Metallic objects (e.g., jewelry, body rings) within the examination field, which may inhibit organ visualization and cause unclear images.
- Patients who are extremely obese may require more radiation to obtain a clear image.
- Patients with extreme claustrophobia unless sedation is given before the study.
- Inability of the patient to cooperate or remain still during the procedure because of age, significant pain, or mental status.

Other considerations

- The procedure may be terminated if chest pain or severe cardiac dysrhythmias occur.
- Failure to follow dietary restrictions and other pretesting preparations may cause the procedure to be canceled or repeated.
- The procedure may be canceled if the patient's weight exceeds the safety limit for the equipment.

NURSING IMPLICATIONS AND PROCEDURE

See Potential Nursing Problems on Fast Find at davispl.us/vanleeuwen7

PRETEST:

- Positively identify the patient using at least two person-specific identifiers before services, treatments, or procedures are performed.
- ***Patient Teaching:*** Inform the patient this procedure can assist in assessing the abdomen and pancreatic area.
- Obtain a history of the patient's health concerns, symptoms, surgical procedures, and results of previously performed laboratory and diagnostic studies. Include a list of known allergens, especially allergies or sensitivities to latex, anesthetics, sedatives, or contrast medium. Ensure results of coagulation testing are obtained and recorded prior to the procedure; a creatinine level is also needed before contrast medium is to be used.
- Note any recent procedures that can interfere with test results, including examinations using barium- or iodine-based contrast medium. Ensure that barium studies were performed more than 4 days before the CT scan.
- Record the date of the last menstrual period and determine the possibility of pregnancy in perimenopausal women.
- Obtain a list of the patient's current medications, including over-the-counter medications, anticoagulants, aspirin and other salicylates, and

dietary supplements (see Effects of Natural Products on Laboratory Values online at Davis*Plus*). Such products should be discontinued by medical direction for the appropriate number of days prior to a surgical procedure. Note the last time and dose of medication taken.

- If iodinated contrast medium is scheduled to be used in patients receiving metformin (Glucophage) for type 2 diabetes, the drug should be discontinued on the day of the test and continue to be withheld for 48 hr after the test. Iodinated contrast can temporarily impair kidney function, and failure to withhold metformin may indirectly result in drug-induced lactic acidosis, a dangerous and sometimes fatal adverse effect of metformin ***related to renal impairment that does not support sufficient excretion of metformin.***
- Review the procedure with the patient. Address concerns about pain and explain that there may be moments of discomfort and some pain experienced during the test. Inform the patient the procedure is usually performed in a radiology suite by a health-care provider (HCP) specializing in this procedure, with support staff, and takes approximately 15 to 30 min depending on factors such as the type of study ordered, whether contrast will be used, and the type of contrast used.
- ***Sensitivity to social and cultural issues,*** as well as concern for modesty, is important in providing psychological support before, during, and after the procedure.
- Explain that an IV line may be inserted to allow infusion of fluids such as saline, anesthetics, contrast medium, or sedatives.
- Inform the patient that he or she may experience nausea, a feeling of warmth, a salty or metallic taste, or a transient headache after injection of contrast medium.
- Advise the patient that he or she may be requested to drink approximately 450 mL of a dilute barium solution (approximately 1% barium) or a water-soluble oral contrast; the oral contrast is given within a specified time period, prior to the study. Oral contrast is administered to distinguish GI organs from the other abdominal organs and to enhance other areas of interest.
- Instruct the patient to remove jewelry and other metallic objects from the area to be examined.
- Inform the patient, as appropriate, that CT studies performed without contrast usually do not require the patient to fast before the procedure. Instruct the patient, if required, to fast and restrict fluids for the specified time period prior to the procedure; fasting may be ordered as a precaution against aspiration related to nausea and vomiting during the administration of contrast. Also instruct the patient to avoid taking anticoagulant medication or to reduce dosage as ordered prior to the procedure due to increased risk of bleeding at the IV insertion site. Protocols may vary among facilities.
- Instruct the patient to remove jewelry and other metallic objects from the area to be examined.
- *Make sure a written and informed consent has been signed prior to the procedure and before administering any medications.*

INTRATEST:

Potential Complications:

Injection of the contrast through IV tubing into a blood vessel is an invasive procedure. Complications are rare but do include risk for allergic reaction ***related to contrast reaction,*** cardiac dysrhythmias, hematoma ***related to blood leakage into the tissue following insertion of the IV needle,*** or infection ***that might occur if bacteria from the skin surface is introduced at the IV needle insertion site.***

- Observe standard precautions, and follow the general guidelines in Patient Preparation and Specimen Collection online at Davis*Plus*. Positively identify the patient.

- Ensure the patient has complied with dietary, fluids, medication restrictions, and other pretesting preparations prior to the study, as instructed.
- Ensure that the patient has removed all external metallic objects from the area to be examined prior to the procedure.
- Administer ordered prophylactic steroids or antihistamines before the procedure if the patient has a history of allergic reactions to any substance or drug.
- Avoid the use of equipment containing latex if the patient has a history of allergic reaction to latex.
- Have emergency equipment readily available.
- Instruct the patient to void prior to the procedure and to change into the gown, robe, and foot coverings provided.
- Instruct the patient to cooperate fully and to follow directions. Instruct the patient to remain still throughout the procedure because movement produces unreliable results.
- Establish an IV fluid line for the injection of contrast medium, emergency drugs, and sedatives.
- Administer an antianxiety drug, as ordered, if the patient has claustrophobia. Administer a sedative to a child or to an adult who is uncooperative, as ordered.
- Place the patient in the supine position on an examination table.
- If IV contrast medium is used, a rapid series of images is taken during and after injection.
- Instruct the patient to inhale deeply and hold his or her breath while the images are taken, and then to exhale after the images are taken.
- Instruct the patient to take slow, deep breaths if nausea occurs during the procedure.
- Monitor the patient for complications related to the procedure (e.g., allergic reaction, anaphylaxis, bronchospasm) if contrast is used.
- The needle is removed, and a pressure dressing is applied over the puncture site.
- Observe/assess the needle site for bleeding, inflammation, or hematoma formation.

POST-TEST:

- Inform the patient that a report of the results will be made available to the requesting HCP, who will discuss the results with the patient.
- Instruct the patient to resume usual diet, fluids, medications, and activity, as directed by the HCP. Kidney function should be assessed before metformin is resumed, if contrast was used.
- Monitor vital signs and neurological status every 15 min for 1 hr, then every 2 hr for 4 hr, and then as ordered by the HCP. Monitor temperature every 4 hr for 24 hr. Monitor intake and output at least every 8 hr. Compare with baseline values. Notify the HCP if temperature is elevated. Protocols may vary among facilities.
- If contrast was used, observe for delayed allergic reactions, such as rash, urticaria, tachycardia, hyperpnea, hypertension, palpitations, nausea, or vomiting. Antihistamines may be ordered and given to alleviate symptoms of allergic reaction.
- Instruct the patient to immediately report symptoms such as fast heart rate, difficulty breathing, skin rash, itching, chest pain, persistent right shoulder pain, or abdominal pain. Immediately report symptoms to the appropriate HCP.
- Observe/assess the needle site for bleeding, inflammation, or hematoma formation.
- Instruct the patient in the care and assessment of the site.
- Instruct the patient to apply cold compresses to the puncture site as needed, to reduce discomfort or edema.
- Instruct the patient to increase fluid intake to help eliminate the contrast medium, if used.
- Inform the patient that diarrhea may occur after ingestion of oral contrast medium.
- Recognize anxiety related to test results. Discuss the implications of

abnormal test results on the patient's lifestyle. Provide teaching and information regarding the clinical implications of the test results, as appropriate.

- Reinforce information given by the patient's HCP regarding further testing, treatment, or referral to another HCP. Answer any questions or address any concerns voiced by the patient or family.
- Depending on the results of this procedure, additional testing may be needed to evaluate or monitor progression of the disease process and determine the need for a change in therapy. Evaluate test results in relation to the patient's symptoms and other tests performed.

Patient Education:

- Teach the patient that the consumption of alcohol can exacerbate the pain due to pancreatic stimulation.
- Facilitate a dietary consultation to assist the patient in managing his or her nutritional status.

Expected Patient Outcomes:

Understanding

- The patient and family acknowledge the importance of progressing the diet slowly to evaluate food tolerance and make adjustments as needed.
- The patient and family acknowledge the importance of taking dietary supplements to support positive nutrition.

Ability

- The patient and family demonstrate the ability to select low-fat foods to include in the diet plan.
- The patient and family demonstrate the ability to accurately record intake and output.

Response

- The patient agrees to avoid drinking alcoholic and caffeinated beverages.
- The patient participates in a pain management plan that provides a level of relief acceptable to the patient.

RELATED STUDIES:

- Related tests include amylase, angiography of the abdomen, biopsy intestinal, BUN, cancer antigens, CBC hemoglobin, creatinine, ERCP, lipase, MRI abdomen, PT/INR, and US pancreas.
- Refer to the Gastrointestinal and Hepatobiliary systems tables online at Davis*Plus* for related tests by body system.

Computed Tomography, Pelvis

SYNONYM/ACRONYM: Computed axial tomography (CAT), computed transaxial tomography (CTT), pelvis CT, helical/spiral CT.

COMMON USE: To visualize and assess pelvic structures and vascularities related to assisting in diagnosing bleeding, infection, masses, and cyst aspiration (needle-guided biopsy). Used to monitor the effectiveness of medical, radiation, and surgical therapeutic interventions.

AREA OF APPLICATION: Pelvis.

DESCRIPTION: Computed tomography (CT) of the pelvis is a noninvasive procedure used to enhance certain anatomic views of the pelvic structures. It becomes an invasive procedure when intravenous (IV) contrast medium is used. During the procedure, the patient lies on a motorized table. The table is moved in and out of a circular opening in a doughnut-like device called a *gantry,* which houses the x-ray tube and associated electronics. A beam of x-rays irradiates the patient as the table moves in and out of the scanner in a series of phases. The x-rays penetrate liquids and solids of different densities by varying degrees. Multiple detectors rotate around the patient to collect numeric data associated with the density coefficients assigned to each degree of tissue density. The imaging system's computer converts the numeric data obtained from the scanner into digital images. Air appears black; bone appears white; and body fluids, fat, and soft tissue structures are represented in various shades between black and white. The cross-sectional views, or *slices,* of the esophagus, pelvis, bladder, prostate (males), uterine structures (females), kidneys, ureters, rectum, and associated mesentery tissue can be reviewed individually or as a three-dimensional image to allow differentiations of solid, cystic, inflammatory, or vascular lesions as well as identification of suspected hematomas. The scan may be repeated after administration of contrast medium given orally, by IV injection, or rectally. Contrast is used to differentiate, enhance, or "light up" areas of interest depending on the type of study to be performed, type of contrast medium to be used, and method of administration. The medium works by creating a contrast between areas of interest based on density; penetration of the x-rays is weaker in areas where the contrast medium is detected by the scanner, showing the blood vessels, organs, and tissue as whitish areas that either outline the area of interest or completely fill it. Oral ingestion of contrast medium can be used for opacification to distinguish the bowel, adjacent abdominal organs, other types of tissue, and blood vessels as the medium moves through the digestive tract. IV injection of contrast medium is used for evaluation of blood flow through vessels and greater enhancement of tissue density and organ visualization. In some cases, scans may be repeated after multiple types of contrast are administered. Multislice or multidetector CT scanners continuously collect images in a helical or spiral fashion instead of a series of individual images as with standard scanners. Helical CT can collect many images over a short period of time (seconds), is sensitive in identifying small abnormalities, and produces high-quality images. Positron emission tomography-computed tomography (PET/CT) is an imaging application that superimposes PET and CT findings. The images are collected and produced by a single gantry system. The co-registered or image fusion PET/CT findings can provide a detailed combination of anatomical and functional images. Images can be recorded on photographic or x-ray film or stored in digital format as digitized computer data. The CT scan can be used to guide biopsy needles into areas of tumors to obtain tissue for laboratory analysis and to guide placement of catheters for drainage of abscesses. Tumor staging and progression, before and after therapy, and effectiveness of medical interventions may be monitored by CT scanning.

The images can be reevaluated and manipulated for further, detailed examination without having to repeat the procedure.

This procedure is contraindicated for

C

- Patients who are pregnant or suspected of being pregnant, unless the potential benefits of a procedure using radiation far outweigh the risk of radiation exposure to the fetus and mother.
- Patients who are claustrophobic.
- Patients with conditions associated with adverse reactions to contrast medium (e.g., asthma, food allergies, or allergy to contrast medium).

Although patients are asked specifically if they have a known allergy to iodine or shellfish, it has been well established that the reaction is not to iodine; an actual iodine allergy would be problematic because iodine is required for the production of thyroid hormones. In the case of shellfish, the reaction is to a muscle protein called tropomyosin; in the case of iodinated contrast medium, the reaction is to the noniodinated part of the contrast molecule. Patients with a known hypersensitivity to the medium may benefit from premedication with corticosteroids and diphenhydramine; the use of nonionic contrast or an alternative noncontrast imaging study, if available, may be considered for patients who have severe asthma or who have experienced moderate to severe reactions to ionic contrast medium.

- Patients with conditions associated with preexisting renal insufficiency (e.g., chronic kidney disease, single kidney transplant, nephrectomy, diabetes, multiple myeloma, treatment with aminoglycosides and NSAIDs) ***because iodinated contrast is nephrotoxic.***
- Patients who are chronically dehydrated before the test, especially older adults and patients whose health is already compromised, ***because of their risk of contrast-induced acute kidney injury.***
- Patients with pheochromocytoma ***because iodinated contrast may cause a hypertensive crisis.***
- Patients with bleeding disorders or receiving anticoagulant therapy ***because the puncture site may not stop bleeding.***

INDICATIONS

- Assist in differentiating between benign and malignant tumors.
- Detect tumor extension of masses and metastasis into the pelvic area.
- Differentiate infectious from inflammatory processes.
- Evaluate pelvic lymph nodes.
- Evaluate cysts, masses, abscesses, ureteral and bladder calculi, gastrointestinal (GI) bleeding and obstruction, and trauma.
- Monitor and evaluate effectiveness of medical, radiation, or surgical therapies.

POTENTIAL MEDICAL DIAGNOSIS

Normal findings

- Normal size, position, and shape of pelvic organs and vascular system

Abnormal findings related to

Identification of abnormal findings is assisted by comparison of parameters such as size, shape, symmetry, density, and location. For example, areas of altered density in either an expected or unexpected location may indicate enlargement of an organ or the presence of blood or other fluids, tumors, or cysts. Comparison by type of abnormal findings may also assist in evaluating areas of altered density. For example, well-defined round or oval areas, smaller in size and having lower density than a primary tumor, may indicate a cyst.

- Bladder calculi
- Ectopic pregnancy
- Fibroid tumors
- Hydrosalpinx
- Ovarian cyst or abscess
- Primary and metastatic neoplasms

CRITICAL FINDINGS:

- Ectopic pregnancy
- Tumor with significant mass effect

Note and immediately report to the requesting health-care provider (HCP) any critical findings and related symptoms. A listing of these findings varies among facilities. Timely notification of a critical finding for laboratory or diagnostic studies is a role expectation of the professional nurse. The notification processes vary among facilities. Upon receipt of the critical finding, the information should be read back to the caller to verify accuracy.

INTERFERING FACTORS

Factors that may alter the results of the study

- Gas or feces in the GI tract resulting from inadequate cleansing or failure to restrict food intake before the study.
- Retained barium from a previous radiological procedure.
- Metallic objects (e.g., jewelry, body rings) within the examination field, which may inhibit organ visualization and can produce unclear images.
- Patients who are extremely obese may require more radiation to obtain a clear image.
- Patients with extreme claustrophobia unless sedation is given before the study.
- Inability of the patient to cooperate or remain still during the procedure because of age, significant pain, or mental status.

Other considerations

- The procedure may be terminated if chest pain or severe cardiac dysrhythmias occur.
- Failure to follow dietary restrictions and other pretesting preparations may cause the procedure to be canceled or repeated.
- The procedure may be canceled if the patient's weight exceeds the safety limit for the equipment.

NURSING IMPLICATIONS AND PROCEDURE

See Potential Nursing Problems on Fast Find at davispl.us/vanleeuwen7

PRETEST:

- Positively identify the patient using at least two person-specific identifiers before services, treatments, or procedures are performed.
- *Patient Teaching:* Inform the patient this procedure can assist in assessing the pelvis and pelvic organs.
- Obtain a history of the patient's health concerns, symptoms, surgical procedures, and results of previously performed laboratory and diagnostic studies. Include a list of known allergens, especially allergies or sensitivities to latex, anesthetics, sedatives, or contrast medium. Ensure results of coagulation testing are obtained and recorded prior to the procedure; a creatinine level is also needed before contrast medium is to be used.
- Note any recent procedures that can interfere with test results, including examinations using barium- or iodine-based contrast medium. Ensure that barium studies were performed more than 4 days before the CT scan.
- Record the date of the last menstrual period and determine the possibility of pregnancy in perimenopausal women.
- Obtain a list of the patient's current medications, including over-the-counter medications, anticoagulants, aspirin and other salicylates, and dietary supplements (see Effects

of Natural Products on Laboratory Values online at Davis*Plus*). Such products should be discontinued by medical direction for the appropriate number of days prior to a surgical procedure. Note the last time and dose of medication taken.

- If iodinated contrast medium is scheduled to be used in patients receiving metformin (Glucophage) for type 2 diabetes, the drug should be discontinued on the day of the test and continue to be withheld for 48 hr after the test. Iodinated contrast can temporarily impair kidney function, and failure to withhold metformin may indirectly result in drug-induced lactic acidosis, a dangerous and sometimes fatal adverse effect of metformin ***related to renal impairment that does not support sufficient excretion of metformin.***
- Review the procedure with the patient. Address concerns about pain and explain that there may be moments of discomfort and some pain experienced during the test. Inform the patient the procedure is usually performed in a radiology suite by an HCP specializing in this procedure, with support staff, and takes approximately 15 to 30 min depending on factors such as the type of study ordered, whether contrast will be used, and the type of contrast used.
- *Sensitivity to social and cultural issues,* as well as concern for modesty, is important in providing psychological support before, during, and after the procedure.
- Explain that an IV line may be inserted to allow infusion of fluids such as saline, anesthetics, contrast medium, or sedatives.
- Inform the patient that he or she may experience nausea, a feeling of warmth, a salty or metallic taste, or a transient headache after injection of contrast medium.
- Advise the patient that he or she may be requested to drink approximately 450 mL of a dilute barium solution (approximately 1% barium) or a water-soluble oral contrast; the oral contrast is given within a specified time period prior to the study. Oral contrast is administered to distinguish GI organs from the other abdominal organs and to enhance other areas of interest.
- Instruct the patient to remove jewelry and other metallic objects from the area to be examined.
- Inform the patient, as appropriate, that CT studies performed without contrast usually do not require the patient to fast before the procedure. Instruct the patient, if required, to fast and restrict fluids for the specified time period, prior to the procedure; fasting may be ordered as a precaution against aspiration related to nausea and vomiting during the administration of contrast. Also instruct the patient to avoid taking anticoagulant medication or to reduce dosage as ordered prior to the procedure due to increased risk of bleeding at the IV insertion site. Protocols may vary among facilities.
- *Make sure a written and informed consent has been signed prior to the procedure and before administering any medications.*

INTRATEST:

Potential Complications:

Injection of the contrast through IV tubing into a blood vessel is an invasive procedure. Complications are rare but do include risk for allergic reaction ***related to contrast reaction,*** cardiac dysrhythmias, hematoma ***related to blood leakage into the tissue following insertion of the IV needle,*** or infection ***that might occur if bacteria from the skin surface is introduced at the IV needle insertion site.***

- Observe standard precautions, and follow the general guidelines in Patient Preparation and Specimen Collection online at Davis*Plus*. Positively identify the patient.
- Ensure the patient has complied with dietary, fluids, medication restrictions, and other pretesting preparations prior to the study, as instructed.
- Ensure the patient has removed all external metallic objects from the

area to be examined prior to the procedure.
- Administer ordered prophylactic steroids or antihistamines before the procedure if the patient has a history of allergic reactions to any substance or drug.
- Avoid the use of equipment containing latex if the patient has a history of allergic reaction to latex.
- Have emergency equipment readily available.
- Instruct the patient to void prior to the procedure and to change into the gown, robe, and foot coverings provided.
- Instruct the patient to cooperate fully and to follow directions. Instruct the patient to remain still throughout the procedure because movement produces unreliable results.
- Establish an IV fluid line for the injection of contrast, emergency drugs, and sedatives.
- Administer an antianxiety drug, as ordered, if the patient has claustrophobia. Administer a sedative to a child or to an adult who is uncooperative, as ordered.
- Place the patient in the supine position on an examination table.
- If IV contrast medium is used, a rapid series of images is taken during and after injection.
- Instruct the patient to inhale deeply and hold his or her breath while the images are taken, and then to exhale after the images are taken.
- Instruct the patient to take slow, deep breaths if nausea occurs during the procedure.
- Monitor the patient for complications related to the procedure (e.g., allergic reaction, anaphylaxis, bronchospasm) if contrast is used.
- The needle is removed, and a pressure dressing is applied over the puncture site.
- Observe/assess the needle site for bleeding, inflammation, or hematoma formation.

POST-TEST:

- Inform patient that a report of the results will be made available to the requesting HCP, who will discuss the results with the patient.
- Instruct the patient to resume usual diet, fluids, medications, and activity, as directed by the HCP. Kidney function should be assessed before metformin is resumed, if contrast was used.
- Monitor vital signs and neurological status every 15 min for 1 hr, then every 2 hr for 4 hr, and then as ordered by the HCP. Monitor temperature every 4 hr for 24 hr. Monitor intake and output at least every 8 hr. Compare with baseline values. Notify the HCP if temperature is elevated. Protocols may vary among facilities.
- If contrast was used, observe for delayed allergic reactions, such as rash, urticaria, tachycardia, hyperpnea, hypertension, palpitations, nausea, or vomiting. Antihistamines may be ordered and given to alleviate symptoms of allergic reaction.
- Instruct the patient to immediately report symptoms such as fast heart rate, difficulty breathing, skin rash, itching, chest pain, persistent right shoulder pain, or abdominal pain. Immediately report symptoms to the appropriate HCP.
- Observe/assess the needle insertion site for bleeding, inflammation, or hematoma formation.
- Instruct the patient in the care and assessment of the site.
- Instruct the patient to apply cold compresses to the insertion site as needed, to reduce discomfort or edema.
- Instruct the patient to increase fluid intake to help eliminate the contrast medium, if used.
- Inform the patient that diarrhea may occur after ingestion of oral contrast medium.
- Recognize anxiety related to test results. Discuss the implications of abnormal test results on the patient's lifestyle. Provide teaching and information regarding the clinical implications of the test results, as appropriate.
- Reinforce information given by the patient's HCP regarding further

C

testing, treatment, or referral to another HCP. Answer any questions or address any concerns voiced by the patient or family.

- Depending on the results of this procedure, additional testing may be needed to evaluate or monitor progression of the disease process and determine the need for a change in therapy. Evaluate test results in relation to the patient's symptoms and other tests performed.

Patient Education:

- Teach the pathophysiology of the disease process.
- Teach the patient the importance of calling for pain medication as soon as it is needed for effective pain management.

Expected Patient Outcomes:

Understanding

- The patient and family correctly describe treatment options related to disease process.
- The patient and family acknowledge the importance of family or group counseling related to end-of-life issues.

Ability

- The patient and family demonstrate the ability to maintain a quiet environment for emotional and physical rest.
- The patient and family demonstrate successful coping strategies.

Response

- The patient and family agree to family or individual support group counseling related to prognosis and end of life.
- The patient and family agree to all follow-up diagnostic and laboratory studies needed to monitor health status and the effectiveness of treatment modalities.

RELATED STUDIES:

- Related tests include angiography pelvis, barium enema, BUN, calculus kidney stone panel, cancer antigens, CBC, CBC hematocrit, CBC hemoglobin, creatinine, HCG, IVP, KUB film, MRI abdomen, proctosigmoidoscopy, PT/INR, US pelvis, and UA.
- Refer to the Gastrointestinal, Genitourinary, and Reproductive systems tables online at Davis*Plus* for related tests by body system.

Computed Tomography, Pituitary

SYNONYM/ACRONYM: Computed axial tomography (CAT), computed transaxial tomography (CTT), pituitary CT, helical/spiral CT.

COMMON USE: To visualize and assess portions of the brain and pituitary gland for cancer, tumor, and bleeding. Used as an evaluation tool for surgical, radiation, and medical therapeutic interventions.

AREA OF APPLICATION: Pituitary/brain.

DESCRIPTION: Computed tomography (CT) of the pituitary is a noninvasive procedure that enhances certain anatomic views of the pituitary gland and perisellar region. It becomes invasive when a contrast medium is used. During the procedure, the patient lies on a motorized table. The table is moved in and out of a circular opening in a doughnut-like device called a *gantry,* which houses the x-ray tube and associated electronics. A beam of x-rays irradiates the patient as the table moves in and out of the scanner in a series of phases. The x-rays penetrate liquids and solids of different densities by varying degrees. Multiple detectors rotate around the patient to collect numeric data associated with the density coefficients assigned to each degree of tissue density. The imaging system's computer converts the numeric data obtained from the scanner into digital images. Air appears black; bone appears white; and body fluids, fat, and soft tissue structures are represented in various shades between black and white. The cross-sectional views or slices of the pituitary gland and associated vascular system can be reviewed individually or as a three-dimensional image to allow differentiations of solid, cystic, inflammatory, or vascular lesions as well as identification of suspected hematomas and aneurysms. The scan may be repeated after administration of contrast medium given by intravenous (IV) injection. Contrast is used to differentiate, enhance, or "light up" areas of interest depending on the type of study to be performed, type of contrast medium to be used, and method of administration. The medium works by creating a contrast between areas of interest based on density; penetration of the x-rays is weaker in areas where the contrast medium is detected by the scanner, showing the blood vessels, organs, and tissue as whitish areas that either outline the area of interest or completely fill it. An IV injection of contrast medium is used for evaluation of blood flow through vessels and greater enhancement of tissue density and organ visualization. This procedure aids in the evaluation of pituitary adenoma, craniopharyngioma, meningioma, aneurysm, metastatic disease, exophthalmos, and cysts. Visualization of bony septa in the sphenoid sinus and evaluation for nonpneumatization of the sphenoid sinus are best performed with this procedure. Multislice or multidetector CT scanners continuously collect images in a helical or spiral fashion instead of a series of individual images as with standard scanners. Helical CT can collect many images over a short period of time (seconds), is sensitive in identifying small abnormalities, and produces high-quality images. Images can be recorded on photographic or x-ray film or stored in digital format as digitized computer data. The CT scan can be used to guide biopsy needles into areas of suspected tumors to obtain tissue for laboratory analysis. Tumor staging and progression, before and after therapy, and effectiveness of medical interventions may be monitored by CT scanning. The images can be reevaluated and manipulated for further, detailed examination without having to repeat the procedure.

This procedure is contraindicated for

- Patients who are pregnant or suspected of being pregnant, unless the potential benefits of a procedure using radiation far outweigh the risk of radiation exposure to the fetus and mother.
- Patients who are claustrophobic.
- Patients with conditions associated with adverse reactions to contrast medium (e.g., asthma, food allergies, or allergy to contrast medium).

Although patients are asked specifically if they have a known allergy to iodine or shellfish, it has been well established that the reaction is not to iodine, in fact an actual iodine allergy would be problematic because iodine is required for the production of thyroid hormones. In the case of shellfish the reaction is to a muscle protein called tropomyosin; in the case of iodinated contrast medium the reaction is to the noniodinated part of the contrast molecule. Patients with a known hypersensitivity to the medium may benefit from premedication with corticosteroids and diphenhydramine; the use of nonionic contrast or an alternative noncontrast imaging study, if available, may be considered for patients who have severe asthma or who have experienced moderate to severe reactions to ionic contrast medium.

Patients with conditions associated with preexisting renal insufficiency (e.g., chronic kidney disease, single kidney transplant, nephrectomy, diabetes, multiple myeloma, treatment with aminoglycosides and NSAIDs) ***because iodinated contrast is nephrotoxic.***

Patients who are chronically dehydrated before the test, especially older adults and patients whose health is already compromised, ***because of their risk of contrast-induced acute kidney injury.***

Patients with pheochromocytoma ***because iodinated contrast may cause a hypertensive crisis.***

Patients with bleeding disorders or receiving anticoagulant therapy ***because the puncture site may not stop bleeding.***

INDICATIONS

- Assist in differentiating between benign and malignant tumors.
- Detect aneurysms and vascular abnormalities.
- Detect congenital anomalies, such as partially empty sella.
- Detect tumor extension of masses and metastasis.
- Determine pituitary size and location in relation to surrounding structures.
- Evaluate cysts, masses, abscesses, and trauma.
- Monitor and evaluate effectiveness of medical, radiation, or surgical therapies.

POTENTIAL MEDICAL DIAGNOSIS

Normal findings

- Normal size, position, and shape of the pituitary fossa, cavernous sinuses, and vascular system

Abnormal findings related to

Identification of abnormal findings is assisted by comparison of parameters such as size, shape, symmetry, density, and location. For example, areas of altered density in either an expected or unexpected location may indicate enlargement of an organ or the presence of blood or other fluids, tumors, or cysts. Comparison by type of abnormal findings may also assist in evaluating areas of altered density. For example, well-defined round or oval areas, smaller in size and having lower density than a primary tumor, may indicate a cyst.

- Abscess
- Adenoma
- Aneurysm
- Chordoma
- Craniopharyngioma
- Cyst
- Meningioma
- Metastasis
- Pituitary hemorrhage

CRITICAL FINDINGS: N/A

INTERFERING FACTORS

Factors that may alter the results of the study

- Retained contrast from a previous radiological procedure.
- Metallic objects (e.g., jewelry, dentures, body rings) within the

examination field, which may inhibit organ visualization and cause unclear images.

- Patients who are extremely obese may require more radiation to obtain a clear image.
- Patients with extreme claustrophobia unless sedation is given before the study.
- Inability of the patient to cooperate or remain still during the procedure because of age, significant pain, or mental status.

Other considerations

- The procedure may be terminated if chest pain or severe cardiac dysrhythmias occur.
- Failure to follow pretesting preparations may cause the procedure to be canceled or repeated.
- The procedure may be canceled if the patient's weight exceeds the safety limit for the equipment.

NURSING IMPLICATIONS AND PROCEDURE

PRETEST:

- Positively identify the patient using at least two person-specific identifiers before services, treatments, or procedures are performed.
- *Patient Teaching:* Inform the patient this procedure can assist in assessing the brain and pituitary gland.
- Obtain a history of the patient's health concerns, symptoms, surgical procedures, and results of previously performed laboratory and diagnostic studies. Include a list of known allergens, especially allergies or sensitivities to latex, anesthetics, sedatives, or contrast medium. Ensure results of coagulation testing are obtained and recorded prior to the procedure; a creatinine level is also needed before contrast medium is to be used.
- Note any recent procedures that can interfere with test results, including examinations using barium- or iodine-based contrast medium. Ensure that barium studies were performed more than 4 days before the CT scan.
- Record the date of the last menstrual period and determine the possibility of pregnancy in perimenopausal women.
- Obtain a list of the patient's current medications, including over-the-counter medications, anticoagulants, aspirin and other salicylates, and dietary supplements (see Effects of Natural Products on Laboratory Values online at Davis*Plus*). Such products should be discontinued by medical direction for the appropriate number of days prior to a surgical procedure. Note the last time and dose of medication taken.
- If iodinated contrast medium is scheduled to be used in patients receiving metformin (Glucophage) for type 2 diabetes, the drug should be discontinued on the day of the test and continue to be withheld for 48 hr after the test. Iodinated contrast can temporarily impair kidney function, and failure to withhold metformin may indirectly result in drug-induced lactic acidosis, a dangerous and sometimes fatal adverse effect of metformin ***related to renal impairment that does not support sufficient excretion of metformin.***
- Review the procedure with the patient. Address concerns about pain and explain that there may be moments of discomfort and some pain experienced during the test. Inform the patient the procedure is usually performed in a radiology suite by a health-care provider (HCP) specializing in this procedure, with support staff, and takes approximately 15 to 30 min depending on factors such as the type of study ordered, whether contrast will be used, and the type of contrast used.
- ***Sensitivity to social and cultural issues,*** as well as concern for modesty, is important in providing psychological support before, during and after the procedure.
- Explain that an IV line may be inserted to allow infusion of fluids such as saline, anesthetics, contrast medium, or sedatives.

- Inform the patient that he or she may experience nausea, a feeling of warmth, a salty or metallic taste, or a transient headache after injection of contrast medium.
- Instruct the patient to remove dentures and all external metallic objects from the area to be examined.
- Inform the patient, as appropriate, that CT studies performed without contrast usually do not require the patient to fast before the procedure. Instruct the patient, if required, to fast and restrict fluids for the specified time period, prior to the procedure; fasting may be ordered as a precaution against aspiration related to nausea and vomiting during the administration of contrast. Also instruct the patient to avoid taking anticoagulant medication or to reduce dosage as ordered prior to the procedure due to increased risk of bleeding at the IV insertion site. Protocols may vary among facilities.
- *Make sure a written and informed consent has been signed prior to the procedure and before administering any medications.*

INTRATEST:

Potential Complications:

Injection of the contrast through IV tubing into a blood vessel is an invasive procedure. Complications are rare but do include risk for allergic reaction ***related to contrast reaction,*** cardiac dysrhythmias, hematoma ***related to blood leakage into the tissue following insertion of the IV needle,*** or infection ***that might occur if bacteria from the skin surface is introduced at the IV needle insertion site.***

- Observe standard precautions, and follow the general guidelines in Patient Preparation and Specimen Collection online at Davis*Plus.* Positively identify the patient.
- Ensure the patient has complied with dietary, fluids, medication restrictions, and other pretesting preparations prior to the study, as instructed.
- Ensure the patient has removed dentures and all external metallic objects from the area to be examined prior to the procedure.
- Administer ordered prophylactic steroids or antihistamines before the procedure. Use nonionic contrast medium for the procedure if the patient has a history of allergic reactions to any substance or drug.
- Avoid the use of equipment containing latex if the patient has a history of allergic reaction to latex.
- Have emergency equipment readily available.
- Instruct the patient to void prior to the procedure and to change into the gown, robe, and foot coverings provided.
- Instruct the patient to cooperate fully and to follow directions. Instruct the patient to remain still throughout the procedure because movement produces unreliable results.
- Record baseline vital signs, and continue to monitor throughout the procedure. Protocols may vary among facilities.
- Establish an IV fluid line for the injection of contrast medium, emergency drugs, and sedatives.
- Administer an antianxiety drug, as ordered, if the patient has claustrophobia. Administer a sedative to a child or to an adult who is uncooperative, as ordered.
- Place the patient in the supine position on an examination table.
- If IV contrast medium is used, a rapid series of images is taken during and after injection.
- Instruct the patient to inhale deeply and hold his or her breath while the images are taken, and then to exhale after the images are taken.
- Instruct the patient to take slow, deep breaths if nausea occurs during the procedure.
- Monitor the patient for complications related to the procedure (e.g., allergic reaction, anaphylaxis, bronchospasm) if contrast medium is used.
- The needle is removed, and a pressure dressing is applied over the puncture site.

- Observe/assess the needle site for bleeding, inflammation, or hematoma formation.

POST-TEST:

- Inform the patient that a report of the results will be made available to the requesting HCP, who will discuss the results with the patient.
- Instruct the patient to resume usual medications and activity, as directed by the HCP. Kidney function should be assessed before metformin is resumed, if contrast was used.
- Monitor vital signs and neurological status every 15 min for 1 hr, then every 2 hr for 4 hr, and then as ordered by the HCP. Monitor temperature every 4 hr for 24 hr. Monitor intake and output at least every 8 hr. Compare with baseline values. Notify the HCP if temperature is elevated. Protocols may vary among facilities.
- If contrast was used, observe for delayed allergic reactions, such as rash, urticaria, tachycardia, hyperpnea, hypertension, palpitations, nausea, or vomiting. Antihistamines may be ordered and given to alleviate symptoms of allergic reaction.
- Instruct the patient to immediately report symptoms such as fast heart rate, difficulty breathing, skin rash, itching, chest pain, persistent right shoulder pain, or abdominal pain. Immediately report symptoms to the appropriate HCP.
- Observe/assess the needle insertion site for bleeding, inflammation, or hematoma formation.
- Instruct the patient in the care and assessment of the site.
- Instruct the patient to apply cold compresses to the insertion site as needed, to reduce discomfort or edema.
- Instruct the patient to increase fluid intake to help eliminate the contrast medium, if used.
- Recognize anxiety related to test results. Discuss the implications of abnormal test results on the patient's lifestyle. Provide teaching and information regarding the clinical implications of the test results, as appropriate.
- Reinforce information given by the patient's HCP regarding further testing, treatment, or referral to another HCP. Answer any questions or address any concerns voiced by the patient or family.
- Depending on the results of this procedure, additional testing may be needed to evaluate or monitor progression of the disease process and determine the need for a change in therapy. Evaluate test results in relation to the patient's symptoms and other tests performed.

RELATED STUDIES:

- Related tests include ACTH and challenge tests, BUN, CT angiography, CBC, CBC hematocrit, CBC hemoglobin, CT brain, cortisol and challenge tests, creatinine, MRA, MRI brain, PET brain, and PT/INR.
- Refer to the Endocrine System table online at Davis*Plus* for related tests by body system.

Computed Tomography, Spine

SYNONYM/ACRONYM: Computed axial tomography (CAT), computed transaxial tomography (CTT), spine CT, CT myelogram.

COMMON USE: To visualize and assess spinal structure related to tumor, injury, bleeding, and infection. Used as an evaluation tool for surgical, radiation, and medical therapeutic interventions.

AREA OF APPLICATION: Spine.

C

DESCRIPTION: Computed tomography (CT) of the spine is a noninvasive procedure that enhances certain anatomic views of the spinal structures. CT scanning is more versatile than conventional radiography and can easily detect and identify tumors and their types. During the procedure, the patient lies on a motorized table. The table is moved in and out of a circular opening in a doughnut-like device called a *gantry,* which houses the x-ray tube and associated electronics. A beam of x-rays irradiates the patient as the table moves in and out of the scanner in a series of phases. The x-rays penetrate liquids and solids of different densities by varying degrees. Multiple detectors rotate around the patient to collect numeric data associated with the density coefficients assigned to each degree of tissue density. The imaging system's computer converts the numeric data obtained from the scanner into digital images. Air appears black; bone appears white; and body fluids, fat, and soft tissue structures are represented in various shades between black and white. The cross-sectional views, or *slices,* of the spine can be reviewed individually or as a three-dimensional image to allow differentiations of solid, cystic, inflammatory, or vascular lesions as well as identification of suspected hematomas and aneurysms. The scan may be repeated after administration of contrast medium given by intravenous (IV) injection. Contrast is used to differentiate, enhance, or "light up" areas of interest depending on the type of study to be performed, type of contrast medium to be used, and method of administration. The medium works by creating a contrast between areas of interest based on density; penetration of the x-rays is weaker in areas where the contrast medium is detected by the scanner, showing the blood vessels, organs, and tissue as whitish areas that either outline the area of interest or completely fill it. IV injection of contrast medium is used for evaluation of blood flow through vessels and greater enhancement of tissue density and organ visualization. Imaging technology continues to evolve. Multislice or multidetector CT scanners continuously collect images in a helical or spiral fashion instead of a series of individual images as with standard scanners. Helical CT can collect many images over a short period of time (seconds), is sensitive in identifying small abnormalities, and produces high-quality images. Positron emission tomography (PET) and single-photon emission tomography (SPECT) are types of nuclear medicine studies that offer insights into functionality such as movement of blood flow or uptake and distribution of metabolites into tumors. PET/CT and SPECT/CT are imaging applications that superimpose PET or SPECT and CT findings. The images are collected and produced by a single gantry system. The co-registered or image fusion of PET/CT or SPECT/CT findings can provide a detailed combination of anatomical and functional images. Images can be recorded on photographic or x-ray film or stored in digital format as digitized computer data. The CT scan can be used to guide biopsy needles into areas of suspected tumors to obtain tissue for laboratory analysis and to guide placement of catheters for drainage of cysts or abscesses. Tumor staging and progression, before and after therapy, and effectiveness of medical interventions may be monitored by PET/CT, SPECT/CT, or PET scanning. The images can be reevaluated and manipulated for further, detailed examination without having to repeat the procedure.

This procedure is contraindicated for

Patients who are pregnant or suspected of being pregnant, unless the potential benefits of a procedure using radiation far outweigh the risk of radiation exposure to the fetus and mother.

Patients who are claustrophobic.

Patients with conditions associated with adverse reactions to contrast medium (e.g., asthma, food allergies, or allergy to contrast medium).

Although patients are asked specifically if they have a known allergy to iodine or shellfish, it has been well established that the reaction is not to iodine; an actual iodine allergy would be problematic because iodine is required for the production of thyroid hormones. In the case of shellfish, the reaction is to a muscle protein called tropomyosin; in the case of iodinated contrast medium, the reaction is to the noniodinated part of the contrast molecule. Patients with a known hypersensitivity to the medium may benefit from premedication with corticosteroids and diphenhydramine; the use of nonionic contrast or an alternative noncontrast imaging study, if available, may be considered for patients who have severe asthma or who have experienced moderate to severe reactions to ionic contrast medium.

Patients with conditions associated with preexisting renal insufficiency (e.g., chronic kidney disease, single kidney transplant, nephrectomy, diabetes, multiple myeloma, treatment with aminoglycosides and NSAIDs) ***because iodinated contrast is nephrotoxic.***

Patients who are chronically dehydrated before the test, especially older adults and patients whose health is already compromised, ***because of their risk of contrast-induced acute kidney injury.***

Patients with pheochromocytoma ***because iodinated contrast may cause a hypertensive crisis.***

Patients with bleeding disorders or receiving anticoagulant therapy ***because the puncture site may not stop bleeding.***

INDICATIONS

- Assist in differentiating between benign and malignant tumors.
- Detect congenital spinal anomalies, such as spina bifida, meningocele, and myelocele.
- Detect herniated intervertebral disks.
- Detect paraspinal cysts.
- Detect vascular malformations.
- Monitor and evaluate effectiveness of medical, radiation, or surgical therapies.

POTENTIAL MEDICAL DIAGNOSIS

Normal findings

- Normal density, size, position, and shape of spinal structures

Abnormal findings related to

Identification of abnormal findings is assisted by comparison of parameters such as size, shape, symmetry, density, and location. For example, areas of altered density in either an expected or unexpected location may indicate enlargement of an organ or the presence of blood or other fluids, tumors, or cysts. Comparison by type of abnormal findings may also assist in evaluating areas of altered density.

For example, well-defined round or oval areas, smaller in size and having lower density than a primary tumor, may indicate a cyst.

- Congenital spinal malformations, such as meningocele, myelocele, or spina bifida
- Herniated intervertebral disks
- Paraspinal cysts
- Spinal tumors
- Spondylosis (cervical or lumbar)
- Vascular malformations

C

CRITICAL FINDINGS:

- Cord compression
- Fracture
- Tumor with significant mass effect

Note and immediately report to the requesting health-care provider (HCP) any critical findings and related symptoms. A listing of these findings varies among facilities. Timely notification of a critical finding for laboratory or diagnostic studies is a role expectation of the professional nurse. The notification processes vary among facilities. Upon receipt of the critical finding, the information should be read back to the caller to verify accuracy.

INTERFERING FACTORS

Factors that may alter the results of the study

- Gas or feces in the gastrointestinal tract resulting from inadequate cleansing or failure to restrict food intake before the study.
- Retained barium from a previous radiological procedure.
- Metallic objects (e.g., jewelry, body rings) within the examination field, which may inhibit organ visualization and cause unclear images.
- Patients who are extremely obese may require more radiation to obtain a clear image.
- Patients with extreme claustrophobia unless sedation is given before the study.
- Inability of the patient to cooperate or remain still during the procedure because of age, significant pain, or mental status.

Other considerations

- The procedure may be terminated if chest pain or severe cardiac dysrhythmias occur.
- Failure to follow pretesting preparations may cause the procedure to be canceled or repeated.
- The procedure may be canceled if the patient's weight exceeds the safety limit for the equipment.

NURSING IMPLICATIONS AND PROCEDURE

See Potential Nursing Problems on Fast Find at davispl.us/vanleeuwen7

PRETEST:

- Positively identify the patient using at least two person-specific identifiers before services, treatments, or procedures are performed.
- ***Patient Teaching:*** Inform the patient this procedure can assist in assessing the spine.
- Obtain a history of the patient's health concerns, symptoms, surgical procedures, and results of previously performed laboratory and diagnostic studies. Include a list of known allergens, especially allergies or sensitivities to latex, anesthetics, sedatives, or contrast medium. Ensure results of coagulation testing are obtained and recorded prior to the procedure; a creatinine level is also needed before contrast medium is to be used.
- Note any recent procedures that can interfere with test results, including examinations using barium- or iodine-based contrast medium. Ensure that barium studies were performed more than 4 days before the CT scan.
- Record the date of the last menstrual period and determine the possibility of pregnancy in perimenopausal women.

- Obtain a list of the patient's current medications, including over-the-counter medications, anticoagulants, aspirin and other salicylates, and dietary supplements (see Effects of Natural Products on Laboratory Values online at Davis*Plus*). Such products should be discontinued by medical direction for the appropriate number of days prior to a surgical procedure. Note the last time and dose of medication taken.
- If iodinated contrast medium is scheduled to be used in patients receiving metformin (Glucophage) for type 2 diabetes, the drug should be discontinued on the day of the test and continue to be withheld for 48 hr after the test. Iodinated contrast can temporarily impair kidney function, and failure to withhold metformin may indirectly result in drug-induced lactic acidosis, a dangerous and sometimes fatal adverse effect of metformin ***related to renal impairment that does not support sufficient excretion of metformin.***
- Review the procedure with the patient. Address concerns about pain and explain that there may be moments of discomfort and some pain experienced during the test. Inform the patient the procedure is usually performed in a radiology suite by an HCP specializing in this procedure, with support staff, and takes approximately 15 to 30 min depending on factors such as the type of study ordered, whether contrast will be used, and the type of contrast used.
- ***Sensitivity to social and cultural issues,*** as well as concern for modesty, is important in providing psychological support before, during, and after the procedure.
- Explain that an IV line may be inserted to allow infusion of fluids such as saline, anesthetics, contrast medium, or sedatives.
- Inform the patient that he or she may experience nausea, a feeling of warmth, a salty or metallic taste, or a transient headache after injection of contrast medium.
- Instruct the patient to remove all external metallic objects from the area to be examined.
- Inform the patient, as appropriate, that CT studies performed without contrast usually do not require the patient to fast before the procedure. Instruct the patient, if required, to fast and restrict fluids for the specified time period, prior to the procedure; fasting may be ordered as a precaution against aspiration related to nausea and vomiting during the administration of contrast. Also instruct the patient to avoid taking anticoagulant medication or to reduce dosage as ordered prior to the procedure due to increased risk of bleeding at the IV insertion site. Protocols may vary among facilities.
- *Make sure a written and informed consent has been signed prior to the procedure and before administering any medications.*

INTRATEST:

Potential Complications:

Injection of the contrast through IV tubing into a blood vessel is an invasive procedure. Complications are rare but do include risk for allergic reaction ***related to contrast reaction,*** cardiac dysrhythmias, hematoma ***related to blood leakage into the tissue following insertion of the IV needle,*** or infection ***that might occur if bacteria from the skin surface is introduced at the IV needle insertion site.***

- Observe standard precautions, and follow the general guidelines in Patient Preparation and Specimen Collection online at Davis*Plus*. Positively identify the patient.
- Ensure the patient has complied with medication restrictions and pretesting preparations, prior to the study, as instructed.
- Ensure that the patient has removed all external metallic objects from the area to be examined prior to the procedure.
- Administer ordered prophylactic steroids or antihistamines before the procedure if the patient has a history

of allergic reactions to any substance or drug.

- Avoid the use of equipment containing latex if the patient has a history of allergic reaction to latex.
- Have emergency equipment readily available.
- Instruct the patient to void prior to the procedure and to change into the gown, robe, and foot coverings provided.
- Instruct the patient to cooperate fully and to follow directions. Instruct the patient to remain still throughout the procedure because movement produces unreliable results.
- Record baseline vital signs, and continue to monitor throughout the procedure. Protocols may vary among facilities.
- If ordered, establish an IV fluid line for the injection of contrast medium, emergency drugs, and sedatives.
- Administer an antianxiety drug, as ordered, if the patient has claustrophobia. Administer a sedative to a child or to an adult who is uncooperative, as ordered.
- Place the patient in the supine position on an examination table.
- If IV contrast medium is used, a rapid series of images is taken during and after injection.
- Instruct the patient to inhale deeply and hold his or her breath while the images are taken, and then to exhale after the images are taken.
- Instruct the patient to take slow, deep breaths if nausea occurs during the procedure.
- Monitor the patient for complications related to the procedure (e.g., allergic reaction, anaphylaxis, bronchospasm) if contrast is used.
- The needle is removed, and a pressure dressing is applied over the puncture site.
- Observe/assess the needle insertion site for bleeding, inflammation, or hematoma formation.

POST-TEST:

- Inform the patient that a report of the results will be made available to the requesting HCP, who will discuss the results with the patient.
- Instruct the patient to resume usual diet, fluids, medications, and activity, as directed by the HCP. Kidney function should be assessed before metformin is resumed, if contrast was used.
- Monitor vital signs and neurological status every 15 min for 1 hr, then every 2 hr for 4 hr, and then as ordered by the HCP. Monitor temperature every 4 hr for 24 hr. Monitor intake and output at least every 8 hr. Compare with baseline values. Notify the HCP if temperature is elevated. Protocols may vary among facilities.
- If contrast was used, observe for delayed allergic reactions, such as rash, urticaria, tachycardia, hyperpnea, hypertension, palpitations, nausea, or vomiting. Antihistamines may be ordered and given to alleviate symptoms of allergic reaction.
- Instruct the patient to immediately report symptoms such as fast heart rate, difficulty breathing, skin rash, itching, chest pain, persistent right shoulder pain, or abdominal pain. Immediately report symptoms to the appropriate HCP.
- Observe/assess the needle site for bleeding, inflammation, or hematoma formation.
- Instruct the patient in the care and assessment of the site.
- Instruct the patient to apply cold compresses to the puncture site as needed, to reduce discomfort or edema.
- Instruct the patient to increase fluid intake to help eliminate the contrast medium, if used.
- Recognize anxiety related to test results. Discuss the implications of abnormal test results on the patient's lifestyle. Provide teaching and information regarding the clinical implications of the test results, as appropriate.
- Reinforce information given by the patient's HCP regarding further testing, treatment, or referral to another HCP. Answer any questions or address any concerns voiced by the patient or family.

- Depending on the results of this procedure, additional testing may be needed to evaluate or monitor progression of the disease process and determine the need for a change in therapy. Evaluate test results in relation to the patient's symptoms and other tests performed.

Patient Education:

- Teach the patient the pathophysiology associated with the disease process.
- Teach the patient how personal choices affect successful pain management.

Expected Patient Outcomes:

Understanding

- The patient and family acknowledge that weight loss can decrease the stress on the back and decrease pain.
- The patient and family acknowledge the importance of regular exercise to strengthen the back.

Ability

- The patient demonstrates the ability to use proper body mechanics (move without sudden turning, twisting, correct lifting).
- The patient demonstrates the correct use of assistive devices that decrease stress on the back.

Response

- The patient agrees to attend a weight loss program.
- The patient agrees to attend a support group on the management of chronic pain.

RELATED STUDIES:

- Related tests include ALP, BUN, bone scan, CBC, CBC hematocrit, CBC hemoglobin, creatinine, MRI bone, PT/INR, and radiography of the bones.
- Refer to the Musculoskeletal System table online at Davis*Plus* for related tests by body system.

C

Computed Tomography, Spleen

SYNONYM/ACRONYM: Computed axial tomography (CAT), computed transaxial tomography (CTT), helical/spiral CT, splenic CT.

COMMON USE: To visualize and assess the spleen and surrounding structure for tumor, bleeding, infection, and trauma. Used to monitor the effectiveness of medical, surgical, and radiation therapeutic interventions.

AREA OF APPLICATION: Abdomen/spleen.

DESCRIPTION: Computed tomography (CT) of the spleen is a noninvasive procedure that enhances certain anatomic views of the splenic structures. It becomes an invasive procedure with the use of contrast medium. The spleen is not often the organ of interest when abdominal CT scans are obtained. However, a wide variety of splenic variations and abnormalities may be detected on abdominal scans designed to evaluate the liver, pancreas, or retroperitoneum. During the procedure, the patient lies on a motorized table. The table is moved in and out of a circular opening in a doughnut-like device called a *gantry,* which houses the x-ray tube and associated electronics. A beam of x-rays irradiates the patient as the table moves in and out of the scanner in a series of phases. The x-rays penetrate liquids and solids of

C

different densities by varying degrees. Multiple detectors rotate around the patient to collect numeric data associated with the density coefficients assigned to each degree of tissue density. The imaging system's computer converts the numeric data obtained from the scanner into digital images. Air appears black; bone appears white; and body fluids, fat, and soft tissue structures are represented in various shades between black and white. The cross-sectional views, or *slices,* of the spleen, associated abdominal organs, and vascular system can be reviewed individually or as a three-dimensional image to allow differentiations of solid, cystic, inflammatory, or vascular lesions as well as identification of suspected hematomas and aneurysms. The scan may be repeated after administration of contrast medium given orally or by intravenous (IV) injection. Contrast is used to differentiate, enhance, or "light up" areas of interest depending on the type of study to be performed, type of contrast medium to be used, and method of administration. The medium works by creating a contrast between areas of interest based on density; penetration of the x-rays is weaker in areas where the contrast medium is detected by the scanner, showing the blood vessels, organs, and tissue as whitish areas that either outline the area of interest or completely fill it. Oral ingestion of contrast medium can be used for opacification to distinguish the bowel, adjacent abdominal organs, other types of tissue, and blood vessels as the medium moves through the digestive tract. IV injection of contrast medium is used for evaluation of blood flow through vessels and greater enhancement of tissue density and organ visualization. In some cases, scans may be repeated after both types of contrast are administered. Multislice or multidetector CT scanners continuously collect images in a helical or spiral fashion instead of a series of individual images as with standard scanners. Helical CT can collect many images over a short period of time (seconds), is sensitive in identifying small abnormalities, and produces high-quality images. Positron emission tomography–computed tomography (PET/CT) is an imaging application that superimposes PET and CT findings. The images are collected and produced by a single gantry system. The co-registered or image fusion PET/CT findings can provide a detailed combination of anatomical and functional images. Images can be recorded on photographic or x-ray film or stored in digital format as digitized computer data. The CT scan can be used to guide biopsy needles into areas of suspected tumors to obtain tissue for laboratory analysis and to guide placement of catheters for drainage of cysts or abscesses. Tumor staging and progression, before and after therapy, and effectiveness of medical interventions may be monitored by CT scanning. The images can be reevaluated and manipulated for further, detailed examination without having to repeat the procedure.

This procedure is contraindicated for

Patients who are pregnant or suspected of being pregnant, unless the potential benefits of a procedure using radiation far outweigh the risk of radiation exposure to the fetus and mother.

- Patients who are claustrophobic.
- Patients with conditions associated with adverse reactions to contrast medium (e.g., asthma, food allergies, or allergy to contrast medium).

Although patients are asked specifically if they have a known allergy to iodine or shellfish, it has been well established that the reaction is not to iodine; an actual iodine allergy would be problematic because iodine is required for the production of thyroid hormones. In the case of shellfish, the reaction is to a muscle protein called tropomyosin; in the case of iodinated contrast medium, the reaction is to the noniodinated part of the contrast molecule. Patients with a known hypersensitivity to the medium may benefit from premedication with corticosteroids and diphenhydramine; the use of nonionic contrast or an alternative noncontrast imaging study, if available, may be considered for patients who have severe asthma or who have experienced moderate to severe reactions to ionic contrast medium.

- Patients with conditions associated with preexisting renal insufficiency (e.g., chronic kidney disease, single kidney transplant, nephrectomy, diabetes, multiple myeloma, treatment with aminoglycosides and NSAIDs) because iodinated contrast is nephrotoxic
- Patients who are chronically dehydrated before the test, especially older adults and patients whose health is already compromised, ***because of their risk of contrast-induced acute kidney injury.***
- Patients with pheochromocytoma ***because iodinated contrast may cause a hypertensive crisis.***
- Patients with bleeding disorders or receiving anticoagulant therapy ***because the puncture site may not stop bleeding.***

INDICATIONS

- Assist in differentiating between benign and malignant tumors.
- Detect tumor extension of masses and metastasis.
- Differentiate infectious from inflammatory processes.
- Evaluate cysts, masses, abscesses, and trauma.
- Evaluate the presence of an accessory spleen, polysplenia, or asplenia.
- Evaluate splenic vein thrombosis.
- Monitor and evaluate effectiveness of medical, radiation, or surgical therapies.

POTENTIAL MEDICAL DIAGNOSIS

Normal findings

- Normal size, position, and shape of the spleen and associated vascular system

Abnormal findings related to

Identification of abnormal findings is assisted by comparison of parameters such as size, shape, symmetry, density, and location. For example, areas of altered density in either an expected or unexpected location may indicate enlargement of an organ or the presence of blood or other fluids, tumors, or cysts. Comparison by type of abnormal findings may also assist in evaluating areas of altered density. For example, well-defined round or oval areas, smaller in size and having lower density than a primary tumor, may indicate a cyst.

- Abdominal aortic aneurysm
- Hematomas
- Hemoperitoneum
- Primary and metastatic neoplasms
- Splenic cysts or abscesses
- Splenic laceration, tumor, infiltration, and trauma

CRITICAL FINDINGS:

- Abscess
- Hemorrhage
- Laceration

Note and immediately report to the requesting health-care provider (HCP) any critical findings and related symptoms. A listing of these findings varies among facilities. Timely notification of a critical finding for laboratory or diagnostic studies is a role expectation of the professional nurse. The notification processes vary among facilities. Upon receipt of the critical finding, the information should be read back to the caller to verify accuracy.

C

INTERFERING FACTORS

Factors that may alter the results of the study

- Gas or feces in the gastrointestinal (GI) tract resulting from inadequate cleansing or failure to restrict food intake before the study.
- Retained barium from a previous radiological procedure.
- Metallic objects (e.g., jewelry, body rings) within the examination field, which may inhibit organ visualization and cause unclear images.
- Patients who are extremely obese may require more radiation to obtain a clear image.
- Patients with extreme claustrophobia unless sedation is given before the study.
- Inability of the patient to cooperate or remain still during the procedure because of age, significant pain, or mental status.

Other considerations

- The procedure may be terminated if chest pain or severe cardiac dysrhythmias occur.
- Failure to follow dietary restrictions and other pretesting preparations may cause the procedure to be canceled or repeated.
- The procedure may be canceled if the patient's weight exceeds the safety limit for the equipment.

NURSING IMPLICATIONS AND PROCEDURE

PRETEST:

- Positively identify the patient using at least two person-specific identifiers before services, treatments, or procedures are performed.
- *Patient Teaching:* Inform the patient this procedure can assist in assessing the abdomen and spleen.
- Obtain a history of the patient's health concerns, symptoms, surgical procedures, and results of previously performed laboratory and diagnostic studies. Include a list of known allergens, especially allergies or sensitivities to latex, anesthetics, sedatives, or contrast medium. Ensure results of coagulation testing are obtained and recorded prior to the procedure; a creatinine level is also needed before contrast medium is to be used.
- Note any recent procedures that can interfere with test results, including examinations using barium- or iodine-based contrast medium. Ensure that barium studies were performed more than 4 days before the CT scan.
- Record the date of the last menstrual period and determine the possibility of pregnancy in perimenopausal women.
- Obtain a list of the patient's current medications, including over-the-counter medications, anticoagulants, aspirin and other salicylates, and dietary supplements (see Effects of Natural Products on Laboratory Values online at Davis*Plus*). Such products should be discontinued by medical direction for the appropriate number of days prior to a surgical procedure. Note the last time and dose of medication taken.
- If iodinated contrast medium is scheduled to be used in patients receiving metformin (Glucophage) for type 2 diabetes, the drug should be discontinued on the day of the test and continue to be withheld for 48 hr after the test. Iodinated contrast can temporarily impair kidney function, and failure to withhold metformin may

indirectly result in drug-induced lactic acidosis, a dangerous and sometimes fatal adverse effect of metformin ***related to renal impairment that does not support sufficient excretion of metformin.***

- Review the procedure with the patient. Address concerns about pain and explain that there may be moments of discomfort and some pain experienced during the test. Inform the patient the procedure is usually performed in a radiology suite by an HCP specializing in this procedure, with support staff, and takes approximately 15 to 30 min depending on factors such as the type of study ordered, whether contrast will be used, and the type of contrast used.
- Explain that an IV line may be inserted to allow infusion of fluids such as saline, anesthetics, contrast medium, or sedatives.
- *Sensitivity to social and cultural issues,* as well as concern for modesty, is important in providing psychological support before, during, and after the procedure.
- Advise the patient that he or she may be requested to drink approximately 450 mL of a dilute barium solution (approximately 1% barium) or a water-soluble oral contrast; the oral contrast is given within a specified time period, prior to the study. Oral contrast is administered to distinguish GI organs from the other abdominal organs and to enhance other areas of interest.
- Inform the patient that he or she may experience nausea, a feeling of warmth, a salty or metallic taste, or a transient headache after injection of contrast medium.
- Instruct the patient to remove jewelry and other metallic objects from the area to be examined.
- Inform the patient, as appropriate, that CT studies performed without contrast usually do not require the patient to fast before the procedure. Instruct the patient, if required, to fast and restrict fluids for the specified time period prior to the procedure; fasting may be ordered as a precaution against aspiration related to nausea and vomiting during the administration of contrast. Also instruct the patient to avoid taking anticoagulant medication or to reduce dosage as ordered prior to the procedure due to increased risk of bleeding at the IV insertion site. Protocols may vary among facilities.
- *Make sure a written and informed consent has been signed prior to the procedure and before administering any medications.*

INTRATEST:

Potential Complications:

Injection of the contrast through IV tubing into a blood vessel is an invasive procedure. Complications are rare but do include risk for allergic reaction ***related to contrast reaction,*** cardiac dysrhythmias, hematoma ***related to blood leakage into the tissue following insertion of the IV needle,*** or infection ***that might occur if bacteria from the skin surface is introduced at the IV needle insertion site.***

- Observe standard precautions, and follow the general guidelines in Patient Preparation and Specimen Collection online at Davis*Plus*. Positively identify the patient.
- Ensure the patient has complied with dietary, fluids, and medication restrictions, prior to the study, as instructed.
- Ensure the patient has removed all external metallic objects from the area to be examined prior to the procedure.
- Administer ordered prophylactic steroids or antihistamines before the procedure if the patient has a history of allergic reactions to any substance or drug.
- Avoid the use of equipment containing latex if the patient has a history of allergic reaction to latex.
- Have emergency equipment readily available.
- Instruct the patient to void prior to the procedure and to change into

the gown, robe, and foot coverings provided.

- Instruct the patient to cooperate fully and to follow directions. Instruct the patient to remain still throughout the procedure because movement produces unreliable results.
- Record baseline vital signs, and continue to monitor throughout the procedure. Protocols may vary among facilities.
- Establish an IV fluid line for the injection of contrast medium, emergency drugs, and sedatives.
- Administer an antianxiety drug, as ordered, if the patient has claustrophobia. Administer a sedative to a child or to an adult who is uncooperative, as ordered.
- Place the patient in the supine position on an examination table.
- If IV contrast medium is used, a rapid series of images is taken during and after injection.
- Instruct the patient to inhale deeply and hold his or her breath while the images are taken, and then to exhale after the images are taken.
- Instruct the patient to take slow, deep breaths if nausea occurs during the procedure.
- Monitor the patient for complications related to the procedure (e.g., allergic reaction, anaphylaxis, bronchospasm) if contrast medium is used.
- The needle is removed, and a pressure dressing is applied over the puncture site.
- Observe/assess the needle site for bleeding, inflammation, or hematoma formation.

POST-TEST:

- Inform the patient that a report of the results will be made available to the requesting HCP, who will discuss the results with the patient.
- Instruct the patient to resume usual diet, fluids, medications, and activity, as directed by the HCP. Kidney function should be assessed before metformin is resumed, if contrast was used.
- Monitor vital signs and neurological status every 15 min for 1 hr, then every 2 hr for 4 hr, and then as ordered by the HCP. Monitor temperature every 4 hr for 24 hr. Monitor intake and output at least every 8 hr. Compare with baseline values. Notify the HCP if temperature is elevated. Protocols may vary among facilities.
- If contrast was used, observe for delayed allergic reactions, such as rash, urticaria, tachycardia, hyperpnea, hypertension, palpitations, nausea, or vomiting. Antihistamines may be ordered and given to alleviate symptoms of allergic reaction.
- Instruct the patient to immediately report symptoms such as fast heart rate, difficulty breathing, skin rash, itching, chest pain, persistent right shoulder pain, or abdominal pain. Immediately report symptoms to the appropriate HCP.
- Observe/assess the needle site for bleeding, inflammation, or hematoma formation.
- Instruct the patient in the care and assessment of the site.
- Instruct the patient to apply cold compresses to the puncture site as needed, to reduce discomfort or edema.
- Instruct the patient to increase fluid intake to help eliminate the contrast medium, if used.
- Inform the patient that diarrhea may occur after ingestion of oral contrast medium.
- Recognize anxiety related to test results. Discuss the implications of abnormal test results on the patient's lifestyle. Provide teaching and information regarding the clinical implications of the test results, as appropriate.
- Reinforce information given by the patient's HCP regarding further testing, treatment, or referral to another HCP. Answer any questions or address any concerns voiced by the patient or family.
- Depending on the results of this procedure, additional testing may be needed to evaluate or monitor progression of the disease process and determine the need for a change in therapy. Evaluate test results in

relation to the patient's symptoms and other tests performed.

RELATED STUDIES:

- Related tests include angiography abdomen, BUN, CBC, CBC hematocrit, CBC hemoglobin, creatinine, KUB film, MRI abdomen, PT/INR, and US liver.
- Refer to the Hematopoietic System table online at Davis*Plus* for related tests by body system.

C

Computed Tomography, Thoracic

SYNONYM/ACRONYM: Chest CT, computed axial tomography (CAT), computed transaxial tomography (CTT), helical/spiral CT.

COMMON USE: To visualize and assess structures within the thoracic cavity such as the heart, lungs, and mediastinal structures to evaluate for aneurysm, cancer, tumor, and infection. Used as an evaluation tool for surgical, radiation, and medical therapeutic interventions.

AREA OF APPLICATION: Thorax.

DESCRIPTION: Computed tomography (CT) of the thorax is more detailed than a chest x-ray. It is a noninvasive procedure used to enhance certain anatomic views of the lungs, heart, and mediastinal structures. It becomes invasive when a contrast medium is used. During the procedure, the patient lies on a motorized table. The table is moved in and out of a circular opening in a doughnut-like device called a *gantry,* which houses the x-ray tube and associated electronics. A beam of x-rays irradiates the patient as the table moves in and out of the scanner in a series of phases. The x-rays penetrate liquids and solids of different densities by varying degrees. Multiple detectors rotate around the patient to collect numeric data associated with the density coefficients assigned to each degree of tissue density. The imaging system's computer converts the numeric data obtained from the scanner into digital images. Air appears black; bone appears white; and body fluids, fat, and soft tissue structures are represented in various shades between black and white. The cross-sectional views, or *slices,* of the thoracic region, including the mediastinal area (heart and cardiac vessels, trachea, esophagus, thyroid gland, thymus, lymph nodes), ribs, lungs, and spine, can be reviewed individually or as a three-dimensional image to allow differentiations of solid, cystic, inflammatory, or vascular lesions as well as identification of suspected hematomas and aneurysms. The scan may be repeated after administration of contrast medium given by intravenous (IV) injection. Contrast is used to differentiate, enhance, or "light up" areas of interest depending on the type of study to be performed, type of contrast medium to be used, and method of administration. The medium works by creating a contrast between areas of interest based on density; penetration of the x-rays is weaker in areas where the contrast medium is detected by the scanner, showing the blood vessels, organs, and tissue as whitish areas that either outline the area of interest or completely fill it. IV injection of contrast medium is used for evaluation of blood flow through vessels and greater enhancement of tissue density and organ visualization. Multislice or multidetector CT scanners continuously collect images in a helical or spiral fashion instead of a series of individual images as with standard scanners. Helical CT can collect many images over a short period of time (seconds), is sensitive in identifying small abnormalities, and produces high-quality images. Positron emission tomography–computed tomography (PET/CT) is an imaging application that superimposes PET and CT findings. The images are collected and produced by a single gantry system. The co-registered or image fusion PET/CT findings can provide a detailed combination of anatomical and functional images. Images can be recorded on photographic or x-ray film or stored in digital format as digitized computer data. The CT scan can be used to guide biopsy needles into areas of suspected tumors to obtain tissue for laboratory analysis and to guide placement of catheters for drainage of cysts or abscesses. Tumor staging and progression, before and after therapy, and effectiveness of medical interventions may be monitored by CT scanning. The images can be reevaluated and manipulated for further, detailed examination without having to repeat the procedure.

This procedure is contraindicated for

- Patients who are pregnant or suspected of being pregnant, unless the potential benefits of a procedure using radiation far outweigh the risk of radiation exposure to the fetus and mother.
- Patients who are claustrophobic.
- Patients with conditions associated with adverse reactions to contrast medium (e.g., asthma, food allergies, or allergy to contrast medium).

  Although patients are asked specifically if they have a known allergy to iodine or shellfish, it has been well established that the reaction is not to iodine; an actual iodine allergy would be problematic because iodine is required for the production of thyroid hormones. In the case of shellfish, the reaction is to a muscle protein called tropomyosin; in the case of iodinated contrast medium, the reaction is to the noniodinated part of the contrast molecule. Patients with a known hypersensitivity to the medium may benefit from premedication with corticosteroids and diphenhydramine; the use of nonionic contrast or an alternative noncontrast imaging study, if available, may be considered for patients who have severe asthma or who have experienced moderate to severe reactions to ionic contrast medium.
- Conditions associated with preexisting renal insufficiency (e.g., chronic kidney disease, single kidney transplant, nephrectomy, diabetes, multiple myeloma, treatment with aminoglycosides and NSAIDs) ***because iodinated contrast is nephrotoxic.***
- Patients who are chronically dehydrated before the test, especially older adults and patients whose health is already compromised, ***because of their risk of contrast-induced acute kidney injury.***

Patients with pheochromocytoma ***because iodinated contrast may cause a hypertensive crisis.***

Patients with bleeding disorders or receiving anticoagulant therapy ***because the puncture site may not stop bleeding.***

INDICATIONS

- Detect aortic aneurysms.
- Detect bronchial abnormalities, such as stenosis, dilation, or tumor.
- Detect lymphomas, especially Hodgkin's disease.
- Detect mediastinal and hilar lymphadenopathy.
- Detect primary and metastatic pulmonary, esophageal, or mediastinal tumors.
- Detect tumor extension of neck mass to thoracic area.
- Determine blood, fluid, or fat accumulation in tissues, pleuritic space, or vessels.
- Differentiate aortic aneurysms from tumors near the aorta.
- Differentiate between benign and malignant tumors.
- Differentiate infectious from inflammatory processes.
- Differentiate tumor from tuberculosis.
- Evaluate cardiac chambers and pulmonary vessels.
- Evaluate the presence of plaque in cardiac vessels.
- Identify or rule out thymoma in cases of diagnosed myasthenia gravis.
- Monitor and evaluate effectiveness of medical or surgical therapeutic regimen.

POTENTIAL MEDICAL DIAGNOSIS

Normal findings

- Normal size, position, and shape of thoracic organs, tissues, and structures

Abnormal findings related to

Identification of abnormal findings is assisted by comparison of parameters such as size, shape, symmetry, density, and location. For example, areas of altered density in either an expected or unexpected location may indicate enlargement of an organ or the presence of blood or other fluids, tumors, or cysts. Comparison by type of abnormal findings may also assist in evaluating areas of altered density. For example, well-defined round or oval areas, smaller in size and having lower density than a primary tumor, may indicate a cyst.

- Aortic aneurysm
- Chest, mediastinal, spine, or rib lesions
- Cysts or abscesses
- Enlarged lymph nodes
- Esophageal pathology, including tumors
- Hodgkin's disease
- Pleural effusion
- Pneumonitis
- Pneumothorax
- Pulmonary embolism

CRITICAL FINDINGS:

- Aortic aneurysm
- Aortic dissection
- Pneumothorax
- Pulmonary embolism

Note and immediately report to the requesting health-care provider (HCP) any critical findings and related symptoms. A listing of these findings varies among facilities. Timely notification of a critical finding for laboratory or diagnostic studies is a role expectation of the professional nurse. The notification processes vary among facilities. Upon receipt of the critical finding, the information should be read back to the caller to verify accuracy.

INTERFERING FACTORS

Factors that may alter the results of the study

- Metallic objects (e.g., jewelry, body rings) within the examination field,

which may inhibit organ visualization and cause unclear images.
- Patients who are extremely obese may require more radiation to obtain a clear image.
- Patients with extreme claustrophobia unless sedation is given before the study.
- Inability of the patient to cooperate or remain still during the procedure because of age, significant pain, or mental status.

C

Other considerations
- The procedure may be terminated if chest pain or severe cardiac dysrhythmias occur.
- Failure to follow dietary restrictions and other pretesting preparations may cause the procedure to be canceled or repeated.
- The procedure may be canceled if the patient's weight exceeds the safety limit for the equipment.

NURSING IMPLICATIONS AND PROCEDURE

PRETEST:

- Positively identify the patient using at least two person-specific identifiers before services, treatments, or procedures are performed.
- *Patient Teaching:* Inform the patient this procedure can assist in assessing the chest.
- Obtain a history of the patient's health concerns, symptoms, surgical procedures, and results of previously performed laboratory and diagnostic studies. Include a list of known allergens, especially allergies or sensitivities to latex, anesthetics, sedatives, or contrast medium. Ensure results of coagulation testing are obtained and recorded prior to the procedure; a creatinine level is also needed before contrast medium is to be used.
- Note any recent procedures that can interfere with test results, including examinations using barium- or iodine-based contrast medium. Ensure that barium studies were performed more than 4 days before the CT scan.
- Record the date of the last menstrual period and determine the possibility of pregnancy in perimenopausal women.
- Obtain a list of the patient's current medications, including over-the-counter medications, anticoagulants, aspirin and other salicylates, and dietary supplements (see Effects of Natural Products on Laboratory Values online at Davis*Plus*). Such products should be discontinued by medical direction for the appropriate number of days prior to a surgical procedure. Note the last time and dose of medication taken.
- If iodinated contrast medium is scheduled to be used in patients receiving metformin (Glucophage) for type 2 diabetes, the drug should be discontinued on the day of the test and continue to be withheld for 48 hr after the test. Iodinated contrast can temporarily impair kidney function, and failure to withhold metformin may indirectly result in drug-induced lactic acidosis, a dangerous and sometimes fatal adverse effect of metformin ***related to renal impairment that does not support sufficient excretion of metformin.***
- Review the procedure with the patient. Address concerns about pain and explain that there may be moments of discomfort and some pain experienced during the test. Inform the patient the procedure is usually performed in a radiology suite by an HCP specializing in this procedure, with support staff, and takes approximately 15 to 30 min depending on factors such as the type of study ordered, whether contrast will be used, and the type of contrast used.
- Explain that an IV line may be inserted to allow infusion of fluids such as saline, anesthetics, contrast medium, or sedatives.
- ***Sensitivity to social and cultural issues,*** as well as concern for modesty, is

important in providing psychological support before, during, and after the procedure.

- Inform the patient that he or she may experience nausea, a feeling of warmth, a salty or metallic taste, or a transient headache after injection of contrast medium.
- Instruct the patient to remove jewelry and other metallic objects from the area to be examined.
- Inform the patient, as appropriate, that CT studies performed without contrast usually do not require the patient to fast before the procedure. Instruct the patient, if required, to fast and restrict fluids for the specified time period prior to the procedure; fasting may be ordered as a precaution against aspiration related to nausea and vomiting during the administration of contrast. Also instruct the patient to avoid taking anticoagulant medication or to reduce dosage as ordered prior to the procedure due to increased risk of bleeding at the IV insertion site. Protocols may vary among facilities.
- *Make sure a written and informed consent has been signed prior to the procedure and before administering any medications.*

INTRATEST:

Potential Complications:

Injection of the contrast through IV tubing into a blood vessel is an invasive procedure. Complications are rare but do include risk for allergic reaction ***related to contrast reaction,*** cardiac dysrhythmias, hematoma ***related to blood leakage into the tissue following insertion of the IV needle,*** or infection ***that might occur if bacteria from the skin surface is introduced at the IV needle insertion site.***

- Observe standard precautions, and follow the general guidelines in Patient Preparation and Specimen Collection online at Davis*Plus*. Positively identify the patient.
- Ensure the patient has complied with dietary, fluids, medication restrictions, prior to the study, as instructed.
- Ensure the patient has removed all external metallic objects from the area to be examined prior to the procedure.
- Administer ordered prophylactic steroids or antihistamines before the procedure if the patient has a history of allergic reactions to any substance or drug.
- Avoid the use of equipment containing latex if the patient has a history of allergic reaction to latex.
- Have emergency equipment readily available.
- Instruct the patient to void prior to the procedure and to change into the gown, robe, and foot coverings provided.
- Instruct the patient to cooperate fully and to follow directions. Instruct the patient to remain still throughout the procedure because movement produces unreliable results.
- Record baseline vital signs, and continue to monitor throughout the procedure. Protocols may vary among facilities.
- Establish an IV fluid line for the injection of contrast medium, emergency drugs, and sedatives.
- Administer an antianxiety drug, as ordered, if the patient has claustrophobia. Administer a sedative to a child or to an adult who is uncooperative, as ordered.
- Place the patient in the supine position on an examination table.
- If IV contrast medium is used, a rapid series of images is taken during and after injection.
- Ask the patient to inhale deeply and hold his or her breath while the images are taken, and then to exhale after the images are taken.
- Instruct the patient to take slow, deep breaths if nausea occurs during the procedure. Monitor and administer an antiemetic drug if ordered. Ready an emesis basin for use.
- Monitor the patient for complications related to the procedure (e.g., allergic reaction, anaphylaxis, bronchospasm) if contrast is used.
- The needle is removed, and a pressure dressing is applied over the puncture site.

- Observe/assess the needle insertion site for bleeding, inflammation, or hematoma formation.

POST-TEST:

- Inform the patient that a report of the results will be made available to the requesting HCP, who will discuss the results with the patient.
- Instruct the patient to resume usual medications and activity, as directed by the HCP. Kidney function should be assessed before metformin is resumed, if contrast was used.
- Monitor vital signs and neurological status every 15 min for 1 hr, then every 2 hr for 4 hr, and then as ordered by the HCP. Monitor temperature every 4 hr for 24 hr. Monitor intake and output at least every 8 hr. Compare with baseline values. Notify the HCP if temperature is elevated. Protocols may vary among facilities.
- If contrast was used, observe for delayed allergic reactions, such as rash, urticaria, tachycardia, hyperpnea, hypertension, palpitations, nausea, or vomiting. Antihistamines may be ordered and given to alleviate symptoms of allergic reaction.
- Instruct the patient to immediately report symptoms such as fast heart rate, difficulty breathing, skin rash, itching, chest pain, persistent right shoulder pain, or abdominal pain. Immediately report symptoms to the appropriate HCP.
- Observe/assess the needle site for bleeding, inflammation, or hematoma formation.
- Instruct the patient in the care and assessment of the site.
- Instruct the patient to apply cold compresses to the insertion site as needed, to reduce discomfort or edema.
- Instruct the patient to increase fluid intake to help eliminate the contrast medium, if used.
- Recognize anxiety related to test results. Discuss the implications of abnormal test results on the patient's lifestyle. Provide teaching and information regarding the clinical implications of the test results, as appropriate.
- Reinforce information given by the patient's HCP regarding further testing, treatment, or referral to another HCP. Answer any questions or address any concerns voiced by the patient or family.
- Depending on the results of this procedure, additional testing may be needed to evaluate or monitor progression of the disease process and determine the need for a change in therapy. Evaluate test results in relation to the patient's symptoms and other tests performed.

RELATED STUDIES:

- Related tests include acetylcholine receptor antibody, biopsy bone marrow, BUN, chest x-ray, CBC, CBC hematocrit, CBC hemoglobin, creatinine, echocardiogram, gallium scan, lung scan, MRI chest, mediastinoscopy, MRI venography, pleural fluid analysis, and PT/INR.
- Refer to the Respiratory System table online at Davis*Plus* for related tests by body system.

Coombs' Antiglobulin, Direct

SYNONYM/ACRONYM: Direct antiglobulin testing (DAT).

COMMON USE: To detect associated conditions or drug therapies that can result in cell hemolysis, such as found in hemolytic disease of newborns, and hemolytic transfusion reactions.

SPECIMEN: Serum collected in a red-top tube and whole blood collected in a lavender-top (EDTA) tube.

NORMAL FINDINGS: (Method: Agglutination) Negative (no agglutination).

DESCRIPTION: Direct antiglobulin testing (DAT) detects in vivo antibody sensitization of red blood cells (RBCs). Immunoglobulin G (IgG) produced in certain disease states or in response to certain drugs can coat the surface of RBCs, resulting in cellular damage and hemolysis. When DAT is performed, RBCs are taken from the patient's blood sample, washed with saline to remove residual globulins, and mixed with anti–human globulin reagent. If the anti–human globulin reagent causes agglutination of the patient's RBCs, specific antiglobulin reagents can be used to determine whether the patient's RBCs are coated with IgG, complement, or both. (See study titled "Blood Groups and Antibodies" and Transfusion Reactions: Laboratory Findings and Potential online at Davis*Plus* for more information regarding transfusion reactions.)

This procedure is contraindicated for: N/A

INDICATIONS

- Detect autoimmune hemolytic anemia or hemolytic disease of the newborn.
- Evaluate hemolytic anemia (autoimmune or induced by drugs or other substances).
- Evaluate transfusion reaction.

POTENTIAL MEDICAL DIAGNOSIS

Positive findings in

Antibodies formed during these circumstances or conditions attach to the patient's RBCs, and hemolysis occurs. Agglutination is graded from 1+ to 4+ in manual testing systems, with 4+ being the strongest degree of agglutination. Automated testing systems can report 1+ to 4+ graded results, provide images of the tested material so laboratory professionals can interpret the results, or provide computer-assisted interpretation of the test results as positive or negative findings.

- Anemia ***(autoimmune hemolytic, drug-induced)***
- Hemolytic disease of the newborn ***(related to ABO or Rh incompatibility)***
- Infectious mononucleosis
- Lymphomas
- Mycoplasma pneumonia
- Paroxysmal cold hemoglobinuria ***(idiopathic or disease related)***
- Passively acquired antibodies from plasma products
- Post–cardiac vascular surgery ***(increased incidence of positive DAT has been reported in patients following cardiac surgery, possibly related to mechanical RBC destruction while the patient is on cardiac bypass)***
- Systemic lupus erythematosus and other connective tissue immune disorders
- Transfusion reactions ***(related to blood incompatibility)***

Negative findings in

- Samples in which sensitization of erythrocytes has not occurred

CRITICAL FINDINGS: N/A

INTERFERING FACTORS

- Drugs and other substances that may cause a positive DAT include

acetaminophen, aminosalicylic acid, ampicillin, antihistamines, aztreonam, cephalosporins, chlorinated hydrocarbon insecticides, chlorpromazine, chlorpropamide, cisplatin, clonidine, dipyrone, ethosuximide, hydralazine, hydrochlorothiazide, ibuprofen, insulin, isoniazid, levodopa, mefenamic acid, melphalan, methadone, methicillin, methyldopa, moxalactam, penicillin, phenytoin, probenecid, procainamide, quinidine, quinine, rifampin, stibophen, streptomycin, sulfonamides, and tetracycline.
- Wharton's jelly may cause a false-positive DAT.
- Cold agglutinins and large amounts of paraproteins in the specimen may cause false-positive results.
- Newborns' cells may give negative results in ABO hemolytic disease.
- Tube methods for DAT are less sensitive than gel methods, and false-negative findings are possible in cases where weak, incompletely developed antigen sites on newborns' RBCs may not allow detectable amounts of anti-A and/or anti-B to bind to the RBC membrane. Neonates who have received multiple intrauterine transfusions of antigen-negative (group O) cells may also have a negative DAT because the results represent circulating donated red blood cells rather than the neonate's native red blood cells.

C

NURSING IMPLICATIONS AND PROCEDURE

POTENTIAL NURSING PROBLEMS:

Problem	Signs & Symptoms	Interventions
Injury risk ***(related to Rh incompatibility; blood incompatibility)***	Jaundice in newborn; infant cardiac stress (heart failure); infant death	Administer prescribed Rh(D) immune globulin RhoGAM intramuscular (IM) or Rhophylac IM or intravenous 🍁 to mother; obtain maternal blood type and crossmatch; use bilirubin light for newborn; use infant treatment with prescribed erythropoietin and iron supplements; administer prescribed blood transfusion to infant; follow blood transfusion guidelines; monitor degree of jaundice and associated laboratory results (bilirubin); monitor hemoglobin (Hgb) and hematocrit (Hct)

Problem	Signs & Symptoms	Interventions
Fear ***(related to possible loss of newly born child; long-term effects of elevated bilirubin)***	Expression of fear; preoccupation with fear; increased tension; parental complaints of diarrhea, nausea; parental expressions of fatigue or insomnia; crying; withdrawal; panic attacks	Access social services; provide specific and culturally appropriate education; assist the patient and family to recognize effective coping strategies; assist the patient to acknowledge fear; provide a safe environment to decease fear; explore cultural influences that may enhance fear; utilize therapeutic touch as appropriate to decrease fear
Gas exchange ***(related to destruction of red cells secondary to maternal-child Rh incompatibility)***	Shortness of breath; orthopnea; cyanosis; increased heart rate; increased respiratory rate; use of respiratory accessory muscles	Auscultate and trend breath sounds; use pulse oximetry to monitor oxygenation; administer oxygen as ordered; collaborate with health-care provider (HCP) to consider intubation and/or mechanical ventilation; elevate the infant's head; administer ordered blood or blood products; monitor Hgb and Hct

PRETEST:

- Positively identify the patient using at least two person-specific identifiers before services, treatments, or procedures are performed.
- ***Patient Teaching:*** Inform the patient/parent this test can assist in assessing for disorders that break down red blood cells.
- Obtain a history of the patient's health concerns, symptoms, surgical procedures, and results of previously performed laboratory and diagnostic studies. Include a list of known allergens, especially allergies or sensitivities to latex.
- Obtain a list of the patient's current medications, including over-the-counter medications and dietary supplements (see Effects of Natural Products on Laboratory Values online at Davis*Plus*).
- Review the procedure with the patient. Inform the patient that specimen collection takes approximately 5 to 10 min. Address concerns about pain and explain that there may be some discomfort during the venipuncture. If a cord sample is to be taken from a newborn, inform parents that the sample will be obtained at the time of delivery and will not result in blood loss to the infant.

- ***Sensitivity to social and cultural issues,*** as well as concern for modesty, is important in providing psychological support before, during, and after the procedure.
- There are no food, fluid, or medication restrictions unless by medical direction.

C

INTRATEST:

Potential Complications:

Acute hemolytic reactions can be immediate and life threatening for patients of any age. Chronic hemolytic anemia is also a significant condition that requires timely identification of the problem in order to treat the condition.

Assess the newborn's bilirubin and hematocrit levels. Increased bilirubin and decreased hematocrit may be indicative of RBC breakdown. Kernicterus, or deposition of bilirubin in the brain, is a serious and significant development that can lead to permanent brain damage or death.

- Avoid the use of equipment containing latex if the patient has a history of allergic reaction to latex.
- Instruct the patient to cooperate fully and to follow directions. Direct the patient to breathe normally and to avoid unnecessary movement.
- Observe standard precautions, and follow the general guidelines in Patient Preparation and Specimen Collection online at Davis*Plus*. Positively identify the patient, and label the appropriate specimen container with the corresponding patient demographics, initials of the person collecting the specimen, date, and time of collection. Perform a venipuncture. Cord specimens are obtained by inserting a needle attached to a syringe into the umbilical vein. The specimen is drawn into the syringe and gently expressed into the appropriate collection container.
- Remove the needle and apply direct pressure with dry gauze to stop bleeding. Observe/assess venipuncture site for bleeding or hematoma formation and secure gauze with adhesive bandage.
- Promptly transport the specimen to the laboratory for processing and analysis.

POST-TEST:

- Inform the patient that a report of the results will be made available to the requesting HCP, who will discuss the results with the patient.
- Recognize anxiety related to test results, and inform the postpartum patient of the implications of positive test results in cord blood; also assess newborn's bilirubin and hematocrit levels. The results may indicate the need for immediate exchange transfusion of fresh whole blood that has been typed and crossmatched with the mother's serum in order to identify the presence of unusual antibodies. Observation of the neonatal patient, especially for the development of jaundice, is an important way to identify a hemolytic process. Facilities not equipped for neonatal exchange transfusion may elect to transfer the neonate to a facility where the appropriate level of care can be provided. Hand-Off communication is a standardized approach to sharing information in an effort to minimize the risk of error or injury during transition between caregivers. The SBAR-R format (situation, background, assessment, recommendation, and read-back) may be used as a communication tool to ensure mutual understanding of the clinical situation.
- Depending on the results of this procedure, additional testing may be performed to evaluate or monitor progression of the disease process and determine the need for a change in therapy. Evaluate test results in relation to the patient's symptoms and other tests performed.

Patient Education:

- Inform the postpartum patient of the implications of positive test results in cord blood.
- Prepare the newborn for exchange transfusion, on medical direction.

- Reinforce information given by the patient's HCP regarding further testing, treatment, or referral to another HCP.
- Answer any questions or address any concerns voiced by the patient or family.

Expected Patient Outcomes:

Understanding

- Parents state the purpose for the recommended infant blood transfusion.
- Mother states the purpose of RhIG (Rh immune globulin) or RhoGam 🍁 injection in relation to future pregnancies.

Ability

- Parents demonstrate proficiency in placing the infant under the bilirubin light and adhering to identified precautions.
- Parents demonstrate proficiency in administering prescribed iron supplements to infant.

Response

- Parents comply with the request to bring the infant in for bilirubin blood checks as designated by the HCP.
- Patient/mother complies with the recommendation to receive RhIG (Rh immune globulin) or RhoGam.

RELATED STUDIES:

- Related tests include bilirubin, blood groups and antibodies, CBC hematocrit, CBC hemoglobin, Coombs' indirect antiglobulin (IAT), Ham's test, and haptoglobin.
- Refer to Transfusion Reactions: Laboratory Findings and Potential online at Davis*Plus* for further information regarding laboratory studies used in the investigation of transfusion reactions, findings, and potential nursing interventions associated with types of transfusion reactions.
- Refer to the Hematopoietic System table online at Davis*Plus* for related tests by body system.

Coombs' Antiglobulin, Indirect

SYNONYM/ACRONYM: Indirect antiglobulin test (IAT), antibody screen.

COMMON USE: To check recipient serum for antibodies prior to blood transfusion.

SPECIMEN: Serum collected in a red-top tube.

NORMAL FINDINGS: (Method: Agglutination) Negative (no agglutination).

DESCRIPTION: The indirect antiglobulin test (IAT) detects and identifies unexpected circulating complement molecules or antibodies in the patient's serum. The first use of this test was for the detection and identification of anti-D using an indirect method. The test is now commonly used to screen a patient's serum for the presence of antibodies that may react against transfused red blood cells (RBCs). During testing, the patient's serum is allowed to incubate with reagent RBCs. The reagent RBCs used are from group O donors and have most of the clinically significant antigens present (D, C, E, c, e, K, M, N, S, s, Fy^a, Fy^b, Jk^a, and Jk^b). Antibodies present in the patient's serum coat antigenic sites on the RBC membrane. The reagent cells are washed with saline to remove any unbound antibody. Antihuman globulin is added in the final step of the test. If the patient's serum contains antibodies, the antihuman globulin will cause the antibody-coated RBCs to stick together or agglutinate. (See study titled "Blood Groups and Antibodies" and Transfusion Reactions: Laboratory Findings and Potential online at Davis*Plus* for more information regarding transfusion reactions.)

This procedure is contraindicated for: N/A

INDICATIONS

- Detect other antibodies in maternal blood that can be potentially harmful to the fetus.
- Determine antibody titers in Rh-negative women sensitized by an Rh-positive fetus.
- Screen for antibodies before blood transfusions.
- Test for the weak Rh-variant antigen D^u. Development of anti-D antibodies occur when Rh-negative women become sensitized by an Rh-positive fetus. Antibody titers should be performed as soon as a subsequent pregnancy becomes known in order to appropriately anticipate management of hemolytic disease of the newborn. The IAT has also been used to test for the weak Rh-variant antigen D^u. Modern technology and more potent reagents provide better sensitivity, and for this reason women who have the D^u variant will likely be typed as Rh-positive. For this reason, the AABB has determined weak D testing is no longer necessary to be used on obstetric patients. Women who have the weak D variant are tested using less sensitive reagents, and those typed as Rh-negative will be candidates for immunization with Rh(D) immune globulin RhoGAM IM or Rhophylac intramuscular (IM) or intravenous (IV). 🍁 Administration of RhIG (Rh immune globulin) or RhoGam 🍁 to these candidates is not harmful. Whether the test is used currently varies among facilities.

POTENTIAL MEDICAL DIAGNOSIS

Positive findings in

Circulating antibodies or medications attach to the patient's RBCs, and hemolysis occurs. Agglutination is graded from 1+ to 4+ in manual testing systems; with 4+ being the strongest degree of agglutination. Automated testing systems are capable of reporting 1+ to 4+ graded results, or providing images of the tested material so laboratory professionals can interpret the results, or providing computer assisted interpretation of the test results as positive or negative findings.

- Hemolytic anemia ***(autoimmune or induced by drugs or other substances)***
- Hemolytic disease of the newborn ***(related to ABO or Rh incompatibility)***
- Incompatible crossmatch
- Infections (mycoplasma pneumonia, mononucleosis)

Negative findings in

- Samples in which the patient's antibodies exhibit dosage effects (i.e., stronger reaction with homozygous than with heterozygous expression of an antigen) and reagent erythrocyte antigens contain single-dose expressions of the corresponding antigen (heterozygous)
- Samples in which reagent erythrocyte antigens are unable to detect low-prevalence antibodies
- Samples in which sensitization of erythrocytes has not occurred (true negative, complete absence of antibodies)

CRITICAL FINDINGS: N/A

INTERFERING FACTORS

- Drugs and other substances that may cause a positive IAT include meropenem, methyldopa, penicillin, quinidine, and rifampin.
- Recent administration of dextran, whole blood or fractions, or IV contrast media can result in a false-positive reaction.

NURSING IMPLICATIONS AND PROCEDURE

PRETEST:

- Positively identify the patient using at least two person-specific identifiers before services, treatments, or procedures are performed.
- *Patient Teaching:* Inform the patient this test can assist in assessing for blood compatibility prior to transfusion.
- Obtain a history of the patient's health concerns, symptoms, surgical procedures, and results of previously performed laboratory and diagnostic studies. Include a list of known allergens, especially allergies or sensitivities to latex.
- Note any recent procedures that can interfere with test results.
- Obtain a list of the patient's current medications, including over-the-counter medications and dietary supplements (see Effects of Natural Products on Laboratory Values online at Davis*Plus*).
- Review the procedure with the patient. Inform the patient that specimen collection takes approximately 5 to 10 min. Address concerns about pain and explain that there may be some discomfort during the venipuncture. Prenatal mothers may be concerned about blood collection from their newborn. Explain that a cord sample of blood taken from the infant at the time of delivery does not result in infant blood loss.
- ***Sensitivity to social and cultural issues,*** as well as concern for modesty, is important in providing psychological support before, during, and after the procedure.
- There are no food, fluid, or medication restrictions unless by medical direction.

INTRATEST:

Potential Complications:

Acute hemolytic reactions, whether immune mediated or developed due to sensitivities to drugs or other substances, can be immediate and life threatening. Chronic hemolytic anemia is also a significant condition that requires timely identification of the problem in order to treat the condition.

Positive findings in the pregnant patient may require further investigation by amniocentesis. Any sampling method that involves penetration of natural tissue barriers carries the risk of infection.

- Avoid the use of equipment containing latex if the patient has a history of allergic reaction to latex.
- Instruct the patient to cooperate fully and to follow directions. Direct the patient to breathe normally and to avoid unnecessary movement.
- Observe standard precautions, and follow the general guidelines in Patient Preparation and Specimen Collection online at Davis*Plus*. Positively identify the patient, and label the appropriate specimen container with the corresponding patient demographics, initials of the person collecting the specimen, date, and time of collection. Perform a venipuncture.
- Remove the needle and apply direct pressure with dry gauze to stop bleeding. Observe/assess venipuncture site for bleeding or hematoma formation and secure gauze with adhesive bandage.
- Promptly transport the specimen to the laboratory for processing and analysis.

POST-TEST:

- Inform the patient that a report of the results will be made available to the requesting health-care provider

(HCP), who will discuss the results with the patient. It is important for the patient to be made aware of the presence of unusual antibodies. A person may have circulating antibodies, other than ABO/Rh group antibodies, which may respond to transfused blood. The antibodies attach to the person's red blood cells, damaging the integrity of the cell wall, and hemolysis occurs. Therefore, it is important to screen for the presence of antibodies in the recipient's serum prior to transfusion. Unexpected antibodies, other than ABO/Rh, can develop at any time. If present in maternal blood, they can be potentially harmful to the fetus, which makes antibody screening an important test in prenatal care.

- Inform pregnant women that negative tests during the first 12 wk of gestation should be repeated at 28 wk to rule out the presence of an antibody.
- Positive test results in pregnant women after 28 wk of gestation indicate the need for antibody identification testing.
- Reinforce information given by the patient's HCP regarding further testing, treatment, or referral to another HCP. Answer any questions or address any concerns voiced by the patient or family.
- Depending on the results of this procedure, additional testing may be performed to evaluate or monitor progression of the disease process and determine the need for a change in therapy. Evaluate test results in relation to the patient's symptoms and other tests performed.

RELATED STUDIES:

- Related tests include bilirubin, blood groups and antibodies, CBC hematocrit, CBC hemoglobin, Coombs' direct antiglobulin (DAT), and haptoglobin.
- Refer to Transfusion Reactions: Laboratory Findings and Potential online at Davis*Plus* for further information regarding laboratory studies used in the investigation of transfusion reactions, findings and potential nursing interventions associated with types of transfusion reactions.
- Refer to the Hematopoietic System table online at Davis*Plus* for related tests by body system.

C

Copper

SYNONYM/ACRONYM: Cu.

COMMON USE: To evaluate and monitor exposure to copper and to assist in diagnosing Wilson's disease.

SPECIMEN: Serum collected in a royal blue-top, trace element–free tube.

NORMAL FINDINGS: (Method: Inductively coupled plasma-mass spectrometry)

Age	Conventional Units	SI Units (Conventional Units × 0.157)
Newborn–5 d	9–46 mcg/dL	1.4–7.2 micromol/L
1–5 yr	80–150 mcg/dL	12.6–23.6 micromol/L
6–9 yr	84–136 mcg/dL	13.2–21.4 micromol/L
10–14 yr	80–120 mcg/dL	12.6–18.8 micromol/L

Age	Conventional Units	SI Units (Conventional Units × 0.157)
15–19 yr	80–171 mcg/dL	12.6–26.8 micromol/L
Adult		
Male	71–141 mcg/dL	11.1–22.1 micromol/L
Female	80–155 mcg/dL	12.6–24.3 micromol/L
Pregnant female	118–302 mcg/dL	18.5–47.4 micromol/L

Values for African Americans are 8% to 12% higher. Values increase in older adults.

C

POTENTIAL MEDICAL DIAGNOSIS

Increased in:

Ceruloplasmin is an acute-phase reactant protein and the main protein binder of copper; therefore, copper levels will be increased in many inflammatory conditions, including cancer. Estrogens increase levels of binding protein; therefore, copper is elevated in pregnancy and estrogen therapy.

- Anemias ***(related to increased RBC production)***
- Ankylosing rheumatoid spondylitis
- Biliary cirrhosis ***(related to release from damaged liver tissue)***
- Collagen diseases
- Complications of hemodialysis ***(trace element disturbances related to contamination from dialysate fluid and the disease process itself can be significant and can compound over time)***
- Hodgkin's disease
- Infections
- Inflammation
- Leukemia
- Malignant neoplasms
- Myocardial infarction (MI) ***(a correlation exists among copper levels, creatine kinase, and lactate dehydrogenase in myocardial infarction (MI); the pathophysiology is unclear, but some studies indicate a relationship between trace metal levels and risk of acute MI)***
- Pellagra ***(related to niacin deficiency; niacin is an essential cofactor in reactions involving copper)***
- Poisoning from copper-contaminated solutions or insecticides ***(related to excessive accumulation due to environmental exposure)***
- Pregnancy
- Pulmonary tuberculosis
- Rheumatic fever
- Rheumatoid arthritis
- Systemic lupus erythematosus
- Thalassemias ***(related to zinc deficiency of thalassemia and increased rate of release from hemolyzed RBCs; copper and zinc compete for the same binding sites so that a deficiency in one results in an increase of the other)***
- Thyroid disease (hypothyroid or hyperthyroid) ***(related to stimulation of thyroid hormone production by copper)***
- Trauma
- Typhoid fever
- Use of copper intrauterine device ***(related to copper leaching from the device)***

Decreased in:

- Burns ***(related to loss of stores in tissue and possibly to competitive inhibition of zinc-containing medications or vitamins administered as part of burn therapy)***
- Cystic fibrosis ***(related to inadequate intake and absorption)***
- Dysproteinemia ***(related to decreased transport to and from stores)***

- Infants ***(related to inadequate intake of milk or consumption of milk deficient in copper; especially premature infants)***
- Iron-deficiency anemias (some) ***(related to decreased absorption of iron from the intestines and transfer from tissues to plasma; it is essential to hemoglobin formation)***
- Long-term total parenteral nutrition ***(related to inadequate intake)***
- Malabsorption disorders (celiac disease, tropical sprue) ***(related to inadequate absorption)***
- Malnutrition ***(related to inadequate intake)***
- Menkes' disease ***(evidenced by a severe genetic X-linked defect causing failed transport to the liver and tissues)***
- Nephrotic syndrome ***(related to loss of transport proteins)***
- Occipital horn syndrome ***(evidenced by an inherited disorder of copper metabolism; similar to Menkes' disease)***
- Wilson's disease ***(evidenced by a genetic defect causing failed transport to the liver and tissues)***

CRITICAL FINDINGS: N/A

Find and print out the full study on Fast Find at davispl.us/vanleeuwen7.

Cortisol and Challenge Tests

SYNONYM/ACRONYM: Hydrocortisone, compound F.

COMMON USE: To assist in diagnosing adrenocortical insufficiency such as found in Cushing's syndrome and Addison's disease.

SPECIMEN: Serum collected in a red- or red/gray-top tube. Plasma collected in a green-top (heparin) tube is also acceptable. Care must be taken to use the same type of collection container if serial measurements are to be taken.

Procedure	Indications	Medication Administered	Recommended Collection Times
ACTH stimulation, rapid test	Suspect adrenal insufficiency (Addison's disease) or congenital adrenal hyperplasia	1 mcg (low-dose physiologic protocol) cosyntropin intramuscular (IM) or intravenous (IV); 250 mcg (standard pharmacologic protocol) cosyntropin IM or IV	3 cortisol levels: baseline immediately before bolus, 30 min after bolus, and 60 min after bolus. Note: Baseline and 30-min levels are adequate for accurate diagnosis using

Procedure	Indications	Medication Administered	Recommended Collection Times
			either dosage; low-dose protocol sensitivity is most accurate for 30 min level only
CRH stimulation	Differential diagnosis between ACTH-dependent conditions such as Cushing's disease (pituitary source) or Cushing's syndrome (ectopic source) and ACTH-independent conditions such as Cushing's syndrome (adrenal source)	IV dose of 1 mg/kg ovine or human CRH	0800 cortisol and 0800 ACTH levels: baseline collected 15 min before injection, 0 min before injection, and then 5, 15, 30, 60, 120, and 180 min after injection
Dexamethasone suppression (overnight)	Differential diagnosis between ACTH-dependent conditions such as Cushing's disease (pituitary source) or Cushing's syndrome (ectopic source) and ACTH-independent conditions such as Cushing's syndrome (adrenal source)	Oral dose of 1 mg dexamethasone (Decadron) at 2300	Collect cortisol at 0800 on the morning after the dexamethasone dose
Metyrapone stimulation (overnight)	Suspect hypothalamic/pituitary disease such as adrenal insufficiency,	Oral dose of 30 mg/kg metyrapone with snack at midnight	Collect cortisol and ACTH at 0800 on the morning after the metyrapone dose

(table continues on page 612)

C

Procedure	Indications	Medication Administered	Recommended Collection Times
	ACTH-dependent conditions such as Cushing's disease (pituitary source) or Cushing's syndrome (ectopic source), and ACTH-independent conditions such as Cushing's syndrome (adrenal source)		

ACTH = adrenocorticotropic hormone; CRH = corticotropin-releasing hormone.

NORMAL FINDINGS: (Method: Immunochemiluminescent assay)

Cortisol

Time	Conventional Units	SI Units (Conventional Units × 27.6)
0800		
Birth–1 wk	2–11 mcg/dL	55–304 nmol/L
1 wk–Adult/older adult	5–25 mcg/dL	138–690 nmol/L
1600		
1 wk–Adult/older adult	3–16 mcg/dL	83–442 nmol/L

Long-term use of corticosteroids in patients, especially older adults, may be reflected by elevated cortisol levels. After the first week of life, cortisol levels approach adult levels.

ACTH Challenge Tests

ACTH (Cosyntropin) Stimulated, Rapid Test	Conventional Units	SI Units (Conventional Units × 27.6)
Baseline	Cortisol greater than 5 mcg/dL	Greater than 138 nmol/L
30- or 60-min response	Cortisol 18–20 mcg/dL or incremental increase of 7 mcg/dL over baseline value	497–552 nmol/L or incremental increase of 193 nmol/L over baseline value

Corticotropin-Releasing Hormone Stimulated Test	Conventional Units	SI Units (Conventional Units × 27.6)
	Cortisol peaks at greater than 20 mcg/dL within 30–60 min	Greater than 552 nmol/L
		SI Units (Conventional Units × 0.22)
	ACTH increases twofold to fourfold within 30–60 min	Twofold to fourfold increase within 30–60 min

Dexamethasone Suppressed Overnight Test	Conventional Units	SI Units (Conventional Units × 27.6)
	Cortisol less than 1.8 mcg/dL next day	Less than 49.7 nmol/L

Metyrapone Stimulated Overnight Test	Conventional Units	SI Units (Conventional Units × 27.6)
	Cortisol less than 3 mcg/dL next day	Less than 83 nmol/L
		SI Units (Conventional Units × 0.22)
	ACTH greater than 75 pg/mL	Greater than 16.5 pmol/L
		SI Units (Conventional Units × 28.9)
	11-deoxycortisol greater than 7 mcg/dL	Greater than 202 nmol/L

DESCRIPTION: Cortisol (hydrocortisone) is the predominant glucocorticoid secreted by the adrenal glands in response to pituitary adrenocorticotropic hormone (ACTH). Cortisol is responsible for a number of regulatory functions which include stimulation of gluconeogenesis (generation of glucose from amino acids by the liver), breaking down fats to generate energy, acting as an insulin antagonist by increasing glucose levels, responding to stress, and suppressing inflammation. Measuring levels of cortisol in blood is the best indicator of adrenal function. Cortisol secretion varies diurnally, with highest levels occurring on awakening and lowest levels occurring late in the day, although bursts of cortisol excretion can occur at night. This pattern may be reversed in individuals who sleep during daytime hours and are active during nighttime hours. Cortisol and ACTH test results are evaluated together because they each control the other's concentrations (i.e., any change in one causes a change in the other). ACTH levels exhibit a diurnal variation, peaking between 0600 and 0800 and reaching the lowest point between 1800 and 2300. (See study titled "Adrenocorticotropic Hormone [and Challenge Tests].") Salivary cortisol levels are known to parallel blood levels and can be used to screen for Cushing's disease and Cushing's syndrome.

There are three main conditions that can result from an imbalance in cortisol levels. Cushing's syndrome is a complex condition that results from excessive levels of cortisol, regardless of the cause. Cushing's disease is a condition in which the pituitary gland releases too much ACTH resulting in overproduction of cortisol. Addison's disease is caused by failure of the adrenal glands to produce cortisol.

This procedure is contraindicated for

Patients with suspected adrenal insufficiency should not undergo the metyrapone stimulation test because it may induce an acute adrenal crisis, a life-threatening condition, in patients whose adrenal function is already compromised.

INDICATIONS

- Detect adrenal hyperfunction (Cushing's syndrome).
- Detect adrenal hypofunction (Addison's disease).

POTENTIAL MEDICAL DIAGNOSIS

The dexamethasone suppression test is useful in differentiating the causes for increased cortisol levels. Dexamethasone is a synthetic steroid that suppresses secretion of ACTH. With this test, a baseline morning cortisol level is collected, and the patient is given a 1-mg dose of dexamethasone at bedtime. A second specimen is collected the following morning. If cortisol levels have not been suppressed, adrenal adenoma may be suspected. The dexamethasone suppression test also produces abnormal results in patients with mental health disorders.

The corticotropin-releasing hormone (CRH) stimulation test works as well as the dexamethasone suppression test in distinguishing Cushing's disease from conditions in which ACTH is secreted ectopically. In this test, cortisol levels are measured after an injection of CRH. A fourfold increase in cortisol levels above baseline is seen in Cushing's disease. No increase in cortisol is seen if ectopic ACTH secretion is the cause.

The ACTH (cosyntropin)-stimulated rapid test is used when adrenal insufficiency is suspected. Cosyntropin is a synthetic form of ACTH. A baseline cortisol level is collected before the injection of cosyntropin. Specimens are subsequently collected at 30- and 60-min intervals. If the adrenal glands are functioning normally, cortisol levels rise

significantly after administration of cosyntropin.

The metyrapone stimulation test is used to distinguish corticotropin-dependent (pituitary Cushing's disease and ectopic Cushing's disease) from corticotropin-independent (carcinoma of the lung or thyroid) causes of increased cortisol levels. Metyrapone inhibits the conversion of 11-deoxycortisol to cortisol. Cortisol levels should decrease to less than 3 mcg/dL (SI: 83 nmol/L) if normal pituitary stimulation by ACTH occurs after an oral dose of metyrapone. Specimen collection and administration of the medication are performed as with the overnight dexamethasone test.

Increased in:

Conditions that result in excessive production of cortisol.

- Adrenal adenoma
- Cushing's syndrome
- Ectopic ACTH production
- Hyperglycemia
- Pregnancy
- Stress

Decreased in:

Conditions that result in adrenal hypofunction and corresponding low levels of cortisol.

- Addison's disease
- Adrenogenital syndrome
- Hypopituitarism

Summary of the Relationship Between Cortisol and ACTH Levels in Conditions Affecting the Adrenal and Pituitary Glands

Disease	Cortisol Level	ACTH Level
Addison's disease (adrenal insufficiency)	Decreased	Increased
Cushing's disease (pituitary adenoma)	Increased	Increased
Cushing's syndrome related to ectopic source of ACTH	Increased	Increased
Cushing's syndrome (ACTH independent; adrenal cancer or adenoma)	Increased	Decreased
Congenital adrenal hyperplasia	Decreased	Increased

CRITICAL FINDINGS: N/A

INTERFERING FACTORS

- Drugs and other substances that may increase cortisol levels include anticonvulsants, clomipramine, corticotropin, cortisone, CRH, ether, gemfibrozil, hydrocortisone, insulin, lithium, methadone, metoclopramide, mifepristone, naloxone, opiates, oral contraceptives, ranitidine, tetracosactrin, and vasopressin.
- Drugs and other substances that may decrease cortisol levels include barbiturates, beclomethasone, betamethasone, clonidine, desoximetasone, dexamethasone, ephedrine, etomidate, fluocinolone, ketoconazole, levodopa, lithium, methylprednisolone, metyrapone, midazolam, morphine, nitrous oxide, oxazepam, phenytoin, ranitidine, and trimipramine.
- Test results are affected by the time this test is done because cortisol levels vary diurnally.
- Stress and excessive physical activity can produce elevated levels.
- Normal values can be obtained in the presence of partial pituitary deficiency.
- Metyrapone may cause gastrointestinal distress and/or confusion. Administer oral dose of metyrapone with milk and snack.

C

NURSING IMPLICATIONS AND PROCEDURE

POTENTIAL NURSING PROBLEMS:

Problem	Signs & Symptoms	Interventions
Body image ***(related to increased androgen production [virilism, hirsutism]; wasting of muscle and bone matrix; capillary fragility; purple striae; slender limbs; abnormal fat distribution [buffalo hump])***	Negative verbalization of altered physical appearance; preoccupation with physical body changes; distress and refusal to talk about changed appearance; negative verbalization about changes in appearance; using clothing to conceal body changes	Assess the patient's perception of physical changes; note the frequency of negative comments about changed physical state; assist in the identification of positive coping strategies to address changed physical appearance; provide reassurance that changes in physical appearance will improve as hormones return to normal level; provide a referral to local support groups
Infection risk ***(related to impaired immune response secondary to elevated cortisol level)***	Delayed wound healing; inhibited collagen formation; impaired blood flow to edematous tissues; symptoms of infection (temperature, increased heart rate, increased blood pressure, shaking, chills, mottled skin, lethargy, fatigue, swelling, edema, pain, localized pressure, diaphoresis, night sweats, confusion, vomiting, nausea, headache)	Decrease exposure to environment by placing the patient in a private room; monitor and trend vital signs; monitor and trend laboratory values that would indicate an infection (white blood cells, C-reactive protein); promote good hygiene; assist with hygiene as needed; administer prescribed antibiotics, antipyretics; provide cooling measures; administer prescribed IV fluids; monitor vital signs and trend temperatures; encourage oral fluids; adhere to standard or universal precautions; isolate as appropriate; obtain cultures as ordered; encourage use of lightweight clothing and bedding

Problem	Signs & Symptoms	Interventions
Fluid volume (water) ***(related to sodium and water retention secondary to elevated cortisol levels)***	**Overload:** Edema, shortness of breath, increased weight, ascites, rales, rhonchi, and diluted laboratory values	Record daily weight and monitor trends; record accurate intake and output; monitor laboratory values that reflect alterations in fluid status (potassium, blood urea nitrogen, creatinine, calcium, hemoglobin, and hematocrit, sodium); manage underlying cause of fluid alteration; monitor urine characteristics and respiratory status; establish baseline assessment data; assess and trend heart rate and blood pressure; assess for symptoms of fluid overload such as jugular venous distention, shortness of breath, dyspnea, crackles; encourage low-sodium diet; administer prescribed diuretic; administer prescribed antihypertensive; elevate feet when sitting; monitor oxygenation with pulse oximetry
Injury risk ***(related to poor wound healing; decreased bone density; capillary fragility)***	Easy bruising; blood in stool; skin breakdown; fracture; poor wound healing	Assess for bruising; assess stool for occult blood; assess for skin breakdown; assess wound for healing progress; facilitate ordered bone density screening

PRETEST:

- Positively identify the patient using at least two person-specific identifiers before services, treatments, or procedures are performed.
- *Patient Teaching:* Inform the patient this test can assist in assessing for the amount of cortisol in the blood.
- Obtain a history of the patient's health concerns, symptoms, surgical procedures, and results of previously performed laboratory and diagnostic studies. Include a list of known allergens, especially allergies or sensitivities to latex.
- Obtain a list of the patient's current medications, including over-the-counter medications and dietary supplements (see Effects of Natural Products on Laboratory Values online at Davis*Plus*).

- Weigh patient and report weight to pharmacy for dosing of metyrapone (30 mg/kg body weight to a maximum dose of 3 g).
- Review the procedure with the patient. Inform the patient that multiple specimens may be required. Inform the patient that specimen collection takes approximately 5 to 10 min. Address concerns about pain and explain that there may be some discomfort during the venipuncture.
- *Sensitivity to social and cultural issues,* as well as concern for modesty, is important in providing psychological support before, during, and after the procedure.
- Note that there are no food, fluid, or medication restrictions unless by medical direction.
- Drugs that enhance steroid metabolism may be withheld by medical direction prior to metyrapone stimulation testing.
- Instruct the patient to minimize stress to avoid raising cortisol levels.

C

INTRATEST:

Potential Complications:

Adverse reactions to metyrapone include nausea and vomiting (N/V), abdominal pain, headache, dizziness, sedation, allergic rash, decreased white blood cell count, or bone marrow depression. Monitor the patient for hypotension, rapid and weak pulse, rapid respiratory rate, pallor, and extreme weakness that may indicate the patient is in acute adrenocortical insufficiency (addisonian crisis). Other signs and symptoms include cardiac arrhythmias, hypotension, dehydration, anxiety, confusion, impairment of consciousness, N/V, epigastric pain, diarrhea, hyponatremia, and hyperkalemia.

- Have emergency equipment readily available.
- Avoid the use of equipment containing latex if the patient has a history of allergic reaction to latex.
- Instruct the patient to cooperate fully and to follow directions. Direct the patient to breathe normally and to avoid unnecessary movement.
- Observe standard precautions, and follow the general guidelines in Patient Preparation and Specimen Collection online at Davis*Plus*. Positively identify the patient, and label the appropriate specimen container with the corresponding patient demographics, initials of the person collecting the specimen, date, and time of collection. Perform a venipuncture. Collect specimen between 0600 and 0800, when cortisol levels are highest.
- Remove the needle and apply direct pressure with dry gauze to stop bleeding. Observe/assess venipuncture site for bleeding or hematoma formation and secure gauze with adhesive bandage.
- Promptly transport the specimen to the laboratory for processing and analysis.

POST-TEST:

- Inform the patient that a report of the results will be made available to the requesting health-care provider (HCP), who will discuss the results with the patient.
- Recognize anxiety related to test results, and offer support.
- Observe/assess the patient who has been administered metyrapone for signs and symptoms of an acute adrenal (addisonian) crisis which may include abdominal pain, nausea, vomiting, hypotension, tachycardia, tachypnea, dehydration, excessively increased perspiration of the face and hands, sudden and significant fatigue or weakness, confusion, loss of consciousness, shock, coma. Potential interventions include immediate corticosteroid replacement (intravenous [IV] or IM), airway protection and maintenance, administration of dextrose for hypoglycemia, correction of electrolyte imbalance, and rehydration with IV fluids.
- Depending on the results of this procedure, additional testing

may be performed to evaluate or monitor progression of the disease process and determine the need for a change in therapy. Evaluate test results in relation to the patient's symptoms and other tests performed.

Patient Education:

- Instruct the patient to resume usual medications, as directed by the HCP.
- Discuss the implications of abnormal test results on the patient's lifestyle.
- Provide teaching and information regarding the clinical implications of the test results, as appropriate.
- Assess the patient with regard to the effects of abnormal cortisol levels, and monitor blood glucose levels to identify hyperglycemia associated with elevated cortisol.
- Educate the patient regarding access to counseling services.
- Provide contact information, if desired, for the Cushing's Support and Research Foundation (www.csrf.net).
- Reinforce information given by the patient's HCP regarding further testing, treatment, or referral to another HCP.
- Recognize anxiety related to test results and answer any questions or address any concerns voiced by the patient or family.
- Teach patient to use devices that will decrease injury risk such as soft toothbrush or electric rather than steel blade razor.

Expected Patient Outcomes:

Understanding

- The patient and family state that precautions should be taken with activity to prevent injury.
- The patient and family state the importance of reporting difficulty breathing promptly for timely intervention and prevention of respiratory distress.

Ability

- The patient identifies and selects a diet that is high in fiber and drinks plenty of fluids to prevent constipation and potential GI bleed.
- The patient demonstrates performance of good personal hygiene, including moisturizing of skin to prevent breakdown.

Response

- The patient complies with HCP's recommendation to increase the intake of calcium and vitamin D.
- The patient and family comply with the request to maintain good personal hygiene, including frequent hand hygiene.

RELATED STUDIES:

- Related tests include ACTH and challenge tests, angiography adrenal, chloride, CT abdomen, CT pituitary, DHEA, glucagon, glucose, glucose tolerance test, growth hormone, insulin, MRI abdomen, MRI pituitary, renin, sodium, testosterone, and US abdomen.
- Refer to the Endocrine System table online at Davis*Plus* for related tests by body system.

C-Peptide

SYNONYM/ACRONYM: Connecting peptide insulin, insulin C-peptide, proinsulin C-peptide.

COMMON USE: To evaluate hypoglycemia, assess beta cell function, and distinguish between type 1 and type 2 diabetes.

SPECIMEN: Serum collected in a red-top tube.

NORMAL FINDINGS: (Method: Immunochemiluminometric assay, ICMA)

Age	Conventional Units	SI Units (Conventional Units × 0.333)
9 yr	0–3.3 ng/mL	0–1.1 nmol/L
10–16 yr	0.4–3.3 ng/mL	0.1–1.1 nmol/L
Greater than 16 yr	0.8–3.5 ng/mL	0.3–1.2 nmol/L
1-hr response to glucose	2.3–11.8 ng/mL	0.8–3.9 nmol/L

C

DESCRIPTION: C-peptide is a biologically inactive peptide formed when beta cells of the pancreas convert proinsulin to insulin. Most of C-peptide is excreted by the kidneys. C-peptide levels usually correlate with insulin levels and provide a reliable indication of how well the pancreatic beta cells secrete insulin. Release of C-peptide is not affected by exogenous insulin administration. C-peptide values double after stimulation with glucose or glucagon, and measurement of C-peptide levels are very useful in the evaluation of hypoglycemia. An insulin/C-peptide ratio less than 1 indicates endogenous insulin secretion, whereas a ratio greater than 1 indicates an excess of exogenous insulin. An elevated C-peptide level in the presence of plasma glucose less than 40 mg/dL (SI: 2.22 mmol/L) supports a diagnosis of pancreatic islet cell tumor.

This procedure is contraindicated for: N/A

INDICATIONS

- Assist in the diagnosis of insulinoma: serum levels of insulin and C-peptide are elevated.
- Detect suspected factitious cause of hypoglycemia (excessive insulin administration): an increase in blood insulin from injection does not increase C-peptide levels.
- Determine beta cell function when insulin antibodies preclude accurate measurement of serum insulin production.
- Distinguish between type 1 and type 2 diabetes (with C-peptide–stimulating test): Patients with diabetes whose C-peptide stimulation level is greater than 18 ng/mL (SI: 6 nmol/L) can be managed without insulin treatment.
- Evaluate hypoglycemia.
- Evaluate viability of pancreatic transplant.

POTENTIAL MEDICAL DIAGNOSIS

Increased in:

- Chronic kidney disease or end stage renal disease ***(increase in circulating levels of C-peptide related to decreased renal excretion)***
- Islet cell tumor ***(related to excessive endogenous insulin production)***
- Pancreas or beta cell transplants ***(related to increased insulin production)***
- Type 2 diabetes ***(related to increased insulin production)***

Decreased in:

- Factitious hypoglycemia ***(related to decrease in blood glucose levels in response to insulin injection)***
- Pancreatectomy ***(evidenced by absence of the pancreas)***
- Type 1 diabetes ***(evidenced by insufficient production of insulin by the pancreas)***

CRITICAL FINDINGS: N/A

INTERFERING FACTORS

- Drugs and other substances that may increase C-peptide levels include betamethasone, chloroquine, danazol, deferoxamine, ethinyl estradiol, glibenclamide, glimepiride, indapamide, oral contraceptives, piretanide, prednisone, and rifampin.
- Drugs and other substances that may decrease C-peptide levels include atenolol and calcitonin.
- C-peptide and endogenous insulin levels do not always correlate in obese patients.
- Failure to follow dietary restrictions before the procedure may cause the procedure to be canceled or repeated.

NURSING IMPLICATIONS AND PROCEDURE

PRETEST:

- Positively identify the patient using at least two person-specific identifiers before services, treatments, or procedures are performed.
- *Patient Teaching:* Inform the patient this test can assist in assessing for low blood sugar.
- Obtain a history of the patient's health concerns, symptoms, surgical procedures, and results of previously performed laboratory and diagnostic studies. Include a list of known allergens, especially allergies or sensitivities to latex.
- Obtain a list of the patient's current medications, including over-the-counter medications and dietary supplements (see Effects of Natural Products on Laboratory Values online at Davis*Plus*).
- Review the procedure with the patient. Inform the patient that specimen collection takes approximately 5 to 10 min. Address concerns about pain and explain that there may be some discomfort during the venipuncture.
- *Sensitivity to social and cultural issues,* as well as concern for modesty, is important in providing psychological support before, during, and after the procedure.
- Instruct the patient to fast for at least 10 hr before specimen collection. Protocols may vary among facilities.
- Note that there are no fluid or medication restrictions unless by medical direction.

INTRATEST:

Potential Complications: N/A

- Ensure that the patient has complied with dietary restrictions and pretesting preparations prior to the study, as instructed.
- Avoid the use of equipment containing latex if the patient has a history of allergic reaction to latex.
- Instruct the patient to cooperate fully and to follow directions. Direct the patient to breathe normally and to avoid unnecessary movement.
- Observe standard precautions, and follow the general guidelines in Patient Preparation and Specimen Collection online at Davis*Plus*. Positively identify the patient, and label the appropriate specimen container with the corresponding patient demographics, initials of the person collecting the specimen, date, and time of collection. Perform a venipuncture.
- Remove the needle and apply direct pressure with dry gauze to stop bleeding. Observe/assess venipuncture site for bleeding or hematoma formation and secure gauze with adhesive bandage.
- Promptly transport the specimen to the laboratory for processing and analysis.

POST-TEST:

- Inform the patient that a report of the results will be made available to the requesting health-care provider (HCP), who will discuss the results with the patient.

C

- Instruct the patient to resume usual diet as directed by the HCP.
- *Nutritional Considerations:* Abnormal C-peptide levels may be associated with diabetes. There is no "diabetic diet"; however, many meal-planning approaches with nutritional goals are endorsed by the American Diabetes Association (ADA). 🍁 Patients who adhere to dietary recommendations report a better general feeling of health, better weight management, greater control of glucose and lipid values, and improved use of insulin. Instruct the patient, as appropriate, in nutritional management of diabetes. A variety of dietary patterns are beneficial for people with diabetes. The Mediterranean-style diet emphasizes inclusion of vegetables, whole grains, fruits, low-fat dairy, nuts, legumes, and nontropical vegetable oils (e.g., olive, canola, peanut, sunflower, flaxseed) along with fish and lean poultry. A similar dietary pattern known as the Dietary Approaches to Stop Hypertension (DASH) diet makes additional recommendations for the reduction of dietary sodium. Both dietary styles emphasize a reduction in consumption of red meats, which are high in saturated fats and cholesterol, and other foods containing sugar, saturated fats, trans fats, and sodium. A vegetarian diet as well as other potential weight loss diets, such as Weight Watchers, are also supported by the ADA. 🍁 If triglycerides also are elevated, the patient should be advised to eliminate or reduce alcohol. The nutritional needs of each patient with diabetes need to be determined individually (especially during pregnancy) with the appropriate HCPs, particularly professionals educated in nutrition.
- Instruct the patient and caregiver to report signs and symptoms of hypoglycemia (weakness, confusion, diaphoresis, rapid pulse) or hyperglycemia (thirst, polyuria, hunger, lethargy). Emphasize, as appropriate, that good control of glucose levels delays the onset and slows the progression of diabetic retinopathy, nephropathy, and neuropathy.
- Recognize anxiety related to test results, and be supportive of perceived loss of independence and fear of shortened life expectancy. Discuss the implications of abnormal test results on the patient's lifestyle. Provide teaching and information regarding the clinical implications of the test results, as appropriate. Emphasize, if indicated, that good glycemic control delays the onset and slows the progression of diabetic retinopathy, nephropathy, and neuropathy. Educate the patient regarding access to counseling services, as appropriate. Provide contact information, if desired, for the American Heart Association (www.americanheart.org), National Heart, Lung, and Blood Institute (www.nhlbi.nih.gov), Institute of Medicine of the National Academies (www.iom.edu), or USDA's resource for nutrition (www.choosemyplate.gov). 🍁
- Reinforce information given by the patient's HCP regarding further testing, treatment, or referral to another HCP. Answer any questions or address any concerns voiced by the patient or family.
- Depending on the results of this procedure, additional testing may be performed to evaluate or monitor progression of the disease process and determine the need for a change in therapy. Evaluate test results in relation to the patient's symptoms and other tests performed.

RELATED STUDIES:

- Related tests include CT cardiac scoring, cortisol, creatinine, creatinine clearance, EMG, ENG, fluorescein angiography, fructose, fundoscopy, glucagon, glucose, glucose tolerance tests, glycated hemoglobin, insulin, insulin antibodies, microalbumin, plethysmography, and visual fields test.
- Refer to the Endocrine System table online at Davis*Plus* for related tests by body system.

C-Reactive Protein

SYNONYM/ACRONYM: CRP.

COMMON USE: Conventional assay indicates a nonspecific inflammatory response; the high-sensitivity test is used to assess risk for cardiovascular and peripheral arterial disease.

SPECIMEN: Serum collected in a gold-, red-, or red/gray-top tube.

NORMAL FINDINGS: (Method: Nephelometry)

High-Sensitivity Immunoassay (Cardiac Applications)	Conventional and SI Units
Low risk	Less than 1 mg/L
Average risk	1–3 mg/L
High risk	Greater than 3 mg/L (after repeat testing)

Conventional Assay	Conventional and SI Units
Adult	Less than 10 mg/L

DESCRIPTION: C-reactive protein (CRP) is a glycoprotein produced by the liver in response to acute inflammation. The CRP assay is a nonspecific test that determines the presence (not the cause) of inflammation; it is often ordered in conjunction with erythrocyte sedimentation rate (ESR). CRP assay is a more sensitive and rapid indicator of the presence of an inflammatory process than ESR. CRP disappears from the serum rapidly when inflammation has subsided. The inflammatory process and its association with atherosclerosis make the presence of CRP, as detected by highly sensitive CRP assays, a potential marker for coronary artery disease. It is believed that the inflammatory process may instigate the conversion of a stable plaque to a weaker one that can rupture and occlude an artery.

This procedure is contraindicated for: N/A

INDICATIONS

Conventional assay

- Assist in the differential diagnosis of appendicitis and acute pelvic inflammatory disease.
- Assist in the differential diagnosis of Crohn's disease and ulcerative colitis.
- Assist in the differential diagnosis of rheumatoid arthritis and uncomplicated systemic lupus erythematosus (SLE).
- Detect the presence or exacerbation of inflammatory processes.
- Monitor response to therapy for autoimmune disorders such as rheumatoid arthritis.

High-sensitivity assay
- Assist in the evaluation of coronary artery disease.
- Detect the presence or exacerbation of inflammatory processes.

POTENTIAL MEDICAL DIAGNOSIS

Increased in:

Conditions associated with an inflammatory response stimulate production of CRP.

- Acute bacterial infections
- Crohn's disease
- Inflammatory bowel disease
- Metabolic syndrome ***(inflammation of the coronary vessels is associated with increased CRP levels and increased risk for coronary vessel injury, which may result in distal vessel plaque occlusions)***
- Myocardial infarction ***(inflammation of the coronary vessels is associated with increased CRP levels and increased risk for coronary vessel injury, which may result in distal vessel plaque occlusions)***
- Pregnancy (second half)
- Rheumatic fever
- Rheumatoid arthritis
- SLE

Decreased in: N/A

CRITICAL FINDINGS: N/A

INTERFERING FACTORS

- Drugs and other substances that may increase CRP levels include chemotherapy, interleukin-2, oral contraceptives, and pamidronate.
- Drugs and other substances that may decrease CRP levels include aurothiomalate, dexamethasone, gemfibrozil, leflunomide, methotrexate, NSAIDs, oral contraceptives (progestogen effect), penicillamine, pentopril, prednisolone, prinomide, and sulfasalazine.
- NSAIDs, salicylates, and steroids may cause false-negative results because of suppression of inflammation.
- Falsely elevated levels may occur with the presence of an intrauterine device.
- Lipemic samples that are turbid in appearance may be rejected for analysis when nephelometry is the test method.

NURSING IMPLICATIONS AND PROCEDURE

POTENTIAL NURSING PROBLEMS:

Problem	Signs & Symptoms	Interventions
Infection ***(related to metabolic or endocrine dysfunction; chronic debilitating illness; cirrhosis; trauma; vectors; decreased tissue perfusion)***	Temperature; increased heart rate; increased blood pressure; shaking; chills; mottled skin; lethargy; fatigue; swelling; edema; pain; localized pressure; diaphoresis; night sweats; confusion; vomiting; nausea; headache	Promote good hygiene; assist with hygiene as needed; administer prescribed antibiotics, antipyretics; provide cooling measures; administer prescribed intravenous fluids; monitor vital signs and trend temperatures; encourage oral fluids; adhere to standard or universal precautions; isolate as appropriate; obtain cultures as ordered; encourage use of lightweight clothing and bedding

Problem	Signs & Symptoms	Interventions
Fear ***(related to loss of control; ineffective coping; change in life expectancy; unfamiliar surroundings; illness; disease; unknown)***	Expression of fear; preoccupation with fear; increased tension; increased blood pressure; increased heart rate; vomiting; diarrhea; nausea; fatigue; weakness; insomnia; shortness of breath; increased respiratory rate; withdrawal; panic attacks	Access social services; provide specific and culturally appropriate education; assist the patient and family to recognize effective coping strategies; assist the patient to acknowledge his or her fear; provide a safe environment to decrease fear; explore cultural influences that may enhance fear; utilize therapeutic touch as appropriate to decrease fear; collaborate with social services, respiratory services, physical therapy, occupational therapy to address specific medical problems associated with fear
Tissue perfusion ***(related to hypovolemia; decreased hemoglobin; interrupted arterial flow; interrupted venous flow)***	Hypotension; dizziness; cool extremities; pallor; capillary refill greater than 3 sec in fingers and toes; weak pedal pulses; altered level of consciousness; altered sensation	Monitor blood pressure; assess for dizziness; assess extremities for skin temperature, color, warmth; assess capillary refill; assess pedal pulses; monitor for numbness, tingling, hyperesthesia, hypoesthesia; monitor for deep vein thrombosis; carefully use heat and cold on affected areas; use foot cradle to keep pressure off of affected body parts
Activity ***(related to inflammation; altered tissue perfusion; deconditioned state)***	Weakness; verbal report of fatigue; altered sleep pattern; altered blood pressure, heart rate, or respiratory rate in response to activity; oxygen desaturation with activity	Assess current level of activity and weakness; identify the patient's perception of the cause of weakness; assess the need for the use of assistive devices; observe and document the patient's tolerance to activity; provide ordered oxygen; limit energy expenditure to necessary activities

PRETEST:

- Positively identify the patient using at least two person-specific identifiers before services, treatments, or procedures are performed.
- *Patient Teaching:* Inform the patient this test can assist in assessing for inflammation.
- Obtain a history of the patient's health concerns, symptoms, surgical

procedures, and results of previously performed laboratory and diagnostic studies. Include a list of known allergens, especially allergies or sensitivities to latex.

- Obtain a list of the patient's current medications, including over-the-counter medications and dietary supplements (see Effects of Natural Products on Laboratory Values online at Davis*Plus*).
- Review the procedure with the patient. Inform the patient that specimen collection takes approximately 5 to 10 min. Address concerns about pain and explain that there may be some discomfort during the venipuncture.
- ***Sensitivity to social and cultural issues,*** as well as concern for modesty, is important in providing psychological support before, during, and after the procedure.
- Note that there are no food, fluid, or medication restrictions unless by medical direction.

INTRATEST:

Potential Complications:

- Avoid the use of equipment containing latex if the patient has a history of allergic reaction to latex.
- Instruct the patient to cooperate fully and to follow directions. Direct the patient to breathe normally and to avoid unnecessary movement.
- Observe standard precautions, and follow the general guidelines in Patient Preparation and Specimen Collection online at Davis*Plus*. Positively identify the patient, and label the appropriate specimen container with the corresponding patient demographics, initials of the person collecting the specimen, date, and time of collection. Perform a venipuncture.
- Remove the needle and apply direct pressure with dry gauze to stop bleeding. Observe/assess venipuncture site for bleeding or hematoma formation and secure gauze with adhesive bandage.
- Promptly transport the specimen to the laboratory for processing and analysis.

POST-TEST:

- Inform the patient that a report of the results will be made available to the requesting health-care provider (HCP), who will discuss the results with the patient.
- Recognize anxiety related to test results, and assist with pain management as ordered. Ensure the patient receives a referral for physical therapy as appropriate. Explain the importance of maintaining an upright position when standing, sitting, and walking to maximize joint function and mobility. Discuss the proper mix of rest and activity and the importance of taking regular rest periods throughout the day to prevent exhaustion.
- Depending on the results of this procedure, additional testing may be performed to evaluate or monitor progression of the disease process and determine the need for a change in therapy. Evaluate test results in relation to the patient's symptoms and other tests performed.

Patient Education:

- Answer any questions or address any concerns voiced by the patient or family.
- Teach the patient to use pillows to properly position himself or herself and provide relief to stressed joints.
- Explain the signs and symptoms of infection to the patient and family, including what to report and when to report concerns.
- Teach the appropriate use of environmental aids to facilitate safe activity such as lowering and raising the bed, moving from bed to chair, and using assistive devices in the bathroom.

Expected Patient Outcomes:

Understanding

- The patient and family formulate a plan that will decrease fall risk.
- The patient and family describe symptoms that may occur as a result of physical overactivity.

Ability

- The patient and family accurately demonstrate how to take and record a temperature.

- The patient and family proficiently demonstrate the proper use of assistive devices.

Response

- The patient and family comply with the request to obtain appropriate immunizations.
- The patient joins a counseling group to address ongoing anxiety and associated fears.

RELATED STUDIES:

- Related tests include antidysrhythmic drugs, antibodies anticyclic citrullinated peptide, ANA, apolipoprotein A and B, arthroscopy, ANP, blood gases, BMD, bone scan, BNP, calcium, cholesterol (total, HDL, and LDL), CBC, CBC WBC count and differential, CT, cardiac scoring, CK and isoenzymes, echocardiography, ESR, glucose, glycated hemoglobin, Holter monitor, homocysteine, ketones, LDH and isoenzymes, MRI chest, MRI musculoskeletal, MI scan, myocardial perfusion scan, myoglobin, PET heart, potassium, procalcitonin, radiography bone, RF, synovial fluid analysis, triglycerides, and troponin.
- Refer to the Cardiovascular and Immune systems tables online at Davis*Plus* for related tests by body system.

Creatine Kinase and Isoenzymes

SYNONYM/ACRONYM: CK and isoenzymes.

COMMON USE: To monitor myocardial infarction and some disorders of the musculoskeletal system such as Duchenne's muscular dystrophy.

SPECIMEN: Serum collected in a red- or red/gray-top tube. Serial specimens are highly recommended. Care must be taken to use the same type of collection container if serial measurements are to be taken.

NORMAL FINDINGS: (Method: Enzymatic for CK, electrophoresis for isoenzymes; enzyme immunoassay techniques are in common use for CK-MB)

	Conventional & SI Units
Total CK	
Newborn–1 yr	Up to 2 × adult values
Male (children and adults)	50–204 units/L
Female (children and adults)	36–160 units/L
CK Isoenzymes by Electrophoresis	
CK-BB	Absent
CK-MB	0–4%
CK-MM	96–100%
CK-MB by Immunoassay	0–5 ng/mL
CK-MB Index	0–2.5

CK = creatine kinase; CK-BB = CK isoenzyme in brain; CK-MB = CK isoenzyme in heart; CK-MM = CK isoenzyme in skeletal muscle.
The CK-MB index is the CK-MB (by immunoassay) divided by the total CK and then multiplied by 100. For example, a CK-MB by immunoassay of 25 ng/mL with a total CK of 250 units/L would have a CK-MB index of 10.
Elevations in total CK occur after exercise. Values in older adults may decline slightly related to loss of muscle mass.

C

DESCRIPTION: Creatine kinase (CK) is an enzyme that exists almost exclusively in skeletal muscle, heart muscle, and, in smaller amounts, in the brain and lungs. This enzyme is important for intracellular storage and release of energy. Three isoenzymes, based on primary location, have been identified by electrophoresis: brain and lungs CK-BB, cardiac CK-MB, and skeletal muscle CK-MM. When injury to these tissues occurs, the enzymes are released into the bloodstream. Levels increase and decrease in a predictable time frame. Measuring the serum levels can help determine the extent and timing of the damage. Noting the presence of the specific isoenzyme helps determine the location of the tissue damage. Atypical forms of CK can be identified. Macro-CK, an immunoglobulin complex of normal CK isoenzymes, has no clinical significance. Mitochondrial-CK is sometimes identified in the sera of seriously ill patients, especially those with metastatic carcinoma.

Acute myocardial infarction (MI) releases CK into the serum within the first 48 hr; values return to normal in about 3 days. The isoenzyme CK-MB appears in the first 4 to 6 hr, peaks in 24 hr, and usually returns to normal in 72 hr. Recurrent elevation of CK suggests reinfarction or extension of ischemic damage. Significant elevations of CK are expected in early phases of muscular dystrophy, even before the clinical signs and symptoms appear. CK elevation diminishes as the disease progresses and muscle mass decreases. Differences in total CK with age and gender relate to the fact that the predominant isoenzyme is muscular in origin. Body builders have higher values, whereas older individuals have lower values because of deterioration of muscle mass.

Serial use of the mass assay for CK-MB with serial cardiac troponin I, myoglobin, and serial electrocardiograms in the assessment of MI has largely replaced the use of CK isoenzyme assay by electrophoresis. CK-MB mass assays are more sensitive and rapid than electrophoresis. Studies have demonstrated a high positive predictive value for acute MI when the CK-MB (by immunoassay) is greater than 10 ng/mL with a relative CK-MB index greater than 3.

Timing for Appearance and Resolution of Serum/Plasma Cardiac Markers in Acute MI

Cardiac Marker	Appearance (hr)	Peak (hr)	Resolution (d)
CK (total)	4–6	24	2–3
CK-MB	4–6	15–20	2–3
LDH	12	24–48	10–14
Myoglobin	1–3	4–12	1
Troponin I	2–6	15–20	5–7

This procedure is contraindicated for: N/A

INDICATIONS

- Assist in the diagnosis of acute MI and evaluate cardiac ischemia (CK-MB).
- Detect musculoskeletal disorders that do not have a neurological basis, such as dermatomyositis or Duchenne's muscular dystrophy (CK-MM).
- Determine the success of coronary artery reperfusion after fibrinolytic therapy or percutaneous transluminal angioplasty, as evidenced by a decrease in CK-MB.

POTENTIAL MEDICAL DIAGNOSIS

Increased in:

CK is released from any damaged cell in which it is stored, so conditions that affect the brain, heart, or skeletal muscle and cause cellular destruction demonstrate elevated CK levels and correlating isoenzyme source CK-BB, CK-MB, CK-MM.

- Alcoholism ***(CK-MM)***
- Brain infarction (extensive) ***(CK-BB)***
- Delirium tremens ***(CK-MM)***
- Dermatomyositis ***(CK-MM)***
- Gastrointestinal (GI) tract infarction ***(CK-MM)***
- Head injury ***(CK-BB)***
- Heart failure ***(CK-MB)***
- Hypothyroidism ***(CK-MM related to metabolic effect on and damage to skeletal muscle tissue)***
- Hypoxic shock ***(CK-MM related to muscle damage from lack of oxygen)***
- Loss of blood supply to any muscle ***(CK-MM)***
- Malignant hyperthermia ***(CK-MM related to skeletal muscle injury)***
- MI ***(CK-MB)***
- Muscular dystrophies ***(CK-MM)***
- Myocarditis ***(CK-MB)***
- Neoplasms of the prostate, bladder, and GI tract ***(CK-MM)***
- Polymyositis ***(CK-MM)***
- Pregnancy; during labor ***(CK-MM)***
- Prolonged hypothermia ***(CK-MM)***
- Pulmonary edema ***(CK-MM)***
- Pulmonary embolism ***(CK-MM)***
- Reye's syndrome ***(CK-BB)***
- Rhabdomyolysis ***(CK-MM)***
- Surgery ***(CK-MM)***
- Tachycardia ***(CK-MB)***
- Tetanus ***(CK-MM related to muscle injury from injection)***
- Trauma ***(CK-MM)***

Decreased in:

- Small stature ***(related to lower muscle mass than average stature)***
- Sedentary lifestyle ***(related to decreased muscle mass)***

CRITICAL FINDINGS: N/A

INTERFERING FACTORS

- Drugs and other substances that may increase total CK levels include aspirin, captopril, clofibrate, ethyl alcohol, propranolol, statins, and any intramuscularly injected preparations will increase CK levels because of tissue trauma caused by the injection.
- Drugs and other substances that may decrease total CK levels include dantrolene.

C

NURSING IMPLICATIONS AND PROCEDURE

POTENTIAL NURSING PROBLEMS:

Problem	Signs & Symptoms	Interventions
Coping ***(related to a feeling of threat; inadequate support system; inadequate problem-solving ability; disease process; poor self-confidence)***	Inability to cope with the situation; inability to make decisions; inability to ask for help; fatigue; sleep disturbance; lack of confidence; inappropriate self-defense strategies	Assess for specific stressors that alter coping; identify the patient's perception of stressors; assess for use of positive coping mechanisms; provide opportunities to express fear and anxiety in a safe, nonjudgmental environment; avoid false reassurance; convey acceptance and understanding; encourage patient to identify his or her own strengths; assist the patient to accurately evaluate current situation; reduce environmental stimuli that could be misunderstood as threatening; provide a safe outlet for personal feelings; use relaxation techniques; administer prescribed medication
Sleep ***(related to perceived wellness and diagnosis; fear; anxiety; inadequate coping; medication adverse effect)***	Report of lack of sleep or rest; fatigue; decreased energy; restlessness; decreased level of concentration; irritability; listlessness; lethargy; malaise; daytime drowsiness; confusion	Avoid loud noises; decrease lighting to a preferred restful level; administer prescribed medication; minimize interruptions; provide single-patient room if possible (if not possible, a compatible roommate); assist the patient to identify the cause of his or her fear that results in insomnia; facilitate as much as possible the patient's normal bedtime routine; limit daytime sleeping; collaborate with health-care provider (HCP) to revise medications that may be causing sleeplessness

Problem	Signs & Symptoms	Interventions
Cardiac output ***(related to prolonged myocardial ischemia; acute myocardial infarction; reduced cardiac muscle contractility; ruptured papillary muscle; mitral insufficiency)***	Weak peripheral pulses; slow capillary refill; decreased urinary output; cool, clammy skin; tachypnea; dyspnea; altered level of consciousness; abnormal heart sounds; fatigue; hypoxia; loud holosystolic murmur; EKG changes; increased jugular venous distention	Assess peripheral pulses and capillary refill; monitor blood pressure and check for orthostatic changes; assess respiratory rate, breath sounds, and orthopnea; assess skin color and temperature; assess level of consciousness; monitor urinary output; use pulse oximetry to monitor oxygenation; monitor EKG; administer ordered inotropic and peripheral vasodilator medications, nitrates; provide oxygen administration
Pain ***(related to myocardial ischemia; myocardial infarction)***	Reports of chest pain; new onset of angina; shortness of breath; pallor; weakness; diaphoresis; palpitations; nausea; vomiting; epigastric pain or discomfort; increased blood pressure; increased heart rate	Assess pain characteristics, squeezing pressure, location in substernal back, neck, or jaw; assess pain duration and onset (minimal exertion, sleep, or rest); identify pain modalities that have relieved pain in the past; monitor cardiac biomarkers (CK-MB, troponin, myoglobin); collaborate with ancillary departments to complete ordered echocardiography, exercise stress testing, pharmacological stress testing; administer prescribed pain medication; monitor and trend vital signs; administer prescribed oxygen; administer prescribed anticoagulants, antiplatelets, beta blockers, calcium channel blockers, angiotensin-converting enzyme inhibitors, Angiotensin II receptor blockers, thrombolytic drugs

C

PRETEST:

- Positively identify the patient using at least two person-specific identifiers before services, treatments, or procedures are performed.
- *Patient Teaching:* Inform the patient this test can assist in assessing for heart muscle cell damage.
- Obtain a history of the patient's health concerns, symptoms, surgical procedures, and results of previously performed laboratory and diagnostic studies. Include a list of known allergens, especially allergies or sensitivities to latex.
- Obtain a list of the patient's current medications, including over-the-counter medications and dietary supplements (see Effects of Natural Products on Laboratory Values online at Davis*Plus*).
- Review the procedure with the patient. Inform the patient that a series of samples will be required. (Samples at time of admission and 2 to 4 hr, 6 to 8 hr, and 12 hr after admission are the minimal recommendations. Protocols may vary among facilities. Additional samples may be requested.) Inform the patient that specimen collection takes approximately 5 to 10 min. Address concerns about pain and explain that there may be some discomfort during the venipuncture.
- Note that there are no food, fluid, or medication restrictions unless by medical direction.

INTRATEST:

Potential Complications: N/A

- Avoid the use of equipment containing latex if the patient has a history of allergic reaction to latex.
- Instruct the patient to cooperate fully and to follow directions. Direct the patient to breathe normally and to avoid unnecessary movement.
- Observe standard precautions, and follow the general guidelines in Patient Preparation and Specimen Collection online at Davis*Plus*. Positively identify the patient, and label the appropriate specimen container with the corresponding patient demographics, initials of the person collecting the specimen, date, and time of collection. Perform a venipuncture.
- Remove the needle and apply direct pressure with dry gauze to stop bleeding. Observe/assess venipuncture site for bleeding or hematoma formation and secure gauze with adhesive bandage.
- Promptly transport the specimen to the laboratory for processing and analysis.

POST-TEST:

- Inform the patient that a report of the results will be made available to the requesting HCP, who will discuss the results with the patient.
- *Nutritional Considerations:* Increased CK levels may be associated with coronary artery disease (CAD). Nutritional therapy is recommended for the patient identified to be at risk for developing CAD or for individuals who have specific risk factors and/or existing medical conditions (e.g., elevated LDL cholesterol levels, other lipid disorders, type 1 diabetes, type 2 diabetes, insulin resistance, or metabolic syndrome). Other changeable risk factors warranting patient education include strategies to encourage patients, especially those who are overweight and with high blood pressure, to safely decrease sodium intake, achieve a normal weight, ensure regular participation in moderate aerobic physical activity three to four times per week, eliminate tobacco use, and adhere to a heart-healthy diet. If triglycerides also are elevated, the patient should be advised to eliminate or reduce alcohol. A variety of dietary patterns are beneficial for people with CAD, and there are many meal-planning approaches with nutritional goals endorsed by the American Diabetes Association (ADA). The Guideline on Lifestyle Management to Reduce Cardiovascular Risk published by the American College of Cardiology (ACC) and the American Heart Association (AHA) in conjunction

with the National Heart, Lung, and Blood Institute (NHLBI) recommends a Mediterranean-style diet rather than a low-fat diet. The guideline emphasizes inclusion of vegetables, whole grains, fruits, low-fat dairy, nuts, legumes, and nontropical vegetable oils (e.g., olive, canola, peanut, sunflower, flaxseed) along with fish and lean poultry. 🍁 A similar dietary pattern known as the Dietary Approaches to Stop Hypertension (DASH) diet makes additional recommendations for the reduction of dietary sodium. Both dietary styles emphasize a reduction in consumption of red meats, which are high in saturated fats and cholesterol, and other foods containing sugar, saturated fats, trans fats, and sodium. The ADA also includes a vegetarian diet as well as other potential weight loss diets such as Weight Watchers. 🍁 The nutritional needs of each patient need to be determined individually (especially during pregnancy) with the appropriate HCPs, particularly professionals educated in nutrition.

- Recognize anxiety related to test results, and be supportive of fear of shortened life expectancy.
- Depending on the results of this procedure, additional testing may be performed to evaluate or monitor progression of the disease process and determine the need for a change in therapy. Evaluate test results in relation to the patient's symptoms and other tests performed.

Patient Education:

- Discuss the implications of abnormal test results on the patient's lifestyle.
- Provide teaching and information regarding the clinical implications of the test results, as appropriate.
- Educate the patient regarding access to counseling services.
- Provide contact information, if desired, for the AHA (www.americanheart.org), NHLBI (www.nhlbi.nih.gov), Institute of Medicine of the National Academies (www.iom.edu), or USDA's resource for nutrition (www.choosemyplate.gov). 🍁
- Reinforce information given by the patient's HCP regarding further testing, treatment, or referral to another HCP.
- Answer any questions or address any concerns voiced by the patient or family.
- Teach the patient and family the importance of adequate rest in relation to their overall health.
- Discuss with the patient and family factors that can interfere with adequate rest such as fear or anxiety.

Expected Patient Outcomes:

Understanding

- The patient and family recognize that irritability and mood changes are common with sleep deprivation
- The patient and family recognize that there are safe medications available that can be used to enhance sleep.

Ability

- The patient and family identify measures that will increase the ability to obtain sleep or rest.
- The patient and family identify nighttime foods or drinks that interfere with sleep.

Response

- The patient complies with the recommendation to limit daytime sleeping in order to enhance nighttime rest.
- The patient complies with the recommendation to take prescribed medication to enhance sleep if necessary.

RELATED STUDIES:

- Related tests include antidysrhythmic drugs, apolipoprotein A and B, ANP, blood gases, BNP, calcium, cholesterol (total, HDL and LDL), CRP, CT cardiac scoring, echocardiography, glucose, glycated hemoglobin, Holter monitor, homocysteine, ketones, LDH and isoenzymes, lipoprotein electrophoresis, magnesium, MRI chest, MRI venography, MI scan, myocardial perfusion scan, myoglobin, pericardial fluid, PET heart, potassium, triglycerides, and troponin.
- Refer to the Cardiovascular and Musculoskeletal systems tables online at Davis*Plus* for related tests by body system.

Creatinine, Blood

SYNONYM/ACRONYM: N/A

COMMON USE: To assess kidney function found in acute kidney injury and chronic kidney disease, related to drug reaction and disease such as diabetes.

C

SPECIMEN: Serum collected in a red- or red/gray-top tube. Plasma collected in a green-top (heparin) tube is also acceptable.

NORMAL FINDINGS: (Method: Spectrophotometry)

Age	Conventional Units	SI Units (Conventional Units × 88.4)
Newborn	0.31–1.21 mg/dL	27–107 micromol/L
Infant	0.31–0.71 mg/dL	27–63 micromol/L
1–5 yr	0.31–0.51 mg/dL	27–45 micromol/L
6–10 yr	0.51–0.81 mg/dL	45–72 micromol/L
Adult male	0.61–1.21 mg/dL	54–107 micromol/L
Adult female	0.51–1.11 mg/dL	45–98 micromol/L

Values in older adults remain relatively stable after a period of decline related to loss of muscle mass during the transition from adult to older adult.

The National Kidney Foundation recommends the use of two decimal places in reporting serum creatinine for use in calculating estimated glomerular filtration rate.

DESCRIPTION: Creatine resides almost exclusively in skeletal muscle, where it participates in energy-requiring metabolic reactions. A small amount of creatine is irreversibly converted to creatinine by the liver, which then circulates to the kidneys and is excreted. The amount of creatinine generated in an individual is proportional to the mass of skeletal muscle present and remains fairly constant throughout the life span; its consistency in production and clearance is the reason that creatinine is used as an indicator of kidney function. Creatinine values normally decrease with age owing to diminishing muscle mass. Conditions involving degenerative muscle wasting or massive muscle trauma from a crushing injury will also result in decreased creatinine levels. Blood urea nitrogen (BUN) is often ordered with creatinine for comparison. The BUN/creatinine ratio is also a useful indicator of kidney disease. The ratio should be between 10:1 and 20:1. The creatinine clearance test measures a blood sample and a urine sample to determine the rate at which the kidneys are clearing creatinine from the blood; this reflects the glomerular filtration rate, or GFR (see study titled "Creatinine, Urine, and Creatinine Clearance, Urine").

Chronic kidney disease (CKD) is a significant health concern worldwide. International studies have been undertaken to evaluate the risk factors common to cardiovascular disease, diabetes, and hypertension; these three diseases are all associated with CKD. Albuminuria, which can result from increased glomerular permeability to proteins, is considered an independent risk factor predictive of kidney or cardiovascular disease. There has also been an international effort by the National Kidney Disease Education Program (NKDEP), International Confederation of Clinical Chemistry and Laboratory Medicine, and European Communities Confederation of Clinical Chemistry (since renamed *European Federation of Clinical Chemistry and Laboratory Medicine*) to standardize methods to identify and monitor CKD. International efforts have resulted in development of an isotope dilution mass spectrometry (IDMS) reference method for standardized measurement of creatinine and use of equations to estimate glomerular filtration rate (eGFR) for both adults and children under the age of 18 yr. The equation for adults is based on factors identified in either the National Kidney Foundation (NKF)'s Modification of Diet in Renal Disease study or the Chronic Kidney Disease Epidemiology Collaboration equation using creatinine results from a method that has calibration traceable to IDMS. The equation includes four factors: serum or plasma creatinine value, age in years, gender, and race. The equation for adults is valid only for patients between the ages of 18 and 70. A correction factor is incorporated in the equation if the patient is African American because CKD is more prevalent in African Americans; results are approximately 20% higher. An IDMS-traceable equation using serum creatinine results from a method that has a calibration traceable to the IDMS, referred to as the *bedside Schwartz equation*, is recommended for estimating GFR for children under 18 yr of age. The formula uses the patient's height in centimeters and the serum creatinine value where the GFR (mL/min/1.73 m2) = (0.41 × height cm)/serum creatinine mg/dL (SI Units: GFR (mL/min/1.73 m2) = (36.2 × height cm)/serum creatinine micromol/L. For consistency in the interpretation of test results, it is important to know whether the creatinine has been measured using IDMS-traceable test methods and equations. The equations have not been validated for pregnant women (GFR is significantly increased in pregnancy); patients older than 70; patients with serious comorbidities; or patients with extremes in body size, muscle mass, or nutritional status. eGFR calculators can be found at the NKDEP (www.nkdep.nih.gov/professionals/gfr_calculators/index.htm).

Cystatin C, also known as cystatin 3 and CST3, is now recognized as a useful marker for kidney damage and monitor of function in transplanted kidneys. It is a low molecular weight molecule belonging in the family of proteinase inhibitors. Cystatin C is produced by all nucleated cells in the body and is freely filtered by the glomerular membrane in the kidney. It is not secreted by the kidney tubules and although a small amount is reabsorbed by the kidney tubules, it is metabolized in the tubules and does not re-enter circulation. Therefore, its serum concentration is directly proportional to kidney function. It is believed to be a better marker of kidney function than creatinine because levels are independent of weight and height, diet, muscle mass, age, and sex. Normal values for individuals aged 1 to 50 yr are 0.56 to 0.9 mg/L (SI: 41.9–67.4 nmol/L, conversion factor = 74.9) for individuals aged 1 to 50 yr and 0.58 to 1.08 mg/L (SI: 43.4–80.9 nmol/L, conversion factor = 74.9) for those aged 50 yr and older.

This procedure is contraindicated for: N/A

INDICATIONS

- Assess a known or suspected disorder involving muscles in the absence of kidney disease.
- Evaluate known or suspected impairment of kidney function.

POTENTIAL MEDICAL DIAGNOSIS

Increased in:

- Acromegaly ***(related to increased muscle mass)***
- Dehydration ***(related to hemoconcentration)***
- Gigantism ***(related to increased muscle mass)***
- Heart failure ***(related to decreased renal blood flow)***
- Kidney disease, acute kidney injury, and CKD ***(related to decreased urinary excretion)***
- Poliomyelitis ***(related to increased release from damaged muscle)***
- Pregnancy induced hypertension ***(related to reduced GFR and decreased urinary excretion)***
- Renal calculi ***(related to decreased kidney excretion due to obstruction)***
- Rhabdomyolysis ***(related to increased release from damaged muscle)***
- Shock ***(related to increased release from damaged muscle)***

Decreased in:

- Decreased muscle mass ***(related to debilitating disease or increasing age)***
- Hyperthyroidism ***(related to increased GFR)***
- Inadequate protein intake ***(related to decreased muscle mass)***
- Liver disease (severe) ***(related to fluid retention)***
- Muscular dystrophy ***(related to decreased muscle mass)***
- Pregnancy ***(related to increased GFR and renal clearance)***
- Small stature ***(related to decreased muscle mass)***

CRITICAL FINDINGS:

Adults

Potential critical finding is greater than 7.4 mg/dL (SI: 654.2 micromol/L) (patient not on dialysis).

Children

Potential critical finding is greater than 3.8 mg/dL (SI: 336 micromol/L) (patient not on dialysis).

Note and immediately report to the requesting health-care provider (HCP) any critical findings and related symptoms. A listing of these findings varies among facilities. Timely notification of a critical finding for laboratory or diagnostic studies is a role expectation of the professional nurse. The notification processes vary among facilities. Upon receipt of the critical finding, the information should be read back to the caller to verify accuracy.

Consideration may be given to verification of critical findings before action is taken. Policies vary among facilities and may include requesting immediate recollection and retesting by the laboratory or retesting using a rapid point-of-care testing instrument at the bedside, if available.

Chronic renal insufficiency is identified by creatinine levels between

1.5 and 3 mg/dL (SI: 132.6 and 265.2 micromol/L); CKD is present at levels greater than 3 mg/dL (SI: 265.2 micromol/L).

Possible interventions may include renal or peritoneal dialysis and organ transplant, but early discovery of the cause of elevated creatinine levels might avoid such drastic interventions.

INTERFERING FACTORS

- Drugs and other substances that may increase creatinine levels include acebutolol, acetaminophen (overdose), acetylsalicylic acid, amikacin, amiodarone, amphotericin B, arginine, arsenicals, ascorbic acid, asparaginase, barbiturates, capreomycin, captopril, carbutamide, carvedilol, cephalothin, chlorthalidone, cimetidine, cisplatin, clofibrate, colistin, corn oil (Lipomul), cyclosporine, dextran, doxycycline, enalapril, ethylene glycol, gentamicin, indomethacin, ipodate, kanamycin, levodopa, mannitol, methicillin, mitomycin, neomycin, netilmicin, nitrofurantoin, NSAIDs, oxyphenbutazone, paromomycin, penicillin, pentamidine, phosphorus, plicamycin, radiographic medium, semustine, streptokinase, streptozocin, tetracycline, thiazides, tobramycin, triamterene, vancomycin, vasopressin, viomycin, and vitamin D.
- Drugs and other substances that may decrease creatinine levels include citrates, dopamine, ibuprofen, and lisinopril.
- High blood levels of bilirubin and glucose can cause false decreases in creatinine.
- A diet high in meat can cause increased creatinine levels.
- Ketosis can cause a significant increase in creatinine.
- Hemolyzed specimens are unsuitable for analysis.

C

NURSING IMPLICATIONS AND PROCEDURE

POTENTIAL NURSING PROBLEMS:

Problem	Signs & Symptoms	Interventions
Fluid volume (water) ***(related to excess fluid and sodium intake; compromised renal function)***	**Excess:** Edema, shortness of breath, increased weight, ascites, rales, rhonchi, and diluted laboratory values; distended neck veins; tachycardia; restlessness	Record daily weight and monitor trends; ensure accurate intake and output; monitor laboratory values that reflect alterations in fluid status (potassium, blood urea nitrogen, creatinine, calcium, hemoglobin, and hematocrit, sodium); manage underlying cause of fluid alteration; monitor urine characteristics and respiratory status; establish baseline assessment data; assess and trend heart rate and blood pressure; assess for

(table continues on page 638)

Problem	Signs & Symptoms	Interventions
		symptoms of fluid overload such as jjugular venous distension (JVD), shortness of breath, dyspnea, crackles; ensure low-sodium diet; administer prescribed diuretic; administer prescribed antihypertensive; elevate feet when sitting; monitor oxygenation with pulse oximetry; administer oxygen as appropriate; elevate the head of the bed; administer prescribed antihypertensives
Cardiac output ***(related to excess fluid volume; pericarditis; electrolyte imbalance; toxin accumulation)***	Weak peripheral pulses; slow capillary refill; decreased urinary output; cool clammy skin; tachypnea; dyspnea; altered level of consciousness; abnormal heart sounds; fatigue; hypoxia; loud holosystolic murmur; EKG changes; increased JVD	Assess peripheral pulses and capillary refill; monitor blood pressure and check for orthostatic changes; assess respiratory rate, breath sounds, and orthopnea; assess skin color and temperature; assess level of consciousness; monitor urinary output; use pulse oximetry to monitor oxygenation; monitor EKG; administer ordered inotropic and peripheral vasodilator medications, nitrates; provide oxygen administration; administer as prescribed (sodium bicarbonate, glucose, insulin drip, potassium excretion resin, calcium salt)
Protection ***(anemia related to bone marrow suppression secondary to renal insufficiency [erythropoietic]; red cell destruction secondary to altered plasma***	Pallor; fatigue; weakness; shortness of breath; anxiety; easy bruising; increased clotting time	Assess for symptoms of anemia (fatigue, pallor, decreased activity); observe for prolonged bleeding associated with ineffective clotting; use pulse oximetry or arterial blood gases to assess oxygenation; administer oxygen as required; administer blood or blood products as required; administer prescribed epoetin

Problem	Signs & Symptoms	Interventions
environment; nutritional deficiency; decreased and defective platelets; blood loss; ineffective clotting)		alfa; use bleeding precautions (avoid aspirin products, trauma, constipation, and forceful nose blowing that could cause nosebleed)
Sexuality ***(related to amenorrhea; decreased libido; lack of ovulation; testicular atrophy; impotence; psychological impairment secondary to physical effects of renal insufficiency)***	Reduced sexual function; decreased sexual satisfaction; alteration in the relationship with partner	Assess perception of reported change in sexual function; assess the emotional impact of decreased libido (depression, altered self-esteem, altered personal relationships); assess for need of counseling; encourage verbalization of feelings; discuss alternative forms of intimate expression; discuss medical treatments that may improve sexual function

PRETEST:

- Positively identify the patient using at least two person-specific identifiers before services, treatments, or procedures are performed.
- *Patient Teaching:* Inform the patient this test can assist in assessing kidney function.
- Obtain a history of the patient's health concerns, symptoms, surgical procedures, and results of previously performed laboratory and diagnostic studies. Include a list of known allergens, especially allergies or sensitivities to latex.
- Obtain a list of the patient's current medications, including over-the-counter medications and dietary supplements (see Effects of Natural Products on Laboratory Values online at Davis*Plus*).
- Review the procedure with the patient. Inform the patient that specimen collection takes approximately 5 to 10 min. Address concerns about pain and explain that there may be some discomfort during the venipuncture.
- *Sensitivity to social and cultural issues,* as well as concern for modesty, is important in providing psychological support before, during, and after the procedure.
- Note that there are no food, fluid, or medication restrictions unless by medical direction.
- Instruct the patient to refrain from excessive exercise for 8 hr before the test.

INTRATEST:

Potential Complications: N/A

- Ensure that the patient has complied with activity restrictions; assure that activity has been restricted prior to the study, as instructed.
- Avoid the use of equipment containing latex if the patient has a history of allergic reaction to latex.
- Instruct the patient to cooperate fully and to follow directions. Direct the

patient to breathe normally and to avoid unnecessary movement.

- Observe standard precautions, and follow the general guidelines in Patient Preparation and Specimen Collection online at Davis*Plus*. Positively identify the patient, and label the appropriate specimen container with the corresponding patient demographics, initials of the person collecting the specimen, date, and time of collection. Perform a venipuncture.
- Remove the needle and apply direct pressure with dry gauze to stop bleeding. Observe/assess venipuncture site for bleeding or hematoma formation and secure gauze with adhesive bandage.
- Promptly transport the specimen to the laboratory for processing and analysis.

POST-TEST:

- Inform the patient that a report of the results will be made available to the requesting HCP, who will discuss the results with the patient.
- *Nutritional Considerations:* Increased creatinine levels may be associated with kidney disease. The nutritional needs of patients with kidney disease vary widely and are in constant flux. Anorexia, nausea, and vomiting commonly occur, prompting the need for continuous monitoring for malnutrition, especially among patients receiving long-term hemodialysis therapy.
- Recognize anxiety related to test results and be supportive of impaired activity related to fear of shortened life expectancy. Help the patient to cope with long-term implications. Recognize that anticipatory anxiety and grief related to potential lifestyle changes may be expressed when someone is faced with a chronic disorder.
- Depending on the results of this procedure, additional testing may be performed to evaluate or monitor progression of the disease process and determine the need for a change in therapy. Evaluate test results in relation to the patient's symptoms and other tests performed.

Patient Education:

- Discuss the implications of abnormal test results on the patient's lifestyle.
- Provide teaching and information regarding the clinical implications of the test results, as appropriate.
- Educate the patient regarding access to counseling services.
- Provide contact information, if desired, for the American Diabetes Association (www.diabetes.org), NKF (www.kidney.org), or NKDEP (www.nkdep.nih.gov). 🍁

Expected Patient Outcomes:

- Reinforce information given by the patient's HCP regarding further testing, treatment, or referral to another HCP.
- Answer any questions or address any concerns voiced by the patient or family.
- Instruct the patient to resume usual activity as directed by the HCP.

Understanding

- The patient states causes of decreased libido.
- The patient and family identify causes of anemia.

Ability

- The patient demonstrates proficiency in taking prescribed medication accurately.
- The patient and family demonstrate proficiency in selecting activities that decrease bleeding risk.

Response

- The patient discusses the efficacy of counseling to repair personal relationship secondary to intimacy concerns.
- The patient states approach to care planning for sexual dysfunction is realistic.

RELATED STUDIES:

- Related tests include anion gap, antimicrobial drugs, ANF, BNP, biopsy muscle, blood gases, BUN, calcium, calculus kidney stone panel, CT abdomen, CT kidney, CK and isoenzymes, creatinine clearance, cystoscopy, echocardiography, echocardiography transesophageal, electrolytes, EMG, ENG, glucagon, glucose, glycolated hemoglobin, insulin, IVP, KUB studies, lung perfusion scan, MRI venography, microalbumin, osmolality, phosphorus, renogram, retrograde ureteropyelography, TSH, thyroxine, US abdomen, uric acid, and UA.

- Refer to the Genitourinary and Musculoskeletal systems tables online at Davis*Plus* for related tests by body system.

Creatinine, Urine, and Creatinine Clearance, Urine

SYNONYM/ACRONYM: N/A

COMMON USE: To assess and monitor kidney function related to acute kidney injury or chronic kidney disease.

SPECIMEN: Urine from an unpreserved random or timed specimen collected in a clean plastic collection container.

NORMAL FINDINGS: (Method: Spectrophotometry)

Normal Urine Volume per 24 Hours	
These ranges are very general averages and were not calculated on the basis of normal average body weights. Literature shows that expected urinary output can be estimated by a formula in which the expected output is as follows: Infants: 1–2 mL/kg/hr Children and adolescents: 0.5–1 mL/kg/hr Adults and older adults: 1 mL/kg/hr	
Newborns	15–60 mL
Infants	
3–10 d	100–300 mL
11–59 d	250–450 mL
2–12 months	400–500 mL
Children and Adolescents	
13 months–4 years	500–700 mL
5–7 years	650–1000 mL
8–14 years	800–1400 mL
Adults and Older Adults	800–2500 mL (average 1200 mL)

Normally, more urine is produced during the day than at night. With advancing age, the reverse often occurs. The total expected outcome for adults appears to remain the same regardless of age.

Urine Creatinine		
Age	**Conventional Units**	**SI Units**
		Urine Creatinine (Conventional Units × 8.84)
2–3 yr	6–22 mg/kg/24 hr	53–194 micromol/kg/24 hr
4–18 yr	12–30 mg/kg/24 hr	106–265 micromol/kg/24 hr
Adult male	14–26 mg/kg/24 hr	124–230 micromol/kg/24 hr
Adult female	11–20 mg/kg/24 hr	97–177 micromol/kg/24 hr
	Creatinine Clearance	***Creatinine Clearance (Conventional Units × 0.0167)***
Children	70–140 mL/min/1.73 m^2	1.17–2.33 mL/s/1.73 m^2
Adult male	85–125 mL/min/1.73 m^2	1.42–2.08 mL/s/1.73 m^2
Adult female	75–115 mL/min/1.73 m^2	1.25–1.92 mL/s/1.73 m^2
For each decade after 40 yr	Decrease of 6–7 mL/min/1.73 m^2	Decrease of 0.06–0.07 mL/s/1.73 m^2

The 24-hr urine volume is recorded and provided with the results of the creatinine measurement.

DESCRIPTION: Creatinine is the end product of creatine metabolism. Creatine resides almost exclusively in skeletal muscle, where it participates in energy-requiring metabolic reactions. In these processes, a small amount of creatine is irreversibly converted to creatinine, which then circulates to the kidneys and is excreted. The amount of creatinine generated in an individual is proportional to the mass of skeletal muscle present and remains fairly constant, unless there is massive muscle damage resulting from crushing injury or degenerative muscle disease. Creatinine values decrease with advancing age owing to diminishing muscle mass. Although the measurement of urine creatinine is an effective indicator of kidney function, the creatinine clearance test is more precise. The creatinine clearance test measures a blood sample and a urine sample to determine the rate at which the kidneys are clearing creatinine from the blood; this reflects the glomerular filtration rate (GFR) and is based on an estimate of body surface.

Chronic kidney disease (CKD) is a significant health concern worldwide. International studies have been undertaken to evaluate the risk factors common to cardiovascular disease, diabetes, and hypertension; these three diseases are all associated with CKD. Albuminuria, which can result from increased glomerular permeability to proteins, is considered an independent risk factor predictive of kidney or cardiovascular disease. There has also been an international effort by the National Kidney Disease Education Program (NKDEP), International Confederation of Clinical Chemistry and Laboratory Medicine, and European Communities Confederation of Clinical Chemistry (since renamed *European Federation of Clinical Chemistry and Laboratory Medicine*) to standardize methods to identify and monitor CKD. International efforts have resulted in development of an isotope dilution mass spectrometry (IDMS) reference method for standardized measurement of creatinine and use of equations to estimate glomerular filtration rate (eGFR) for both adults and children under the age of 18 yr. The equation for adults is based on factors identified in either the National Kidney Foundation (NKF)'s Modification of Diet in Renal Disease study or the Chronic Kidney Disease Epidemiology Collaboration (CKD-EPI) equation using creatinine results from a method that has calibration traceable to IDMS. The equation includes four factors: serum or plasma creatinine value, age in years, gender, and race. The equation for adults is valid only for patients between the ages of 18 and 70. A correction factor is incorporated in the equation if the patient is African American because CKD is more prevalent in African Americans; results are approximately 20% higher. An ADMS-traceable equation using serum creatinine results from a method that has a calibration traceable to the IDMS, referred to as the *bedside Schwartz equation,* is recommended for estimating GFR for children under 18 yr of age. The formula uses the patient's height in centimeters and the serum creatinine value where the GFR (mL/min/1.73 m2) = (0.41 × height cm)/serum creatinine mg/dL (SI Units: GFR (mL/min/1.73 m2) = (36.2 × height cm)/serum creatinine micromol/L. For consistency in the interpretation of test results, it is important to know whether the creatinine has been measured using IDMS-traceable test methods and equations. The equations have not been validated for pregnant women (GFR is significantly increased in pregnancy); patients older than 70; patients with serious comorbidities; or patients with extremes in body size, muscle mass, or nutritional status. eGFR calculators can be found at the NKDEP (www.nkdep.nih.gov/professionals/gfr_calculators/index.htm).

- **Creatinine clearance can be estimated from a blood creatinine level:**

  Creatinine clearance = [1.2 × (140 – age in years) × (weight in kg)]/blood creatinine level.

The result is multiplied by 0.85 if the patient is female; the result is multiplied by 1.18 if the patient is African American.

This procedure is contraindicated for: N/A

INDICATIONS

- Determine the extent of nephron damage in known kidney disease (at least 50% of functioning nephrons must be lost before values are decreased).
- Determine renal function before administering nephrotoxic drugs.
- Evaluate accuracy of a 24-hr urine collection based on the constant level of creatinine excretion.
- Evaluate glomerular function.
- Monitor effectiveness of treatment in kidney disease.

POTENTIAL MEDICAL DIAGNOSIS

Increased in:

- Acromegaly ***(related to increased muscle mass)***
- Carnivorous diets ***(related to increased intake of creatine,***

which is metabolized to creatinine and excreted by the kidneys)
- Exercise ***(related to muscle damage; increased renal blood flow)***
- Gigantism ***(related to increased muscle mass)***

C

Decreased in:
Conditions that decrease GFR, impair kidney function, or reduce renal blood flow will decrease renal excretion of creatinine

- Acute or chronic glomerulonephritis
- Chronic bilateral pyelonephritis
- Leukemia
- Muscle wasting diseases ***(related to abnormal creatinine production; decreased production reflected in decreased excretion)***
- Paralysis ***(related to abnormal creatinine production; decreased production reflected in decreased excretion)***
- Polycystic kidney disease
- Pregnancy induced hypertension ***(related to reduced GFR)***
- Shock
- Urinary tract obstruction (e.g., from calculi)
- Vegetarian diets ***(evidenced by diets that exclude intake of animal muscle, the creatine source metabolized to creatinine and excreted by the kidneys)***

CRITICAL FINDINGS:

- Degree of impairment:
  Borderline: 62.5–80 mL/min/1.73 m^2 (SI: 1–1.3 mL/s/1.73 m^2)
  Slight: 52–62.5 mL/min/1.73 m^2 (SI: 0.9–1 mL/s/1.73 m^2)
  Mild: 42–52 mL/min/1.73 m^2 (SI: 0.7–0.9 mL/s/1.73 m^2)
  Moderate: 28–42 mL/min/1.73 m^2 (SI: 0.5–0.7 mL/s/1.73 m^2)
  Marked: Less than 28 mL/min/1.73 m^2 (SI: Less than 0.5 mL/s/1.73 m^2)

Note and immediately report to the requesting health-care provider (HCP) any critical findings and related symptoms. A listing of these findings varies among facilities. Timely notification of a critical finding for laboratory or diagnostic studies is a role expectation of the professional nurse. The notification processes vary among facilities. Upon receipt of the critical finding, the information should be read back to the caller to verify accuracy.

INTERFERING FACTORS

- Drugs and other substances that may increase urine creatinine levels include ascorbic acid, cefoxitin, cephalothin, corticosteroids, levodopa, methotrexate, methyldopa, nitrofurans (including nitrofurazone), phenolphthalein, and prednisone.
- Drugs and other substances that may increase urine creatinine clearance include enalapril, oral contraceptives, prednisone, and ramipril.
- Drugs and other substances that may decrease urine creatinine levels include anabolic steroids, androgens, captopril, and thiazides.
- Drugs and other substances that may decrease the urine creatinine clearance include acetylsalicylic acid, amphotericin B, chlorthalidone, cimetidine, cisplatin, cyclosporine, guancidine, ibuprofen, indomethacin, mitomycin, oxyphenbutazone, probenecid (coadministered with digoxin), puromycin, and thiazides.
- Excessive ketones in urine may cause falsely decreased values.
- Failure to follow proper technique in collecting 24-hr specimen may invalidate test results.
- Failure to refrigerate specimen throughout urine collection period allows decomposition of creatinine, causing falsely decreased values.

- **Consumption of large amounts of meat, excessive exercise, and stress should be avoided for 24 hr before the test. Protocols may vary among facilities.**
- **Failure to follow dietary restrictions before the procedure may cause the procedure to be canceled or repeated.**

NURSING IMPLICATIONS AND PROCEDURE

PRETEST:

- Positively identify the patient using at least two person-specific identifiers before services, treatments, or procedures are performed.
- *Patient Teaching:* Inform the patient this test can assist in assessing kidney function.
- Obtain a history of the patient's health concerns, symptoms, surgical procedures, and results of previously performed laboratory and diagnostic studies. Include a list of known allergens, especially allergies or sensitivities to latex.
- Obtain a list of the patient's current medications, including over-the-counter medications and dietary supplements (see Effects of Natural Products on Laboratory Values online at Davis*Plus*).
- Review the procedure with the patient. Provide a nonmetallic urinal, bedpan, or toilet-mounted collection device. Address concerns about pain and explain to the patient that there should be no discomfort during the urine collection procedure. Inform the patient that a blood sample for creatinine will be required on the day urine collection begins or at some point during the 24 hr collection period (see study titled "Creatinine, Blood" for additional information).
- *Sensitivity to social and cultural issues,* as well as concern for modesty, is important in providing psychological support before, during, and after the procedure.
- Usually a 24-hr time frame for urine collection is ordered. Inform the patient that all urine must be saved during that 24-hr period. Instruct the patient not to void directly into the laboratory collection container. Instruct the patient to avoid defecating in the collection device and to keep toilet tissue out of the collection device to prevent contamination of the specimen. Place a sign in the bathroom to remind the patient to save all urine.
- Instruct the patient to void all urine into the collection device and then to pour the urine into the laboratory collection container. Alternatively, the specimen can be left in the collection device for a health-care staff member to add to the laboratory collection container.
- Note that there are no fluid or medication restrictions unless by medical direction.
- Instruct the patient to refrain from eating meat during the test. Protocols may vary among facilities.

INTRATEST:

Potential Complications: N/A

- Ensure that the patient has complied with dietary and activity restrictions for 24 hr prior to the procedure; assure that ingestion of meat has been restricted during the test.
- Avoid the use of equipment containing latex if the patient has a history of allergic reaction to latex.
- Instruct the patient to cooperate fully and to follow directions.
- Observe standard precautions, and follow the general guidelines in Patient Preparation and Specimen Collection online at Davis*Plus*. Positively identify the patient, and label the appropriate specimen container with the corresponding patient demographics, initials of the person collecting the specimen, date, and time of collection. Perform a venipuncture as appropriate.

Random Specimen (Collect in Early Morning) Clean-Catch Specimen

- Instruct the male patient to (1) thoroughly wash his hands, (2) cleanse the meatus, (3) void a small amount into the toilet, and (4) void directly into the specimen container.

- Instruct the female patient to (1) thoroughly wash her hands; (2) cleanse the labia from front to back; (3) while keeping the labia separated, void a small amount into the toilet; and (4) without interrupting the urine stream, void directly into the specimen container.

C

Pediatric Urine Collector

- Put on gloves. Appropriately cleanse the genital area and allow the area to dry. Remove the covering over the adhesive strips on the collector bag and apply over the genital area. Diaper the child. When specimen is obtained, place the entire collection bag in a sterile urine container.

Indwelling Catheter

- Put on gloves. Empty drainage tube of urine. It may be necessary to clamp off the catheter for 15 to 30 min before specimen collection. Cleanse specimen port with antiseptic swab, and then aspirate 5 mL of urine with a 21- to 25-gauge needle and syringe. Transfer urine to a sterile container.

Urinary Catheterization

- Place female patient in lithotomy position or male patient in supine position. Using sterile technique, open the straight urinary catheterization kit and perform urinary catheterization. Place the retained urine in a sterile specimen container.

Suprapubic Aspiration

- Place the patient in a supine position. Cleanse the area with antiseptic and drape with sterile drapes. A needle is inserted through the skin into the bladder. A syringe attached to the needle is used to aspirate the urine sample. The needle is then removed and a sterile dressing is applied to the site. Place the sterile sample in a sterile specimen container.
- Do not collect urine from the pouch from the patient with a urinary diversion (e.g., ileal conduit). Instead, perform catheterization through the stoma.

Timed Specimen

- Obtain a clean 3-L urine specimen container, toilet-mounted collection device, and plastic bag (for transport of the specimen container). The specimen must be refrigerated or kept on ice throughout the entire collection period. If an indwelling urinary catheter is in place, the drainage bag must be kept on ice.
- Begin the test between 0600 and 0800 if possible. Collect first voiding and discard. Record the time the specimen was discarded as the beginning of the timed collection period. The next morning, ask the patient to void at the same time the collection was started and add this last voiding to the container. Urinary output should be recorded throughout the collection time.
- If an indwelling catheter is in place, replace the tubing and container system at the start of the collection time. Keep the container system on ice during the collection period, or empty the urine into a larger container periodically during the collection period; monitor to ensure continued drainage, and conclude the test the next morning at the same time the collection was begun.
- At the conclusion of the test, compare the quantity of urine with the urinary output record for the collection; if the specimen contains less than what was recorded as output, some urine may have been discarded, invalidating the test.
- Include on the collection container's label the amount of urine, test start and stop times, and any foods or medications that can affect test results.
- Promptly transport the specimen to the laboratory for processing and analysis.

POST-TEST:

- Inform the patient that a report of the results will be made available to the requesting HCP, who will discuss the results with the patient.

- Instruct the patient to resume usual diet, medications, and activity, as directed by the HCP.
- Recognize anxiety related to test results and be supportive of impaired activity related to fear of shortened life expectancy. Discuss the implications of abnormal test results on the patient's lifestyle. Provide teaching and information regarding the clinical implications of the test results, as appropriate. Educate the patient regarding access to counseling services. Help the patient to cope with long-term implications. Recognize that anticipatory anxiety and grief related to potential lifestyle changes may be expressed when someone is faced with a chronic disorder.
- Provide contact information, if desired, for the American Diabetes Association (www.diabetes.org), NKF (www.kidney.org), or NKDEP (www.nkdep.nih.gov). 🍁
- Reinforce information given by the patient's HCP regarding further testing, treatment, or referral to another HCP. Answer any questions or address any concerns voiced by the patient or family.
- Depending on the results of this procedure, additional testing may be performed to evaluate or monitor progression of the disease process and determine the need for a change in therapy. Evaluate test results in relation to the patient's symptoms and other tests performed.

RELATED STUDIES:

- Related tests include anion gap, antimicrobial drugs, antibodies antiglomerular basement membrane, ANF, biopsy kidney, biopsy muscle, blood gases, BNP, BUN, calcium, calculus kidney stone analysis, C4, CT abdomen, CT kidneys, CK and isoenzymes, creatinine, culture urine, cytology urine, cystoscopy, echocardiography, echocardiography transesophageal, electrolytes, EMG, ENG, EPO, gallium scan, glucagon, glucose, haptoglobin, insulin, IVP, KUB studies, lung perfusion scan, microalbumin, osmolality, phosphorus, renogram, retrograde ureteropyelography, TSH, thyroxine, US kidney, uric acid, and UA.
- Refer to the Genitourinary System table online at Davis*Plus* for related tests by body system.

Cryoglobulin

SYNONYM/ACRONYM: Cryo.

COMMON USE: To assist in identifying the presence of certain immunological disorders such as Reynaud's phenomenon.

SPECIMEN: Serum collected in a red-top tube.

NORMAL FINDINGS: (Method: Visual observation for changes in appearance) Negative.

POTENTIAL MEDICAL DIAGNOSIS

Increased in:

Cryoglobulins are present in varying degrees in associated conditions.

Type I cryoglobulin (monoclonal)

- Chronic lymphocytic leukemia
- Lymphoma
- Multiple myeloma

Type II cryoglobulin (mixtures of monoclonal immunoglobulin [Ig] M and polyclonal IgG)

- Autoimmune hepatitis
- Rheumatoid arthritis

- Sjögren's syndrome
- Waldenström's macroglobulinemia

Type III cryoglobulin (mixtures of polyclonal IgM and IgG)

- Acute post-streptococcal glomerulonephritis
- Chronic infection (especially hepatitis C)
- Cirrhosis
- Endocarditis
- Infectious mononucleosis
- Polymyalgia rheumatica
- Rheumatoid arthritis
- Sarcoidosis
- Systemic lupus erythematosus

Decreased in: N/A

CRITICAL FINDINGS: N/A

Find and print out the full study on Fast Find at davispl.us/vanleeuwen7.

Culture and Molecular Testing, Fungal

SYNONYM/ACRONYM: N/A

COMMON USE: To identify the pathogenic fungal organisms causing infection.

SPECIMEN: Hair, skin, nail, pus, sterile fluids, blood, bone marrow, stool, bronchial washings, sputum, or tissue samples collected in a sterile plastic, tightly capped container.

NORMAL FINDINGS: (Method: Culture on selective media; macroscopic and microscopic examination) No presence of fungi.

DESCRIPTION: Fungi, organisms that normally live in soil, can be introduced into humans through the accidental inhalation of spores or inoculation of spores into tissue through trauma. Yeast are classified as single-celled fungi. Individuals most susceptible to fungal infection usually are debilitated by chronic disease, are receiving prolonged antibiotic therapy, or have impaired immune systems. Fungal diseases may be classified according to the involved tissue type: dermatophytoses involve superficial and cutaneous tissue; there are also subcutaneous and systemic mycoses. Culture is a method commonly used to identify the cause of a fungal infection. However, fungal growth occurs slowly, and it can take days to weeks before culture and susceptibility results are available. Systemic fungal infections, especially those caused by fluconazole-resistant fungi, can be life threatening. Identification of the infectious agent and effective therapeutic treatment can be more time sensitive than what is required for the natural course of growth by culture. Rapid, direct testing platforms are not yet widely available, but molecular-based blood assays are being developed and approved for use in clinical situations. For example, the T2Candida panel employs a combination of molecular technology (DNA amplification) with magnetic resonance technology to identify five common yeast species from a single blood sample in 3 to 5 hr.

This procedure is contraindicated for: N/A

INDICATIONS

- Determine antimicrobial sensitivity of the organism.
- Isolate and identify organisms responsible for neonatal thrush.
- Isolate and identify organisms responsible for nail infections or abnormalities.
- Isolate and identify organisms responsible for skin eruptions, drainage, or other evidence of infection.
- Isolate and identify organisms responsible for systemic infection and sepsis.

POTENTIAL MEDICAL DIAGNOSIS

Positive findings in

- Blood
  Candida albicans
  Histoplasma capsulatum
- Cerebrospinal fluid
  Coccidioides immitis
  Cryptococcus neoformans
  Members of the order Mucorales
  Paracoccidioides brasiliensis
  Sporothrix schenckii
- Hair
  Epidermophyton
  Microsporum
  Trichophyton
- Nails
  C. albicans
  Cephalosporium
  Epidermophyton
  Trichophyton
- Skin
  Actinomyces israelii
  C. albicans
  C. immitis
  Epidermophyton
  Microsporum
  Trichophyton
- Tissue
  A. israelii
  Aspergillus
  C. albicans
  Nocardia
  P. brasiliensis

CRITICAL FINDINGS:

- Positive findings in any sterile body fluid such as blood or cerebrospinal fluid.

Note and immediately report to the requesting health-care provider (HCP) any critical findings and related symptoms. A listing of these findings varies among facilities. Timely notification of a critical finding for laboratory or diagnostic studies is a role expectation of the professional nurse. The notification processes vary among facilities. Upon receipt of the critical finding, the information should be read back to the caller to verify accuracy. Lists of specific organisms may vary among facilities; specific organisms are required to be reported to local, state, and national departments of health. 🍁

INTERFERING FACTORS

- Prompt and proper specimen processing, storage, and analysis are important to achieve accurate results.

NURSING IMPLICATIONS AND PROCEDURE

PRETEST:

- Positively identify the patient using at least two person-specific identifiers before services, treatments, or procedures are performed.
- ***Patient Teaching:*** Inform the patient this test can assist in identification of the organism causing infection.
- Obtain a history of the patient's health concerns, symptoms, surgical procedures, and results of previously performed laboratory and diagnostic studies. Include a list of known allergens, especially allergies or sensitivities to latex.
- Obtain a list of the patient's current medications, including over-the-counter medications and dietary supplements (see Effects of Natural Products on Laboratory Values online at Davis*Plus*).

- Note any recent medications, especially antifungals, that can interfere with test results.
- Review the procedure with the patient. Inform the patient that specimen collection takes approximately 5 min. Address concerns about pain and explain that there may be some discomfort during the specimen collection.
- *Sensitivity to social and cultural issues,* as well as concern for modesty, is important in providing psychological support before, during, and after the procedure.
- Note that there are no food or fluid restrictions unless by medical direction.

INTRATEST:

Potential Complications: N/A

- Instruct the patient to cooperate fully and to follow directions. Direct the patient to breathe normally and to avoid unnecessary movement.
- Observe standard precautions, and follow the general guidelines in Patient Preparation and Specimen Collection online at Davis*Plus*. Instructions regarding the appropriate transport materials for blood, bone marrow, bronchial washings, sputum, sterile fluids, stool, and tissue samples should be obtained from the laboratory. Positively identify the patient, and label the appropriate collection containers with the corresponding patient demographics, initials of the person collecting the specimen, date, and time of collection.
- Promptly transport the specimen to the laboratory for processing and analysis.

Skin

- Clean the collection site with 70% alcohol. Scrape the peripheral margin of the collection site with a sterile scalpel or wooden spatula. Place the scrapings in a sterile collection container.

Hair

- Fungi usually grow at the base of the hair shaft. Infected hairs can be identified by using a Wood's lamp in a darkened room. A Wood's lamp provides rays of ultraviolet light at a wavelength of 366 nm, or 3,660 Å. Infected hairs fluoresce a bright yellow-green when exposed to light from the Wood's lamp. Using tweezers, pluck hair from skin.

Nails

- Ideally, softened material from the nailbed is sampled from beneath the nail plate. Alternatively, shavings from the deeper portions of the nail itself can be collected.
- Results of a conventional fungal culture may take up to 4 wk. Results of fungal antibody tests are available within a few days of collection and may be ordered when there is a strong suspicion of a particular pathogen. Most often, results indicating the presence or absence of fungi can be obtained in moments by looking at small amounts of the specimen under a microscope. A portion of the sample or swab is placed in sterile saline, and a drop from the diluted sample is placed on a glass slide, also called a wet prep. Another portion of the sample or a second swab is mixed with 15% potassium hydroxide (KOH), and a drop from the KOH sample is placed on a glass slide. A coverslip is placed over each specimen on the slide. The slides are examined under a microscope for the presence of fungal elements: mycelium, mycelial fragments, spores, or budding yeast cells. The KOH test is used in conjunction with the wet prep because the KOH destroys bacterial and epithelial cells while leaving fungal elements clearly visible, if present.

POST-TEST:

- Inform the patient that a report of the results will be made available to the requesting HCP, who will discuss the results with the patient.
- Instruct patient to begin antifungal therapy, as prescribed. Instruct the patient in the importance of completing the entire course of antifungal therapy even if no symptoms are present.
- Recognize anxiety related to test results. Discuss the implications of

abnormal test results on the patient's lifestyle. Provide teaching and information regarding the clinical implications of the test results, as appropriate.

- Reinforce information given by the patient's HCP regarding further testing, treatment, or referral to another HCP. Emphasize the importance of reporting continued signs and symptoms of the infection. Answer any questions or address any concerns voiced by the patient or family. Educate the adult patient regarding good oral and personal hygiene. Educate the parents or caregivers of infants or children with thrush (oral *Candida* infection) regarding the mechanism for transmission of the infection; stress the importance of keeping bottle-feeding equipment (especially nipples), pacifiers, and toys, cleaned and disinfected or sterilized, as appropriate, on a regular basis. Stress the importance of good hand hygiene for all who come in contact with the infant/child whose immune system is still developing and may be at higher risk for infection. Diaper rash, or diaper candidiasis, may be instigated by changes in diet or frequent stools that affect the integrity of the infant or child's delicate skin and allow an opportunity for infection to occur. Discuss the importance of frequent diaper changes and proper cleansing of the genital area with the parents or caregivers of infants or children with diaper rash.
- Depending on the results of this procedure, additional testing may be performed to evaluate or monitor progression of the disease process and determine the need for a change in therapy. Evaluate test results in relation to the patient's symptoms and other tests performed.

RELATED STUDIES:

- Related tests include relevant biopsies (lung, lymph node, skin), bronchoscopy, cultures (blood, mycobacteria, throat, sputum, viral), CSF analysis, gallium scan, HIV-1/2 antibodies, pulmonary function tests, and TB tests.
- Refer to the Immune System table online at Davis*Plus* for related tests by body system.

Culture and Smear, Mycobacteria

SYNONYM/ACRONYM: Acid-fast bacilli (AFB) culture and smear, tuberculosis (TB) culture and smear, *Mycobacterium* culture and smear.

COMMON USE: To assist in the diagnosis of tuberculosis.

SPECIMEN: Sputum, bronchopulmonary lavage, tissue, material from fine-needle aspiration, bone marrow, cerebrospinal fluid (CSF), gastric aspiration, urine, and stool.

NORMAL FINDINGS: (Method: Culture on selected media, microscopic examination of sputum by acid-fast or auramine-rhodamine fluorochrome stain) Rapid methods include: chemiluminescent-labelled DNA probes that target ribosomal RNA of the *Mycobacterium* radiometric carbon dioxide detection from ^{14}C-labelled media, polymerase chain reaction/amplification techniques.

Culture: No growth
Smear: Negative for AFB
Rapid Testing Method: Mycobacterium

POTENTIAL MEDICAL DIAGNOSIS

Identified Organism	Primary Specimen Source	Condition
Mycobacterium avium intracellulare	CSF, lymph nodes, semen, sputum, urine	Opportunistic pulmonary infection
M. fortuitum	Bone, body fluid, sputum, surgical wound, tissue	Opportunistic infection (usually pulmonary)
M. leprae	CSF, skin scrapings, lymph nodes	Hanson's disease (leprosy)
M. kansasii	Joint, lymph nodes, skin, sputum	Pulmonary tuberculosis
M. marinum	Joint	Granulomatous skin lesions
M. tuberculosis	CSF, gastric washing, sputum, urine	Pulmonary tuberculosis
M. xenopi	Sputum	Pulmonary tuberculosis

CRITICAL FINDINGS:

- *Smear:* Positive for AFB
- *Rapid Testing Method:* Positive for *Mycobacterium*
- *Culture:* Growth of pathogenic bacteria

Note and immediately report to the requesting health-care provider (HCP) any critical findings and related symptoms. A listing of these findings varies among facilities. Timely notification of a critical finding for laboratory or diagnostic studies is a role expectation of the professional nurse. The notification processes vary among facilities. Upon receipt of the critical finding the information should be read back to the caller to verify accuracy. Lists of specific organisms may vary among facilities; specific organisms are required to be reported to local, state, and national departments of health. 🍁

Find and print out the full study on Fast Find at davispl.us/vanleeuwen7.

Culture, Bacterial, Anal/Genital, Ear, Eye, Skin, and Wound

SYNONYM/ACRONYM: N/A

COMMON USE: To identify pathogenic bacterial organisms as an indicator for appropriate therapeutic interventions for multiple sites of infection.

SPECIMEN: Sterile fluid or swab from affected area placed in transport media tube provided by laboratory.

NORMAL FINDINGS: (Method: Culture aerobic and/or anaerobic on selected media; cell culture followed by use of direct immunofluorescence, nucleic acid amplification, polymerase chain reaction [PCR], and DNA probe assays [e.g., Gen-Probe] are available for identification of *Neisseria gonorrhoeae*, *Streptococcus agalactiae* (group B streptococcus), and *Chlamydia trachomatis*.) Culture, negative: No growth of pathogens. Culture-enhanced PCR or other DNA assays, negative: None detected.

DESCRIPTION: When indicated by patient history, anal and genital cultures may be performed to isolate the organism responsible for sexually transmitted infections (STIs). Chlamydia, gonorrhea, and syphilis are reportable STIs. Anal and genital cultures may also be performed on pregnant women to identify the presence of group B streptococcus (GBS), a significant and serious neonatal infection transmitted as the newborn passes through the birth canal of colonized mothers. Neonatal GBS is the most common cause of sepsis, pneumonia, and meningitis in newborns. The disease is classified as either early onset (first week of life) or late onset (after the first week of life). The Centers for Disease Control and Prevention (CDC), American Academy of Family Physicians, American Academy of Pediatrics, American College of Nurse-Midwives, and American College of Obstetricians and Gynecologists recommend universal screening for all pregnant women at 35 to 37 weeks' gestation. 🍁 Pregnant patients with positive results for a GBS urinary tract infection at any time during pregnancy should receive appropriate medical treatment at the time of diagnosis and also receive intrapartum antibiotic prophylaxis to offer continued protection in the absence of complete eradication of the infection at the time of delivery. Rapid GBS test kits can provide results within minutes on vaginal or rectal fluid swab specimens submitted in a sterile red-top tube. Negative rapid test findings should be followed up with culture and Gram stain or culture-enhanced molecular methods.

Ear and eye cultures are performed to isolate the organism responsible for chronic or acute infectious disease of the ear and eye.

Skin and soft tissue samples from infected sites must be collected carefully to avoid contamination from the surrounding normal skin flora. Skin and tissue infections may be caused by both aerobic and anaerobic organisms. Therefore, a portion of the sample should be placed in aerobic and a portion in anaerobic transport media. Care must be taken to use transport media that are approved by the laboratory performing the testing.

Sterile fluids can be collected from the affected site. Refer to related body fluid studies (i.e., amniotic fluid, cerebrospinal fluid, pericardial fluid, peritoneal fluid, pleural fluid, synovial fluid) for specimen collection.

A wound culture involves collecting a specimen of exudates, drainage, or tissue so that the causative organism can be isolated and pathogens identified. Specimens can be obtained from superficial and deep wounds.

Optimally, specimens should be obtained before antibiotic use. The method used to culture and grow the organism depends on the suspected infectious organism. There are transport media specifically for bacterial organisms. The laboratory will select the appropriate media for suspect organisms and will initiate antibiotic sensitivity testing if indicated by test results. Sensitivity testing identifies the antibiotics to which organisms are susceptible to ensure an effective treatment plan.

C

This procedure is contraindicated for: N/A

INDICATIONS

Anal/Genital

- Assist in the diagnosis of STIs.
- Determine the cause of genital itching or purulent drainage.
- Determine effective antimicrobial therapy specific to the identified pathogen.
- Routine prenatal screening for vaginal and rectal GBS colonization.

Ear

- Isolate and identify organisms responsible for ear pain, drainage, or changes in hearing.
- Isolate and identify organisms responsible for outer-, middle-, or inner-ear infection.
- Determine effective antimicrobial therapy specific to the identified pathogen.

Eye

- Isolate and identify pathogenic microorganisms responsible for infection of the eye.
- Determine effective antimicrobial therapy specific to identified pathogen.

Skin

- Isolate and identify organisms responsible for skin eruptions, drainage, or other evidence of infection.
- Determine effective antimicrobial therapy specific to the identified pathogen.

Sterile Fluids

- Isolate and identify organisms before surrounding tissue becomes infected.
- Determine effective antimicrobial therapy specific to the identified pathogen.

Wound

- Detect abscess or deep-wound infectious process.
- Determine if an infectious organism is the cause of wound redness, warmth, or edema with drainage at a site.
- Determine presence of infectious organisms in a stage 3 and stage 4 decubitus ulcer.
- Isolate and identify organisms responsible for the presence of pus or other exudate in an open wound.
- Determine effective antimicrobial therapy specific to the identified pathogen.

POTENTIAL MEDICAL DIAGNOSIS

Positive findings in

Anal/Endocervical/Genital

Infections or carrier states are caused by the following organisms: *C. trachomatis,* obligate intracellular bacteria without a cell wall, gram-variable *Gardnerella vaginalis,* gram-negative *N. gonorrhoeae, Treponema pallidum,* and toxin-producing strains of gram-positive *Staphylococcus aureus* and gram-positive GBS.

Ear

Commonly identified gram-negative organisms include *Escherichia coli, Proteus* spp., *Pseudomonas aeruginosa,* gram-positive *S. aureus,* and β-hemolytic streptococci.

Eye

Commonly identified organisms include *C. trachomatis* (transmitted to newborns from infected mothers), gram-negative

Haemophilus influenzae (transmitted to newborns from infected mothers), *H. aegyptius, N. gonorrhoeae* (transmitted to newborns from infected mothers), *P. aeruginosa,* gram-positive *S. aureus,* and *Streptococcus pneumoniae*.

Skin

Commonly identified gram-negative organisms include *Bacteroides, Pseudomonas,* gram-positive *Clostridium, Corynebacterium,* staphylococci, and group A streptococci.

Sterile Fluids

Commonly identified pathogens include gram-negative *Bacteroides, E. coli, P. aeruginosa,* gram-positive *Enterococcus* spp., and *Peptostreptococcus* spp.

Wound

Aerobic and anaerobic microorganisms can be identified in wound culture specimens. Commonly identified gram-negative organisms include *Klebsiella, Proteus,* and *Pseudomonas* and gram-positive *Clostridium perfringens, S. aureus,* and group A streptococci.

CRITICAL FINDINGS:

- *Listeria* in genital cultures; listeriosis in pregnant women may result in premature birth, miscarriage, or stillbirth. The earlier in pregnancy the infection occurs, the more likely that it will lead to miscarriage or fetal death. After 20 weeks' gestation, listeriosis is more likely to cause premature labor and birth.
- Methicillin-resistant *S. aureus* in skin or wound cultures
- GBS in urine or anal/genital cultures

Note and immediately report to the requesting health-care provider (HCP) any critical findings and related symptoms. A listing of these findings varies among facilities; specific organisms are required to be reported to local, state, and national departments of health. Timely notification of a critical finding for laboratory or diagnostic studies is a role expectation of the professional nurse. The notification processes vary among facilities. Upon receipt of the critical finding, the information should be read back to the caller to verify accuracy.

INTERFERING FACTORS

- Failure to collect adequate specimen, improper collection or storage technique, and failure to transport specimen in a timely fashion are causes for specimen rejection.
- Pretest antimicrobial therapy will delay or inhibit the growth of pathogens.
- Testing specimens more than 1 hr after collection may result in decreased growth or no growth of organisms.

NURSING IMPLICATIONS AND PROCEDURE

PRETEST:

- Positively identify the patient using at least two person-specific identifiers before services, treatments, or procedures are performed.
- *Patient Teaching:* Inform the patient that test can assist in identification of the organism causing infection.
- Obtain a history of the patient's health concerns, as appropriate, a history of sexual activity, symptoms, surgical procedures, and results of previously performed laboratory and diagnostic studies. Include a list of known allergens, especially allergies or sensitivities to latex.
- Obtain a list of the patient's current medications, including over-the-counter medications and dietary supplements (see Effects of Natural Products on Laboratory Values online at Davis*Plus*).

- Note any recent medications that can interfere with test results.
- Review the procedure with the patient. Inform the patient that specimen collection takes approximately 5 min. Address concerns about pain and explain that there may be some discomfort during the specimen collection. Instruct female patients not to douche for 24 hr before a cervical or vaginal specimen is to be obtained.
- ***Sensitivity to social and cultural issues,*** as well as concern for modesty, is important in providing psychological support before, during, and after the procedure.
- Note that there are no food or fluid restrictions unless by medical direction.

C

INTRATEST:

Potential Complications: N/A

- Ensure that the patient has complied with medication restrictions prior to the procedure.
- Instruct the patient to cooperate fully and to follow directions. Direct the patient to breathe normally and to avoid unnecessary movement.
- Observe standard precautions, and follow the general guidelines in Patient Preparation and Specimen Collection online at Davis*Plus*. Positively identify the patient, and label the appropriate specimen containers with the corresponding patient demographics, specify the exact specimen source/origin (e.g., vaginal lesion or ear, left or right, as appropriate), patient age and gender, date and time of collection, and any medication the patient is taking that may interfere with the test results (e.g., antibiotics). Do not freeze the specimen or allow it to dry. Chlamydia is an intracellular obligate pathogen. Culture of infected epithelial cells is considered the gold standard for the identification of chlamydia because of the higher sensitivity of nucleic acid amplification or DNA probe assays relative to antibody assays. Therefore, culture should always be the test of choice in cases of suspected or known child abuse.

Anal

- Place the patient in a lithotomy or side-lying position and drape for privacy. Insert the swab 1 in. into the anal canal and rotate, moving it from side to side to allow it to come into contact with the microorganisms. Remove the swab. Place the swab in the Culturette tube, and squeeze the bottom of the tube to release the transport medium. Ensure that the end of the swab is immersed in the medium. Repeat with a clean swab if the swab is pushed into feces.

Genital

Female Patient

- Position the patient on the gynecological examination table with the feet up in stirrups. Drape the patient's legs to provide privacy and reduce chilling.
- Cleanse the external genitalia and perineum from front to back with towelettes provided in culture kit. Using a Culturette swab, obtain a sample of the lesion or discharge from the urethra or vulva. Place the swab in the Culturette tube, and squeeze the bottom of the tube to release the transport medium. Ensure that the end of the swab is immersed in the medium.
- To obtain a vaginal and endocervical culture, insert a water-lubricated vaginal speculum. Insert the swab into the cervical orifice and rotate the swab to collect the secretions containing the microorganisms. Remove and place in the appropriate culture medium or Gen-Probe transport tube. Material from the vagina can be collected by moving a swab along the sides of the vaginal mucosa. The swab is removed and then placed in a tube of saline medium.

Male Patient

- To obtain a urethral culture, cleanse the penis (retracting the foreskin), have the patient milk the penis to express discharge from the urethra. Insert a swab into the urethral orifice and rotate the swab to obtain a sample of the discharge. Place the swab in the Culturette or Gen-Probe transport tube, and squeeze the bottom of the tube to release the transport medium. Ensure that the end of the swab is immersed in the medium.

Ear

- Cleanse the area surrounding the site with a swab containing cleaning solution to remove any contaminating material or flora that have collected in the ear canal. If needed, assist the appropriate HCP in removing any cerumen that has collected.
- Insert a Culturette swab approximately 1/4 in. into the external ear canal. Rotate the swab in the area containing the exudate. Carefully remove the swab, ensuring that it does not touch the side or opening of the ear canal.
- Place the swab in the Culturette tube, and squeeze the bottom of the tube to release the transport medium. Ensure that the end of the swab is immersed in the medium.

Eye

- Pass a moistened swab over the appropriate site, avoiding eyelid and eyelashes unless those areas are selected for study. Collect any visible pus or other exudate. Place the swab in the Culturette or Gen-Probe transport tube, and squeeze the bottom of the tube to release the transport medium. Ensure that the end of the swab is immersed in the medium.
- An appropriate HCP should perform procedures requiring eye culture.

Skin

- Assist the appropriate HCP in obtaining a skin sample from several areas of the affected site. If indicated, the dark, moist areas of the folds of the skin and outer growing edges of the infection where microorganisms are most likely to flourish should be selected. Place the scrapings in a collection container or spread on a slide. Aspirate any fluid from a pustule or vesicle using a sterile needle and tuberculin syringe. The exudate will be flushed into a sterile collection tube. If the lesion is not fluid filled, open the lesion with a scalpel and swab the area with a sterile cotton-tipped swab. Place the swab in the Culturette tube, and squeeze the bottom of the tube to release the transport medium. Ensure that the end of the swab is immersed in the medium.

Sterile Fluid

- Refer to related body fluid studies (i.e., amniotic fluid, cerebrospinal fluid, pericardial fluid, peritoneal fluid, pleural fluid, synovial fluid, urine) for specimen collection.

Wound

- Place the patient in a comfortable position, and drape the site to be cultured. Cleanse the area around the wound to remove flora indigenous to the skin.
- Place a Culturette swab in a superficial wound where the exudate is the most excessive without touching the wound edges. Place the swab in the Culturette tube, and squeeze the bottom of the tube to release the transport medium. Ensure that the end of the swab is immersed in the medium. Use more than one swab and Culturette tube to obtain specimens from other areas of the wound.
- To obtain a deep wound specimen, insert a sterile syringe and needle into the wound and aspirate the drainage. Following aspiration, inject the material into a tube containing an anaerobic culture medium.

General

- Promptly transport the specimen to the laboratory for processing and analysis.

POST-TEST:

- Instruct the patient to resume usual medication as directed by the HCP.
- Instruct the patient to report symptoms such as pain related to tissue inflammation or irritation.
- Instruct the patient to begin antibiotic therapy, as prescribed. Instruct the patient in the importance of completing the entire course of antibiotic therapy even if no symptoms are present.

- Inform the patient that a repeat culture may be needed in 1 wk after completion of the antimicrobial regimen.
- Advise the patient that final test results may take 24 to 72 hr depending on the method used and organism suspected but that antibiotic therapy may be started immediately.

C

Anal/Endocervical/Genital
- Advise the patient to avoid sexual contact until test results are available.
- Instruct the patient in vaginal suppository and medicated cream installation and administration of topical medication to treat specific conditions, as indicated.
- Inform infected patients that all sexual partners must be tested for the microorganism.
- Inform the patient that positive culture findings for certain organisms must be reported to a local health department official, who will question him or her regarding sexual partners.
- ***Social and Cultural Considerations:*** Offer support, as appropriate, to patients who may be the victims of sexual assault. Educate the patient regarding access to counseling services. Provide a nonjudgmental, nonthreatening atmosphere for discussing the risks of STIs. It is also important to address problems the patient may experience (e.g., guilt, depression, anger).

Wound
- Instruct the patient in wound care and nutritional requirements (e.g., protein, vitamin C) to promote wound healing.

General
- Inform the patient that a report of the results will be made available to the requesting HCP, who will discuss the results with the patient.
- Recognize anxiety related to test results. Discuss the implications of abnormal test results on the patient's lifestyle. Provide teaching and information regarding the clinical implications of the test results, as appropriate.
- Reinforce information given by the patient's HCP regarding further testing, treatment, or referral to another HCP. Emphasize the importance of reporting continued signs and symptoms of the infection. Provide information regarding vaccine-preventable diseases, as indicated (e.g., cervical cancer, hepatitis A and B, human papillomavirus). Provide contact information, if desired, for the CDC (www.cdc.gov/vaccines/vpd-vac) 🍁 for guidelines on vaccine-preventable diseases. Answer any questions or address any concerns voiced by the patient or family.
- Instruct the patient in the use of any ordered medications (oral, topical, drops). Instruct the patient in the proper use of sterile technique for cleansing the affected site and application of dressings, as directed. Explain the importance of adhering to the therapy regimen. As appropriate, instruct the patient in significant adverse effects associated with the prescribed medication. Encourage him or her to review corresponding literature provided by a pharmacist.
- Depending on the results of this procedure, additional testing may be performed to evaluate or monitor progression of the disease process and determine the need for a change in therapy. Evaluate test results in relation to the patient's symptoms and other tests performed.

RELATED STUDIES:
- Related tests include relevant amniotic fluid analysis, antimicrobial drugs, audiometry hearing loss, biopsy site, CSF analysis, culture viral, Gram stain, otoscopy, pericardial fluid analysis, Pap smear, peritoneal fluid analysis, pleural fluid analysis, procalcitonin, spondee speech reception threshold, synovial fluid analysis, syphilis serology, tuning fork tests, vitamin C, and zinc.
- Refer to the Immune System table online at Davis*Plus* for related tests by body system.

Culture, Bacterial, Blood

SYNONYM/ACRONYM: N/A

COMMON USE: To identify pathogenic bacterial organisms in the blood as an indicator for appropriate therapeutic interventions for sepsis.

SPECIMEN: Whole blood collected in bottles containing standard aerobic and anaerobic culture media.

NORMAL FINDINGS: (Method: Growth of organisms in standard culture media identified by radiometric or infrared automation, by manual reading of subculture, or polymerase chain reaction [PCR].) Negative: no growth of pathogens.

DESCRIPTION: Pathogens can enter the bloodstream from soft-tissue infection sites, contaminated intravenous lines, or invasive procedures (e.g., surgery, tooth extraction, cystoscopy). Blood cultures are collected whenever bacteremia (bacterial infection of the blood) or septicemia (a condition of systemic infection caused by pathogenic organisms or their toxins) is suspected. Although mild bacteremia is found in many infectious diseases, a persistent, continuous, or recurrent bacteremia indicates a more serious condition that may require immediate treatment. Early detection of pathogens in the blood may aid in making clinical and etiological diagnoses.

Blood cultures can detect the presence of bacteria and fungi. Organisms can be classified in a number of ways; blood culture findings use oxygen requirements to categorize findings into one of two groups. Blood culture begins with the introduction of a blood specimen into 2 types of culture medium. The medium is designed to promote the growth of organisms; one group of organisms require oxygen (aerobic) and the other either requires sparing amounts to no oxygen at all (anaerobic).

A blood culture may also be done with an antimicrobial removal device (ARD) if antibiotic therapy is initiated prior to specimen collection. This involves transferring some of the blood sample into a special vial containing absorbent resins that remove antibiotics from the sample before the culture is performed.

Traditional automated culture methods entail incubation of inoculated culture containers for a specific length of time, at a specific temperature, and under other conditions suitable for growth. If organisms are present, they will produce carbon dioxide as they metabolize the nutrients in the culture media. The presence of carbon dioxide in the culture is detected when the culture bottles are "read" by an instrument at specified intervals over a period of time. There are a number of automated blood culture systems with sophisticated computerized algorithms. The complex software allows for frequent monitoring of growth throughout the day and rapid interpretation of culture findings.

With these systems, as soon as a positive culture is detected, usually within 24 to 72 hr, the bottle can be removed from the system and a Gram stain performed to provide a preliminary identification of the bacteria present. This preliminary report provides an opportunity for the health-care provider (HCP) to initiate therapy. A sample from the positive blood culture bottle is then subcultured on the appropriate plated media for growth, isolation, and positive identification of the organism. The plated organisms are also used for sensitivity testing, if indicated. Sensitivity testing identifies the antibiotics to which the organisms are susceptible to ensure an effective treatment plan and can take several days. Negative cultures are generally removed from the automated culture system after 5 days and finalized as having "no growth." The subspecialty of microbiology has been revolutionized by molecular diagnostics. Molecular diagnostics involves the identification of specific sequences of DNA. The application of molecular diagnostics techniques, such as PCR, has led to the development of automated instruments that can identify a single infectious organism or multiple pathogens from a small amount of blood in less than 2 hr. The instruments can detect the presence of gram-negative bacteria, gram-positive bacteria, and yeast commonly associated with bloodstream infections. The instruments can also detect mutations in the genetic material of specific pathogens that code for antibiotic resistance.

This procedure is contraindicated for

If the patient has a history of severe allergic reaction to any of the materials in the iodine disinfectant solution, care should be taken to avoid the use of iodine disinfectant solutions.

INDICATIONS

- Determine sepsis in the newborn as a result of prolonged labor, early rupture of membranes, maternal infection, or neonatal aspiration.
- Evaluate chills and fever in patients with infected burns, urinary tract infections, rapidly progressing tissue infection, postoperative wound sepsis, and indwelling venous or arterial catheter.
- Evaluate intermittent or continuous temperature elevation of unknown origin.
- Evaluate persistent, intermittent fever associated with a heart murmur.
- Evaluate a sudden change in pulse and temperature with or without chills and diaphoresis.
- Evaluate suspected bacteremia after invasive procedures.
- Identify the cause of shock in the postoperative period.

POTENTIAL MEDICAL DIAGNOSIS

Positive findings in

- Bacteremia or septicemia: Gram-negative organisms such as *Aerobacter, Bacteroides, Brucella, Escherichia coli* and other coliform bacilli, *Haemophilus influenzae, Klebsiella, Pseudomonas aeruginosa,* and *Salmonella*.
- Bacteremia or septicemia: Gram-positive organisms such as *Clostridium perfringens, Enterococci, Listeria monocytogenes, Staphylococcus aureus, S. epidermidis*, and β-hemolytic streptococci.
- Plague

- Malaria (by special request, a stained capillary smear would be examined)
- Typhoid fever

Note: *Candida albicans* is a yeast that can cause disease and can be isolated by blood culture.

CRITICAL FINDINGS:

- Positive findings in any sterile body fluid such as blood

Note and immediately report to the requesting health-care provider (HCP) any critical findings and related symptoms. A listing of these findings varies among facilities. Timely notification of a critical finding for laboratory or diagnostic studies is a role expectation of the professional nurse. The notification processes vary among facilities. Upon receipt of the critical finding, the information should be read back to the caller to verify accuracy.

Assess for signs and symptoms of sepsis or development of septic shock to include change in body temperature (greater than 101.3°F or less than 95°F 🍁); decreased systolic blood pressure (less than 90 mm Hg); increased heart rate (greater than 90 beats per minute); sudden change in mental status (restlessness, agitation or confusion); significantly decreased urine output (less than 30 mL/hr); increased respirations (greater than 20 breaths/min); change in extremities (pale, mottled, and/or cyanotic in appearance); decreased or absent peripheral pulses.

INTERFERING FACTORS

- Pretest antimicrobial therapy will delay or inhibit growth of pathogens.
- Contamination of the specimen by the skin's resident flora may invalidate interpretation of test results.
- An inadequate amount of blood or number of blood specimens drawn for examination may invalidate interpretation of results.
- Testing specimens more than 1 hr after collection may result in decreased growth or no growth of organisms. Delay in transport of specimen to the laboratory may result in specimen rejection. Verify submission requirements with the laboratory prior to specimen collection.
- Collection of the specimen in an expired media tube will result in specimen rejection.
- Negative findings do not ensure the absence of infection.

NURSING IMPLICATIONS AND PROCEDURE

PRETEST:

- Positively identify the patient using at least two person-specific identifiers before services, treatments, or procedures are performed.
- ***Patient Teaching:*** Inform the patient this test can assist in identification of the organism causing infection.
- Obtain a history of the patient's health concerns, symptoms, surgical procedures, and results of previously performed laboratory and diagnostic studies. Include a list of known allergens, especially allergies or sensitivities to latex or iodine disinfectant solutions.
- Obtain a list of the patient's current medications, including over-the-counter medications and dietary supplements (see Effects of Natural Products on Laboratory Values online at Davis*Plus*).
- Note any recent medications that can interfere with test results.
- Review the procedure with the patient. Inform the patient that specimen collection takes approximately 5 min. Inform the patient that multiple specimens may be required at timed intervals. Address concerns about pain and explain to the patient that there may be some discomfort during the venipuncture. Consider the use of pediatric culture tubes, if appropriate for the patient's age.

- ***Sensitivity to social and cultural issues,*** as well as concern for modesty, is important in providing psychological support before, during, and after the procedure.
- Note that there are no food or fluid restrictions unless by medical direction.

C

INTRATEST:

Potential Complications: N/A

- Ensure that the patient has complied with medication restrictions prior to the study, as instructed.
- Avoid the use of iodine solutions if the patient has a history of severe allergic reaction to any of the materials in the iodine solution.
- Instruct the patient to cooperate fully and to follow directions. Direct the patient to breathe normally and to avoid unnecessary movement.
- Observe standard precautions, and follow the general guidelines in Patient Preparation and Specimen Collection online at Davis*Plus*. Positively identify the patient, and label the appropriate specimen containers with the corresponding patient demographics, date and time of collection, and any medication the patient is taking that may interfere with test results (e.g., antibiotics). Perform a venipuncture; collect the specimen in the appropriate blood culture collection container.
- The high risk for contamination of blood cultures by skin and other flora can be dramatically reduced by careful preparation of the puncture site and collection containers before specimen collection. Cleanse the rubber stoppers of the collection containers with the appropriate disinfectant as recommended by the laboratory, allow to air-dry, and cleanse with 70% alcohol. Once the vein has been located by palpation, cleanse the site with 70% alcohol followed by swabbing with an iodine disinfectant solution. The iodine disinfectant solution should be swabbed in a circular, concentric motion, moving outward or away from the puncture site. The iodine disinfectant solution should be allowed to completely dry before the sample is collected. If the patient is sensitive to iodine disinfectant solutions, a double alcohol scrub or green soap may be substituted.
- If collection is performed by directly drawing the sample into a culture tube, fill the aerobic culture tube first.
- If collection is performed using a syringe, transfer the blood sample directly into each culture bottle.
- Remove the needle and apply direct pressure with a dry gauze to stop bleeding. Observe/assess venipuncture site for bleeding and secure gauze with adhesive bandage.
- Promptly transport the specimen to the laboratory for processing and analysis.
- More than three sets of cultures per day do not significantly add to the likelihood of pathogen capture. Capture rates are more likely affected by obtaining a sufficient volume of blood per culture.
- The use of ARDs or resin bottles is costly and controversial with respect to their effectiveness versus standard culture techniques. They may be useful in selected cases, such as when septicemia or bacteremia is suspected after antimicrobial therapy has been initiated.

Disease Suspected	Recommended Collection
Bacterial pneumonia, fever of unknown origin, meningitis, osteomyelitis, sepsis	Two sets of cultures, each collected from a separate site, 30 min apart
Acute or subacute endocarditis	Three sets of cultures, each collected from a separate site, 30–40 min apart. If cultures are negative after 24–48 hr, repeat collections

Disease Suspected	Recommended Collection
Septicemia, fungal or mycobacterial infection in immunocompromised patient	Two sets of cultures, each collected from a separate site, 30–60 min apart (laboratory may use a lysis concentration technique to enhance recovery)
Septicemia, bacteremia after therapy has been initiated, or request to monitor effectiveness of antimicrobial therapy	Two sets of cultures, each collected from a separate site, 30–60 min apart (consider use of ARD to enhance recovery)

POST-TEST:

- Inform the patient that a report of the results will be made available to the requesting HCP, who will discuss the results with the patient.
- Instruct the patient to resume usual medication as directed by the HCP.
- Cleanse the iodine solution from the collection site.
- Instruct the patient to report symptoms such as pain related to tissue inflammation or irritation.
- Instruct the patient to report fever, chills, and other signs and symptoms of acute infection to the HCP.
- Instruct the patient to begin antibiotic therapy, as prescribed. Instruct the patient in the importance of completing the entire course of antibiotic therapy even if no symptoms are present.
- Inform the patient that preliminary results should be available in 24 to 72 hr, but final culture results are not available for 5 to 7 days. Test results for PCR methods are generally available a few hours after testing is completed.
- Recognize anxiety related to test results. Discuss the implications of abnormal test results on the patient's lifestyle. Provide teaching and information regarding the clinical implications of the test results, as appropriate.
- Reinforce information given by the patient's HCP regarding further testing, treatment, or referral to another HCP. Emphasize the importance of reporting continued signs and symptoms of the infection. Provide information regarding vaccine-preventable diseases, as indicated (e.g., *Haemophilus influenza,* meningococcal disease). Provide contact information, if desired, for the Centers for Disease Control and Prevention (www.cdc.gov/vaccines/vpd-vac) 🍁 for guidelines on vaccine-preventable diseases. Answer any questions or address any concerns voiced by the patient or family.
- Depending on the results of this procedure, additional testing may be performed to evaluate or monitor progression of the disease process and determine the need for a change in therapy. Evaluate test results in relation to the patient's symptoms and other tests performed.

RELATED STUDIES:

- Related tests include bone scan, bronchoscopy, CBC, cultures (fungal, mycobacteria, throat, sputum, viral), CSF analysis, ESR, gallium scan, Gram stain, HIV-1/2 antibodies, MRI musculoskeletal, procalcitonin, PFT, radiography bone, and TB tests.
- Refer to the Immune System table online at Davis*Plus* for related tests by body system.

Culture, Bacterial, Sputum

SYNONYM/ACRONYM: Routine culture of sputum.

COMMON USE: To identify pathogenic bacterial organisms in the sputum as an indicator for appropriate therapeutic interventions for respiratory infections.

SPECIMEN: Sputum.

NORMAL FINDINGS: (Method: Aerobic culture on selective and enriched media; microscopic examination of sputum by Gram stain.) The presence of normal upper respiratory tract flora should be expected. Tracheal aspirates and bronchoscopy samples can be contaminated with normal flora, but transtracheal aspiration specimens should show no growth. Normal respiratory flora include *Neisseria catarrhalis, Candida albicans,* diphtheroids, α-hemolytic streptococci, and some staphylococci. The presence of normal flora does not rule out infection. A normal Gram stain of sputum contains polymorphonuclear leukocytes, alveolar macrophages, and a few squamous epithelial cells.

DESCRIPTION: This test involves collecting a sputum specimen so the pathogen can be isolated and identified. The test results will reflect the type and number of organisms present in the specimen as well as the antibiotics to which the identified pathogenic organisms are susceptible. Sputum collected by expectoration or suctioning with catheters and by bronchoscopy cannot be cultured for anaerobic organisms; instead, transtracheal aspiration or lung biopsy must be used. The laboratory will initiate antibiotic sensitivity testing if indicated by test results. Sensitivity testing identifies antibiotics to which the organisms are susceptible to ensure an effective treatment plan.

This procedure is contraindicated for: N/A

INDICATIONS

Culture

- Assist in the diagnosis of respiratory infections, as indicated by the presence or absence of organisms in culture.

Gram Stain

- Assist in the differentiation of gram-positive from gram-negative bacteria in respiratory infection.
- Assist in the differentiation of sputum from upper respiratory tract secretions, the latter being indicated by excessive squamous cells or absence of polymorphonuclear leukocytes.

POTENTIAL MEDICAL DIAGNOSIS

- The major difficulty in evaluating results is in distinguishing organisms infecting the lower respiratory tract from organisms that have colonized but not infected the lower respiratory tract. Review of the Gram stain assists in this process. The presence of greater than 25 squamous epithelial cells per low-power field indicates oral contamination, and the specimen should be rejected. The presence of many polymorphonuclear neutrophils and few squamous epithelial cells indicates that the specimen was collected from an area of infection and is satisfactory for further analysis.

- Bacterial pneumonia can be caused by *Streptococcus pneumoniae, Haemophilus influenzae,* staphylococci, and some gram-negative bacteria. Other pathogens that can be identified by culture are *Corynebacterium diphtheriae, Klebsiella pneumoniae,* and *Pseudomonas aeruginosa*. Some infectious agents, such as *C. diphtheriae,* are more fastidious in their growth requirements and cannot be cultured and identified without special treatment. Suspicion of infection by less commonly identified and/or fastidious organisms must be communicated to the laboratory to ensure selection of the proper procedure required for identification.

CRITICAL FINDINGS:

- *C. diphtheriae*
- *Legionella*

Note and immediately report to the requesting health-care provider (HCP) any critical findings and related symptoms. A listing of these findings varies among facilities; specific organisms are required to be reported to local, state, and national departments of health. Timely notification of a critical finding for laboratory or diagnostic studies is a role expectation of the professional nurse. The notification processes vary among facilities. Upon receipt of the critical finding, the information should be read back to the caller to verify accuracy.

INTERFERING FACTORS

- Contamination with oral flora may invalidate results.
- Specimen collection after antibiotic therapy has been initiated may result in inhibited or no growth of organisms.

NURSING IMPLICATIONS AND PROCEDURE

PRETEST:

- Positively identify the patient using at least two person-specific identifiers before services, treatments, or procedures are performed.
- *Patient Teaching:* Inform the patient this test can assist in identification of the organism causing infection.
- Obtain a history of the patient's health concerns, symptoms, surgical procedures, and results of previously performed laboratory and diagnostic studies. Include a list of known allergens, especially allergies or sensitivities to latex.
- Obtain a list of the patient's current medications, including over-the-counter medications and dietary supplements (see Effects of Natural Products on Laboratory Values online at Davis*Plus*).
- Note any recent medications that can interfere with test results.
- Review the procedure with the patient. Reassure the patient that he or she will be able to breathe during the procedure if specimen collection is accomplished via suction method. Ensure that oxygen has been administered 20 to 30 min before the procedure if the specimen is to be obtained by tracheal suctioning. Address concerns about pain related to the procedure. Atropine is usually given before bronchoscopy examinations to reduce bronchial secretions and prevent vagally induced bradycardia. A sedative may be given to promote relaxation. Lidocaine is sprayed in the patient's throat to reduce discomfort caused by the presence of the tube.
- Explain to the patient that the time it takes to collect a proper specimen varies according to the level of cooperation of the patient and the specimen collection site. Emphasize that sputum and saliva are not the same. Inform the patient that multiple specimens may be required at timed intervals.

- *Sensitivity to social and cultural issues,* as well as concern for modesty, is important in providing psychological support before, during, and after the procedure.

Bronchoscopy

- *Make sure a written and informed consent has been signed prior to the bronchoscopy/biopsy procedure and before administering any medications.*
- Other than antimicrobial drugs, there are no medication restrictions, unless by medical direction.
- Instruct the patient that to reduce the risk of aspiration related to nausea and vomiting, solid food and milk or milk products have been restricted for at least 6 hr, and clear liquids have been restricted for at least 2 hr prior to general anesthesia, regional anesthesia, or sedation/analgesia (monitored anesthesia). The American Society of Anesthesiologists has fasting guidelines for risk levels according to patient status. More information can be located at www.asahq.org. 🍁 Patients on beta blockers before the surgical procedure should be instructed to take their medication as ordered during the perioperative period. Protocols may vary among facilities.

Expectorated Specimen

- Additional liquids the night before may assist in liquefying secretions during expectoration the following morning.
- Assist the patient with oral cleaning before sample collection to reduce the amount of sample contamination by organisms that normally inhabit the mouth.
- Instruct the patient not to touch the edge or inside of the container with the hands or mouth.
- Other than antimicrobial drugs, there are no medication restrictions, unless by medical direction.
- There are no food or fluid restrictions, unless by medical direction.

Tracheal Suctioning

- Assist in providing extra fluids, unless contraindicated, and proper humidification to decrease tenacious secretions. Inform the patient that increasing fluid intake before retiring on the night before the test aids in liquefying secretions and may make it easier to expectorate in the morning. Also explain that humidifying inspired air also helps liquefy secretions.
- Other than antimicrobial drugs, there are no medication restrictions, unless by medical direction.
- There are no food or fluid restrictions, unless by medical direction.
- If the specimen is collected by expectoration or tracheal suctioning, there are no food, fluid, or medication restrictions (except antibiotics), unless by medical direction.

INTRATEST:

Potential Complications:

Complications associated with bronchoscopy are rare but may include bleeding, bronchial perforation, bronchospasm, infection, laryngospasm, and pneumothorax.

- Ensure that the patient has complied with dietary and medication restrictions prior to the bronchoscopy procedure, as instructed.
- Have patient remove dentures, contact lenses, eyeglasses, and jewelry. Notify the HCP if the patient has permanent crowns on teeth. Have the patient remove clothing and change into a gown for the procedure.
- Avoid the use of equipment containing latex if the patient has a history of allergic reaction to latex.
- Have emergency equipment readily available. Keep resuscitation equipment on hand in case of respiratory impairment or laryngospasm after the procedure.
- Avoid using morphine sulfate in patients with asthma or other pulmonary disease. This drug can further exacerbate bronchospasms and respiratory impairment.
- Avoid the use of equipment containing latex if the patient has a history of allergic reaction to latex.
- Assist the patient to a comfortable position and direct the patient to

breathe normally during the beginning of the general anesthesia and to avoid unnecessary movement during the local anesthetic and the procedure. Instruct the patient to cooperate fully and to follow directions.

- Observe standard precautions, and follow the general guidelines in Patient Preparation and Specimen Collection online at Davis*Plus*. Positively identify the patient, and label the appropriate tubes with the corresponding patient demographics, date and time of collection, and any medication the patient is taking that may interfere with test results (e.g., antibiotics). Collect the specimen in the appropriate sterile collection container.

Bronchoscopy

- Record baseline vital signs.
- The patient is positioned in relation to the type of anesthesia being used. If local anesthesia is used, the patient is seated and the tongue and oropharynx are sprayed and swabbed with anesthetic before the bronchoscope is inserted. For general anesthesia, the patient is placed in a supine position with the neck hyperextended. After anesthesia, the patient is kept in supine or shifted to a side-lying position and the bronchoscope is inserted. After inspection, the samples are collected from suspicious sites by bronchial brush or biopsy forceps.

Expectorated Specimen

- Ask the patient to sit upright, with assistance and support (e.g., with an overbed table) as needed.
- Ask the patient to take two or three deep breaths and cough deeply. Any sputum raised should be expectorated directly into a sterile sputum collection container.
- If the patient is unable to produce the desired amount of sputum, several strategies may be attempted. One approach is to have the patient drink two glasses of water, and then assume the position for postural drainage of the upper and middle lung segments. Effective coughing may be assisted by placing either the hands or a pillow over the diaphragmatic area and applying slight pressure.
- Another approach is to place a vaporizer or other humidifying device at the bedside. After sufficient exposure to adequate humidification, postural drainage of the upper and middle lung segments may be repeated before attempting to obtain the specimen.
- Other methods may include obtaining an order for an expectorant to be administered with additional water approximately 2 hr before attempting to obtain the specimen. Chest percussion and postural drainage of all lung segments may also be employed. If the patient is still unable to raise sputum, the use of an ultrasonic nebulizer ("induced sputum") may be necessary; this is usually done by a respiratory therapist.

Tracheal Suctioning

- Obtain the necessary equipment, including a suction device, suction kit, and Lukens tube or in-line trap.
- Position the patient with head elevated as high as tolerated.
- Put on sterile gloves. Maintain the dominant hand as sterile and the nondominant hand as clean.
- Using the sterile hand, attach the suction catheter to the rubber tubing of the Lukens tube or in-line trap. Then attach the suction tubing to the male adapter of the trap with the clean hand. Lubricate the suction catheter with sterile saline.
- Ask patients who are not intubated to protrude the tongue and to take a deep breath as the suction catheter is passed through the nostril. When the catheter enters the trachea, a reflex cough is stimulated; immediately advance the catheter into the trachea and apply suction. Maintain suction for approximately 10 sec, but never longer than 15 sec. Withdraw the catheter without applying suction. Separate the suction catheter and suction tubing from the trap, and place the rubber tubing over the male adapter to seal the unit.

C

- For patients who are intubated or patients with a tracheostomy, the previous procedure is followed except that the suction catheter is passed through the existing endotracheal or tracheostomy tube rather than through the nostril. The patient should be hyperoxygenated before and after the procedure in accordance with standard protocols for suctioning these patients.
- Generally, a series of three to five early morning sputum samples are collected in sterile containers.

General

- Monitor the patient for complications related to the procedure (e.g., allergic reaction, anaphylaxis, bronchospasm).
- Promptly transport the specimen to the laboratory for processing and analysis.

POST-TEST:

- Inform the patient that a report of the results will be made available to the requesting HCP, who will discuss the results with the patient.
- Instruct the patient to resume preoperative diet, as directed by the HCP. Assess the patient's ability to swallow before allowing the patient to attempt liquids or solid foods.
- Inform the patient that he or she may experience some throat soreness and hoarseness. Instruct patient to treat throat discomfort with lozenges and warm gargles when the gag reflex returns.
- Monitor vital signs and compare with baseline values every 15 min for 1 hr, then every 2 hr for 4 hr, and then as ordered by the HCP. Monitor temperature every 4 hr for 24 hr. Notify the HCP if temperature is elevated. Protocols may vary among facilities.
- Emergency resuscitation equipment should be readily available if the vocal cords become spastic after intubation.
- Observe for delayed allergic reactions, such as rash, urticaria, tachycardia, hyperpnea, hypertension, palpitations, nausea, or vomiting.
- Observe the patient for hemoptysis, dyspnea, cough, air hunger, excessive coughing, pain, or absent breathing sounds over the affected area. Report any symptoms to the HCP.
- Evaluate the patient for symptoms indicating the development of pneumothorax, such as dyspnea, tachypnea, anxiety, decreased breathing sounds, or restlessness. A chest x-ray may be ordered to check for the presence of this complication.
- Evaluate the patient for symptoms of empyema, such as fever, tachycardia, malaise, or elevated white blood cell count.
- Administer antibiotic therapy if ordered. Remind the patient of the importance of completing the entire course of antibiotic therapy, even if signs and symptoms disappear before completion of therapy.
- ***Nutritional Considerations:*** Malnutrition is commonly seen in patients with severe respiratory disease for numerous reasons, including fatigue, lack of appetite, and gastrointestinal distress. Adequate intake of Vitamins A and C are also important to prevent pulmonary infection and to decrease the extent of lung tissue damage.
- Recognize anxiety related to test results. Discuss the implications of abnormal test results on the patient's lifestyle. Provide teaching and information regarding the clinical implications of the test results, as appropriate. Educate the patient regarding access to counseling services.
- Reinforce information given by the patient's HCP regarding further testing, treatment, or referral to another HCP. Instruct the patient to use lozenges or gargle for throat discomfort. Inform the patient of smoking cessation programs as appropriate. The importance of following the prescribed diet should be stressed to the patient/caregiver. Educate the patient regarding access to counseling services, as appropriate. Provide information regarding vaccine preventable diseases

where indicated (e.g., H1N1 flu, *Haemophilus influenzae*, seasonal influenza, pertussis, pneumococcal disease). Provide contact information, if desired, for the Centers for Disease Control and Prevention (www.cdc.gov/vaccines/vpd-vac) for guidelines on vaccine-preventable diseases. Answer any questions or address any concerns voiced by the patient or family.

- Instruct the patient in the use of any ordered medications. Explain the importance of adhering to the therapy regimen. As appropriate, instruct the patient in significant adverse effects and systemic reactions associated with the prescribed medication. Encourage him or her to review corresponding literature provided by a pharmacist.
- Depending on the results of this procedure, additional testing may be needed to evaluate or monitor progression of the disease process and determine the need for a change in therapy. Evaluate test results in relation to the patient's symptoms and other tests performed.

RELATED STUDIES:

- Related tests include antibodies, antiglomerular basement membrane, arterial/alveolar oxygen ratio, biopsy lung, blood gases, bronchoscopy, chest x-ray, CBC, CT thoracic, culture (fungal, mycobacterium, throat, viral), cytology sputum, gallium scan, Gram stain/acid-fast stain, HIV-1/2 antibodies, lung perfusion scan, lung ventilation scan, MRI chest, mediastinoscopy, pleural fluid analysis, PFT, and TB tests.
- Refer to the Immune and Respiratory systems tables online at Davis*Plus* for related tests by body system.

Culture, Bacterial, Stool

SYNONYM/ACRONYM: N/A

COMMON USE: To identify pathogenic bacterial organisms in the stool as an indicator for appropriate therapeutic interventions to treat organisms such as *Clostridium difficile* and *Escherichia coli.*

SPECIMEN: Fresh, random stool collected in a clean plastic container.

NORMAL FINDINGS: (Method: Culture on selective media for identification of pathogens usually to include *Salmonella. Shigella, Escherichia coli* O157:H7, *Yersinia enterocolitica,* and *Campylobacter*; latex agglutination or enzyme immunoassay for *Clostridium* A and B toxins). Polymerase chain reaction (PCR) may be used to identify bacterial, protozoan, or viral pathogens. Negative: No growth of pathogens. Normal fecal flora is 96% to 99% anaerobes and 1% to 4% aerobes. Normal flora present may include *Bacteroides, Candida albicans, Clostridium, Enterococcus, E. coli, Proteus, Pseudomonas,* and *Staphylococcus aureus*.

DESCRIPTION: Stool culture involves collecting a sample of feces so that organisms present can be isolated and identified. Certain bacteria are normally found in feces. However, when overgrowth of these organisms occurs or pathological organisms are present, diarrhea or other signs and symptoms of systemic infection occur. These symptoms are the result of damage to the intestinal tissue by the pathogenic organisms. Routine stool culture normally screens for a small number of common pathogens associated with food poisoning, such as *S. aureus, Salmonella,* and *Shigella*. Identification of other bacteria is initiated by special request or upon consultation with a microbiologist when there is knowledge of special circumstances. An example of this situation is an outbreak of *C. difficile* in a long-term care facility or hospital unit where the infection can spread rapidly from one person to the next. A life-threatening *C. difficile* infection of the bowel may occur in patients who are immunocompromised or are receiving broad-spectrum antibiotic therapy (e.g., clindamycin, ampicillin, cephalosporins). The bacteria release a toxin that causes necrosis of the colon tissue. The toxin can be more rapidly identified from a stool sample using an immunochemical method than from a routine culture. Appropriate interventions can be quickly initiated and might include intravenous replacement of fluid and electrolytes, cessation of broad-spectrum antibiotic administration, and institution of vancomycin or metronidazole antibiotic therapy. The laboratory will initiate antibiotic sensitivity testing if indicated by test results. Sensitivity testing identifies the antibiotics to which organisms are susceptible to ensure an effective treatment plan. The subspecialty of microbiology has been revolutionized by molecular diagnostics. Molecular diagnostics involves the identification of specific sequences of DNA. The application of molecular diagnostics techniques, such as PCR, has led to the development of automated instruments that can identify a single infectious agent or multiple pathogens from a small amount of stool in less than 2 hr. The instruments can detect the presence of bacteria, viruses, or protozoans commonly associated with gastrointestinal infections.

This procedure is contraindicated for: N/A

INDICATIONS

- Assist in establishing a diagnosis for diarrhea of unknown etiology.
- Identify pathogenic organisms causing gastrointestinal disease and carrier states.

POTENTIAL MEDICAL DIAGNOSIS

Positive findings in

- Bacterial infection: Gram-negative organisms such as *Aeromonas* spp., *Campylobacter, E. coli* including serotype O157: H7, *Plesiomonas shigelloides, Salmonella, Shigella, Vibrio,* and *Yersinia*
- Bacterial infection: Gram-positive organisms such as *Bacillus cereus, C. difficile,* and *Listeria*. Isolation of *Staphylococcus aureus* may indicate infection or a carrier state
- Botulism: *Clostridium botulinum* (the bacteria must also be isolated from the food or the presence of toxin confirmed in the stool specimen)
- Parasitic enterocolitis

CRITICAL FINDINGS:

- Bacterial pathogens: *Campylobacter, C. difficile, E. coli* including 0157:H7, *Listeria, Rotavirus* (especially in pediatric patients), *Salmonella, Shigella, Vibrio, Yersinia,* or parasites *Acanthamoeba,*

Ascaris (hookworm), *Cyclospora, Cryptosporidium, Entamoeba histolytica, Giardia,* and *Strongyloides* (tapeworm), parasitic ova, proglottid, and larvae.

Note and immediately report to the requesting health-care provider (HCP) any critical findings and related symptoms. A listing of these findings varies among facilities. Timely notification of a critical finding for laboratory or diagnostic studies is a role expectation of the professional nurse. The notification processes vary among facilities. Upon receipt of the critical finding, the information should be read back to the caller to verify accuracy.

INTERFERING FACTORS

- A rectal swab does not provide an adequate amount of specimen for evaluating the carrier state and should be avoided in favor of a standard stool specimen.
- A rectal swab should never be submitted for *Clostridium* toxin studies. Specimens for *Clostridium* toxins should be refrigerated if they are not immediately transported to the laboratory because toxins degrade rapidly.
- A rectal swab should never be submitted for *Campylobacter* culture. Excessive exposure of the sample to air or room temperature may damage this bacterium so that it will not grow in the culture.
- Therapy with antibiotics before specimen collection may decrease the type and the amount of bacteria.
- Failure to transport the culture within 1 hr of collection or urine contamination of the sample may affect results.
- Barium and laxatives used less than 1 wk before the test may reduce bacterial growth.

NURSING IMPLICATIONS AND PROCEDURE

PRETEST:

- Positively identify the patient using at least two person-specific identifiers before services, treatments, or procedures are performed.
- ***Patient Teaching:*** Inform the patient this test can assist in identification of the organism causing infection.
- Obtain a history of the patient's health concerns, symptoms, surgical procedures, and results of previously performed laboratory and diagnostic studies. Include a list of known allergens, especially allergies or sensitivities to latex.
- Obtain a history of the patient's travel to foreign countries.
- Obtain a list of the patient's current medications, including over-the-counter medications and dietary supplements (see Effects of Natural Products on Laboratory Values online at Davis*Plus*.
- Note any recent medications that can interfere with test results.
- Review the procedure with the patient. Address concerns about pain and explain that there may be some discomfort during the specimen collection. Inform the patient that specimen collection takes approximately 5 min.
- ***Sensitivity to social and cultural issues,*** as well as concern for modesty, is important in providing psychological support before, during, and after the procedure.
- Note that there are no food or fluid restrictions unless by medical direction.

INTRATEST:

Potential Complications: N/A

- Ensure that the patient has complied with medication restrictions prior to the study, as instructed.
- Instruct the patient to cooperate fully and to follow directions. Direct the patient to breathe normally and to avoid unnecessary movement.

C

- Observe standard precautions, and follow the general guidelines in Patient Preparation and Specimen Collection online at Davis*Plus*. Positively identify the patient, and label the appropriate collection containers with the corresponding patient demographics, date and time of collection, and any medication the patient is taking that may interfere with test results (e.g., antibiotics).
- Collect a stool specimen directly into a clean container. If the patient requires a bedpan, make sure it is clean and dry, and use a tongue blade to transfer the specimen to the container. Make sure representative portions of the stool are sent for analysis. Note specimen appearance on collection container label.
- Promptly transport the specimen to the laboratory for processing and analysis.

POST-TEST:

- Inform the patient that a report of the results will be made available to the requesting HCP, who will discuss the results with the patient.
- Instruct the patient to resume usual medication as directed by the HCP.
- Instruct the patient to report symptoms such as pain related to tissue inflammation or irritation.
- Advise the patient that final test results for culture may take up to 72 hr but that antibiotic therapy may be started immediately. Test results for PCR methods are generally available a few hours after testing is completed. Instruct the patient about the importance of completing the entire course of antibiotic therapy even if no symptoms are present. Note: Antibiotic therapy is frequently contraindicated for *Salmonella* infection unless the infection has progressed to a systemic state.
- Recognize anxiety related to test results. Discuss the implications of abnormal test results on the patient's lifestyle. Provide teaching and information regarding the clinical implications of the test results, as appropriate.
- Reinforce information given by the patient's HCP regarding further testing, treatment, or referral to another HCP. Emphasize the importance of reporting continued signs and symptoms of the infection. Answer any questions or address any concerns voiced by the patient or family.
- Depending on the results of this procedure, additional testing may be performed to evaluate or monitor progression of the disease process and determine the need for a change in therapy. Evaluate test results in relation to the patient's symptoms and other tests performed.

RELATED STUDIES:

- Related tests include capsule endoscopy, colonoscopy, fecal analysis, Gram stain, ova and parasites, and proctosigmoidoscopy.
- Refer to the Gastrointestinal and Immune systems tables online at Davis*Plus* for related tests by body system.

Culture, Bacterial, Throat or Nasopharyngeal

SYNONYM/ACRONYM: Routine throat culture.

COMMON USE: To identify pathogenic bacterial organisms in the throat and nares as an indicator for appropriate therapeutic interventions. Treat infections such as pharyngitis, thrush, strep throat, and screen for methicillin-resistant *Staphylococcus aureus* (MRSA).

SPECIMEN: Throat or nasopharyngeal swab.

NORMAL FINDINGS: (Method: Aerobic culture) No growth.

DESCRIPTION: The routine throat culture is a commonly ordered test to screen for the presence of group A β-hemolytic streptococci. *Streptococcus pyogenes* is the gram-positive organism that most commonly causes acute pharyngitis. The more dangerous sequelae of scarlet fever, rheumatic heart disease, and glomerulonephritis are less frequently seen because of the early treatment of infection at the pharyngitis stage. There are a number of other bacterial organisms responsible for pharyngitis. Specific cultures can be set up to detect other pathogens such as *Bordetella* (gram negative), *Corynebacteria* (gram positive), *Haemophilus* (gram negative), or *Neisseria* (gram negative) if they are suspected or by special request from the health-care provider (HCP). *Corynebacterium diphtheriae* is the causative pathogen of diphtheria. *Neisseria gonorrhoeae* is a sexually transmitted pathogen. In children, a positive throat culture for *Neisseria* usually indicates sexual abuse. The laboratory will initiate antibiotic sensitivity testing if indicated by test results. Sensitivity testing identifies the antibiotics to which the organisms are susceptible to ensure an effective treatment plan.

This procedure is contraindicated for

Patients with epiglottitis. In cases of acute epiglottitis, the throat culture may need to be obtained in the operating room or other appropriate location where the required emergency equipment and trained personnel can safely perform the procedure.

INDICATIONS

- Assist in the diagnosis of bacterial infections such as tonsillitis, diphtheria, gonorrhea, or pertussis.
- Assist in the diagnosis of upper respiratory infections resulting in bronchitis, pharyngitis, croup, and influenza.
- Isolate and identify group A β-hemolytic streptococci as the cause of strep throat, acute glomerulonephritis, scarlet fever, or rheumatic fever.

POTENTIAL MEDICAL DIAGNOSIS

Reports on cultures that are positive for group A β-hemolytic streptococci are generally available within 24 to 48 hr. Cultures that report on normal respiratory flora are issued after 48 hr. Culture results of no growth for *Corynebacterium* require 72 hr to report; 48 hr are required to report negative *Neisseria* cultures.

CRITICAL FINDINGS:

- Culture: Growth of *Corynebacterium* or MRSA

Note and immediately report to the requesting HCP any critical findings and related symptoms. A listing of these findings varies among facilities. Timely notification of a critical finding for laboratory or diagnostic studies is a role expectation of the professional nurse. The notification processes vary among facilities. Upon receipt of the critical finding, the information should be read back to the caller to verify accuracy. Lists of specific organisms may vary among facilities; specific organisms are required to be reported to local, state, and national departments of health. 🍁

INTERFERING FACTORS

- Contamination with oral flora may invalidate results.
- Specimen collection after antibiotic therapy has been initiated may result in inhibited or no growth of organisms.

C

NURSING IMPLICATIONS AND PROCEDURE

PRETEST:

- Positively identify the patient using at least two person-specific identifiers before services, treatments, or procedures are performed.
- ***Patient Teaching:*** Inform the patient this test can assist in identification of the organism causing infection.
- Obtain a history of the patient's health concerns, symptoms, surgical procedures, and results of previously performed laboratory and diagnostic studies. Include a list of known allergens, especially allergies or sensitivities to latex.
- Obtain a list of the patient's current medications, including over-the-counter medications and dietary supplements (see Effects of Natural Products on Laboratory Values online at Davis*Plus*.
- Note any recent medications, especially antibiotics, that can interfere with test results.
- Review the procedure with the patient. Address concerns about pain and explain that there may be some discomfort during the specimen collection. The time it takes to collect a proper specimen varies according to the level of cooperation of the patient. Inform the patient that specimen collection takes approximately 5 min.
- Note that there are no food or fluid restrictions unless by medical direction.
- ***Sensitivity to social and cultural issues,*** as well as concern for modesty, is important in providing psychological support before, during, and after the procedure.

INTRATEST:

Potential Complications:

In cases of epiglottitis, do not swab the throat. This can cause a laryngospasm resulting in a loss of airway. Symptoms associated with epiglottitis include sore throat, difficulty swallowing, difficulty breathing ***(related to blocked airway),*** blue skin (especially around the lips), confusion, irritability, and sluggishness ***(related to decreased oxygen levels).*** Potential interactions include stabilizing the airway, monitoring vital signs, and administering the appropriate medications which may include antibiotics. Antibiotics may be administered before the results of the culture are obtained.

- Ensure that the patient has complied with medication restrictions prior to the procedure.
- Have emergency equipment readily available. Keep resuscitation equipment on hand in case of respiratory impairment or laryngospasm after the procedure.
- Instruct the patient to cooperate fully and to follow directions. Direct the patient to breathe normally and to avoid unnecessary movement.
- Observe standard precautions, and follow the general guidelines in Patient Preparation and Specimen Collection online at Davis*Plus*. Positively identify the patient, and label the appropriate collection containers with the corresponding patient demographics, date and time of collection, and any medication the patient is taking that may interfere with test results (e.g., antibiotics).
- To collect the throat culture, tilt the patient's head back. Swab both tonsillar pillars and oropharynx with the sterile Culturette. A tongue depressor can be used to ensure that contact with the tongue and uvula is avoided.
- A nasopharyngeal specimen is collected through the use of a flexible

probe inserted through the nose and directed toward the back of the throat.
- Place the swab in the Culturette tube and squeeze the bottom of the Culturette tube to release the liquid transport medium. Ensure that the end of the swab is immersed in the liquid transport medium.
- Promptly transport the specimen to the laboratory for processing and analysis.

POST-TEST:

- Inform the patient that a report of the results will be made available to the requesting HCP, who will discuss the results with the patient.
- Instruct the patient to resume usual medication as directed by the HCP.
- Instruct the patient to notify the HCP immediately if difficulty in breathing or swallowing occurs or if bleeding occurs.
- Instruct the patient to perform mouth care after the specimen has been obtained.
- Provide comfort measures and treatment such as antiseptic gargles; inhalants; and warm, moist applications as needed. A cool beverage may aid in relieving throat irritation caused by coughing or suctioning.
- Administer antibiotic therapy if ordered. Remind the patient of the importance of completing the entire course of antibiotic therapy, even if signs and symptoms disappear before completion of therapy.
- *Nutritional Considerations:* Dehydration can been seen in patients with a bacterial throat infection due to pain with swallowing. Pain medications reduce patient's dysphagia and allow for adequate intake of fluids and foods.
- Recognize anxiety related to test results. Discuss the implications of abnormal test results on the patient's lifestyle. Provide teaching and information regarding the clinical implications of the test results, as appropriate.
- Reinforce information given by the patient's HCP regarding further testing, treatment, or referral to another HCP. Instruct the patient to use lozenges or gargle for throat discomfort. Inform the patient of smoking cessation programs as appropriate. Emphasize the importance of reporting continued signs and symptoms of the infection. Provide information regarding vaccine-preventable diseases where indicated (e.g., diphtheria H1N1 flu, *Haemophilus influenza,* seasonal influenza, pneumococcal disease). Provide contact information, if desired, for the Centers for Disease Control and Prevention (www.cdc.gov/vaccines/vpd-vac) 🍁 for guidelines on vaccine-preventable diseases. Answer any questions or address any concerns voiced by the patient or family.
- Depending on the results of this procedure, additional testing may be performed to evaluate or monitor progression of the disease process and determine the need for a change in therapy. Evaluate test results in relation to the patient's symptoms and other tests performed.

RELATED STUDIES:

- Related tests include CBC, Gram stain, and group A streptococcal (rapid) screen.
- Refer to the Immune and Respiratory systems tables online at Davis*Plus* for related tests by body system.

Culture, Bacterial, Urine

SYNONYM/ACRONYM: Routine urine culture.

COMMON USE: To identify the pathogenic bacterial organisms in the urine as an indicator for appropriate therapeutic interventions to treat urinary tract infections.

SPECIMEN: Urine collected in a sterile plastic collection container. Transport tubes containing a preservative are highly recommended if testing will not occur within 2 hr of collection.

NORMAL FINDINGS: (Method: Culture on selective and enriched media) Negative: no growth.

C

DESCRIPTION: A urine culture involves collecting a urine specimen so that the organism causing disease can be isolated and identified. Urine can be collected by clean catch, urinary catheterization, or suprapubic aspiration. The severity of the infection or contamination of the specimen can be determined by knowing the type and number of organisms (colonies) present in the specimen. The laboratory will initiate sensitivity testing if indicated by test results. Sensitivity testing identifies the antibiotics to which the organisms are susceptible to ensure an effective treatment plan.

Commonly detected organisms are those normally found in the genitourinary tract, including gram negative *Enterococci, Escherichia coli, Klebsiella, Proteus,* and *Pseudomonas*. A culture showing multiple organisms indicates a contaminated specimen.

Colony counts of 100,000/mL or more indicate urinary tract infection (UTI).

Colony counts of 1,000/mL or less suggest contamination resulting from poor collection technique.

Colony counts between 1,000 and 10,000/mL may be significant depending on a variety of factors, including patient's age, gender, number of types of organisms present, method of specimen collection, and presence of antibiotics.

This procedure is contraindicated for: N/A

INDICATIONS

- Assist in the diagnosis of suspected UTI.
- Determine the sensitivity of significant organisms to antibiotics.
- Monitor the response to UTI treatment.

POTENTIAL MEDICAL DIAGNOSIS

Positive findings in

- UTIs

Negative findings in: N/A

CRITICAL FINDINGS:

- Gram-negative extended spectrum beta lactamases *E. coli* or *Klebsiella*
- Gram-negative *Legionella*
- Gram-positive Vancomycin-resistant *Enterococci*

Note and immediately report to the requesting health-care provider (HCP) any critical findings and related symptoms. A listing of these findings varies among facilities. Timely notification of a critical finding for laboratory or diagnostic studies is a role expectation of the professional nurse. The notification processes vary among facilities. Upon receipt of the critical finding, the information should be read back to the caller to verify accuracy. Lists of specific organisms may vary among facilities; specific organisms are required to be reported to local, state, and national departments of health. 🍁

INTERFERING FACTORS

- Antibiotic therapy initiated before specimen collection may produce false-negative results.

- Improper collection techniques may result in specimen contamination.
- Specimen storage for longer than 2 hr at room temperature or 24 hr at refrigerated temperature may result in overgrowth of bacteria and false-positive results. Such specimens may be rejected for analysis.
- Results of urine culture are often interpreted along with routine urinalysis findings.
- Discrepancies between culture and urinalysis may be reason to recollect the specimen.
- Specimens submitted in expired urine transport tubes will be rejected for analysis.

NURSING IMPLICATIONS AND PROCEDURE

PRETEST:

- Positively identify the patient using at least two person-specific identifiers before services, treatments, or procedures are performed.
- ***Patient Teaching:*** Inform the patient this test can assist in identification of the organism causing infection.
- Obtain a history of the patient's health concerns, symptoms, surgical procedures, and results of previously performed laboratory and diagnostic studies. Include a list of known allergens, especially allergies or sensitivities to latex.
- Obtain a list of the patient's current medications, including over-the-counter medications and dietary supplements (see Effects of Natural Products on Laboratory Values online at Davis*Plus*).
- Note any recent medications, especially antibiotics, that can interfere with test results.
- Review the procedure with the patient. Address concerns about pain and explain that there should be no discomfort during the specimen collection. Inform the patient that specimen collection depends on patient cooperation and usually takes approximately 5 to 10 min.
- ***Sensitivity to social and cultural issues,*** as well as concern for modesty, is important in providing psychological support before, during, and after the procedure.
- Note that there are no food or fluid restrictions, unless by medical direction.
- Instruct the patient on clean-catch procedure and provide necessary supplies.

INTRATEST:

Potential Complications: N/A

- Ensure that the patient has complied with medication restrictions prior to the study, as instructed.
- Instruct the patient to cooperate fully and to follow directions. Direct the patient to breathe normally and to avoid unnecessary movement.
- Observe standard precautions, and follow the general guidelines in Patient Preparation and Specimen Collection online at Davis*Plus*. Positively identify the patient, and label the appropriate collection containers with the corresponding patient demographics, date and time of collection, method of specimen collection, and any medications the patient has taken that may interfere with test results (e.g., antibiotics).
- Avoid the use of equipment containing latex if the patient has a history of allergic reaction to latex.

Clean-Catch Specimen

- Instruct the male patient to (1) thoroughly wash his hands, (2) cleanse the meatus, (3) void a small amount into the toilet, and (4) void directly into the specimen container.
- Instruct the female patient to (1) thoroughly wash her hands; (2) cleanse the labia from front to back; (3) while keeping the labia separated, void a small amount into the toilet; and (4) without interrupting the urine stream, void directly into the specimen container.

Pediatric Urine Collector

- Put on gloves. Appropriately cleanse the genital area, and allow the area to dry. Remove the covering over the adhesive strips on the collector bag and apply over the genital area. Diaper the child. When specimen is obtained, place the entire collection bag in a sterile urine container.

Indwelling Catheter

- Put on gloves. Empty drainage tube of urine. It may be necessary to clamp off the catheter for 15 to 30 min before specimen collection. Cleanse specimen port with antiseptic swab, and then aspirate 5 mL of urine with a 21- to 25-gauge needle and syringe. Transfer urine to a sterile container.

Urinary Catheterization

- Place female patient in lithotomy position or male patient in supine position. Using sterile technique, open the straight urinary catheterization kit and perform urinary catheterization. Place the retained urine in a sterile specimen container.

Suprapubic Aspiration

- Place the patient in supine position. Cleanse the area with antiseptic, and drape with sterile drapes. A needle is inserted through the skin into the bladder. A syringe attached to the needle is used to aspirate the urine sample. The needle is then removed and a sterile dressing is applied to the site. Place the sterile sample in a sterile specimen container.
- Do not collect urine from the pouch from a patient with a urinary diversion (e.g., ileal conduit). Instead, perform catheterization through the stoma.

General

- Promptly transport the specimen to the laboratory for processing and analysis. If a delay in transport is expected, an aliquot of the specimen into a special tube containing a preservative is recommended. Urine transport tubes can be requested from the laboratory.

POST-TEST:

- Inform the patient that a report of the results will be made available to the requesting HCP, who will discuss the results with the patient.
- Instruct the patient to resume usual medication as directed by the HCP.
- Instruct the patient to report symptoms such as pain related to tissue inflammation, pain or irritation during void, bladder spasms, or alterations in urinary elimination.
- Observe for signs of inflammation if the specimen is obtained by suprapubic aspiration.
- Administer antibiotic therapy as ordered. Remind the patient of the importance of completing the entire course of antibiotic therapy, even if signs and symptoms disappear before completion of therapy.
- ***Nutritional Considerations:*** Instruct the patient to increase water consumption by drinking 8 to 12 glasses of water to assist in flushing the urinary tract. Instruct the patient to avoid alcohol, caffeine, and carbonated beverages, which can cause bladder irritation.
- Prevention of UTIs includes increasing daily water consumption, urinating when urge occurs, wiping the perineal area from front to back after urination/defecation, and urinating immediately after intercourse. Prevention also includes maintaining the normal flora of the body. Patients should avoid using spermicidal creams with diaphragms or condoms (when recommended by an HCP), becoming constipated, douching, taking bubble baths, wearing tight-fitting garments, and using deodorizing feminine hygiene products that alter the body's normal flora and increase susceptibility to UTIs.
- Recognize anxiety related to test results. Discuss the implications of abnormal test results on the patient's lifestyle. Provide teaching and information regarding the clinical implications of the test results, as appropriate.
- Reinforce information given by the patient's HCP regarding further testing, treatment, or referral to another HCP. Emphasize the importance of reporting continued signs and symptoms of the infection. Instruct patient on the proper technique for wiping the perineal area (front to back) after

a bowel movement. Answer any questions or address any concerns voiced by the patient or family.
- Depending on the results of this procedure, additional testing may be performed to evaluate or monitor progression of the disease process and determine the need for a change in therapy. Evaluate test results in relation to the patient's symptoms and other tests performed.

RELATED STUDIES:
- Related tests include CBC, CBC WBC count and differential, cystometry, cystoscopy, cystourethrography voiding, cytology urine, Gram stain, renogram, and UA.
- Refer to the Genitourinary and Immune systems tables online at Davis*Plus* for related tests by body system.

Culture, Viral

SYNONYM/ACRONYM: N/A

COMMON USE: To identify infection caused by pathogenic viral organisms as evidenced by ocular, genitourinary, intestinal, or respiratory symptoms. Commonly identified are cytomegalovirus (CMV), Epstein-Barr virus, herpes simplex virus (HSV), H1N1 (swine flu), HIV, human papillomavirus (HPV), respiratory syncytial virus (RSV), and severe acute respiratory syndrome (SARS)–associated coronavirus, varicella zoster virus.

SPECIMEN: Urine, semen, blood, body fluid, stool, tissue, or swabs from the affected site

NORMAL FINDINGS: (Method: Culture in special media, enzyme-linked immunoassays, direct fluorescent antibody techniques, latex agglutination, immunoperoxidase, polymerase chain reaction [PCR] techniques) No virus isolated.

DESCRIPTION: Viruses, the most common cause of human infection, are submicroscopic organisms that invade living cells. They can be classified as either RNA- or DNA-type viruses. Viral titers are highest in the early stages of disease before the host has begun to manufacture significant antibodies against the invader. Specimens need to be collected as early as possible in the disease process. The subspecialty of microbiology has been revolutionized by molecular diagnostics. Molecular diagnostics involves the identification of specific sequences of DNA. The application of molecular diagnostics techniques, such as PCR, has led to the development of automated instruments that can identify a single pathogen or multiple pathogens from a small amount of specimen in less than 2 hr. The instruments can detect the presence of bacteria and viruses commonly associated with viral infections.

This procedure is contraindicated for: N/A

INDICATIONS

Assist in the identification of viral infection.

C

POTENTIAL MEDICAL DIAGNOSIS

Positive findings in

- **AIDS**
  HIV
- **Acute respiratory failure**
  Hantavirus
- **Anorectal infections**
  HSV
  HPV
- **Bronchitis**
  Parainfluenza virus
  RSV
- **Cervical cancer**
  HPV
- **Condylomata**
  HPV
- **Conjunctivitis/keratitis**
  Adenovirus
  Epstein-Barr virus
  HSV
  Measles virus
  Parvovirus
  Rubella virus
  Varicella zoster virus (shingles)
- **Croup**
  Parainfluenza virus
  RSV
- **Cutaneous infection with rash**
  Enteroviruses
  HSV
  Varicella zoster virus
- **Encephalitis**
  Enteroviruses
  Flaviviruses
  HSV
  HIV
  Measles virus
  Rabies virus
  Togaviruses
  West Nile virus (mosquito-borne arbovirus)
- **Febrile illness with rash**
  Coxsackieviruses
  Echovirus
- **Gastroenteritis**
  Norwalk virus
  Rotavirus
- **Genital herpes**
  HSV-1
  HSV-2
- **Genital warts**
  HPV
- **Hemorrhagic cystitis**
  Adenovirus
- **Hemorrhagic fever**
  Ebola virus
  Hantavirus
  Lassa virus
  Marburg virus
- **Herpangina**
  Coxsackievirus (group A)
- **Infectious mononucleosis**
  CMV
  Epstein-Barr virus
- **Meningitis**
  Coxsackieviruses
  Echovirus
  HSV-2
  Lymphocytic choriomeningitis virus
- **Myocarditis/pericarditis**
  Coxsackievirus
  Echovirus
- **Parotitis**
  Mumps virus
  Parainfluenza virus
- **Pharyngitis**
  Adenovirus
  Coxsackievirus (group A)
  Epstein-Barr virus
  HSV
  H1N1 influenza virus (swine flu)
  Influenza virus
  Parainfluenza virus
  Rhinovirus
- **Pleurodynia**
  Coxsackievirus (group B)
- **Pneumonia**
  Adenovirus
  H1N1 influenza virus (swine flu)
  Influenza virus
  Parainfluenza virus
  RSV
  SARS-associated corona virus
- **Upper respiratory tract infection**
  Adenovirus
  Coronavirus
  H1N1 influenza virus (swine flu)
  Influenza virus
  Parainfluenza virus
  RSV
  Rhinovirus

CRITICAL FINDINGS:

Note and immediately report to the requesting health-care provider (HCP) any critical findings and related symptoms. A listing of these findings varies among facilities. Timely notification of a critical finding for laboratory or diagnostic studies is a role expectation of the professional nurse. The notification processes vary among facilities. Upon receipt of the critical finding, the information should be read back to the caller to verify accuracy. Positive RSV, influenza, and varicella zoster cultures should be reported immediately to the requesting HCP. Lists of specific organisms may vary among facilities; specific organisms are required to be reported to local, state, and national departments of health. 🍁

INTERFERING FACTORS

- Viral specimens are unstable. Prompt and proper specimen processing, storage, and analysis are important to achieve accurate results.

NURSING IMPLICATIONS AND PROCEDURE

PRETEST:

- Positively identify the patient using at least two person-specific identifiers before services, treatments, or procedures are performed.
- ***Patient Teaching:*** Inform the patient this test can assist in identification of the organism causing infection.
- Obtain a history of the patient's health concerns, symptoms, surgical procedures, and results of previously performed laboratory and diagnostic studies. Include a list of known allergens, especially allergies or sensitivities to latex.
- Obtain a list of the patient's current medications, including over-the-counter medications and dietary supplements (see Effects of Natural Products on Laboratory Values online at Davis*Plus*).
- Note any recent medications, especially antivirals, that can interfere with test results.
- Review the procedure with the patient. Inform the patient that specimen collection takes approximately 5 min. Address concerns about pain and explain that there may be some discomfort during the specimen collection.
- Note that there are no food, fluid, or medication restrictions unless by medical direction.
- ***Sensitivity to social and cultural issues,*** as well as concern for modesty, is important in providing psychological support before, during, and after the procedure.

INTRATEST:

Potential Complications: N/A

- Instruct the patient to cooperate fully and to follow directions. Direct the patient to breathe normally and to avoid unnecessary movement.
- Observe standard precautions, and follow the general guidelines in Patient Preparation and Specimen Collection online at Davis*Plus*. Positively identify the patient, and label the appropriate collection containers with the corresponding patient demographics, date and time of collection, exact site, contact person for notification of results, and other pertinent information (e.g., patient immunocompromised owing to organ transplant, radiation, or chemotherapy).
- Avoid the use of equipment containing latex if the patient has a history of allergic reaction to latex.
- Instructions regarding the appropriate transport materials for blood, bronchial washings, sputum, sterile fluids, stool, and tissue samples should be obtained from the laboratory. The type of applicator used to obtain swabs should be verified by consultation with the testing laboratory personnel.

- The appropriate viral transport material should be obtained from the laboratory. Nasopharyngeal washings or swabs for RSV testing should be immediately placed in cold viral transport media.
- Promptly transport the specimen to the laboratory for processing and analysis.

C

POST-TEST:

- Inform the patient that a report of the results will be made available to the requesting HCP, who will discuss the results with the patient.
- ***Nutritional Considerations:*** Dehydration can been seen in patients with viral infections due to loss of fluids through fever, diarrhea, and/or vomiting. Antipyretic medication includes acetaminophen to decrease fever and allow for adequate intake of fluids and foods. Do not give acetylsalicylic acid to pediatric patients with a viral illness because it increases the risk of Reye's syndrome.
- *Sensitivity to social and cultural issues:* Offer support, as appropriate, to patients who may be the victims of sexual assault. Educate the patient regarding access to counseling services. Provide a nonjudgmental, nonthreatening atmosphere for discussing the risks of sexually transmitted infections. It is also important to address problems the patient may experience (e.g., guilt, depression, anger).
- Recognize anxiety related to test results. Discuss the implications of abnormal test results on the patient's lifestyle. Provide teaching and information regarding the clinical implications of the test results, as appropriate.
- Reinforce information given by the patient's HCP regarding further testing, treatment, or referral to another HCP. Explain that multiple specimens may be required during the course of the infection, as directed by the HCP. The time frame for serial sample collection may vary depending on the viral organism involved. Provide information regarding vaccine-preventable diseases where indicated (e.g., encephalitis, H1N1 flu, seasonal influenza). Provide contact information, if desired, for the Centers for Disease Control and Prevention (www.cdc.gov/vaccines/vpd-vac) 🍁 for guidelines on vaccine-preventable diseases. Answer any questions or address any concerns voiced by the patient or family.
- Depending on the results of this procedure, additional testing may be performed to evaluate or monitor progression of the disease process and determine the need for a change in therapy. Evaluate test results in relation to the patient's symptoms and other tests performed.

RELATED STUDIES:

- Related tests include alveolar/arterial gradient, β-2-microglobulin, barium enema, biopsy (cervical, intestinal, kidney, liver, lung, lymph node, muscle, skin), blood gases, bronchoscopy, CD4/CD8 ratio, CSF analysis, *Chlamydia* group antibody, chest x-ray, cultures (anal, blood, ear, eye, fungal, genital, mycobacteria, skin, sputum, stool, throat, urine, wound), CBC, cytology (sputum, urine), gallium scan, gastric emptying scan, lung perfusion scan, lung ventilation scan, Pap smear, pericardial fluid analysis, plethysmography, pulse oximetry, PFT, slit-lamp biomicroscopy, syphilis serology, TB tests, and viral serology tests (hepatitis, HIV, HTLV, infectious mononucleosis, mumps, rubella, rubeola, varicella).
- Refer to the Gastrointestinal, Genitourinary, Immune, Reproductive, and Respiratory systems tables online at Davis*Plus* for related tests by body system.

Cystometry

SYNONYM/ACRONYM: Cystometrography (CMG), urodynamic testing of bladder function.

COMMON USE: To assess bladder function related to obstruction, neurogenic pathology, and infection including evaluation of surgical, and medical management.

AREA OF APPLICATION: Bladder, urethra.

DESCRIPTION: Cystometry evaluates the motor and sensory function of the bladder when incontinence is present or neurological bladder dysfunction is suspected and monitors the effects of treatment for the abnormalities. This manometric study measures the bladder pressure and volume characteristics in milliliters of water (cm H_2O) during the filling and emptying phases. The test provides information about bladder structure and function that can lead to uninhibited bladder contractions, sensations of bladder fullness and need to void, and ability to inhibit voiding. These abnormalities cause incontinence and other impaired patterns of micturition. Cystometry can be performed with EEG (sleep studies for nocturnal incontinence), cystoscopy, and electromyography pelvic floor sphincter.

A post-void residual measurement can also be done at the bedside to measure how much urine is left in the bladder after the patient voids. Completion of this test requires catheterization of the patient directly after voiding. The amount of urine remaining is measured and reported as the post-void or residual urine. Normal post-void residual is less than 30 to 50 mL of urine. This may be adjusted to less than 100 mL for those over the age of 65.

This procedure is contraindicated for

- Patients with acute urinary tract infections (UTIs) because the study can cause infection to spread to the kidneys.
- Patients with urethral obstruction.
- Patients who are unable to be catheterized.
- Patients with cervical cord lesions ***because they may exhibit autonomic dysreflexia, as seen by bradycardia, flushing, hypertension, diaphoresis, and headache.***

INDICATIONS

- Detect congenital urinary abnormalities.
- Determine cause of bladder dysfunction and pathology.
- Determine cause of recurrent UTIs.
- Determine cause of urinary retention.
- Determine type of incontinence: *functional* (involuntary and unpredictable), *reflex* (involuntary when a specific volume is reached), *stress* (weak pelvic muscles), *total* (continuous and unpredictable), *urge* (involuntary when urgency is sensed),

and *psychological* (e.g., dementia, confusion affecting awareness).
- Determine type of neurogenic bladder (motor or sensory).
- Evaluate the management of neurological bladder before surgical intervention.
- Evaluate postprostatectomy incontinence.
- Evaluate signs and symptoms of urinary elimination pattern dysfunction.
- Evaluate urinary obstruction in male patients experiencing urinary retention.
- Evaluate the usefulness of drug therapy on detrusor muscle function and tonicity and on internal and external sphincter function.
- Evaluate voiding disorders associated with spinal cord injury.

C

POTENTIAL MEDICAL DIAGNOSIS

Normal findings

- Normal filling pattern
- Normal sensory perception of bladder fullness, desire to void, and ability to inhibit urination; appropriate response to temperature (hot and cold)
- Normal bladder capacity: 250 to 450 mL. Bladder size and corresponding capacity vary with gender and age; in the pediatric patient, the normal bladder stretches to maximum capacity without an increase in pressure
- Amount of postvoid residual urine is less than 30 to 50 mL
- Normal functioning bladder pressure: 8 to 15 cm H_2O
- Normal bladder pressure increases 30 to 40 cm H_2O during voiding
- Normal detrusor pressure: less than 10 cm H_2O
- Normal first urge to void: 175 to 250 mL; sensation of fullness and need to empty the bladder: 350 to 450 mL
- Urethral pressure that is higher than bladder pressure, ensuring continence

Abnormal findings related to

Bladder Dysfunction Related to Disorders of the Nervous System
- Diabetic neuropathy
- Multiple sclerosis
- Parkinson's disease
- Spinal cord injury
- Stroke
- Tabes dorsalis

Bladder Dysfunction Related to Urinary Incontinence
- Emotional or psychological origin
- Hyperreflexia
- Urinary tract infection

Bladder Dysfunction Related to Urinary Retention
- Bladder obstruction (e.g., congenital origin, tumor)
- Enlarged prostate
- UTI

CRITICAL FINDINGS: N/A

INTERFERING FACTORS

Factors that may impair the results of the examination

- Inability of the patient to cooperate or remain still during the procedure because of age, significant pain, or mental status.
- Inability of the patient to void in a supine position or straining to void during the study.
- A high level of patient anxiety or embarrassment, which may interfere with the study, making it difficult to distinguish whether the results are due to stress or organic pathology.
- Administration of drugs that affect bladder function, such as muscle relaxants or antihistamines.

NURSING IMPLICATIONS AND PROCEDURE

See Potential Nursing Problems on Fast Find at davispl.us/vanleeuwen7

PRETEST:

- Positively identify the patient using at least two person-specific identifiers before services, treatments, or procedures are performed.
- ***Patient Teaching:*** Inform the patient this procedure can assist in assessing bladder function.
- Obtain a history of the patient's health concerns, symptoms, surgical procedures, and results of previously performed laboratory and diagnostic studies. Include a list of known allergens, especially allergies or sensitivities to latex.
- Record the date of the last menstrual period and determine the possibility of pregnancy in perimenopausal women.
- Obtain a list of the patient's current medications, including over-the-counter medications, dietary supplements, anticoagulants, aspirin and other salicylates (see Effects of Natural Products on Laboratory Values online at Davis*Plus*). Such products should be discontinued by medical direction for the appropriate number of days prior to a surgical procedure. Note the last time and dose of medication taken.
- Review the procedure with the patient. Address concerns about pain and explain that there may be moments of discomfort and some pain experienced during the test. Inform the patient that the procedure is performed in a special urology room or in a clinic setting by the health-care provider (HCP), with support staff, and takes approximately 30 to 45 min.
- ***Sensitivity to social and cultural issues,*** as well as concern for modesty, is important in providing psychological support before, during, and after the procedure.
- Instruct the patient to report pain, sweating, nausea, headache, and the urge to void during the study.
- Note that there are no food, fluid, or medication restrictions unless by medical direction.
- *Make sure a written and informed consent has been signed prior to the procedure and before administering any medications.*

INTRATEST:

Potential Complications:

UTI ***related to use of a catheter***

- Observe standard precautions, and follow the general guidelines in Patient Preparation and Specimen Collection online at Davis*Plus*. Positively identify the patient.
- Avoid the use of equipment containing latex if the patient has a history of allergic reaction to latex.
- Have emergency equipment readily available.
- Instruct the patient to change into the gown, robe, and foot coverings provided, but not to void.
- Position the patient in a supine or lithotomy position on the examination table. If spinal cord injury is present, the patient can remain on a stretcher in a supine position and be draped appropriately.
- Ask the patient to void. During voiding, note characteristics such as start time; force and continuity of the stream; volume voided; presence of dribbling, straining, or hesitancy; and stop time.
- Instruct the patient to cooperate fully and to follow directions. Instruct the patient to remain still during the procedure.
- A urinary catheter is inserted into the bladder under sterile conditions, and residual urine is measured and recorded. A test for sensory response to temperature is done by instilling 30 mL of room-temperature sterile water followed by 30 mL of warm sterile water. Sensations are assessed and recorded.
- Fluid is removed from the bladder, and the catheter is connected to a

cystometer that measures the pressure. Sterile normal saline, distilled water, or carbon dioxide gas is instilled in controlled amounts into the bladder. When the patient indicates the urge to void, the bladder is considered full. The patient is instructed to void, and urination amounts as well as start and stop times are then recorded.

- Pressure and volume readings are recorded and graphed for response to heat, full bladder, urge to void, and ability to inhibit voiding. The patient is requested to void without straining, and pressures are taken and recorded during this activity.
- After completion of voiding, the bladder is emptied of any other fluid, and the catheter is withdrawn, unless further testing is planned.
- Further testing may be done to determine if abnormal bladder function is being caused by muscle incompetence or interruption in innervation; anticholinergic medication (e.g., atropine) or cholinergic medication (e.g., bethanechol [Urecholine]) can be administered and the study repeated in 20 or 30 min.

POST-TEST:

- Inform the patient that a report of the results will be made available to the requesting HCP, who will discuss the results with the patient.
- Monitor fluid intake and urinary output for 24 hr after the procedure.
- Monitor vital signs after the procedure every 15 min for 2 hr or as directed. Monitor intake and output at least every 8 hr. Elevated temperature may indicate infection. Notify the HCP if temperature is elevated. Protocols may vary among facilities.
- Instruct the patient to immediately report symptoms such as fast heart rate, difficulty breathing, skin rash, itching, chest pain, persistent right shoulder pain, or abdominal pain. Immediately report symptoms to the appropriate HCP.
- Inform the patient that he or she may experience burning or discomfort on urination for a few voidings after the procedure.
- Persistent flank or suprapubic pain, fever, chills, blood in the urine, difficulty urinating, or change in urinary pattern must be reported immediately to the HCP.
- Recognize anxiety related to test results. Discuss the implications of abnormal test results on the patient's lifestyle. Provide teaching and information regarding the clinical implications of the test results, as appropriate.
- Reinforce information given by the patient's HCP regarding further testing, treatment, or referral to another HCP. Answer any questions or address any concerns voiced by the patient or family.
- Depending on the results of this procedure, additional testing may be needed to evaluate or monitor progression of the disease process and determine the need for a change in therapy. Evaluate test results in relation to the patient's symptoms and other tests performed.

Patient Education:

- Teach the patient symptoms that would indicate bladder distention.
- Teach the patient to request pain medication as soon as needed for adequate pain management.

Expected Patient Outcomes:

Understanding

- The patient and family state treatment options related to urinary retention (surgical, medical).
- The patient and family state the pathophysiology related to the disease process.

Ability

- The patient and family demonstrate the ability to measure and document urine output accurately.
- The patient demonstrates how to place pressure on the bladder to stimulate urination.

Response

- The patient and family take positive measures to prevent social isolation.

- The patient agrees to discuss concerns related to health issues with a support group.

RELATED STUDIES:

- Related tests include bladder cancer markers, calculus kidney stone panel, *Chlamydia* group antibody, CBC, CBC hematocrit, CBC hemoglobin, CT pelvis, culture urine, cytology urine, IVP, MRI pelvis, PT/INR, US pelvis, and UA.
- Refer to the Genitourinary System table online at Davis*Plus* for related tests by body system.

Cystoscopy

SYNONYM/ACRONYM: Cystoureterography, prostatography.

COMMON USE: To assess the urinary tract for bleeding, cancer, tumor, and prostate health.

AREA OF APPLICATION: Bladder, urethra, ureteral orifices.

DESCRIPTION: Cystoscopy provides direct visualization of the urethra, urinary bladder, and ureteral orifices—areas not usually visible with x-ray procedures. This procedure is also used to obtain specimens and treat pathology associated with the aforementioned structures. Cystoscopy is accomplished by transurethral insertion of a cystoscope into the bladder. Rigid cystoscopes contain an obturator and a telescope with a lens and light system; there are also flexible cystoscopes, which use fiberoptic technology. The procedure may be performed during or after ultrasonography or radiography, or during urethroscopy or retrograde pyelography.

This procedure is contraindicated for

Patients who are pregnant or suspected of being pregnant, unless the potential benefits of a procedure using radiation far outweigh the risk of radiation exposure to the fetus and mother.

Patients with bleeding disorders ***because instrumentation may lead to excessive bleeding from the lower urinary tract.***

Patients with acute cystitis or urethritis ***because instrumentation could allow bacteria to enter the bloodstream, resulting in septicemia.***

INDICATIONS

- Coagulate bleeding areas.
- Determine the possible source of persistent urinary tract infections.
- Determine the source of hematuria of unknown cause.
- Differentiate, through tissue biopsy, between benign and cancerous lesions involving the bladder.
- Dilate the urethra and ureters.
- Evacuate blood clots and perform fulguration of bleeding sites within the lower urinary tract.
- Evaluate changes in urinary elimination patterns.
- Evaluate the extent of prostatic hyperplasia and degree of obstruction.
- Evaluate the function of each kidney by obtaining urine samples via ureteral catheters.

- Evaluate urinary tract abnormalities such as dysuria, frequency, retention, inadequate stream, urgency, and incontinence.
- Identify and remove polyps and small tumors (including by fulguration) from the bladder.
- Identify and remove foreign body.
- Identify congenital anomalies, such as duplicate ureters, ureteroceles, urethral or ureteral strictures, diverticula, and areas of inflammation or ulceration.
- Implant radioactive seeds.
- Place ureteral catheters to drain urine from the renal pelvis or for retrograde pyelography.
- Place ureteral stents and resect prostate gland tissue (transurethral resection of the prostate).
- Remove renal calculi from the bladder or ureters.
- Resect small tumors.

POTENTIAL MEDICAL DIAGNOSIS

Normal findings

- Normal ureter, bladder, and urethral structure

Abnormal findings related to

- Bladder cancer
- Diverticulum of the bladder, fistula, stones, and strictures
- Foreign body
- Inflammation or infection
- Obstruction
- Polyps
- Prostatic hyperplasia
- Prostatitis
- Renal calculi
- Tumors
- Ureteral calculi
- Ureteral reflux
- Ureteral or urethral stricture
- Ureterocele
- Urinary fistula
- Urinary tract malformation and congenital anomalies

CRITICAL FINDINGS: N/A

INTERFERING FACTORS

Other considerations

- Failure to follow dietary restrictions before the procedure may cause the procedure to be canceled or repeated.
- Inability of the patient to cooperate or remain still during the procedure because of age, significant pain, or mental status.

NURSING IMPLICATIONS AND PROCEDURE

See Potential Nursing Problems on Fast Find at davispl.us/vanleeuwen7

PRETEST:

- Positively identify the patient using at least two person-specific identifiers before services, treatments, or procedures are performed.
- ***Patient Teaching:*** Inform the patient this procedure can assist in assessing the urinary tract.
- Obtain a history of the patient's health concerns, symptoms, surgical procedures, and results of previously performed laboratory and diagnostic studies. Include a list of known allergens, especially allergies or sensitivities to latex, anesthetics, sedatives, or contrast medium. Ensure results of coagulation testing are obtained and recorded prior to the procedure; a creatinine level is also needed before contrast medium is to be used.
- Record the date of the last menstrual period and determine the possibility of pregnancy in perimenopausal women.
- Obtain a list of the patient's current medications, including over-the-counter medications, dietary supplements, anticoagulants, aspirin and other salicylates (see Effects of Natural Products on Laboratory Values online at Davis*Plus*). Such products should be discontinued by medical direction for the appropriate number of days prior to a surgical procedure. Note the last time and dose of medication taken.

- Review the procedure with the patient. Address concerns about pain and explain that there may be moments of discomfort and some pain experienced during the test. Inform the patient that the procedure is usually performed in a special cystoscopy suite near or in the surgery department by a health-care provider (HCP), with support staff, and takes approximately 10 to 30 min. The procedure can also be performed in a urologist's office; pediatric cystoscopy is performed in the surgery unit.
- ***Sensitivity to social and cultural issues,*** as well as concern for modesty, is important in providing psychological support before, during, and after the procedure.
- Explain that an intravenous (IV) line may be inserted to allow infusion of fluids such as saline, anesthetics, sedatives, or emergency medications.
- Instruct the patient that to reduce the risk of aspiration related to nausea and vomiting, solid food and milk or milk products have been restricted for at least 6 hr, and clear liquids have been restricted for at least 2 hr prior to general anesthesia, regional anesthesia, or sedation/analgesia (monitored anesthesia). The American Society of Anesthesiologists has fasting guidelines for risk levels according to patient status. More information can be located at www.asahq.org. 🍁 Patients on beta blockers before the surgical procedure should be instructed to take their medication as ordered during the perioperative period. Protocols may vary among facilities.
- Obtain and record the patient's vital signs.
- *Make sure a written and informed consent has been signed prior to the procedure and before administering any medications.*

INTRATEST:

Potential Complications:

Infection ***related to the use of the endoscope*** or bleeding

- Observe standard precautions, and follow the general guidelines in Patient Preparation and Specimen Collection online at Davis*Plus*. Positively identify the patient, and label the appropriate specimen container with the corresponding patient demographics, initials of the person collecting the specimen, date, and time of collection.
- Ensure that the patient has complied with dietary restrictions prior to the study, as instructed.
- Administer ordered prophylactic steroids or antihistamines before the procedure if the patient has a history of allergic reactions to any substance or drug to be used in the study.
- Avoid the use of equipment containing latex if the patient has a history of allergic reaction to latex.
- Have emergency equipment readily available.
- Establish an IV fluid line for the injection of saline, anesthetics, sedatives, or emergency medications.
- Administer ordered preoperative sedation.
- Instruct the patient to void prior to the procedure and to change into the gown, robe, and foot coverings provided.
- Position patient on the examination table, draped and with legs in stirrups. If general or spinal anesthesia is to be used, it is administered before positioning the patient on the table.
- Cleanse external genitalia with antiseptic solution. If local anesthetic is used, it is instilled into the urethra and retained for 5 to 10 min. A penile clamp may be used for male patients to aid in retention of anesthetic.
- The HCP inserts a cystoscope or a urethroscope to examine the urethra before cystoscopy. The urethroscope has a sheath that may be left in place, and the cystoscope is inserted through it, avoiding multiple instrumentations.
- After insertion of the cystoscope, a sample of residual urine may be obtained for culture or other analysis.
- The bladder is irrigated via an irrigation system attached to the scope. The irrigation fluid aids in bladder visualization.

- If a prostatic tumor is found, a biopsy specimen may be obtained by means of a cytology brush or biopsy forceps inserted through the scope. If the tumor is small and localized, it can be excised and fulgurated. This procedure is termed *transurethral resection of the bladder*. Polyps can also be identified and excised.
- Ulcers or bleeding sites can be fulgurated using electrocautery.
- Renal calculi can be crushed and removed from the ureters and bladder.
- Ureteral catheters can be inserted via the scope to obtain urine samples from each kidney for comparative analysis and radiographic studies.
- Ureteral and urethral strictures can also be dilated during this procedure.
- Upon completion of the examination and related procedures, the cystoscope is withdrawn.
- Place obtained specimens in proper containers, label them properly, and immediately transport them to the laboratory.

POST-TEST:

- Inform the patient that a report of the results will be made available to the requesting HCP, who will discuss the results with the patient.
- Instruct the patient to resume his or her usual diet and medications, as directed by the HCP.
- Encourage the patient to drink increased amounts of fluids (125 mL/hr for 24 hr) after the procedure.
- Monitor vital signs and neurological status every 15 min for 1 hr, then every 2 hr for 4 hr, and then as ordered by the HCP. Take the temperature every 4 hr for 24 hr. Monitor intake and output at least every 8 hr. Compare with baseline values. Notify the HCP if temperature is elevated. Protocols may vary among facilities.
- Instruct the patient to immediately report symptoms such as fast heart rate, difficulty breathing, skin rash, itching, chest pain, persistent right shoulder pain, or abdominal pain. Immediately report symptoms to the appropriate HCP.
- Inform the patient that burning or discomfort on urination can be experienced for a few voidings after the procedure and that the urine may be blood-tinged for the first and second voidings after the procedure.
- Persistent flank or suprapubic pain, fever, chills, blood in the urine, difficulty urinating, or change in urinary pattern must be reported immediately to the HCP.
- Recognize anxiety related to test results. Discuss the implications of abnormal test results on the patient's lifestyle. Provide teaching and information regarding the clinical implications of the test results, as appropriate.
- Reinforce information given by the patient's HCP regarding further testing, treatment, or referral to another HCP. Answer any questions or address any concerns voiced by the patient or family.
- Depending on the results of this procedure, additional testing may be needed to evaluate or monitor progression of the disease process and determine the need for a change in therapy. Evaluate test results in relation to the patient's symptoms and other tests performed.

Patient Education:

- Teach the patient the pathophysiology of the disease process and its effects on lifestyle.
- Teach the patient the importance of taking all prescribed medications to support health maintenance.

Expected Patient Outcomes:

Understanding

- The patient states the importance of emptying the bladder every 3 to 4 hr.
- The patient and family state the importance of monitoring the urine for blood and reporting an occurrence to the HCP.

Ability

- The patient and family accurately measure and document intake and output.

- The patient and family describe lifestyle changes that can decrease urinary retention (avoid alcohol, decongestants).

Response

- The patient agrees to complete any follow-up diagnostic or laboratory studies to maintain health.
- The patient agrees to avoid alcohol consumption to decrease urinary retention.

RELATED STUDIES:

- Related tests include biopsy kidney, biopsy prostate, calculus kidney stone panel, *Chlamydia* group antibody, CT pelvis, culture urine, cytology urine, IVP, MRI pelvis, PSA, US pelvis, and UA.
- Refer to the Genitourinary System table online at Davis*Plus* for related tests by body system.

C

Cystourethrography, Voiding

SYNONYM/ACRONYM: Voiding cystourethrography (VCU), voiding cystourethrogram (VCUG), micturating cystourethrogram (MCUG).

COMMON USE: To visualize and assess the bladder during voiding for evaluation of chronic urinary tract infections.

AREA OF APPLICATION: Bladder, urethra.

DESCRIPTION: Voiding cystourethrography involves visualization of the bladder filled with contrast medium instilled through a catheter by use of a syringe or gravity, and, after the catheter is removed, the excretion of the contrast medium. Excretion or micturition is recorded electronically or on videotape for confirmation or exclusion of ureteral reflux and evaluation of the urethra. Fluoroscopic or plain images may also be taken to record bladder filling and emptying. This procedure is often used to evaluate chronic urinary tract infections (UTIs).

This procedure is contraindicated for

Patients who are pregnant or suspected of being pregnant, unless the potential benefits of a procedure using radiation far outweigh the risk of radiation exposure to the fetus.

Patients with conditions associated with adverse reactions to contrast medium (e.g., asthma, food allergies, or allergy to contrast medium).

Although patients are asked specifically if they have a known allergy to iodine or shellfish, it has been well established that the reaction is not to iodine, in fact an actual iodine allergy would be problematic because iodine is required for the production of thyroid hormones. In the case of shellfish, the reaction is to a muscle protein called tropomyosin; in the case of iodinated contrast medium, the reaction is to the noniodinated part of the contrast molecule. Patients with a known hypersensitivity to the medium may benefit from premedication with corticosteroids and diphenhydramine; the use of nonionic contrast or an alternative noncontrast imaging study, if available, may be considered for patients who have severe asthma or who have experienced moderate to severe reactions to ionic contrast medium.

- Patients with conditions associated with preexisting renal insufficiency (e.g., chronic kidney disease, single kidney transplant, nephrectomy, diabetes, multiple myeloma, treatment with aminoglycosides and NSAIDs) ***because iodinated contrast is nephrotoxic.***
- Patients who are chronically dehydrated before the test, especially older adults and patients whose health is already compromised, ***because of their risk of contrast-induced acute kidney injury.***
- Patients with bleeding disorders ***because the puncture site may not stop bleeding.***
- Patients with an active urinary tract infection, obstruction, or injury.

C

INDICATIONS

- Assess the degree of compromise of a stenotic prostatic urethra.
- Assess hypertrophy of the prostate lobes.
- Assess ureteral stricture.
- Confirm the diagnosis of congenital lower urinary tract anomaly.
- Evaluate abnormal bladder emptying and incontinence.
- Evaluate the effects of bladder trauma.
- Evaluate possible cause of frequent UTIs.
- Evaluate the presence and extent of ureteral reflux.
- Evaluate the urethra for obstruction and strictures.

POTENTIAL MEDICAL DIAGNOSIS

Normal findings

- Normal bladder and urethra structure and function

Abnormal findings related to

- Bladder trauma
- Bladder tumors
- Hematomas
- Neurogenic bladder
- Pelvic tumors
- Prostatic enlargement
- Ureteral stricture
- Ureterocele
- Urethral diverticula
- Vesicoureteral reflux

CRITICAL FINDINGS: N/A

INTERFERING FACTORS

Factors that may alter the results of the study

- Metallic objects within the examination field, which may inhibit organ visualization and cause unclear images.
- Inability of the patient to cooperate or remain still during the procedure because of age, significant pain, or mental status.
- Gas or feces in the gastrointestinal tract resulting from inadequate cleansing or failure to restrict food intake before the study.
- Retained barium from a previous radiological procedure.

NURSING IMPLICATIONS AND PROCEDURE

PRETEST:

- Positively identify the patient using at least two person-specific identifiers before services, treatments, or procedures are performed.
- *Patient Teaching:* Inform the patient this procedure can assist in assessing the urinary tract.
- Obtain a history of the patient's health concerns, symptoms, surgical procedures, and results of previously performed laboratory and diagnostic studies. Include a list of known allergens, especially allergies or sensitivities to latex, anesthetics, sedatives, or contrast medium. Ensure results of coagulation testing are obtained and recorded prior to the procedure; a creatinine level is also needed before contrast medium is to be used.

- Ensure that this procedure is performed before an upper gastrointestinal study or barium swallow.
- Record the date of the last menstrual period and determine the possibility of pregnancy in perimenopausal women.
- Obtain a list of the patient's current medications, including over-the-counter medications, dietary supplements, anticoagulants, aspirin and other salicylates (see Effects of Natural Products on Laboratory Values online at Davis*Plus*). Such products should be discontinued by medical direction for the appropriate number of days prior to a surgical procedure. Note the last time and dose of medication taken.
- If iodinated contrast medium is scheduled to be used in patients receiving metformin for type 2 diabetes, the drug should be discontinued on the day of the test and continue to be withheld for 48 hr after the test. Iodinated contrast can temporarily impair kidney function, and failure to withhold metformin may indirectly result in drug-induced lactic acidosis, a dangerous and sometimes fatal adverse effect of metformin ***(related to renal impairment that does not support sufficient excretion of metformin).***
- Review the procedure with the patient. Address concerns about pain and explain that there may be moments of discomfort and some pain experienced during the test. Inform the patient that the procedure is usually performed in the radiology department by a health-care provider (HCP), with support staff, and takes approximately 30 to 60 min. **Pediatric Considerations** There is no specific pediatric patient preparation for cystourethrography. Encourage parents to be truthful about unpleasant sensations (pinching or pushing) the child may experience during catheter insertion and to use words that they know their child will understand. Toddlers and preschool-age children have a very short attention span, so the best time to talk about the test is right before the procedure. The pediatric patient should be assured that he or she will be allowed to bring a favorite comfort item into the examination room, and if appropriate, that a parent will be with the child during the procedure. Infants and small children may be wrapped tightly in a blanket to assist in keeping them still during the procedure.
- *Sensitivity to social and cultural issues,* as well as concern for modesty, is important in providing psychological support before, during, and after the procedure.
- Inform the patient that he or she may receive a laxative the night before the test or an enema or a cathartic the morning of the test, as ordered.
- Instruct the patient to increase fluid intake the day before the test and to have only clear fluids 8 hr before the test.
- *Make sure a written and informed consent has been signed prior to the procedure and before administering any medications.*

INTRATEST:

Potential Complications:

Complications include dysuria, injury to the urethra, and urinary infection ***related to use of a catheter.*** Allergic reaction to contrast media is another potential complication.

- Observe standard precautions, and follow the general guidelines in Patient Preparation and Specimen Collection online at Davis*Plus*. Positively identify the patient.
- Ensure that the patient has complied with dietary restrictions prior to the study, as instructed. Assess for completion of bowel preparation if ordered.
- Ensure that the patient has removed all external metallic objects from the area to be examined prior to the procedure.
- Administer ordered prophylactic steroids or antihistamines before the procedure if the patient has a history of allergic reactions to any substance or drug.

- Avoid the use of equipment containing latex if the patient has a history of allergic reaction to latex.
- Have emergency equipment readily available.
- Instruct the patient to void prior to the procedure and to change into the gown, robe, and foot coverings provided.
- Insert a urinary catheter before the procedure, if ordered. Inform the patient that he or she may feel some pressure when the catheter is inserted and when the contrast medium is instilled through the catheter.
- Place the patient on the table in a supine or lithotomy position.
- A kidney, ureter, and bladder radiograph is taken to ensure that no barium or stool obscures visualization of the urinary system.
- A catheter is filled with contrast medium to eliminate air pockets and is inserted until the balloon reaches the meatus if not previously inserted in the patient.
- When three-fourths of the contrast medium has been injected, a radiographic exposure is made while the remainder of the contrast medium is injected.
- When the patient is able to void, the catheter is removed and the patient is asked to urinate while images of the bladder and urethra are recorded.
- Monitor the patient for complications related to the procedure (e.g., allergic reaction, anaphylaxis, bronchospasm).

POST-TEST:

- Inform the patient that a report of the results will be made available to the requesting HCP, who will discuss the results with the patient.
- Instruct the patient to resume usual diet and medications, as directed by the HCP. Kidney function should be assessed before metformin is resumed.
- Monitor vital signs and neurological status every 15 min for 1 hr, then every 2 hr for 4 hr, and then as ordered by the HCP. Take the temperature every 4 hr for 24 hr. Monitor intake and output at least every 8 hr. Compare with baseline values. Notify the HCP if temperature is elevated. Protocols may vary among facilities.
- Monitor for reaction to iodinated contrast medium, including rash, urticaria, tachycardia, hyperpnea, hypertension, palpitations, nausea, or vomiting.
- Instruct the patient to immediately report symptoms such as fast heart rate, difficulty breathing, skin rash, itching, chest pain, persistent right shoulder pain, or abdominal pain. Immediately report symptoms to the appropriate HCP.
- Maintain the patient on adequate hydration after the procedure. Encourage the patient to drink increased amounts of fluids (125 mL/hr for 24 hr) after the procedure to prevent stasis and bacterial buildup.
- Recognize anxiety related to test results. Discuss the implications of abnormal test results on the patient's lifestyle. Provide teaching and information regarding the clinical implications of the test results, as appropriate.
- Reinforce information given by the patient's HCP regarding further testing, treatment, or referral to another HCP. Answer any questions or address any concerns voiced by the patient or family.
- Depending on the results of this procedure, additional testing may be needed to evaluate or monitor progression of the disease process and determine the need for a change in therapy. Evaluate test results in relation to the patient's symptoms and other tests performed.

RELATED STUDIES:

- Related tests include biopsy prostate, bladder cancer markers, BUN, CT pelvis, creatinine cytology urine, IVP, MRI pelvis, PSA, PT/INR, and US pelvis.
- Refer to the Genitourinary System table online at Davis*Plus* for related tests by body system.

Cytology, Sputum

SYNONYM/ACRONYM: N/A

COMMON USE: To identify cellular changes associated with neoplasms or organisms that result in respiratory tract infections, such as *Pneumocystis jiroveci*.

SPECIMEN: Sputum collected on three to five consecutive first-morning, deep-cough expectorations.

NORMAL FINDINGS: (Method: Macroscopic and microscopic examination) Negative for abnormal cells, fungi, ova, and parasites.

DESCRIPTION: Cytology is the study of the origin, structure, function, and pathology of cells. In clinical practice, cytological examinations are generally performed to detect cell changes resulting from neoplastic or inflammatory conditions. Sputum specimens for cytological examinations may be collected by expectoration alone, by suctioning, by lung biopsy, during bronchoscopy, or by expectoration after bronchoscopy. A description of the method of specimen collection by bronchoscopy and biopsy is found in the study titled "Biopsy, Lung."

This procedure is contraindicated for: N/A

INDICATIONS

- Assist in the diagnosis of lung cancer.
- Assist in the identification of *Pneumocystis jiroveci* in persons with AIDS.
- Detect known or suspected fungal or parasitic infection involving the lung.
- Detect known or suspected viral disease involving the lung.
- Screen cigarette smokers for neoplastic (nonmalignant) cellular changes.
- Screen patients with history of acute or chronic inflammatory or infectious lung disorders, which may lead to benign atypical or metaplastic changes.

POTENTIAL MEDICAL DIAGNOSIS

(Method: Microscopic examination) The method of reporting results of cytology examinations varies according to the laboratory performing the test. Terms used to report results may include *negative* (no abnormal cells seen), *inflammatory, benign atypical, suspect for neoplasm,* and *positive for neoplasm.*

Positive findings in

- Infections caused by fungi, ova, or parasites
- Lipoid or aspiration pneumonia, as seen by lipid droplets contained in macrophages
- Neoplasms
- Viral infections and lung disease

CRITICAL FINDINGS:

- Identification of malignancy

Note and immediately report to the requesting health-care provider (HCP) any critical findings and related symptoms. A listing of these findings varies among facilities. Timely notification of a critical finding for laboratory or diagnostic studies is a role expectation of the professional nurse. The notification processes vary among facilities. Upon receipt of the critical finding, the information should be read back to the caller to verify accuracy.

If the patient becomes hypoxic or cyanotic, remove catheter immediately and administer oxygen.

If patient has asthma or chronic bronchitis, watch for aggravated bronchospasms with use of normal saline or acetylcysteine in an aerosol.

C

INTERFERING FACTORS

- Improper specimen fixation may be cause for specimen rejection.
- Improper technique used to obtain bronchial washing may be cause for specimen rejection.
- Failure to follow dietary restrictions before the procedure may cause the procedure to be canceled or repeated.

NURSING IMPLICATIONS AND PROCEDURE

PRETEST:

- Positively identify the patient using at least two person-specific identifiers before services, treatments, or procedures are performed.
- *Patient Teaching:* Inform the patient this test can assist in identification of the organism causing infection.
- Obtain a history of the patient's health concerns, symptoms, surgical procedures, and results of previously performed laboratory and diagnostic studies. Include a list of known allergens, especially allergies or sensitivities to latex, anesthetics, or sedatives.
- Obtain a list of the patient's current medications, including over-the-counter medications and dietary supplements (see Effects of Natural Products on Laboratory Values online at Davis*Plus*).
- Note any recent procedures that can interfere with test results.
- Review the procedure with the patient. If the laboratory has provided a container with fixative, instruct the patient that the fixative contents of the specimen collection container should not be ingested or otherwise removed. Instruct the patient not to touch the edge or inside of the specimen container with the hands or mouth. Inform the patient that three samples may be required, on three separate mornings, either by passing a small tube (tracheal catheter) and adding suction or by expectoration. The time it takes to collect a proper specimen varies according to the level of cooperation of the patient and the specimen collection procedure. Address concerns about pain related to the procedure. Explain that a sedative and/or analgesia may be administered to promote relaxation and reduce discomfort prior to the procedure. Atropine is usually given before bronchoscopy examinations to reduce bronchial secretions and prevent vagally induced bradycardia. Lidocaine is sprayed in the patient's throat to reduce discomfort caused by the presence of the tube.
- Reassure the patient that he or she will be able to breathe during the procedure if specimen is collected via suction method. Ensure that oxygen has been administered 20 to 30 min before the procedure if the specimen is to be obtained by tracheal suctioning.
- Assist in providing extra fluids, unless contraindicated, and proper humidification to loosen tenacious secretions. Inform the patient that increasing fluid intake before retiring on the night before the test aids in liquefying secretions and may make it easier to expectorate in the morning. Also explain that humidifying inspired air also helps to liquefy secretions.
- Assist with mouth care (brushing teeth or rinsing mouth with water), if needed, before collection so as not to contaminate the specimen by oral secretions.

- *Sensitivity to social and cultural issues,* as well as concern for modesty, is important in providing psychological support before, during and after the procedure.
- For specimens collected by suctioning or expectoration without bronchoscopy, there are no food, fluid, or medication restrictions unless by medical direction.
- If bronchoscopy or biopsy is to be performed, instruct the patient that to reduce the risk of aspiration related to nausea and vomiting, solid food and milk or milk products are restricted for at least 6 hr, and clear liquids are restricted for at least 2 hr prior to general anesthesia, regional anesthesia, or sedation/analgesia (monitored anesthesia). The American Society of Anesthesiologists has fasting guidelines for risk levels according to patient status. More information can be located at www.asahq.org. 🍁 Patients on beta blockers before the surgical procedure should be instructed to take their medication as ordered during the perioperative period. Protocols may vary among facilities.
- *Make sure a written and informed consent has been signed prior to the bronchoscopy or biopsy procedure and before administering any medications.*

INTRATEST:

Potential Complications:

Bleeding ***(related to a bleeding disorder, or the effects of natural products and medications with known anticoagulant, antiplatelet, or thrombolytic properties),*** bronchospasm, pneumothorax, or hemoptysis.

- Ensure that the patient has complied with dietary restrictions prior to the study, as instructed.
- Have patient remove dentures, contact lenses, eyeglasses, and jewelry. Notify the HCP if the patient has permanent crowns on teeth. Have the patient remove clothing and change into a gown for the procedure.
- Have emergency equipment readily available. Keep resuscitation equipment on hand in the case of respiratory impairment or laryngospasm after the procedure.
- Avoid using morphine sulfate in those with asthma or other pulmonary disease. This drug can further exacerbate bronchospasms and respiratory impairment.
- Avoid the use of equipment containing latex if the patient has a history of allergic reaction to latex.
- Assist the patient to a comfortable position, and direct the patient to breathe normally during the beginning of the general anesthesia and to avoid unnecessary movement during the local anesthetic and the procedure. Instruct the patient to cooperate fully and to follow directions.
- Observe standard precautions, and follow the general guidelines in Patient Preparation and Specimen Collection online at Davis*Plus.* Positively identify the patient, and label the appropriate collection container with the corresponding patient demographics, date and time of collection, and any medication the patient is taking that may interfere with test results (e.g., antibiotics). Cytology specimens may also be expressed onto a glass slide and sprayed with a fixative or 95% alcohol.

Bronchoscopy

- Record baseline vital signs.
- The patient is positioned in relation to the type of anesthesia being used. If local anesthesia is used, the patient is seated, and the tongue and oropharynx are sprayed and swabbed with anesthetic before the bronchoscope is inserted. For general anesthesia, the patient is placed in a supine position with the neck hyperextended. After anesthesia, the patient is kept in supine or shifted to side-lying position, and the bronchoscope is inserted. After inspection, the samples are collected from suspicious sites by bronchial brush or biopsy forceps.

C

Expectorated Specimen

- Ask the patient to sit upright, with assistance and support (e.g., with an overbed table) as needed.
- Ask the patient to take two or three deep breaths and cough deeply. Any sputum raised should be expectorated directly into a sterile sputum collection container.
- If the patient is unable to produce the desired amount of sputum, several strategies may be attempted. One approach is to have the patient drink two glasses of water, and then assume the position for postural drainage of the upper and middle lung segments. Effective coughing may be assisted by placing either the hands or a pillow over the diaphragmatic area and applying slight pressure.
- Another approach is to place a vaporizer or other humidifying device at the bedside. After sufficient exposure to adequate humidification, postural drainage of the upper and middle lung segments may be repeated before attempting to obtain the specimen.
- Other methods may include obtaining an order for an expectorant to be administered with additional water approximately 2 hr before attempting to obtain the specimen. Chest percussion and postural drainage of all lung segments may also be employed. If the patient is still unable to raise sputum, the use of an ultrasonic nebulizer ("induced sputum") may be necessary; this is usually done by a respiratory therapist.

Tracheal Suctioning

- Obtain the necessary equipment, including a suction device, suction kit, and Lukens tube or in-line trap.
- Position the patient with head elevated as high as tolerated.
- Put on sterile gloves. Maintain the dominant hand as sterile and the nondominant hand as clean.
- Using the sterile hand, attach the suction catheter to the rubber tubing of the Lukens tube or in-line trap. Then attach the suction tubing to the male adapter of the trap with the clean hand. Lubricate the suction catheter with sterile saline.
- Ask patients who are nonintubated to protrude the tongue and to take a deep breath as the suction catheter is passed through the nostril. When the catheter enters the trachea, a reflex cough is stimulated; immediately advance the catheter into the trachea and apply suction. Maintain suction for approximately 10 sec, but never longer than 15 sec. Withdraw the catheter without applying suction. Separate the suction catheter and suction tubing from the trap, and place the rubber tubing over the male adapter to seal the unit.
- For patients who are intubated or patients with a tracheostomy, the previous procedure is followed except that the suction catheter is passed through the existing endotracheal or tracheostomy tube rather than through the nostril. The patient should be hyperoxygenated before and after the procedure in accordance with standard protocols for suctioning these patients.
- Generally, a series of three to five early-morning sputum samples are collected in sterile containers.

General

- Monitor the patient for complications related to the procedure (e.g., allergic reaction, anaphylaxis, bronchospasm).
- Promptly transport the specimen to the laboratory for processing and analysis.

POST-TEST:

- Inform the patient that a report of the results will be made available to the requesting HCP, who will discuss the results with the patient.
- Instruct the patient to resume usual diet, as directed by the HCP. Assess the patient's ability to swallow before allowing the patient to attempt liquids or solid foods.
- Inform the patient that he or she may experience some throat soreness and hoarseness. Instruct patient to treat

throat discomfort with lozenges and warm gargles when the gag reflex returns.

- Monitor vital signs and compare with baseline values every 15 min for 1 hr, then every 2 hr for 4 hr, and then as ordered by the HCP. Monitor temperature every 4 hr for 24 hr. Notify the HCP if temperature is elevated. Protocols may vary among facilities.
- Emergency resuscitation equipment should be readily available if the vocal cords become spastic after intubation.
- Observe/assess for delayed allergic reactions, such as rash, urticaria, tachycardia, hyperpnea, hypertension, palpitations, nausea, or vomiting.
- Observe/assess the patient for hemoptysis, dyspnea, cough, air hunger, excessive coughing, pain, or absent breathing sounds over the affected area. Report any symptoms to the HCP.
- Evaluate the patient for symptoms indicating the development of pneumothorax, such as dyspnea, tachypnea, anxiety, decreased breathing sounds, or restlessness. A chest x-ray may be ordered to check for the presence of this complication.
- Evaluate the patient for symptoms of empyema, such as fever, tachycardia, malaise, or elevated white blood cell count.
- Administer antibiotic therapy if ordered. Remind the patient of the importance of completing the entire course of antibiotic therapy, even if signs and symptoms disappear before completion of therapy.
- ***Nutritional Considerations:*** Malnutrition is commonly seen in patients with severe respiratory disease for numerous reasons including fatigue, lack of appetite, and gastrointestinal distress. Adequate intake of Vitamins A and C are also important to prevent pulmonary infection and to decrease the extent of lung tissue damage.
- Recognize anxiety related to test results, and be supportive of impaired activity related to perceived loss of independence and fear of shortened life expectancy. Discuss the implications of abnormal test results on the patient's lifestyle. Provide teaching and information regarding the clinical implications of the test results, as appropriate. Educate the patient regarding access to counseling services. Provide contact information, if desired, for the American Lung Association (www.lungusa.org). ✦
- Reinforce information given by the patient's HCP regarding further testing, treatment, or referral to another HCP. Inform the patient of smoking cessation programs, as appropriate. Inform the patient with abnormal findings of the importance of medical follow-up, and suggest ongoing support resources to assist in coping with chronic illness and possible early death. Answer any questions or address any concerns voiced by the patient or family.
- Instruct the patient in the use of any ordered medications. Explain the importance of adhering to the therapy regimen. As appropriate, instruct the patient in significant adverse effects associated with the prescribed medication. Encourage him or her to review corresponding literature provided by a pharmacist.
- Depending on the results of this procedure, additional testing may be performed to evaluate or monitor progression of the disease process and determine the need for a change in therapy. Evaluate test results in relation to the patient's symptoms and other tests performed.

RELATED STUDIES:

- Related tests include arterial/alveolar oxygen ratio, biopsy lung, blood gases, bronchoscopy, CBC, CT thoracic, relevant cultures (fungal, mycobacteria, sputum, throat, viral), gallium scan, Gram/acid-fast stain, lung perfusion scan, lung ventilation scan, MRI chest, mediastinoscopy, pleural fluid analysis, pulmonary function tests, and TB tests.
- Refer to the Immune and Respiratory systems tables online at Davis*Plus* for related tests by body system.

Cytology, Urine

C

SYNONYM/ACRONYM: N/A

COMMON USE: To identify the presence of neoplasms of the urinary tract and assist in the diagnosis of urinary tract infections.

SPECIMEN: Urine collected in a clean wide-mouth plastic container.

NORMAL FINDINGS: (Method: Microscopic examination) No abnormal cells or inclusions seen.

DESCRIPTION: Cytology is the study of the origin, structure, function, and pathology of cells. In clinical practice, cytological examinations are generally performed to detect cell changes resulting from neoplastic or inflammatory conditions. Cells from the epithelial lining of the urinary tract can be found in the urine. Examination of these cells for abnormalities is useful with suspected infection, inflammatory conditions, or malignancy.

This procedure is contraindicated for: N/A

INDICATIONS

- Assist in the diagnosis of urinary tract diseases, such as cancer, cytomegalovirus infection, and other inflammatory conditions.

POTENTIAL MEDICAL DIAGNOSIS

Positive findings in

- Cancer of the urinary tract
- Cytomegalic inclusion disease
- Inflammatory disease of the urinary tract

Negative findings in: N/A

CRITICAL FINDINGS:

- Identification of malignancy

Note and immediately report to the requesting health-care provider (HCP) any critical findings and related symptoms. A listing of these findings varies among facilities. Timely notification of a critical finding for laboratory or diagnostic studies is a role expectation of the professional nurse. The notification processes vary among facilities. Upon receipt of the critical finding, the information should be read back to the caller to verify accuracy.

INTERFERING FACTORS: N/A

NURSING IMPLICATIONS AND PROCEDURE

PRETEST:

- Positively identify the patient using at least two person-specific identifiers before services, treatments, or procedures are performed.
- ***Patient Teaching:*** Inform the patient this test can assist in identification of the organism causing infection or the presence of a tumor in the urinary tract.
- Obtain a history of the patient's health concerns, symptoms, surgical procedures, and results of previously performed laboratory and diagnostic studies. Include a list of known allergens, especially allergies or sensitivities to latex.
- Obtain a list of the patient's current medications, including over-the-counter medications and dietary supplements (see Effects of Natural

Products on Laboratory Values online at Davis*Plus*).

- Note any recent procedures that can interfere with test results.
- Review the procedure with the patient. If a catheterized specimen is to be collected, explain this procedure to the patient and obtain a catheterization tray. Address concerns about pain and explain that there may be some discomfort during the catheterization.
- ***Sensitivity to social and cultural issues,*** as well as concern for modesty, is important in providing psychological support before, during, and after the procedure.
- Note that there are no food, fluid, or medication restrictions, unless by medical direction.

INTRATEST:

Potential Complications: N/A

- Avoid the use of equipment containing latex if the patient has a history of allergic reaction to latex.
- Instruct the patient to cooperate fully and to follow directions.
- Observe standard precautions, and follow the general guidelines in Patient Preparation and Specimen Collection online at Davis*Plus*. Positively identify the patient, and label the appropriate tubes with the corresponding patient demographics, date and time of collection, method of specimen collection, and any medications the patient has taken that may interfere with test results (e.g., antibiotics).

Clean-Catch Specimen

- Instruct the male patient to (1) thoroughly wash his hands, (2) cleanse the meatus, (3) void a small amount into the toilet, and (4) void directly into the specimen container.
- Instruct the female patient to (1) thoroughly wash her hands; (2) cleanse the labia from front to back; (3) while keeping the labia separated, void a small amount into the toilet; and (4) without interrupting the urine stream, void directly into the specimen container.

Pediatric Urine Collector

- Put on gloves. Appropriately cleanse the genital area, and allow the area to dry. Remove the covering over the adhesive strips on the collector bag and apply over the genital area. Diaper the child. After obtaining the specimen, place the entire collection bag in a sterile urine container.

Indwelling Catheter

- Put on gloves. Empty drainage tube of urine. It may be necessary to clamp off the catheter for 15 to 30 min before specimen collection. Cleanse specimen port with antiseptic swab, and then aspirate 5 mL of urine with a 21- to 25-gauge needle and syringe. Transfer urine to a sterile container.

Urinary Catheterization

- Place female patient in lithotomy position or male patient in supine position. Using sterile technique, open the straight urinary catheterization kit and perform urinary catheterization. Place the retained urine in a sterile specimen container.

Suprapubic Aspiration

- Place the patient in supine position. Cleanse the area with antiseptic, and drape with sterile drapes. A needle is inserted through the skin into the bladder. A syringe attached to the needle is used to aspirate the urine sample. The needle is then removed and a sterile dressing is applied to the site. Place the sterile sample in a sterile specimen container.
- Do not collect urine from the pouch from a patient with a urinary diversion (e.g., ileal conduit). Instead perform catheterization through the stoma.

General

- Promptly transport the specimen to the laboratory for processing and analysis. If a delay in transport is expected, add an equal volume of 50% alcohol to the specimen as a preservative.

POST-TEST:

- Inform the patient that a report of the results will be made available to the requesting HCP, who will discuss the results with the patient.
- Instruct the patient to resume usual medication as directed by the HCP.

- Instruct the patient to report symptoms such as pain related to tissue inflammation, pain or irritation during void, bladder spasms, or alterations in urinary elimination.
- Observe for signs of inflammation if the specimen is obtained by suprapubic aspiration.
- Administer antibiotic therapy as ordered. Remind the patient of the importance of completing the entire course of antibiotic therapy, even if signs and symptoms disappear before completion of therapy.
- Recognize anxiety related to test results, and be supportive of fear of shortened life expectancy. Discuss the implications of abnormal test results on the patient's lifestyle. Provide teaching and information regarding the clinical implications of the test results, as appropriate. Educate the patient regarding access to counseling services.
- Reinforce information given by the patient's HCP regarding further testing, treatment, or referral to another HCP. Answer any questions or address any concerns voiced by the patient or family.
- Depending on the results of this procedure, additional testing may be performed to evaluate or monitor progression of the disease process and determine the need for a change in therapy. Evaluate test results in relation to the patient's symptoms and other tests performed.

RELATED STUDIES:

- Related tests include biopsy kidney, bladder cancer markers, cystoscopy, CMV IgG and IgM, Pap smear, UA, and US bladder.
- Refer to the Genitourinary and Immune systems tables online at Davis*Plus* for related tests by body system.

Cytomegalovirus, Immunoglobulin G, and Immunoglobulin M

SYNONYM/ACRONYM: CMV.

COMMON USE: To assist in diagnosing cytomegalovirus infection.

SPECIMEN: Serum collected in a plain red-top tube.

NORMAL FINDINGS: (Method: Enzyme immunoassay)

	IgM & IgG	Interpretation
Negative	0.9 index or less	No significant level of detectable antibody
Indeterminate	0.91–1.09 index	Equivocal results; retest in 10–14 d
Positive	1.1 index or greater	Antibody detected; indicative of recent immunization, current or recent infection

DESCRIPTION: Cytomegalovirus (CMV) is a double-stranded DNA herpesvirus. The Centers for Disease Control and Prevention estimates that 50% to 85% of adults are infected by age 40. The incubation period for primary infection is 4 to 8 wk. Transmission may occur by direct contact with oral, respiratory, or venereal secretions and excretions. CMV infection is of primary concern in pregnant or immunocompromised patients or patients who have recently received an organ transplant. Blood units are sometimes tested for the presence of CMV if patients in these high-risk categories are the transfusion recipients. CMV serology is part of the TORCH (*t*oxoplasmosis, *o*ther [congenital syphilis and viruses], *r*ubella, *CMV*, and *h*erpes simplex type 2) panel used to test pregnant women. CMV, as well as these other infectious organisms, can cross the placenta and result in congenital malformations, abortion, or stillbirth. The presence of immunoglobulin (Ig) M antibodies indicates acute infection. The presence of IgG antibodies indicates current or past infection. There are numerous methods for detection of CMV. The methodology selected is based on both the test purpose and specimen type. Other types of assays used to detect CMV include direct fluorescent assays used to identify CMV in tissue, sputum, and swab specimens; hemagglutination assays, cleared by the FDA for testing blood prior to transfusion; polymerase chain reaction, used to test a wide variety of specimen types, including amniotic fluid, plasma, urine, CSF, and whole blood; and cell tissue culture, which remains the gold standard for the identification of CMV.

This procedure is contraindicated for: N/A

INDICATIONS

- Assist in the diagnosis of congenital CMV infection in newborns.
- Determine susceptibility, particularly in pregnant women, immunocompromised patients, and patients who recently have received an organ transplant.
- Screen blood for high-risk-category transfusion recipients.

POTENTIAL MEDICAL DIAGNOSIS

Positive findings in

- CMV infection

Negative findings in: N/A

CRITICAL FINDINGS: N/A

INTERFERING FACTORS

- False-positive results may occur in the presence of rheumatoid factor.
- False-negative results may occur if treatment was begun before antibodies developed or if the test was done less than 6 days after exposure to the virus.

NURSING IMPLICATIONS AND PROCEDURE

POTENTIAL NURSING PROBLEMS:

Problem	Signs & Symptoms	Interventions
Infection ***(related to viral infection secondary to blood transfusion; organ transplant; sexual contact; exposure to respiratory droplets)***	Fever, fatigue, loss of appetite; malaise; muscle aches; headache; irregular heartbeat; stiff neck; shortness of	Promote good hygiene; assist with hygiene as needed; administer prescribed antivirals as appropriate, antipyretics; administer cooling measures; monitor

(table continues on page 704)

Problem	Signs & Symptoms	Interventions
	breath; swollen liver or spleen; tachycardia; rash; sore throat; increased blood pressure; elevated IgM, IgG	vital signs and trend temperatures; encourage oral fluids; adhere to standard or universal precautions; provide isolation as appropriate; obtain cultures as ordered; assess nutritional status and provide supplements as needed
Fatigue ***(related to infection and inflammation)***	Report of tiredness; inability to maintain activities of daily living at current level; inability to restore energy after rest or sleep	Discuss the implementation of energy conservation activities (even pace when working, frequent rest periods, frequent items in easy reach, push items instead of pulling); limit naps to increase nighttime sleeping; set priorities for energy expenditures; administer ordered antibiotics
Sexuality ***(related to positive CMV [herpes virus])***	Reduced sexual function; decreased sexual satisfaction; reports of alteration in relationship with partner	Assess perception of reported change in sexual function; assess emotional impact of herpes diagnosis (depression, altered self-esteem, altered personal relationships); assess need for counseling; encourage verbalization of feelings; discuss alternative forms of intimate expression; discuss medical treatments that may improve sexual interaction

PRETEST:

- Positively identify the patient using at least two person-specific identifiers before services, treatments, or procedures are performed.
- ***Patient Teaching:*** Inform the patient this test can assist in identification of the organism causing infection.
- Obtain a history of the patient's health concerns and history of exposure. Obtain a list of known allergens, especially allergies or sensitivities to latex.
- Obtain a history of the patient's immune and reproductive systems, symptoms, and results of previously

performed laboratory tests and diagnostic and surgical procedures.
- Obtain a list of the patient's current medications, including over-the-counter medications and dietary supplements (see Effects of Natural Products on Laboratory Values online at Davis*Plus*).
- Review the procedure with the patient. Inform the patient that multiple specimens may be required. Any individual positive result should be repeated in 7 to 14 days to monitor a change in titer. Inform the patient that specimen collection takes approximately 5 to 10 min. Address concerns about pain and explain that there may be some discomfort during the venipuncture.
- ***Sensitivity to social and cultural issues,*** as well as concern for modesty, is important in providing psychological support before, during, and after the procedure.
- Note that there are no food, fluid, or medication restrictions, unless by medical direction.

INTRATEST:

Potential Complications: N/A
- Avoid the use of equipment containing latex if the patient has a history of allergic reaction to latex.
- Instruct the patient to cooperate fully and to follow directions. Direct the patient to breathe normally and to avoid unnecessary movement.
- Observe standard precautions, and follow the general guidelines in Patient Preparation and Specimen Collection online at Davis*Plus*. Positively identify the patient, and label the appropriate specimen container with the corresponding patient demographics, initials of the person collecting the specimen, date, and time of collection. Perform a venipuncture.
- Remove the needle and apply direct pressure with dry gauze to stop bleeding. Observe/assess venipuncture site for bleeding or hematoma formation and secure gauze with adhesive bandage.
- Promptly transport the specimen to the laboratory for processing and analysis.

POST-TEST:
- Inform the patient that a report of the results will be made available to the requesting health-care provider (HCP), who will discuss the results with the patient. Some HCPs may take additional precautions in the case of CMV antibody negative immunocompromised or pregnant patients by requesting CMV antibody negative blood products or organs in the event those interventions are required.
- Instruct the patient in isolation precautions during time of communicability or contagion.
- Emphasize the need to return to have a convalescent blood sample taken in 7 to 14 days.
- Warn the patient that there is a possibility of false-negative or false-positive results.
- Recognize anxiety related to test results if the patient is pregnant, and offer support. Discuss the implications of abnormal test results on the patient's lifestyle. Provide teaching and information regarding the clinical implications of the test results, as appropriate. Educate the patient regarding access to counseling services.
- Reinforce information given by the patient's HCP regarding further testing, treatment, or referral to another HCP. Answer any questions or address any concerns voiced by the patient or family.
- Depending on the results of this procedure, additional testing may be performed to evaluate or monitor progression of the disease process and determine the need for a change in therapy. Evaluate test results in relation to the patient's symptoms and other tests performed.

Patient Education:
- Provide emotional support if the patient is pregnant and if results are positive.

- Reinforce information given by the patient's HCP regarding further testing, treatment, or referral to another HCP.
- Answer any questions or address any concerns voiced by the patient or family.

Expected Patient Outcomes:

Understanding

- The patient and family state that it may take up to 6 wk for full recovery from the diagnosed viral infection.
- The patient and family state that once CMV virus is in an individual, it will remain present for the rest of his or her life.
- The patient and family state emergency response number and understand to call for severe abdominal pain that could indicate a ruptured spleen requiring emergency surgery.

Ability

- The patient demonstrates proficiency in using warm saltwater gargles for comfort with sore throat.

Response

- The patient complies with the recommendation of infected persons to refrain from kissing or other sexual contact to prevent infecting others.
- The patient complies with the request to stay at home while infectious to avoid exposing others.

RELATED STUDIES:

- Related tests include β_2-microglobulin, bronchoscopy, *Chlamydia* group antibody, culture viral, cytology urine, HIV-1/2 antibodies, Pap smear, rubella antibody, and *Toxoplasma* antibody.
- Refer to the Immune and Reproductive systems tables online at Davis*Plus* for related tests by body system.

D-Dimer

SYNONYM/ACRONYM: Dimer, fibrin degradation fragment.

COMMON USE: To assist in diagnosing a diffuse state of hypercoagulation as seen in disseminated intravascular coagulation (DIC), acute myocardial infarction (MI), deep venous thrombosis (DVT), and pulmonary embolism (PE).

SPECIMEN: Plasma collected in a completely filled blue-top (3.2% sodium citrate) tube. If the patient's hematocrit exceeds 55%, the volume of citrate in the collection tube must be adjusted.

NORMAL FINDINGS: (Method: Immunoturbidimetric)

Conventional Units (FEU = Fibrinogen Equivalent Units)	SI Units (Conventional Units × 5.476)
0–0.5 mcg/mL FEU	0–2.7 nmol/L

Levels increase with age.

DESCRIPTION: Activated Factor II or thrombin serves two functions. It helps convert fibrinogen to fibrin during the process of hemostasis and simultaneously activates the fibrinolytic system to provide a balance between blood clotting and vessel occlusion. D-dimers are crosslinked fragments of fibrin produced during fibrinolysis or dissolution of a clot. It is for this reason that increased D-dimers are utilized as an indication of the presence of a thrombus or clot. The test is not specific to the presence of a clot as other factors, to include infection, inflammation, and pregnancy can increase D-dimer concentration. A negative test can largely rule out presence of a new blood clot. A positive test is presumptive evidence of disseminated intravascular coagulation (DIC), deep vein thrombosis (DVT) or pulmonary embolism (PE) which must be confirmed using other tests. The D-dimer is specific to secondary fibrinolysis because it involves fibrin rather than fibrinogen. This test may be used in combination with fibrinogen split or fibrinogen degradation products to differentiate primary fibrinolysis from secondary fibrinolysis. The treatment for primary fibrinolysis would require antifibrinolytic therapy while the treatment for secondary fibrinolysis (DIC) might include transfusion to replace consumed coagulation factors and platelets and anticoagulant therapy to prevent recurrent clot formation.

This procedure is contraindicated for: N/A

INDICATIONS

- Assist in the detection of DIC and DVT.
- Assist in the evaluation of myocardial infarction (MI) and unstable angina.
- Assist in the evaluation of possible veno-occlusive disease associated with sequelae of bone marrow transplant.
- Assist in the evaluation of PE.

POTENTIAL MEDICAL DIAGNOSIS

The sensitivity and specificity of the assay varies among test kits and between test methods.

Increased in:

D-Dimers are formed in inflammatory conditions where plasmin carries out its fibrinolytic action on a fibrin clot.

D

- Arterial or venous thrombosis
- DVT
- DIC
- Neoplastic disease
- Pre-eclampsia
- Pregnancy (late and postpartum)
- PE
- Recent surgery (within 2 days)
- Secondary fibrinolysis
- Thrombolytic or fibrinolytic therapy

Decreased in: N/A

CRITICAL FINDINGS: N/A

INTERFERING FACTORS

- High rheumatoid factor titers can cause a false-positive result.
- Increased CA 125 levels can cause a false-positive result; patients with cancer may demonstrate increased levels.
- Drugs and other substances that may cause an increase in plasma D-dimer include those administered for antiplatelet therapy.
- Drugs and other substances that may cause a decrease in plasma D-dimer include pravastatin and warfarin.
- Placement of tourniquet for longer than 1 min can result in venous stasis and changes in the concentration of plasma proteins to be measured. Platelet activation may also occur under these conditions, causing erroneous results.
- Vascular injury during phlebotomy can activate platelets and coagulation factors, causing erroneous results.
- Hemolyzed specimens must be rejected because hemolysis is an indication of platelet and coagulation factor activation.
- Hematocrit greater than 55% may cause falsely prolonged results because of anticoagulant excess relative to plasma volume.
- Incompletely filled collection tubes, specimens contaminated with heparin, clotted specimens, or unprocessed specimens not delivered to the laboratory within 1 to 2 hr of collection should be rejected.
- Icteric or lipemic specimens interfere with optical testing methods, producing erroneous results.

NURSING IMPLICATIONS AND PROCEDURE

POTENTIAL NURSING PROBLEMS:

Problem	Signs & Symptoms	Interventions
Bleeding ***(related to alerted clotting factors secondary to anticoagulant therapy; depleted clotting factors)***	Altered level of consciousness; hypotension; increased heart rate; decreased hemoglobin (Hgb) and hematocrit (Hct); capillary refill greater than 3 sec; cool extremities	Increase frequency of vital sign assessment with variances in results; monitor for vital sign trends; administer blood or blood products as ordered; administer stool softeners as needed; monitor stool for blood; encourage

Problem	Signs & Symptoms	Interventions
		intake of foods rich in vitamin K; monitor and trend Hgb/Hct; assess skin for petechiae, purpura, hematoma; monitor for blood in emesis, or sputum; institute bleeding precautions (prevent unnecessary venipuncture; avoid intramuscular injections; prevent trauma; be gentle with oral care, suctioning; avoid use of a sharp razor); administer prescribed medications (recombinant human activated protein C; epsilon aminocaproic acid)
Protection ***(related to increased bleeding risk associated with the hemorrhagic possibility with DIC protection; red cell destruction secondary to altered plasma environment; decreased and defective platelets; blood loss; ineffective clotting)***	Pallor; fatigue; weakness; shortness of breath; anxiety; admits easily bruising; increased clotting time	Assess for symptoms of blood loss (fatigue, pallor, decreased activity); observe for prolonged bleeding associated with ineffective clotting; use pulse oximetry or arterial blood gases to assess oxygenation; administer oxygen as required; administer blood or blood products as required; administer prescribed epoetin alfa; use bleeding precautions (avoid aspirin products, trauma, constipation, and forceful nose blowing that could cause nosebleed)
Tissue perfusion (cerebral, peripheral, renal) ***(related to altered blood flow associated with platelet clumping)***	Hypotension; dizziness; cool extremities; capillary refill greater than 3 sec; weak pedal pulses; altered level of consciousness	Monitor blood pressure; assess for dizziness; check skin temperature for warmth; assess capillary refill; assess pedal pulses; monitor level of consciousness; administer prescribed vasodilators and inotropic drugs; provide oxygen as required

(table continues on page 710)

Problem	Signs & Symptoms	Interventions
Fear ***(related to the possibility of death secondary to diagnosis of DIC, MI, PE, DVT, or other associated diagnoses)***	Verbalization of fear; restlessness; increased tension; continuous questioning; increased blood pressure, heart rate, respiratory rate; diarrhea; anorexia; nausea; pallor; vomiting; fatigue; dry mouth	Evaluate verbal and nonverbal indicators of fear; assess for the cause of fear; acknowledge the patient's awareness of fear; explain all procedures with simple age and culturally appropriate language; administer prescribed mild tranquilizer; maintain a confident, assured, professional manner in all patient interactions

D

PRETEST:

- Positively identify the patient using at least two person-specific identifiers before services, treatments, or procedures are performed.
- *Patient Teaching:* Inform the patient this test can assist in diagnosing and evaluating conditions affecting normal blood clot formation.
- Obtain a history of the patient's health concerns, symptoms, surgical procedures, and results of previously performed laboratory and diagnostic studies. Include a list of known allergens, especially allergies or sensitivities to latex.
- Obtain a list of the patient's current medications, including over-the-counter medications and dietary supplements (see Effects of Natural Products on Laboratory Values online at Davis*Plus*).
- Review the procedure with the patient. Inform the patient that specimen collection takes approximately 5 to 10 min. Address concerns about pain and explain that there may be some discomfort during the venipuncture.
- ***Sensitivity to social and cultural issues,*** as well as concern for modesty, is important in providing psychological support before, during, and after the procedure.
- Note that there are no food, fluid, or medication restrictions unless by medical direction.

INTRATEST:

Potential Complications: N/A

- Avoid the use of equipment containing latex if the patient has a history of allergic reaction to latex.
- Instruct the patient to cooperate fully and to follow directions. Direct the patient to breathe normally and to avoid unnecessary movement.
- Observe standard precautions, and follow the general guidelines in Patient Preparation and Specimen Collection online at Davis*Plus*. Positively identify the patient, and label the appropriate specimen container with the corresponding patient demographics, initials of the person collecting the specimen, date, and time of collection. Perform a venipuncture. Fill tube completely. *Important note:* When multiple specimens are drawn, the blue-top tube should be collected after sterile (i.e., blood culture) tubes. Otherwise, when using a standard vacutainer system, the blue top is the first tube collected. When a butterfly is used and due to the added tubing, an extra red-top tube should be collected before the blue-top tube to ensure complete filling of the blue-top tube.

- Remove the needle and apply direct pressure with dry gauze to stop bleeding. Observe/assess venipuncture site for bleeding or hematoma formation and secure gauze with adhesive bandage.
- Promptly transport the specimen to the laboratory for processing and analysis. The recommendation for processed and unprocessed samples stored in unopened tubes is that testing should be completed within 1 to 4 hr of collection.

POST-TEST:

- Inform the patient that a report of the results will be made available to the requesting health-care provider (HCP), who will discuss the results with the patient.
- Depending on the results of this procedure, additional testing may be performed to evaluate or monitor progression of the disease process and determine the need for a change in therapy. Evaluate test results in relation to the patient's symptoms and other tests performed.

Patient Education:

- Reinforce information given by the patient's HCP regarding further testing, treatment, or referral to another HCP.
- Teach the patient and family about bleeding precautions that can be used to decrease injury risk.
- Answer any questions or address any concerns voiced by the patient or family.

Expected Patient Outcomes:

Understanding

- The patient and family state that support groups are available to address fears and concerns.
- The patient and family state the disease process and treatment plan.

Ability

- The patient and family participate in discussions related to distinguishing between rational and irrational fears.
- The patient and family demonstrate proficiency with the use of positive coping techniques.

Response

- The patient and family express fear related to diagnosis appropriately.
- The patient complies with the request for psychological evaluation related to fear management.

RELATED STUDIES:

- Related tests include aPTT, alveolar/arterial gradient, angiography pulmonary, antibodies anticardiolipin, AT-III, blood gases, coagulation factors, CBC platelet count, FDP, fibrinogen, lactic acid, lung perfusion scan, MRI venography, plasminogen, plethysmography, protein S, PT/INR, US venous Doppler extremity studies, and venography lower extremity studies.
- Refer to the Cardiovascular, Hematopoietic, and Respiratory systems tables online at Davis*Plus* for related tests by body system.

Dehydroepiandrosterone Sulfate

SYNONYM/ACRONYM: DHEAS.

COMMON USE: To assist in identifying the cause of infertility, amenorrhea, or hirsutism.

SPECIMEN: Serum collected in a red- or red/gray-top tube. Plasma collected in a lavender-top (EDTA) tube is also acceptable. Place separated serum into a standard transport tube within 2 hr of collection.

NORMAL FINDINGS: (Method: Immunochemiluminometric assay [ICMA])

Age	Male Conventional Units mcg/dL	Male SI Units micromol/L (Conventional Units × 0.027)	Female Conventional Units mcg/dL	Female SI Units micromol/L (Conventional Units × 0.027)
Newborn	108–607	2.9–16.4	108–607	2.9–16.4
7–30 d	32–431	0.9–11.6	32–431	0.9–11.6
1–5 mo	3–124	0.1–3.3	3–124	0.1–3.3
6–35 mo	0–30	0–0.8	0–30	0–0.8
3–6 yr	0–50	0–1.4	0–50	0–1.4
7–9 yr	5–115	0.1–3.1	5–94	0.1–2.5
10–14 yr	22–332	0.6–9	22–255	0.6–6.9
15–19 yr	88–483	2.4–13	63–373	1.7–10
20–29 yr	280–640	7.6–17.3	65–380	1.8–10.3
30–39 yr	120–520	3.2–14	45–270	1.2–7.3
40–49 yr	95–530	2.6–14.3	32–240	0.9–6.5
50–59 yr	70–310	1.9–8.4	26–200	0.7–5.4
60–69 yr	42–290	1.1–7.8	13–130	0.4–3.5
70 yr and older	28–175	0.8–4.7	10–90	0.3–2.4

D

POTENTIAL MEDICAL DIAGNOSIS

Increased in:

DHEAS is produced by the adrenal cortex and testis; therefore, any condition stimulating these organs or associated feedback mechanisms will result in increased levels.

- Anovulation
- Cushing's syndrome
- Ectopic ACTH-producing tumors
- Hirsutism
- Hyperprolactinemia
- Polycystic ovary (Stein-Leventhal syndrome)
- Virilizing adrenal tumors

Decreased in:

DHEAS is produced by the adrenal cortex and testis; therefore, any condition suppressing the normal function of these organs or associated feedback mechanisms will result in decreased levels.

- Addison's disease
- Adrenal insufficiency (primary or secondary)
- Aging adults ***(related to natural decline in production with age)***
- Hyperlipidemia
- Pregnancy ***(related to DHEAS produced by fetal adrenals and converted to estrogens in the placenta)***
- Psoriasis ***(some potent topical medications used for long periods of time can result in chronic adrenal insufficiency)***
- Psychosis ***(related to acute adrenal insufficiency)***

CRITICAL FINDINGS: N/A

Find and print out the full study on Fast Find at davispl.us/vanleeuwen7.

Drugs of Abuse

Amphetamines
Opiates
Ethanol (Alcohol)
Cocaine
Cannabinoids
Phencyclidine

SYNONYM/ACRONYM: Amphetamines, cannabinoids (THC), cocaine, ethanol (alcohol, ethyl alcohol, ETOH), phencyclidine (PCP), opiates (heroin).

COMMON USE: To assist in rapid identification of commonly abused drugs in suspected drug overdose or for workplace drug screening.

SPECIMEN: For ethanol, serum collected in a red-top tube; plasma collected in a gray-top (sodium fluoride/potassium oxalate) tube is also acceptable. For drug screen, urine collected in a clean plastic container. Gastric contents may also be submitted for testing.

Workplace drug-screening programs, because of the potential medicolegal consequences associated with them, require collection of urine and blood specimens using a *chain of custody protocol.* Analysis is performed in laboratories that are specially certified to perform workplace drug testing. The protocol provides securing the sample in a sealed transport device in the presence of the donor and a representative of the donor's employer, such that tampering would be obvious. The protocol also provides a written document of specimen transfer from donor to specimen collection personnel, to storage, to analyst, and to disposal.

NORMAL FINDINGS: (Method: Spectrophotometry for ethanol; immunoassay for drugs of abuse)
Ethanol: None detected
Drug screen: None detected

POTENTIAL MEDICAL DIAGNOSIS

A urine screen merely identifies the presence of these substances in urine; it does not indicate time of exposure, amount used, quality of the source used, or level of impairment. Positive screens should be considered presumptive. Drug-specific confirmatory methods should be used to investigate questionable results of a positive urine screen.

CRITICAL FINDINGS:

Note and immediately report to the requesting health-care provider (HCP) any critical findings and related symptoms. A listing of these findings varies among facilities. Timely notification of a critical finding for laboratory or diagnostic studies is a role expectation of the professional nurse. The notification processes vary among facilities. Upon receipt of the critical finding, the information should be read back to the caller to verify accuracy.

The legal limit for ethanol intoxication varies by state, but in most places, greater than 80 mg/dL (0.08 %) is considered impaired for driving. Levels greater than 300 mg/dL are associated with amnesia, vomiting, double vision, and hypothermia. Levels of 80 to 400 mg/dL are associated with coma and may be fatal. Possible interventions for ethanol toxicity include administration of tap water or 3% sodium bicarbonate lavage, breathing support, and hemodialysis (usually indicated only if levels exceed 300 mg/dL).

Amphetamine intoxication (greater than 200 ng/mL) causes psychoses, tremors, convulsions, insomnia, tachycardia, dysrhythmias, impotence, cerebrovascular accident, and respiratory failure. Possible interventions include emesis (if orally ingested and if the patient has a gag reflex and normal central nervous system [CNS] function), administration of activated charcoal followed by magnesium citrate cathartic, acidification of the urine to promote excretion, and administration of liquids to promote urinary output.

Cocaine intoxication (greater than 1,000 ng/mL) causes short-term symptoms of CNS stimulation, hypertension, tachypnea, mydriasis, and tachycardia. Possible interventions include emesis (if orally ingested and if the patient has a gag reflex and normal CNS function), gastric lavage (if orally ingested), whole-bowel irrigation (if packs of the drug were ingested), airway protection, cardiac support, and administration of diazepam or phenobarbital for convulsions. The use of beta blockers is contraindicated.

Heroin and morphine are opiates that at toxic levels (greater than 200 ng/mL) cause bradycardia, flushing, itching, hypotension, hypothermia, and respiratory depression. Possible interventions include airway protection and the administration of naloxone (Narcan).

PCP intoxication (greater than 100 ng/mL) causes a variety of symptoms depending on the stage of intoxication. Stage I includes psychiatric signs, muscle spasms, fever, tachycardia, flushing, small pupils, salivation, nausea, and vomiting. Stage II includes stupor, convulsions, hallucinations, increased heart rate, and increased blood pressure. Stage III includes further increases of heart rate and blood pressure that may culminate in cardiac and respiratory failure. Possible interventions may include providing respiratory support, administration of activated charcoal with a cathartic such as sorbitol, gastric lavage and suction, administration of intravenous nutrition and electrolytes, and acidification of the urine to promote PCP excretion.

Find and print out the full study on Fast Find at davispl.us/vanleeuwen7.

Ductography

SYNONYM/ACRONYM: Breast ductoscopy, fiberoptic ductoscopy, galactography.

COMMON USE: To visualize and assess the breast ducts for disease and malignancy in women with nipple discharge.

AREA OF APPLICATION: Breast.

POTENTIAL MEDICAL DIAGNOSIS

Normal findings
- Normal breast tissue

Abnormal findings related to
- Ductal thickening
- Papillary lesions

CRITICAL FINDINGS:
- Ductal carcinoma in situ
- Invasive breast cancer

Note and immediately report to the requesting health-care provider (HCP) any critical findings and related symptoms. A listing of these findings varies among facilities. Timely notification of a critical finding for laboratory or diagnostic studies is a role expectation of the professional nurse. The notification processes vary among facilities. Upon receipt of the critical finding, the information should be read back to the caller to verify accuracy.

Find and print out the full study on Fast Find at davispl.us/vanleeuwen7.

D

D-Xylose Tolerance Test

SYNONYM/ACRONYM: N/A

COMMON USE: To assist in the differential diagnosis of small intestine malabsorption syndromes such as celiac, tropical sprue, and Crohn's diseases.

SPECIMEN: Plasma collected in a gray-top (fluoride/oxalate) tube and urine (from a 5-hr collection) in a clean amber plastic container.

NORMAL FINDINGS: (Method: Spectrophotometry)

Dose Given	Conventional Units	SI Units (Conventional Units × 0.0666)
	Plasma	
Infant dose 0.5 g/kg (max. 25 g)	Greater than 15 mg/dL after 2 hr	Greater than 1 mmol/L
Pediatric dose 0.5 g/kg (max. 25 g)	Greater than 20 mg/dL after 2 hr	Greater than 1.3 mmol/L
Adult dose		
25 g	Greater than 25 mg/dL after 2 hr	Greater than 1.7 mmol/L
5 g (given if patient is known or expected to have severe symptoms)	Greater than 20 mg/dL after 2 hr	Greater than 1.3 mmol/L

	Urine
Children	Greater than 16%–40% of dose in 5-hr urine sample
Adults	Greater than 16% or greater than 4 g of dose in 5-hr urine sample
Older adults (65 yr and older)	Greater than 14% or greater than 3.5 g of dose in 5-hr urine sample

POTENTIAL MEDICAL DIAGNOSIS

Increased in: N/A

Decreased in:

Conditions that involve defective mucosal absorption of carbohydrates and other nutrients.

- Amyloidosis
- Bacterial overgrowth ***(sugar is consumed by bacteria)***
- Eosinophilic gastroenteritis
- Lymphoma
- Nontropical sprue (celiac disease, gluten-induced enteropathy)
- Parasitic infestations (Giardia, schistosomiasis, hookworm)
- Postoperative period after massive resection of the intestine
- Radiation enteritis
- Scleroderma
- Small bowel ischemia
- Tropical sprue
- Whipple's disease
- Zollinger-Ellison syndrome

CRITICAL FINDINGS: N/A

D

Find and print out the full study on Fast Find at davispl.us/vanleeuwen7.

Echocardiography

SYNONYM/ACRONYM: Doppler echo, Doppler ultrasound of the heart, echo, sonogram of the heart, transthoracic echocardiogram (TTE).

COMMON USE: To assist in diagnosing cardiovascular disorders such as defect, heart failure, tumor, infection, and bleeding.

AREA OF APPLICATION: Chest/thorax.

DESCRIPTION: Echocardiography, a noninvasive ultrasound (US) procedure, uses high-frequency sound waves of various intensities to assist in diagnosing cardiovascular disorders. The procedure records the echoes created by the deflection of an ultrasonic beam off the cardiac structures and allows visualization of the size, shape, position, thickness, and movement of all four valves, atria, ventricular and atria septa, papillary muscles, chordae tendineae, and ventricles. This study can also determine blood-flow velocity and direction and the presence of pericardial effusion during the movement of the transducer over areas of the chest. Electrocardiography and phonocardiography can be done simultaneously to correlate the findings with the cardiac cycle. These procedures can be done at the bedside or in a specialized department, health-care provider's (HPC's) office, or clinic.

Included in the study are the M-mode method, which produces a linear tracing of timed motions of the heart, its structures, and associated measurements over time; and the two-dimensional grayscale method, or two-dimensional real-time Doppler color-flow imaging with pulsed and continuous-wave Doppler spectral tracings, which produces a cross-section of the structures of the heart and their relationship to one another, including changes in the coronary vasculature, velocity and direction of blood flow, and areas of eccentric blood flow. Red and blue colors are assigned to represent the direction of blood flow, and the intensity of the color is an indication of velocity. Doppler color-flow imaging may also be helpful in depicting the function of biological and prosthetic valves.

Echocardiography has become the method of choice for cardiac stress testing and evaluation of chest pain. Congenital heart disease such as atrial or ventricular septal defects are frequently evaluated with echocardiography. Cardiac contrast medium, composed of nonIodinated lipid microspheres, such as DEFINITY or Optison may be used to improve the visualization of the heart.

This procedure is contraindicated for: N/A

INDICATIONS

- Detect atrial tumors (myxomas).
- Detect subaortic stenosis as evidenced ***either by displacement of the anterior atrial leaflet or by a reduction in aortic valve flow, depending on the obstruction.***
- Detect ventricular or atrial mural thrombi and evaluate cardiac wall motion after myocardial infarction.
- Determine the presence of pericardial effusion, tamponade, and pericarditis.
- Determine the severity of valvular abnormalities such as stenosis, prolapse, and regurgitation.

- Evaluate congenital heart disorders.
- Evaluate endocarditis.
- Evaluate or monitor prosthetic valve function.
- Evaluate the presence of shunt flow and continuity of the aorta and pulmonary artery.
- Evaluate unexplained chest pain, electrocardiographic changes, and abnormal chest x-ray ***(evidenced by an enlarged cardiac silhouette).***
- Evaluate ventricular aneurysms and/or thrombus.
- Measure the size of the heart's chambers and determine if hypertrophic cardiomyopathy or heart failure is present.

E

POTENTIAL MEDICAL DIAGNOSIS

Normal findings

- Normal appearance in the size, position, structure, and movements of the heart valves visualized and recorded in a combination of ultrasound modes; and normal heart muscle walls of both ventricles and left atrium, with adequate blood filling. Established values for the measurement of heart activities obtained by the study may vary by HCP and institution.

Abnormal findings related to

- Aortic aneurysm
- Aortic valve abnormalities
- Cardiac neoplasm
- Cardiomyopathy
- Congenital heart defect
- Coronary artery disease (CAD)
- Endocarditis
- Heart failure
- Mitral valve abnormalities
- Myxoma
- Pericardial effusion, tamponade, and pericarditis
- Pulmonary hypertension
- Pulmonary valve abnormalities
- Septal defects
- Ventricular hypertrophy
- Ventricular or atrial mural thrombi

CRITICAL FINDINGS:

- Aortic aneurysm
- Infection
- Obstruction
- Tumor with significant mass effect (rare)

Note and immediately report to the requesting HCP any critical findings and related symptoms. A listing of these findings varies among facilities. Timely notification of a critical finding for laboratory or diagnostic studies is a role expectation of the professional nurse. The notification processes vary among facilities. Upon receipt of the critical finding, the information should be read back to the caller to verify accuracy.

INTERFERING FACTORS

Factors that may alter the results of the study

- Incorrect placement of the transducer over the desired test site.
- Patients who are dehydrated, resulting in failure to demonstrate the boundaries between organs and tissue structures.
- Metallic objects (e.g., jewelry, body rings) within the examination field, which may inhibit organ visualization and cause unclear images.
- The presence of chronic obstructive pulmonary disease or use of mechanical ventilation, which increases the air between the heart and chest wall (hyperinflation) and can attenuate the ultrasound waves.
- Obese patients due to the enlarged space between the transducer and the heart and because fatty tissue may distort the sound waves.
- Inability of the patient to cooperate or remain still during the procedure because of age, significant pain, or mental status.
- The presence of dysrhythmias.

NURSING IMPLICATIONS AND PROCEDURE

See Potential Nursing Problems on Fast Find at davispl.us/vanleeuwen7.

PRETEST:

- Positively identify the patient using at least two person-specific identifiers before services, treatments, or procedures are performed.
- ***Patient Teaching:*** Inform the patient this procedure can assist in assessing heart function.
- Obtain a history of the patient's health concerns, symptoms, surgical procedures, and results of previously performed laboratory and diagnostic studies. Include a list of known allergens, especially allergies or sensitivities to latex, anesthetics, or sedatives.
- Record the date of the last menstrual period and determine the possibility of pregnancy in perimenopausal women.
- Obtain a list of the patient's current medications, including over-the-counter medications and dietary supplements (see Effects of Natural Products on Laboratory Values online at Davis*Plus*).
- Review the procedure with the patient. Address concerns about pain related to the procedure and explain that there should be no discomfort during the procedure. Inform the patient the procedure is performed in a US or cardiology department, usually by an HCP, and takes approximately 30 to 45 min.
- Explain that an intravenous (IV) line may be inserted to allow infusion of fluids such as saline, anesthetics, sedatives, contrast medium, or emergency medications.
- ***Sensitivity to social and cultural issues,*** as well as concern for modesty, is important in providing psychological support before, during, and after the procedure.
- Instruct the patient to remove jewelry, and other metallic objects from the area to be examined.
- Note that there are no food or fluid restrictions unless by medical direction.

INTRATEST:

Potential Complications: N/A

- Observe standard precautions, and follow the general guidelines in Patient Preparation and Specimen Collection online at Davis*Plus*. Positively identify the patient.
- Ensure the patient has removed all external metallic objects from the area to be examined prior to the procedure.
- Avoid the use of equipment containing latex if the patient has a history of allergic reaction to latex.
- Have emergency equipment readily available.
- Instruct the patient to void prior to the procedure and to change into the gown, robe, and foot coverings provided.
- Instruct the patient to cooperate fully and to follow directions. Instruct the patient to remain still throughout the procedure because movement produces unreliable results.
- Place the patient in a supine position on a flat table with foam wedges to help maintain position and immobilization.
- Establish an IV fluid line for the injection of saline, anesthetics, sedatives, contrast medium, or emergency medications.
- Expose the chest, and attach electrocardiogram leads for simultaneous tracings, if desired.
- Apply conductive gel to the chest. Place the transducer on the chest surface along the left sternal border, the subxiphoid area, suprasternal notch, and supraclavicular areas to obtain views and tracings of the portions of the heart. Scan the areas by systematically moving the probe in a perpendicular position to direct the ultrasound waves to each part of the heart.
- To obtain different views or information about heart function, position the patient on the left side and/or sitting

up, or request that the patient breathe slowly or hold the breath during the procedure. To evaluate heart function changes, the patient may be asked to inhale amyl nitrate (vasodilator).
- Administer contrast medium, if ordered. A second series of images is obtained.

POST-TEST:

- Inform the patient that a report of the results will be made available to the requesting HCP, who will discuss the results with the patient.
- When the study is completed, remove the gel from the skin.
- Recognize anxiety related to test results, and offer support. Discuss the implications of abnormal test results on the patient's lifestyle. Provide teaching and information regarding the clinical implications of the test results, as appropriate.
- ***Nutritional Considerations:*** Abnormal findings may be associated with cardiovascular disease. Nutritional therapy is recommended for the patient identified to be at risk for developing CAD or for individuals who have specific risk factors and/or existing medical conditions (e.g., elevated LDL cholesterol levels, other lipid disorders, type 1 diabetes, type 2 diabetes, insulin resistance, or metabolic syndrome). Other changeable risk factors warranting patient education include strategies to encourage patients, especially those who are overweight and with high blood pressure, to safely decrease sodium intake, achieve a normal weight, ensure regular participation in moderate aerobic physical activity three to four times per week, eliminate tobacco use, and adhere to a heart-healthy diet. If triglycerides also are elevated, the patient should be advised to eliminate or reduce alcohol. A variety of dietary patterns are beneficial for people with CAD, and there are many meal-planning approaches with nutritional goals endorsed by the American Diabetes Association (ADA). The Guideline on Lifestyle Management to Reduce Cardiovascular Risk published by the American College of Cardiology and the American Heart Association (AHA) in conjunction with the National Heart, Lung, and Blood Institute (NHLBI) recommends a Mediterranean-style diet rather than a low-fat diet. The guideline emphasizes inclusion of vegetables, whole grains, fruits, low-fat dairy, nuts, legumes, and nontropical vegetable oils (e.g., olive, canola, peanut, sunflower, flaxseed) along with fish and lean poultry. 🍁 A similar dietary pattern known as the Dietary Approaches to Stop Hypertension (DASH) diet makes additional recommendations for the reduction of dietary sodium. Both dietary styles emphasize a reduction in consumption of red meats, which are high in saturated fats and cholesterol, and other foods containing sugar, saturated fats, trans fats, and sodium. The ADA also includes a vegetarian diet as well as other potential weight loss diets such as Weight Watchers. 🍁 The nutritional needs of each patient need to be determined individually (especially during pregnancy) with the appropriate HCPs, particularly professionals educated in nutrition.
- ***Social and Cultural Considerations:*** Numerous studies point to the prevalence of excess body weight in American children and adolescents. Experts estimate that obesity is present in 25% of the population aged 6 to 11 yr. The medical, social, and emotional consequences of excess body weight are significant. Special attention should be given to instructing the pediatric patient and caregiver regarding health risks and weight control education. 🍁
- Recognize anxiety related to test results, and be supportive of fear of shortened life expectancy. Discuss the implications of abnormal test results on the patient's lifestyle. Provide teaching and information regarding the clinical implications of the test results, as appropriate. Educate the patient regarding access to counseling services. Provide contact

information, if desired, for the AHA (www.americanheart.org), NHLBI (www.nhlbi.nih.gov), and Legs for Life (www.legsforlife.org). 🍁

- Reinforce information given by the patient's HCP regarding further testing, treatment, or referral to another HCP. Answer any questions or address any concerns voiced by the patient or family.
- Depending on the results of this procedure, additional testing may be needed to evaluate or monitor progression of the disease process and determine the need for a change in therapy. Evaluate test results in relation to the patient's symptoms and other tests performed.

Patient Education:

- Teach the patient to report any dizziness when getting up and down or ambulating.
- Teach the patient to weigh himself or herself at the same time each day and record the weight to report to the HCP.

Expected Patient Outcomes:

Understanding

- The patient and family verbalize that weight gain is an indicator of fluid retention that should be reported to the HCP.
- The patient and family state the importance of pacing activities to meet energy stores.

Ability

- The patient demonstrates weighing self and recording the results accurately.
- The patient demonstrates the ability to take prescribed medications accurately.

Response

- The patient agrees to limit fluids as recommend by the HCP.
- The patient agrees to use assistive devices that may support energy conservation.

RELATED STUDIES:

- Related tests include antidysrhythmic drugs, apolipoprotein A and B, atrial natriuretic peptide, BNP, blood gases, blood pool imaging, calcium, chest x-ray, cholesterol (total, HDL, LDL), CT cardiac scoring, CT thorax, CRP, CK and isoenzymes, echocardiography, echocardiography transesophageal, electrocardiogram, exercise stress test, glucose, glycated hemoglobin, Holter monitor, homocysteine, ketones, LDH and isos, lipoprotein electrophoresis, lung perfusion scan, magnesium, MRI chest, MI infarct scan, myocardial perfusion heart scan, myoglobin, PET heart, potassium, pulse oximetry, sodium, triglycerides, and troponin.
- Refer to the Cardiovascular System table online at Davis*Plus* for related tests by body system.

Echocardiography, Transesophageal

SYNONYM/ACRONYM: Echo, TEE.

COMMON USE: To assess and visualize cardiovascular structures toward diagnosing disorders such as tumors, congenital defects, valve disorders, chamber disorders, and bleeding.

AREA OF APPLICATION: Chest/thorax.

DESCRIPTION: Transesophageal echocardiography (TEE) is performed to assist in the diagnosis of cardiovascular disorders when noninvasive echocardiography is contraindicated or does not reveal enough information to confirm a diagnosis. Noninvasive echocardiography may be an inadequate procedure for patients who are obese, have chest wall structure abnormalities, or have chronic obstructive pulmonary disease (COPD). TEE provides a better view of the posterior aspect of the heart, including the atrium and aorta. It is done with a transducer attached to a gastroscope that is inserted into the esophagus. The transducer and the ultrasound (US) instrument allow the beam to be directed to the back of the heart. The echoes are amplified and recorded on a screen for visualization and recorded on graph paper or videotape. The depth of the endoscope and movement of the transducer is controlled to obtain various images of the heart structures. TEE is usually performed during surgery; it is also used on patients who are in the intensive care unit, in whom the transmission of waves to and from the chest has been compromised and more definitive information is needed. The images obtained by TEE have better resolution than those obtained by routine transthoracic echocardiography because TEE uses higher frequency sound waves and offers closer proximity of the transducer to the cardiac structures. Cardiac contrast medium, composed of noniodinated lipid microspheres, such as DEFINITY or Optison, is used to improve the visualization of viable myocardial tissue within the heart.

This procedure is contraindicated for: N/A

A variety of circumstances that may be considered absolute or relative depending on the facility's providers:

- Barrett esophagus
- Bleeding disorders
- Esophageal obstruction (e.g., spasm, stricture, tumor)
- Esophageal trauma (e.g., laceration, perforation)
- Esophageal varices
- Known upper esophagus disease
- Tracheoesophageal fistula
- Recent esophageal surgery (e.g., esophagectomy or esophagogastrectomy)
- Unstable cardiac or respiratory status
- Zenker diverticulum

INDICATIONS

- Confirm diagnosis if conventional echocardiography does not correlate with other findings.
- Detect and evaluate congenital heart disorders.
- Detect atrial tumors (myxomas).
- Detect or determine the severity of valvular abnormalities and regurgitation.
- Detect subaortic stenosis as evidenced by displacement of the anterior atrial leaflet and reduction in aortic valve flow, depending on the obstruction.
- Detect thoracic aortic dissection and coronary artery disease (CAD).
- Detect ventricular or atrial mural thrombi and evaluate cardiac wall motion after myocardial infarction.
- Determine the presence of pericardial effusion.
- Evaluate aneurysms and ventricular thrombus.
- Evaluate or monitor biological and prosthetic valve function.
- Evaluate septal defects.
- Measure the size of the heart's chambers and determine if hypertrophic cardiomyopathy or congestive heart failure is present.
- Monitor cardiac function during open heart surgery (most sensitive method for monitoring ischemia).
- Reevaluate after inadequate visualization with conventional echocardiography as a result of obesity,

trauma to or deformity of the chest wall, or lung hyperinflation associated with COPD.

POTENTIAL MEDICAL DIAGNOSIS

Normal findings

- Normal appearance of the size, position, structure, movements of the heart valves and heart muscle walls, and chamber blood filling; no evidence of valvular stenosis or insufficiency, cardiac tumor, foreign bodies, or CAD. The established values for the measurement of heart activities obtained by the study may vary by health-care provider (HCP) and institution.

Abnormal findings related to

- Aortic aneurysm
- Aortic valve abnormalities
- CAD
- Cardiomyopathy
- Congenital heart defects
- Heart failure
- Mitral valve abnormalities
- Myocardial infarction
- Myxoma
- Pericardial effusion
- Pulmonary hypertension
- Pulmonary valve abnormalities
- Septal defects
- Shunting of blood flow
- Thrombus
- Ventricular hypertrophy
- Ventricular or atrial mural thrombi

CRITICAL FINDINGS:

- Aortic aneurysm
- Aortic dissection

Note and immediately report to the requesting HCP any critical findings and related symptoms. A listing of these findings varies among facilities. Timely notification of a critical finding for laboratory or diagnostic studies is a role expectation of the professional nurse. The notification processes vary among facilities. Upon receipt of the critical finding, the information should be read back to the caller to verify accuracy.

INTERFERING FACTORS

Factors that may alter the results of the study

- Incorrect placement of the transducer over the desired test site.
- Patients who are dehydrated, resulting in failure to demonstrate the boundaries between organs and tissue structures.
- Large diaphragmatic hernia.
- Unknown upper esophageal pathology.
- Conditions such as esophageal dysphagia and irradiation of the mediastinum ***related to difficulty manipulating the US probe once it has been inserted in the esophagus.***
- The presence of COPD or use of mechanical ventilation, which increases the air between the heart and chest wall (hyperinflation) and can attenuate the US waves.
- Obese patients due to the enlarged space between the transducer and the heart and because fatty tissue can distort the sound waves.
- The presence of dysrhythmias.
- Inability of the patient to cooperate or remain still during the procedure because of age, significant pain, or mental status.

Other considerations

- Failure to follow dietary restrictions before the procedure may cause the procedure to be canceled or repeated.

NURSING IMPLICATIONS AND PROCEDURE

See Potential Nursing Problems on Fast Find at davispl.us/vanleeuwen7.

PRETEST:

- Positively identify the patient using at least two person-specific identifiers before services, treatments, or procedures are performed.

- ***Patient Teaching:*** Inform the patient this procedure can assist in assessing cardiac (heart) function.
- Obtain a history of the patient's health concerns, symptoms, surgical procedures, and results of previously performed laboratory and diagnostic studies. Include a list of known allergens, especially allergies or sensitivities to latex, anesthetics, or sedatives.
- Record the date of the last menstrual period and determine the possibility of pregnancy in perimenopausal women.
- Obtain a list of the patient's current medications, including over-the-counter medications, dietary supplements, anticoagulants, aspirin and other salicylates (see Effects of Natural Products on Laboratory Values online at Davis*Plus*). Such products should be discontinued by medical direction for the appropriate number of days prior to a surgical procedure. Note the last time and dose of medication taken.
- Review the procedure with the patient. Address concerns about pain related to the procedure. Explain that some pain may be experienced during the test, and there may be moments of discomfort during insertion of the scope. Lidocaine is sprayed in the patient's throat to reduce discomfort caused by the presence of the endoscope. Inform the patient that the procedure is performed in a US or cardiology department, usually by an HCP, and takes approximately 20 to 30 min.
- Explain that an intravenous (IV) line may be inserted to allow infusion of fluids such as saline, anesthetics, sedatives, or emergency medications.
- ***Sensitivity to social and cultural issues,*** as well as concern for modesty, is important in providing psychological support before, during, and after the procedure.
- Instruct the patient to remove jewelry and other metallic objects from the area to be examined.
- Instruct the patient that to reduce the risk of aspiration related to nausea and vomiting, solid food and milk or milk products are restricted for at least 6 hr and clear liquids are restricted for at least 2 hr prior to sedation/analgesia (monitored anesthesia). The American Society of Anesthesiologists has fasting guidelines for risk levels according to patient status. More information can be located at www.asahq.org. 🍁 Protocols may vary among facilities.
- *Make sure a written and informed consent has been signed prior to the procedure and before administering any medications.*

INTRATEST:

Potential Complications:

While complications are rare, trauma to the upper GI tract (e.g., esophageal bleeding, perforation, or rupture) may occur. Other potential complications include undiagnosed esophageal pathology, laryngospasm, or bronchospasm.

- Observe standard precautions, and follow the general guidelines in Patient Preparation and Specimen Collection online at Davis*Plus*. Positively identify the patient.
- Ensure that the patient has complied with dietary and fluid restriction prior to the procedure, as instructed.
- Ensure the patient has removed all external metallic objects from the area to be examined prior to the procedure.
- Avoid the use of equipment containing latex if the patient has a history of allergic reaction to latex.
- Have emergency equipment readily available.
- Instruct the patient to void prior to the procedure and to change into the gown, robe, and foot coverings provided.
- Obtain and record the patient's vital signs.
- Instruct the patient to cooperate fully and to follow directions. Instruct the patient to remain still throughout the procedure because movement produces unreliable results.

- Ask the patient, as appropriate, to remove his or her dentures.
- Monitor pulse oximetry to determine oxygen saturation in sedated patients.
- Establish an IV fluid line for the injection of saline, sedatives, contrast medium, or emergency medications.
- Expose the chest, and attach electrocardiogram leads for simultaneous tracings, if desired.
- Spray or swab the patient's throat with a local anesthetic, and place the oral bridge device in the mouth to to protect the patient's mouth and teeth and to prevent accidental damage to the endoscope from biting.
- Place the patient in a left side-lying position on a flat table with foam wedges to help maintain position and immobilization. The pharyngeal area is anesthetized, and the endoscope with the ultrasound device attached to its tip is inserted 30 to 50 cm to the posterior area of the heart, as in any esophagogastroduodenoscopy procedure.
- Ask the patient to swallow as the scope is inserted. When the transducer is in place, the scope is manipulated by controls on the handle to obtain scanning that provides real-time images of the heart motion and recordings of the images for viewing. Actual scanning is usually limited to 15 min or until the desired number of image planes is obtained at different depths of the scope.
- Administer contrast medium, if ordered. A second series of images is obtained.

POST-TEST:

- Inform the patient that a report of the results will be made available to the requesting HCP, who will discuss the results with the patient.
- Monitor vital signs and neurological status every 15 min for 1 hr, then every 2 hr for 4 hr, and as ordered. Take temperature every 4 hr for 24 hr. Monitor intake and output at least every 8 hr. Compare with baseline values. Notify the HCP if temperature is elevated. Protocols may vary among facilities.
- Instruct the patient to resume usual diet and activity 4 to 6 hr after the test, as directed by the HCP.
- Instruct the patient to treat throat discomfort with lozenges and warm gargles when the gag reflex returns.
- Recognize anxiety related to test results, and offer support. Discuss the implications of abnormal test results on the patient's lifestyle. Provide teaching and information regarding the clinical implications of the test results, as appropriate.
- ***Nutritional Considerations:*** Abnormal findings may be associated with cardiovascular disease. Nutritional therapy is recommended for the patient identified to be at risk for developing CAD or for individuals who have specific risk factors and/or existing medical conditions (e.g., elevated LDL cholesterol levels, other lipid disorders, type 1 diabetes, type 2 diabetes, insulin resistance, or metabolic syndrome). Other changeable risk factors warranting patient education include strategies to encourage patients, especially those who are overweight and with high blood pressure, to safely decrease sodium intake, achieve a normal weight, ensure regular participation in moderate aerobic physical activity three to four times per week, eliminate tobacco use, and adhere to a heart-healthy diet. If triglycerides also are elevated, the patient should be advised to eliminate or reduce alcohol. A variety of dietary patterns are beneficial for people with CAD, and there are many meal-planning approaches with nutritional goals endorsed by the American Diabetes Association (ADA). The Guideline on Lifestyle Management to Reduce Cardiovascular Risk published by the American College of Cardiology and the American Heart Association (AHA) in conjunction with the National Heart, Lung, and Blood Institute (NHLBI) recommends a Mediterranean-style diet rather than a low-fat diet. The guideline emphasizes inclusion of vegetables, whole grains, fruits, low-fat dairy,

nuts, legumes, and nontropical vegetable oils (e.g., olive, canola, peanut, sunflower, flaxseed) along with fish and lean poultry. 🍁 A similar dietary pattern known as the Dietary Approaches to Stop Hypertension (DASH) diet makes additional recommendations for the reduction of dietary sodium. Both dietary styles emphasize a reduction in consumption of red meats, which are high in saturated fats and cholesterol, and other foods containing sugar, saturated fats, trans fats, and sodium. The ADA also includes a vegetarian diet as well as other potential weight loss diets such as Weight Watchers. 🍁 The nutritional needs of each patient need to be determined individually (especially during pregnancy) with the appropriate HCPs, particularly professionals educated in nutrition.

- ***Social and Cultural Considerations:*** Numerous studies point to the prevalence of excess body weight in American children and adolescents. Experts estimate that obesity is present in 25% of the population aged 6 to 11 yr. The medical, social, and emotional consequences of excess body weight are significant. Special attention should be given to instructing the pediatric patient and caregiver regarding health risks and weight control education. 🍁
- Recognize anxiety related to test results, and be supportive of fear of shortened life expectancy. Discuss the implications of abnormal test results on the patient's lifestyle. Provide teaching and information regarding the clinical implications of the test results, as appropriate. Educate the patient regarding access to counseling services. Provide contact information, if desired, for the AHA (www.americanheart.org), NHLBI (www.nhlbi.nih.gov), and Legs for Life (www.legsforlife.org). 🍁
- Reinforce information given by the patient's HCP regarding further testing, treatment, or referral to another HCP. Answer any questions or address any concerns voiced by the patient or family.
- Depending on the results of this procedure, additional testing may be needed to evaluate or monitor progression of the disease process and determine the need for a change in therapy. Evaluate test results in relation to the patient's symptoms and other tests performed.

Patient Education:

- Teach the patient to weigh himself or herself at the same time each day and record the weight to report to the HCP.
- Teach the patient regarding normal heart function.

Expected Patient Outcomes:

Understanding

- The patient and family verbalize that restlessness, sleeplessness, and irritability can be symptoms of poor oxygenation that should be reported to the HCP.
- The patient and family verbalize that shortness of breath and activity intolerance are symptoms of diminished cardiac output that should be reported to the HCP.

Ability

- The patient and family correctly describe symptoms of fluid retention.
- The patient and family correctly identify foods high in potassium that can be included in the diet to offset lost stores secondary to diuretic use.

Response

- The patient agrees to limit dietary sodium intake.
- The patient agrees to use assistive devices that may support energy conservation.

RELATED STUDIES:

- Related tests include antidysrhythmic drugs, apolipoprotein A and B, atrial natriuretic peptide, BNP, blood gases, blood pool imaging, calcium, chest x-ray, cholesterol (total, HDL, LDL), CT cardiac scoring, CT thorax, CRP, CK and isoenzymes, echocardiography, electrocardiogram, exercise stress test, glucose, glycated hemoglobin, Holter monitor, homocysteine, ketones, LDH and isos, lipoprotein electrophoresis, lung perfusion scan, magnesium, MRI chest, MI infarct scan, myocardial perfusion heart scan, myoglobin, PET heart, potassium, pulse oximetry, sodium, triglycerides, and troponin.

- Refer to the Cardiovascular System table online at Davis*Plus* for related tests by body system.

Electrocardiogram

SYNONYM/ACRONYM: ECG, EKG.

COMMON USE: To evaluate the electrical impulses generated by the heart during the cardiac cycle to assist with diagnosis of cardiac dysrhythmias, blocks, damage, infection, or enlargement.

AREA OF APPLICATION: Heart.

DESCRIPTION: The cardiac muscle consists of three layers of cells: the inner *endocardium,* the middle *myocardium,* and the outer *epicardium*. The systolic phase of the cardiac cycle reflects the contraction of the myocardium, whereas the diastolic phase takes place when the heart relaxes to allow blood to rush in. All muscle cells have a characteristic rate of contraction called *depolarization*. Therefore, the heart will maintain a predetermined heart rate unless other stimuli are received.

The monitoring of pulse and blood pressure evaluates only the mechanical activity of the heart. The electrocardiogram (ECG), a noninvasive study, measures the electrical currents or impulses that the heart generates during a cardiac cycle (see figure of a normal ECG at end of study). Electrical impulses travel through a conduction system beginning with the sinoatrial (SA) node, moving to the atrioventricular (AV) node via internodal pathways. From the AV node, the impulses travel to the bundle of His and onward to the right and left bundle branches. These bundles are located within the right and left ventricles. The impulses continue to the cardiac muscle cells by terminal fibers called *Purkinje fibers*. The ECG is a graphic display of the electrical activity of the heart, which is analyzed by time intervals and segments. Continuous tracing of the cardiac cycle activity is captured as heart cells are electrically stimulated, causing depolarization and movement of the activity through the cells of the myocardium.

The ECG study is completed by using 12, 15, or 18 electrodes attached to the skin surface to obtain the total electrical activity of the heart. Each lead records the electrical potential between the limbs or between the heart and limbs. The ECG machine records and marks the 12 leads (most common system used) on the strip of paper in the machine in proper sequence, usually 6 in. ✦ of the strip for each lead. Leads I, II, and III, known as *extremity leads* in a 12-lead ECG, form a triangle known as the *Einthoven triangle* when placed on the body.

The ECG pattern, called a *heart rhythm,* is recorded by a machine as a series of waves, intervals, and segments, each of which pertains to a specific occurrence during the contraction of the heart. The ECG tracings are recorded on graph paper using vertical and horizontal lines for analysis and calculations of time, measured by the vertical lines (1 mm apart and 0.04 sec per line), and of voltage, measured by the horizontal lines (1 mm apart and 0.5 mV per 5 squares). A pulse rate can be calculated from the ECG strip to obtain the beats per minute. The P wave represents the depolarization of the atrial myocardium; the QRS complex represents the depolarization of the ventricular myocardium; the PR interval represents the time from beginning of the excitation of the atrium to the beginning of the ventricular excitation; the ST segment, which represents the time between the end of depolarization and initiation of repolarization, has no deflection from baseline but in an abnormal state may be elevated or depressed; and the T wave represents the repolarization of the ventricular myocardium. An abnormal rhythm is called a *dysrhythmia*.

Microvolt T wave alternans (MTWA) is a type of noninvasive testing that identifies variations or alterations in electrical activity of the T wave. These alterations are associated with sudden cardiac death from ventricular dysrhythmias. Specialized electrodes are used to reduce background noise from natural internal movement such as respirations or external movement such as caused by the friction of electrodes on skin. Research has shown that the extent of MTWA becomes more demonstrable as heart rate increases, which is why the test includes a period of controlled exercise. MTWA occurs at a rate that is specific to each individual and is reproducible at a rate above the initial threshold for an individual. The two main methods of interpreting the beat-to-beat data, or ECG T-wave data, collected from electrodes placed on the patient's chest at rest prior to a period of activity, during an interval of controlled exercise, and during the recovery period after exercise are the spectral and modified moving average methods. Either of the two methods can be combined with a computer program to produce printable reports from the study results, which are interpreted by a cardiologist as positive, negative, or indeterminate. Spectral analysis is considered the preferred method for measurement and comparison of T wave activity based on the availability of documented studies using spectral analysis.

Another modification of the ECG, used to evaluate for ventricular dysrhythmias, is the *signal-averaged ECG*. Heart rhythms in patients who have coronary artery disease (CAD), nonischemic dilated cardiomyopathy, left ventricular aneurysm, ventricular tachycardia, or healed ventricular incisions or who are recovering from an myocardial infarction (MI) may demonstrate abnormally slow electrical conduction, called *late potentials,* through the heart. The late potentials are believed to be the result of delayed conduction through areas of plaque, fibrous scarring, or inflammation and can reliably predict significant and sudden ventricular dysrhythmias.

The abnormal changes in conduction are too small to be detected by standard ECG equipment and require specially designed computer software. The test takes 15 to 20 min and analyzes hundreds of cardiac cycles to detect the presence of late potentials.

The ankle-brachial index (ABI) can also be assessed during this study. This noninvasive, simple comparison of blood pressure measurements in the arms and legs can be used to detect peripheral arterial disease (PAD). A Doppler stethoscope is used to obtain the systolic pressure in either the dorsalis pedis or the posterior tibial artery. This ankle pressure is then divided by the highest brachial systolic pressure acquired after taking the blood pressure in both arms of the patient. This index should be greater than 1. When the index falls below 0.5, blood flow impairment is considered significant. Patients should be scheduled for a vascular consult for an abnormal ABI. Patients with diabetes or kidney disease, as well as some older adult patients, may have a falsely elevated ABI due to calcifications of the vessels in the ankle causing an increased systolic pressure. The ABI test approaches 95% accuracy in detecting PAD. However, a normal ABI value does not absolutely rule out the possibility of PAD for some individuals, and additional tests should be done to evaluate symptoms.

This procedure is contraindicated for: N/A

INDICATIONS

- Assess the extent of congenital heart disease.
- Assess the extent of MI or ischemia, as indicated by abnormal ST segment, interval times, and amplitudes.
- Assess the function of heart valves.
- Assess global cardiac function.
- Detect dysrhythmias, as evidenced by abnormal wave deflections.
- Detect PAD.
- Detect pericarditis, shown by ST segment changes or shortened PR interval.
- Determine electrolyte imbalances, as evidenced by short or prolonged QT interval.
- Determine hypertrophy of the heart chamber, as evidenced by P- or R-wave deflections, atrial biphasic P waves in V1, and ventricular exaggerated R waves in V leads.
- Evaluate and monitor cardiac pacemaker function.
- Evaluate and monitor the effect of drugs, such as digoxin, antidysrhythmics, or vasodilating drugs.
- Monitor ECG changes during an exercise test.
- Monitor rhythm changes during the recovery phase after MI.

POTENTIAL MEDICAL DIAGNOSIS

Normal findings

Normal Resting Heart Rate by Age

Age	Beats/Min
Newborns (0–1 mo)	70–180
Infants (2–11 mo)	80–160
1–2 yr	80–130
3–4 yr	75–140
5–7 yr	70–130
8–9 yr	70–120
10 years and older, adults, older adults	60–100

- Normal resting heart rate for trained athletes is in the range of 40 to 60 beats/min.

- Normal, regular rhythm and wave deflections with normal measurement of ranges of cycle components and height, depth, and duration of complexes are as follows:
  P wave: 0.12 sec, or three small blocks with amplitude of 2.5 mm
  Q wave: Less than 0.04 mm
  R wave: 5 to 27 mm amplitude, depending on lead
  T wave: 1 to 13 mm amplitude, depending on lead
  QRS complex: 0.1 sec or two and a half small blocks
  ST segment: 1 mm

E

Abnormal findings related to

- Atrial or ventricular hypertrophy
- Bundle branch block
- Dysrhythmias
- Electrolyte imbalances
- Heart rate of 40 to 60 beats/min in adults
- Ischemia or MI
- PAD
- Pericarditis
- Pulmonary infarction
- P wave: An enlarged P-wave deflection could indicate atrial enlargement; an absent or altered P wave could suggest that the electrical impulse did not come from the SA node
- PR interval: An increased interval could imply a conduction delay in the AV node
- QRS complex: An enlarged Q wave may indicate an old infarction; an enlarged deflection could indicate ventricular hypertrophy; increased time duration may indicate a bundle branch block
- ST segment: A depressed ST segment indicates myocardial ischemia; an elevated ST segment may indicate an acute MI or pericarditis; a prolonged ST segment (or prolonged QT) may indicate hypocalcemia. A shortened ST segment may indicate hypokalemia
- Tachycardia greater than 120 beats/min
- T wave: A flat or inverted T wave may indicate myocardial ischemia, infarction, or hypokalemia; a tall, peaked T wave with a shortened QT interval may indicate hyperkalemia

CRITICAL FINDINGS:

Adult

- Acute changes in ST elevation are usually associated with acute MI or pericarditis
- Asystole
- Heart block, second- and third-degree with bradycardia less than 60 beats/min
- Pulseless electrical activity
- Pulseless ventricular tachycardia
- Premature ventricular contractions greater than three in a row, pauses greater than 3 sec, or identified blocks
- Unstable tachycardia
- Ventricular fibrillation

Pediatric

- Asystole
- Bradycardia less than 60 beats/min
- Pulseless electrical activity
- Pulseless ventricular tachycardia
- Supraventricular tachycardia
- Ventricular fibrillation

Note and immediately report to the requesting health-care provider (HCP) any critical findings and related symptoms. A listing of these findings varies among facilities. Timely notification of a critical finding for laboratory or diagnostic studies is a role expectation of the professional nurse. The notification processes vary among facilities. Upon receipt of the critical finding, the information should be read back to the caller to verify accuracy.

INTERFERING FACTORS

Factors that may impair the results of the examination

- Anatomic variation of the heart (i.e., the heart may be rotated in both the horizontal and frontal planes).
- Distortion of cardiac cycles due to age, gender, weight, or a medical condition (e.g., infants, women [may exhibit slight ST segment depression], patients who are obese, patients who are pregnant, patients with ascites).
- High intake of carbohydrates or electrolyte imbalances of potassium or calcium.
- Improper placement of electrodes or inadequate contact between skin and electrodes because of insufficient conductive gel or poor placement, which can cause ECG tracing problems.
- ECG machine malfunction or interference from electromagnetic waves in the vicinity.
- Inability of the patient to remain still during the procedure, because movement, muscle tremor, or twitching can affect accurate test recording.
- Increased patient anxiety, resulting in hyperventilation or deep respirations.
- Medications such as barbiturates and digoxin.
- Strenuous exercise before the procedure.

NURSING IMPLICATIONS AND PROCEDURE

See Potential Nursing Problems on Fast Find at davispl.us/vanleeuwen7.

PRETEST:

- Positively identify the patient using at least two person-specific identifiers before services, treatments, or procedures are performed.
- *Patient Teaching:* Inform the patient this procedure can assist in assessing cardiac (heart) function.
- Obtain a history of the patient's health concerns, symptoms, surgical procedures, and results of previously performed laboratory and diagnostic studies. Include a list of known allergens, especially allergies or sensitivities to latex, anesthetics, or sedatives. Ask if the patient has had a heart transplant, implanted pacemaker, or internal cardiac defibrillator.
- Obtain a list of the patient's current medications, including over-the-counter medications and dietary supplements (see Effects of Natural Products on Laboratory Values online at Davis*Plus*).
- Review the procedure with the patient. Inform the patient that it may be necessary to remove hair from the site before the procedure. Address concerns about pain related to the procedure and explain that there should be no discomfort related to the procedure. Inform the patient that the procedure is performed by an HCP and takes approximately 15 min.
- ***Sensitivity to social and cultural issues,*** as well as concern for modesty, is important in providing psychological support before, during, and after the procedure.
- Instruct the patient to remove jewelry and other metallic objects from the area to be examined.
- Note that there are no food, fluid, or medication restrictions unless by medical direction.

INTRATEST:

Potential Complications: N/A

- Observe standard precautions, and follow the general guidelines in Patient Preparation and Specimen Collection online at Davis*Plus*. Positively identify the patient.
- Ensure the patient has complied with pretesting preparations.
- Ensure the patient has removed all external metallic objects from the area to be examined prior to the procedure.

- Instruct the patient to void prior to the procedure and to change into the gown, robe, and foot coverings provided.
- Record baseline values.
- Place patient in a supine position. Expose and appropriately drape the chest, arms, and legs.
- Instruct the patient to cooperate fully and to follow directions. Instruct the patient to remain still throughout the procedure because movement produces unreliable results.
- Prepare the skin surface with alcohol and remove excess hair. Use clippers to remove hair from the site, if appropriate. Dry skin sites.
- Avoid the use of equipment containing latex if the patient has a history of allergic reaction to latex.
- Apply the electrodes in the proper position. When placing the six unipolar chest leads, place V_1 at the fourth intercostal space at the border of the right sternum, V_2 at the fourth intercostal space at the border of the left sternum, V_3 between V_2 and V_4, V_4 at the fifth intercostal space at the midclavicular line, V_5 at the left anterior axillary line at the level of V_4 horizontally, and V_6 at the level of V_4 horizontally and at the left midaxillary line. The wires are connected to the matched electrodes and the ECG machine. Chest leads (V_1, V_2, V_3, V_4, V_5, and V_6) record data from the horizontal plane of the heart.
- Place three limb bipolar leads (two electrodes combined for each) on the arms and legs. Lead I is the combination of two arm electrodes, lead II is the combination of right arm and left leg electrodes, and lead III is the combination of left arm and left leg electrodes. Limb leads (I, II, III, aVL, aVF, and aVR) record data from the frontal plane of the heart.
- The machine is set and turned on after the electrodes, grounding, connections, paper supply, computer, and data storage device are checked.
- If the patient has any chest discomfort or pain during the procedure, mark the ECG strip indicating that occurrence.

POST-TEST:

- Inform the patient that a report of the results will be made available to the requesting HCP, who will discuss the results with the patient.
- When the procedure is complete, remove the electrodes and clean the skin where the electrode was applied.
- Evaluate the results in relation to previously performed ECGs. Denote cardiac rhythm abnormalities on the strip.
- Monitor vital signs and compare with baseline values. Protocols may vary among facilities.
- Instruct the patient to immediately notify an HCP of chest pain, changes in pulse rate, or shortness of breath.
- Recognize anxiety related to the test results and be supportive of perceived loss of independence and fear of shortened life expectancy. Discuss the implications of abnormal test results on the patient's lifestyle. Provide teaching and information regarding the clinical implications of the test results, as appropriate.
- ***Nutritional Considerations:*** Abnormal findings may be associated with cardiovascular disease. Nutritional therapy is recommended for the patient identified to be at risk for developing CAD or for individuals who have specific risk factors and/or existing medical conditions (e.g., elevated LDL cholesterol levels, low HDL cholesterol levels, other lipid disorders, type 1 diabetes, type 2 diabetes, insulin resistance, or metabolic syndrome). Other changeable risk factors warranting patient education include strategies to encourage patients, especially those who are overweight and with high blood pressure, to safely decrease sodium intake, achieve a normal weight, ensure regular participation of moderate aerobic physical activity three to four times per week, eliminate tobacco use, and adhere to a heart-healthy diet. If triglycerides also are elevated, the patient should be advised to eliminate or reduce alcohol. A variety of dietary patterns are beneficial for people with CAD,

and there are many meal-planning approaches with nutritional goals endorsed by the American Diabetes Association (ADA). The Guideline on Lifestyle Management to Reduce Cardiovascular Risk published by the American College of Cardiology and the American Heart Association (AHA) in conjunction with the National Heart, Lung, and Blood Institute (NHLBI) recommends a Mediterranean-style diet rather than a low-fat diet. The guideline emphasizes inclusion of vegetables, whole grains, fruits, low-fat dairy, nuts, legumes, and nontropical vegetable oils (e.g., olive, canola, peanut, sunflower, flaxseed) along with fish and lean poultry. 🍁 A similar dietary pattern known as the Dietary Approaches to Stop Hypertension (DASH) diet makes additional recommendations for the reduction of dietary sodium. Both dietary styles emphasize a reduction in consumption of red meats, which are high in saturated fats and cholesterol, and other foods containing sugar, saturated fats, trans fats, and sodium. The ADA also includes a vegetarian diet as well as other potential weight loss diets such as Weight Watchers. 🍁 The nutritional needs of each patient need to be determined individually (especially during pregnancy) with the appropriate HCPs, particularly professionals educated in nutrition.

- ***Sensitivity to social and cultural issues:*** Numerous studies point to the prevalence of excess body weight in American children and adolescents. Experts estimate that obesity is present in 25% of the population aged 6 to 11 yr. The medical, social, and emotional consequences of excess body weight are significant. Special attention should be given to instructing the pediatric patient and caregiver regarding health risks and weight control education. 🍁
- Recognize anxiety related to test results, and be supportive of fear of shortened life expectancy. Discuss the implications of abnormal test results on the patient's lifestyle. Provide teaching and information regarding the clinical implications of the test results, as appropriate. Educate the patient regarding access to counseling services. Provide contact information, if desired, for the AHA (www.americanheart.org), NHLBI (www.nhlbi.nih.gov), Institute of Medicine of the National Academies (www.iom.edu) or USDA's resource for nutrition (www.choosemyplate.gov). 🍁
- Reinforce information given by the patient's HCP regarding further testing, treatment, or referral to another HCP. Answer any questions or address any concerns voiced by the patient or family.
- Depending on the results of this procedure, additional testing may be performed to evaluate or monitor progression of the disease process and determine the need for a change in therapy. Evaluate test results in relation to the patient's symptoms and other tests performed.

Patient Education:

- Teach the patient the importance of wearing oxygen to decrease cardiac ischemia.
- Teach the patient to rest with the head of the bed elevated to improve oxygenation.

Expected Patient Outcomes:

Understanding

- The patient and family acknowledge that invasive procedures (angiogram; arterial line) may be necessary to fully evaluate cardiac health.
- The patient and family state the treatment options and how cardiac disease effects health status.

Ability

- The patient and family take measures to maintain a quiet environment to decrease energy demands.
- The patient and family describe lifestyle changes that need to be made to support cardiac health (diet, smoking, activity).

Response

- The patient agrees to smoking cessation.

- The patient agrees to attend a cardiac rehabilitation program.

RELATED STUDIES:

- Related tests include antidysrhythmic drugs, apolipoprotein A and B, atrial natriuretic peptide, BNP, blood gases, blood pool imaging, calcium, chest x-ray, cholesterol (total, HDL, LDL), CT cardiac scoring, CT thorax, CRP, CK and isoenzymes, echocardiography, echocardiography transesophageal, exercise stress test, glucose, glycated hemoglobin, Holter monitor, homocysteine, ketones, LDH and isos, lipoprotein electrophoresis, lung perfusion scan, magnesium, MRI chest, MI scan, myocardial perfusion heart scan, myoglobin, PET heart, potassium, pulse oximetry, sodium, triglycerides, and troponin.
- Refer to the Cardiovascular System table online at Davis*Plus* for related tests by body system.

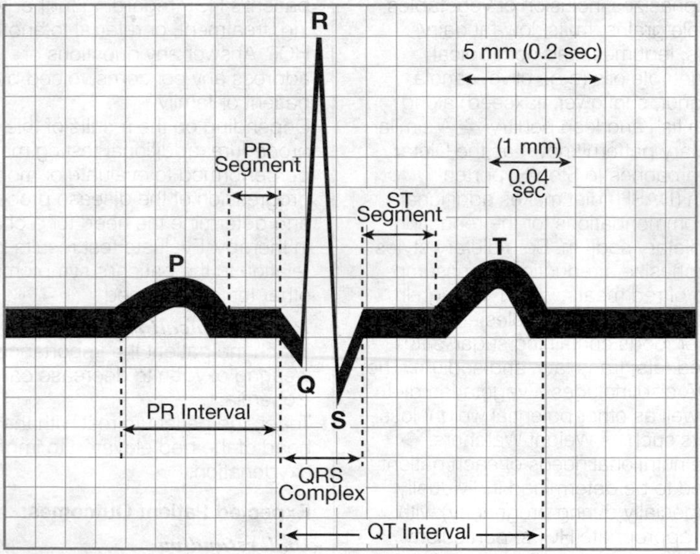

Electroencephalography

SYNONYM/ACRONYM: Electrical activity (for sleep disturbances), EEG.

COMMON USE: To assess the electrical activity in the brain toward assisting in diagnosis of brain death, injury, infection, and bleeding.

AREA OF APPLICATION: Brain.

DESCRIPTION: Electroencephalography (EEG) is a noninvasive study that measures the brain's electrical activity and records that activity on graph paper. These electrical impulses arise from the brain cells of the cerebral cortex. Electrodes, placed on the patient's scalp according to the International 10/20 system, transmit the different frequencies and amplitudes of the brain's electrical activity to the EEG equipment, which records the results in graph form on a moving paper strip or a computerized system for retrieval and review or comparison at a later date. Guidelines for the performance and evaluation of an EEG are set by the American Clinical Neurophysiology Society. The EEG can evaluate responses to various stimuli, such as flickering light, hyperventilation, auditory signals, or somatosensory signals generated by skin electrodes. The procedure is usually performed in a room designed to eliminate electrical interference and minimize distractions. An EEG can be done at the bedside, and a health-care provider (HCP) analyzes the waveforms. The test is used to detect epilepsy, intracranial abscesses, or tumors; to evaluate cerebral involvement due to head injury or meningitis; and to monitor for cerebral tissue ischemia during surgery when cerebral vessels must be occluded (e.g., carotid endarterectomy). EEG is also used to confirm brain death, which can be defined as absence of electrical activity in the brain. To evaluate abnormal EEG waves further, the patient may be connected to an ambulatory EEG system similar to a Holter monitor for the heart.

This procedure is contraindicated for: N/A

INDICATIONS

- Confirm brain death.
- Confirm suspicion of increased intracranial pressure caused by trauma or disease.
- Detect cerebral ischemia during endarterectomy.
- Detect intracranial cerebrovascular lesions, such as hemorrhages and infarcts.
- Detect seizure disorders and identify focus of seizure and seizure activity, as evidenced by abnormal spikes and waves recorded on the graph.
- Determine the presence of tumors, abscesses, or infection.
- Evaluate the effect of drug intoxication on the brain.
- Evaluate sleeping disorders, such as sleep apnea and narcolepsy.
- Identify area of abnormality in dementia.

POTENTIAL MEDICAL DIAGNOSIS

Normal findings

- Normal occurrences of alpha, beta, theta, and delta waves (rhythms varying depending on the patient's age)
- Normal frequency, amplitude, and characteristics of brain waves

Abnormal findings related to

- Abscess
- Alzheimer's disease
- Brain death
- Cerebral infarct
- Encephalitis
- Glioblastoma and other brain tumors
- Head injury
- Hematoma
- Hypocalcemia or hypoglycemia
- Infarct
- Intracranial hemorrhage
- Meningitis
- Migraine headaches
- Narcolepsy
- Parkinson's disease
- Seizure disorders (epilepsy, grand mal, focal, temporal lobe, myoclonic, petit mal)
- Sleep apnea

CRITICAL FINDINGS:

- Abscess
- Brain death

- Head injury
- Hemorrhage
- Intracranial hemorrhage

Note and immediately report to the requesting HCP any critical findings and related symptoms. A listing of these findings varies among facilities. Timely notification of a critical finding for laboratory or diagnostic studies is a role expectation of the professional nurse. The notification processes vary among facilities. Upon receipt of the critical finding, the information should be read back to the caller to verify accuracy.

E

INTERFERING FACTORS

Factors that may impair the results of the examination

- Inability of the patient to cooperate or remain still during the procedure because of age, significant pain, or mental status.
- Drugs and other substances such as sedatives, anticonvulsants, anxiolytics, alcohol, and stimulants such as caffeine and nicotine.
- Hypoglycemic or hypothermic states.
- Hair that is dirty, oily, or sprayed or treated with hair preparations.

NURSING IMPLICATIONS AND PROCEDURE

See Potential Nursing Problems on Fast Find at davispl.us/vanleeuwen7.

PRETEST:

- Positively identify the patient using at least two person-specific identifiers before services, treatments, or procedures are performed.
- ***Patient Teaching:*** Inform the patient/family this procedure can assist in measuring the electrical activity in the brain.
- Obtain a history of the patient's health concerns, symptoms, surgical procedures, and results of previously performed laboratory and diagnostic studies. Include a list of known allergens, especially allergies or sensitivities to latex, anesthetics, or sedatives.
- Obtain a history of the patient's musculoskeletal system, symptoms, and results of previously performed laboratory tests and diagnostic and surgical procedures.
- Obtain a list of the patient's current medications, including over-the-counter medications and dietary supplements (see Effects of Natural Products on Laboratory Values online at Davis*Plus*).
- Review the procedure with the patient. Address concerns about pain related to the procedure and assure the patient there is no discomfort during the procedure, but if needle electrodes are used, a slight pinch may be felt. Explain that electricity flows from the patient's body, not into the body, during the procedure. Explain that the procedure reveals brain activity only, not thoughts, feelings, or intelligence. Inform the patient the procedure is performed in a neurodiagnostic department, usually by an HCP and support staff, and takes approximately 30 to 120 min, depending on the purpose of the study.
- Inform the patient that he or she may be asked to alter breathing pattern; be asked to follow simple commands such as opening or closing eyes, blinking, or swallowing; be stimulated with bright light; or be given a drug to induce sleep during the study.
- ***Sensitivity to social and cultural issues,*** as well as concern for modesty, is important in providing psychological support before, during, and after the procedure.
- Instruct the patient to clean the hair and to refrain from using hair sprays, creams, or solutions before the test.
- Instruct the patient to limit sleep to 5 hr for an adult and 7 hr for a child the night before the study. Young infants and children should not be allowed to nap before the study.
- Instruct the patient to eat a meal before the study and to avoid stimulants such as caffeine and nicotine

for 8 hr prior to the procedure. Under medical direction, the patient should avoid sedatives, anticonvulsants, anxiolytics, and alcohol for 24 to 48 hr before the test.

- *Make sure a written and informed consent has been signed prior to the procedure and before administering any medications.*

INTRATEST:

Potential Complications: N/A

- Observe standard precautions, and follow the general guidelines in Patient Preparation and Specimen Collection online at Davis*Plus*. Positively identify the patient.
- Ensure the patient has complied with pretesting preparations prior to the study, as instructed.
- Ensure that all substances with the potential to interfere with test results were withheld for 24 to 48 hr before the test.
- Ensure that the patient is able to relax; report any extreme anxiety or restlessness.
- Ensure that hair is clean and free of hair sprays, creams, or solutions.
- Avoid the use of equipment containing latex if the patient has a history of allergic reaction to latex.
- Place the patient in the supine position in a bed or in a semi-Fowler's position on a recliner in a special room protected from any noise or electrical interferences that could affect the tracings.
- Remind the patient to relax and not to move any muscles or parts of the face or head. The HCP should be able to observe the patient for movements or other interferences through a window into the test room.
- The electrodes are prepared and applied to the scalp. Electrodes are applied to the prefrontal, frontal, temporal, parietal, and occipital areas of both sides of the head, and amplifier wires are attached. An electrode is also attached to each earlobe as grounding electrodes. At this time, a baseline recording can be made with the patient at rest.
- Recordings are made with the patient at rest and with eyes closed. Recordings are stopped about every 5 min to allow the patient to move. Recordings are also made during a drowsy and sleep period, depending on the patient's clinical condition and symptoms.
- Procedures (e.g., stroboscopic light stimulation, hyperventilation to induce alkalosis, and sleep induction by administration of sedative to detect abnormalities that occur only during sleep) may be done to bring out abnormal electrical activity or other brain abnormalities.
- Observations for seizure activity are carried out during the study, and a description and time of activity is noted by the HCP.

POST-TEST:

- Inform the patient that a report of the results will be made available to the requesting HCP, who will discuss the results with the patient.
- When the procedure is complete, remove electrodes from the hair and remove paste by cleansing with oil or witch hazel.
- Allow the patient to recover if a sedative was given during the test. Bedside rails are put in the raised position for safety.
- Instruct the patient to resume medications, as directed by the HCP.
- Instruct the patient to report any seizure activity.
- Recognize anxiety related to test results, and be supportive of perceived loss of independent function. Discuss the implications of abnormal test results on the patient's lifestyle. Provide teaching and information regarding the clinical implications of the test results, as appropriate. Provide contact information, if desired, for the Epilepsy Foundation (www.epilepsyfoundation.org), Alzheimer's Association of America (www.alzfdn.org), or U.S. Government Information on Organ and Tissue Donation and Transplantation (www.organdonor.gov/index.html). 🍁

E

- Reinforce information given by the patient's HCP regarding further testing, treatment, or referral to another HCP. Answer any questions or address any concerns voiced by the patient or family.
- Depending on the results of this procedure, additional testing may be performed to evaluate or monitor progression of the disease process and determine the need for a change in therapy. Evaluate test results in relation to the patient's symptoms and other tests performed.

Patient Education:

- Provide simple-to-understand information related to head injury treatment and outcome (may need to be provided to the family or significant other).
- Explain the importance of maintaining a system of continuous communication to meet health-care needs in a timely manner.

Expected Patient Outcomes:

Understanding

- The patient and family state that there may be personality changes with brain injury.
- The patient and family state that there may be speech deficits with brain injury.

Ability

- Family or significant other demonstrates the performance of activities recommended by the occupational therapist that will be necessary for home rehabilitation.
- Family or significant other demonstrates correct body mechanics when moving the patient or assisting with ambulation.

Response

- The patient and family participate in the discussion regarding treatment options, thereby reducing fear of the unknown.
- The patient and family state the importance of having a spokesperson for the family to streamline communications.

RELATED STUDIES:

- Related tests include CSF analysis, CT brain, evoked brain potentials (SER, VER), MRI brain, and PET brain.
- Refer to the Musculoskeletal System table online at Davis*Plus* for related tests by body system.

Electromyography

SYNONYM/ACRONYM: Electrodiagnostic study, EMG, neuromuscular junction testing.

COMMON USE: To assess the electrical activity within the skeletal muscles to assist in diagnosing diseases such as muscular dystrophy, Guillain-Barré, polio, and other myopathies.

AREA OF APPLICATION: Muscles.

DESCRIPTION: Electromyography (EMG) measures skeletal muscle activity during rest, voluntary contraction, and electrical stimulation. Percutaneous extracellular needle electrodes containing fine wires are inserted into selected muscle groups to detect neuromuscular abnormalities and measure nerve and electrical conduction properties of skeletal muscles. The electrical potentials are amplified, displayed on a screen in waveforms, and electronically recorded, similar to electrocardiography. Comparison and analysis of the amplitude, duration, number, and configuration of the muscle activity provide diagnostic information about the extent of nerve and muscle involvement in the detection of primary muscle diseases, including lower motor neuron, anterior horn cell, or neuromuscular junction diseases; defective transmission at the neuromuscular junction; and peripheral nerve damage or disease. The responses of a relaxed muscle are electrically silent, but spontaneous muscle movement such as fibrillation and fasciculation can be detected in a relaxed, denervated muscle. Muscle action potentials are detected with minimal or maximal muscle contractions and the differences in the size and numbers of activity potentials during voluntary contractions determine whether the muscle weakness is a disease of the striated muscle fibers or cell membranes (myogenic) or a disease of the lower motor neuron (neurogenic). Nerve conduction studies (electroneurography) are commonly done in conjunction with electromyelography; the combination of the procedures is known as electromyoneurography. The major use of the examination lies in differentiating among the following disease classes: primary myopathy, peripheral motor neuron disease, and disease of the neuromuscular junction.

EMG can aid with the diagnosis of nerve compression or injury such as carpal tunnel syndrome, nerve root injury such as sciatica, or other problems on the muscles or nerves. An EMG uses tiny devices called electrodes which are inserted directly into a muscle to transmit or detect electrical signals. A nerve conduction study or nerve conduction velocity test, which is another part of an EMG, uses electrodes taped to the skin to measure the strength and speed of the signals traveling between two or more points.

This procedure is contraindicated for

Patients with extensive skin infection or with an infection at the sites of electrode placement, ***to avoid risk of spreading infection into the muscle*** or patients who are receiving anticoagulant therapy, ***to avoid bleeding.***

INDICATIONS

- Assess primary muscle diseases affecting striated muscle fibers or cell membrane, such as muscular dystrophy or myasthenia gravis.
- Detect muscle disorders caused by diseases of the lower motor neuron involving the motor neuron on the anterior horn of the spinal cord, such as anterior poliomyelitis, amyotrophic lateral sclerosis, amyotonia, and spinal tumors.
- Detect muscle disorders caused by diseases of the lower motor neuron involving the nerve root, such as Guillain-Barré syndrome, herniated disk, or spinal stenosis.
- Detect neuromuscular disorders, such as peripheral neuropathy caused by diabetes or alcoholism, and locate the site of the abnormality.
- Determine if a muscle abnormality is caused by the toxic effects of drugs (e.g., antibiotics, chemotherapy) or toxins (e.g., Clostridium botulinum, snake venom, heavy metals).
- Differentiate between primary and secondary muscle disorders or between neuropathy and myopathy.
- Differentiate secondary muscle disorders caused by polymyositis, sarcoidosis, hypocalcemia, thyroid toxicity, tetanus, and other disorders.

- Monitor and evaluate progression of myopathies or neuropathies, including confirmation of diagnosis of carpal tunnel syndrome.

POTENTIAL MEDICAL DIAGNOSIS

Normal findings

- Normal muscle electrical activity during rest and contraction states

Abnormal findings related to

- Evidence of neuromuscular disorders or primary muscle disease (*Note:* Findings must be correlated with the patient's history, clinical features, and results of other neurodiagnostic tests.):
  - Amyotrophic lateral sclerosis
  - Bell's palsy
  - Beriberi
  - Carpal tunnel syndrome
  - Dermatomyositis
  - Diabetic peripheral neuropathy
  - Eaton-Lambert syndrome
  - Guillain-Barré syndrome
  - Multiple sclerosis
  - Muscular dystrophy
  - Myasthenia gravis
  - Myopathy
  - Polymyositis as indicated by fast, small spontaneous waveforms
  - Radiculopathy
  - Traumatic injury

CRITICAL FINDINGS: N/A

INTERFERING FACTORS

Factors that may impair the results of the examination

- Inability of the patient to cooperate or remain still during the procedure because of age, significant pain, or mental status.
- Age-related decreases in electrical activity.
- Medications such as muscle relaxants, cholinergics, and anticholinergics.
- Improper placement of surface or needle electrodes.

NURSING IMPLICATIONS AND PROCEDURE

PRETEST:

- Positively identify the patient using at least two person-specific identifiers before services, treatments, or procedures are performed.
- *Patient Teaching:* Inform the patient this procedure can assist in measuring the electrical activity of the muscles.
- Obtain a history of the patient's health concerns, symptoms, surgical procedures, and results of previously performed laboratory and diagnostic studies. Include a list of known allergens, especially allergies or sensitivities to latex, anesthetics, or sedatives.
- Obtain a list of the patient's current medications, including over-the-counter medications and dietary supplements (see Effects of Natural Products on Laboratory Values online at Davis*Plus*).
- Review the procedure with the patient. Address concerns about pain related to the procedure and warn the patient the procedure may be uncomfortable, but an analgesic or sedative will be administered. Inform the patient that as many as 10 electrodes may be inserted at various locations on the body. Inform the patient the procedure is performed in a special laboratory by a health-care provider (HCP) and takes approximately 1 to 3 hr to complete, depending on the patient's condition.
- *Sensitivity to social and cultural issues,* as well as concern for modesty, is important in providing psychological support before, during, and after the procedure.
- Assess for the ability to comply with directions given for exercising during the test.
- Instruct the patient to remove jewelry and other metallic objects from the area to be examined.
- Under medical direction, the patient should avoid muscle relaxants, cholinergics, and anticholinergics for 3 to 6 days before the test.

- Instruct the patient to refrain from smoking and drinking caffeine-containing beverages for 3 hr before the procedure. Protocols may vary among facilities.
- *Make sure a written and informed consent has been signed prior to the procedure and before administering any medications.*

INTRATEST:

Potential Complications:

EMG is a low-risk procedure, and complications are rare. There is a small risk of bleeding and infection or nerve injury where the needle electrodes are inserted.

- Observe standard precautions, and follow the general guidelines in Patient Preparation and Specimen Collection online at Davis*Plus*. Positively identify the patient.
- Ensure the patient has refrained from smoking and drinking caffeine-containing beverages for 3 hr before the procedure.
- Ensure medications such as muscle relaxants, cholinergics, and anticholinergics have been withheld, as ordered.
- Ensure the patient has removed all external metallic objects from the area to be examined prior to the procedure.
- Instruct the patient to void prior to the procedure and to change into the gown, robe, and foot coverings provided.
- Avoid the use of equipment containing latex if the patient has a history of allergic reaction to latex.
- Place the patient in a supine or sitting position depending on the location of the muscle to be tested. Ensure that the area or room is protected from noise or metallic interference that may affect the test results.
- Ask the patient to remain still and relaxed and to cooperate with instructions given to contract muscles during the procedure.
- Administer mild analgesic (adult) or sedative (children), as ordered, to promote a restful state before the procedure.
- Cleanse the skin thoroughly with alcohol pads, as necessary.
- Observe that a small needle is inserted into the muscle being examined and acts as a recording electrode. A second electrode, a reference electrode, is placed on the skin surface near the recording electrode. An oscilloscope displays any spontaneous electrical activity while the patient keeps the muscle at rest. The electrical waves produced will be examined for the number, amplitude, and form.
- Ask the patient to alternate between a relaxed and a contracted muscle state or to perform progressive muscle contractions while the potentials are being measured.
- Note that this sequence may be repeated up to four times.
- When the procedure is complete, remove the electrodes and clean the skin where the electrode was applied. Apply pressure for 1 to 2 min to control any bleeding. Observe electrode sites for bleeding, hematoma, or inflammation.

POST-TEST:

- Inform the patient that a report of the results will be made available to the requesting HCP, who will discuss the results with the patient.
- If residual pain is noted after the procedure, instruct the patient to apply warm compresses and to take analgesics, as ordered.
- Instruct the patient to resume usual diet, medication, and activity, as directed by the HCP.
- Reinforce information given by the patient's HCP regarding further testing, treatment, or referral to another HCP. Answer any questions or address any concerns voiced by the patient or family.
- Depending on the results of this procedure, additional testing may be performed to evaluate or monitor progression of the disease process and determine the need for a change in therapy. Evaluate test results in relation to the patient's symptoms and other tests performed.

RELATED STUDIES:

- Related tests include acetylcholine receptor antibody, biopsy muscle, CSF analysis, CT brain, CK, ENG, evoked brain potentials (SER, VER), MRI brain, plethysmography, and PET brain.
- Refer to the Musculoskeletal System table online at Davis*Plus* for related tests by body system.

Electromyography, Pelvic Floor Sphincter

SYNONYM/ACRONYM: Electrodiagnostic study, rectal electromyography.

E

COMMON USE: To assess urinary sphincter electrical activity to assist with diagnosis of urinary incontinence.

AREA OF APPLICATION: Sphincter muscles.

DESCRIPTION: Pelvic floor sphincter electromyography, also known as rectal electromyography, is performed to measure electrical activity of the external urinary sphincter. This procedure, often done in conjunction with cystometry and voiding urethrography as part of a full urodynamic study, helps to diagnose neuromuscular dysfunction and incontinence.

This procedure is contraindicated for

Patients with bleeding disorders ***because the puncture sites may not stop bleeding.***

INDICATIONS

Evaluate neuromuscular dysfunction and incontinence.

POTENTIAL MEDICAL DIAGNOSIS

Normal findings

- Normal urinary and anal sphincter muscle function; increased electromyographic signals during the filling of the urinary bladder and at the conclusion of voiding; absence of signals during the actual voiding; no incontinence

Abnormal findings related to

Neuromuscular dysfunction of lower urinary sphincter, pelvic floor muscle, or anal sphincter is evidenced by diminished electrical activity as measured by the electrodes. Pelvic muscle weakness is commonly seen in older females as a result of muscles that become overstretched during pregnancy and childbirth; muscle weakness can also occur as a result of neurologic injury.

- Anal incontinence
- Urinary incontinence
- Uterine prolapse

CRITICAL FINDINGS: N/A

INTERFERING FACTORS

Factors that may impair the results of the examination

- Inability of the patient to cooperate or remain still during the procedure because of age, significant pain, or mental status.
- Age-related decreases in electrical activity.
- Medications such as muscle relaxants, cholinergics, and anticholinergics.

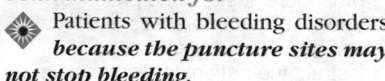

Other considerations

- **Failure to follow dietary restrictions before the procedure may cause the procedure to be canceled or repeated.**

NURSING IMPLICATIONS AND PROCEDURE

PRETEST:

- Positively identify the patient using at least two person-specific identifiers before services, treatments, or procedures are performed.
- *Patient Teaching:* Inform the patient this procedure can assist in measuring the electrical activity of the pelvic floor muscles.
- Obtain a history of the patient's health concerns, symptoms, surgical procedures, and results of previously performed laboratory and diagnostic studies. Include a list of known allergens, especially allergies or sensitivities to latex, anesthetics, or sedatives.
- Obtain a list of the patient's current medications, including over-the-counter medications and dietary supplements (see Effects of Natural Products on Laboratory Values online at Davis*Plus*).
- Review the procedure with the patient. Address concerns about pain related to the procedure. Warn the patient the procedure may be uncomfortable, but an analgesic or sedative will be administered. Assure the patient the pain is minimal during the catheter insertion. Inform the patient the procedure is performed in a special laboratory by a health-care provider (HCP) and takes about 30 min to complete.
- *Sensitivity to social and cultural issues,* as well as concern for modesty, is important in providing psychological support before, during, and after the procedure.
- Instruct the patient to remove jewelry and other metallic objects from the area to be examined.
- Assess for ability to comply with directions given for exercising during the test.
- Under medical direction, the patient should avoid muscle relaxants, cholinergics, and anticholinergics for 3 to 6 days before the test.
- Instruct the patient to abstain from smoking and drinking caffeine-containing beverages for 3 hr before the procedure. Protocols may vary among facilities.
- *Make sure a written and informed consent has been signed prior to the procedure and before administering any medications.*

INTRATEST:

Potential Complications:

Complications are rare but include bleeding ***related to a bleeding disorder or the effects of natural products and medications with known anticoagulant, antiplatelet, or thrombolytic properties*** and urinary infection ***related to use of a catheter.***

- Observe standard precautions, and follow the general guidelines in Patient Preparation and Specimen Collection online at Davis*Plus*. Positively identify the patient.
- Ensure the patient has complied with dietary, fluid, tobacco, and medication restrictions and pretesting preparations.
- Record baseline vital signs.
- Instruct the patient to void prior to the procedure and to change into the gown, robe, and foot coverings provided.
- Avoid the use of equipment containing latex if the patient has a history of allergic reaction to latex.
- Place the patient in a supine position on the examining table and place a drape over the patient, exposing the perianal area.
- Ask the patient to remain very still and relaxed and to cooperate when instructed to contract muscles during the procedure.
- Two skin electrodes are positioned slightly to the left and right of the

perianal area and a grounding electrode is placed on the thigh.
- If needle electrodes are used, they are inserted into the muscle surrounding the urethra.
- Muscle activity signals are recorded as waves, which are interpreted for number and configurations in diagnosing urinary abnormalities.
- An indwelling urinary catheter is inserted, and the bulbocavernosus reflex is tested; the patient is instructed to cough while the catheter is gently pulled.
- Voluntary control is tested by requesting the patient to contract and relax the muscle. Electrical activity is recorded during this period of relaxation with the bladder empty.
- The bladder is filled with sterile water at a rate of 100 mL/min while the electrical activity during filling is recorded.
- The catheter is removed; the patient is then placed in a position to void and is asked to urinate and empty the full bladder. This voluntary urination is then recorded until completed. The complete procedure includes recordings of electrical signals before, during, and at the end of urination.

POST-TEST:

- Inform the patient that a report of the results will be made available to the requesting HCP, who will discuss the results with the patient.
- Instruct the patient to resume usual diet, fluids, medications, and activity, as directed by the HCP.
- Monitor vital signs and neurological status every 15 min for 1 hr, then every 2 hr for 4 hr, and as ordered. Take temperature every 4 hr for 24 hr. Monitor intake and output at least every 8 hr. Compare with baseline values. Protocols may vary among facilities.
- Instruct the patient to increase fluid intake unless contraindicated.
- If tested with needle electrodes, warn female patients to expect hematuria after the first voiding.
- Advise the patient to report symptoms of urethral irritation, such as dysuria, persistent or prolonged hematuria, and urinary frequency.
- Recognize anxiety related to test results, and be supportive of perceived loss of independent function. Discuss the implications of abnormal test results on the patient's lifestyle. Provide teaching and information regarding the clinical implications of the test results, as appropriate.
- Reinforce information given by the patient's HCP regarding further testing, treatment, or referral to another HCP. Answer any questions or address any concerns voiced by the patient or family.
- Depending on the results of this procedure, additional testing may be needed to evaluate or monitor progression of the disease process and determine the need for a change in therapy. Evaluate test results in relation to the patient's symptoms and other tests performed.

RELATED STUDIES:

- Related tests include CT pelvis, cystometry, cystoscopy, cystourethrography voiding, IVP, and US bladder.
- Refer to the Genitourinary System table online at Davis*Plus* for related tests by body system.

Electroneurography

SYNONYM/ACRONYM: Electrodiagnostic study, nerve conduction study.

COMMON USE: To assess peripheral nerve conduction to assist in the diagnosis of diseases such as diabetic neuropathy and muscular dystrophy.

AREA OF APPLICATION: Muscles.

POTENTIAL MEDICAL DIAGNOSIS

Normal findings

- No evidence of peripheral nerve injury or disease. Variable readings depend on the nerve being tested. For patients aged 3 yr and older, the maximum conduction velocity is 40 to 80 milliseconds; for infants and the elderly, the values are divided by 2.

Abnormal findings related to

- Carpal tunnel syndrome
- Diabetic neuropathy
- Guillain-Barré syndrome
- Herniated disk disease
- Muscular dystrophy
- Myasthenia gravis
- Poliomyelitis
- Tarsal tunnel syndrome indicated by decreased conduction time
- Thoracic outlet syndrome

CRITICAL FINDINGS: N/A

Find and print out the full study on Fast Find at davispl.us/vanleeuwen7.

Endoscopy, Sinus

SYNONYM/ACRONYM: N/A

COMMON USE: To facilitate diagnosis and treatment of recurring sinus infections or infections resulting from unresolved sinus infection, including incursion into the brain, eye orbit, or eyeball.

AREA OF APPLICATION: Sinuses.

DESCRIPTION: Sinus endoscopy, done with a narrow flexible tube, is used to help diagnose damage to the sinuses, nose, and throat. The tube contains an optical device with a magnifying lens with a bright light; the tube is inserted through the nose and threaded through the sinuses to the throat. A camera, monitor, or other viewing device is connected to the endoscope to record areas being examined. Sinus endoscopy helps to diagnose structural defects (e.g., polyps or other abnormal growths), damage, and acute or recurring infection to the nose, sinuses, and throat. Cultures can be obtained during the procedure to assist in the identification of infectious organisms and to determine appropriate treatments. Therapeutic applications include drainage of infected sinuses and administration of medications directly to the site of infection. The procedure is usually done in a health-care provider's (HCP's) office, but if done as a surgical procedure, the endoscope may be used to remove polyps from the nose or throat.

This procedure is contraindicated for: N/A

INDICATIONS

- Identify nasal obstruction.
- Assess recurrent sinusitis.

POTENTIAL MEDICAL DIAGNOSIS

Normal findings

- Normal soft tissue appearance

Abnormal findings related to

- Foreign bodies in the nose
- Growths in the nasal passages

- Polyps
- Sinusitis

CRITICAL FINDINGS: N/A

INTERFERING FACTORS

- **Inability of the patient to cooperate or remain still during the test because of age, significant pain, or mental status may interfere with the test results.**

E

NURSING IMPLICATIONS AND PROCEDURE

PRETEST:

- Positively identify the patient using at least two person-specific identifiers before services, treatments, or procedures are performed.
- *Patient Teaching:* Inform the patient this procedure can assist in locating and treating infection of the sinus or surrounding areas.
- Obtain a history of the patient's health concerns, symptoms, surgical procedures, and results of previously performed laboratory and diagnostic studies. Include a list of known allergens, especially allergies or sensitivities to latex, anesthetics, or sedatives.
- Obtain a list of the patient's current medications, including over-the-counter medications and dietary supplements (see Effects of Natural Products on Laboratory Values online at Davis*Plus*).
- Instruct the patient to remove contact lenses or glasses, as appropriate.
- Review the procedure with the patient. Inform the patient that the procedure is usually done with the patient awake and seated upright in a chair. Address concerns about pain and explain that a local anesthetic spray or liquid may be applied to the throat to ease with insertion of the endoscope. Inform the patient that the procedure is usually performed in the office of an HCP and takes about 10 min.
- *Sensitivity to social and cultural issues,* as well as concern for modesty, is important in providing psychological support before, during, and after the procedure.
- Note that there are no food, fluid, or medication restrictions unless by medical direction.
- *Make sure a written and informed consent has been signed prior to the procedure and before administering any medications.*

INTRATEST:

Potential Complications:

Bleeding; cerebrospinal fluid leakage from the ethmoid sinus

- Instruct the patient to cooperate fully and to follow directions. Instruct the patient to remain still throughout the procedure because movement produces unreliable results.
- Avoid the use of equipment containing latex if the patient has a history of allergic reaction to latex.
- Seat the patient comfortably. Instill ordered topical anesthetic in the throat, as ordered, and allow time for it to work.
- Observe that the endoscope is inserted and the structures inside the nose are examined.
- Observe standard precautions, and follow the general guidelines in Patient Preparation and Specimen Collection online at Davis*Plus*. Positively identify the patient, and label the appropriate specimen container with the corresponding patient demographics, initials of the person collecting the specimen, date, and time of collection, if cultures are to be obtained on aspirated sinus material.

POST-TEST:

- Inform the patient that a report of the results will be made available to the requesting HCP, who will discuss the results with the patient.
- Instruct the patient to wait until the numbness in the throat wears off

before attempting to eat or drink following the procedure.
- Recognize anxiety related to test results. Discuss the implications of abnormal test results on the patient's lifestyle. Provide teaching and information regarding the clinical implications of the test results, as appropriate.
- Reinforce information given by the patient's HCP regarding further testing, treatment, or referral to another HCP. Answer any questions or address any concerns voiced by the patient or family.
- Depending on the results of this procedure, additional testing may be needed to evaluate or monitor progression of the disease process and determine the need for a change in therapy. Evaluate test results in relation to the patient's symptoms and other tests performed.

RELATED STUDIES:
- Related tests include CT brain.
- Refer to the Respiratory System table online at Davis*Plus* for related tests by body system.

Eosinophil Count

SYNONYM/ACRONYM: Eos count, total eosinophil count.

COMMON USE: To assist in diagnosing conditions related to immune response such as asthma, dermatitis, and hay fever. Also used to assist in identification of parasitic infections.

SPECIMEN: Whole blood collected in a lavender-top (EDTA) tube.

NORMAL FINDINGS: (Method: Manual count using eosinophil stain and hemocytometer or automated analyzer)
Absolute count: 50 to 500 cells/microL [SI units ($0.05–0.5 \times 10^9$/L)]
Relative percentage: 1% to 4%

POTENTIAL MEDICAL DIAGNOSIS

Increased in:

Eosinophils are released and migrate to inflammatory sites in response to numerous environmental, chemical/drug, or immune-mediated triggers. T cells, mast cells, and macrophages release cytokines like interlukin-3 (IL3), interlukin-5 (IL5), granulocyte/macrophage colony–stimulating factor, and chemokines like the eotaxins, which can result in the activation of eosinophils.

- Addison's disease ***(most commonly related to autoimmune destruction of adrenal glands)***
- Allergy
- Asthma
- Cancer
- Dermatitis
- Drug reactions
- Eczema
- Hay fever
- Hodgkin's disease
- Hypereosinophilic syndrome (rare and idiopathic)
- Löffler's syndrome ***(pulmonary eosinophilia due to allergic reaction or infection from a fungus or parasite)***
- Myeloproliferative disorders ***(related to abnormal changes in the bone marrow)***

- Parasitic infection (visceral larva migrans)
- Rheumatoid arthritis ***(possibly related to medications used in therapy)***
- Rhinitis
- Sarcoidosis
- Splenectomy
- Tuberculosis

Decreased in:

- Aplastic anemia ***(bone marrow failure)***
- Eclampsia ***(shift to the left; relative to significant production of neutrophils)***
- Infections ***(shift to the left; relative to significant production of neutrophils)***
- Stress ***(release of cortisol suppresses eosinophils)***

CRITICAL FINDINGS: N/A

Find and print out the full study on Fast Find at davispl.us/vanleeuwen7.

Erythrocyte Protoporphyrin, Free

SYNONYM/ACRONYM: Free erythrocyte protoporphyrin (FEP).

COMMON USE: To assist in diagnosing anemias related to chronic disease, hemolysis, iron deficiency, and lead toxicity.

SPECIMEN: Whole blood collected in a lavender-top (EDTA), royal blue-top (EDTA), or a pink-top (EDTA) tube.

NORMAL FINDINGS: (Method: Fluorometry)

Conventional Units	SI Units (Conventional Units × 0.0178)
Adult	
Male	
Less than 30 mcg/dL	Less than 0.534 micromol/L
Female	
Less than 40 mcg/dL	Less than 0.712 micromol/L

POTENTIAL MEDICAL DIAGNOSIS

Increased in:

- Anemia of chronic disease ***(related to accumulation of protoporphyrin in the absence of available iron)***
- Conditions with marked erythropoiesis (e.g., hemolytic anemias) ***(related to increased cell destruction)***
- Erythropoietic protoporphyria ***(related to abnormal increased secretion)***
- Iron-deficiency anemias ***(related to accumulation of protoporphyrin in the absence of available iron)***
- Lead poisoning ***(possibly related to inactivation of enzymes involved in iron binding or transfer)***
- Some sideroblastic anemias

Decreased in: N/A

CRITICAL FINDINGS: N/A

Find and print out the full study on Fast Find at davispl.us/vanleeuwen7.

Erythrocyte Sedimentation Rate

SYNONYM/ACRONYM: Sed rate, ESR.

COMMON USE: To assist in diagnosing acute infection in diseases such as tissue necrosis, chronic infection, and acute inflammation.

SPECIMEN: Whole blood collected in a completely filled lavender-top (EDTA) tube for the modified Westergren method or a completely filled gray-top (3.8% sodium citrate) tube for the original Westergren method.

NORMAL FINDINGS: (Method: Westergren or modified Westergren)

Age	Male	Female
Newborn	0–2 mm/hr	0–2 mm/hr
Less than 50 yr	0–15 mm/hr	0–25 mm/hr
50 yr and older	0–20 mm/hr	0–30 mm/hr

DESCRIPTION: The erythrocyte sedimentation rate (ESR) is a measure of the rate of sedimentation of red blood cells (RBCs) in an anticoagulated whole blood sample over a specified period of time. The basis of the ESR test is the alteration of blood proteins by inflammatory and necrotic processes that cause the RBCs to stick together, become heavier, and rapidly settle at the bottom of a vertically held, calibrated tube over time. The most common promoter of rouleaux is an increase in circulating fibrinogen levels. In general, relatively little settling occurs in normal blood because normal RBCs do not form rouleaux and would not stack together. The sedimentation rate is proportional to the size or mass of the falling RBCs and is inversely proportional to plasma viscosity. The test is a nonspecific indicator of disease but is fairly sensitive and is frequently the earliest indicator of widespread inflammatory reaction due to infection or autoimmune disorders. Prolonged elevations are also present in malignant disease. The ESR can also be used to monitor the course of a disease and the effectiveness of therapy. The most commonly used method to measure the ESR is the Westergren (or modified Westergren) method.

This procedure is contraindicated for: N/A

INDICATIONS

- Assist in the diagnosis of acute infection, such as tuberculosis or tissue necrosis.
- Assist in the diagnosis of acute inflammatory processes.
- Assist in the diagnosis of chronic infections.
- Assist in the diagnosis of rheumatoid or autoimmune disorders.
- Assist in the diagnosis of temporal arthritis and polymyalgia rheumatica.
- Monitor inflammatory and malignant disease.

E

POTENTIAL MEDICAL DIAGNOSIS

Increased in:

Increased rouleaux formation is associated with increased levels of fibrinogen and/or production of cytokines and other acute-phase reactant proteins in response to inflammation. Anemia of chronic disease as well as acute anemia influence the ESR because the decreased number of RBCs falls faster with the relatively increased plasma volume.

- Acute myocardial infarction
- Anemia ***(RBCs fall faster with increased plasma volume)***
- Carcinoma
- Cat scratch fever (Bartonella henselae)
- Collagen diseases, including systemic lupus erythematosus (SLE)
- Crohn's disease ***(due to anemia or related to acute-phase reactant proteins)***
- Elevated blood glucose ***(hyperglycemia in older adult patients can induce production of cytokines responsible for the inflammatory response; hyperglycemia related to insulin resistance can cause hepatocytes to shift protein synthesis from albumin to production of acute-phase reactant proteins)***
- Endocarditis
- Heavy metal poisoning ***(related to anemia affecting size and shape of RBCs)***
- Increased plasma protein level ***(RBCs fall faster with increased plasma viscosity)***
- Infections (e.g., pneumonia, syphilis)
- Inflammatory diseases
- Lymphoma
- Lymphosarcoma
- Multiple myeloma ***(RBCs fall faster with increased plasma viscosity)***
- Nephritis
- Pregnancy ***(related to anemia)***
- Pulmonary embolism
- Rheumatic fever
- Rheumatoid arthritis
- Subacute bacterial endocarditis
- Temporal arteritis
- Toxemia
- Tuberculosis
- Waldenström's macroglobulinemia ***(RBCs fall faster with increased plasma viscosity)***

Decreased in:

- Conditions resulting in high hemoglobin and RBC count

CRITICAL FINDINGS: N/A

INTERFERING FACTORS

- Some drugs and other substances cause an SLE-like syndrome that results in a physiological increase in ESR. These include anticonvulsants, hydrazine derivatives, nitrofurantoin, procainamide, and quinidine. Other drugs and substances that may cause an increased ESR include acetylsalicylic acid, cephalothin, cyclosporin A, dextran, and oral contraceptives.
- Drugs and other substances that may cause a decrease in ESR include aurothiomalate, corticotropin, cortisone, dexamethasone, methotrexate, minocycline, NSAIDs, penicillamine, prednisolone, prednisone, quinine, sulfasalazine, tamoxifen, and trimethoprim.
- Menstruation may cause falsely increased test results.
- Prolonged tourniquet constriction around the arm may cause hemoconcentration and falsely low values.
- The Westergren and modified Westergren methods are affected by heparin, which causes a false elevation in values.
- Bubbles in the Westergren tube or pipette, or tilting the measurement

column more than 3° from vertical, will falsely increase the values.

- Movement or vibration of the surface on which the test is being conducted will affect the results.
- Inaccurate timing or a delay in performing the test once the specimen has been collected will invalidate test results.
- Specimens that are clotted, hemolyzed, or insufficient in volume should be rejected for analysis.
- The test should be performed within 4 hr of collection when the specimen has been stored at room temperature; delays in testing may result in decreased values. If a delay in testing is anticipated, refrigerate the sample at 2°C to 4°C; stability at refrigerated temperature is reported to be extended up to 12 hr. Refrigerated specimens should be brought to room temperature before testing.

E

NURSING IMPLICATIONS AND PROCEDURE

POTENTIAL NURSING PROBLEMS:

Problem	Signs & Symptoms	Interventions
Infection ***(related to inadequate defense mechanism; insufficient nutrition; chronic disease; intravenous (IV) access devices; pathogen exposure; indwelling urinary catheter; compromised immune system; mechanical intubation)***	Fever; increased heart rate; increased blood pressure; shaking; chills; mottled skin; lethargy; fatigue; swelling; edema; pain; localized pressure; diaphoresis; night sweats; confusion; vomiting; nausea; headache; cloudy, foul smelling urine with sediment; elevated white blood cell (WBC) count; elevated ESR	Promote good hygiene; assist with hygiene as needed; administer prescribed antibiotics, antipyretics; provide cooling measures; administer prescribed IV fluids; monitor vital signs and trend temperatures; encourage oral fluids; adhere to standard or universal precautions; isolate as appropriate; obtain cultures as ordered; encourage use of lightweight clothing and bedding; assess nutritional status and provide supplements as needed; assess for exposure to infections; monitor sputum color and viscosity; assess urine characteristics (color, clarity); monitor and trend WBC and ESR rate; monitor for symptoms of infection (redness, swelling, purulent drainage, pain from wound or incisions); provide aseptic tracheal care; perform dressing changes with sterile or aseptic technique; perform vigilant hand hygiene

(table continues on page 752)

Problem	Signs & Symptoms	Interventions
Tissue integrity ***(related to infection)***	Area on the skin that is warm or tender to touch; skin that turns red, purple, or black; localized pain; swelling of affected area; elevated WBC count; elevated ESR	Perform baseline skin assessment and frequent reassessment using a standardized scale (Braden); monitor and note the presence of herpes lesions; encourage the use of hypoallergenic soap and lanolin products, pat rather than rub skin dry; avoid bed wrinkles; ensure sheets are soft and gentle on skin; encourage adequate nutrition; administer prescribed vitamin supplements; encourage and assist range of motion; assess the characteristics of a wound (color, size, length, width, depth, drainage, and odor); monitor for fever; identify the cause of the tissue damage; monitor and trend WBC and ESR
Nutrition ***(related to nutrition due to inability to digest foods, metabolize foods, ingest foods; refusal to eat; increased metabolic needs associated with disease process; lack of understanding)***	Unintended weight loss; current weight is 20% below ideal weight; pale dry skin; dry mucous membranes; documented inadequate caloric intake; subcutaneous tissue loss; hair pulls out easily; paresthesia	Record accurate daily weight at the same time each day with the same scale; obtain an accurate nutritional history; assess attitude toward eating; promote a dietary consult to evaluate current eating habits and best method of nutritional supplementation; develop short-term and long-term eating strategies; monitor nutritional laboratory values such as albumin; assess swallowing ability; encourage cultural home foods; provide a pleasant environment for eating; alter food seasoning to enhance flavor; provide parenteral or enteral nutrition as prescribed

Problem	Signs & Symptoms	Interventions
Activity ***(related to inflammation; infection; altered tissue perfusion; deconditioned state)***	Weakness; verbal report of fatigue; altered sleep pattern; altered blood pressure, heart rate, or respiratory rate in response to activity; oxygen desaturation with activity	Assess current level of activity and weakness; identify the patient's perception of the cause of weakness; assess the need for the use of assistive devices; observe and document the patient's tolerance to activity; provide ordered oxygen; limit energy expenditure to necessary activities

PRETEST:

- Positively identify the patient using at least two person-specific identifiers before services, treatments, or procedures are performed.
- ***Patient Teaching:*** Inform the patient this test can assist in identification of inflammation.
- Obtain a history of the patient's health concerns, symptoms, surgical procedures, and results of previously performed laboratory and diagnostic studies. Include a list of known allergens, especially allergies or sensitivities to latex.
- Obtain a list of the patient's current medications, including over-the-counter medications and dietary supplements (see Effects of Natural Products on Laboratory Values online at Davis*Plus*).
- Review the procedure with the patient. Inform the patient that specimen collection takes approximately 5 to 10 min. Address concerns about pain and explain that there may be some discomfort during the venipuncture.
- ***Sensitivity to social and cultural issues,*** as well as concern for modesty, is important in providing psychological support before, during, and after the procedure.
- Note that there are no food, fluid, or medication restrictions unless by medical direction.

INTRATEST:

Potential Complications: N/A

- Avoid the use of equipment containing latex if the patient has a history of allergic reaction to latex.
- Instruct the patient to cooperate fully and to follow directions. Direct the patient to breathe normally and to avoid unnecessary movement.
- Observe standard precautions, and follow the general guidelines in Patient Preparation and Specimen Collection online at Davis*Plus*. Positively identify the patient, and label the appropriate tubes with the corresponding patient demographics, date, and time of collection. Perform a venipuncture; collect the specimen in a gray-top (sodium citrate) tube if the Westergren method will be used. Collect the specimen in a purple-top (EDTA) tube if the modified Westergren method will be used.
- Remove the needle and apply direct pressure with dry gauze to stop bleeding. Observe/assess venipuncture site for bleeding or hematoma formation and secure gauze with adhesive bandage.
- Promptly transport the specimen to the laboratory for processing and analysis.

POST-TEST:

- Inform the patient that a report of the results will be made available to the requesting health-care provider (HCP), who will discuss the results with the patient.

- Depending on the results of this procedure, additional testing may be performed to evaluate or monitor progression of the disease process and determine the need for a change in therapy. Evaluate test results in relation to the patient's symptoms and other tests performed.

Patient Education:

- Provide teaching and information regarding the clinical implications of the test results, as appropriate.
- Educate the patient regarding access to counseling services, as appropriate.
- Provide contact information, if desired, for the American College of Rheumatology (www.rheumatology.org) or the Arthritis Foundation (www.arthritis.org). 🍁
- Reinforce information given by the patient's HCP regarding further testing, treatment, or referral to another HCP.
- Answer any questions or address any concerns voiced by the patient or family.

Expected Patient Outcomes:

Understanding

- The patient and family state the signs and symptoms of infection including what to report and when to report concerns.
- The patient and family state the importance of follow-up ESR to monitor the effectiveness of therapeutic interventions.

Ability

- The patient effectively paces activities to manage energy expenditures and increase participation in activities of daily living.
- The patient increases dietary intake by 50% and is validated with increased weight.

Response

- The patient and family comply with the request to perform vigilant hand hygiene to decrease infection risk.
- The patient and family comply with the request to monitor temperature and report elevation to the HCP.

RELATED STUDIES:

- Related tests include antibodies, anticyclic citrullinated peptide, ANA, arthroscopy, arthrogram, blood pool imaging, BMD, bone scan, CBC, CBC hematocrit, CBC hemoglobin, CBC RBC indices, CBC RBC morphology, CT cardiac scoring, copper, CRP, D-dimer, exercise stress test, fibrinogen, glucose, iron, lead, MRI musculoskeletal, MRI venography, microorganism-specific serologies and related cultures, myocardial perfusion heart scan, procalcitonin, radiography bone, RF, synovial fluid analysis, and troponin.
- Refer to the Cardiovascular, Hematopoietic, Immune, and Respiratory systems tables online at Davis*Plus* for related tests by body system.

Erythropoietin

SYNONYM/ACRONYM: EPO.

COMMON USE: To evaluate the effectiveness of erythropoietin (EPO) administration as a treatment for anemia, especially related to chemotherapy and kidney disease.

SPECIMEN: Serum collected in a gold-, red-, or red/gray-top tube.

NORMAL FINDINGS: (Method: Immunochemiluminometric assay)

Age	Conventional & SI Units	Conventional & SI Units
	Male	*Female*
0–3 yr	1.7–17.9 milli-international units/mL	2.1–15.9 milli-international units/mL
4–6 yr	3.5–21.9 milli-international units/mL	2.9–8.5 milli-international units/mL
7–9 yr	1.1–13.5 milli-international units/mL	2.1–8.2 milli-international units/mL
10–12 yr	1.1–14.1 milli-international units/mL	1.1–9.1 milli-international units/mL
13–15 yr	2.2–14.4 milli-international units/mL	3.8–20.5 milli-international units/mL
16–18 yr	1.5–15.2 milli-international units/mL	2.1–14.2 milli-international units/mL
Adult	4.2–27.8 milli-international units/mL	4.2–27.8 milli-international units/mL

Based on normal hemoglobin and hematocrit. Values may be decreased in older adults due to the effects of medications and the presence of multiple chronic or acute diseases with or without muted symptoms.

DESCRIPTION: Erythropoietin (EPO) is a glycoprotein produced mainly by the kidney. Its function is to stimulate the bone marrow to make red blood cells (RBCs). EPO levels fall after removal of the kidney but do not disappear completely. Small amounts of EPO are produced by the liver. Erythropoiesis is regulated by EPO and tissue Po_2. When Po_2 is normal, EPO levels decrease; when Po_2 falls, EPO secretion occurs and EPO levels increase.

This procedure is contraindicated for: N/A

INDICATIONS
- Assist in assessment of anemia of chronic kidney disease.
- Assist in the diagnosis of EPO-producing tumors.
- Evaluate the possibility of EPO abuse by athletes.
- Evaluate the presence of rare anemias.
- Monitor patients receiving EPO therapy.

POTENTIAL MEDICAL DIAGNOSIS

Increased in:
- After moderate bleeding in an otherwise healthy patient ***(related to loss of RBCs, which stimulates production)***
- AIDS ***(related to anemia, which stimulates production)***
- Anemias (e.g., hemolytic, iron deficiency, megaloblastic) ***(related to low RBC count, which stimulates production)***
- Blood doping ***(enhancement of athletic performance and stamina, related to increased production of RBCs)***
- Hepatoma ***(related to EPO-producing tumors)***
- Kidney transplant rejection ***(15% of cases respond with an exaggerated secretion of EPO and a transient post-transplantation erythrocytosis)***
- Nephroblastoma ***(related to EPO-producing tumors)***

- Pheochromocytoma ***(related to EPO-producing tumors)***
- Polycystic kidney disease ***(related to EPO-producing tumors or cysts)***
- Pregnancy ***(related to anemia of pregnancy, which stimulates production)***
- Secondary polycythemia where low oxygen levels stimulate production ***(high-altitude hypoxia, chronic obstructive pulmonary disease, pulmonary fibrosis)***

Decreased in:

- Chemotherapy ***(related to therapy, which can be toxic to the kidney)***
- Chronic kidney disease ***(related to decreased production and excessive loss through excretion by damaged kidneys)***
- Primary polycythemia ***(related to feedback loop response to elevated RBC count)***

CRITICAL FINDINGS: N/A

INTERFERING FACTORS

- Drugs and other substances that may increase EPO levels include adrenocorticotropic hormone, anabolic steroids, androgens, angiotensin, epinephrine, daunorubicin, fenoterol, growth hormone, thyroid-stimulating hormone, and xenon (gas).
- Phlebotomy may increase EPO levels.
- Drugs and other substances that may decrease EPO levels include amphotericin B, cisplatin, enalapril, estrogens, furosemide, and theophylline.
- Blood transfusions may also decrease EPO levels.

NURSING IMPLICATIONS AND PROCEDURE

PRETEST:

- Positively identify the patient using at least two person-specific identifiers before services, treatments, or procedures are performed.
- *Patient Teaching:* Inform the patient this test can assist in evaluation of anemia.
- Obtain a history of the patient's health concerns, symptoms, surgical procedures, and results of previously performed laboratory and diagnostic studies. Include a list of known allergens, especially allergies or sensitivities to latex.
- Note any recent procedures that can interfere with test results.
- Obtain a list of the patient's current medications, including over-the-counter medications and dietary supplements (see Effects of Natural Products on Laboratory Values online at Davis*Plus*).
- Review the procedure with the patient. Inform the patient that specimen collection takes approximately 5 to 10 min. Address concerns about pain and explain to the patient that there may be some discomfort during the venipuncture.
- *Sensitivity to social and cultural issues,* as well as concern for modesty, is important in providing psychological support before, during, and after the procedure.
- Note that there are no food, fluid, or medication restrictions unless by medical direction.

INTRATEST:

Potential Complications: N/A

- Avoid the use of equipment containing latex if the patient has a history of allergic reaction to latex.
- Instruct the patient to cooperate fully and to follow directions. Direct the patient to breathe normally and to avoid unnecessary movement.
- Observe standard precautions, and follow the general guidelines in Patient Preparation and Specimen Collection online at Davis*Plus*. Positively identify the patient, and label the appropriate specimen container with the corresponding patient demographics, initials of the person collecting the specimen, date, and time of collection. Perform a venipuncture.

- Remove the needle and apply direct pressure with dry gauze to stop bleeding. Observe/assess venipuncture site for bleeding or hematoma formation and secure gauze with adhesive bandage.
- Promptly transport the specimen to the laboratory for processing and analysis.

POST-TEST:

- Inform the patient that a report of the results will be made available to the requesting health-care provider (HCP), who will discuss the results with the patient.
- Reinforce information given by the patient's HCP regarding further testing, treatment, or referral to another HCP. Answer any questions or address any concerns voiced by the patient or family.
- Depending on the results of this procedure, additional testing may be performed to evaluate or monitor progression of the disease process and determine the need for a change in therapy. Evaluate test results in relation to the patient's symptoms and other tests performed.

RELATED STUDIES:

- Related tests include biopsy bone marrow, BUN, CBC, CBC hematocrit, CBC hemoglobin, CBC RBC count, CBC RBC indices, CBC RBC morphology and inclusions, CT kidneys, creatinine, creatinine clearance, ferritin, iron/TIBC, microalbumin, retrograde ureteropyelography, US kidney, and vitamin B_{12}.
- Refer to the Hematopoietic and Genitourinary systems tests online at Davis*Plus* for related tests by body system.

E

Esophageal Manometry

SYNONYM/ACRONYM: Esophageal function study, esophageal acid study (Tuttle test), acid reflux test, Bernstein test (acid perfusion), esophageal motility study.

COMMON USE: To evaluate potential ineffectiveness of the esophageal muscle and structure in swallowing, vomiting, and regurgitation in diseases such as scleroderma, infection, and gastric esophageal reflux.

AREA OF APPLICATION: Esophagus.

DESCRIPTION: Esophageal manometry (EM) consists of a group of invasive studies performed to assist in diagnosing abnormalities of esophageal muscle function and esophageal structure. These studies measure esophageal pressure, the effects of gastric acid in the esophagus, lower esophageal sphincter pressure, and motility patterns that result during swallowing. EM can be used to document and quantify gastroesophageal reflux disease (GERD). It is indicated when a patient is experiencing difficulty swallowing, heartburn, regurgitation, or vomiting or has chest pain for which no diagnosis has been found. Tests performed in combination with EM include the acid reflux, acid clearing, and acid perfusion (Bernstein) tests.

This procedure is contraindicated for

Patients with unstable cardiopulmonary status, blood coagulation defects, recent gastrointestinal surgery, esophageal varices, or bleeding.

INDICATIONS

- Aid in the diagnosis of achalasia, evidenced by increased pressure in EM.
- Aid in the diagnosis of achalasia in children, evidenced by decreased pressure in EM.
- Aid in the diagnosis of esophageal scleroderma, evidenced by decreased pressure in EM.
- Aid in the diagnosis of esophagitis, evidenced by decreased motility.
- Aid in the diagnosis of GERD, evidenced by low pressure in EM, decreased pH in acidity test, and pain in acid reflux and perfusion tests.
- Differentiate between esophagitis or cardiac condition as the cause of epigastric pain.
- Evaluate pyrosis and dysphagia to determine if the cause is GERD or esophagitis.

POTENTIAL MEDICAL DIAGNOSIS

Normal findings

- Acid clearing: fewer than 10 swallows
- Acid perfusion: no GERD
- Acid reflux: no regurgitation into the esophagus
- Bernstein test: negative (no discomfort or pain following instillation of hydrochloric acid)
- Esophageal secretions: pH 5 to 6
- Esophageal sphincter pressure: 10 to 20 mm Hg

Abnormal findings related to

- Achalasia (sphincter pressure of 50 mm Hg)
- Chalasia
- Esophageal scleroderma
- Esophagitis
- GERD (sphincter pressure of 0 to 5 mm Hg, pH of 1 to 3)
- Hiatal hernia
- Progressive systemic sclerosis (scleroderma)
- Spasms

CRITICAL FINDINGS: N/A

INTERFERING FACTORS

Factors that may impair the results of the examination

- Inability of the patient to cooperate or remain still during the procedure because of age, significant pain, or mental status.
- Administration of medications (e.g., sedatives, antacids, anticholinergics, cholinergics, corticosteroids) that can change pH or relax the sphincter muscle, causing inaccurate results.

Other considerations

- Failure to follow dietary restrictions before the procedure may cause the procedure to be canceled or repeated.

NURSING IMPLICATIONS AND PROCEDURE

See Potential Nursing Problems on Fast Find at davispl.us/vanleeuwen7.

PRETEST:

- Positively identify the patient using at least two person-specific identifiers before services, treatments, or procedures are performed.
- *Patient Teaching:* Inform the patient this procedure can assist in assessing the esophagus.
- Obtain a history of the patient's health concerns, symptoms, surgical procedures, and results of previously performed laboratory and diagnostic studies. Include a list of known allergens, especially allergies or sensitivities to latex, anesthetics or sedatives.
- Note any recent barium or other radiological contrast procedures. Ensure that barium studies were performed more than 4 days before the EM.
- Record the date of the last menstrual period and determine the possibility of pregnancy in perimenopausal women.

- Obtain a list of the patient's current medications, including over-the-counter medications, dietary supplements, anticoagulants, aspirin and other salicylates (see Effects of Natural Products on Laboratory Values online at Davis*Plus*). Such products should be discontinued by medical direction for the appropriate number of days prior to a surgical procedure. Note the last time and dose of medication taken.
- Review the procedure with the patient. Address concerns about pain related to the procedure and explain that some pain may be experienced during the test; there may be moments of discomfort and gagging when the scope is inserted, but there are no complications resulting from the procedure; and the throat will be anesthetized with a spray or swab. Inform the patient that he or she will not be able to speak during the procedure but breathing will not be affected. Inform the patient that the procedure is performed in an endoscopy suite by a health-care provider (HCP), under local anesthesia, and takes approximately 30 to 45 min.
- ***Sensitivity to social and cultural issues,*** as well as concern for modesty, is important in providing psychological support before, during, and after the procedure.
- Explain that an intravenous (IV) line may be inserted to allow infusion of fluids such as saline, anesthetics, sedatives, or emergency medications.
- Instruct the patient to remove dentures and eyewear.
- Under medical direction, the patient should withhold medications for 24 hr before the study; special arrangements may be necessary for diabetic patients.
- Instruct the patient to fast and restrict fluids for 6 hr prior to the procedure to reduce the risk of aspiration related to nausea and vomiting. The American Society of Anesthesiologists has fasting guidelines for risk levels according to patient status. More information can be located at www.asahq.org. 🍁 Protocols may vary among facilities.
- Obtain and record baseline vital signs.
- *Make sure a written and informed consent has been signed prior to the procedure and before administering any medications.*

INTRATEST:

Potential Complications:

Establishing an IV site and injection of contrast medium by catheter are invasive procedures. Complications are rare but do include risk for bleeding from the puncture site ***related to a bleeding disorder or the effects of natural products and medications with known anticoagulant, antiplatelet, or thrombolytic properties;*** hematoma ***related to blood leakage into the tissue following needle insertion;*** or infection ***that might occur if bacteria from the skin surface is introduced at the puncture site.***

- Observe standard precautions, and follow the general guidelines in Patient Preparation and Specimen Collection online at Davis*Plus*. Positively identify the patient.
- Ensure that the patient has complied with dietary, fluids, and medication restrictions and pretesting preparations prior to the study, as instructed.
- Ensure the patient has removed dentures and eyewear prior to the procedure.
- Avoid using morphine sulfate in patients with asthma or other pulmonary disease. This drug can further exacerbate bronchospasms and respiratory impairment.
- Avoid the use of equipment containing latex if the patient has a history of allergic reaction to latex.
- Have emergency equipment readily available.
- Instruct the patient to void prior to the procedure and to change into the gown, robe, and foot coverings provided.
- Instruct the patient to cooperate fully and to follow directions. Instruct the patient to remain still throughout the procedure because movement produces unreliable results.

- Establish an IV fluid line for the injection of saline, anesthetics, sedatives, or emergency medications.
- Spray or swab the oropharynx with a topical local anesthetic.
- Provide an emesis basin for the increased saliva and encourage the patient to spit out saliva since the gag reflex may be impaired.
- Monitor the patient for complications related to the procedure (e.g., aspiration of stomach contents into the lungs, dyspnea, tachypnea, adventitious sounds).
- Suction the mouth, pharynx, and trachea, and administer oxygen as ordered.

Esophageal Manometry

- One or more small tubes are inserted through the nose into the esophagus and stomach.
- A small transducer is attached to the ends of the tubes to measure lower esophageal sphincter pressure, intraluminal pressures, and regularity and duration of peristaltic contractions.
- Instruct the patient to swallow small amounts of water or flavored gelatin.

Esophageal Acid and Clearing (Tuttle Test)

- With the tube in place, a pH electrode probe is inserted into the esophagus with Valsalva maneuvers performed to stimulate reflux of stomach contents into the esophagus.
- If acid reflux is absent, 100 mL of 0.1% hydrochloric acid is instilled into the stomach during a 3-min period, and the pH measurement is repeated.
- To determine acid clearing, hydrochloric acid is instilled into the esophagus and the patient is asked to swallow while the probe measures the pH.

Acid Perfusion (Bernstein Test)

- A catheter is inserted through the nose into the esophagus, and the patient is asked to inform the HCP when pain is experienced.
- Normal saline solution is allowed to drip into the catheter at about 10 mL/min. Then hydrochloric acid is allowed to drip into the catheter.
- Pain experienced when the hydrochloric acid is instilled determines the presence of an esophageal abnormality. If no pain is experienced, symptoms are the result of some other condition.

POST-TEST:

- Inform the patient that a report of the results will be made available to the requesting HCP, who will discuss the results with the patient.
- Monitor the patient for signs of respiratory depression (less than 15 respirations/min) every 15 min for 2 hr. Resuscitation equipment should be available.
- ***Observe the patient for indications of perforation:*** painful swallowing with neck movement, substernal pain with respiration, shoulder pain, dyspnea, abdominal or back pain, cyanosis, and fever.
- Instruct the patient not to eat or drink until the gag reflex returns and then to eat lightly for 12 to 24 hr.
- Instruct the patient to resume usual activity, medication, and diet 24 hr after the examination or as tolerated, as directed by the HCP.
- Inform the patient to expect some throat soreness and possible hoarseness. Advise the patient to use warm gargles, lozenges, or ice packs to the neck and to drink cool fluids to alleviate throat discomfort.
- Emphasize that any severe pain, fever, difficulty breathing, or expectoration of blood must be reported to the HCP immediately.
- Recognize anxiety related to test results, and offer support. Discuss the implications of abnormal test results on the patient's lifestyle. Provide teaching and information regarding the clinical implications of the test results, as appropriate.
- Reinforce information given by the patient's HCP regarding further testing, treatment, or referral to another HCP. Answer any questions or address any concerns voiced by the patient or family.
- Depending on the results of this procedure, additional testing may be needed to evaluate or monitor progression of the disease process

and determine the need for a change in therapy. Evaluate test results in relation to the patient's symptoms and other tests performed.

Patient Education:

- Teach the patient and family symptoms of low Hgb and Hct associated with anemia and blood loss.
- Teach the patient and family the pathophysiology associated with esophageal disease.

Expected Patient Outcomes:

Understanding

- The patient and family verbalize the purpose of blood transfusion within the context of a low Hgb and Hct.
- The patient and family verbalize the importance of reporting symptoms of anemia and blood loss to the HCP.

Ability

- The patient demonstrates observing and evaluating stool for color, consistency, and odor.
- The patient demonstrates taking prescribed medications to decrease pain and improve nutrition.

Response

- The patient agrees to monitor stools at home for color, consistency, and amount.
- The patient agrees to alter diet selections to support esophageal healing.

RELATED STUDIES:

- Related tests include ANA, barium swallow, biopsy skin, capsule endoscopy, chest x-ray, CT thoracic, esophagogastroduodenoscopy, fecal analysis, gastric emptying scan, GERD scan, lung perfusion scan, mediastinoscopy, and upper GI series.
- Refer to the Gastrointestinal System table online at Davis*Plus* for related tests by body system.

E

Esophagogastroduodenoscopy

SYNONYM/ACRONYM: Esophagoscopy, gastroscopy, upper GI endoscopy, EGD.

COMMON USE: To visualize and assess the esophagus, stomach, and upper portion of the duodenum to assist in diagnosis of bleeding, ulcers, inflammation, tumor, and cancer.

AREA OF APPLICATION: Esophagus, stomach, and upper duodenum.

DESCRIPTION: Esophagogastroduodenoscopy (EGD) allows direct visualization of the upper gastrointestinal (GI) tract mucosa, which includes the esophagus, stomach, and upper portion of the duodenum, by means of a flexible endoscope. The standard flexible fiberoptic endoscope contains three channels that allow passage of the instruments needed to perform therapeutic or diagnostic procedures, such as biopsies or cytology washings. The endoscope, a multichannel instrument, allows visualization of the GI tract linings, insufflation of air, aspiration of fluid, removal of foreign bodies by suction or by snare or forceps, and passage of a laser beam for obliteration of abnormal tissue or control of bleeding. Direct visualization yields greater diagnostic data than is possible through radiological procedures, and therefore EGD is rapidly replacing upper GI series as the diagnostic procedure of choice.

This procedure is contraindicated for

- Patients who have had surgery involving the stomach or duodenum, which can make locating the duodenal papilla difficult.
- Patients with a bleeding disorder.
- Patients with unstable cardiopulmonary status, blood coagulation defects, or cholangitis, unless the patient received prophylactic antibiotic therapy before the test (otherwise the examination must be rescheduled).
- Patients with known aortic arch aneurysm, large esophageal Zenker's diverticulum, recent GI surgery, esophageal varices, or known esophageal perforation.

E

INDICATIONS

- Assist in differentiating between benign and neoplastic tumors.
- Detect gastric or duodenal ulcers.
- Detect upper GI inflammatory disease.
- Determine the presence and location of acute upper GI bleeding.
- Evaluate the extent of esophageal injury after ingestion of chemicals.
- Evaluate stomach or duodenum after surgical procedures.
- Evaluate suspected gastric outlet obstruction.
- Identify tissue abnormalities and obtain biopsy specimens.
- Investigate the cause of dysphagia, dyspepsia, and epigastric pain.

POTENTIAL MEDICAL DIAGNOSIS

Normal findings

- Esophageal mucosa is normally yellow-pink. At about 9 in. from the incisor teeth, a pulsation indicates the location of the aortic arch. The gastric mucosa is orange-red and contains rugae. The proximal duodenum is reddish and contains a few longitudinal folds, whereas the distal duodenum has circular folds lined with villi. No abnormal structures or functions are observed in the esophagus, stomach, or duodenum.

Abnormal findings related to

- Acute and chronic gastric and duodenal ulcers
- Diverticular disease
- Duodenitis
- Esophageal varices
- Esophageal or pyloric stenosis
- Esophagitis or strictures
- Gastritis
- Hiatal hernia
- Mallory-Weiss syndrome
- Tumors (benign or malignant)

CRITICAL FINDINGS:

- Presence and location of acute GI bleed

Note and immediately report to the requesting health-care provider (HCP) any critical findings and related symptoms. A listing of these findings varies among facilities. Timely notification of a critical finding for laboratory or diagnostic studies is a role expectation of the professional nurse. The notification processes vary among facilities. Upon receipt of the critical finding, the information should be read back to the caller to verify accuracy.

INTERFERING FACTORS

Factors that may alter the results of the study

- Gas or food in the GI tract resulting from inadequate cleansing or failure to restrict food intake before the study.
- Retained barium from a previous radiological procedure.
- Inability of the patient to cooperate or remain still during the procedure because of age, significant pain, or mental status.

Other considerations

- The procedure may be terminated if chest pain or severe cardiac dysrhythmias occur.

- **Failure to follow dietary restrictions and other pretesting preparations may cause the procedure to be canceled or repeated.**

NURSING IMPLICATIONS AND PROCEDURE

See Potential Nursing Problems on Fast Find at davispl.us/vanleeuwen7.

PRETEST:

- Positively identify the patient using at least two person-specific identifiers before services, treatments, or procedures are performed.
- *Patient Teaching:* Inform the patient this procedure can assist in assessing the esophagus and gastrointestinal tract.
- Obtain a history of the patient's health concerns, symptoms, surgical procedures, and results of previously performed laboratory and diagnostic studies. Include a list of known allergens, especially allergies or sensitivities to latex, anesthetics or sedatives.
- Note any recent barium or other radiological contrast procedures ordered. Ensure that barium studies are performed after this study.
- Record the date of the last menstrual period and determine the possibility of pregnancy in perimenopausal women.
- Obtain a list of the patient's current medications, including over-the-counter medications, dietary supplements, anticoagulants, aspirin and other salicylates (see Effects of Natural Products on Laboratory Values online at Davis*Plus*). Such products should be discontinued by medical direction for the appropriate number of days prior to a surgical procedure. Note the last time and dose of medication taken.
- Review the procedure with the patient. Address concerns about pain related to the procedure and explain that some pain may be experienced during the test, and there may be moments of discomfort, but the throat will be anesthetized with a spray or swab. Inform the patient that he or she will not be able to speak during the procedure, but breathing will not be affected. Inform the patient that the procedure is performed in a GI laboratory or radiology department, usually by an HCP and support staff, and takes approximately 30 to 60 min.
- ***Sensitivity to social and cultural issues,*** as well as concern for modesty, is important in providing psychological support before, during, and after the procedure.
- Explain that an intravenous (IV) line may be inserted to allow infusion of fluids such as saline, anesthetics, sedatives, or emergency medications.
- Inform the patient that a laxative and cleansing enema may be needed the day before the procedure, with cleansing enemas on the morning of the procedure, depending on the institution's policy.
- Inform the patient that dentures and eyewear will be removed before the test.
- Instruct the patient to remove jewelry and other metallic objects from the area to be examined.
- Instruct the patient to fast and restrict fluids for 6 hr prior to the procedure to reduce the risk of aspiration related to nausea and vomiting. The American Society of Anesthesiologists has fasting guidelines for risk levels according to patient status. More information can be located at www.asahq.org. 🍁 Protocols may vary among facilities.
- *Make sure a written and informed consent has been signed prior to the procedure and before administering any medications.*

INTRATEST:

Potential Complications:

May include bleeding and cardiac dysrhythmias.

- Ensure the patient has complied with dietary and medication restrictions and pretesting preparations prior to the study, as instructed.
- Ensure the patient has removed all external metallic objects from the

area to be examined prior to the procedure.

- Assess for completion of bowel preparation according to the institution's procedure.
- Avoid the use of equipment containing latex if the patient has a history of allergic reaction to latex.
- Have emergency equipment readily available.
- Instruct the patient to void prior to the procedure and to change into the gown, robe, and foot coverings provided.
- Instruct the patient to cooperate fully and to follow directions. Instruct the patient to remain still throughout the procedure because movement produces unreliable results.
- Observe standard precautions, and follow the general guidelines in Patient Preparation and Specimen Collection online at Davis*Plus*. Positively identify the patient, and label the appropriate specimen container with the corresponding patient demographics, initials of the person collecting the specimen, date, and time of collection.
- Obtain and record baseline vital signs.
- Establish an IV fluid line for the injection of saline, sedatives, or emergency medications. Administer ordered sedation.
- Spray or swab the oropharynx with a topical local anesthetic.
- Provide an emesis basin for the increased saliva and encourage the patient to spit out the saliva because the gag reflex may be impaired.
- Place the patient on an examination table in the left lateral decubitus position with the neck slightly flexed forward.
- The endoscope is passed through the mouth with a dental suction device in place to drain secretions. A side-viewing flexible, fiberoptic endoscope is advanced, and visualization of the GI tract is started.
- Air is insufflated to distend the upper GI tract, as needed. Biopsy specimens are obtained and/or endoscopic surgery is performed.
- Promptly transport the specimens to the laboratory for processing and analysis.
- At the end of the procedure, excess air and secretions are aspirated through the scope and the endoscope is removed.
- The needle or catheter is removed, and a pressure dressing is applied over the puncture site.
- Observe/assess the needle/catheter insertion site for bleeding, inflammation, or hematoma formation.

POST-TEST:

- Inform the patient that a report of the results will be made available to the requesting HCP, who will discuss the results with the patient.
- Observe the patient for indications of esophageal perforation (i.e., painful swallowing with neck movement, substernal pain with respiration, shoulder pain or dyspnea, abdominal or back pain, cyanosis, or fever).
- Do not allow the patient to eat or drink until the gag reflex returns; then allow the patient to eat lightly for 12 to 24 hr.
- Monitor vital signs and neurological status every 15 min for 1 hr, then every 2 hr for 4 hr, and as ordered by the HCP. Take temperature every 4 hr for 24 hr. Monitor intake and output at least every 8 hr. Compare with baseline values. Notify the HCP if temperature is elevated. Protocols may vary among facilities.
- Instruct the patient to resume usual activity and diet in 24 hr or as tolerated after the examination, as directed by the HCP.
- Observe/assess the needle/catheter insertion site for bleeding, inflammation, or hematoma formation.
- Instruct the patient in the care and assessment of the injection site.
- Inform the patient that he or she may experience some throat soreness and hoarseness. Instruct patient to treat throat discomfort with lozenges and warm gargles when the gag reflex returns.

- Inform the patient that any belching, bloating, or flatulence is the result of air insufflation and is temporary.
- Instruct the patient to report any severe pain, fever, difficulty breathing, or expectoration of blood. Immediately report symptoms to the appropriate HCP.
- Recognize anxiety related to test results, and offer support. Discuss the implications of abnormal test results on the patient's lifestyle. Provide teaching and information regarding the clinical implications of the test results, as appropriate.
- Reinforce information given by the patient's HCP regarding further testing, treatment, or referral to another HCP. Answer any questions or address any concerns voiced by the patient or family.
- Depending on the results of this procedure, additional testing may be needed to evaluate or monitor progression of the disease process and determine the need for a change in therapy. Evaluate test results in relation to the patient's symptoms and other tests performed.

Patient Education:
- Teach the patient and family how to correctly evaluate the amount of food eaten.
- Teach the patient and family nonpharmacological pain options to relieve discomfort (diversion, imagery, relaxation, music).

Expected Patient Outcomes:

Understanding
- The patient and family verbalize that caffeinated drinks can increase gastric acid production in increase distress.
- The patient and family verbalize the pathophysiology related to the specific disease process.

Ability
- The patient identifies and avoids foods that cause gastric upset.
- The patient and family make lifestyle changes that will support health and wellness.

Response
- The patient agrees to avoid caffeinated drinks as a beverage choice.
- The patient agrees to avoid excessive alcohol use.

RELATED STUDIES:
- Related tests include barium enema, barium swallow, capsule endoscopy, colonoscopy, CT abdomen, esophageal manometry, fecal analysis, gastric acid emptying scan, gastric fluid analysis and gastric acid stimulation test, gastrin and gastrin stimulation test, GI blood loss scan, Helicobacter pylori, MRI abdomen, proctosigmoidoscopy, US pelvis, and upper GI series.
- Refer to the Gastrointestinal System table online at Davis*Plus* for related tests by body system.

Estradiol

SYNONYM/ACRONYM: E_2.

COMMON USE: To assist in diagnosing female fertility problems that may occur from tumor or ovarian failure.

SPECIMEN: Serum collected in a gold-, red-, or red/gray-top tube. Plasma collected in green-top (heparin) tube is also acceptable.

NORMAL FINDINGS: (Method: Immunoassay)

Age	Conventional Units	SI Units (Conventional Units × 3.67)
6 mo–10 yr		
Male and female	Less than 15 pg/mL	Less than 55 pmol/L
11–15 yr		
Male	Less than 40 pg/mL	Less than 147 pmol/L
Female	10–300 pg/mL	37–1,100 pmol/L
Adult male	10–50 pg/mL	37–184 pmol/L
Adult female		
Early follicular phase	20–150 pg/mL	73–551 pmol/L
Late follicular phase	40–350 pg/mL	147–1,285 pmol/L
Midcycle peak	150–750 pg/mL	551–2,753 pmol/L
Luteal phase	30–450 pg/mL	110–1,652 pmol/L
Postmenopause	Less than 20 pg/mL	Less than 73 pmol/L

POTENTIAL MEDICAL DIAGNOSIS

Increased in:

- Adrenal tumors ***(related to overproduction by tumor cells)***
- Estrogen-producing tumors
- Feminization in children ***(related to increased production)***
- Gynecomastia ***(newborns may demonstrate swelling of breast tissue in response to maternal estrogens; somewhat common and transient in pubescent males)***
- Hepatic cirrhosis ***(accumulation occurs due to lack of liver function)***
- Hyperthyroidism ***(related to primary increases in estrogen or response to increased levels of sex hormone–binding globulin)***

Decreased in:

- Ovarian failure ***(resulting in lack of estrogen synthesis)***
- Primary and secondary hypogonadism ***(related to lack of estrogen synthesis)***
- Turner's syndrome ***(genetic abnormality in females in which there is only one X chromosome, resulting in varying degrees of underdeveloped sexual characteristics)***

CRITICAL FINDINGS: N/A

Find and print out the full study on Fast Find at davispl.us/vanleeuwen7.

Evoked Brain Potentials

SYNONYM/ACRONYM: Brainstem auditory evoked potentials (BAEP), brainstem auditory evoked responses (BAER), EP studies.

COMMON USE: To assist in diagnosing sensory deficits related to nervous system lesions manifested by visual defects, hearing defects, neuropathies, and cognitive disorders.

AREA OF APPLICATION: Brain.

DESCRIPTION: Evoked brain potentials, also known as evoked potential (EP) responses, are electrophysiological studies performed to measure the brain's electrical responses to various visual, auditory, and somatosensory stimuli. EP studies help diagnose lesions of the nervous system by evaluating the integrity of the visual, somatosensory, and auditory nerve pathways. Three response types are measured: visual evoked response (VER), auditory brainstem response (ABR), and somatosensory evoked response (SER). The stimuli activate the nerve tracts that connect the stimulated (receptor) area with the cortical (visual and somatosensory) or midbrain (auditory) sensory area. A number of stimuli are given, and then responses are electronically displayed in waveforms, recorded, and computer analyzed. Abnormalities are determined by a delay in time, measured in milliseconds, between the stimulus and the response. This is known as ***increased latency.*** VER provides information about visual pathway function to identify lesions of the optic nerves, optic tracts, and demyelinating diseases such as multiple sclerosis. ABR provides information about auditory pathways to identify hearing loss and lesions of the brainstem. SER provides information about the somatosensory pathways to identify lesions at various levels of the central nervous system (spinal cord and brain) and peripheral nerve disease. EP studies are especially useful in patients with problems related to the nervous system and those unable to speak or respond to instructions during the test, because these studies do not require voluntary cooperation or participation in the activity. This allows collection of objective diagnostic information about visual or auditory disorders affecting infants and children and allows differentiation between organic brain and psychological disorders in adults. EP studies are also used to monitor the progression of or the effectiveness of treatment for deteriorating neurological diseases such as multiple sclerosis.

This procedure is contraindicated for: N/A

INDICATIONS

VER (potentials)

- Detect cryptic or past retrobulbar neuritis.
- Detect lesions of the eye or optic nerves.
- Detect neurological disorders such as multiple sclerosis, Parkinson's disease, and Huntington's chorea.
- Evaluate binocularity in infants.
- Evaluate optic pathway lesions and visual cortex defects.

ABR (potentials)

- Detect abnormalities or lesions in the brainstem or auditory nerve areas.
- Detect brainstem tumors and acoustic neuromas.
- Screen or evaluate neonates, infants, children, and adults for auditory problems.
- EP studies may be indicated when a child falls below growth chart norms.
- Evaluate patients in comatose states.

SER (potentials)

- Detect multiple sclerosis and Guillain-Barré syndrome.
- Detect sensorimotor neuropathies and cervical pathology.

- Evaluate spinal cord and brain injury and function.
- Monitor sensory potentials to determine spinal cord function during a surgical procedure or medical regimen.

ERP (potentials)

- Detect suspected psychosis or dementia.
- Differentiate between organic brain disorder and cognitive function abnormality.

E

POTENTIAL MEDICAL DIAGNOSIS

Normal findings

- ***VER and ABR:*** Normal latency in recorded cortical and brainstem waveforms depending on age, gender, and stature
- ***ERP:*** Normal recognition and attention span
- ***SER:*** No loss of consciousness or presence of weakness

Abnormal findings related to

- VER (extended latencies):
  Absence of biocular vision
  Amblyopias
  Blindness
  Demyelinating diseases such as multiple sclerosis
  Huntington chorea
  Lesions or disease of the optic nerve and eye (e.g., anterior optic chiasm, neuritis)
  Lesions or disease of the optic tract
  Optic nerve neuritis
  Parkinson disease
  Visual field defects
- ABR (extended latencies):
  Acoustic neuroma
  Auditory nerve or brain stem damage or disease
  Cerebrovascular accidents
  Demyelinating diseases such as multiple sclerosis
- SER (extended latencies):
  Abnormal upper limb latencies suggest cervical spondylosis or intracerebral lesions.
  Abnormal lower limb latencies suggest peripheral nerve root disease such as Guillain-Barré syndrome, multiple sclerosis, transverse myelitis, or traumatic spinal cord injuries.

CRITICAL FINDINGS: N/A

INTERFERING FACTORS

Factors that may impair the results of the examination

- Inability of the patient to cooperate or remain still during the procedure because of age, significant pain, or mental status. (*Note:* Significant behavioral problems may limit the ability to complete the test.)
- Improper placement of electrodes.
- Patient stress, which can affect brain chemistry, thus making it difficult to distinguish whether the results are due to the patient's emotional reaction or to organic pathology.
- Extremely poor visual acuity, which can hinder accurate determination of VER.
- Severe hearing loss, which can interfere with accurate determination of ABR.

NURSING IMPLICATIONS AND PROCEDURE

PRETEST:

- Positively identify the patient using at least two person-specific identifiers before services, treatments, or procedures are performed.
- ***Patient Teaching:*** Inform the patient this procedure measures electrical activity in the nervous system.
- Obtain a history of the patient's health concerns, symptoms, surgical procedures, and results of previously performed laboratory and diagnostic studies. Include a list of known allergens, especially allergies or sensitivities to latex.
- Obtain a list of the patient's current medications, including

over-the-counter medications and dietary supplements (see Effects of Natural Products on Laboratory Values online at Davis*Plus*).

- Review the procedure with the patient. Address concerns about pain related to the procedure and explain that the procedure is painless and harmless. Inform the patient that the procedure is performed in a special laboratory by a health-care provider (HCP) and takes approximately 30 min to 2 hr, depending on the type of studies required.
- ***Sensitivity to social and cultural issues,*** as well as concern for modesty, is important in providing psychological support before, during, and after the procedure.
- Instruct the patient to clean the hair and to refrain from using hair sprays, creams, or solutions before the test.
- Instruct the patient to remove jewelry and other metallic objects from the area to be examined.
- Note that there are no food, fluid, or medication restrictions unless by medical direction.
- *Make sure a written and informed consent has been signed prior to the procedure and before administering any medications.*

INTRATEST:

Potential Complications: N/A

- Observe standard precautions, and follow the general guidelines in Patient Preparation and Specimen Collection online at Davis*Plus*. Positively identify the patient.
- Ensure the patient is able to relax; report any extreme anxiety or restlessness.
- Ensure that hair is clean and free of hair sprays, creams, or solutions.
- Ensure the patient has removed all external metallic objects from the area to be examined prior to the procedure.
- Avoid the use of equipment containing latex if the patient has a history of allergic reaction to latex.

Visual Evoked Potentials

- Place the patient in a comfortable position about 1 m from the stimulation source. Attach electrodes to the occipital and vertex lobe areas and a reference electrode to the ear. Placement of electrodes for VER generally follows the International 10/20 system. A light-emitting stimulation or a checkerboard pattern is projected on a screen at a regulated speed. This procedure is done for each eye (with the opposite eye covered) as the patient looks at a dot on the screen without any change in the gaze while the stimuli are delivered. A computer interprets the brain's responses to the stimuli and records them in waveforms.

Auditory Evoked Potentials

- Place the patient in a comfortable position, and place the electrodes on the scalp at the vertex lobe area and on each earlobe. Earphones are placed on the patient's ears, and a clicking noise stimulus is delivered into one ear while a continuous tone is delivered to the opposite ear. Responses to the stimuli are recorded as waveforms for analysis.

Somatosensory Evoked Potentials

- Place the patient in a comfortable position, and place the electrodes at the nerve sites of the wrist, knee, and ankle and on the scalp at the sensory cortex of the hemisphere on the opposite side (the electrode that picks up the response and delivers it to the recorder). Additional electrodes can be positioned at the cervical or lumbar vertebrae for upper or lower limb stimulation. The rate at which the electric shock stimulus is delivered to the nerve electrodes and travels to the brain is measured, computer analyzed, and recorded in waveforms for analysis. Both sides of the area being examined can be tested by switching the electrodes and repeating the procedure.

Event-Related Potentials

- Place the patient in a sitting position in a chair in a quiet room. Earphones are placed on the patient's ears and auditory cues administered. The patient is asked to push a button when the tones are recognized. Flashes of light are also used as visual cues, with the patient pushing a button when cues are noted. Results are compared to normal EP waveforms for correct, incorrect, or absent responses.

POST-TEST:

- Inform the patient that a report of the results will be made available to the requesting HCP, who will discuss the results with the patient.
- When the procedure is complete, remove the electrodes and clean the skin where the electrodes were applied.
- Recognize anxiety related to test results, and be supportive of perceived loss of independent function. Discuss the implications of abnormal test results on the patient's lifestyle. Provide teaching and information regarding the clinical implications of the test results, as appropriate. Provide contact information, if desired, for the National Multiple Sclerosis Society (www.nationalmssociety.org). 🍁
- Reinforce information given by the patient's HCP regarding further testing, treatment, or referral to another HCP. Answer any questions or address any concerns voiced by the patient or family.
- Depending on the results of this procedure, additional testing may be needed to evaluate or monitor progression of the disease process and determine the need for a change in therapy. Evaluate test results in relation to the patient's symptoms and other tests performed.

RELATED STUDIES:

- Related tests include acetylcholine receptor antibody, Alzheimer's disease markers, biopsy muscle, CSF analysis, CT brain, CK, EEG, electroneurography, MRI brain, plethysmography, and PET brain.
- Refer to the Musculoskeletal System table online at Davis*Plus* for related tests by body system.

Exercise Stress Test

SYNONYM/ACRONYM: Exercise electrocardiogram, ECG, EKG, graded exercise tolerance test, cardiac stress testing, stress testing, treadmill test.

COMMON USE: To assess cardiac function in relation to increased workload, evidenced by dysrhythmia or pain during exercise.

AREA OF APPLICATION: Heart.

DESCRIPTION: The exercise stress test is a noninvasive study to measure cardiac function during physical stress. Exercise electrocardiography is primarily useful in determining the extent of coronary artery occlusion by the heart's ability to meet the need for additional oxygen in response to the stress of exercising in a safe environment. The patient exercises on a treadmill or pedals a stationary bicycle to increase the heart rate to 80% to 90% of maximal heart rate determined by age and gender, known as the *target heart rate*. Every 2 to 3 min, the speed and/or grade of the treadmill is increased to yield an increment of stress. The patient's electrocardiogram (ECG) and blood pressure are monitored during the test. The test proceeds until the patient reaches the target heart rate or experiences chest pain or fatigue. The risks involved in the procedure are possible myocardial infarction (1 in 500) and death (1 in 10,000) in patients experiencing frequent angina episodes before the test. Although useful, this procedure is not as accurate as cardiac nuclear scans for diagnosing coronary artery disease (CAD).

For patients unable to complete the test, pharmacological stress testing can be done. Medications used to pharmacologically exercise the patient's heart include vasodilators such as dipyridamole and adenosine or dobutamine (which stimulates heart rate and pumping force). Stress testing should be discontinued when maximal performance has been reached or if certain criteria occur as noted in the Contraindications section. The patient's ECG and blood pressure are monitored during the exercise phase. The test proceeds until the stimulated exercise portion is completed when a radiotracer, such as technetium-99m or sestamibi, is injected and images are taken by a gamma camera during the stimulated portion to compare with images taken at rest.

This procedure is contraindicated for

A variety of circumstances that may be considered absolute or relative depending on the facility's providers:

- Abnormal EKG changes causing symptoms ***related to the possibility of stress-induced infarction.***
- Acute myocardial infarction (within 2 days) ***related to the possibility of stress-induced reinfarction.***
- Acute myocarditis ***related to low stress tolerance.***
- Aortic dissection ***related to the possibility of stress-induced tears and rupture.***
- Chest pain ***related to the possibility of stress-induced infarction.***
- Heart failure with symptoms (e.g., shortness of breath) ***related to low stress tolerance.***
- Mental or physical (e.g., severe leg claudication) impairment that prevents the patient from performing the required exercise.
- Significant hypertension or hypotension.
- Stenotic valvular disease with symptoms ***related to low stress tolerance from having the heart work harder to pump blood through the narrow valve.***
- Very fast (tachydysrhythmia) or very slow (bradydysrhythmia) heart rate.

INDICATIONS

- Detect dysrhythmias during exercising, as evidenced by ECG changes.
- Detect peripheral arterial disease (PAD), as evidenced by leg pain or cramping during exercising.
- Determine exercise-induced hypertension.
- Evaluate cardiac function after myocardial infarction or cardiac surgery to determine safe exercise levels for cardiac rehabilitation as well as work limitations.
- Evaluate effectiveness of medication regimens, such as antianginals or antidysrhythmics.
- Evaluate suspected CAD in the presence of chest pain and other symptoms.
- Screen for CAD in the absence of pain and other symptoms in patients at risk.

POTENTIAL MEDICAL DIAGNOSIS

Normal findings

- Normal heart rate during physical exercise. Heart rate and systolic blood pressure rise in direct proportion to workload and to metabolic oxygen demand, which is based on age and exercise protocol. Maximal heart rate for adults is estimated by subtracting the age in years from 220 (e.g., estimated maximal heart rate for a 45-year-old adult is 220–45 or 170 beats/min.

Abnormal findings related to

- Activity intolerance related to oxygen supply and demand imbalance
- Bradycardia
- CAD
- Chest pain related to ischemia or inflammation
- Decreased cardiac output
- Dysrhythmias
- Hypertension
- PAD
- ST segment depression of 1 mm (considered a positive test), indicating myocardial ischemia
- Tachycardia

CRITICAL FINDINGS: N/A

INTERFERING FACTORS

The following factors may impair interpretation of examination results because they create an artificial state that makes it difficult to determine true physiological function:

- Anxiety or panic attack.
- Drugs such as beta blockers, cardiac glycosides, calcium channel blockers, coronary vasodilators, and barbiturates.
- High food intake or smoking before testing.
- Hypertension, hypoxia, left bundle branch block, and ventricular hypertrophy.
- Improper electrode placement.
- Potassium or calcium imbalance.
- Viagra should not be taken in combination with nitroglycerin or other nitrates 24 hr prior to the procedure because it may result in a dangerously low blood pressure.
- Wolff-Parkinson-White syndrome (anomalous atrioventricular excitation).

NURSING IMPLICATIONS AND PROCEDURE

See Potential Nursing Problems on Fast Find at davispl.us/vanleeuwen7.

PRETEST:

- Positively identify the patient using at least two person-specific identifiers before services, treatments, or procedures are performed.
- ***Patient Teaching:*** Inform the patient this procedure can assist in assessing the heart's ability to respond to an increasing workload.
- Obtain a history of the patient's health concerns, symptoms, surgical procedures, and results of previously performed laboratory and diagnostic studies. Include a list of known allergens, especially allergies or sensitivities to latex.
- Inquire if the patient has had any chest pain within the past 48 hr or has a history of anginal attacks; if either of these has occurred, inform the health-care provider (HCP) immediately because the stress test may be too risky and should be rescheduled in 4 to 6 wk.
- Obtain a list of the patient's current medications, including over-the-counter medications and dietary supplements (see Effects of Natural Products on Laboratory Values online at Davis*Plus*).
- Review the procedure with the patient. Address concerns about pain related to the procedure and explain that some discomfort may be experienced during the stimulated portion of the test. Inform the patient that the procedure is performed in a special department by an HCP specializing in this procedure and takes approximately 30 to 60 min.

- *Sensitivity to social and cultural issues,* as well as concern for modesty, is important in providing psychological support before, during, and after the procedure.
- Record a baseline 12-lead ECG and vital signs.
- Instruct the patient to wear comfortable shoes and clothing for the exercise.
- Instruct the patient to fast, restrict fluids, and avoid tobacco products for 4 to 6 hr prior to the procedure. Protocols may vary among facilities.
- *Make sure a written and informed consent has been signed prior to the procedure and before administering any medications.*

INTRATEST:

Potential Complications:

Myocardial infarction (MI)

- Observe standard precautions, and follow the general guidelines in Patient Preparation and Specimen Collection online at Davis*Plus*. Positively identify the patient.
- Ensure the patient has complied with dietary and tobacco restrictions prior to the study, as instructed.
- An intravenous access may be established for emergency use.
- Avoid the use of equipment containing latex if the patient has a history of allergic reaction to latex.
- Have emergency equipment readily available.
- Instruct the patient to void prior to the procedure and to change into the gown provided.
- Place electrodes in appropriate positions on the patient and connect a blood pressure cuff to a monitoring device. If the patient's oxygen consumption is to be continuously monitored, connect the patient to a machine via a mouthpiece or to a pulse oximeter via a finger lead.
- Instruct the patient to walk on a treadmill (most commonly used) and use the handrails to maintain balance or to peddle a bicycle. As stress is increased, inform the patient to report any symptoms, such as chest or leg pain, difficulty breathing, or fatigue.
- Turn the treadmill on at a slow speed, and increase in speed and elevation to raise the patient's heart rate. Increase the stress until the patient's predicted target heart rate is reached.
- Instruct the patient to report symptoms such as dizziness, sweating, breathlessness, or nausea, which can be normal, as speed increases. The test is terminated if pain or fatigue is severe; maximum heart rate under stress is attained; signs of ischemia are present; maximum effort has been achieved; or dyspnea, hypertension (systolic blood pressure greater than 200 mm Hg, diastolic blood pressure greater than 110 mm Hg, or both), tachycardia (greater than 200 beats/min minus person's age), new dysrhythmias, chest pain that begins or worsens, faintness, extreme dizziness, or confusion develops.
- After the exercise period, allow a 3- to 15-min rest period with the patient in a sitting position. During this period, the ECG, blood pressure, and heart rate monitoring is continued.
- Remove the electrodes and cleanse the skin of any remaining gel or ECG electrode adhesive.

POST-TEST:

- Inform the patient that a report of the results will be made available to the requesting HCP, who will discuss the results with the patient.
- Instruct the patient to resume usual activity, as directed by the HCP.
- Instruct the patient to contact the HCP to report any anginal pain or other discomforts experienced after the test.
- ***Nutritional Considerations:*** Abnormal findings may be associated with cardiovascular disease. Nutritional therapy is recommended for the patient identified to be at risk for developing CAD or for individuals who have specific risk factors and/or existing medical conditions (e.g., elevated LDL cholesterol levels, other lipid disorders, type 1 diabetes, type 2 diabetes, insulin resistance, or metabolic syndrome). Other

E

changeable risk factors warranting patient education include strategies to encourage patients, especially those who are overweight and with high blood pressure, to safely decrease sodium intake, achieve a normal weight, ensure regular participation of moderate aerobic physical activity three to four times per week, eliminate tobacco use, and adhere to a heart-healthy diet. If triglycerides also are elevated, the patient should be advised to eliminate or reduce alcohol. A variety of dietary patterns are beneficial for people with CAD, and there are many meal-planning approaches with nutritional goals endorsed by the American Diabetes Association (ADA). The Guideline on Lifestyle Management to Reduce Cardiovascular Risk published by the American College of Cardiology and the American Heart Association (AHA) in conjunction with the National Heart, Lung, and Blood Institute (NHLBI) recommends a Mediterranean-style diet rather than a low-fat diet. The guideline emphasizes inclusion of vegetables, whole grains, fruits, low-fat dairy, nuts, legumes, and nontropical vegetable oils (e.g., olive, canola, peanut, sunflower, flaxseed) along with fish and lean poultry. 🍁 A similar dietary pattern known as the Dietary Approaches to Stop Hypertension (DASH) diet makes additional recommendations for the reduction of dietary sodium. Both dietary styles emphasize a reduction in consumption of red meats, which are high in saturated fats and cholesterol, and other foods containing sugar, saturated fats, trans fats, and sodium. The ADA also includes a vegetarian diet as well as other potential weight loss diets such as Weight Watchers. 🍁 The nutritional needs of each patient need to be determined individually (especially during pregnancy) with the appropriate HCPs, particularly professionals educated in nutrition.

- ***Sensitivity to social and cultural issues:*** Numerous studies point to the prevalence of excess body weight in American children and adolescents. Experts estimate that obesity is present in 25% of the population aged 6 to 11 yr. The medical, social, and emotional consequences of excess body weight are significant. Special attention should be given to instructing the pediatric patient and caregiver regarding health risks and weight control education. 🍁
- Recognize anxiety related to test results, and be supportive of fear of shortened life expectancy. Discuss the implications of abnormal test results on the patient's lifestyle. Provide teaching and information regarding the clinical implications of the test results, as appropriate. Educate the patient regarding access to counseling services. Provide contact information, if desired, for the AHA (www.americanheart.org), NHLBI (www.nhlbi.nih.gov), Institute of Medicine of the National Academies (www.iom.edu), or USDA's resource for nutrition (www.choosemyplate.gov). 🍁 Reinforce information given by the patient's HCP regarding further testing, treatment, or referral to another HCP. Answer any questions or address any concerns voiced by the patient or family.
- Depending on the results of this procedure, additional testing may be performed to evaluate or monitor progression of the disease process and determine the need for a change in therapy. Evaluate test results in relation to the patient's symptoms and other tests performed.

Patient Education:

- Teach the patient how to pace activities to better manage oxygen demand and improve gas exchange.
- Provide information on the pathophysiology of cardiac disease and physical limitations that are appropriate to the disease process.

Expected Patient Outcomes:

Understanding

- The patient verbalizes that sexual relations may need to be limited during healing of a cardiac injury.
- The patient and family verbalize that assistance may be required at home until regular activity can be restored.

Ability

- The patient reports chest pain as soon as it occurs to receive prompt medical attention.
- The patient and family bundle activities to place the least amount of stress on the heart.

Response

- The patient agrees to attend cardiac rehabilitation support as recommended by the HCP.
- The patient and family agree to make lifestyle changes that will improve cardiac health.

RELATED STUDIES:

- Related tests include antidysrhythmic drugs, apolipoprotein A and B, atrial natriuretic peptide, BNP, blood gases, blood pool imaging, calcium, chest x-ray, cholesterol (total, HDL, LDL), CT cardiac scoring, CT thorax, CRP, CK and isoenzymes, echocardiography, echocardiography transesophageal, electrocardiogram, glucose, glycated hemoglobin, Holter monitor, homocysteine, ketones, LDH and isos, lipoprotein electrophoresis, lung perfusion scan, magnesium, MRI chest, MI infarct scan, myocardial perfusion heart scan, myoglobin, PET heart, potassium, pulse oximetry, sodium, triglycerides, and troponin.
- Refer to the Cardiovascular System table online at Davis*Plus* for related tests by body system.

E

Fecal Analysis

SYNONYM/ACRONYM: N/A

COMMON USE: To assess for the presence of blood in the stool toward diagnosing gastrointestinal bleeding, cancer, inflammation, and infection.

SPECIMEN: Stool.

NORMAL FINDINGS: (Method: Macroscopic examination, for appearance and color; microscopic examination, for cell count and presence of meat fibers; leukocyte esterase, for leukocytes; Bendict's solution (copper sulfate) for reducing substances; guaiac, for occult blood; x-ray paper, for trypsin.)

Characteristic	Normal Result
Appearance	Solid and formed
Color	Brown
Epithelial cells	Few to moderate
Fecal fat	See "Fecal Fat" study
Leukocytes (white blood cells)	Negative
Meat fibers	Negative
Occult blood	Negative
Reducing substances	Negative
Trypsin	2+ to 4+

F

DESCRIPTION: Feces consist mainly of cellulose and other undigested foodstuffs, bacteria, and water. Other substances normally found in feces include epithelial cells shed from the gastrointestinal (GI) tract, small amounts of fats, bile pigments in the form of urobilinogen, GI and pancreatic secretions, electrolytes, and trypsin. Trypsin is a proteolytic enzyme produced in the pancreas. The average adult excretes 100 to 300 g of fecal material per day, the residue of approximately 10 L of liquid material that enters the GI tract each day. The laboratory analysis of feces includes macroscopic examination (volume, odor, shape, color, consistency, presence of mucus), microscopic examination (leukocytes, epithelial cells, meat fibers), and chemical tests for specific substances (occult blood, trypsin, estimation of carbohydrate). Detection of occult blood is the most common test performed on stool. The prevalence of colorectal adenoma is greater than 30% in people aged 60 and older. Progression from adenoma to carcinoma occurs over a period of 5 to 12 yr; from carcinoma to metastatic disease in 2 to 3 yr.

This procedure is contraindicated for: N/A

INDICATIONS

- Assist in diagnosing disorders associated with GI bleeding or drug therapy that leads to bleeding.
- Assist in the diagnosis of pseudomembranous enterocolitis after use of broad-spectrum antibiotic therapy.

- Assist in the diagnosis of suspected inflammatory bowel disorder.
- Detect altered protein digestion.
- Detect intestinal parasitic infestation, as indicated by diarrhea of unknown cause.
- Investigate diarrhea of unknown cause.
- Monitor effectiveness of therapy for intestinal malabsorption or pancreatic insufficiency.
- Screen for colorectal cancer.
- Screen for cystic fibrosis.

POTENTIAL MEDICAL DIAGNOSIS

Unusual Appearance

- Bloody: ***Excessive intestinal wall irritation or malignancy***
- Bulky or frothy: ***Malabsorption***
- Mucous: ***Inflammation of intestinal walls***
- Slender or ribbonlike: ***Obstruction***

Unusual Color

- Black: ***Bismuth (antacid) or charcoal ingestion, iron therapy, upper GI bleeding***
- Grayish white: ***Barium ingestion, bile duct obstruction***
- Green: ***Antibiotics, biliverdin, green vegetables***
- Red: ***Beets and food coloring, lower GI bleed, phenazopyridine hydrochloride compounds, rifampin***
- Yellow: ***Rhubarb***

Increased

- Blood ***related to bleeding in the digestive tract***
- Carbohydrates/reducing substances: ***Malabsorption syndromes, inability to digest some sugars***
- Epithelial cells: ***Inflammatory bowel disorders***
- Fat ***pancreatitis, sprue (celiac disease), cystic fibrosis related to malabsorption***
- Leukocytes: ***inflammation of the intestines related to bacterial infections of the intestinal wall, salmonellosis, shigellosis, or ulcerative colitis***
- Meat fibers: ***Altered protein digestion, pancreatitis***
- Occult blood: ***Anal fissure, diverticular disease, esophageal varices, esophagitis, gastritis, hemorrhoids, infectious diarrhea, inflammatory bowel disease, Mallory-Weiss tears, polyps, tumors, ulcers*** pH: ***related to inflammation in the intestine from colitis, cancer, or antibiotic use***

Decreased

- Carbohydrates/reducing substances ***sprue, cystic fibrosis, malnutrition, medications such as colchicine (gout) or birth control pills***
- Leukocytes: ***Amebic colitis, cholera, disorders resulting from toxins, parasites, viral diarrhea***
- pH: ***Related to poor absorption of carbohydrate or fat***
- Trypsin: ***Cystic fibrosis, malabsorption syndromes, pancreatic deficiency***

CRITICAL FINDINGS: N/A

INTERFERING FACTORS

- Drugs that can cause positive results for occult blood include acetylsalicylic acid, anticoagulants, colchicine, corticosteroids, iron preparations, and phenylbutazone.
- Ingestion of a diet high in red meat, certain vegetables, and bananas can cause false-positive results for occult blood.
- Large doses of vitamin C can cause false-negative occult blood.
- Constipated stools may not indicate any trypsin activity owing to extended exposure to intestinal bacteria.

F

NURSING IMPLICATIONS AND PROCEDURE

POTENTIAL NURSING PROBLEMS:

Problem	Signs & Symptoms	Interventions
Bleeding ***(related to bowel inflammation; irritation; infection; chronic disease)***	Altered level of consciousness; hypotension; increased heart rate; decreased hemoglobin (Hgb) and hematocrit (Hct); capillary refill greater than 3 sec; cool extremities	Monitor and trend Hgb/Hct, platelet count; increase frequency of vital sign assessment with variances in results; monitor for vital sign trends; administer blood or blood products as ordered; assess diet for iron-rich foods, and foods with vitamin K; discuss the importance of reporting black or tarry stools that are indicative of GI bleeding; assess for cultural or religious barriers to blood transfusion
Pain ***(related to infection; inflammation; contractions of diseased bowel)***	Colicky intermittent abdominal pain; bloating; cramping; distention; self-report of pain; abdominal tenderness; hyperactive bowel sounds; increased pain and cramping with eating	Assess the degree in cramping, colicky abdominal pain, and bloating with eating; auscultate bowel sounds; evaluate tolerance of dairy products in the diet; identify successful pain management strategies that have been used in the past; administer prescribed medications (sulfasalazine, corticosteriods, immunosuppressants, immunomodulators, anticholinergics, antidiarrheal); recommend diversional activities as a pain management modality; collaborate to make necessary dietary alterations that will decrease bowel irritation
Nutrition ***(related to inadequate absorption; decreased caloric intake; nausea; diarrhea with nitrogen loss)***	Decreased weight; poor wound healing; pedal edema; decreased calcium, potassium, vitamins, zinc, folic acid; skin lesions; muscle wasting	Monitor and trend serum calcium, potassium, vitamin K and B_{12}, zinc, and folic acid; take an accurate actual weight daily (not verbally reported or estimated); assess for skin lesions; assess current dietary habits and caloric intake; arrange dietary consult and collaboration to

Problem	Signs & Symptoms	Interventions
		develop an appropriate diet; administer ordered vitamin supplements; discuss the possibility of using total parenteral nutrition if oral intake is not sufficient
Fluid volume ***(related to nausea; vomiting; diarrhea)***	Hypotension; decreased cardiac output; decreased urinary output; dry skin/mucous membranes; poor skin turgor; sunken eyeballs; increased urine specific gravity; hemoconcentration	Assess current hydration status, skin turgor, check for the presence of dry mucous membranes, assess for decreased urine output, dark urine, hypotension; check stools for occult blood; assess for tarry or black stools (indicative of bleeding); administer intravenous fluids, blood and blood products as ordered; encourage oral intake

F

PRETEST:

- Positively identify the patient using at least two person-specific identifiers before services, treatments, or procedures are performed.
- ***Patient Teaching:*** Inform the patient this test can assist in the diagnosis of intestinal disorders.
- Obtain a history of the patient's health concerns, symptoms, surgical procedures, and results of previously performed laboratory and diagnostic studies. Include a list of known allergens, especially allergies or sensitivities to latex.
- Obtain a list of the patient's current medications, including over-the-counter medications and dietary supplements (see Effects of Natural Products on Laboratory Values online at Davis*Plus*).
- Review the procedure with the patient. Inform the patient of the procedure for collecting a stool sample, including the importance of good hand-washing techniques. The patient should place the sample in a tightly covered container. Instruct the patient not to contaminate the specimen with urine, water, or toilet tissue. Address concerns about pain and explain that there should be no discomfort during the procedure.
- ***Sensitivity to social and cultural issues,*** as well as concern for modesty, is important in providing psychological support before, during, and after the procedure.
- Instruct the patient not to use laxatives, enemas, or suppositories for 3 days before the test.
- Instruct the patient to follow a normal diet. If the test is being performed to identify blood, instruct the patient to follow a special diet that includes small amounts of chicken, turkey, and tuna (no red meats), raw and cooked vegetables and fruits, and bran cereal for several days before the test. Foods to avoid with the special diet include beets, turnips, cauliflower, broccoli, bananas, parsnips, and cantaloupe, because these foods can interfere with the occult blood test.

INTRATEST:

Potential Complications: N/A

- Ensure that the patient has complied with dietary, medication, and other pretesting preparation prior to the study, as instructed.

- Instruct the patient to cooperate fully and to follow directions.
- Observe standard precautions, and follow the general guidelines in Patient Preparation and Specimen Collection online at Davis*Plus*. Positively identify the patient, and label the appropriate specimen container with the corresponding patient demographics, initials of the person collecting the specimen, date and time of collection, and suspected cause of enteritis; note any current or recent antibiotic therapy.
- Collect a stool specimen in a waterproof container with a tight-fitting lid; if the patient is not ambulatory, collect it in a clean, dry bedpan. Use a tongue blade to transfer the specimen to the container, and include any mucoid and bloody portions. Collect specimen from the first, middle, and last portion of the stool. The specimen should be refrigerated if it will not be transported to the laboratory within 4 hr after collection.
- To collect specimen by rectal swab, insert the swab past the anal sphincter, rotate gently, and withdraw. Place the swab in the appropriate container.
- Promptly transport the specimen to the laboratory for processing and analysis.

POST-TEST:

- Inform the patient that a report of the results will be made available to the requesting health-care provider (HCP), who will discuss the results with the patient.
- The American Cancer Society recommends regular screening for colon cancer, beginning at age 50 yr for individuals without identified risk factors; sooner for those with identified risk factors. Its recommendations for frequency of screening are as follows: annually for occult blood testing (fecal occult blood testing or fecal immunochemical testing); or every 5 yr for flexible sigmoidoscopy, double contrast barium enema, or computed tomography colonography; or every 10 yr for colonoscopy; or every 3 yr for stool DNA testing. 🍁 Abnormal findings should be followed up by colonoscopy. There are both advantages and disadvantages to the screening tests that are available today. Methods to use DNA testing of stool are being investigated and are designed to identify abnormal changes in DNA from the cells in the lining of the colon that are normally shed and excreted in stool. The DNA tests under development use multiple markers to identify colon cancers that demonstrate different, abnormal DNA changes. Unlike some of the current screening methods, the DNA tests would be able to detect precancerous polyps. The most current guidelines for colon cancer screening of the general population as well as of individuals with increased risk are available from the American Cancer Society (www.cancer.org), U.S. Preventive Services Task Force (www.uspreventiveservicestaskforce.org), and the American College of Gastroenterology (www.gi.org). 🍁 Answer any questions or address any concerns voiced by the patient or family.
- Depending on the results of this procedure, additional testing may be performed to evaluate or monitor progression of the disease process and determine the need for a change in therapy. Evaluate test results in relation to the patient's symptoms and other tests performed.

Patient Education:

- Recognize anxiety related to test results.
- Discuss the implications of abnormal test results on the patient's lifestyle.
- Provide teaching and information regarding the clinical implications of the test results, as appropriate.
- Reinforce information given by the patient's HCP regarding further testing, treatment, or referral to another HCP.

- Note that decisions regarding the need for and frequency of occult blood testing, colonoscopy, or other cancer screening procedures should be made after consultation.

Expected Patient Outcomes:

Understanding

- The patient and family state the importance of notifying the HCP of black or tarry stools.
- The patient and family state that untreated disease could result in colon cancer.

Ability

- The patient demonstrates proficiency in the self-administration of ordered vitamin supplements.
- The patient and family demonstrate the ability to select a diet that will support bowel health and decrease gastric irritation.

Response

- The patient complies with the request to adjust diet to decrease abdominal pain and improve caloric intake.
- The patient complies with the request to provide a stool specimen for analysis in a timely manner.

RELATED STUDIES:

- Related tests include α_1-antitrypsin/phenotyping, barium enema, biopsy intestine, capsule endoscopy, cancer antigens, chloride sweat, colonoscopy, CT colonoscopy, culture stool, D-xylose tolerance, fecal fat, genetic testing, gliadin antibody, lactose tolerance test, ova and parasites, and proctosigmoidoscopy.
- Refer to the Gastrointestinal System table online at Davis*Plus* for related tests by body system.

F

Fecal Fat

SYNONYM/ACRONYM: Stool fat, fecal fat stain.

COMMON USE: To assess for the presence of fat in the stool toward diagnosing malabsorption disorders such as Crohn's disease and cystic fibrosis.

SPECIMEN: Stool aliquot from an unpreserved and homogenized 24- to 72-hr timed collection. Random specimens may also be submitted.

NORMAL FINDINGS: (Method: Stain with Sudan black or oil red O. Treatment with ethanol identifies neutral fats; treatment with acetic acid identifies fatty acids.)

	Random, Semiquantitative
Neutral fat	Less than 60 fat globules/hpf*
Fatty acids	Less than 100 fat globules/hpf
	72-hr, Quantitative
Age (normal diet)	
Infant (breast milk)	Less than 1 g/24 hr
0–6 yr	Less than 2 g/24 hr
Adult	2–7 g/24 hr; less than 20% of total solids
Adult (fat-free diet)	Less than 4 g/24 hr

*hpf = high-power field.

POTENTIAL MEDICAL DIAGNOSIS

Increased in:

- Abetalipoprotein deficiency ***(related to lack of transport proteins for absorption)***
- Addison's disease ***(related to impaired transport)***
- Amyloidosis ***(increased rate of excretion related to malabsorption)***
- Bile salt deficiency ***(related to lack of bile salts required for proper fat digestion)***
- Carcinoid syndrome ***(increased rate of excretion related to malabsorption)***
- Celiac disease ***(increased rate of excretion related to malabsorption)***
- Crohn's disease ***(increased rate of excretion related to malabsorption)***
- Cystic fibrosis ***(related to insufficient digestive enzymes)***
- Diabetes ***(abnormal motility related to primary condition)***
- Enteritis ***(increased rate of excretion related to malabsorption)***
- Malnutrition ***(related to detrimental effects on organs and systems responsible for digestion, transport, and absorption)***
- Multiple sclerosis ***(abnormal motility related to primary condition)***
- Pancreatic insufficiency or obstruction ***(related to insufficient digestive enzymes)***
- Peptic ulcer disease ***(related to improper digestion due to low pH)***
- Pernicious anemia ***(related to bacterial overgrowth that decreases overall absorption and results in vitamin*** B_{12} ***deficiency)***
- Progressive systemic sclerosis ***(abnormal motility related to primary condition)***
- Thyrotoxicosis ***(abnormal motility related to primary condition)***
- Tropical sprue ***(increased rate of excretion related to malabsorption)***
- Viral hepatitis ***(related to insufficient production of digestive enzymes and bile)***
- Whipple's disease ***(increased rate of excretion related to malabsorption)***
- Zollinger-Ellison syndrome ***(related to improper digestion due to low pH)***

Decreased in: N/A

CRITICAL FINDINGS: N/A

Find and print out the full study on Fast Find at davispl.us/vanleeuwen7.

F

Ferritin

SYNONYM/ACRONYM: N/A

COMMON USE: To assist in diagnosing and monitoring various forms of anemia related to ferritin levels such as iron-deficiency anemia, anemia of malnourishment related to alcoholism, hemolytic anemia, chronic anemia of inflammation, and anemia related to long-term kidney dialysis.

SPECIMEN: Serum collected in a gold-, red-, or red/gray-top tube.

NORMAL FINDINGS: (Method: Immunoassay)

Age	Conventional Units	SI Units (Conventional Units × 1)
Newborn	25–200 ng/mL	25–200 mcg/L
1 mo	200–600 ng/mL	200–600 mcg/L
2–5 mo	50–200 ng/mL	50–200 mcg/L
6 mo–15 yr	7–140 ng/mL	7–140 mcg/L
Adult		
Males	20–250 ng/mL	20–250 mcg/L
Females (18–39 yr)	10–120 ng/mL	10–120 mcg/L
Females (40 yr and older)	12–263 ng/mL	12–263 mcg/L

DESCRIPTION: Ferritin, a protein manufactured in the liver, spleen, and bone marrow, consists of a protein shell, apoferritin, and an iron core. The amount of ferritin in the circulation is usually proportional to the amount of stored iron (ferritin and hemosiderin) in body tissues. Levels vary according to age and gender, but they are not affected by exogenous iron intake or subject to diurnal variations. Compared to iron and total iron-binding capacity, ferritin is a more sensitive and specific test for diagnosing iron-deficiency anemia. Iron-deficiency anemia in adults is indicated at ferritin levels less than 10 ng/mL (SI = 10 mcg/L); hemochromatosis or hemosiderosis is indicated at levels greater than 400 ng/mL (SI = 400 mcg/L).

This procedure is contraindicated for: N/A

INDICATIONS

- Assist in the diagnosis of iron-deficiency anemia.
- Assist in the differential diagnosis of microcytic, hypochromic anemias.
- Monitor hematological responses during pregnancy, when serum iron is usually decreased and ferritin may be decreased.
- Support diagnosis of hemochromatosis or other disorders of iron metabolism and storage.

POTENTIAL MEDICAL DIAGNOSIS

Increased in:

- Alcoholism ***(active misuse, as evidenced by release of ferritin into the circulation from damaged hepatocytes and red blood cells [RBCs])***
- Breast cancer ***(acute, related to release of ferritin as an acute-phase reactant protein; chronic, pathophysiology is uncertain)***
- Hemochromatosis ***(related to increased iron deposits in the liver, which stimulate ferritin production)***
- Hemolytic anemia ***(related to increased iron levels from hemolyzed RBCs, which stimulate ferritin production)***
- Hemosiderosis ***(related to increased iron levels, which stimulate ferritin production)***
- Hepatocellular disease ***(acute, related to release of ferritin as an acute-phase reactant protein; chronic, related to release of ferritin into the circulation from damaged hepatocytes)***
- Hodgkin's disease ***(acute, related to release of ferritin as an acute-phase reactant protein; chronic, pathophysiology is uncertain)***

- Hyperthyroidism ***(possibly related to the stimulating effect of thyroid-stimulating hormone on ferritin production)***
- Infection ***(acute, related to release of ferritin as an acute-phase reactant protein; chronic, pathophysiology is uncertain)***
- Inflammatory diseases ***(related to release of ferritin as an acute-phase reactant protein)***
- Leukemias ***(acute, related to release of ferritin as an acute-phase reactant protein; chronic, pathophysiology is uncertain)***
- Oral or parenteral administration of iron ***(evidenced by an increased circulating iron level, which stimulates ferritin production)***
- Thalassemia ***(related to increased iron levels from hemolyzed RBCs, which stimulate ferritin production)***

Decreased in:

Conditions that decrease iron stores result in corresponding low levels of ferritin.

- Hemodialysis
- Iron-deficiency anemia

CRITICAL FINDINGS: N/A

INTERFERING FACTORS

- Drugs and other substances that may increase ferritin levels include ethanol, ferric polymaltose, iron, and oral contraceptives.
- Drugs and other substances that may decrease ferritin levels include erythropoietin and methimazole.
- Recent transfusion can elevate serum ferritin.

NURSING IMPLICATIONS AND PROCEDURE

PRETEST:

- Positively identify the patient using at least two person-specific identifiers before services, treatments, or procedures are performed.
- *Patient Teaching:* Inform the patient this test can assist in the diagnosis of anemia.
- Obtain a history of the patient's health concerns, symptoms, surgical procedures, and results of previously performed laboratory and diagnostic studies. Include a list of known allergens, especially allergies or sensitivities to latex.
- Note any recent procedures that can interfere with test results.
- Obtain a list of the patient's current medications, including over-the-counter medications and dietary supplements (see Effects of Natural Products on Laboratory Values online at Davis*Plus*).
- Review the procedure with the patient. Inform the patient that specimen collection takes approximately 5 to 10 min. Address concerns about pain and explain that there may be some discomfort during the venipuncture.
- *Sensitivity to social and cultural issues,* as well as concern for modesty is important in providing psychological support before, during, and after the procedure.
- Note that there are no food, fluid, or medication restrictions unless by medical direction.

INTRATEST:

Potential Complications: N/A

- Avoid the use of equipment containing latex if the patient has a history of allergic reaction to latex.
- Instruct the patient to cooperate fully and to follow directions. Direct the patient to breathe normally and to avoid unnecessary movement.
- Observe standard precautions, and follow the general guidelines in Patient Preparation and Specimen Collection online at Davis*Plus*. Positively identify the patient, and label the appropriate specimen container with the corresponding patient demographics, initials of the person collecting the specimen, date, and time of collection. Perform a venipuncture.

- Remove the needle and apply direct pressure with dry gauze to stop bleeding. Observe/assess venipuncture site for bleeding or hematoma formation and secure gauze with adhesive bandage.
- Promptly transport the specimen to the laboratory for processing and analysis.

POST-TEST:

- Inform the patient that a report of the results will be made available to the requesting health-care provider (HCP), who will discuss the results with the patient.
- ***Nutritional Considerations:*** Nutritional therapy may be indicated for patients with decreased ferritin values because this may indicate corresponding iron deficiency. Instruct these patients in the dietary inclusion of iron-rich foods and in the administration of iron supplements, including adverse effects, as appropriate.
- Reinforce information given by the patient's HCP regarding further testing, treatment, or referral to another HCP. Answer any questions or address any concerns voiced by the patient or family.
- Depending on the results of this procedure, additional testing may be performed to evaluate or monitor progression of the disease process and determine the need for a change in therapy. Evaluate test results in relation to the patient's symptoms and other tests performed.

RELATED STUDIES:

- Related tests include biopsy bone marrow, biopsy liver, complement, CBC, CBC hematocrit, CBC hemoglobin, CBC platelet count, CBC RBC count, CBC RBC indices, CBC RBC morphology and inclusions, CBC WBC count and differential, Coomb's antiglobulin direct and indirect, erythropoietin, FEP, G6PD, Ham's test, Hgb electrophoresis, hemosiderin, iron/TIBC, osmotic fragility, PK, sickle cell screen, and transferrin.
- Refer to the Hematopoietic System table online at Davis*Plus* for related tests by body system.

F

Fetal Fibronectin

SYNONYM/ACRONYM: fFN.

COMMON USE: To assist in assessing for premature labor.

SPECIMEN: Swab of vaginal secretions.

NORMAL FINDINGS: (Method: Immunoassay) Negative (Less than 0.05 mcg/mL).

DESCRIPTION: Fibronectin is a protein found in fetal connective tissue, amniotic fluid, and the placenta of pregnant women. Placental fetal fibronectin (fFN) is concentrated in the area where the placenta and its membranes are in contact with the uterine wall. It is first secreted early in pregnancy and is believed to help implantation of the fertilized egg to the uterus. Fibronectin is not detectable again until just before delivery, at approximately 37 wk. If it is detected in vaginal secretions at 22 to 34 wk of gestation, delivery may happen prematurely. The test is a useful marker for impending membrane rupture within 7 to 14 days if the level rises to greater than 0.05 mcg/mL.

This procedure is contraindicated for: N/A

INDICATIONS

Investigate signs of premature labor.

POTENTIAL MEDICAL DIAGNOSIS

Positive findings in

- Premature labor ***(possibly initiated by mechanical or infectious processes, the membranes pull away from the uterine wall and amniotic fluid containing fFN leaks into endocervical fluid)***

F

CRITICAL FINDINGS: N/A

INTERFERING FACTORS

If signs and symptoms persist in light of negative test results, repeat testing may be necessary.

NURSING IMPLICATIONS AND PROCEDURE

PRETEST:

- Positively identify the patient using at least two person-specific identifiers before services, treatments, or procedures are performed.
- ***Patient Teaching:*** Inform the patient this test can assess for risk of preterm delivery.
- Obtain a history of the patient's health concerns, symptoms, surgical procedures, and results of previously performed laboratory and diagnostic studies. Include a list of known allergens, especially allergies or sensitivities to latex.
- Ensure that the patient knows the symptoms of premature labor, which include uterine contractions (with or without pain) lasting 20 sec or longer or increasing in frequency, menstrual-like cramping (intermittent or continuous), pelvic pressure, lower back pain that does not dissipate with a change in position, persistent diarrhea, intestinal cramps, changes in vaginal discharge, or a feeling that something is wrong.
- The health-care provider (HCP) should be informed if contractions occur more frequently than four times per hour.
- Obtain a list of the patient's current medications, including over-the-counter medications and dietary supplements (see Effects of Natural Products on Laboratory Values online at Davis*Plus*).
- Review the procedure with the patient. Inform the patient that specimen collection takes approximately 5 to 10 min and will be performed by an HCP specializing in this branch of medicine. Address concerns about pain related to the procedure. Explain to the patient that there should be minimal to no discomfort during the procedure.
- ***Sensitivity to social and cultural issues,*** as well as concern for modesty, is important in providing psychological support before, during, and after the procedure.
- Note that there are no food, fluid, or medication restrictions unless by medical direction.

INTRATEST:

Potential Complications: N/A

- Avoid the use of equipment containing latex if the patient has a history of allergic reaction to latex.
- Instruct the patient to cooperate fully and to follow directions. Direct the patient to breathe normally and to avoid unnecessary movement.
- Observe standard precautions, and follow the general guidelines in Patient Preparation and Specimen Collection online at Davis*Plus*. Positively identify the patient, and label the appropriate specimen container with the corresponding patient demographics, initials of the person collecting the specimen, date, and time of collection.
- Position the patient on the gynecological examination table with the feet up in stirrups. Drape the patient's legs to provide privacy and to reduce chilling. Collect a small amount of vaginal secretion using a special swab from a fetal fibronectin kit.
- Promptly transport the specimen to the laboratory for processing and analysis.

POST-TEST:

- Inform the patient that a report of the results will be made available to the requesting HCP, who will discuss the results with the patient.
- Recognize anxiety related to test results. Discuss the implications of abnormal test results on the patient's lifestyle. Provide teaching and information regarding the clinical implications of the test results, as appropriate. Educate the patient regarding access to counseling services.
- Reinforce information given by the patient's HCP regarding further testing, treatment, or referral to another HCP. Explain the possible causes and increased risks associated with premature labor and delivery. Reinforce education on signs and symptoms of labor, as appropriate. Inform the patient that hospitalization or more frequent prenatal checks may be ordered. Other therapies may also be administered, such as antibiotics, corticosteroids, and intravenous tocolytics. Instruct the patient in the importance of completing the entire course of antibiotic therapy, if ordered, even if no symptoms are present. Answer any questions or address any concerns voiced by the patient or family.
- Depending on the results of this procedure, additional testing may be performed to evaluate or monitor progression of the disease process and determine the need for a change in therapy. Evaluate test results in relation to the patient's symptoms and other tests performed.

RELATED STUDIES:

- Related tests include amniotic fluid analysis (nitrazine and fern test) and L/S ratio, biopsy chorionic villus, chromosome analysis, estradiol, α_1-fetoprotein, HCG, progesterone, and US biophysical profile obstetric.
- Refer to the Reproductive System table online at Davis*Plus* for related tests by body system.

F

α_1-Fetoprotein

SYNONYM/ACRONYM: AFP.

COMMON USE: To assist in the evaluation of fetal health related to neural tube defects and some forms of liver cancer.

SPECIMEN: Serum collected in a gold-, red-, or red/gray-top tube. For maternal triple- or quad-marker testing, include human chorionic gonadotropin and free estriol measurement.

NORMAL FINDINGS: (Method: Immunochemiluminometric assay)

α_1-Fetoprotein as a Tumor Marker: Males, Females, and Children

	Males (Conventional Units)	SI Units (Conventional Units × 1)	Females (Conventional Units)	SI Units (Conventional Units × 1)
Less than 1 mo	0.5–16,387 ng/mL	0.5–16,387 mcg/L	0.5–18,964 ng/mL	0.5–18,964 mcg/L
1–11 mo	0.5–28.3 ng/mL	0.5–28.3 mcg/L	0.5–77 ng/mL	0.5–77 mcg/L
1–3 yr	0.5–7.9 ng/mL	0.5–7.9 mcg/L	0.5–11.1 ng/mL	0.5–11.1 mcg/L
4 yr and older	Less than 6.1 ng/mL	Less than 6.1 mcg/L	Less than 6.1 ng/mL	Less than 6.1 mcg/L

Values may be higher for premature newborns.

	α_1-Fetoprotein (AFP) in Maternal Serum for Triple or Quad Marker			
	White (AFP Median)	African American (AFP Median)	Hispanic (AFP Median)	Asian (AFP Median)
Low risk	Less than 2 MoM	Less than 2 MoM	Less than 2 MoM	Less than 2 MoM

MoM = multiples of the median. Serum values vary with maternal race, weight, weeks of gestation, diabetic status, and number of fetuses, and variations exist between test methods. Serial testing should be determined using the same test method.

Gestational Age (wk)	HCG (Conventional Units)	SI Units (Conventional Units × 1)
2 wk	5–100 milli-international units/mL	5–100 international units/L
3 wk	200–3,000 milli-international units/mL	200–3,000 international units/L
4 wk	10,000–80,000 milli-international units/mL	10,000–80,000 international units/L
5–12 wk	10,000–200,000 milli-international units/mL	10,000–200,000 international units/L
13–24 wk	5,000–80,000 milli international units/mL	5,000–80,000 international units/L
26–28 wk	3,000–15,000 milli-international units/mL	3,000–15,000 international units/L
	Pregnancy-Associated Plasma Protein A	
8 wk	90–7,000 milli-international units/L	
9 wk	0–5,800 milli-international units/L	
10 wk	140–7,000 milli-international units/L	
11 wk	575–7,250 milli-international units/L	
12 wk	900–9,000 milli-international units/L	
13 wk	550–11,500 milli-international units/L	
14 wk	2,200–39,500 milli-international units/L	
	Unconjugated Estriol (E3) (Conventional Units)	**SI Units (Conventional Units × 3.467)**
30 wk	3.5–19 ng/mL	12.1–65.9 nmol/L
34 wk	5.3–18.3 ng/mL	18.4–63.4 nmol/L
35 wk	5.2–26.4 ng/mL	18–91.5 nmol/L
36 wk	8.2–28.1 ng/mL	28.4–97.4 nmol/L
37 wk	8–30.1 ng/mL	27.7–104.4 nmol/L
38 wk	8.6–38 ng/mL	29.8–131.9 nmol/L
39 wk	7.2–34.3 ng/mL	25–118.9 nmol/L
40 wk	9.6–28.9 ng/mL	33.3–100.2 nmol/L

Results vary widely among laboratories and methods.
HCG = human chorionic gonadotropin.

DESCRIPTION: Maternal blood screening for birth defects is optimally performed between 16 and 18 wk but may be done as early as 15 wk or as late as 22.9 wk. A number of serum and amniotic fluid markers can be used in collaboration to screen for Down syndrome, neural tube defects, and trisomy 18. These markers include α_1-fetoprotein (AFP), human chorionic gonadotropin (HCG), unconjugated estriol, dimeric inhibin-A (DIA), and pregnancy-associated plasma protein A. Ultrasound (nuchal translucency [NT] ultrasound measurements of the fluid-filled space in the back of the fetus's neck, larger-than-normal NT measurements are found in Down syndrome), maternal age, race, weight, diabetic status, and number of fetuses are also factors used to calculate risk. The algorithm used to calculate risk depends on whether gestational age is based on ultrasound findings or date of last menstrual period. Diagnostic tests that include AFP, acetylcholinesterase, chromosome analysis, and fetal hemoglobin testing performed on amniotic fluid are discussed in the studies "Amniotic Fluid Analysis" and "Biopsy, Chorionic Villus."

AFP is a glycoprotein produced in the fetal liver, gastrointestinal tract, and yolk sac. AFP is the major serum protein produced for 10 wk in early fetal life. (See "Amniotic Fluid Analysis" study for measurement of AFP levels in amniotic fluid.) After 10 wk of gestation, levels of fetal AFP can be detected in maternal blood, with peak levels occurring at 16 to 18 wk. Elevated maternal levels of AFP on two tests taken 1 wk apart suggest further investigation into fetal well-being by ultrasound or amniocentesis. HCG, a hormone secreted by the placenta, stimulates secretion of progesterone by the corpus luteum. (The use of HCG as a triple marker is also discussed in the study titled "Human Chorionic Gonadotropin.") During intrauterine development, the normal fetus and placenta produce estriol, a portion of which passes into maternal circulation. Decreased estriol levels are an independent indicator of neural tube defects. DIA is the fourth biochemical marker used in prenatal quad screening. It is a glycoprotein secreted by the placenta. Maternal blood levels of DIA normally remain fairly stable during the 15th to 18th weeks of pregnancy. Blood levels are twice as high in the second trimester of pregnancies affected by Down syndrome. The incidence of Down syndrome is 1 in 750 live births. The triple screen detection rate for Down syndrome is 67%. The Down syndrome detection rate increases to 76% and maintains a false-positive rate of 5% when DIA is included. The incidence of neural tube defects is 1 in 1,300 pregnancies; anencephaly is almost always fatal at, or within a very short time after, birth. The incidence of trisomy 18 is 1 in 4,100 live births; most die within the first year after birth.

The presence of AFP in excessive amounts is abnormal in adults and children. AFP measurements are used as a tumor marker to assist in the diagnosis of cancer.

This procedure is contraindicated for: N/A

INDICATIONS

- Assist in the diagnosis of primary hepatocellular carcinoma or

F

metastatic lesions involving the liver, as indicated by highly elevated levels (30% to 50% of Americans with liver cancer do not have elevated AFP levels).

- Investigate suspected hepatitis or cirrhosis, indicated by slightly to moderately elevated levels.
- Monitor response to treatment for hepatic carcinoma, with successful treatment indicated by an immediate decrease in levels.
- Monitor for recurrence of hepatic carcinoma, with elevated levels occurring 1 to 6 mo before the patient becomes symptomatic.
- Investigate suspected intrauterine fetal death, as indicated by elevated levels.
- Routine prenatal screening at 15 to 16 wk of pregnancy for fetal neural tube defects and other disorders, as indicated by elevated levels in maternal serum and amniotic fluid.
- Support diagnosis of embryonal gonadal teratoblastoma, hepatoblastoma, and testicular or ovarian carcinomas.

POTENTIAL MEDICAL DIAGNOSIS

Maternal serum AFP test results report actual values and multiples of the median (MoM) by gestational age (in weeks). MoM are calculated by dividing the patient's AFP by the midpoint (or median) of values expected for a large population of unaffected women at the same gestational age in weeks. MoM should be corrected for maternal weight. The MoM should also be corrected for maternal insulin requirement (achieved by dividing MoM by 1.1 for diabetic African American patients and by 0.8 for patients with diabetes of other ethnicities) and multiple fetuses (multiply by 2.13 for twins). Some laboratories also provide additional statistical information regarding Down syndrome risk.

Increased in:

- Pregnant women:
  - Congenital nephrosis ***(related to defective renal reabsorption)***
  - Fetal abdominal wall defects ***(related to release of AFP from open body wall defect)***
  - Fetal distress
  - Fetal neural tube defects (e.g., anencephaly, spina bifida, myelomeningocele) ***(related to release of AFP from open body wall defect)***
  - Low birth weight ***(related to inaccurate estimation of gestational age)***
  - Multiple pregnancy ***(related to larger quantities from multiple fetuses)***
  - Polycystic kidneys ***(related to defective renal reabsorption)***
  - Underestimation of gestational age ***(related to the expectation of a lower value based on incorrect prediction of gestational age, i.e., AFP increases with age; therefore, if the age is believed to be less than it is actually, the expectation of the corresponding AFP value will be lower than it is actually, and the result appears to be elevated)***
- Men, nonpregnant women, and children (the cancer cells contain undifferentiated hepatocytes that produce glycoproteins of fetal origin):
  - Cirrhosis
  - Hepatic carcinoma
  - Hepatitis
  - Metastatic lesions involving the liver

Decreased in:

- Pregnant women:
  - Down syndrome (trisomy 21)
  - Edwards' syndrome (trisomy 18)
  - Fetal demise (undetected over a lengthy period of time) ***(related to cessation of AFP production)***
  - Hydatidiform moles ***(partial mole may secrete some AFP)***
  - Overestimation of gestational age ***(related to the expectation of a higher value based on incorrect prediction of gestational age; i.e., AFP increases with age; therefore, if the age is believed to be greater than it actually is, the expectation of the corresponding AFP value***

will be greater than it actually is, and the result appears to be decreased)

Pseudopregnancy ***(there is no fetus to produce AFP)***

Spontaneous abortion ***(there is no fetus to produce AFP)***

CRITICAL FINDINGS: N/A

INTERFERING FACTORS

- Drugs and other substances that may decrease AFP levels in pregnant women include acetaminophen and acetylsalicylic acid.
- Multiple fetuses can cause increased levels.
- Gestational age must be between 15 and 22 wk for initial and follow-up testing. The most common cause of an abnormal MoM is inaccurate estimation of gestational age (defined as weeks from the first day of the last menstrual period).
- Maternal AFP levels vary by ethnicity.

NURSING IMPLICATIONS AND PROCEDURE

F

POTENTIAL NURSING PROBLEMS:

Problem	Signs & Symptoms	Interventions
Fear ***(related to prognosis secondary to diagnosis [cancer]; disabled child; ability to function in caregiver role; risk of death [cancer]; loss of control; ineffective coping; unfamiliar therapeutic regime; unknown)***	Expression of fear; preoccupation with fear; increased tension; increased blood pressure; increased heart rate; vomiting; diarrhea, nausea; fatigue; weakness; insomnia; shortness of breath; increased respiratory rate; withdrawal; panic attacks	Provide specific education related to disease process (neural tube defect, liver disease); provide specific information related to treatment based on diagnosis or defect; access social services; ensure education is culturally appropriate; assist the patient and family to recognize effective coping strategies; assist the patient and family to acknowledge their fear; provide a safe environment to discuss fear; explore cultural influences that may enhance fear; utilize therapeutic touch as appropriate to decrease fear
Fatigue ***(related to hepatic disease process; malnutrition; anemia; chemotherapy; radiation therapy)***	Decreased concentration; increased physical complaints; inability to restore energy with sleep; report of being tired; inability to maintain normal routine	Assess for physical cause of fatigue; pace activities to preserve energy stores; rate fatigue on a numeric scale to trend degree of fatigue over time; identify what aggravates and decreases fatigue; assess for related emotional factors such as depression; evaluate current medications in relation to fatigue; assess for physiologic factors such as anemia

(table continues on page 792)

Problem	Signs & Symptoms	Interventions
Confusion; altered sensory perception ***(related to an alteration in fluid and electrolytes, hepatic disease and encephalopathy; acute alcohol consumption; hepatic metabolic insufficiency)***	Disorganized thinking, restless, irritable, altered concentration and attention span, changeable mental function over the day, hallucinations; altered attention span; unable to follow directions; disoriented to person, place, time, and purpose; inappropriate affect	Treat the medical condition; correlate confusion with the need to reverse altered electrolytes; evaluate medications; prevent falls and injury through appropriate use of postural support, bed alarm, or restraints; consider pharmacological interventions; record accurate intake and output to assess fluid status; monitor blood ammonia level; determine last alcohol use; assess for symptoms of hepatic encephalopathy such as confusion, sleep disturbances, incoherence; protect the patient from physical harm; administer lactulose as prescribed
Spirituality ***(related to significant loss; fear of death; debilitation disease process; diagnosed child disability)***	Forgiveness; acceptance; anger at spiritual leaders; expressed feelings of hopeless, powerlessness, abandonment; refusal or inability to participate in spiritual activities (prayer); expresses feelings over lack of meaning with life or serenity	Encourage the verbalization of feelings in a safe, nonjudgmental environment; assess the desire for contact from associated spiritual advisor; foster a supportive relationship with the patient and family; encourage a display of objects (spiritual, religious) that provide emotional relief; assess for expressions of hope

PRETEST:

- Positively identify the patient using at least two person-specific identifiers before services, treatments, or procedures are performed.
- *Patient Teaching:* Inform the patient this test can assist in evaluating fetal health.
- Obtain a history of the patient's health concerns, symptoms, surgical procedures, and results of previously performed laboratory and diagnostic studies. Include a list of known allergens, especially allergies or sensitivities to latex.
- Note any recent procedures that can interfere with test results.
- Provide required information to laboratory for triple-marker testing, including maternal birth date, weight, age, race, calculated gestational age, gestational age by ultrasound, gestational date by physical examination, first day of last menstrual

period, estimated date of delivery, and whether the patient has type 1 diabetes.

- Obtain a list of the patient's current medications, including over-the-counter medications and dietary supplements (see Effects of Natural Products on Laboratory Values online at Davis*Plus*).
- Review the procedure with the patient. Inform the patient that specimen collection takes approximately 5 to 10 min. Address concerns about pain and explain that there may be some discomfort during the venipuncture.
- Note that there are no food, fluid, or medication restrictions unless by medical direction.
- *Consent may be required for this type of testing. As appropriate make sure a written and informed consent has been signed prior to the venipuncture procedure.*

INTRATEST:

Potential Complications: N/A

- Avoid the use of equipment containing latex if the patient has a history of allergic reaction to latex.
- Instruct the patient to cooperate fully and to follow directions. Direct the patient to breathe normally and to avoid unnecessary movement.
- Observe standard precautions, and follow the general guidelines in Patient Preparation and Specimen Collection online at Davis*Plus*. Positively identify the patient, and label the appropriate specimen container with the corresponding patient demographics, initials of the person collecting the specimen, date, and time of collection. Perform a venipuncture.
- The sample may be collected directly from the cord using a syringe and transferred to a red-top tube.
- Remove the needle and apply direct pressure with dry gauze to stop bleeding. Observe/assess venipuncture site for bleeding or hematoma formation and secure gauze with adhesive bandage.
- Promptly transport the specimen to the laboratory for processing and analysis.

POST-TEST:

- Inform the patient that a report of the results will be made available to the requesting health-care provider (HCP), who will discuss the results with the patient.
- ***Nutritional Considerations:*** Hyperhomocysteinemia resulting from folate deficiency in pregnant women is believed to increase the risk of neural tube defects. Elevated levels of homocysteine are thought to chemically damage the exposed neural tissue of the developing fetus. As appropriate, instruct pregnant patients to eat foods rich in folate, such as liver, salmon, eggs, asparagus, green leafy vegetables, broccoli, sweet potatoes, beans, and whole wheat.
- ***Social and Cultural Considerations:*** In pregnant patients, recognize anxiety related to test results, and encourage the family to seek counseling if concerned with pregnancy termination or to seek genetic counseling if a chromosomal abnormality is determined. Discuss the implications of abnormal test results on the patient's lifestyle. Provide teaching and information regarding the clinical implications of the test results, as appropriate. Decisions regarding elective abortion should take place in the presence of both parents. Provide a nonjudgmental, nonthreatening atmosphere for discussing the risks and difficulties of delivering and raising a developmentally challenged infant, as well as exploring other options (termination of pregnancy or adoption). It is also important to discuss feelings the mother and father may experience (e.g., guilt, depression, anger) if fetal abnormalities are detected. Educate the patient regarding access to counseling services.
- In patients with carcinoma, recognize anxiety related to test results, and offer support. Discuss the implications of abnormal test results on the patient's lifestyle.

- Depending on the results of this procedure, additional testing may be performed to evaluate or monitor progression of the disease process and determine the need for a change in therapy. Inform the pregnant patient that an ultrasound may be performed and AFP levels in amniotic fluid may be analyzed if maternal blood levels are elevated in two samples obtained 1 wk apart. Evaluate test results in relation to the patient's symptoms and other tests performed.

Patient Education:

- Reinforce information given by the patient's HCP regarding further testing, treatment, or referral to another HCP.
- Answer any questions or address any concerns voiced by the patient or family.
- Provide teaching and information regarding the clinical implications of the test results, as appropriate.
- Educate the patient regarding access to counseling services, as appropriate.

Expected Patient Outcomes:

Understanding

- The patient and family state that neural tube defect is a causative factor in birth disabilities.
- The patient and family state the specifics of the care plan developed to support the health of the disabled child.

Ability

- The patient and family design a plan to support the home care of the disabled child while meeting own basic needs.
- The patient and family demonstrate proficiency in administering medication to the disabled child.

Response

- The patient and family comply with the request to attend a support group for parents of disabled children.
- The patient and family comply with the recommendation to abstain from alcohol use, as it can exacerbate liver disease.

RELATED STUDIES:

- Related tests include amniotic fluid analysis and L/S ratio, biopsy chorionic villus, cancer antigens, estradiol, fetal fibronectin, folic acid, hexosaminidase, homocysteine, HCG, and US biophysical profile obstetric.
- Refer to the Immune and Reproductive systems tables online at Davis*Plus* for related tests by body system.

F

Fetoscopy

SYNONYM/ACRONYM: Endoscopic fetal surgery, fetal endoscopy.

COMMON USE: To facilitate diagnosis and treatment of the fetus. Evaluate for disorders such as neural tube defects and congenital blood disorders, and assist with fetal karyotyping.

AREA OF APPLICATION: Fetus, uterus.

DESCRIPTION: Fetoscopy is usually performed around the 18th week of pregnancy or later when the fetus is developed sufficiently for diagnosis of potential problems. It is done to evaluate or treat the fetus during pregnancy. Fetoscopy can be accomplished externally using a stethoscope with an attached headpiece, which is placed on the mother's abdomen to assess the fetal heart tones. Endoscopic fetoscopy is accomplished using an instrument called a fetoscope, a thin, 1-mm flexible scope, which is placed with the aid of sonography. The fetoscope is inserted into the uterus through a thin incision in the abdominal wall (transabdominally) or through the cervix (transcervically) in earlier stages of pregnancy. Fetal tissue and blood samples can be obtained through the fetoscope. In addition, fetal surgery can be performed for such procedures as the repair of a fetal congenital diaphragmatic hernia, enlarged bladder, and spina bifida.

This procedure is contraindicated for: N/A

INDICATIONS

- Assess the fetus for birth defects during pregnancy; areas examined include the amniotic fluid, umbilical cord, and fetal side of the placenta.

POTENTIAL MEDICAL DIAGNOSIS

Normal findings

- Absence of birth defects

Abnormal findings related to

- Acardiac twin
- Congenital diaphragmatic hernia
- Hemophilia
- Neural tube defects
- Spinal bifida

CRITICAL FINDINGS: N/A

INTERFERING FACTORS

Factors that may alter the results of the study

- Activity of fetus.
- Amniotic fluid that is extremely cloudy.
- Inability of patient to remain still during the procedure.
- Obesity or very overweight patient.

NURSING IMPLICATIONS AND PROCEDURE

PRETEST:

- Positively identify the patient using at least two person-specific identifiers before services, treatments, or procedures are performed.
- ***Patient Teaching:*** Inform the patient this procedure can assist in locating and treating fetal abnormalities.
- Obtain a history of the patient's health concerns, including a list of known allergens, especially allergies or sensitivities to latex, anesthetics, or sedatives.
- Obtain a history of the patient's health concerns, symptoms, surgical procedures, and results of previously performed laboratory and diagnostic studies. Include a list of known allergens, especially allergies or sensitivities to latex.
- Record the date of last menstrual period and determine the age of the fetus.
- Obtain a list of the patient's current medications, including over-the-counter medications and dietary supplements (see Effects of Natural Products on Laboratory Values online at Davis*Plus*).
- Instruct the patient to remove jewelry and other metallic objects in the area to be examined.
- Review the procedure with the patient. Address concerns about pain and explain that a local anesthetic will be applied to the abdomen to ease with insertion of the fetoscope. Inform the patient that the procedure is performed in an ultrasound department, by a health-care provider (HCP) specializing in this procedure, with support staff, and takes approximately 60 min.
- ***Sensitivity to social and cultural issues,*** as well as concern for modesty, is important in providing psychological support before, during, and after the procedure.
- Instruct patient that food and fluid should be withheld for 8 hr prior to the endoscopic procedure. There are no medication restrictions unless by medical direction.

- *Make sure a written and informed consent has been signed prior to the procedure and before administering any medications.*

INTRATEST:

Potential Complications: N/A

- Ensure that the patient has complied with dietary restrictions prior to the study, as instructed.
- Ensure that the patient has removed external metallic objects prior to the procedure.
- Instruct the patient to void prior to the procedure and to change into the gown, robe, and foot coverings provided.
- Avoid the use of equipment containing latex if the patient has a history of allergic reaction to latex.
- Instruct the patient to cooperate fully and to follow directions. Instruct the patient to remain still throughout the procedure because movement produces unreliable results.
- Instruct the patient to lie on her back.
- Observe standard precautions, and follow the general guidelines in Patient Preparation and Specimen Collection online at Davis*Plus*. Positively identify the patient.

Endoscopic procedure

- The lower abdomen area is cleaned, and a local anesthetic is administered in the area where the incision will be made. Label the appropriate specimen container with the corresponding patient demographics, initials of the person collecting the specimen, date, and time of collection if samples are to be obtained on aspirated amniotic fluid or fetal material.
- Conductive gel is applied to the skin, and a Doppler transducer is moved over the skin to locate the position of the fetus.
- Ask the patient to breathe normally during the examination. If necessary for better fetal visualization, ask the patient to inhale deeply and hold her breath.

POST-TEST:

- Inform the patient that a report of the results will be made available to the requesting HCP, who will discuss the results with the patient.
- When the study is completed, remove the gel from the skin.
- Observe/assess the incision for redness or leakage of fluid or blood following the endoscopic procedure.
- Instruct the patient in the care of the incision and to contact her HCP immediately if she is experiencing chills, fever, dizziness, moderate or severe abdominal cramping, or fluid or blood loss from the vagina or incision.
- Inform the patient that a follow-up ultrasound will be completed the next day to assess the fetus and placenta.
- Recognize anxiety related to test results. Discuss the implications of abnormal test results on the patient's lifestyle. Provide teaching and information regarding the clinical implications of the test results, as appropriate.
- Reinforce information given by the patient's HCP regarding further testing, treatment, or referral to another HCP. Answer any questions or address any concerns voiced by the patient or family.
- Depending on the results of this procedure, additional testing may be needed to evaluate or monitor progression of the disease process and determine the need for a change in therapy. Evaluate test results in relation to the patient's symptoms and other tests performed.

RELATED STUDIES:

- Related tests include amniotic fluid analysis and L/S ratio, biopsy chorionic villus, blood groups and antibodies, chromosome analysis, culture bacterial anal/genital, culture viral, fetal fibronectin, α_1-fetoprotein, hexosaminidase A and B, human chorionic gonadotropin, KUB, Kleihauer-Betke test, prolactin, MRI abdomen, and ultrasound biophysical profile obstetric.
- Refer to the Reproductive System table online at Davis*Plus* for related tests by body system.

Fibrinogen

SYNONYM/ACRONYM: Factor I.

COMMON USE: Commonly used to evaluate fibrinolytic activity as well as identify congenital deficiency, disseminated intravascular coagulation (DIC), and severe liver disease.

SPECIMEN: Plasma collected in a completely filled blue-top (3.2% sodium citrate) tube. If the patient's hematocrit exceeds 55%, the volume of citrate in the collection tube must be adjusted.

NORMAL FINDINGS: (Method: Photo-optical clot detection)

Age	Conventional Units	SI Units (Conventional Units × 0.0294)
Newborn	200–500 mg/dL	5.9–14.7 micromol/L
Adult	200–400 mg/dL	5.9–11.8 micromol/L

Values are higher in older adults.

DESCRIPTION: Fibrinogen (factor I) is an acute-phase reactant protein synthesized in the liver. It is an essential component in the process of hemostasis or clot formation. In the common final pathway of the coagulation process, thrombin converts fibrinogen to fibrin, which then become crosslinked fibrin monomers, and ultimately a stable fibrin clot. The use of fibrinogen levels is not limited to coagulation studies. The role of fibrinogen in the inflammatory response has also established an association between elevated levels and vascular diseases like coronary heart disease, myocardial infarction, stroke, and peripheral arterial disease.

This procedure is contraindicated for: N/A

INDICATIONS

- Assist in the diagnosis of suspected disseminated intravascular coagulation (DIC), as indicated by decreased fibrinogen levels.
- Evaluate congenital or acquired dysfibrinogenemias.
- Monitor hemostasis in disorders associated with low fibrinogen levels or elevated levels that can predispose patients to excessive thrombosis.

POTENTIAL MEDICAL DIAGNOSIS

Increased in:

Fibrinogen is an acute-phase reactant protein and will be increased in inflammatory conditions.

- Acute myocardial infarction
- Cancer
- Eclampsia
- Hodgkin's disease
- Inflammation
- Multiple myeloma
- Nephrotic syndrome
- Pregnancy
- Stroke
- Tissue necrosis

Decreased in:

- Congenital fibrinogen deficiency (rare) ***(related to deficient synthesis)***

- DIC ***(related to rapid consumption as fibrinogen is converted to fibrin)***
- Dysfibrinogenemia ***(related to an inherited abnormality in fibrinogen synthesis)***
- Liver disease (severe) ***(related to decreased synthesis)***
- Primary fibrinolysis ***(related to rapid conversion during fibrinolysis; plasmin breaks down fibrinogen and fibrin)***

CRITICAL FINDINGS:

- Less than 80 mg/dL (SI: Less than 2.4 micromol/L)

Note and immediately report to the requesting health-care provider (HCP) any critical findings and related symptoms. A listing of these findings varies among facilities. Timely notification of a critical finding for laboratory or diagnostic studies is a role expectation of the professional nurse. The notification processes vary among facilities. Upon receipt of the critical finding, the information should be read back to the caller to verify accuracy.

Signs and symptoms of microvascular thrombosis include cyanosis, ischemic tissue necrosis, hemorrhagic necrosis, tachypnea, dyspnea, pulmonary emboli, venous distention, abdominal pain, and oliguria. Possible interventions include identification and treatment of the underlying cause, support through administration of required blood products (cryoprecipitate or fresh frozen plasma), and administration of heparin. Cryoprecipitate may be a more effective product than fresh frozen plasma in cases where the fibrinogen level is less than 100 mg/dL (SI = 2.94 micromol/L), the minimum level required for adequate hemostasis, because it delivers a concentrated amount of fibrinogen without as much plasma volume.

INTERFERING FACTORS

- Drugs and other substances that may increase fibrinogen levels include acetylsalicylic acid and oral contraceptives.
- Drugs and other substances that may decrease fibrinogen levels include anabolic steroids, asparaginase, bezafibrate, danazol, dextran, fenofibrate, fish oils, gemfibrozil, lovastatin, pentoxifylline, phosphorus, and ticlopidine.
- Considerations for draw times after transfusion include the type of product, the amount of product transfused, and the patient's clinical situation. The circulating half-life of fibrinogen is 3 to 5 days. Generally, specimens are collected 30 to 60 min after a massive transfusion to provide guidance regarding the need for administration of additional units.
- Placement of tourniquet for longer than 60 sec can result in venous stasis and changes in the concentration of plasma proteins to be measured. Platelet activation may also occur under these conditions, causing erroneous results.
- Vascular injury during phlebotomy can activate platelets and coagulation factors, causing erroneous results.
- Hemolyzed specimens must be rejected because hemolysis is an indication of platelet and coagulation factor activation.
- Hematocrit greater than 55% may cause falsely prolonged results because of anticoagulant excess relative to plasma volume.
- Incompletely filled collection tubes, specimens contaminated with heparin, clotted specimens, or unprocessed specimens not delivered to the laboratory within 1 to 2 hr of collection should be rejected.

- **Icteric or lipemic specimens interfere with optical testing methods, producing erroneous results.**
- **Traumatic venipuncture and excessive agitation of the sample can alter test results.**

NURSING IMPLICATIONS AND PROCEDURE

PRETEST:

- Positively identify the patient using at least two person-specific identifiers before services, treatments, or procedures are performed.
- *Patient Teaching:* Inform the patient that this laboratory study can assist in diagnosing diseases associated with clotting disorders.
- Obtain a history of the patient's health concerns, symptoms, surgical procedures, and results of previously performed laboratory and diagnostic studies. Include a list of known allergens, especially allergies or sensitivities to latex.
- Note any recent procedures that can interfere with test results.
- Obtain a list of the patient's current medications, including over-the-counter medications, dietary supplements, anticoagulants, aspirin and other salicylates (see Effects of Natural Products on Laboratory Values online at Davis*Plus*). Such products should be discontinued by medical direction for the appropriate number of days prior to a surgical procedure. Note the last time and dose of medication taken.
- Review the procedure with the patient. Inform the patient that specimen collection takes approximately 5 to 10 min. Address concerns about pain and explain that there may be some discomfort during the venipuncture.
- ***Sensitivity to social and cultural issues,*** as well as concern or modesty, is important in providing psychological support before, during, and after the procedure.
- Note that there are no food, fluid, or medication restrictions unless by medical direction.

INTRATEST:

Potential Complications: N/A

- Avoid the use of equipment containing latex if the patient has a history of allergic reaction to latex.
- Instruct the patient to cooperate fully and to follow directions. Direct the patient to breathe normally and to avoid unnecessary movement.
- Observe standard precautions, and follow the general guidelines in Patient Preparation and Specimen Collection online at Davis*Plus*. Positively identify the patient, and label the appropriate specimen container with the corresponding patient demographics, initials of the person collecting the specimen, date, and time of collection. Perform a venipuncture. Fill tube completely. *Important note:* When multiple specimens are drawn, the blue-top tube should be collected after sterile (i.e., blood culture) tubes. Otherwise, when using a standard vacutainer system, the bluo top tube is the first tube collected. When a butterfly is used, due to the added tubing, an extra red-top tube should be collected before the blue-top tube to ensure complete filling of the blue top tube.
- Remove the needle and apply direct pressure with dry gauze to stop bleeding. Observe/assess venipuncture site for bleeding or hematoma formation and secure gauze with adhesive bandage.
- Promptly transport the specimen to the laboratory for processing and analysis. The recommendation for processed and unprocessed samples stored in unopened tubes is that testing should be completed within 1 to 4 hr of collection.

POST-TEST:

- Inform the patient that a report of the results will be made available to the requesting HCP, who will discuss the results with the patient.

- Instruct the patient to report bruising, petechiae, and bleeding from mucous membranes, hematuria, and occult blood.
- Inform the patient with a decreased fibrinogen level of the importance of taking precautions against bruising and bleeding, including the use of a soft bristle toothbrush, use of an electric razor, avoidance of constipation, avoidance of acetylsalicylic acid and similar products, and avoidance of intramuscular injections.
- Reinforce information given by the patient's HCP regarding further testing, treatment, or referral to another HCP. Answer any questions or address any concerns voiced by the patient or family.
- Depending on the results of this procedure, additional testing may be performed to evaluate or monitor progression of the disease process and determine the need for a change in therapy. Evaluate test results in relation to the patient's symptoms and other tests performed.

RELATED STUDIES:

- Related tests include ALT, albumin, ALP, AT-III, AST, bilirubin, biopsy bone, biopsy bone marrow, biopsy liver, clot retraction, coagulation factors, CBC platelet count, CT cardiac scoring, CK and isoenzymes, CRP, D-dimer, echocardiography, echocardiography transesophageal, ECG, ESR, exercise stress test, FDP, GGT, Holter monitor, IFE, immunoglobulins, myocardial perfusion heart scan, aPTT, plasminogen, procalcitonin, protein S, and PT/INR.
- Refer to the Hematopoietic and Hepatobiliary systems tables online at Davis*Plus* for related tests by body system.

F

Fibrinogen Degradation Products

SYNONYM/ACRONYM: Fibrin split products, fibrin breakdown products, FDP, FSP, FBP.

COMMON USE: To evaluate conditions associated with abnormal fibrinolytic and fibrinogenolytic activity such as disseminated intravascular coagulation (DIC), deep vein thrombosis (DVT), and pulmonary embolism (PE).

SPECIMEN: Plasma collected in a completely filled blue-top (3.2% sodium citrate) tube. If the patient's hematocrit exceeds 55%, the volume of citrate in the collection tube must be adjusted.

NORMAL FINDINGS: (Method: Latex agglutination)

Conventional Units	SI Units (Conventional Units × 1)
Less than 5 mcg/mL	Less than 5 mg/dL

DESCRIPTION: This coagulation test evaluates fibrin split products or fibrin/fibrinogen degradation products (FDPs) that interfere with normal coagulation and formation of the hemostatic platelet plug. As thrombin initiates the formation of the fibrin clot, it also activates the fibrinolytic system to limit the size of clot formation and prevent venous occlusion. The D-dimer is specific to secondary fibrinolysis because it detects the disintegration of fibrin rather than fibrinogen. The FDP test detects degradation products of primary fibrinolysis generated by the action of thrombin on fibrinogen as well as degradation products of secondary fibrinolysis by the action of plasmin on fibrin. The two tests together can be useful for differentiation and treatment of suspected cases of fibrinolysis. In the case of primary fibrinolysis, the FDP will be positive while the D-dimer is normal. In DIC, or secondary fibrinolysis, both will be elevated. FDPs are normally cleared rapidly from circulation, however increased circulating levels can interfere with hemostasis by interfering with fibrin polymerization and adhering to platelet cell membranes thereby inhibiting their normal function.

This procedure is contraindicated for: N/A

INDICATIONS

- Assist in the diagnosis of suspected DIC.
- Evaluate response to therapy with fibrinolytic drugs.
- Monitor the effects on hemostasis of trauma, extensive surgery, obstetric complications, and disorders such as liver or kidney disease.

POTENTIAL MEDICAL DIAGNOSIS

Increased in:

- DIC ***(FDP can be positive in a number of conditions in which the coagulation system has been excessively stimulated as a result of tissue injury and fibrin and/or fibrinogen is being degraded by plasmin)***
- Excessive bleeding ***(clot formation related to depletion of platelets and clotting factors will stimulate fibrinolysis and increase circulation of fibrin breakdown products)***
- Kidney disease ***(FDP can be positive in a number of conditions in which the coagulation system has been excessively stimulated as a result of tissue injury and fibrin and/or fibrinogen is being degraded by plasmin)***
- Kidney transplant rejection
- Liver disease ***(related to decreased hepatic clearance)***
- Myocardial infarction ***(FDP can be positive in a number of conditions in which the coagulation system has been excessively stimulated as a result of tissue injury and fibrin and/or fibrinogen is being degraded by plasmin)***
- Obstetric complications, such as pre-eclampsia, abruptio placentae, intrauterine fetal death ***(excessive stimulation of the coagulation system; microthrombi are formed and plasminogen is released to dissolve the fibrin clots)***
- Post–cardiothoracic surgery period ***(FDP can be positive in a number of conditions in which the coagulation system has been excessively stimulated as a result of tissue injury and fibrin and/or fibrinogen is being degraded by plasmin)***
- Pulmonary embolism ***(FDP can be positive in a number of conditions in which the coagulation system has been excessively stimulated as a result of tissue injury and fibrin and/or fibrinogen is being degraded by plasmin)***

Decreased in: N/A

CRITICAL FINDINGS: N/A

F

INTERFERING FACTORS

- Traumatic venipunctures and excessive agitation of the sample can alter test results.
- Drugs and other substances that may increase fibrin degradation product levels include heparin and fibrinolytic drugs such as streptokinase and urokinase.
- The presence of rheumatoid factor may falsely elevate results with some test kits.
- The test should not be ordered on patients receiving heparin therapy.
- Hematocrit greater than 55% may cause falsely prolonged results because of anticoagulant excess relative to plasma volume.
- Incompletely filled collection tubes, specimens contaminated with heparin, clotted specimens, or unprocessed specimens not delivered to the laboratory within 1 to 2 hr of collection should be rejected.

NURSING IMPLICATIONS AND PROCEDURE

F

POTENTIAL NURSING PROBLEMS:

Problem	Signs & Symptoms	Interventions
Bleeding ***(related to anticoagulant therapy; altered clotting factors; depleted clotting factors)***	Altered level of consciousness; hypotension; increased heart rate; decreased hemoglobin (Hgb) and hematocrit (Hct); capillary refill greater than 3 sec; cool extremities	Increase frequency of vital sign assessment with variances in results; monitor for vital sign trends; administer blood or blood products as ordered; administer stool softeners as needed; monitor stool for blood; encourage intake of foods rich in vitamin K; monitor and trend Hgb and Hct; assess skin for petechiae, purpura, hematoma; monitor for blood in emesis, or sputum; institute bleeding precautions (prevent unnecessary venipuncture; avoid intramuscular [IM] injections; prevent trauma; be gentle with oral care, suctioning; avoid use of a sharp razor); administer prescribed medications (recombinant human activated protein C; epsilon aminocaproic acid)

Problem	Signs & Symptoms	Interventions
Gas exchange ***(related to decreased lung tissue perfusion secondary to embolic obstruction; aveolar dead space; increased shunting secondary to alveolar collapse; ventilation perfusion mismatch)***	Cyanosis; increased respiratory rate; anxiety; restlessness; confusion; irritability; tachycardia; dyspnea; headache; abnormal arterial blood gases (ABG); lethargy; somnolence; decreased oxygen saturation (less than 90%); adventitious breath sounds (crackles); areas of decreased lung ventilation; cough, hemoptysis, pleuritic pain in the presence of pulmonary infarct	Monitor and trend ABG results; monitor respiratory rate and effort; monitor and trend pulse oximetry; monitor and trend vital signs; ensure patient does not cross legs while lying or sitting; assess lung sounds frequently; use pulse oximetry to monitor oxygen saturation; collaborate with physician to administer oxygen as needed; elevate the head of the bed 30 degrees; assess for hypoxia symptoms; administer prescribed anticoagulant therapy
Bleeding ***(related to altered clotting factors secondary to anticoagulant therapy)***	Altered level of consciousness; hypotension; increased heart rate; decreased Hgb and Hct; capillary refill greater than 3 sec; cool extremities	Increase frequency of vital sign assessment with variances in results; monitor for vital sign trends; administer blood or blood products as ordered; monitor stool for blood; encourage intake of foods rich in vitamin K; monitor and trend Hgb/Hct, INR, prothrombin time (PT), activated partial thromboplastin time (aPTT); ensure that anticoagulant therapy is accurately administered (intravenous, PO); assess skin for petechiae, purpura, hematoma; monitor for blood in emesis, or sputum; institute bleeding precautions (prevent unnecessary venipuncture; avoid IM injections; prevent trauma; be gentle with oral care, suctioning; avoid use of a sharp razor)

(table continues on page 804)

F

Problem	Signs & Symptoms	Interventions
Tissue perfusion ***(related to vessel wall injury; blood hypercoagulability)***	Femoral, popliteal, or small calf vein tenderness, warmth at involved area, pain with leg palpation, edema; it is possible to be asymptomatic if the deep vein thrombosis (DVT) is located in a distal vein	Assess for symptoms of DVT; assess for contributing factors (trauma, recent surgery, smoking, varicose veins, age, venous stasis, obesity, pregnancy, oral contraceptive use); monitor diagnostic test results (D-dimer, ultrasound, impedance plethysmography); monitor and trend coagulation studies (PT, INR, PTT); encourage bedrest with leg elevation; administer prescribed anticoagulant therapy; institute bleeding precautions (avoid IM injections, prevent trauma, be gentle with oral care and suctioning, avoid use of a sharp razor); apply moist heat at affected area; apply leg compression devices as prescribed; prepare for potential adjunct therapy (thrombolytic, vena cava filter, thrombectomy)

F

PRETEST:

- Positively identify the patient using at least two person-specific identifiers before services, treatments, or procedures are performed.
- ***Patient Teaching:*** Inform the patient this test can assist in diagnosing diseases associated with clotting disorders.
- Obtain a history of the patient's health concerns (especially any bleeding disorders), symptoms, surgical procedures, and results of previously performed laboratory and diagnostic studies. Include a list of known allergens, especially allergies or sensitivities to latex.
- Note any recent procedures that can interfere with test results.
- Obtain a list of the patient's current medications, including over-the-counter medications, dietary supplements, anticoagulants, aspirin and other salicylates (see Effects of Natural Products on Laboratory Values online at Davis*Plus*). Such products should be discontinued by medical direction for the appropriate number of days prior to a surgical procedure. Note the last time and dose of medication taken.
- Review the procedure with the patient. Inform the patient that

specimen collection takes approximately 5 to 10 min. Address concerns about pain and explain that there may be some discomfort during the venipuncture.

- *Sensitivity to social and cultural issues,* as well as concern for modesty, is important in providing psychological support before, during, and after the procedure.
- Note that there are no food, fluid, or medication restrictions unless by medical direction.

INTRATEST:

Potential Complications: N/A

- Avoid the use of equipment containing latex if the patient has a history of allergic reaction to latex.
- Instruct the patient to cooperate fully and to follow directions. Direct the patient to breathe normally and to avoid unnecessary movement.
- Observe standard precautions, and follow the general guidelines in Patient Preparation and Specimen Collection online at Davis*Plus*. Positively identify the patient, and label the appropriate specimen container with the corresponding patient demographics, initials of the person collecting the specimen, date, and time of collection. Perform a venipuncture. Fill tube completely. *Important note:* When multiple specimens are drawn, the blue-top tube should be collected after sterile (i.e., blood culture) tubes. Otherwise, when using a standard vacutainer system, the blue-top tube is the first tube collected. When a butterfly is used, due to the added tubing, an extra red-top tube should be collected before the blue-top tube to ensure complete filling of the blue top tube.
- Remove the needle and apply direct pressure with dry gauze to stop bleeding. Observe/assess venipuncture site for bleeding or hematoma formation and secure gauze with adhesive bandage.
- Promptly transport the specimen to the laboratory for processing and analysis. The recommendation for processed and unprocessed samples stored in unopened tubes is that testing should be completed within 1 to 4 hr of collection.

POST-TEST:

- Inform the patient that a report of the results will be made available to the requesting HCP, who will discuss the results with the patient.
- Depending on the results of this procedure, additional testing may be performed to evaluate or monitor progression of the disease process and determine the need for a change in therapy. Evaluate test results in relation to the patient's symptoms and other tests performed.

Patient Education:

- Instruct the patient to report bleeding from skin or mucous membranes, ecchymosis, petechiae, hematuria, and occult blood.
- Inform the patient with increased levels of fibrin degradation products of the importance of taking precautions against bruising and bleeding, including the use of a soft bristle toothbrush, use of an electric razor, avoidanoc of constipation, avoidance of acetylsalicylic acid and similar products, and avoidance of IM injections.
- Reinforce information given by the patient's HCP regarding further testing, treatment, or referral to another HCP.
- Answer any questions or address any concerns voiced by the patient or family.
- Teach patient that crossing legs increases DVT risk.

Expected Patient Outcomes:

Understanding

- The patient and family state the purpose of anticoagulant therapy is to prevent more clot formation.
- The patient and family state the purpose of heat application to the affected area is to relieve pain and inflammation.

Ability

- The patient demonstrates proficiency with deep breathing exercises.

- The patient demonstrates proficiency in self-administration of ordered anti-coagulant therapy.

Response

- The patient complies with the request to maintain bedrest until the HCP deems it is safe to resume activity.
- The patient complies with the request to refrain from risky activities to prevent injury.

RELATED STUDIES:

- Related tests include aPTT, ALT, alveolar/arterial gradient, angiography pulmonary, AT-III, AST, bilirubin, biopsy liver, blood pool imaging, BUN, coagulation factors, CT cardiac scoring, creatinine, CBC, CBC platelet count, CK and isoenzymes, CRP, D-dimer, exercise stress test, FDP, fibrinogen, GGT, lung perfusion scan, lung ventilation scan, myoglobin, plasminogen, PET heart, procalcitonin, protein S, PT/INR, troponin, US venous Doppler extremity studies, and venography lower extremity studies.
- Refer to the Hematopoietic System table online at Davis*Plus* for related tests by body system.

F

Fluorescein Angiography

SYNONYM/ACRONYM: FA.

COMMON USE: To assist in detecting vascular changes in the eyes affecting vision related to diseases such as diabetic retinopathy and macular degeneration.

AREA OF APPLICATION: Eyes.

DESCRIPTION: Fluorescein angiography (FA) involves the color radiographic examination of the retinal vasculature following rapid intravenous (IV) injection of a sodium fluorescein contrast medium. A special camera allows images to be taken in sequence and manipulated by a computer to provide views of the retinal vessels during filling and emptying of the dye. The camera allows only light waves in the blue range to strike the fundus of the eye. When the fluorescein reaches the blood vessels in the eye, blue light excites the dye molecules to a higher state of activity and causes them to emit a greenish-yellow fluorescence that is recorded.

This procedure is contraindicated for

- Patients with a past history of hypersensitivity to radiographic dyes. Address concerns about nausea and vomiting, as appropriate.
- Patients with narrow-angle glaucoma if pupil dilation is performed; dilation can initiate a severe and sight-threatening open-angle attack.
- Patients with allergies to mydriatics if pupil dilation using mydriatics is performed.

INDICATIONS

- Detect arterial or venous occlusion evidenced by the reduced, delayed, or absent flow of the contrast medium through the vessels or possible vessel leakage of the medium.
- Detect possible vascular disorders affecting visual acuity.
- Detect presence of microaneurysms caused by hypertensive retinopathy.
- Detect the presence of tumors, retinal edema, or inflammation, as evidenced by abnormal patterns or degree of fluorescence.

- Diagnose and manage diabetic retinopathy.
- Diagnose past reduced flow or patency of the vascular circulation of the retina, as evidenced by neovascularization.
- Diagnose presence of macular degeneration and any other degeneration and any associated hemorrhaging.
- Observe ocular effects resulting from the long-term use of high-risk medications.

POTENTIAL MEDICAL DIAGNOSIS

Normal findings

- No leakage of dye from retinal blood vessels
- Normal retina and retinal and choroidal vessels
- No evidence of vascular abnormalities, such as hemorrhage, retinopathy, aneurysms, or obstructions caused by stenosis and resulting in collateral circulation

Abnormal findings related to

- Aneurysm
- Arteriovenous shunts
- Diabetic retinopathy
- Macular degeneration
- Neovascularization
- Obstructive disorders of the arteries or veins that lead to collateral circulation
- Ocular histoplasmosis
- Retinal vascular occlusion

CRITICAL FINDINGS: N/A

INTERFERING FACTORS

Factors that may impair the results of the examination

- Inability of the patient to cooperate or remain still during the test because of age, significant pain, or mental status may interfere with the test results.
- Presence of cataracts may interfere with fundal view.
- Ineffective dilation of the pupils may impair clear imaging.
- Allergic reaction to radiographic dye, including nausea and vomiting, may interrupt the procedure.
- Failure to follow medication restrictions before the procedure may cause the procedure to be canceled or repeated.

NURSING IMPLICATIONS AND PROCEDURE

PRETEST:

- Positively identify the patient using at least two person-specific identifiers before services, treatments, or procedures are performed.
- *Patient Teaching:* Inform the patient this procedure can assist in detecting changes in the eye that affect vision. It may also be used as a preoperative assessment tool prior to retinal laser procedures.
- Obtain a history of the patient's health concerns (especially known or suspected vision loss; changes in visual acuity, including type and cause; use of glasses or contact lenses; and eye conditions with treatment regimens), symptoms, surgical procedures, and results of previously performed laboratory and diagnostic studies. Include a list of known allergens, especially allergies or sensitivities to latex or radiographic dyes. Ensure results of coagulation testing are obtained and recorded prior to the procedure; a creatinine level is also needed before contrast medium is to be used.
- Obtain a list of the patient's current medications, including over-the-counter medications and dietary supplements (see Effects of Natural Products on Laboratory Values online at Davis*Plus*).
- Instruct the patient to remove contact lenses or glasses, as appropriate. Instruct the patient regarding the importance of keeping the eyes open for the test.
- Review the procedure with the patient. Explain that the patient will be

requested to fixate the eyes during the procedure. Address concerns about pain and explain that mydriatics, if used, may cause blurred vision and sensitivity to light. There may also be a brief stinging sensation when the drop is put in the eye. Explain to the patient that some discomfort may be experienced during the insertion of the IV. Inform the patient that when fluorescein dye is injected, it may cause facial flushing or nausea and vomiting. Inform the patient that a health-care provider (HCP) performs the test, in a quiet, darkened room, and that to dilate and evaluate both eyes, the test can take up 60 min.

F

- ***Sensitivity to social and cultural issues,*** as well as concern for modesty, is important in providing psychological support before, during, and after the procedure.
- Explain that an IV line will be inserted to allow intermittent infusion of dye.
- Note that there are no food or fluid restrictions unless by medical direction.
- Instruct the patient to avoid eye medications (particularly miotic eye drops which may constrict the pupil preventing a clear view of the fundus and mydriatic eyedrops in order to avoid instigation of an acute open angle attack in patients with narrow angle glaucoma) for at least 1 day prior to the test.
- Ensure that the patient understands that he or she must refrain from driving until the pupils return to normal (about 4 hr) after the test and has made arrangements to have someone else be responsible for transportation after the test.
- *Make sure a written and informed consent has been signed prior to the procedure and before administering any medications.*

INTRATEST:

Potential Complications:

- Dilation can initiate a severe and sight-threatening open-angle attack in patients with narrow-angle glaucoma if pupil dilation is performed.
- A number of complications are associated with venipuncture. Pain is commonly associated with needles, and although pain experienced during venipuncture is usually mild, on a rare occasion the needle may strike a nerve, causing severe and lasting pain. Hematoma results when blood leaks into the tissue during or after a venipuncture, as evidenced by pain, bruising, and/or swelling at the venipuncture site. The swelling can cause temporary or permanent injury by compressing the surrounding nerves. Hematomas occur more often in older adults or frail patients or those with difficult veins to access. Prolonged bleeding is a complication that occurs with patients who are taking blood thinners, such as aspirin or warfarin, or who have coagulopathies such as hemophilia. Bleeding or bruising can be prevented by applying direct pressure to the site, once the needle has been removed, with gauze for a minute or two. The site should then be observed/assessed for bleeding or bruising. If no further action is required, the site can be covered by the gauze and an adhesive bandage or paper tape. Some patients experience a vasovagal reaction during the venipuncture procedure, evidenced by sweating (diaphoresis), low blood pressure (hypotension), fainting (syncope), or near fainting (near syncope). The potential for a fall injury is a significant concern related to vasovagal reactions. Other, more unusual complications of venipuncture include cellulitis, phlebitis, seizures, inadvertent arterial puncture, and sepsis. Sepsis can be caused by introduction of bacteria from the surface of the skin into the blood as the result of improper cleansing of the venipuncture site. Immunocompromised patients are at higher risk for developing this complication.
- Anaphylaxis, bronchospasm, cardiac arrest, laryngeal edema, myocardial infarction, nausea, pruritus, urticaria, or vomiting can occur in response to the dye, and extravasation of the dye can occur during injection.

- Observe standard precautions, and follow the general guidelines in Patient Preparation and Specimen Collection online at Davis*Plus*. Positively identify the patient.
- Ensure that the patient has complied with medication restrictions prior to the study, as instructed.
- Avoid the use of equipment containing latex if the patient has a history of allergic reaction to latex.
- Have emergency equipment readily available.
- Instruct the patient to cooperate fully and to follow directions. Instruct the patient to remain still during the procedure because movement produces unreliable results.
- Seat the patient in a chair that faces the camera. Instruct the patient to look at a directed target while the eyes are examined.
- Administer the ordered mydriatic to each eye, and repeat in 5 to 15 min if dilation is to be performed. Drops are placed in the eye with the patient looking up and the solution directed at the six o'clock position of the sclera (white of the eye) near the limbus (gray, semitransparent area of the eyeball where the cornea and sclera meet). Neither dropper nor bottle should touch the eyelashes.
- Insert an intermittent infusion device, as ordered, for subsequent injection of the contrast media or emergency medications.
- After the eyedrops are administered but before the dye is injected, color fundus photographs are taken.
- Instruct the patient to place the chin in the chin rest and gently press the forehead against the support bar. Instruct the patient to open his or her eyes wide and look at the desired target.
- Fluorescein dye is injected into the brachial vein using the intermittent infusion device, and a rapid sequence of photographs is taken and repeated after the dye has reached the retinal vascular system. Follow-up photographs are taken in 20 to 30 min.
- At the conclusion of the procedure, remove the IV needle and apply direct pressure with dry gauze to stop bleeding. Observe venipuncture site for bleeding or hematoma formation and secure gauze with adhesive bandage.
- Observe for hypersensitive reaction to the dye. The patient may become nauseous and vomit.

POST-TEST:

- Inform the patient that a report of the results will be made available to the requesting HCP, who will discuss the results with the patient.
- Instruct the patient to resume usual medications, as directed by the HCP.
- ***Nutritional Considerations:*** Increased glucose levels may be associated with diabetes. There is no "diabetic diet"; however, many meal-planning approaches with nutritional goals are endorsed by the American Diabetes Association (ADA). 🍁 Patients who adhere to dietary recommendations report a better general feeling of health, better weight management, greater control of glucose and lipid values, and improved use of insulin. Instruct the patient, as appropriate, in nutritional management of diabetes. A variety of dietary patterns are beneficial for people with diabetes. The Mediterranean-style diet emphasizes inclusion of vegetables, whole grains, fruits, low-fat dairy, nuts, legumes, and nontropical vegetable oils (e.g., olive, canola, peanut, sunflower, flaxseed) along with fish and lean poultry. A similar dietary pattern known as the Dietary Approaches to Stop Hypertension (DASH) diet makes additional recommendations for the reduction of dietary sodium. Both dietary styles emphasize a reduction in consumption of red meats, which are high in saturated fats and cholesterol, and other foods containing sugar, saturated fats, trans fats, and sodium. A vegetarian diet as well as other potential weight loss diets such as Weight Watchers are also supported by the ADA. 🍁 If triglycerides also are elevated, the patient should be advised to eliminate or reduce alcohol. The nutritional needs of each patient with diabetes need to be

determined individually (especially during pregnancy) with the appropriate HCPs, particularly professionals educated in nutrition.

- Recognize anxiety related to test results, and be supportive of impaired activity related to vision loss or anticipated loss of driving privileges. Discuss the implications of abnormal test results on the patient's lifestyle. Provide teaching and information regarding the clinical implications of the test results, as appropriate. Emphasize, as appropriate, that good glycemic control delays the onset of and slows the progression of diabetic retinopathy, nephropathy, and neuropathy. Provide education regarding smoking cessation, as appropriate. Provide contact information regarding vision aids, if desired, for the American Heart Association (www.americanheart.org), American Macular Degeneration Foundation (www.macular.org), Glaucoma Research Foundation (www.glaucoma.org), ABLEDATA (sponsored by the National Institute on Disability and Rehabilitation Research [NIDRR], www.abledata.com), and ADA (www.diabetes.org). 🍁
- Reinforce information given by the patient's HCP regarding further testing, treatment, or referral to another HCP. Inform the patient that visual acuity and responses to light may change. Suggest that the patient wear dark glasses after the test until the pupils return to normal size. Inform the patient that yellow discoloration of the skin and urine from the radiographic dye is normally present for up to 2 days. Answer any questions or address any concerns voiced by the patient or family.
- Depending on the results of this procedure, additional testing may be performed to evaluate or monitor progression of the disease process and determine the need for a change in therapy. Evaluate test results in relation to the patient's symptoms and other tests performed.

RELATED STUDIES:

- Related tests include fructosamine, fundoscopy, glucagon, glucose, glycated hemoglobin, gonioscopy, insulin, intraocular pressure, microalbumin, plethysmography, refraction, slit-lamp biomicroscopy, and visual field testing.
- Refer to the Ocular System table online at Davis*Plus* for related tests by body system.

Folate

SYNONYM/ACRONYM: Folic acid, vitamin B_9.

COMMON USE: To assist in evaluation of diagnoses that are related to fluctuations in folate levels such as vitamin B_{12} deficiency and malabsorption.

SPECIMEN: Serum collected in a gold-, red-, or red/gray-top tube.

NORMAL FINDINGS: (Method: Immunochemiluminometric assay [ICMA])

	Conventional Units	SI Units (Conventional Units × 2.265)
Normal	Greater than 5.4 ng/mL	Greater than 12.2 nmol/L
Intermediate	3.4–5.4 ng/mL	7.7–12.2 nmol/L
Deficient	Less than 3.4 ng/mL	Less than 7.7 nmol/L

Values may be slightly decreased in older adults due to the effects of medications and the presence of multiple chronic or acute diseases with or without muted symptoms.

DESCRIPTION: Folate, a water-soluble vitamin, is produced by bacteria in the intestines and stored in small amounts in the liver. Dietary folate is absorbed through the intestinal mucosa and stored in the liver. Folate is necessary for normal red blood cell (RBC) and white blood cell function, DNA replication, and cell division. Folate levels are often measured in association with serum vitamin B_{12} determinations because vitamin B_{12} is required for folate to enter tissue cells. Folate is an essential coenzyme in the conversion of homocysteine to methionine. Hyperhomocysteinemia resulting from folate deficiency in pregnant women is believed to increase the risk of neural tube defects. Hyperhomocysteinemia related to low folic acid levels is also associated with increased risk for cardiovascular disease.

This procedure is contraindicated for: N/A

INDICATIONS

- Assist in the diagnosis of megaloblastic anemia resulting from deficient folate intake or increased folate requirements, such as in pregnancy and hemolytic anemia.
- Monitor the effects of prolonged parenteral nutrition.
- Monitor response to disorders that may lead to folate deficiency or decreased absorption and storage.

POTENTIAL MEDICAL DIAGNOSIS

Increased in:

- Blind loop syndrome ***(related to malabsorption in a segment of the intestine due to competition for absorption of folate produced by bacterial overgrowth)***
- Excessive dietary intake of folate or folate supplements
- Pernicious anemia ***(related to inadequate levels of vitamin B_{12}, due to impaired absorption, resulting in increased circulating folate levels)***
- Vitamin B_{12} deficiency ***(related to vitamin B_{12} levels inadequate to metabolize folate, resulting in increased circulating folate levels)***

Decreased in:

- Chronic alcoholism ***(related to insufficient intake combined with malabsorption)***
- Crohn's disease ***(related to malabsorption)***
- Exfoliative dermatitis ***(related to increased demand)***
- Hemolytic anemias ***(related to increased demand due to shortened RBC life span caused by folate deficiency)***
- Liver disease ***(related to increased excretion)***
- Malnutrition ***(related to insufficient intake)***
- Megaloblastic anemia ***(related to folate deficiency, which affects development of RBCs and results in anemia)***
- Myelofibrosis ***(related to increased demand)***
- Neoplasms ***(related to increased demand)***
- Pregnancy ***(related to increased demand possibly combined with insufficient dietary intake)***
- Regional enteritis ***(related to malabsorption)***
- Scurvy ***(related to insufficient intake)***
- Sideroblastic anemias ***(evidenced by an acquired anemia resulting from folate deficiency; iron enters and accumulates in the RBCs but cannot become incorporated in hemoglobin)***

- Sprue ***(related to malabsorption)***
- Ulcerative colitis ***(related to malabsorption)***
- Whipple's disease ***(related to malabsorption)***

CRITICAL FINDINGS: N/A

INTERFERING FACTORS

- Drugs and other substances that may decrease folate levels include aminopterin, ampicillin, antacids, anticonvulsants, barbiturates, chloramphenicol, chloroguanide, erythromycin, ethanol, lincomycin, metformin, methotrexate, nitrofurans, oral contraceptives, penicillins, pentamidine, phenytoin, pyrimethamine, tetracycline, and triamterene.
- Hemolysis may falsely increase folate levels.

NURSING IMPLICATIONS AND PROCEDURE

F

POTENTIAL NURSING PROBLEMS:

Problem	Signs & Symptoms	Interventions
Confusion; altered sensory perception ***(related to hepatic disease and encephalopathy; acute alcohol consumption; hepatic metabolic insufficiency)***	Disorganized thinking, restlessness, irritability, altered concentration and attention span, changeable mental function over the day, hallucinations; unable to follow directions; disoriented to person, place, time, and purpose; inappropriate affect	Treat the medical condition; evaluate medications; prevent falls and injury through appropriate use of postural support, bed alarm, or restraints; consider pharmacological interventions; record accurate intake and output to assess fluid status; monitor blood ammonia level; monitor and trend electrolytes; determine last alcohol use; assess for symptoms of hepatic encephalopathy; assess for sleep disturbances, incoherence; protect from physical harm; administer prescribed medication, blood, blood products to treat disease
Fatigue ***(related to hepatic disease process; malnutrition; anemia; chemotherapy; radiation therapy)***	Decreased concentration; increased physical complaints; unable to restore energy with sleep; reports being tired; unable to maintain normal routine	Assess for physical cause of fatigue; pace activities to preserve energy stores; rate fatigue on a numeric scale to trend degree of fatigue over time; identify what aggravates and decreases fatigue; assess for related emotional factors such as depression; evaluate current medications in relation to fatigue; assess for physiologic factors such as anemia

Problem	Signs & Symptoms	Interventions
Nutrition ***(related to poor eating habits; excessive alcohol use; altered liver function; nausea; vomiting)***	Known inadequate caloric intake; weight loss; muscle wasting in arms and legs; stool that is pale or gray colored; skin that is flaky with loss of elasticity	Document food intake with possible calorie count; assess barriers to eating; consider using a food diary; monitor continued alcohol use as it is a barrier to adequate nutrition; monitor glucose levels; monitor daily weight; provide dietary consult with assessment of cultural food selections; administer multivitamin as prescribed; provide parenteral and enteral nutrition as needed; assess liver function tests alanine aminotransferase (ALT), aspartate aminotransferase (AST), alkaline phosphatase (ALP), glucose, protein, albumin, bilirubin, folic acid, thiamine, electrolytes
Gas exchange ***(related to deficient oxygen capacity of the blood)***	Irregular breathing pattern, use of accessory muscles; altered chest excursion; adventitious breath sounds (crackles, rhonchi, wheezes, diminished breath sounds); signs of hypoxia; altered blood gas results; confusion; lethargy; cyanosis	Monitor respiratory rate and effort based on assessment of patient condition; assess lung sounds frequently; use pulse oximetry to monitor oxygen saturation; collaborate with physician to administer oxygen as needed; elevate the head of the bed 30 degrees or higher; monitor intravenous fluids and avoid aggressive fluid resuscitation; assess level of consciousness; anticipate the need for possible intubation

PRETEST:

- Positively identify the patient using at least two person-specific identifiers before services, treatments, or procedures are performed.
- *Patient Teaching:* Inform the patient this test can assist in detecting folate deficiency and monitoring folate therapy.
- Obtain a history of the patient's health concerns, symptoms, surgical procedures, and results of previously performed laboratory and diagnostic studies. Include a list of known allergens, especially allergies or sensitivities to latex.
- Obtain a list of the patient's current medications, including over-the-counter medications and dietary supplements (see Effects of Natural Products on Laboratory Values online at Davis*Plus*).
- Review the procedure with the patient. Inform the patient that specimen collection takes approximately

5 to 10 min. Address concerns about pain and explain that there may be some discomfort during the venipuncture.

- *Sensitivity to social and cultural issues,* as well as concern for modesty, is important in providing psychological support before, during, and after the procedure.
- Note that there are no food, fluid, or medication restrictions unless by medical direction.

INTRATEST:

Potential Complications: N/A

- Avoid the use of equipment containing latex if the patient has a history of allergic reaction to latex.
- Instruct the patient to cooperate fully and to follow directions. Direct the patient to breathe normally and to avoid unnecessary movement.
- Observe standard precautions, and follow the general guidelines in Patient Preparation and Specimen Collection online at Davis*Plus*. Positively identify the patient, and label the appropriate specimen container with the corresponding patient demographics, initials of the person collecting the specimen, date, and time of collection. Perform a venipuncture. Protect the specimen from light.
- Remove the needle and apply direct pressure with dry gauze to stop bleeding. Observe/assess venipuncture site for bleeding or hematoma formation and secure gauze with adhesive bandage.
- Promptly transport the specimen to the laboratory for processing and analysis.

POST-TEST:

- Inform the patient that a report of the results will be made available to the requesting health-care provider (HCP), who will discuss the results with the patient.
- *Nutritional Considerations:* Instruct the patient who is folate-deficient (especially pregnant women), as appropriate, to eat foods rich in folate, such as liver, salmon, eggs, asparagus, green leafy vegetables, broccoli, sweet potatoes, beans, and whole wheat.
- Depending on the results of this procedure, additional testing may be performed to evaluate or monitor progression of the disease process and determine the need for a change in therapy. Evaluate test results in relation to the patient's symptoms and other tests performed.

Patient Education:

- Reinforce information given by the patient's HCP regarding further testing, treatment, or referral to another HCP.
- Answer any questions or address any concerns voiced by the patient or family.
- Educate the patient regarding access to nutritional counseling services.
- Provide contact information, if desired, for the Institute of Medicine of the National Academies (www.iom.edu) or the USDA's resource for nutrition (www.choosemyplate.gov). 🍁

Expected Patient Outcomes:

Understanding

- The patient and family verbalize the importance of reporting any difficulty breathing to facilitate timely interventions.
- The patient and family state information provided to support lifestyle changes that will be necessary to manage disease process.

Ability

- The patient and family design a dietary strategy that encompasses the concept of six small meals a day to better manage caloric needs.
- The patient and family describe ways to conserve energy and prevent fatigue.

Response

- The patient complies with the request to abstain from alcohol use.
- The patient complies with the HCP recommendation of a dietary consult to assist in managing caloric needs appropriately.

RELATED STUDIES:

- Related tests include antibodies antithyroglobulin, biopsy intestinal, capsule endoscopy, CBC, CBC RBC indices, complete blood count, RBC morphology, complete blood count, WBC count and differential, eosinophil count, fecal analysis, gastric acid emptying scan, gastric acid stimulation test, gastrin, G6PD, hemosiderin, homocysteine, intrinsic factor antibodies, thyroid, and vitamin B_{12}.
- Refer to the Gastrointestinal and Hematopoietic systems tables online at Davis*Plus* for related tests by body system.

Follicle-Stimulating Hormone

SYNONYM/ACRONYM: Follitropin, FSH.

COMMON USE: To distinguish primary causes of gonadal failure from secondary causes, evaluate menstrual disturbances, and assist in infertility evaluations.

SPECIMEN: Serum collected in a gold-, red-, or red/gray-top tube.

NORMAL FINDINGS: (Method: Immunoassay)

Age	Conventional Units and SI Units
Child	
Prepuberty	Less than 10 international units/mL
Adult	
Male	1.4–15.5 international units/mL
Female	
Follicular phase	1.4–9.9 international units/mL
Ovulatory peak	6.2–17.2 international units/mL
Luteal phase	1.1–9.2 international units/mL
Postmenopause	19–100 international units/mL

DESCRIPTION: Follicle-stimulating hormone (FSH) is produced and stored in the anterior portion of the pituitary gland. In women, FSH promotes maturation of the graafian (germinal) follicle, causing estrogen secretion and allowing the ovum to mature. In men, FSH partially controls spermatogenesis, but the presence of testosterone is also necessary. Gonadotropin-releasing hormone secretion is stimulated by a decrease in estrogen and testosterone levels. Gonadotropin-releasing hormone secretion stimulates FSH secretion. FSH production is inhibited by an increase in estrogen and testosterone levels. FSH production is pulsatile, episodic, and cyclic and is subject to diurnal variation. Serial measurement is often required.

This procedure is contraindicated for: N/A

INDICATIONS

- Assist in distinguishing between primary and secondary (pituitary or hypothalamic) gonadal failure.
- Define menstrual cycle phases as a part of infertility testing.
- Evaluate ambiguous sexual differentiation in infants.
- Evaluate early sexual development in girls younger than age 9 or boys younger than age 10 (precocious puberty associated with elevated levels).
- Evaluate failure of sexual maturation in adolescence.
- Evaluate testicular dysfunction.
- Investigate impotence, gynecomastia, and menstrual disturbances.

F

POTENTIAL MEDICAL DIAGNOSIS

Increased in:

- Castration ***(oversecretion related to feedback mechanism involving decreased testosterone levels)***
- Gonadal failure ***(oversecretion related to feedback mechanism involving decreased estrogen or testosterone levels)***
- Gonadotropin-secreting pituitary tumors ***(related to oversecretion by tumor cells)***
- Klinefelter's syndrome ***(oversecretion related to feedback mechanism involving decreased estrogen or testosterone levels)***
- Menopause ***(oversecretion related to feedback mechanism involving decreased estrogen levels)***
- Orchitis ***(oversecretion related to feedback mechanism involving decreased testosterone levels)***
- Precocious puberty in children ***(related to oversecretion from the pituitary gland)***
- Primary hypogonadism ***(oversecretion related to feedback mechanism involving decreased estrogen or testosterone levels; failure of testes or ovaries to produce sex hormones)***
- Reifenstein's syndrome ***(oversecretion related to feedback mechanism involving familial partial resistance to testosterone levels)***
- Turner's syndrome ***(oversecretion related to feedback mechanism involving decreased estrogen or testosterone levels)***

Decreased in:

- Anorexia nervosa ***(related to suppressive effects of severe caloric restriction on the hypothalamic-pituitary axis)***
- Anterior pituitary hypofunction ***(underproduction resulting from dysfunctional pituitary gland)***
- Hemochromatosis ***(hypogonadotropic hypogonadism related to absence of the gonadal stimulating pituitary hormones, estrogen, and testosterone; iron deposits in pituitary may affect normal production of FSH)***
- Hyperprolactinemia ***(related to suppressive effect on estrogen production)***
- Hypothalamic disorders ***(decreased production in response to lack of hypothalamic stimulators)***
- Polycystic ovary disease (Stein-Leventhal syndrome) ***(suppressed secretion related to feedback mechanism involving increased estrogen levels)***
- Pregnancy ***(related to elevated estrogen levels)***
- Sickle cell anemia ***(although primary testicular dysfunction is mainly associated with sickle cell disease, related to testicular microinfarcts, hypogonadotropic hypogonadism has been reported in some men with sickle cell disease)***

CRITICAL FINDINGS: N/A

INTERFERING FACTORS

- Drugs and other substances that may increase FSH levels include bicalutamide, bombesin, cimetidine, clomiphene, digoxin, erythropoietin, exemestane, finasteride, gonadotropin-releasing hormone, ketoconazole, levodopa, metformin, nafarelin, naloxone, nilutamide, oxcarbazepine, pravastatin, and tamoxifen.
- Drugs and other substances that may decrease FSH levels include anabolic steroids, anticonvulsants, buserelin, estrogens, corticotropin-releasing hormone, danazol, diethylstilbestrol, goserelin, megestrol, mestranol, oral contraceptives, phenothiazine, pravastatin, progesterone, tamoxifen, toremifene, and valproic acid.
- In women who are menstruating, values vary in relation to the phase of the menstrual cycle. Values are higher in women who are postmenopausal.

NURSING IMPLICATIONS AND PROCEDURE

F

POTENTIAL NURSING PROBLEMS:

Problem	Signs & Symptoms	Interventions
Family process ***(related to altered role performance secondary to disease progression [testicular, ovarian])***	Inability to perform in supportive family role; diagnosed infertility; alterations in intimacy	Refer to family counseling; facilitate opportunities for the patient and family to express their feelings; assess the patient and family perception of the problems; evaluate patient and family weaknesses, strengths, and coping strategies; help the family and patient break down concerns into manageable parts
Self-esteem ***(related to altered view of self secondary to altered ability to participate in sexual intimacy; infertility; altered body image)***	Verbalizes feelings that express being a failure as a man or woman; dissatisfaction with present state of intimacy with significant other	Monitor for negative self-statements; assess for withdrawal; monitor for real or perceived rejection of others; encourage verbalization of self-worth; encourage a discussion of perceived changes in family role; monitor for anxiety; recommend personal and family counseling; facilitate support group participation
Fear ***(related to diagnosis of infertility; permanently altered sexual function [castration];***	Expression of fear; preoccupation with fear; increased tension; increased blood pressure; increased heart rate; vomiting;	Provide specific and culturally appropriate education; assist the patient and family to recognize effective coping strategies; assist the patient to acknowledge fear; provide a safe environment to decease

(table continues on page 818)

Problem	Signs & Symptoms	Interventions
ineffective coping; unfamiliar therapeutic regime; unknown treatment outcome)	diarrhea; nausea; fatigue; weakness; insomnia; shortness of breath; increased respiratory rate; withdrawal; panic attacks	fear; explore cultural influences that may enhance fear; utilize therapeutic touch as appropriate to decrease fear; collaborate with social services to addresses specific medical problems associated with fear; discuss fertility counseling, adoption
Sexuality ***(related to altered sexual desire, activity; diminished intimacy; testicular, ovarian disease)***	Decreased sexual satisfaction; diminished sexual function; ongoing infertility	Discuss the possibility of sperm banking or harvesting ovum for future fertility needs; suggest counseling for patient and family and provide contact information; facilitate a discussion of realistic changes to sexual intimacy associated with altered estrogen and testosterone levels; provide a relaxed atmosphere to discuss sexuality concerns; provide contact information for a support group

F

PRETEST:

- Positively identify the patient using at least two person-specific identifiers before services, treatments, or procedures are performed.
- ***Patient Teaching:*** Inform the patient this test can assist in evaluating disturbances in hormone levels.
- Obtain a history of the patient's health concerns, phase of menstrual cycle, symptoms, surgical procedures, and results of previously performed laboratory and diagnostic studies. Include a list of known allergens, especially allergies or sensitivities to latex.
- Obtain a list of the patient's current medications, including over-the-counter medications and dietary supplements (see Effects of Natural Products on Laboratory Values online at Davis*Plus*).
- Review the procedure with the patient. Inform the patient that specimen collection takes approximately 5 to 10 min. Address concerns about pain and explain that there may be some discomfort during the venipuncture.
- ***Sensitivity to social and cultural issues,*** as well as concern for modesty, is important in providing psychological support before, during, and after the procedure.
- Note that there are no food, fluid, or medication restrictions unless by medical direction.

INTRATEST:

Potential Complications: N/A

- Avoid the use of equipment containing latex if the patient has a history of allergic reaction to latex.
- Instruct the patient to cooperate fully and to follow directions. Direct the patient to breathe normally and to avoid unnecessary movement.

- Observe standard precautions, and follow the general guidelines in Patient Preparation and Specimen Collection online at Davis*Plus*. Positively identify the patient, and label the appropriate specimen container with the corresponding patient demographics, initials of the person collecting the specimen, date, and time of collection. Perform a venipuncture.
- Remove the needle and apply direct pressure with dry gauze to stop bleeding. Observe/assess venipuncture site for bleeding or hematoma formation and secure gauze with adhesive bandage.
- Promptly transport the specimen to the laboratory for processing and analysis.

POST-TEST:

- Inform the patient that a report of the results will be made available to the requesting health-care provider (HCP), who will discuss the results with the patient.
- Recognize anxiety related to test results and provide a supportive, nonjudgmental environment when assisting a patient through the process of fertility testing. Osteoporosis, which can result in a tendency to develop bone fractures, can occur in both female and male patients with this hormone deficiency. Encourage patients to discuss their feelings about the impact test results may have on their life and the life of their partner.
- Depending on the results of this procedure, additional testing may be performed to evaluate or monitor progression of the disease process and determine the need for a change in therapy. Evaluate test results in relation to the patient's symptoms and other tests performed.

Patient Education:

- Discuss the implications of abnormal test results on the patient's lifestyle.
- Provide teaching and information regarding the clinical implications of the test results, as appropriate.
- Educate the patient and partner regarding access to counseling services, as appropriate.
- Educate the female patient regarding the potential effects of FSH deficiency, which may include an absence of menstrual cycles, infertility, decreased sex drive, and vaginal dryness; educate male patients regarding decreased sex drive, erectile dysfunction, and infertility.
- Reinforce information given by the patient's HCP regarding further testing, treatment, or referral to another HCP.
- Inform the patient that multiple specimens may be required.
- Answer any questions or address any concerns voiced by the patient or family.

Expected Patient Outcomes:

Understanding

- The patient acknowledges family planning information provided.
- The patient states osteoporosis can occur with this hormone deficiency and takes recommended calcium replacement.

Ability

- The patient demonstrates proficient self-administration of medication to treat infertility.
- The patient describes the benefits of attending an infertility support group.

Response

- The patient agrees to abstain from alcohol use.
- The patient shares anxieties related to possible treatment to decrease barriers to the plan of care.

RELATED STUDIES:

- Related tests include antibodies antisperm, BMD, Chlamydia group antibody, chromosome analysis, CT pituitary, estradiol, laparoscopy gynecologic, LH, MRI pituitary, prolactin, testosterone, semen analysis, and US scrotal.
- Refer to the Endocrine and Reproductive systems tables online at Davis*Plus* for related tests by body system.

F

Fructosamine

SYNONYM/ACRONYM: Glycated albumin.

COMMON USE: To assist in assessing long-term glucose control in diabetes.

SPECIMEN: Serum collected in a gold-, red-, or red/gray-top tube.

NORMAL FINDINGS: (Method: Spectrophotometry)

Status	Conventional Units	SI Units (Conventional Units × 0.01)
Normal	174–286 micromol/L	1.74–2.86 mmol/L
Diabetic (values vary with degree of control)	210–563 micromol/L	2.10–5.63 mmol/L

F

POTENTIAL MEDICAL DIAGNOSIS

Increased in:

- Patients with diabetes with poor glucose control

Decreased in:

- Severe hypoproteinemia

CRITICAL FINDINGS: N/A

Find and print out the full study on Fast Find at davispl.us/vanleeuwen7.

Fundoscopy With or Without Photography

SYNONYM/ACRONYM: Funduscopy, ophthalmoscopy.

COMMON USE: To evaluate vascular and structural changes in the eye in assessing the progression of diseases such as glaucoma, diabetic retinopathy, and macular degeneration.

AREA OF APPLICATION: Eyes.

DESCRIPTION: Fundoscopy is performed as part of a routine eye examination. This test involves the examination of the structures of the eye to document the condition of the eye, detect abnormalities, and assist in following the progress of treatment. The fundus is the inner lining of the eye. The retina, optic disc, and macula can be visualized directly or indirectly by fundoscopic examination. Photographic images may be taken through dilated pupils to document findings for review and comparison. The Amsler grid is an additional test that may be included in the eye examination, especially if macular degeneration is suspected. This simple test for central vision can be performed using a grid with instructions printed from a home computer.

This procedure is contraindicated for

- Patients with acute narrow-angle glaucoma if pupil dilation is performed; dilation can initiate a severe and sight-threatening open-angle attack.
- Patients with allergies to mydriatics if pupil dilation using mydriatics is performed.

INDICATIONS

- Detect the presence of choroidal nevus.
- Detect various types and stages of glaucoma.
- Document the presence of diabetic retinopathy.
- Document the presence of macular degeneration and any other degeneration and any associated hemorrhaging.
- Observe ocular effects resulting from the long-term use of high-risk medications.

POTENTIAL MEDICAL DIAGNOSIS

Normal findings

- Normal optic nerve and vessels
- No evidence of other ocular abnormalities

Abnormal findings related to

- Aneurysm
- Atrial hypertension
- Benign intracranial hypertension from brain tumor
- Choroidal nevus
- Color vision deficiencies
- Diabetic retinopathy
- Disorders of the optic nerve
- Glaucoma
- Histoplasmosis
- Macular degeneration
- Obstructive disorders of the arteries or veins that lead to collateral circulation
- Papilledema
- Raised intracranial pressure associated with hydrocephalus
- Retinal detachment or tear
- Sickle cell anemia
- Stroke

CRITICAL FINDINGS:

- Detached retina

Flashers, floaters, or a veil that moves across the field of vision may indicate detached retina or retinal tear. This condition requires immediate examination by an ophthalmologist. Untreated, full retinal detachment can result in irreversible and complete loss of vision in the affected eye.

Note and immediately report to the requesting health-care provider (HCP) any critical findings and related symptoms. A listing of these findings varies among facilities. Timely notification of a critical finding for laboratory or diagnostic studies is a role expectation of the professional nurse. The notification processes vary among facilities. Upon receipt of the critical finding, the information should be read back to the caller to verify accuracy.

INTERFERING FACTORS

Factors that may impair the results of the examination

- Inability of the patient to cooperate or remain still during the test because of age, significant pain, or mental status may interfere with the test results.
- Presence of cataracts may interfere with fundal view.
- Ineffective dilation of the pupils may impair clear imaging.
- Rubbing or squeezing the eyes may affect results.
- Failure to follow medication restrictions before the procedure may cause the procedure to be canceled or repeated.

NURSING IMPLICATIONS AND PROCEDURE

PRETEST:

- Positively identify the patient using at least two person-specific identifiers before services, treatments, or procedures are performed.
- ***Patient Teaching:*** Inform the patient this procedure assists in detecting changes in the eye that effect vision.
- Obtain a history of the patient's health concerns (especially known or suspected vision loss; changes in visual acuity, including type and cause; use of glasses or contact lenses; and eye conditions with treatment regimens), symptoms, surgical procedures, and results of previously performed laboratory and diagnostic studies. Include a list of known allergens, especially allergies or sensitivities to latex or mydriatics (if dilation is to be performed).
- Obtain a list of the patient's current medications, including over-the-counter medications and dietary supplements (see Effects of Natural Products on Laboratory Values online at Davis*Plus*).
- Instruct the patient to remove contact lenses or glasses, as appropriate. Instruct the patient regarding the importance of keeping the eyes open for the test.
- Review the procedure with the patient. Explain that the patient will be requested to fixate the eyes during the procedure. Address concerns about pain and explain that mydriatics, if used, may cause blurred vision and sensitivity to light. There may also be a brief stinging sensation when the drop is put in the eye, but no discomfort will be experienced during the examination. Inform the patient that an HCP performs the test, in a quiet, darkened room, and that to dilate and evaluate both eyes, the test can take up to 60 min or longer if photographs are included.
- ***Sensitivity to social and cultural issues,*** as well as concern for modesty, is important in providing psychological support before, during, and after the procedure.
- Note that there are no food or fluid restrictions, unless by medical direction.
- Instruct the patient to avoid eye medications (particularly miotic eye drops which may constrict the pupil preventing a clear view of the fundus and mydriatic eyedrops in order to avoid instigation of an acute open angle attack in patients with narrow angle glaucoma) for at least 1 day prior to the test.
- Ensure that the patient understands that he or she must refrain from driving until the pupils return to normal (about 4 hr) after the test and has made arrangements to have someone else be responsible for transportation after the test.

INTRATEST:

Potential Complications:

Dilation can initiate a severe and sight-threatening open-angle attack in patients with narrow-angle glaucoma.

- Observe standard precautions, and follow the general guidelines in Patient Preparation and Specimen Collection online at Davis*Plus*. Positively identify the patient.
- Ensure that the patient has complied with medication restrictions; ensure that eye medications, especially miotics and mydriatics, have been restricted for at least 1 day prior to the test.
- Instruct the patient to cooperate fully and to follow directions. Instruct the patient to remain still during the procedure because movement produces unreliable results.
- Seat the patient in a chair that faces the camera. Instruct the patient to look at a directed target while the eyes are examined.
- Administer the ordered mydriatic to each eye and repeat in 5 to 15 min if dilation is to be performed. Drops are placed in the eye with the patient looking up and the solution directed at the six o'clock position of the

sclera (white of the eye) near the limbus (gray, semitransparent area of the eyeball where the cornea and sclera meet). Neither dropper nor bottle should touch the eyelashes.

- Instruct the patient to place the chin in the chin rest and gently press the forehead against the support bar. Instruct the patient to open his or her eyes wide and look at desired target while the HCP examines the fundus, with or without dilation. The examination is performed at a variety of prescribed levels of gaze. The patient should be encouraged to maintain a constant gaze but informed that he or she can blink as needed. The direct examination is performed using an instrument called an *ophthalmoscope*. The instrument is about the size of a penlight through which a beam of light is directed into the pupil while the HCP uses magnifying lenses to visualize the interior of the fundus. The indirect examination is carried out using either a binocular indirect ophthalmoscope, a slit-lamp microscope and hand lens, or a hand lens with the light source affixed to the HCP's head.

POST-TEST:

- Inform the patient that a report of the results will be made available to the requesting HCP, who will discuss the results with the patient.
- Instruct the patient to resume usual medications, as directed by the HCP.
- ***Nutritional Considerations:*** Increased glucose levels may be associated with diabetes. There is no "diabetic diet"; however, many meal-planning approaches with nutritional goals are endorsed by the American Diabetes Association (ADA). 🍁 Patients who adhere to dietary recommendations report a better general feeling of health, better weight management, greater control of glucose and lipid values, and improved use of insulin. Instruct the patient, as appropriate, in nutritional management of diabetes. A variety of dietary patterns are beneficial for people with diabetes. The Mediterranean-style diet emphasizes inclusion of vegetables, whole grains, fruits, low-fat dairy, nuts, legumes, and nontropical vegetable oils (e.g., olive, canola, peanut, sunflower, flaxseed) along with fish and lean poultry. A similar dietary pattern known as the Dietary Approaches to Stop Hypertension (DASH) diet makes additional recommendations for the reduction of dietary sodium. Both dietary styles emphasize a reduction in consumption of red meats, which are high in saturated fats and cholesterol, and other foods containing sugar, saturated fats, trans fats, and sodium. A vegetarian diet as well as other potential weight loss diets such as Weight Watchers are also supported by the ADA. 🍁 If triglycerides also are elevated, the patient should be advised to eliminate or reduce alcohol. The nutritional needs of each patient with diabetic patient need to be determined individually (especially during pregnancy) with the appropriate HCPs, particularly professionals educated in nutrition.
- ***Social and Cultural Considerations:*** Studies comparing risk for developing diabetes demonstrate that certain populations are disproportionately affected by type 2 diabetes and complications of type 2 diabetes as compared to the general population. Nonmodifiable risk factors include age, ethnicity, and family history of diabetes or metabolic syndrome. The risk of developing type 2 diabetes increases with age. In the United States, affected populations include African Americans, Asian Americans, Hispanics, native Hawaiians and Pacific Islanders, American Indians, and Alaska natives. 🍁 Modifiable risk factors include lifestyle choices related to making healthy dietary choices, maintaining a healthy body weight, and meeting recommended levels of physical activity. The financial and emotional burdens of diabetes and related complications continue to grow at an alarming rate. A system for the prevention, management, and support of patients with type 2 diabetes should be provided

F

through the coordinated efforts of multidisciplinary partners using strategies that are culturally appropriate.

- Recognize anxiety related to test results, and be supportive of impaired activity related to vision loss or anticipated loss of driving privileges. Discuss the implications of abnormal test results on the patient's lifestyle. Provide teaching and information regarding the clinical implications of the test results, as appropriate. The American Optometric Association's recommendations for the frequency of eye examinations can be accessed at (www.aoa.org). 🍁 Emphasize, as appropriate, that good glycemic control delays the onset of and slows the progression of diabetic retinopathy, nephropathy, and neuropathy. Provide education regarding smoking cessation, as appropriate. Provide contact information regarding vision aids, if desired, for ABLEDATA (sponsored by the National Institute on Disability and Rehabilitation Research, available at www.abledata.com), the American Macular Degeneration Foundation (www.macular.org), American Heart Association (www.americanheart.org), American Diabetes Association (www.diabetes.org), the National Heart, Lung, and Blood Institute (www.nhlbi.nih.gov), Institute of Medicine of the National Academies (www.iom.edu), or the USDA's resource for nutrition (www.choosemyplate.gov). 🍁
- Instruct the patient to avoid strenuous physical activities, like lifting heavy objects, that may increase pressure in the eye, as ordered.
- Reinforce information given by the patient's HCP regarding further testing, treatment, or referral to another HCP. Inform the patient that visual acuity and responses to light may change. Suggest that the patient wear dark glasses after the test until the pupils return to normal size. Answer any questions or address any concerns voiced by the patient or family.
- Depending on the results of this procedure, additional testing may be performed to evaluate or monitor progression of the disease process and determine the need for a change in therapy. Evaluate test results in relation to the patient's symptoms and other tests performed.

RELATED STUDIES:

- Related tests include fluorescein angiography, fructosamine, glucagon, glucose, glycated hemoglobin, gonioscopy, insulin, intraocular pressure, microalbumin, plethysmography, refraction, slit-lamp biomicroscopy, and visual field testing.
- Refer to the Ocular System table online at Davis*Plus* for related tests by body system.

Gallium Scan

SYNONYM/ACRONYM: Ga scan.

COMMON USE: To assist in diagnosing, evaluating, and staging tumors and in detecting areas of infection, inflammation, and abscess.

AREA OF APPLICATION: Whole body.

DESCRIPTION: Gallium imaging is a nuclear medicine study that assists in diagnosing neoplasm and inflammation activity. Gallium, which has 90% sensitivity for inflammatory disease, is readily distributed throughout plasma and body tissues. Gallium imaging is sensitive in detecting abscesses, pneumonia, pyelonephritis, active sarcoidosis, and active tuberculosis. In immunocompromised patients, such as patients with AIDS, gallium imaging can detect complications such as *Pneumocystis jiroveci* pneumonitis. Gallium imaging is useful but less commonly performed in the diagnosis and staging of some neoplasms, including Hodgkin's disease, lymphoma, melanoma, and leukemia. Imaging can be performed 6 to 72 hr after injection of the gallium, and a gamma camera detects the radiation emitted from the injected radioactive material. A representative image of the distribution of the radioactive material is then obtained. Single-photon emission computed tomography (SPECT) has significantly improved the resolution and accuracy of gallium scanning and may or may not be included as part of the examination. SPECT enables images to be recorded from multiple angles around the body and reconstructs them by a computer to produce images, or *slices,* representing the area of interest at different levels. Generally, the nonspecificity of gallium imaging requires correlation with other diagnostic studies, such as computed tomography, CT/PET (positron emission tomography), magnetic resonance imaging, and ultrasonography.

This procedure is contraindicated for

Patients who are pregnant or suspected of being pregnant, unless the potential benefits of a procedure using radiation far outweigh the risk of radiation exposure to the fetus and mother.

INDICATIONS
- Aid in the diagnosis of infectious or inflammatory diseases.
- Evaluate lymphomas.
- Evaluate recurrent lymphomas or tumors after radiation therapy or chemotherapy.
- Perform as a screening examination for fever of undetermined origin.

POTENTIAL MEDICAL DIAGNOSIS

Normal findings
- Normal distribution of gallium; some localization of the radionuclide within the liver, spleen, bone, nasopharynx, lacrimal glands, breast, and bowel is expected

Abnormal findings related to
- Abscess
- Infection
- Inflammation
- Lymphoma
- Tumor

CRITICAL FINDINGS: N/A

INTERFERING FACTORS

Factors that may alter the results of the study

- Inability of the patient to cooperate or remain still during the procedure because of age, significant pain, or mental status.
- Metallic objects (e.g., jewelry, body rings) within the examination field, which may inhibit organ visualization and cause unclear images.
- Performance of other nuclear scans within the preceding 24 to 48 hr.
- Administration of certain medications (e.g., gastrin, cholecystokinin), which may interfere with gastric emptying.

G

Other considerations

- Improper injection of the radionuclide may allow the tracer to seep deep into the muscle tissue, producing erroneous hot spots.

NURSING IMPLICATIONS AND PROCEDURE

See Potential Nursing Problems on Fast Find at davispl.us/vanleeuwen7.

PRETEST:

- Positively identify the patient using at least two person-specific identifiers before services, treatments, or procedures are performed.
- *Patient Teaching:* Inform the patient this procedure can assist in identifying infection or other disease.
- Obtain a history of the patient's health concerns, symptoms, surgical procedures, and results of previously performed laboratory and diagnostic studies. Include a list of known allergens, especially allergies or sensitivities to latex, anesthetics, sedatives, or radionuclides. Ensure results of coagulation testing are obtained and recorded prior to the procedure; a creatinine level is also needed before contrast medium is to be used.
- Note any recent procedures that can interfere with test results, including examinations using iodine-based contrast medium.
- Record the date of the last menstrual period and determine the possibility of pregnancy in perimenopausal women.
- Obtain a list of the patient's current medications, including over-the-counter medications and dietary supplements (see Effects of Natural Products on Laboratory Values online at Davis*Plus*).
- Review the procedure with the patient. Address concerns about pain related to the procedure and explain that some pain may be experienced during the test, or there may be moments of discomfort. Reassure the patient that the radionuclide poses no radioactive hazard and rarely produces adverse effects. Inform the patient that the procedure is performed in a nuclear medicine department by an HCP specializing in this procedure, with support staff, and takes approximately 60 min. **Pediatric Considerations:** Preparing children for a gallium scan depends on the age of the child. Encourage parents to be truthful about what the child may experience during the procedure (e.g., the child may feel a pinch or minor discomfort when the intravenous (IV) needle is inserted) and to use words that they know their child will understand. Toddlers and preschool-age children have a very short attention span, so the best time to talk about the test is right before the procedure. The child should be assured that he or she will be allowed to bring a favorite comfort item into the examination room, and if appropriate, that a parent will be with the child during the procedure. Explain the importance of remaining still while the images are taken.
- *Sensitivity to social and cultural issues,* as well as concern for modesty, is important in providing psychological support before, during, and after the procedure.
- Explain that an IV line may be inserted to allow infusion of IV

fluids such as saline, anesthetics, sedatives, radionuclides, medications used in the procedure, or emergency medications.

- Instruct the patient to remove jewelry and other metallic objects from the area to be examined.
- Note that there are no food, fluid, or medication restrictions unless by medical direction.
- *Make sure a written and informed consent has been signed prior to the procedure and before administering any medications.*

INTRATEST:

Potential Complications:

Although it is rare, there is the possibility of allergic reaction to the radionuclide. Have emergency equipment and medications readily available. If the patient has a history of allergic reactions to any substance or drug, administer ordered prophylactic steroids or antihistamines before the procedure.

Establishing an IV site and injection of radionuclides is an invasive procedure. Complications are rare but do include bleeding from the puncture site ***related to a bleeding disorder, or the effects of natural products and medications with known anticoagulant, antiplatelet, or thrombolytic properties,*** hematoma ***related to blood leakage into the tissue following needle insertion,*** infection ***that might occur if bacteria from the skin surface is introduced at the puncture site,*** or nerve injury ***that might occur if the needle strikes a nerve.***

- Observe standard precautions, and follow the general guidelines in Patient Preparation and Specimen Collection online at Davis*Plus.* Positively identify the patient.
- Ensure that the patient has removed all external metallic objects from the area to be examined prior to the procedure.
- Administer ordered prophylactic steroids or antihistamines before the procedure if the patient has a history of allergic reactions to any substance or drug.
- Avoid the use of equipment containing latex if the patient has a history of allergic reaction to latex.
- Have emergency equipment readily available.
- Instruct the patient to void prior to the procedure and to change into the gown, robe, and foot coverings provided.
- Record baseline vital signs and assess neurological status. Protocols may vary among facilities.
- Establish an IV fluid line for the injection of saline, anesthetics, sedatives, radionuclides, or emergency medications.
- Instruct the patient to cooperate fully and to follow directions. Instruct the patient to lie still during the procedure because movement produces unclear images.
- Administer a sedative to a child or to an uncooperative adult, as ordered.
- Place the patient in a supine position on a flat table with foam wedges, which help maintain position and immobilization.
- IV radionuclide is administered, and the patient is instructed to return for scanning at a designated time after injection. Typical scanning occurs at 6, 24, 48, 72, 96, and/or 120 hr postinjection depending on diagnosis.
- If an abdominal abscess or infection is suspected, laxatives or enemas may be ordered before imaging at 48 or 72 hr after the injection.
- Monitor the patient for complications related to the procedure (e.g., allergic reaction, anaphylaxis, bronchospasm).
- The needle or catheter is removed, and a pressure dressing is applied over the puncture site.
- Observe the needle/catheter insertion site for bleeding, inflammation, or hematoma formation.

POST-TEST:

- Inform the patient that a report of the results will be made available

G

to the requesting HCP, who will discuss the results with the patient.

- Unless contraindicated, advise the patient to drink increased amounts of fluids for 24 to 48 hr to eliminate the radionuclide from the body. Inform the patient that radionuclide is eliminated from the body within 6 to 24 hr.
- Instruct the patient to resume usual medication or activity, as directed by the HCP.
- Instruct the patient in the care and assessment of the injection site.
- If a woman who is breastfeeding must have a nuclear scan, she should not breastfeed the infant until the radionuclide has been eliminated. This could take as long as 3 days. She should be instructed to express the milk and discard it during the 3-day period to prevent cessation of milk production.
- Instruct the patient to immediately flush the toilet and to meticulously wash hands with soap and water after each voiding for 24 hr after the procedure.
- Instruct all caregivers to wear gloves when discarding urine for 48 hr after the procedure. Wash gloved hands with soap and water before removing gloves; then wash ungloved hands.
- Recognize anxiety related to test results, and be supportive of perceived loss of independent function. Discuss the implications of abnormal test results on the patient's lifestyle. Provide teaching and information regarding the clinical implications of the test results, as appropriate.
- Reinforce information given by the patient's HCP regarding further testing, treatment, or referral to another HCP. Answer any questions or address any concerns voiced by the patient or family.
- Depending on the results of this procedure, additional testing may be needed to evaluate or monitor progression of the disease process and determine the need for a change in therapy. Evaluate test results in relation to the patient's symptoms and other tests performed.

Patient Education:

- Explain to the patient that talking about his or her fears and concerns can be beneficial to assist coping.
- Teach the patient the pathophysiology associated with the disease process.

Expected Patient Outcomes:

Understanding

- The patient and family acknowledge the importance of adequate rest to facilitate the healing process.
- The patient and family acknowledge the importance of taking all ordered medications to improve health.

Ability

- The patient seeks spiritual guidance to address personal fears and anxieties.
- The patient keeps a diary to catalog the amount of sleep each night and the number of times awakened.

Response

- The patient agrees to maintain an appropriate caloric intake.
- The patient agrees to counseling for anxiety and withdrawal.

RELATED STUDIES:

- Related tests include angiotensin converting enzyme, biopsy bone marrow, biopsy kidney, biopsy lung, blood gases, bronchoscopy, CBC, CBC WBC and differential, chest x-ray, CT abdomen, CT pelvis, CT thoracic, culture blood, culture and smear mycobacteria, culture viral, cytology sputum, cytology urine, ESR, HIV-1/2 antibodies, IVP, lung perfusion scan, MRI chest, MRI abdomen, mediastinoscopy, pleural fluid analysis, plethysmography, PFT, pulse oximetry, renogram, US kidney, and US lymph node.
- Refer to the Immune System table online at Davis*Plus* for related tests by body system.

γ-Glutamyltranspeptidase

SYNONYM/ACRONYM: Serum γ-glutamyltransferase, γ-glutamyl transpeptidase, GGT, SGGT.

COMMON USE: To assist in diagnosing and monitoring liver disease.

SPECIMEN: Serum collected in a gold-, red-, or red/gray-top tube. Plasma collected in a green-top (heparin) tube is also acceptable.

NORMAL FINDINGS: (Method: Enzymatic spectrophotometry)

Age	Conventional & SI Units
Newborn–6 mo	12–122 units/L
7 mo and older	
Male	0–30 units/L
Female	0–24 units/L

Values may be elevated in older adults due to the effects of medications and the presence of multiple chronic or acute diseases with or without muted symptoms.

DESCRIPTION: Glutamyltransferase (GGT) assists with the reabsorption of amino acids and peptides from the glomerular filtrate and intestinal lumen. Hepatobiliary, renal tubular, and pancreatic tissues contain large amounts of GGT. Other sources include the prostate gland, brain, and heart. GGT is elevated in all types of liver disease and is more responsive to biliary obstruction, cholangitis, or cholecystitis than any of the other enzymes used as markers for liver disease.

This procedure is contraindicated for: N/A

INDICATIONS
- Assist in the diagnosis of obstructive jaundice in neonates.
- Detect the presence of liver disease.
- Evaluate and monitor patients with known or suspected alcohol abuse (levels rise after ingestion of small amounts of alcohol).

POTENTIAL MEDICAL DIAGNOSIS

Increased in:

GGT is released from any damaged cell in which it is stored, so conditions that affect the liver, kidneys, or pancreas and cause cellular destruction demonstrate elevated GGT levels.

- Cirrhosis
- Diabetes with hypertension
- Hepatitis
- Hepatobiliary tract disorders
- Hepatocellular carcinoma
- Hyperthyroidism ***(there is a strong association with concurrent liver abnormalities)***
- Infectious mononucleosis
- Kidney transplantation
- Obstructive liver disease
- Pancreatitis
- Significant alcohol ingestion

G

Decreased in:

- Hypothyroidism ***(related to decreased enzyme production by the liver)***

CRITICAL FINDINGS: N/A

INTERFERING FACTORS

- Drugs and other substances that may increase GGT levels include acetaminophen, alcohol, aminoglutethimide, anticonvulsants, aurothioglucose, barbiturates, captopril, cetirizine, dactinomycin, dantrolene, estrogens, flucytosine, halothane, labetalol, medroxyprogesterone, meropenem, methyldopa, naproxen, niacin, nortriptyline, oral contraceptives, pegaspargase, phenothiazines, piroxicam, probenecid, rifampin, streptokinase, tocainide, and trifluoperazine.
- Drugs and other substances that may decrease GGT levels include clofibrate, conjugated estrogens, and ursodiol.

NURSING IMPLICATIONS AND PROCEDURE

G

POTENTIAL NURSING PROBLEMS:

Problem	Signs & Symptoms	Interventions
Fatigue ***(related to hepatic disease process; malnutrition; anemia; chemotherapy; radiation therapy)***	Decreased concentration; increased physical complaints; inability to restore energy with sleep; reports being tired; inability to maintain normal routine	Assess for physical cause of fatigue; pace activities to preserve energy stores; rate fatigue on a numeric scale to trend degree of fatigue over time; identify what aggravates and decreases fatigue; assess for related emotional factors such as depression; evaluate current medications in relation to fatigue; assess for physiologic factors such as anemia
Confusion ***(related to an alteration in fluid and electrolytes, hepatic disease, and encephalopathy; acute alcohol consumption; hepatic metabolic insufficiency)***	Disorganized thinking, restlessness, irritability, altered concentration and attention span, changeable mental function over the day, hallucinations; inability to follow directions; disoriented to person, place, time, and purpose; inappropriate affect	Treat the medical condition; correlate confusion with the need to reverse altered electrolytes; evaluate medications; prevent falls and injury through appropriate use of postural support, bed alarm, or restraints; consider pharmacological interventions; record accurate intake and output to assess fluid status; monitor blood ammonia level; determine last alcohol use; assess for symptoms of hepatic encephalopathy such as confusion, sleep

Problem	Signs & Symptoms	Interventions
		disturbances, incoherence; protect the patient from physical harm; administer lactulose as prescribed
Fluid volume (water) ***(related to vomiting; decreased intake; compromised kidney function; overly aggressive fluid resuscitation; overly aggressive diuresis)***	**Overload:** Edema, shortness of breath, increased weight, ascites, rales, rhonchi, and diluted laboratory values. **Deficient:** Decreased urinary output, fatigue, and sunken eyes, dark urine, decreased blood pressure, increased heart rate, and altered mental status	Record daily weight and monitor trends; record accurate intake and output; collaborate with health-care provider (HCP) with administration of intravenous (IV) fluids to support hydration; monitor laboratory values that reflect alterations in fluid status (potassium, blood urea nitrogen, creatinine, calcium, hemoglobin, and hematocrit); manage underlying cause of fluid alteration; monitor urine characteristics and respiratory status; establish baseline assessment data; collaborate with HCP to adjust oral and IV fluids to provide optimal hydration status; administer replacement electrolytes as ordered
Skin ***(related to jaundice and elevated bilirubin levels; excessive scratching)***	Jaundiced skin and sclera; dry skin; itching skin; damage to skin associated with scratching	Apply lotion to keep the skin moisturized; avoid alkaline soaps; discourage scratching; apply mittens if patient is not able to follow direction to avoid scratching; administer antihistamines as ordered

PRETEST:

- Positively identify the patient using at least two person-specific identifiers before services, treatments, or procedures are performed.
- *Patient Teaching:* Inform the patient this test can assist in assessing liver function.
- Obtain a history of the patient's health concerns, symptoms, surgical procedures, and results of previously performed laboratory and diagnostic studies. Include a list of known allergens, especially allergies or sensitivities to latex.
- Obtain a history of IV drug use, alcohol use, high-risk sexual activity, and occupational exposure.
- Obtain a list of the patient's current medications, including over-the-counter medications and dietary supplements (see Effects of Natural Products on Laboratory Values online at Davis*Plus*).
- Review the procedure with the patient. Inform the patient that specimen collection takes approximately 5 to 10 min. Address concerns about pain and explain that there may be some discomfort during the venipuncture.

- ***Sensitivity to social and cultural issues,*** as well as concern for modesty, is important in providing psychological support before, during, and after the procedure.
- Note that there are no food, fluid, or medication restrictions unless by medical direction.

INTRATEST:

Potential Complications: N/A

- Avoid the use of equipment containing latex if the patient has a history of allergic reaction to latex.
- Instruct the patient to cooperate fully and to follow directions. Direct the patient to breathe normally and to avoid unnecessary movement.
- Observe standard precautions, and follow the general guidelines in Patient Preparation and Specimen Collection online at Davis*Plus*. Positively identify the patient, and label the appropriate specimen container with the corresponding patient demographics, initials of the person collecting the specimen, date, and time of collection. Perform a venipuncture.
- Remove the needle and apply direct pressure with dry gauze to stop bleeding. Observe/assess venipuncture site for bleeding or hematoma formation and secure gauze with adhesive bandage.
- Promptly transport the specimen to the laboratory for processing and analysis.

POST-TEST:

- Inform the patient that a report of the results will be sent to the requesting HCP, who will discuss the results with the patient.
- ***Nutritional Considerations:*** Increased GGT levels may be associated with liver disease. Dietary recommendations may be indicated and vary depending on the condition and its severity. Currently, there are specific drugs being used to treat different types of viral hepatitis. For example, there are a number of drugs used to treat hepatitis B such as peglated interferon (adults only), interferon alpha (adults and children), and lamivudine (adults and children); harvoni and solvaldi are examples of drugs used to treat hepatitis C. There are also drugs that can be given to treat and reverse the symptoms of non-viral hepatitis once the primary cause of hepatic inflammation is identified. Elimination of alcohol ingestion and a diet optimized for convalescence are commonly included in the treatment plan. A high-calorie, high-protein, moderate-fat diet with a high fluid intake is often recommended for patients with hepatitis. Treatment of cirrhosis is different because a low-protein diet may be in order if the patient's liver has lost the ability to process the end products of protein metabolism. A diet of soft foods also may be required if esophageal varices have developed. Ammonia levels may be used to determine whether protein should be added to or reduced from the diet. The patient should be encouraged to eat simple carbohydrates and emulsified fats (as in homogenized milk or eggs) rather than complex carbohydrates (e.g., starch, fiber, and glycogen [animal carbohydrates]) and complex fats, which require additional bile to emulsify them so that they can be used. The cirrhotic patient should also be carefully observed for the development of ascites, in which case fluid and electrolyte balance requires strict attention. The alcoholic patient should be encouraged to avoid alcohol and to seek appropriate counseling for substance abuse.
- Recognize anxiety related to test results, and be supportive of impaired activity related to lack of neuromuscular control, perceived loss of independence, and fear of shortened life expectancy.
- Depending on the results of this procedure, additional testing may be performed to evaluate or monitor progression of the disease process and determine the need for a change

in therapy. Evaluate test results in relation to the patient's symptoms and other tests performed.

Patient Education:

- Educate the patient regarding access to counseling services.
- Provide teaching and information regarding the clinical implications of the test results, as appropriate.
- Reinforce information given by the patient's HCP regarding further testing, treatment, or referral to another HCP.
- Answer any questions or address any concerns voiced by the patient or family.
- Discuss the implications of abnormal test results on the patient's lifestyle.
- Explain to the patient that ongoing fatigue can impact his or her ability to meet personal role performance expectations.
- Explain that both physical and emotional factors can contribute to fatigue.

Expected Patient Outcomes:

Understanding

- The patient and family state that untreated chronic fatigue can decrease quality of life.
- The patient and family identify how adequate nutrition may assist to decrease fatigue.

Ability

- The patient independently reviews his or her current list of medications to evaluate if any prescription or nonprescription medications are contributing to fatigue.
- The patient and family accurately develop a list of actions that can be taken to reduce fatigue and promote positive health.

Response

- The patient complies with the recommendation to obtain a sleep-disorder evaluation to assess for other causes of fatigue.
- The patient recognizes that both excess and inadequate exercise can contribute to fatigue and makes an effort to pace physical energy expenditures appropriately.

G

RELATED STUDIES:

- Related tests include ALT, ALP ammonia, AST, bilirubin, cholangiography percutaneous transhepatic, electrolytes, HAV antibody, HBV antigen and antibody, HCV antibody, hepatobiliary scan, infectious mono screen, KUB studies, liver and spleen scan, MRI liver, TSH, US abdomen, and US liver.
- Refer to the Hepatobiliary System table online at Davis*Plus* for related tests by body system.

Gastric Analysis and Gastric Acid Stimulation Test

SYNONYM/ACRONYM: N/A

COMMON USE: To evaluate gastric fluid and the amount of gastric acid secreted toward diagnosing gastrointestinal disorders such as ulcers, cancers, and inflammation.

SPECIMEN: Gastric fluid collected in eight plastic tubes at 15-min intervals.

NORMAL FINDINGS: (Method: Volume measurement and pH by ion-selective electrode)

Basal acid output (BAO)	Male: 0–10.5 mmol/hr Female: 0–5.6 mmol/hr
Peak acid output (PAO)	Male: 12–60 mmol/hr Female: 8–40 mmol/hr
Peak response time	Pentagastrin, intramuscular: 15–45 min Pentagastrin, subcutaneous: 10–30 min
BAO/PAO ratio	Less than 0.2

POTENTIAL MEDICAL DIAGNOSIS

Increased in:

Any alteration in the balance between the digestive and protective functions of the stomach that increases gastric acidity, such as hypersecretion of gastrin, use of NSAIDs, or *Helicobacter pylori* ***infection.***

Appearance

- Color

  Yellow to green indicates the presence of bile ***(related to obstruction in the small intestine distal to the ampulla of Vater)***

  Pink, red, brown indicates the presence of blood ***(related to some type of gastric lesion evidenced by ulcer, gastritis, or carcinoma)***

- Microscopic evaluation

  Red blood cells ***(related to trauma or active bleeding)***

  White blood cells ***(related to inflammation of the gastric mucosa, mouth, paranasal sinuses, or respiratory tract)***

  Epithelial cells ***(related to inflammation of the gastric mucosa)***

  Malignant cells ***(related to gastric carcinoma)***

  Bacteria and yeast ***(related to conditions such as pyloric obstruction, pulmonary tuberculosis)***

  Parasites ***(related to parasitic infestation such as*** *Giardia, H. pylori,* ***hookworm, or*** *Strongyloides)*

Increased Gastric Acid Output

- BAO

  Basophilic leukemia
  Duodenal ulcer
  G-cell hyperplasia
  Recurring peptic ulcer
  Retained antrum syndrome
  Systemic mastocytosis
  Vagal hyperfunction
  Zollinger-Ellison syndrome

- PAO

  Duodenal ulcer
  Zollinger-Ellison syndrome

Decreased in:

Conditions that result in the gradual loss of function of the antrum and G cells, where gastrin is produced, will reflect decreased gastrin levels.

Decreased Gastric Acid Output

- BAO

  Gastric ulcer

- PAO

  Chronic gastritis
  Gastric cancers
  Gastric polyps
  Gastric ulcer
  Myxedema
  Pernicious anemia

CRITICAL FINDINGS: N/A

Find and print out the full study on Fast Find at davispl.us/vanleeuwen7.

Gastric Emptying Scan

SYNONYM/ACRONYM: Gastric emptying quantitation, gastric emptying scintigraphy.

COMMON USE: To visualize and assess the time frame for gastric emptying to assist in the diagnosis of diseases such as gastroenteritis and dumping syndrome.

AREA OF APPLICATION: Esophagus, stomach, small bowel.

DESCRIPTION: A gastric emptying scan quantifies gastric emptying physiology. The procedure is indicated for patients with gastric motility symptoms, including diabetic gastroparesis, anorexia nervosa, gastric outlet obstruction syndromes, postvagotomy and postgastrectomy syndromes, and assessment of medical and surgical treatments for diseases known to affect gastric motility. A radionuclide is administered, and the clearance of solids and liquids may be evaluated. The images are recorded electronically, showing the gastric emptying function over time.

This procedure is contraindicated for

- Patients who are pregnant or suspected of being pregnant, unless the potential benefits of a procedure using radiation far outweigh the risks to the fetus and mother.
- Patients with esophageal motor disorders or swallowing difficulties.

INDICATIONS

- Investigate the cause of rapid or slow rate of gastric emptying.
- Measure gastric emptying rate.

POTENTIAL MEDICAL DIAGNOSIS

Normal findings

- Mean time emptying of liquid phase: 30 min (range, 11–49 min)
- Mean time emptying of solid phase: 40 min (range, 28–80 min)
- No delay in gastric emptying rate

Abnormal findings related to

- Decreased rate of gastric emptying:
  - Amyloidosis
  - Anorexia nervosa
  - Gastric outlet obstruction
  - Gastric ulcer
  - Gastroenteritis
  - Gastroesophageal reflux
  - Gastroparesis (e.g. damage to nerves that control stomach muscles related to diabetes or as a result of surgery)
  - Hypokalemia, hypomagnesemia
  - Postoperative ileus
  - Post–radiation therapy period
  - Scleroderma
- Increased rate of gastric emptying:
  - Dumping syndrome
  - Post–gastric surgery period
  - Zollinger-Ellison syndrome

CRITICAL FINDINGS: N/A

INTERFERING FACTORS

Factors that may alter the results of the study

- Inability of the patient to cooperate or remain still during the procedure because of age, significant pain, or mental status.
- Metallic objects (e.g., jewelry, body rings) within the examination field, which may inhibit organ visualization and cause unclear images.
- Retained barium from a previous radiological procedure.
- Other nuclear scans done within the previous 24 to 48 hr.

- **Administration of certain medications (e.g., gastrin, cholecystokinin), which may interfere with gastric emptying.**

Other considerations

- **Failure to follow dietary restrictions before the procedure may cause the procedure to be canceled or repeated.**

NURSING IMPLICATIONS AND PROCEDURE

PRETEST:

- Positively identify the patient using at least two person-specific identifiers before services, treatments, or procedures are performed.
- *Patient Teaching:* Inform the patient this procedure can assist in evaluating the time it takes for the stomach to empty.
- Obtain a history of the patient's health concerns, symptoms, surgical procedures, and results of previously performed laboratory and diagnostic studies. Include a list of known allergens, especially allergies or sensitivities to latex, anesthetics, sedatives, or radionuclides.
- Note any recent procedures that can interfere with test results, including examinations using barium- or iodine-based contrast medium.
- Record the date of the last menstrual period and determine the possibility of pregnancy in perimenopausal women.
- Obtain a list of the patient's current medications, including over-the-counter medications and dietary supplements (see Effects of Natural Products on Laboratory Values online at Davis*Plus*).
- Review the procedure with the patient. Address concerns about pain related to the procedure and explain that some pain may be experienced during the test, and there may be moments of discomfort. Reassure the patient that the radionuclide poses no radioactive hazard and rarely produces adverse effects. Inform the patient that the procedure is performed in a nuclear medicine department by an health-care provider (HCP) specializing in this procedure, with support staff, and takes approximately 30 to 120 min. **Pediatric Considerations:** Preparing children for a gastric emptying scan depends on the age of the child. Encourage parents to be truthful about what the child may experience during the procedure (e.g., length of time the exam will take and the need to intermittently have scans performed), stressing the importance of eating as much of the "breakfast" as possible so the test is successful, and to use words that they know their child will understand. Toddlers and preschool-age children have a short attention span, so the best time to talk about the test is right before the procedure. The child should be assured that he or she will be allowed to bring a favorite comfort item into the examination room, and if appropriate, that a parent will be with the child during the procedure. Explain the importance of remaining still while the images are taken.
- *Sensitivity to social and cultural issues,* as well as concern for modesty, is important in providing psychological support before, during and after the procedure.
- Instruct the patient to restrict food and fluids for 8 hr before the scan. Inquire about allergic reactions to eggs. Protocols may vary among facilities.
- Instruct the patient to remove jewelry and other metallic objects from the area to be examined.
- *Make sure a written and informed consent has been signed prior to the procedure and before administering any medications.*

INTRATEST:

Potential Complications:

Although it is rare, there is the possibility of allergic reaction to the radionuclide. Have emergency equipment and medications readily available. If the patient has a history of allergic reactions to any substance or drug, administer ordered prophylactic steroids or antihistamines before the procedure.

- Observe standard precautions, and follow the general guidelines in Patient Preparation and Specimen Collection online at Davis*Plus*. Positively identify the patient.
- Ensure the patient has complied with dietary and fluid restrictions prior to the study, as instructed. Ensure that the patient does not have a known allergy to eggs.
- Ensure that the patient has removed all external metallic objects from the area to be examined prior to the procedure.
- Instruct the patient to void prior to the procedure and to change into the gown, robe, and foot coverings provided.
- Record baseline vital signs and neurological status. Protocols may vary among facilities.
- Avoid the use of equipment containing latex if the patient has a history of allergic reaction to latex.
- Instruct the patient to cooperate fully and to follow directions. Instruct the patient to remain still during the procedure because movement produces unclear images.
- Administer a sedative to a child or to an adult who is uncooperative, as ordered.
- Place the patient in an upright or supine position in front of the gamma camera; positioning protocols may vary among facilities.
- Ask the patient to take the radionuclide mixed with water or other liquid orally, or combined with eggs for a solid study. **Pediatric Considerations:** If the patient is an infant, a small amount of radionuclide will be added to the patient's feeding.
- Images are recorded over a period of time (30 to 60 min) and evaluated with regard to the amount of time the stomach takes to empty its contents.

POST-TEST:

- Inform the patient that a report of the results will be made available to the requesting HCP, who will discuss the results with the patient.
- Advise the patient to drink increased amounts of fluids for 24 to 48 hr to eliminate the radionuclide from the body, unless contraindicated. Tell the patient that radionuclide is eliminated from the body within 6 to 24 hr.
- Monitor vital signs every 15 min for 1 hr, then every 2 hr for 4 hr, and then as ordered by the HCP. Monitor intake and output at least every 8 hr. Compare with baseline values. Protocols may vary among facilities.
- Instruct the patient to resume usual diet, fluids, medication, and activity, as directed by the HCP.
- If a woman who is breastfeeding must have a nuclear scan, she should not breastfeed the infant until the radionuclide has been eliminated. This could take as long as 3 days. She should be instructed to express the milk and discard it during the 3-day period to prevent cessation of milk production.
- Instruct the patient to immediately flush the toilet and to meticulously wash hands with soap and water after each voiding for 24 hr after the procedure.
- Instruct all caregivers to wear gloves when discarding urine for 24 hr after the procedure. Wash gloved hands with soap and water before removing gloves; then wash ungloved hands.
- Recognize anxiety related to test results, and be supportive of perceived loss of independent function. Discuss the implications of abnormal test results on the patient's lifestyle. Provide teaching and information regarding the clinical implications of the test results, as appropriate.
- Reinforce information given by the patient's HCP regarding further testing, treatment, or referral to another HCP. Answer any questions or address any concerns voiced by the patient or family.
- Depending on the results of this procedure, additional testing may be needed to evaluate or monitor progression of the disease process

G

and determine the need for a change in therapy. Evaluate test results in relation to the patient's symptoms and other tests performed.

RELATED STUDIES:

- Related tests include barium swallow, biopsy kidney, biopsy liver, biopsy lung, calcitonin stimulation, calcium, capsule endoscopy, CT abdomen, esophageal manometry, EGD, fecal analysis, gastric fluid analysis and gastric acid stimulation test, gastrin and gastrin stimulation test, GI blood loss scan, glucose, glycated hemoglobin, *H. pylori* antibodies, liver and spleen scan, magnesium, PTH, UGI and small bowel series, and vitamin B_{12}.
- Refer to the Gastrointestinal System table online at Davis*Plus* for related tests by body system.

Gastrin and Gastrin Stimulation Test

G

SYNONYM/ACRONYM: N/A

COMMON USE: To evaluate gastric production to assist in diagnosis of gastric disease such as Zollinger-Ellison syndrome and gastric cancer.

SPECIMEN: Serum collected in a red- or red/gray-top tube.

NORMAL FINDINGS: (Method: Immunoassay)

Age	Conventional Units	SI Units (Conventional Units × 0.481)
Child	Less than 125 pg/mL	Less than 60 pmol/L
Adult	Less than 100 pg/mL	Less than 48.1 pmol/L

Values represent fasting levels.

Stimulation Tests	
Gastrin stimulation test with secretin; 0.4 mcg/kg by intravenous bolus	No response or slight increase over baseline; increase of greater than 200 pg/ml (SI Units: 96 pmol/L above baseline is considered abnormal

Calcium may also be used as a stimulant.

POTENTIAL MEDICAL DIAGNOSIS

Increased in:

- Chronic gastritis ***(related to hypersecretion of gastrin, use of NSAIDs, or*** *Helicobacter pylori* ***infection)***
- Chronic kidney disease ***(related to inadequate renal excretion)***
- Gastric and duodenal ulcers ***(related to hypersecretion of gastrin, use of NSAIDs, or*** *H. pylori* ***infection)***
- Gastric carcinoma ***(related to disturbance in pH favoring alkalinity, which stimulates gastrin production)***
- G-cell hyperplasia ***(hyperplastic G cells produce excessive amounts of gastrin)***
- Hyperparathyroidism ***(related to hypercalcemia; calcium is a potent stimulator for the release of gastrin)***

- Pernicious anemia ***(related to antibodies against gastric intrinsic factor [66% of cases] and parietal cells [80% of cases that affect the stomach's ability to secrete acid; achlorhydria is a strong stimulator of gastrin production])***
- Pyloric obstruction ***(related to gastric distention, which stimulates gastrin production)***
- Retained antrum ***(remaining tissue stimulates gastrin production)***
- Zollinger-Ellison syndrome ***(gastrin-producing tumor)***

Decreased in:

- Hypothyroidism ***(related to hypocalcemia)***
- Vagotomy ***(vagus nerve impulses stimulate secretion of digestive secretions; interruptions in these nerve impulses result in decreased gastrin levels)***

CRITICAL FINDINGS: N/A

Find and print out the full study on Fast Find at davispl.us/vanleeuwen7.

Gastroesophageal Reflux Scan

G

SYNONYM/ACRONYM: Aspiration scan, GER scan, GERD scan, milk scan (pediatric patients).

COMMON USE: To assess for gastric reflux in relation to heartburn, difficulty swallowing, vomiting, and aspiration.

AREA OF APPLICATION: Esophagus and stomach.

DESCRIPTION: The gastroesophageal reflux (GER) scan assesses gastric reflux across the esophageal sphincter. Symptoms of GER can include heartburn, regurgitation, vomiting, dysphagia, and a bitter taste in the mouth. This procedure may be used to evaluate the medical or surgical treatment of pediatric and adult patients with GER and to detect aspiration of gastric contents into the lungs. A radionuclide such as technetium-99m sulfur colloid is ingested orally in orange juice and scanning studies are done immediately to assess the amount of liquid that has reached the stomach. An abdominal binder is applied and then tightened gradually to obtain images at increasing degrees of abdominal pressure: 0, 20, 40, 60, 80, and 100 mm Hg. A computer calculation determines the amount of reflux into the esophagus at each of these abdominal pressures as recorded on the images. For aspiration scans, images are taken over the lungs to detect possible tracheoesophageal aspiration of the radionuclide.

In infants, the study distinguishes between vomiting and reflux. Reflux occurs predominantly in infants younger than age 2 who are mainly on a milk diet. This procedure is indicated when an infant has symptoms such as failure to thrive, feeding problems, and episodes of wheezing with chest infection. The radionuclide is added to the infant's milk, images are obtained of the gastric and esophageal area, and the images are evaluated visually and by computer.

This procedure is contraindicated for

- Patients who are pregnant or suspected of being pregnant, unless the potential benefits of a procedure using radiation far outweigh the risk of radiation exposure to the fetus and mother.
- Patients with hiatal hernia, esophageal motor disorders, or swallowing difficulties.

G

INDICATIONS

- Aid in the diagnosis of GER in patients with unexplained nausea and vomiting.
- Distinguish between vomiting and reflux in infants with failure to thrive, feeding problems, and wheezing combined with chest infection.

POTENTIAL MEDICAL DIAGNOSIS

Normal findings

- Reflux less than or equal to 4% across the esophageal sphincter

Abnormal findings related to

- Reflux of greater than 4% at any pressure level
- Pulmonary aspiration

CRITICAL FINDINGS: N/A

INTERFERING FACTORS

Factors that may alter the results of the study

- Inability of the patient to cooperate or remain still during the procedure because of age, significant pain, or mental status.
- Metallic objects (e.g., jewelry, body rings, dentures) within the examination field, which may inhibit organ visualization and cause unclear images.
- Retained barium from a previous radiological procedure.
- Other nuclear scans done within the previous 24 to 48 hr.

Other considerations

- Failure to follow dietary restrictions before the procedure may cause the procedure to be canceled or repeated.

NURSING IMPLICATIONS AND PROCEDURE

See Potential Nursing Problems on Fast Find at davispl.us/vanleeuwen7.

PRETEST:

- Positively identify the patient using at least two person-specific identifiers before services, treatments, or procedures are performed.
- *Patient Teaching:* Inform the patient this procedure can assist in evaluating stomach reflux.
- Obtain a history of the patient's health concerns, symptoms, surgical procedures, and results of previously performed laboratory and diagnostic studies. Include a list of known allergens, especially allergies or sensitivities to latex, anesthetics, sedatives, or radionuclides.
- Note any recent procedures that can interfere with test results, including examinations using barium- or iodine-based contrast medium.
- Record the date of the last menstrual period and determine the possibility of pregnancy in perimenopausal women.
- Obtain a list of the patient's current medications, including over-the-counter medications and dietary supplements (see Effects of Natural Products on Laboratory Values online at Davis*Plus*).
- Review the procedure with the patient. Address concerns about pain related to the procedure and explain that some pain may be experienced during the test, or there may be moments of discomfort. Reassure the patient that the radionuclide

poses no radioactive hazard and rarely produces adverse effects. Inform the patient that the procedure is performed in a nuclear medicine department by a health-care provider (HCP) specializing in this procedure, with support staff, and takes approximately 30 to 60 min. **Pediatric Considerations:** Preparing children for a gastroesophageal reflux scan depends on the age of the child. Encourage parents to be truthful about what the child may experience during the procedure (e.g., the child may feel an upset stomach), stressing the importance of drinking as much of the "juice" as possible so the test is successful, and to use words that they know their child will understand. Toddlers and preschool-age children have a short attention span, so the best time to talk about the test is right before the procedure. The child should be assured that he or she will be allowed to bring a favorite comfort item into the examination room, and if appropriate, that a parent will be with the child during the procedure. Explain the importance of remaining still while the images are taken.

- *Sensitivity to social and cultural issues,* as well as concern for modesty, is important in providing psychological support before, during, and after the procedure.
- Instruct the patient to remove jewelry and other metallic objects from the area to be examined.
- Note that there are no food or fluid restrictions unless by medical direction.
- *Make sure a written and informed consent has been signed prior to the procedure and before administering any medications.*

INTRATEST:

Potential Complications:

Although it is rare, there is the possibility of allergic reaction to the radionuclide. Have emergency equipment and medications readily available. If the patient has a history of allergic reactions to any substance or drug, administer ordered prophylactic steroids or antihistamines before the procedure.

- Observe standard precautions, and follow the general guidelines in Patient Preparation and Specimen Collection online at Davis*Plus*. Positively identify the patient.
- Ensure that the patient has removed all external metallic objects from the area to be examined prior to the procedure.
- Avoid the use of equipment containing latex if the patient has a history of allergic reaction to latex.
- Have emergency equipment readily available.
- Instruct the patient to void prior to the procedure and to change into the gown, robe, and foot coverings provided.
- Record baseline vital signs and assess neurological status. Protocols may vary among facilities.
- Instruct the patient to cooperate fully and to follow directions. Instruct the patient to remain still throughout the procedure because movement produces unreliable results.
- Administer a sedative to a child or to an adult who is uncooperative, as ordered.
- Place the patient in an upright position and instruct him or her to ingest the radionuclide combined with orange juice. **Pediatric Considerations:** If the patient is an infant, a small amount of radionuclide will be added to the patient's feeding.
- Place the patient in a supine position on a flat table 15 min after ingestion.
- An abdominal binder with an attached sphygmomanometer is applied, and scans are taken as the binder is tightened at various pressures.
- If reflux occurs at lower pressures, an additional 30 mL of water may be given to clear the esophagus.
- Instruct the patient to take slow, deep breaths if nausea occurs during the procedure. Monitor and administer an antiemetic drug if ordered. Ready an emesis basin for use.

G

- Monitor the patient for complications related to the procedure (e.g., allergic reaction, anaphylaxis, bronchospasm).

POST-TEST:

- Inform the patient that a report of the results will be made available to the requesting HCP, who will discuss the results with the patient.
- Advise the patient to drink increased amounts of fluids for 24 to 48 hr to eliminate the radionuclide from the body unless contraindicated. Tell the patient that radionuclide is eliminated from the body within 6 to 24 hr.
- Monitor vital signs and neurological status every 15 min for 1 hr, then every 2 hr for 4 hr, and then as ordered by the HCP. Monitor intake and output at least every 8 hr. Compare with baseline values. Protocols may vary among facilities.
- Instruct the patient to resume usual diet, fluids, medication, and activity, as directed by the HCP.
- No other radionuclide tests should be scheduled for 24 to 48 hr after this procedure.
- If a woman who is breastfeeding must have a nuclear scan, she should not breastfeed the infant until the radionuclide has been eliminated. This could take as long as 3 days. She should be instructed to express the milk and discard it during the 3-day period to prevent cessation of milk production.
- Instruct the patient to immediately flush the toilet and to meticulously wash hands with soap and water after each voiding for 24 hr after the procedure.
- Instruct all caregivers to wear gloves when discarding urine for 24 hr after the procedure. Wash gloved hands with soap and water before removing gloves; then wash ungloved hands.
- *Nutritional Considerations:* A low-fat, low-cholesterol, and low-sodium diet should be consumed to reduce current disease processes. High fat consumption increases the amount of bile acids in the colon and should be avoided.
- Recognize anxiety related to test results, and be supportive of expected changes in lifestyle. Discuss the implications of abnormal test results on the patient's lifestyle. Provide teaching and information regarding the clinical implications of the test results, as appropriate.
- Reinforce information given by the patient's HCP regarding further testing, treatment, or referral to another HCP. Answer any questions or address any concerns voiced by the patient or family.
- Depending on the results of this procedure, additional testing may be needed to evaluate or monitor progression of the disease process and determine the need for a change in therapy. Evaluate test results in relation to the patient's symptoms and other tests performed.

Patient Education:

- Teach the patient to wear oxygen at all times to maintain specified oxygen saturation.
- Teach the patient how to design a method to manage gastric reflux.

Expected Patient Outcomes:

Understanding

- The patient and family acknowledge aspiration secondary to gastric reflux and the causal factor in altered gas exchange.
- The patient and family acknowledge the importance of following the established therapeutic regime to improve overall health.

Ability

- The patient describes the proper method and duration of self-administering ordered discharge antibiotics.
- The patient and family keep a food diary to identify foods that trigger gastric reflux.

Response

- The patient agrees to maintain NPO status until swallowing can be evaluated and safely restored.
- The patient agrees to lifestyle modifications to control disease process and symptoms.

RELATED STUDIES:

- Related tests include CT abdomen, esophageal manometry, gastric emptying scan, and upper GI series.
- Refer to the Gastrointestinal System table online at Davis*Plus* for related tests by body system.

Gastrointestinal Blood Loss Scan

SYNONYM/ACRONYM: Gastrointestinal bleed localization study, GI scintigram, GI bleed scintigraphy, lower GI blood loss scan.

COMMON USE: To detect areas of active gastrointestinal bleeding or hemorrhage to facilitate surgical intervention or medical treatment. Usefulness is limited in emergency situations because of time constraints in performing the scan.

AREA OF APPLICATION: Abdomen.

DESCRIPTION: Gastrointestinal (GI) blood loss scan is a nuclear medicine study that assists in detecting and localizing active GI tract bleeding (2 or 3 mL/min) for the purpose of better directing endoscopic or angiographic studies. This procedure can detect bleeding if the rate is greater than 0.5 mL/min, but it is not specific for site localization or cause of bleeding. Esophagogastroduodenoscopy is the procedure of choice for diagnosing upper GI bleeding. After injection of technetium-99m-labelled red blood cells, immediate and delayed images of various views of the abdomen are obtained. The radionuclide remains in the circulation long enough to extravasate and accumulate within the bowel lumen at the site of active bleeding. This procedure is valuable for the detection and localization of recent non-GI intra-abdominal hemorrhage. Images may be taken over an extended period to show intermittent bleeding.

Pediatrics: An upper GI series is usually done in the pediatric population to diagnose the cause of recurrent GI signs (bleeding) and symptoms. The etiology is often related to age. In infants, recurrent symptoms such as vomiting after feeding, poor feeding, poor weight gain, and abdominal pain (evidenced by frequent crying during or after a feeding) may trigger an investigation. The most common causes of upper or lower GI bleeding in infants up to 1 mo include allergies to milk proteins, anorectal fissures, bacterial enteritis, coagulopathy, esophagitis, Hirschsprung's disease, intussusception, peptic ulcer, stenosis, varices, or Meckel's diverticulum. Children between 2 to 23 months are most commonly diagnosed with allergies to milk proteins, anorectal fissures, esophagitis caused by gastroesophageal reflux (GER), gastritis, intussusception, Meckel's diverticulum, NSAID-induced ulcer, and ingested foreign body. Pediatric patients 24 mo and older are most commonly diagnosed with esophageal varices, Mallory Weiss tears, peptic ulcer, related to *Helicobacter* *pylori* infection or peptic ulcer secondary to some other type of systemic disease (e.g., Crohn's disease or inflammatory bowel disease [IBD]). Other abnormal findings in this age group include IBD, polyps, malignancy, sepsis, and Meckel's diverticulum.

This procedure is contraindicated for

Patients who are pregnant or suspected of being pregnant, unless the potential benefits of a procedure using radiation far outweigh the risk of radiation exposure to the fetus and mother.

INDICATIONS

- Diagnose unexplained abdominal pain and GI bleeding.

POTENTIAL MEDICAL DIAGNOSIS

Normal findings

- Normal distribution of radionuclide in the large vessels with no extravascular activity

Abnormal findings related to

The radioactive tracer will accumulate in areas of active bleeding, and "hot spots" will identify specific areas of concern.

- Angiodysplasia
- Aortoduodenal fistula
- Diverticulosis
- GI bleeding
- Inflammatory bowel disease
- Polyps
- Tumor
- Ulcer

CRITICAL FINDINGS:

- Acute GI bleed

Note and immediately report to the requesting health-care provider (HCP) any critical findings and related symptoms. A listing of these findings varies among facilities. Timely notification of a critical finding for laboratory or diagnostic studies is a role expectation of the professional nurse. The notification processes vary among facilities. Upon receipt of the critical finding, the information should be read back to the caller to verify accuracy.

INTERFERING FACTORS

Factors that may alter the results of the study

- Inability of the patient to cooperate or remain still during the procedure because of age, significant pain, or mental status.
- Retained barium from a previous radiological procedure.
- Metallic objects (e.g., jewelry, body rings) within the examination field, which may inhibit organ visualization and cause unclear images.
- Other nuclear scans done within the previous 24 to 48 hr.
- Inaccurate timing of imaging after the radionuclide injection.

Other considerations

- The examination detects only active or intermittent bleeding.
- The procedure is of little value in patients with chronic anemia or slowly decreasing hematocrit.
- The scan is less accurate for localization of bleeding sites in the upper GI tract.
- Improper injection of the radionuclide allows the tracer to seep deep into the muscle tissue, producing erroneous hot spots.
- The test is not specific, does not indicate the exact pathological condition causing the bleeding, and may miss small sites of bleeding (less than 0.5 mL/min) caused by diverticular disease or angiodysplasia.
- Physiologically unstable patients may be unable to be scanned over long periods or may need to go to surgery before the procedure is complete.

NURSING IMPLICATIONS AND PROCEDURE

See Potential Nursing Problems on Fast Find at davispl.us/vanleeuwen7.

PRETEST:

- Positively identify the patient using at least two person-specific identifiers before services, treatments, or procedures are performed.
- ***Patient Teaching:*** Inform the patient this procedure can assist in evaluating for stomach and intestinal bleeding.
- Obtain a history of the patient's health concerns, symptoms, surgical procedures, and results of previously performed laboratory and diagnostic studies. Include a list of known allergens, especially allergies or sensitivities to latex, anesthetics, sedatives, or radionuclides.
- Note any recent procedures that can interfere with test results, including examinations using barium- or iodine-based contrast medium.
- Record the date of the last menstrual period and determine the possibility of pregnancy in perimenopausal women.
- Obtain a list of the patient's current medications, including over-the-counter medications and dietary supplements (see Effects of Natural Products on Laboratory Values online at Davis*Plus*).
- Review the procedure with the patient. Address concerns about pain related to the procedure and explain that some pain may be experienced during the test, or there may be moments of discomfort. Reassure the patient that the radionuclide poses no radioactive hazard and rarely produces adverse effects. Inform the patient that the procedure is performed in a nuclear medicine department by a health-care provider (HCP) specializing in this procedure, with support staff, and takes approximately 60 min to complete, with additional images taken periodically over 24 hr as needed.
- Explain that an intravenous (IV) line may be inserted to allow infusion of fluids such as saline, anesthetics, sedatives, radionuclides, medications used in the procedure, or emergency medications.
- ***Sensitivity to social and cultural issues,*** as well as concern for modesty, is important in providing psychological support before, during, and after the procedure.
- Instruct the patient to remove jewelry and other metallic objects from the area to be examined.
- Note that there are no food or fluid restrictions unless by medical direction.
- *Make sure a written and informed consent has been signed prior to the procedure and before administering any medications.*

INTRATEST:

Potential Complications:

Although it is rare, there is the possibility of allergic reaction to the radionuclide. Have emergency equipment and medications readily available. If the patient has a history of allergic reactions to any substance or drug, administer ordered prophylactic steroids or antihistamines before the procedure.

Establishing an IV site and injection of radionuclides is an invasive procedure. Complications are rare but do include bleeding from the puncture site ***related to a bleeding disorder or the effects of natural products and medications with known anticoagulant, antiplatelet, or thrombolytic properties,*** hematoma ***related to blood leakage into the tissue following needle insertion,*** infection ***that might occur if bacteria from the skin surface is introduced at the puncture site,*** or nerve injury ***that might occur if the needle strikes a nerve.***

- Observe standard precautions, and follow the general guidelines in Patient Preparation and Specimen Collection online at Davis*Plus*. Positively identify the patient.

- Ensure that the patient has removed all external metallic objects from the area to be examined prior to the procedure.
- Instruct the patient to void prior to the procedure and to change into the gown, robe, and foot coverings provided.
- Record baseline vital signs and assess neurological status. Protocols may vary among facilities.
- Establish an IV fluid line for the injection of saline, anesthetics, sedatives, radionuclides, or emergency medications.
- Avoid the use of equipment containing latex if the patient has a history of allergic reaction to latex.
- Have emergency equipment readily available.
- Instruct the patient to cooperate fully and to follow directions. Instruct the patient to remain still throughout the procedure because movement produces unreliable results.
- Administer a sedative to a child or to an adult who is uncooperative, as ordered.
- Place the patient in a supine position on a flat table with foam wedges to help maintain position and immobilization.
- The radionuclide is administered IV, and images are recorded immediately and every 5 min over a period of 60 min in various positions. Additional images may be taken up to 24 hr after injection if initial images do not indicate active bleeding in the presence of clinical signs or symptoms of bleeding.
- The needle or catheter is removed, and a pressure dressing is applied over the puncture site.
- Observe/assess the needle/catheter insertion site for bleeding, inflammation, or hematoma formation.

POST-TEST:

- Inform the patient that a report of the results will be made available to the requesting HCP, who will discuss the results with the patient.
- Advise the patient to drink increased amounts of fluids for 24 to 48 hr to eliminate the radionuclide from the body, unless contraindicated. Tell the patient that radionuclide is eliminated from the body within 6 to 24 hr.
- Monitor vital signs and neurological status every 15 min for 1 hr, then every 2 hr for 4 hr, and then as ordered by the HCP. Monitor intake and output at least every 8 hr. Compare with baseline values. Protocols may vary among facilities.
- No other radionuclide tests should be scheduled for 24 to 48 hr after this procedure.
- Instruct the patient to resume usual diet, fluids, medication, and activity, as directed by the HCP.
- Instruct the patient in the care and assessment of the injection site.
- If a woman who is breastfeeding must have a nuclear scan, she should not breastfeed the infant until the radionuclide has been eliminated. This could take as long as 3 days. She should be instructed to express the milk and discard it during the 3-day period to prevent cessation of milk production.
- Instruct the patient to immediately flush the toilet and to meticulously wash hands with soap and water after each voiding for 24 hr after the procedure.
- Instruct all caregivers to wear gloves when discarding urine for 24 hr after the procedure. Wash gloved hands with soap and water before removing gloves; then wash ungloved hands.
- ***Nutritional Considerations:*** A low-fat, low-cholesterol, and low-sodium diet should be consumed to reduce current disease processes. High fat consumption increases the amount of bile acids in the colon and should be avoided.
- Recognize anxiety related to test results, and be supportive of perceived loss of independent function. Discuss the implications of abnormal test results on the patient's lifestyle. Provide teaching and information regarding the clinical implications of the test results, as appropriate.
- Reinforce information given by the patient's HCP regarding further

testing, treatment, or referral to another HCP. Answer any questions or address any concerns voiced by the patient or family.

- Depending on the results of this procedure, additional testing may be needed to evaluate or monitor progression of the disease process and determine the need for a change in therapy. Evaluate test results in relation to the patient's symptoms and other tests performed.

Patient Education:

- Teach the patient the purpose of blood or blood product transfusion and possible reportable reactions.
- Teach the patient regarding medications that irritate the GI tract and should be avoided (NSAIDs, salicylates).

Expected Patient Outcomes:

Understanding

- The patient and family state the importance of wearing oxygen to support oxygenation until blood volume is restored.
- The patient and family state the purpose of all diagnostic studies ordered to identify the cause of blood loss.

Ability

- The patient and family successfully demonstrate measuring and recording urine output.
- The patient successfully demonstrates relaxation techniques that will decrease anxiety.

Response

- The patient agrees to avoid taking medications that could contribute to gastrointestinal bleeding (NSAIDs, ASA).
- The patient allows family, significant others to stay at the bedside to decrease anxiety and provide emotional support.

RELATED STUDIES:

- Related tests include antibodies antineutrophilic cytoplasmic, angiography abdomen, barium enema, barium swallow, cancer antigens, capsule endoscopy, colonoscopy, CBC, CBC hematocrit, CBC hemoglobin, CT abdomen, EGD, fecal analysis, IgA, MRI abdomen, Meckel's diverticulum scan, proctosigmoidoscopy, upper GI series, and WBC scan.
- Refer to the Gastrointestinal System table online at Davis*Plus* for related tests by body system.

Genetic Testing

SYNONYM/ACRONYM: Related terms: personalized medicine, companion diagnostics, molecular diagnostics.

COMMON USE: To assist in the identification of genetic mutations in humans with implications regarding health and treatment decisions; to assist in the identification of pathogenic organisms.

SPECIMEN: The facility or testing laboratory should be contacted regarding specimen collection requirements. Possible specimen types include whole blood, buccal samples, and tissue samples.

NORMAL FINDINGS: Method: Methods are specific to the study of interest and preferred specimen type. Methods include polymerase chain reaction (PCR), immunohistochemical assay, DNA probe using fluorescence in situ hybridization (FISH), gene amplification using chromogenic in situ hybridization (CISH), cell culture with karyotyping. Absence of findings consistent with genetic abnormalities related to disease or the ability to metabolize medications normally.

DESCRIPTION: Genetic testing has become an important piece of the continuously evolving health-care model. It is now possible to identify diseases before symptoms appear, predict the likelihood of disease development, and implement lifestyle or therapeutic interventions that will reduce or eliminate the effects of disease. Closer investigation into the nature of disease has sometimes revealed a more complex set of interactions than what was previously understood. While human DNA has similarities, there are also many individual differences. Additionally, there are numerous factors such as diet, activity, environment, and stress levels that contribute to variations between one individual and another. These factors in combination with our genetic makeup impact our tendency toward the development of illnesses. Technologies made possible through the accomplishments of the Human Genome Project and a multitude of findings from other collaborative research efforts have resulted in an explosion of diagnostic and prognostic information. The subspecialty of microbiology has been revolutionized by molecular diagnostics. Molecular diagnostics involves the identification of specific sequences of DNA. Molecular methods are used to help identify pathogens that were previously undetectable or inconsistently identified by the culture and biochemical methods available at the time. Molecular methods are also used to examine human samples for genetic disorders that are the result of both simple and complex mutations. Areas of great interest and active development related to genetic testing are in microbiology, virology, oncology, and the development of pharmaceuticals. Diagnostic and biotechnology companies are developing assays to identify gene sequences that code for proteins associated with a specific disease. Notable examples include the following:

- Mutations in the epidermal growth factor receptor (EGFR) gene: The gene encodes a protein (EGFR) associated with many types of cancer, including lung, breast, and colorectal cancer.
- Mutations in the KRAS gene: If mutations are present, specific medications used to treat lung, breast, and colorectal cancers will be rendered ineffective; therefore, other options can more immediately be considered.
- Mutations in HER-2–NEU gene associated with breast cancer: If mutations are present, the cancer risk can be stratified, survival can be predicted, and selection of treatment options can be made.
- Mutations in the BRAF gene: If present, the mutations are used to identify patients, with cancers such as melanoma, who might benefit from treatment with specific drugs that are known to be effective.
- Mutations in the P450 cytochrome series: If present, the mutations are used to predict response to specific drugs—some people will be poor metabolizers (requiring adjustments to higher doses) and some people will be ultrasensitive metabolizers (requiring adjustments to smaller doses).
- Factor V Leiden mutation: If present, this mutation indicates the person has a higher than normal risk for thromboembolism.

G

- Mutations in the BRCA1 and BRCA2 genes: If present, this mutation indicates the person has a high risk for development of hereditary breast or ovarian cancer. This knowledge provides the opportunity to make informed decisions regarding prophylactic mastectomy or oophorectomy.

New assays are either being developed after an effective therapy for the disease has also been developed or at the same time the treatment is being developed, as companion diagnostics. The cost-benefit analysis for the development of companion diagnostics makes a clear case for the simultaneous development of tests and targeted therapies rather than application by trial and error. The companion diagnostics model is based on the development tests that identify diseases or their related pathways, from genetic expression to production and interaction of proteins, and then to development of specific related therapies that are predicted with confidence to be effective.

Personalized medicine is the combination of identifying specific knowledge about an individual's genetic makeup with customized therapeutics or adjustments in lifestyle, for example, genotyping for single nucleotide polymorphisms (SNPs). An SNP, or variation of a single nucleic acid in a DNA sequence, has been identified that causes malfunction of an enzyme needed for the metabolism of warfarin. Identification of this genotype has led to the development of algorithms for safe, tailored dosing and administration based on a patient's genotype, age, weight or body mass index, and gender. Personalization can also be achieved in the customized production or compounding of pharmaceuticals with respect to the strength or formulation of the medication. Customized pharmaceuticals are being used to address dosing issues revealed by the presence of mutations in the CYP 450 series; adverse drug reactions either by undermedication or overmedication are sometimes the result of genetic programming rather than a medication error.

Knowledge of genetics assists the nurse in identifying patients and family members who may benefit from additional education, risk assessment, and counseling. Genetics is the study and identification of genes, genetic mutations, and inheritance. For example, genetics provides some insight into the likelihood of inheriting a trait such as blue eyes or a medical condition such as sickle cell anemia. Genes are segments of DNA arranged on chromosomes and are inherited from each parent. Humans normally have 46 chromosomes, or 23 pairs of chromosomes, in each cell: 23 chromosomes are inherited from the mother, and 23 chromosomes are inherited from the father. Twenty-two of the 23 chromosomes inherited from each parent are called *autosomes*. The 23rd pair of chromosomes is called the *sex chromosomes*: two X chromosomes (an XX pair) are found in females (one X chromosome from each parent) and an X and a Y chromosome (an XY pair) are found in males (one X from the mother and one Y from the father).

Variations in number or structure can be congenital or acquired. Variations can range from a small, single-gene mutation to abnormalities in an entire chromosome or set of chromosomes due to duplication, deletion, substitution, translocation, or other rearrangement. Molecular probe techniques are used to detect smaller, more subtle changes in chromosomes. Chromosomes vary in size and may contain hundreds to thousands of genes. Every gene has a specific location on each of its paired chromosomes. Gene sequences on paired chromosomes are also referred to as *alleles,* and they may be identical or varied. Identical alleles for a gene are termed *homozygous*; variable alleles are termed *heterozygous*. An allele can be demonstrated as either a *dominant* (represented by a capital letter) or a *recessive* (represented by a lowercase letter) trait. Since one allele comes from each parent, the possible combinations are DD, Dd, and dd. Expression of an *autosomal dominant* trait would occur with either DD or Dd; expression of an *autosomal recessive* trait would occur with dd. Expression of a recessive X chromosome–linked trait would always occur in male offspring because there is only a single X chromosome (the father will have contributed a Y chromosome); expression in female offspring would depend on whether the trait was D or d in the X chromosome contributed by the father. Recessive genes are not weaker than dominant genes; rather, expression of the recessive gene is masked by expression of the dominant gene. Some conditions are the result of mutations involving a single gene, and other conditions may involve multiple genes and/or multiple chromosomes. Sickle cell anemia and cystic fibrosis are examples of autosomal recessive, single-gene disorders. Down syndrome is an example of a chromosome disorder in which the cells have three copies of chromosome 21 (trisomy) instead of the normal two copies. Hemophilia is an example of a recessive sex-linked genetic disorder passed from a mother to male children.

Genomic studies evaluate the interaction of groups of genes. The combined activity or combined expression of groups of genes allows assumptions or predictions to be made. As an example, genomic studies measure the levels of activity in multiple genes to predict how they, along with environmental and lifestyle decisions, influence the development of coronary artery disease, type 2 diabetes, or development and growth of a tumor.

The System tables, found online at Davis*Plus*, designate the individual studies that contain information regarding specific genetic testing.

This procedure is contraindicated for

Patients who are not capable of comprehending information presented in the pre- and post-testing genetic counseling sessions. The test should not be performed if the parents of an affected born or unborn child, or if the patient himself or herself, is not emotionally capable of understanding the test results and managing the ramifications of the test results. Written and informed consent, in combination with additional education and a support system, are crucial in order to prepare the patient to make life-altering decisions.

INDICATIONS

- Assist in confirming the diagnosis of conditions associated with genetic disorders before or after associated symptoms are manifested.
- Assist in determining drug selection and appropriate dosing on an individual basis.
- Assist in forensic identifications or paternity determinations.
- Assist in monitoring the efficacy of therapeutic interventions.
- Determine the probability of passing a heritable disease to unborn children; discuss prenatal planning.
- Establish a predisposition for the development of certain diseases.
- Identify matches for organ donation.
- Identify the cause of an infectious disease.
- Provide an explanation of death (e.g., miscarriage, stillbirth).
- Screen for a genetic disease or condition that may affect an embryo, fetus, or neonate.

POTENTIAL MEDICAL DIAGNOSIS

- Identification of a condition or disease based on the results of specific genetic testing.
- Identification or disqualification of therapies related to a condition or disease based on the results of specific genetic testing.

CRITICAL FINDINGS: N/A

INTERFERING FACTORS

- Proper specimen handling and transport are crucial in order to provide accurate results. The laboratory should be consulted regarding specific instructions prior to specimen collection, especially since tissue specimens are considered irretrievable.

NURSING IMPLICATIONS AND PROCEDURE

Potential Nursing Problems: N/A

PRETEST:

- Positively identify the patient using at least two person-specific identifiers before services, treatments, or procedures are performed.
- ***Patient Teaching:*** Inform the patient this test can assist in assessing for infection or disease using genetic testing.
- Obtain a history of the patient's health concerns, symptoms, surgical procedures, and results of previously performed laboratory and diagnostic studies. Include a list of known allergens, especially allergies or sensitivities to latex.
- Obtain a list of the patient's current medications, including over-the-counter medications and dietary supplements (see Effects of Natural Products on Laboratory Values online at Davis*Plus*).
- Review the procedure with the patient. Inform the patient that several tests may be necessary to confirm the diagnosis. Inform the patient that specimen collection depends on the type of specimen required for testing. Address concerns about pain and explain that there may be some discomfort during specimen collection. (See related studies for specific information.)
- ***Sensitivity to social and cultural issues,*** as well as concern for modesty, is important in providing psychological support before, during, and after the procedure.
- See the related studies regarding special instructions for patient preparation.
- *Make sure a written and informed consent, if required, has been signed prior to specimen collection.*

INTRATEST:

Potential Complications: N/A

- Avoid the use of equipment containing latex if the patient has a history of allergic reaction to latex.

G

- Instruct the patient to cooperate fully and to follow directions. Direct the patient to breathe normally and to avoid unnecessary movement.
- Contact the testing laboratory prior to specimen collection in order to obtain accurate information regarding specimen collection containers, sample volumes, and specific transport instructions.
- Observe standard precautions, and follow the general guidelines in Patient Preparation and Specimen Collection online at Davis*Plus*. Positively identify the patient, and label the appropriate specimen container with the corresponding patient demographics, initials of the person collecting the specimen, date, and time of collection. Collect the appropriate specimen as described in the related body fluid analysis or culture study. The facility or testing laboratory should be contacted for guidelines regarding specimen collection requirements, and specimen packaging and shipping instructions.
- Perform a venipuncture if blood is the specimen required for testing. Remove the needle and apply direct pressure with dry gauze to stop bleeding. Observe/assess venipuncture site for bleeding or hematoma formation, and secure gauze with adhesive bandage.
- Promptly transport the specimen to the laboratory for processing and analysis.

POST-TEST:

- Inform the patient that a report of the results will be made available to the requesting health-care provider (HCP), who will discuss the results with the patient.
- Recognize anxiety related to test results, and provide emotional support if results are positive. Discuss the implications of abnormal test results on the patient's lifestyle. Provide teaching and information regarding the clinical implications of the test results, as appropriate. Educate the patient regarding access to counseling services.
- Reinforce information given by the patient's HCP regarding further testing, treatment, or referral to another HCP.
- Note that depending on the results of this procedure, additional testing may be performed to evaluate or monitor progression of the disease process and determine the need for a change in therapy. Evaluate test results in relation to the patient's symptoms and other tests performed. Emphasize the need to return to have additional samples taken, if ordered. Answer any questions or address any concerns voiced by the patient or family.

Patient Education: N/A

Expected Patient Outcomes: N/A

RELATED STUDIES:

- Related tests include α_1-antitrypsin, Alzheimer's disease markers, amino acid screen blood & urine, amniotic fluid analysis, antibodies gliadin, anticonvulsant drugs, angiography coronary, antidepressant drugs, antipsychotic drugs, biopsy breast, biopsy chorionic villus, biopsy skin, biopsy thyroid, bladder cancer markers, cancer antigens, ceruloplasmin, chloride sweat, cholesterol (total and fractionated), chromosome analysis, coagulation factors, collagen crosslinked N-telopeptide, color perception test, CBC platelet count, CT cardiac scoring, copper, fecal analysis, glucose, G6PD, hemoglobin electrophoresis, hexosaminidase A & B, HIV 1/2 antibodies, homocysteine, immunosuppressant drugs, leukocyte alkaline phosphatase enzyme, lipoprotein electrophoresis, mammography, newborn screening, prothrombin time and INR, red blood cell cholinesterase, and sickle cell screen.
- Refer to the Gastrointestinal, Genitourinary, Hematopoietic, Hepatobiliary, Immune, Musculoskeletal, and Respiratory system tables online at Davis*Plus* for related tests by body system.

Glucagon

SYNONYM/ACRONYM: N/A

COMMON USE: To evaluate the amount of circulating glucagon toward diagnosing diseases such as hypoglycemia, glucagon secreting tumor, pancreatic cancer, or inflammation.

SPECIMEN: Plasma collected in chilled, lavender-top (EDTA) tube. Specimen should be transported tightly capped and in an ice slurry.

NORMAL FINDINGS: (Method: Radioimmunoassay)

Age	Conventional Units	SI Units (Conventional Units × 1)
Cord blood	0–215 pg/mL	0–215 ng/L
Newborn	0–1,750 pg/mL	0–1,750 ng/L
Child	0–148 pg/mL	0–148 ng/L
Adult	20–100 pg/mL	20–100 ng/L

POTENTIAL MEDICAL DIAGNOSIS

Increased in:

Glucagon is produced in the pancreas and excreted by the kidneys; conditions that affect the pancreas and cause cellular destruction or conditions that impair the ability of the kidneys to remove glucagon from circulation will result in elevated glucagon levels.

- Acromegaly ***(related to stimulated production of glucagon in response to growth hormone)***
- Acute pancreatitis ***(related to decreased pancreatic function)***
- Burns ***(related to stress-induced release of catecholamines, which stimulates glucagon production)***
- Chronic kidney disease ***(related to decreased renal excretion)***
- Cirrhosis ***(pathophysiology is not well established)***
- Cushing's syndrome ***(evidenced by overproduction of cortisol, which stimulates glucagon production)***
- Diabetes (uncontrolled) ***(pathophysiology is not well established)***
- Glucagonoma ***(related to excessive production by the tumor)***
- Hyperlipoproteinemia ***(pathophysiology is not well established)***
- Hypoglycemia ***(related to response to decreased glucose level)***
- Infection ***(related to feedback loop in response to stress)***
- Kidney transplant rejection ***(related to decreased renal excretion)***
- Pheochromocytoma ***(excessive production of catecholamines stimulates increased glucagon levels)***
- Stress ***(related to stress-induced release of catecholamines, which stimulates glucagon production)***
- Trauma ***(related to stress-induced release of catecholamines, which stimulates glucagon production)***

Decreased in:

Low glucagon levels are related to decreased pancreatic function.

- Chronic pancreatitis
- Cystic fibrosis
- Postpancreatectomy period

CRITICAL FINDINGS: N/A

Find and print out the full study on Fast Find at davispl.us/vanleeuwen7.

Access Canadian content on Fast Find: Lab and Dx at davispl.us/vanleeuwen7

Glucose

SYNONYM/ACRONYM: Blood sugar, fasting blood sugar (FBS), postprandial glucose, 2-hr PC (post cibum).

COMMON USE: To assist in the diagnosis of diabetes and to evaluate disorders of carbohydrate metabolism such as malabsorption syndrome.

SPECIMEN: Serum collected in a gold-, red-, or red/gray-top tube, although plasma is recommended for diagnosis of diabetes. Plasma collected in a gray-top (sodium fluoride) or a green-top (heparin) tube.

NORMAL FINDINGS: (Method: Spectrophotometry)

Age	Conventional Units	SI Units (Conventional Units × 0.0555)
Fasting		
Cord blood	45–96 mg/dL	2.5–5.3 mmol/L
Premature infant	20–80 mg/dL	1.1–4.4 mmol/L
Newborn 2 d–2 yr	30–100 mg/dL	1.7–5.6 mmol/L
Child	60–100 mg/dL	3.3–5.6 mmol/L
Adult-older adult	Less than 100 mg/dL	Less than 5.6 mmol/L
Prediabetes or impaired fasting glucose	100–125 mg/dL	5.6–6.9 mmol/L
2-hr postprandial	65–139 mg/dL	3.6–7.7 mmol/L
Prediabetes or impaired 2-hr sample	140–199 mg/dL	7.8–11 mmol/L
Random	Less than 200 mg/dL	Less than 11.1 mmol/L

The American Diabetes Association and National Institute of Diabetes and Digestive and Kidney Diseases consider a confirmed fasting blood glucose greater than 126 mg/dL to be consistent with a diagnosis of diabetes. Values tend to increase in older adults. 🍁

DESCRIPTION: Glucose, a simple six-carbon sugar (monosaccharide), enters the diet as part of the sugars sucrose, lactose, and maltose and from the complex polysaccharide, dietary starch. The body acquires most of its energy from the oxidative metabolism of glucose. Excess glucose is stored in the liver or in muscle tissue as glycogen. Glucose levels in plasma (one of the components of blood) are generally 10% to 15% higher than glucose measurements in whole blood (and even more after eating). This is important because home blood glucose meters measure the glucose in whole blood, whereas most laboratory tests measure the glucose in either plasma or serum.

Diabetes is a group of diseases characterized by hyperglycemia, or elevated glucose levels. Hyperglycemia results from a defect in insulin secretion due to destruction of the beta cells of the pancreas (type 1 diabetes), a defect in insulin action, or a combination of defects in secretion and action (type 2 diabetes). The chronic hyperglycemia of diabetes over time may lead to damage, dysfunction, and eventually failure of the eyes (retinopathy), kidneys (nephropathy), nerves (neuropathy), heart (cardiovascular disease), and blood vessels (microvascular and macrovascular conditions). The American Diabetes Association (ADA) and National Institute of Diabetes and Digestive and Kidney Disease have 🍁 established criteria for diagnosing diabetes to include any combination of the following findings or confirmation of any of the individual findings by repetition of the same test on a subsequent day:

- Symptoms of diabetes (e.g., polyuria, polydipsia, polyphagia, unexplained weight loss) in addition to a random glucose level greater than 200 mg/dL (SI: 11.1 mmol/L) 🍁
- Fasting blood glucose greater than 126 mg/dL (SI: 7 mmol/L) after fasting for a minimum of 8 hr 🍁
- Glucose level greater than 200 mg/dL (SI: 11.1 mmol/L) 2 hr after glucose challenge with standardized 75-mg load
- An A_{1C}(glycated hemoglobin) in adults equal to or greater than 6.5% (assumes the use of a standardized test as referenced to the National Glycohemoglobin Standardization Program—Diabetes Control and Complications Trial and the absence of clinical conditions such as hemoglobinopathies, anemias, and kidney and liver diseases known to affect the accuracy of the test results)

Glucose measurements have been used for many years as an indicator of short-term glycemic control to identify diabetes and assist in management of the disease. Glycated hemoglobin, or hemoglobin A_{1c}, is used to indicate long-term glycemic control over a period of 3 to 4 months and is used as a diagnostic tool in the diagnosis of type 2 diabetes. The estimated average glucose (eAG) is a mathematical relationship between hemoglobin A_{1c} and glucose levels expressed by the formula eAG =

$$(\text{mg/dL}) = [(A_{1c} \times 28.7) - 46.7]$$

For example, eAG for a patient with an A_{1c} of 6% would be calculated as $[(6 \times 28.7) - 46.7] = 125.5$ mg/dL. Studies have documented the need for markers that reflect intermediate glycemic control, or the period of time between 2 to 4 wk as opposed to hours or months. Many patients who appear to be well controlled according to glucose and A_{1c} values actually have significant postprandial hyperglycemia. Management of postprandial hyperglycemia is considered to be extremely important in preventing or delaying the development of diabetes-related complications. The GlycoMark assay measures serum 1,5-anhydroglucitol is a validated marker of short-term glycemic control and can be used in combination with glucose and hemoglobin A_{1C} measurements to provide a more complete picture of glucose levels over time. GlycoMark values greater than 8 mcg/mL are considered normal for adults. Serum 1,5-anhydroglucitol is a naturally occurring monosaccharide found in most foods. It is not normally metabolized by the body and is excreted by the kidneys. During periods of normal glucose levels, there is an equilibrium between glucose and 1,5-anhydroglucitol concentrations. When blood glucose concentration rises above

180 mg/dL (SI = 10 mmol/L), the renal threshold for glucose, levels of circulating serum 1,5-anhydroglucitol decrease due to competitive inhibition of renal tubular absorption favoring glucose over serum 1,5-anhydroglucitol. As glucose is retained in the circulating blood and levels of glucose increase, correspondingly higher amounts of 1,5-anhydroglucitol are excreted in the urine resulting in lower serum concentrations. The change in serum 1,5-anhydroglucitol levels is directly proportional to the severity and frequency of hyperglycemic episodes. Serum 1,5-anhydroglucitol concentration returns to normal after 2 wk with no recurrence of hyperglycemia. Reports from the medical community indicate that over half of the U.S. population will have diabetes or prediabetes by 2020. The combined use of available markers of glycemic control will greatly improve the ability to achieve tighter, more timely glycemic control.

Comparison of Markers of Glycemic Control to Approximate Blood Glucose Concentration

1,5–Anhydroglucitol Measured Using the GlycoMark Assay	Hemoglobin A_{1c}	Estimated Blood Glucose (mg/dL)	Degree of Diabetic Control
14 mcg/mL or greater	4%–5%	68–97 mg/dL	Normal/ nondiabetic
10–12 mcg/mL	4%–6%	68–126 mg/dL	Well controlled
5–10 mcg/mL	6%–8%	126–183 mg/dL	Moderately well controlled
2–5 mcg/mL	8%–10%	183–240 mg/dL	Poorly controlled
Less than 2 mcg/mL	Greater than 10% (11%–14%)	269–355 mg/dL	Very poorly controlled

Assessment of medications used to manage diabetes is an important facet of controlling the disease and its health-related complications. Drug response is an active area of study to ensure that the medications prescribed are meeting the needs of the patients who are taking them. Insulin and metformin are two commonly prescribed medications for the treatment of diabetes. See the "Insulin Antibodies" study for more detailed information. The AccuType Metformin Assay is a genetic test that identifies individuals who may not respond appropriately or who have a suboptimal response to metformin related to a genetic mutation in the proteins responsible for transporting metformin.

This procedure is contraindicated for: N/A

INDICATIONS

- Assist in the diagnosis of insulinoma.
- Determine insulin requirements.
- Evaluate disorders of carbohydrate metabolism.
- Identify hypoglycemia.
- Screen for diabetes.

POTENTIAL MEDICAL DIAGNOSIS

Increased in:

- Acromegaly, gigantism ***(growth hormone [GH] stimulates the release of glucagon, which in turn increases glucose levels)***
- Acute stress reaction ***(hyperglycemia is stimulated by the release of catecholamines and glucagon)***
- Cerebrovascular accident ***(possibly related to stress)***
- Chronic kidney disease ***(glucagon is degraded by the kidneys; when damaged kidneys cannot metabolize glucagon, glucagon levels in blood rise and result in hyperglycemia)***
- Cushing's syndrome ***(related to elevated cortisol)***
- Diabetes ***(glucose intolerance and elevated glucose levels define diabetes)***
- Glucagonoma ***(glucagon releases stored glucose; glucagon-secreting tumors will increase glucose levels)***
- Hemochromatosis ***(related to iron deposition in the pancreas; subsequent damage to pancreatic tissue releases cell contents, including glucagon, resulting in hyperglycemia)***
- Liver disease (severe) ***(damaged liver tissue releases cell contents, including stored glucose, into circulation)***
- Metabolic syndrome ***(related to the development of diabetes)***
- Myocardial infarction ***(related to stress and/or preexisting diabetes)***
- Pancreatic adenoma ***(damage to pancreatic tissue releases cell contents, including glucagon, resulting in hyperglycemia)***
- Pancreatitis (acute and chronic) ***(damage to pancreatic tissue releases cell contents, including glucagon, resulting in hyperglycemia)***
- Pancreatitis due to mumps ***(damage to pancreatic tissue releases cell contents, including glucagon, resulting in hyperglycemia)***
- Pheochromocytoma ***(related to increased catecholamines, which increase glucagon; glucagon increases glucose levels)***
- Shock, trauma ***(hyperglycemia is stimulated by the release of catecholamines and glucagon)***
- Somatostatinoma ***(somatostatin-producing tumor of pancreatic delta cells, associated with diabetes)***
- Strenuous exercise ***(hyperglycemia is stimulated by the release of catecholamines and glucagon)***
- Thyrotoxicosis ***(related to loss of kidney function)***
- Vitamin B_1 deficiency ***(thiamine is involved in the metabolism of glucose; deficiency results in accumulation of glucose)***

Decreased in:

- Acute alcohol ingestion ***(most glucose metabolism occurs in the liver; alcohol inhibits the liver from making glucose)***
- Addison's disease ***(cortisol affects glucose levels; insufficient levels of cortisol result in diminished glucose levels)***
- Ectopic insulin production from tumors (adrenal carcinoma, carcinoma of the stomach, fibrosarcoma)
- Excess insulin by injection
- Galactosemia ***(inherited enzyme disorder that results in accumulation of galactose in excessive proportion to glucose levels)***
- Glucagon deficiency ***(glucagon controls glucose levels; hypoglycemia occurs in the absence of glucagon)***
- Glycogen storage diseases ***(deficiencies in enzymes involved in conversion of glycogen to glucose)***

G

- Hereditary fructose intolerance ***(inherited disorder of fructose metabolism; phosphates needed for intermediate steps in gluconeogenesis are trapped from further action by the enzyme deficiency responsible for fructose metabolism)***
- Hypopituitarism ***(decreased levels of hormones such as adrenocorticotropic hormone [ACTH] and GH result in decreased glucose levels)***
- Hypothyroidism ***(thyroid hormones affect glucose levels; decreased thyroid hormone levels result in decreased glucose levels)***
- Insulinoma ***(the function of insulin is to decrease glucose levels)***
- Malabsorption syndromes ***(insufficient absorption of carbohydrates)***
- Maple syrup urine disease ***(inborn error of amino acid metabolism; accumulation of leucine is believed to inhibit the rate of gluconeogenesis, independently of insulin, and thereby diminish release of hepatic glucose stores)***
- Poisoning resulting in severe liver disease ***(decreased liver function correlates with decreased glucose metabolism)***
- Postgastrectomy ***(insufficient intake of carbohydrates)***
- Starvation ***(insufficient intake of carbohydrates)***
- von Gierke's disease ***(most common glycogen storage disease; G6PD deficiency)***

G

CRITICAL FINDINGS:

Glucose

Adults & children

- Less than 40 mg/dL (SI: Less than 2.22 mmol/L)
- Greater than 400 mg/dL (SI: Greater than 22.2 mmol/L)

Newborns

- Less than 32 mg/dL (SI: Less than 1.8 mmol/L)
- Greater than 328 mg/dL (SI: Greater than 18.2 mmol/L)

Note and immediately report to the requesting health-care provider (HCP) any critical findings and related symptoms. A listing of these findings varies among facilities. Timely notification of a critical finding for laboratory or diagnostic studies is a role expectation of the professional nurse. The notification processes vary among facilities. Upon receipt of the critical finding, the information should be read back to the caller to verify accuracy.

Consideration may be given to verification of critical findings before action is taken. Policies vary among facilities and may include requesting immediate recollection and retesting by the laboratory or retesting using a rapid point-of-care testing instrument at the bedside, if available.

Glucose monitoring is an important measure in achieving tight glycemic control. The enzymatic GDH-PQQ test method may produce falsely elevated results in patients who are receiving products that contain other sugars (e.g., oral xylose, parenterals containing maltose or galactose, and peritoneal dialysis solutions that contain icodextrin). The GDH-NAD, glucose oxidase, and glucose hexokinase methods can distinguish between glucose and other sugars.

Symptoms of decreased glucose levels include headache, confusion, polyphagia, irritability, nervousness, restlessness, diaphoresis, and weakness. Possible interventions include oral or intravenous (IV) administration of glucose, IV or intramuscular injection of glucagon, and continuous glucose monitoring.

Symptoms of elevated glucose levels include abdominal pain, fatigue, muscle cramps, nausea, vomiting, polyuria, polyphagia, and polydipsia. Possible interventions include fluid replacement in addition to subcutaneous or IV injection of insulin with continuous glucose monitoring.

INTERFERING FACTORS

- Drugs and other substances that may increase glucose levels include acetazolamide, alanine, albuterol, anesthetic drugs, antipyrine, atenolol, betamethasone, cefotaxime, chlorpromazine, chlorprothixene, clonidine, clorexolone, corticotropin, cortisone, cyclic AMP, cyclopropane, dexamethasone, dextroamphetamine, diapamide, epinephrine, enflurane, ethacrynic acid, ether, fludrocortisone, furosemide, glucagon, glucocorticoids, homoharringtonine, hydrochlorothiazide, hydroxydione, isoniazid, maltose, meperidine, meprednisone, methyclothiazide, metolazone, niacin, nifedipine, nortriptyline, octreotide, oral contraceptives, oxyphenbutazone, pancreozymin, phenelzine, phenylbutazone, piperacetazine, polythiazide, prednisone, quinethazone, reserpine, rifampin, ritodrine, secretin, somatostatin, thiazides, thyroid hormone, and triamcinolone.
- Drugs and other substances that may decrease glucose levels include acarbose, acetylsalicylic acid, acipimox, alanine, allopurinol, antimony compounds, arsenicals, ascorbic acid, benzene, buformin, cannabis, captopril, chloroform, clofibrate, enalapril, enprostil, erythromycin, gemfibrozil, glibornuride, glyburide, guanethidine, niceritrol, nitrazepam, oral contraceptives, phentolamine, phosphorus, promethazine, ramipril, rotenone, sulfonylureas, thiocarlide, tolbutamide, tromethamine, and verapamil.
- Elevated urea levels and uremia can lead to falsely elevated glucose levels.
- Extremely elevated white blood cell counts can lead to falsely decreased glucose values.
- Administration of insulin or oral hypoglycemic drugs within 8 hr of a fasting blood glucose can lead to falsely decreased values.
- Specimens should never be collected above an IV line because of the potential for dilution when the specimen and the IV solution combine in the collection container, falsely decreasing the result. There is also the potential of contaminating the sample with the substance of interest, if it is present in the IV solution, falsely increasing the result.
- Failure to follow dietary restrictions before the procedure may cause the procedure to be canceled or repeated; failure to follow dietary restrictions before the fasting test can lead to falsely elevated glucose values.

NURSING IMPLICATIONS AND PROCEDURE

POTENTIAL NURSING PROBLEMS:

Problem	Signs & Symptoms	Interventions
Blood glucose ***(related to sedentary lifestyle,***	**Excess:** Fatigue; mild dehydration; elevated blood glucose; weight	Check blood glucose before meals and at bedtime; administer prescribed insulin or oral drugs; educate and encourage the

(table continues on page 860)

Problem	Signs & Symptoms	Interventions
circulating insulin deficiency secondary to pancreatic insufficiency; excessive dietary intake; insulin resistance)	loss; weakness; polyuria; polydipsia; polyphagia; blurred vision; headache; paresthesia; poor skin turgor; dry mouth; nausea; vomiting; abdominal pain; Kussmaul respirations. **Deficit:** Tremor, diaphoresis, decreased concentration; diaphoresis; elevated blood pressure; palpitations; headache; polyphagia; restlessness; lethargy; altered mental status; combativeness; altered speech; altered coordination	patient to participate in glucose self-check and record results; assess readiness to learn and barriers to learning; collaborate with the HCP and dietitian to support medical nutritional therapy; refer to dietitian to assist the patient to select appropriate cultural foods; develop a plan of exercise commensurate with the patient's physical abilities; discuss lifestyle alterations necessary to support positive health management secondary to disease process; teach good hygiene and infection prevention; monitor laboratory studies that may be impacted by altered glucose and trend results (Hgb A_{1C}; BUN; creatinine; electrolytes; arterial pH; magnesium; urine ketones; urine microalbumin; white blood cell [WBC] count; amylase; Hgb/Hct; C-reactive protein; liver enzymes); facilitate oral hydration; correlate blood glucose with other laboratory values and medical conditions; address the psychosocial aspects of the disease; monitor serum insulin levels
Infection risk ***(related to altered blood glucose; exposure to opportunistic hosts; poor personal hygiene; broken skin; wound presence)***	Increased temperature; increased heart rate and respiratory rate; chills; change in mental status; fatigue; malaise; weakness; anorexia; headache; nausea; elevated blood	Provide standard precautions in the provision of care; correlate symptoms with laboratory values and disease process; trend vital signs and laboratory values to monitor for improvement; administer prescribed antibiotics and medications for fever reduction; provide cooling measures; ensure vigilant hand hygiene;

Problem	Signs & Symptoms	Interventions
	glucose; hypotension; diminished oxygen saturation; elevated WBC; elevated C-reactive protein	educate patient and family regarding good hand hygiene; infuse ordered IV fluids to support adequate hydration; ensure implementation of infection prevention measures with consideration of age and culture such as adequate nutrition; provide aseptic wound care; ensure good skin care; ensure good oral care; ensure adequate rest; instruct patient to avoid exposure to opportunistic hosts; send cultures to the laboratory as ordered; correlate culture findings with selected antibiotics
Noncompliance ***(related to refusal to accept new diagnosis; financial instability; cultural norms; complexity of the medical management; lack of knowledge)***	Insufficient disease management; alterations in blood glucose; poor self-management of medication administration; lack of supplies to support self-management; poor dietary control with inappropriate food selections	Assess the patient's ability to and prior efforts to manage the disease process; evaluate the ability to self-manage the disease, including blood glucose screening, dietary management, exercise, and medication self-administration; assess for personal factors that may limit the patient's ability to self-perform, such as visual, cognitive, and hearing; assess the financial ability to purchase the medication and supplies necessary to provide self-care; assess the level of family support; ensure the patient has the adequate knowledge to perform self-care, and if not, provide the necessary training; ensure the patient knows the signs and symptoms related to the disease process; teach correct dietary selections meeting cultural- and age-appropriate needs; refer to social services or home health care; discuss how to manage diabetes during travel

(table continues on page 862)

Problem	Signs & Symptoms	Interventions
Nutrition ***(related to excessive dietary intake more than body requirements, insulin deficiency, stress; anxiety; depression; cultural lifestyle; unhealthy food sources; financial restrictions)***	Polydipsia, polyuria, weight loss; fatigue; elevated blood glucose levels; inadequate glucose management; polyphagia	Monitor blood glucose results, refer to dietitian for evaluation, administer insulin or oral antihyperglycemic drug; assess the cultural aspects of diet selection; correlate dietary intake with blood glucose and monitor trends; collaborate with a dietitian to develop a cultural- and age-appropriate diet plan; correlate nutritional intake and exercise; ensure that the patient understands the relationship between caloric intake and medication (insulin, oral drug); refer to social services and dietitian as necessary

G

PRETEST:

- Positively identify the patient using at least two person-specific identifiers before services, treatments, or procedures are performed.
- *Patient Teaching:* Inform the patient this test can assist in evaluating blood sugar levels.
- Obtain a history of the patient's health concerns, symptoms, surgical procedures, and results of previously performed laboratory and diagnostic studies. Include a list of known allergens, especially allergies or sensitivities to latex.
- Obtain a list of the patient's current medications, including over-the-counter medications and dietary supplements (see Effects of Natural Products on Laboratory Values online at Davis*Plus*).
- Review the procedure with the patient. Inform the patient that specimen collection takes approximately 5 to 10 min. Address concerns about pain and explain that there may be some discomfort during the venipuncture.
- ***Sensitivity to social and cultural issues,*** as well as concern for modesty, is important in providing psychological support before, during, and after the procedure.
- Instruct the patient to fast for at least 8 hr before specimen collection and not to consume any caffeinated products or chew any type of gum before specimen collection for the fasting glucose test; these factors are known to elevate glucose levels.
- Instruct the patient to follow the instructions given for 2-hr postprandial glucose test. Some HCPs may order administration of a standard glucose solution, whereas others may instruct the patient to eat a meal with a known carbohydrate composition.

INTRATEST:

Potential Complications: N/A

- Ensure that the patient has complied with dietary restrictions and other pretesting preparations prior to the fasting study, as instructed.
- Avoid the use of equipment containing latex if the patient has a history of allergic reaction to latex.
- Instruct the patient to cooperate fully and to follow directions. Direct the

patient to breathe normally and to avoid unnecessary movement.

- Observe standard precautions, and follow the general guidelines in Patient Preparation and Specimen Collection online at Davis*Plus*. Positively identify the patient, and label the appropriate specimen container with the corresponding patient demographics, initials of the person collecting the specimen, date, and time of collection. Perform a venipuncture.
- Remove the needle and apply direct pressure with dry gauze to stop bleeding. Observe/assess venipuncture site for bleeding or hematoma formation and secure gauze with adhesive bandage.
- Promptly transport the specimen to the laboratory for processing and analysis.

POST-TEST:

- Inform the patient that a report of the results will be made available to the requesting HCP, who will discuss the results with the patient.
- Instruct the patient to resume usual diet, as directed by the HCP.
- ***Nutritional Considerations:*** Increased glucose levels may be associated with diabetes. There is no "diabetic diet"; however, many meal-planning approaches with nutritional goals are endorsed by the ADA. 🍁 Patients who adhere to dietary recommendations report a better general feeling of health, better weight management, greater control of glucose and lipid values, and improved use of insulin. Instruct the patient, as appropriate, in nutritional management of diabetes. A variety of dietary patterns are beneficial for people with diabetes. The Mediterranean-style diet emphasizes inclusion of vegetables, whole grains, fruits, low-fat dairy, nuts, legumes, and nontropical vegetable oils (e.g., olive, canola, peanut, sunflower, flaxseed) along with fish and lean poultry. A similar dietary pattern known as the Dietary Approaches to Stop Hypertension (DASH) diet makes additional recommendations for the reduction of dietary sodium. Both dietary styles emphasize a reduction in consumption of red meats, which are high in saturated fats and cholesterol, and other foods containing sugar, saturated fats, trans fats, and sodium. A vegetarian diet as well as other potential weight loss diets such as Weight Watchers are also supported by the ADA. 🍁 If triglycerides also are elevated, the patient should be advised to eliminate or reduce alcohol. The nutritional needs of each patient with diabetic patient need to be determined individually (especially during pregnancy) with the appropriate HCPs, particularly professionals educated in nutrition.
- ***Social and Cultural Considerations:*** Numerous studies point to the prevalence of excess body weight in American children and adolescents. Experts estimate that obesity is present in 25% of the population aged 6 to 11 yr. The medical, social, and emotional consequences of excess body weight are significant. Special attention should be given to instructing the pediatric patient and caregiver regarding health risks and weight control education. 🍁
- ***Social and Cultural Considerations:*** Studies comparing risk for developing diabetes demonstrate that certain populations are disproportionately affected by type 2 diabetes and complications of type 2 diabetes as compared to the general population. Nonmodifiable risk factors include age, ethnicity, and family history of diabetes or metabolic syndrome. The risk of developing type 2 diabetes increases with age. In the United States, affected populations include African Americans, Asian Americans, Hispanics, native Hawaiians and Pacific Islanders, American Indians, and Alaska natives. 🍁 Modifiable risk factors include lifestyle choices related to making healthy dietary choices, maintaining a healthy body weight, and meeting recommended levels of physical activity.

G

The financial and emotional burdens of diabetes and related complications continue to grow at an alarming rate. A system for the prevention, management, and support of patients with type 2 diabetes should be provided through the coordinated efforts of multidisciplinary partners using strategies that are culturally appropriate.

- Recognize anxiety related to test results, and be supportive of perceived loss of independence and fear of shortened life expectancy. The ADA recommends A_{1C} testing four times a year for insulin-dependent type 1 or type 2 diabetes when glycemic targets are not being met or when therapy has changed and twice a year when treatment goals are being met for non–insulin-dependent type 2 diabetes. The ADA also recommends that testing for diabetes commence at age 45 for asymptomatic individuals, be considered for adults of any age who are overweight and have additional risk factors, and continue every 3 yr in the absence of symptoms. 🍁
- Depending on the results of this procedure, additional testing may be performed to evaluate or monitor progression of the disease process and determine the need for a change in therapy. Evaluate test results in relation to the patient's symptoms and other tests performed.

Patient Education:

- Instruct the patient and caregiver to report signs and symptoms of hypoglycemia (weakness, confusion, diaphoresis, rapid pulse) or hyperglycemia (thirst, polyuria, hunger, lethargy).
- Discuss the implications of abnormal test results on the patient's lifestyle.
- Provide teaching and information regarding the clinical implications of the test results, as appropriate.
- Emphasize, if indicated, that good glycemic management delays the onset and slows the progression of diabetic retinopathy, nephropathy, and neuropathy.
- Educate the patient regarding access to counseling services, as appropriate.
- Provide contact information, if desired, for the American Heart Association (www.americanheart.org), National Heart, Lung, and Blood Institute (www.nhlbi.nih.gov), Institute of Medicine of the National Academies (www.iom.edu), and USDA's resource for nutrition (www.choosemyplate.gov). 🍁
- Reinforce information given by the patient's HCP regarding further testing, treatment, or referral to another HCP.
- Instruct the patient in the use of home testing strips or meters approved for glucose, ketones, or A_{1C} by the U.S. Food and Drug Administration, if prescribed. 🍁
- Answer any questions or address any concerns voiced by the patient or family.
- Teach the patient and family the signs and symptoms of hyperglycemia and hypoglycemia.

Expected Patient Outcomes:

Understanding

- The patient and family state the signs and symptoms that could indicate an infection because of the risk for developing ulcers or the potential for limb amputation.
- The patient and family state the value of good glucose management to their overall health and longevity.

Ability

- The patient demonstrates proficiency in the ability to perform accurate self-monitored glucose checks.
- The patient demonstrates proficiency in the ability to perform insulin self-administration correctly or to take oral antihyperglycemic drugs.

Response

- The patient complies with the medication management recommended by the HCP.
- The patient complies with dietary restrictions.

RELATED STUDIES:

- Related tests include ACTH, angiography adrenal, BUN, calcium, catecholamines, cholesterol (HDL, LDL, total), cortisol, C-peptide, CT cardiac scoring, CRP, CK and isoenzymes, creatinine, DHEA, echocardiography, fecal analysis, fecal fat, fluorescein angiography, fructosamine, fundoscopy, gastric emptying scan, glucagon, GTT, glycated hemoglobin, gonioscopy, Holter monitor, HVA, insulin, insulin antibodies, ketones, lactic acid, lipoprotein electrophoresis, MRI chest, metanephrines, microalbumin, myoglobin, MI infarct scan, myocardial perfusion heart scan, plethysmography, PET heart, renin, sodium, troponin, and visual fields test.
- Refer to the Endocrine System table online at Davis*Plus* for related tests by body system.

Glucose-6-Phosphate Dehydrogenase

G

SYNONYM/ACRONYM: G6PD.

COMMON USE: To identify an enzyme deficiency that can result in hemolytic anemia.

SPECIMEN: Whole blood collected in a lavender-top (EDTA) tube.

NORMAL FINDINGS: (Method: Fluorescent) Qualitative assay—enzyme activity detected; quantitative assay—the following table reflects enzyme activity in units per gram of hemoglobin:

Age	Conventional Units	SI Units (Conventional Units × 0.0645)
Newborn	7.8–14.4 international units/g hemoglobin	0.5–0.93 micro units/mol hemoglobin
Adult–older adult	5.5–9.3 international units/g hemoglobin	0.35–0.6 micro units/mol hemoglobin

POTENTIAL MEDICAL DIAGNOSIS

Increased in:

The pathophysiology is not well understood but release of the enzymes from hemolyzed cells increases blood levels.

- Chronic blood loss ***(related to reticulocytosis; replacement of RBCs)***
- Hepatic coma ***(pathophysiology is unclear)***
- Hyperthyroidism ***(possible response to increased basal metabolic rate and role of G6PD in glucose metabolism)***
- Idiopathic thrombocytopenic purpura
- Megaloblastic anemia ***(related to reticulocytosis; replacement of RBCs)***
- Myocardial infarction ***(medications [e.g., salicylates] may aggravate***

or stimulate a hemolytic crisis in G6PD-deficient patients)
- Pernicious anemia ***(related to reticulocytosis; replacement of RBCs)***
- Viral hepatitis ***(pathophysiology is unclear)***

Decreased in:
- Congenital nonspherocytic anemia
- G6PD deficiency
- Nonimmunological hemolytic disease of the newborn

CRITICAL FINDINGS: N/A

Find and print out the full study on Fast Find at davispl.us/vanleeuwen7.

Glucose Tolerance Tests

SYNONYM/ACRONYM: Standard oral tolerance test, standard gestational screen, standard gestational tolerance test, GTT.

COMMON USE: To evaluate blood glucose levels to assist in diagnosing diseases such as diabetes.

SPECIMEN: Plasma collected in a gray-top (sodium fluoride) tube. Serum collected in a gold-, red-, or red/gray-top tube or plasma collected in a green-top (heparin) tube is also acceptable, but plasma is recommended for diagnosis. It is important to use the same type of collection container throughout the entire test.

NORMAL FINDINGS: (Method: Spectrophotometry)

Standard Oral Glucose Tolerance (Up to 75-g Glucose Load)

	Conventional Units	SI Units (Conventional Units × 0.0555)
Fasting sample	Less than 100 mg/dL	Less than 5.6 mmol/L
Prediabetes or impaired fasting sample	100–125 mg/dL	5.6–6.9 mmol/L
2-hr sample	Less than 200 mg/dL	Less than 11.1 mmol/L
Prediabetes or impaired 2-hr sample	140–199 mg/dL	7.8–11 mmol/L

Plasma glucose values are reported to be 10% to 20% higher than serum values. 🍁

Tolerance Tests for Gestational Diabetes

One-Step Approach (75-g Glucose Load)	Conventional and SI Units (SI = Conventional Units × 0.0555)
Fasting sample	Less than 93 mg/dL (SI: Less than 5.2 mmol/L)
1-hr sample	Less than 181 mg/dL (SI: Less than 10 mmol/L)
2-hr sample	Less than 154 mg/dL (SI: Less than 8.5 mmol/L)

A diagnosis of gestational diabetes is made when any of the three thresholds are met or exceeded. Plasma glucose values are reported to be 10% to 20% higher than serum values.

🍁 Access Canadian content on Fast Find: Lab and Dx at davispl.us/vanleeuwen7

Tolerance Tests for Gestational Diabetes

	Two-Step Approach	Conventional and SI Units (SI = Conventional Units × 0.0555)	
Step One	**Standard Gestational Screen (50-g Glucose Load)**		
1-hr sample performed while the patient is not fasting		Less than 141 mg/dL; if results exceed 140 mg/dL, the 100-g GTT should be performed	Less than 7.8 mmol/L; if results exceed 7.7 mmol/L, the 75-g GTT should be performed
Step Two	**Gestational GTT (100-g Glucose Load)**	Carpenter and Coustan	National Diabetes Data Group
Fasting sample		Less than 95 mg/dL (SI: Less than 5.3 mmol/L)	Less than 105 mg/dL (SI: Less than 5.8 mmol/L)
1-hr sample		Less 180 mg/dL (SI: Less than 10 mmol/L)	Less than 190 mg/dL (SI: Less than 10.5 mmol/L)
2-hr sample		Less than 155 mg/dL (SI: Less than 8.6 mmol/L)	Less than 165 mg/dL (SI: Less than 9.2 mmol/L)
3-hr sample		Less than 140 mg/dL (SI: Less than 7.8 mmol/L)	Less than 145 mg/dL (SI: Less than 8 mmol/L)

A diagnosis of gestational diabetes is made when two or more of the four thresholds are met or exceeded.
Plasma glucose values are reported to be 10% to 20% higher than serum values.
GTT = glucose tolerance test. 🍁

DESCRIPTION: The glucose tolerance test (GTT) measures glucose levels after administration of an oral or IV carbohydrate challenge. Patients with diabetes are unable to metabolize glucose at a normal rate. The oral glucose tolerance test (OGTT) is used for individuals who are able to eat and who are not known to have problems with gastrointestinal malabsorption. The intravenous (IV) GTT is used for individuals who are unable to tolerate oral glucose.

Glucose, a simple six-carbon sugar (monosaccharide), enters the diet as part of the sugars sucrose, lactose, and maltose and from the complex polysaccharide, dietary starch. The body acquires most of its energy from the oxidative metabolism of glucose. Excess glucose is stored in the liver or in muscle tissue as glycogen. Glucose levels in plasma (one of the components of blood) are generally 10% to 15% higher than glucose measurements in whole blood (and even more after eating). This is important because home blood glucose meters measure the glucose in whole blood, whereas most laboratory tests measure the glucose in either plasma or serum.

Diabetes is a group of diseases characterized by hyperglycemia, or elevated glucose levels. Hyperglycemia results from a defect in insulin secretion due to destruction of the beta cells of the pancreas (type 1 diabetes), a defect in insulin action, or a combination of defects in secretion and action (type 2 diabetes). The chronic hyperglycemia of diabetes may lead to microvascular changes that include retinopathy, nephropathy, and neuropathy. Chronic hyperglycemia may also cause macrovascular changes resulting in cardiovascular disease. The American Diabetes Association (ADA) and National Institute of Diabetes and Digestive and Kidney Disease have 🍁 established criteria for diagnosing diabetes to include any combination of the following findings or confirmation of any of the individual findings by repetition of the same test on a subsequent day:

Symptoms of diabetes (e.g., polyuria, polydipsia, unexplained weight loss) in addition to a random glucose level greater than 200 mg/dL (SI: 11.1 mmol/L) 🍁
Fasting blood glucose greater than 126 mg/dL (SI: 7 mmol/L) after fasting for a minimum of 8 hr 🍁
Glucose level greater than 200 mg/dL (SI: 11.1 mmol/L) 2 hr after glucose challenge with standardized 75-mg load
A_{1C} in adults equal to or greater than 6.5% (assumes the use of a standardized test as referenced to the National Glycohemoglobin Standardization Program—Diabetes Control and Complications Trial and the absence of clinical conditions such as hemoglobinopathies, anemias, and kidney and liver diseases known to affect the accuracy of the test results)

The American Congress of Obstetricians and Gynecologists (ACOG) and ADA recommend screening for all pregnant women at 24 to 28 wk of gestation using patient history, clinical risk factors, or carbohydrate challenge testing. Protocol recommendations may vary among requesting health-care providers (HCPs). The ADA and International Association of Diabetes and Pregnancy Study Groups recommend that all women not previously diagnosed with diabetes undergo a 75-g OGTT at 24 to 28 wk of gestation because unrecognized glucose intolerance may have existed prior to the pregnancy, glucose intolerance identified during pregnancy may have continued unmonitored after pregnancy, and the frequency of diabetes in women of childbearing age has dramatically increased. The ADA also recommends a diagnosis of overt, rather than gestational, diabetes if test results meet the criteria for diabetes at the initial prenatal visit. 🍁

This procedure is contraindicated for: N/A

INDICATIONS

- Evaluate abnormal fasting or postprandial blood glucose levels that do not clearly indicate diabetes.
- Evaluate glucose metabolism in women of childbearing age, especially women who are pregnant and have (1) a history of previous fetal loss or birth of infants weighing 9 lb or more and/or (2) a family history of diabetes.
- Identify abnormal renal tubular function if glycosuria occurs without hyperglycemia.
- Identify impaired glucose metabolism without overt diabetes.

- Support the diagnosis of hyperthyroidism and alcoholic liver disease, which are characterized by a sharp rise in blood glucose followed by a decline to subnormal levels.

POTENTIAL MEDICAL DIAGNOSIS

Tolerance Increased in

- Decreased absorption of glucose:
  - Adrenal insufficiency (Addison's disease, hypopituitarism)
  - Hypothyroidism
  - Intestinal diseases, such as celiac disease and tropical sprue
  - Whipple's disease
- Increased insulin secretion:
  - Pancreatic islet cell tumor

Tolerance Impaired in

- Increased absorption of glucose:
  - Excessive intake of glucose
  - Gastrectomy
  - Gastroenterostomy
  - Hyperthyroidism
  - Vagotomy
- Decreased usage of glucose:
  - Central nervous system lesions
  - Cushing's syndrome
  - Diabetes
  - Hemochromatosis
  - Hyperlipidemia
- Decreased glycogenesis:
  - Hyperthyroidism
  - Infections
  - Liver disease (severe)
  - Pheochromocytoma
  - Pregnancy
  - Stress
  - Von Gierke's disease

CRITICAL FINDINGS:

Glucose

Adults & Children

- Less than 40 mg/dL (SI: Less than 2.22 mmol/L)
- Greater than 400 mg/dL (SI: Greater than 22.2 mmol/L)

Newborns

- Less than 32 mg/dL (SI: Less than 1.8 mmol/L)
- Greater than 328 mg/dL (SI: Greater than 18.2 mmol/L)

Note and immediately report to the requesting HCP any critical findings and related symptoms. A listing of these findings varies among facilities. Timely notification of a critical finding for laboratory or diagnostic studies is a role expectation of the professional nurse. The notification processes vary among facilities. Upon receipt of the critical finding, the information should be read back to the caller to verify accuracy.

Consideration may be given to verification of critical findings before action is taken. Policies vary among facilities and may include requesting immediate recollection and retesting by the laboratory or retesting using a rapid point-of-care testing instrument at the bedside, if available.

Symptoms of decreased glucose levels include headache, confusion, polyphagia, irritability, nervousness, restlessness, diaphoresis, and weakness. Possible interventions include oral or IV administration of glucose, IV or intramuscular injection of glucagon, and continuous glucose monitoring.

Symptoms of elevated glucose levels include abdominal pain, fatigue, muscle cramps, nausea, vomiting, polyuria, polyphagia, and polydipsia. Possible interventions include fluid replacement in addition to subcutaneous or IV injection of insulin with continuous glucose monitoring.

INTERFERING FACTORS

- Drugs and other substances that may increase GTT values include acetylsalicylic acid, atenolol, bendroflumethiazide, caffeine, clofibrate, glyburide, guanethidine, lisinopril, metoprolol, niceritrol, nifedipine, nitrendipine,

G

norethisterone, phenformin, phenobarbital, prazosin, and terazosin.
- Drugs and other substances that may decrease GTT values include acebutolol, beclomethasone, bendroflumethiazide, betamethasone, calcitonin, catecholamines, chlorothiazide, chlorpromazine, chlorthalidone, cimetidine, corticotropin, cortisone, danazol, deflazacort, dexamethasone, diapamide, diethylstilbestrol, ethacrynic acid, fludrocortisone, furosemide, glucagon, glucocorticosteroids, heroin, hydrochlorothiazide, mestranol, methadone, methylprednisolone, muzolimine, niacin, nifedipine, norethindrone, norethynodrel, oral contraceptives, paramethasone, perphenazine, phenolphthalein, phenothiazine, phenytoin, pindolol, prednisolone, prednisone, propranolol, quinethazone, thiazides, triamcinolone, triamterene, and verapamil.
- The test should be performed on ambulatory patients. Impaired physical activity can lead to falsely increased values.
- Excessive physical activity before or during the test can lead to falsely decreased values.
- Failure of the patient to ingest a diet with sufficient carbohydrate content (e.g., 150 g/day) for at least 3 days before the test can result in falsely decreased values.
- The patient may have difficulty drinking the extremely sweet glucose beverage and become nauseous. Vomiting during the course of the test will cause the test to be canceled.
- Smoking before or during the test can lead to falsely increased values.
- The patient should not be under recent or current physiological stress during the test. If the patient has had recent surgery (less than 2 wk previously), an infectious disease, or a major illness (e.g., myocardial infarction), the test should be delayed or rescheduled.
- Failure to follow dietary restrictions before the procedure may cause the procedure to be canceled or repeated.

G

NURSING IMPLICATIONS AND PROCEDURE

POTENTIAL NURSING PROBLEMS:

Problem	Signs & Symptoms	Interventions
Blood glucose ***(related to sedentary lifestyle, circulating insulin deficiency secondary to pancreatic insufficiency; excessive dietary intake; insulin resistance; pregnancy)***	**Excess:** Fatigue; mild dehydration; elevated blood glucose; weight loss; weakness; polyuria; polydipsia; polyphagia; blurred vision; headache; paresthesia; poor skin turgor; dry mouth; nausea; vomiting; abdominal pain;	Check blood glucose before meals and at bedtime; administer prescribed insulin or oral drugs; educate and encourage the patient to participate in glucose self-check and record results; assess readiness to learn and barriers to learning; collaborate with the HCP and dietitian to support medical nutritional therapy; refer to dietitian to assist the patient to select appropriate cultural

Problem	Signs & Symptoms	Interventions
	Kussmaul respirations. **Deficit:** Tremor, diaphoresis, decreased concentration; elevated blood pressure; palpitations; headache; polyphagia; restlessness; lethargy; altered mental status; combativeness; altered speech; altered coordination	foods; develop a plan of exercise commensurate with the patient's physical abilities; discuss lifestyle alterations necessary to support positive health management secondary to disease process; teach good hygiene and infection prevention; monitor laboratory studies that may be impacted by altered glucose and trend results (Hgb A_{1C}; blood urea nitrogen; creatinine; electrolytes; arterial pH; magnesium; urine ketones; urine microalbumin; white blood cell (WBC) count; amylase; Hgb/Hct; WBC; C-reactive protein; liver enzymes); facilitate oral hydration; correlate blood glucose with other laboratory values and medical condition(s); address the psychosocial aspects of the disease; monitor serum insulin levels
Nutrition ***(related to excessive dietary intake more than body requirements, insulin deficiency, stress; anxiety; depression; cultural lifestyle; unhealthy food sources; financial restrictions)***	Polydipsia, polyuria, weight loss; fatigue; elevated blood glucose levels; inadequate glucose management; polyphagia	Monitor blood glucose results, refer to dietitian for evaluation, administer insulin or oral drug; assess the cultural aspects of diet selection; correlate dietary intake with blood glucose and monitor trends; collaborate with a dietitian to develop a cultural- and age-appropriate diet plan; correlate nutritional intake and exercise; ensure that the patient understands the relationship between caloric intake and medication (insulin, oral antihyperglycemics); refer to social services, dietitian as necessary

(table continues on page 872)

Problem	Signs & Symptoms	Interventions
Infection risk ***(related to altered blood glucose; exposure to opportunistic hosts; poor personal hygiene; broken skin; wound presence)***	Increased temperature; increased heart rate and respiratory rate; chills; change in mental status; fatigue; malaise; weakness; anorexia; headache; nausea; elevated blood glucose; hypotension; diminished oxygen saturation; elevated WBC; elevated C-reactive protein	Provide standard precautions in the provision of care; correlate symptoms with laboratory values and disease process; trend vital signs and laboratory values to monitor for improvement; administer prescribed antibiotics and medications for fever reduction; provide cooling measures; perform vigilant hand hygiene; educate patient and family regarding good hand hygiene; infuse ordered IV fluids to support adequate hydration; ensure implementation of infection prevention measures with consideration of age and culture such as adequate nutrition; provide aseptic wound care; ensure skin care; ensure oral care; ensure adequate rest; instruct patient to avoid exposure to opportunistic hosts; send cultures to the laboratory as ordered; correlate culture findings with selected antibiotics
Noncompliance ***(related to refusal to accept new diagnosis; financial instability; cultural norms; complexity of the medical management; lack of knowledge)***	Insufficient disease management; alterations in blood glucose; poor self-management of medication administration; lack of supplies to support self-management; poor dietary control with inappropriate food selections	Assess the patient's ability to and prior efforts to manage the disease process; evaluate the ability to self-manage the disease including blood glucose screening, dietary management, exercise, and medication self-administration; assess for personal factors that may limit the patient's ability to self-perform such as visual, cognitive, and hearing; assess the financial ability to purchase the medication and supplies necessary to provide self-care; assess the level of family support; ensure the patient has the adequate

Problem	Signs & Symptoms	Interventions
		knowledge to perform self-care and if not provide the necessary training; ensure the patient knows the signs and symptoms related to the disease process; teach correct dietary selections meeting cultural- and age-appropriate needs; refer to social services or home care; discuss how to manage diabetes during travel

PRETEST:

- Positively identify the patient using at least two person-specific identifiers before services, treatments, or procedures are performed.
- ***Patient Teaching:*** Inform the patient this test can assist in evaluating blood sugar levels.
- Obtain a history of the patient's health concerns, symptoms, surgical procedures, and results of previously performed laboratory and diagnostic studies. Include a list of known allergens, especially allergies or sensitivities to latex.
- Obtain a list of the patient's current medications, including over-the-counter medications and dietary supplements (see Effects of Natural Products on Laboratory Values online at Davis*Plus*).
- Review the procedure with the patient. Inform the patient that specimen collection takes approximately 5 to 10 min. Inform the patient that multiple specimens may be required. Address concerns about pain and explain that there may be some discomfort during the venipuncture.
- ***Sensitivity to social and cultural issues,*** as well as concern for modesty, is important in providing psychological support before, during, and after the procedure.
- Instruct the patient to fast for at least 8 hr before the standard oral and standard gestational GTTs and not to consume any caffeinated products or chew any type of gum before specimen collection for the test; these factors are known to elevate glucose levels.
- Note that there are no fluid or medication restrictions unless by medical direction prior to the gestational screen.

INTRATEST:

Potential Complications:

Note that the patient may have difficulty drinking the extremely sweet glucose beverage and become nauseous. Vomiting during the course of the test will cause the test to be canceled.

- Ensure that the patient has complied with dietary and activity restrictions as well as other pretesting preparations prior to the study, as instructed.
- Avoid the use of equipment containing latex if the patient has a history of allergic reaction to latex.
- Instruct the patient to cooperate fully and to follow directions. Direct the patient to breathe normally and to avoid unnecessary movement.
- Observe standard precautions, and follow the general guidelines in Patient Preparation and Specimen Collection online at Davis*Plus*. Positively identify the patient, and label the appropriate specimen container with the corresponding patient demographics, initials of the person collecting the specimen, date, and time of collection. Perform a venipuncture.

- Remove the needle and apply direct pressure with dry gauze to stop bleeding. Observe/assess venipuncture site for bleeding or hematoma formation and secure gauze with adhesive bandage.
- Promptly transport the specimen to the laboratory for processing and analysis. Do not wait until all specimens have been collected to transport.

Standard OGTT

- The standard OGTT takes 2 hr. A fasting blood glucose is determined before administration of an oral glucose load. If the fasting blood glucose is less than 126 mg/dL, the patient is given an oral glucose load.
- An oral glucose load should not be administered before the value of the fasting specimen has been received. If the fasting blood glucose is greater than 126 mg/dL, the standard glucose load is not administered and the test is canceled. The laboratory will follow its protocol as far as notifying the patient of his or her glucose level and the reason the test was canceled. The requesting HCP will then be issued a report indicating the glucose level and the cancellation of the test. A fasting glucose greater than 126 mg/dL indicates diabetes; therefore, the glucose load would never be administered before allowing the requesting HCP to evaluate the clinical situation.
- Adults receive 75 g and children receive 1.75 g/kg ideal weight, not to exceed 75 g. The glucose load should be consumed within 5 min, and time 0 begins as soon as the patient begins to ingest the glucose load. A second specimen is collected at 2 hr, concluding the test. The test is discontinued if the patient vomits before the second specimen has been collected.

Gestational Screen or Challenge Test

- The gestational screen is performed on pregnant women, usually at their first prenatal visit. If results from the screen are abnormal, a gestational GTT is performed. The gestational screen does not require a fast. The patient is given a 50-g oral glucose load. The glucose load should be consumed within 5 min, and time 0 begins as soon as the patient begins to ingest the glucose load. A specimen is collected 1 hr after ingestion. The test is discontinued if the patient vomits before the 1-hr specimen has been collected. If the result is normal, the test may be repeated between 24 and 28 wk gestation.

Gestational GTT

- The gestational GTT takes 3 hr. A fasting blood glucose is determined before administration of a 75-g or 100-g oral glucose load, depending on the order. If the fasting blood glucose is less than 126 mg/dL, the patient is given an oral glucose load.
- An oral glucose load should not be administered before the value of the fasting specimen has been received. *If the fasting blood glucose is greater than 126 mg/dL, the Glucola is not administered and the test is canceled* (see previous explanation).
- The glucose load should be consumed within 5 min, and time 0 begins as soon as the patient begins to ingest the glucose load. Subsequent specimens are collected at 1, 2, and 3 hr, concluding the test. The test is discontinued if the patient vomits before all specimens have been collected.

POST-TEST:

- Inform the patient that a report of the results will be made available to the requesting HCP, who will discuss the results with the patient.
- Instruct the patient to resume usual diet and activity, as directed by the HCP.
- ***Nutritional Considerations:*** Impaired glucose tolerance may be associated with diabetes. There is no "diabetic diet"; however, many meal-planning approaches with nutritional goals are endorsed by the ADA. Patients who adhere to dietary recommendations report a better general feeling

of health, better weight management, greater control of glucose and lipid values, and improved use of insulin. Instruct the patient, as appropriate, in nutritional management of diabetes. A variety of dietary patterns are beneficial for people with diabetes. The Mediterranean-style diet emphasizes inclusion of vegetables, whole grains, fruits, low-fat dairy, nuts, legumes, and nontropical vegetable oils (e.g., olive, canola, peanut, sunflower, flaxseed) along with fish and lean poultry. A similar dietary pattern known as the Dietary Approaches to Stop Hypertension (DASH) diet makes additional recommendations for the reduction of dietary sodium. Both dietary styles emphasize a reduction in consumption of red meats, which are high in saturated fats and cholesterol, and other foods containing sugar, saturated fats, trans fats, and sodium. A vegetarian diet as well as other potential weight loss diets such as Weight Watchers are also supported by the ADA. 🍁 If triglycerides also are elevated, the patient should be advised to eliminate or reduce alcohol. The nutritional needs of each patient with diabetes need to be determined individually (especially during pregnancy) with the appropriate HCPs, particularly professionals educated in nutrition.

- ***Social and Cultural Considerations:*** Studies comparing risk for developing diabetes demonstrate that certain populations are disproportionately affected by type 2 diabetes and complications of type 2 diabetes as compared to the general population. Nonmodifiable risk factors include age, ethnicity, and family history of diabetes or metabolic syndrome. The risk of developing type 2 diabetes increases with age.In the United States, affected populations include African Americans, Asian Americans, Hispanics, native Hawaiians and Pacific Islanders, American Indians, and Alaska natives. 🍁 Modifiable risk factors include lifestyle choices related to making healthy dietary choices, maintaining a healthy body weight, and meeting recommended levels of physical activity. The financial and emotional burdens of diabetes and related complications continue to grow at an alarming rate. A system for the prevention, management, and support of patients with type 2 diabetes should be provided through the coordinated efforts of multidisciplinary partners using strategies that are culturally appropriate.
- Recognize anxiety related to test results, and be supportive of perceived loss of independence and fear of shortened life expectancy. The ADA recommends A_{1C} testing four times a year for type 1 or type 2 diabetes when glycemic targets are not being met or when therapy has changed and twice a year when treatment goals are being met for type 2 diabetes. The ADA also recommends that testing for diabetes commence at age 45 for asymptomatic individuals, be considered for adults of any age who are overweight and have additional risk factors, and continue every 3 yr in the absence of symptoms. 🍁
- Depending on the results of this procedure, additional testing may be performed to evaluate or monitor progression of the disease process and determine the need for a change in therapy. Evaluate test results in relation to the patient's symptoms and other tests performed.

Patient Education:

- Instruct the patient and caregiver to report signs and symptoms of hypoglycemia (weakness, confusion, diaphoresis, rapid pulse) or hyperglycemia (thirst, polyuria, hunger, lethargy).
- Recognize anxiety related to test results, and be supportive of perceived loss of independence and fear of shortened life expectancy.
- Discuss the implications of abnormal test results on the patient's lifestyle.
- Provide teaching and information regarding the clinical implications of the test results, as appropriate.
- Emphasize, if indicated, that good glycemic management delays the

onset and slows the progression of diabetic retinopathy, nephropathy, and neuropathy. Educate the patient regarding access to counseling services, as appropriate.

- Provide contact information, if desired, for the American Heart Association (www.americanheart.org), National Heart, Lung, and Blood Institute (www.nhlbi.nih.gov), Institute of Medicine of the National Academies (www.iom.edu), and USDA's resource for nutrition (www.choosemyplate.gov). 🍁
- Reinforce information given by the patient's HCP regarding further testing, treatment, or referral to another HCP.
- Instruct the patient in the use of home testing strips or meters approved for glucose, ketones, or A_{1C} by the U.S. Food and Drug Administration, if prescribed. 🍁 Answer any questions or address any concerns voiced by the patient or family.
- Teach the pregnant patient that untreated gestational diabetes can increase health risks to self and fetus.
- Teach the patient that gestational diabetes may resolve after the pregnancy is over but that diabetes may reoccur later in life.

Expected Patient Outcomes:

Understanding

- The patient and family state the signs and symptoms of high and low blood sugar that should be reported to the HCP.
- The patient and family collaborate with the dietitian to formulate a meal plan that will support fetal health and control blood glucose.

Ability

- The patient demonstrates proficiency in self-administration of prescribed medications to control blood glucose during pregnancy correctly.
- The patient demonstrates proficiency in the ability to perform a self-check glucose accurately.

Response

- The patient complies with the recommended medication and dietary plan to control blood glucose during pregnancy.
- The patient complies with the recommended follow-up glucose studies necessary to manage disease process.

RELATED STUDIES:

- Related tests include ACTH, ALP, antibodies gliadin, angiography adrenal, biopsy intestinal, biopsy thyroid, BUN, C-peptide, capsule endoscopy, catecholamines, cholesterol (total and HDL), cortisol, creatinine, DHEAS, fecal fat, fluorescein angiography, folate, fructosamine, fundoscopy, gastric acid stimulation, gastrin stimulation, glucagon, glucose, glycated hemoglobin, gonioscopy, 5-HIAA, insulin, insulin antibodies, ketones, metanephrines, microalbumin, oxalate, RAIU, thyroid scan, TSH, thyroxine, triglycerides, VMA, and visual fields test.
- Refer to the Endocrine System table online at Davis*Plus* for related tests by body system.

Glycated Hemoglobin

SYNONYM/ACRONYM: Hemoglobin A_{1c}, A_{1c}.

COMMON USE: To monitor treatment in individuals with diabetes by evaluating their long-term glycemic control.

SPECIMEN: Whole blood collected in a lavender-top (EDTA) tube.

NORMAL FINDINGS: (Method: Chromatography)

A_{1c}	
Nondiabetic	4%–5.5%
Prediabetes	5.7%–6.4%
Diabetes	6.5% or less

Values vary widely by method. The treatment goal assumes the use of a standardized test as referenced to the National Glycohemoglobin Standardization Program—Diabetes Control and Complications Trial and the absence of clinical conditions such as hemoglobinopathies, anemias, and kidney and liver diseases known to affect the accuracy of the test results.
American Diabetes Association.

DESCRIPTION: *Glycosylated* or *glycated hemoglobin* is the combination of glucose and hemoglobin into a ketamine; the rate at which this occurs is proportional to glucose concentration. The average life span of a red blood cell (RBC) is approximately 120 days; measurement of glycated hemoglobin is a way to monitor long-term diabetic management. A change of 1% in the A_{1c} is roughly equivalent to a change in glucose concentration of 29 mg/dL or 1.6 mmol/L. The average plasma glucose can be estimated using the formula (mg/dL) = $[(A_{1c} \times 28.7) - 46.7]$.

The same formula can be used to convert the estimated average glucose (eAG) to glucose in SI units (after multiplying the eAG by 0.555 to convert from mg/dL to mmol/L).

For example, an A_{1c} value of 6% would reflect an average plasma glucose of 125.5 mg/dL or $[(6 \times 28.7) - 46.7]$. Expressed in SI units, $[(6 \times 28.7) - 46.7] = 125.5 \times 0.555 = 7$ mmol/L.

Hemoglobin A_{1c} levels are not age dependent and are not affected by exercise, diabetic medications, or nonfasting state before specimen collection. The hemoglobin A_{1c} assay would not be useful for patients with hemolytic anemia or abnormal hemoglobins (e.g., hemoglobin S) accompanied by abnormal red blood cell (RBC) turnover. These patients would be screened, diagnosed, and managed using symptoms, clinical risk factors, short-term glycemic indicators (glucose), and intermediate glycemic indicators (1,5-anhydroglucitol or glycated albumin).

Diabetes is a group of diseases characterized by hyperglycemia, or elevated glucose levels. Hyperglycemia results from a defect in insulin secretion due to destruction of the beta cells of the pancreas (type 1 diabetes), a defect in insulin action, or a combination of defects in secretion and action (type 2 diabetes). The chronic hyperglycemia of diabetes over time may lead to damage, dysfunction, and eventually failure of the eyes (retinopathy), kidneys (nephropathy), nerves (neuropathy), heart (cardiovascular disease), and blood vessels (micro- and macrovascular conditions). The American Diabetes Association (ADA) and National Institute of Diabetes and Digestive and Kidney Disease have established criteria for diagnosing diabetes to include any combination of the following findings or confirmation of any of the individual findings by repetition of the same test on a subsequent day:

Symptoms of diabetes (e.g., polyuria, polydipsia, polyphagia, unexplained weight loss) in addition to a random glucose level greater than 200 mg/dL (SI: 11.1 mmol/L) 🍁

Fasting blood glucose greater than 126 mg/dL (SI: 7 mmol/L) after fasting for a minimum of 8 hr 🍁

Glucose level greater than 200 mg/dL (SI: 11.1 mmol/L) 2 hr after glucose challenge with standardized 75-mg load

A_{1C} in adults equal to or greater than 6.5% (assumes the use of a standardized test as referenced to the National Glycohemoglobin Standardization Program—Diabetes Control and Complications Trial and the absence of clinical conditions such as hemoglobinopathies, anemias, and kidney and liver diseases known to affect the accuracy of the test results)

This procedure is contraindicated for: N/A

INDICATIONS

Assess long-term glucose control in individuals with diabetes

POTENTIAL MEDICAL DIAGNOSIS

Increased in:

- Diabetes (poorly controlled or uncontrolled) ***(related to and evidenced by elevated glucose levels)***
- Pregnancy ***(evidenced by gestational diabetes)***
- Splenectomy ***(related to prolonged RBC survival, which extends the amount of time hemoglobin is available for glycosylation)***

Decreased in:

- Chronic blood loss ***(related to decreased concentration of RBC-bound glycated hemoglobin due to blood loss)***
- Chronic kidney disease ***(low RBC count associated with this condition reflects corresponding decrease in RBC-bound glycated hemoglobin)***
- Conditions that decrease RBC life span ***(evidenced by anemia and low RBC count, reflecting a corresponding decrease in RBC-bound glycated hemoglobin)***
- Hemolytic anemia ***(evidenced by low RBC count due to hemolysis, reflecting a corresponding decrease in RBC-bound glycated hemoglobin)***
- Pregnancy ***(evidenced by anemia and low RBC count, reflecting a corresponding decrease in RBC-bound glycated hemoglobin)***

CRITICAL FINDINGS: N/A

INTERFERING FACTORS

- Drugs and other substances that may increase glycated hemoglobin values include aspirin (large doses), atenolol, chronic use of opiates, drugs that increase glucose levels, propranolol, and sulfonylureas.
- Drugs and other substances that may decrease glycated hemoglobin values include antiretroviral drugs, aspirin (small doses), cholestyramine, drugs that cause RBC hemolysis (e.g., dapsone), drugs that decrease glucose levels (e.g., metformin), vitamin C, and vitamin E.
- Conditions involving abnormal hemoglobins (hemoglobinopathies) affect the reliability of glycated hemoglobin values, causing (1) falsely increased values, (2) falsely decreased values, or (3) discrepancies in either direction depending on the method.

NURSING IMPLICATIONS AND PROCEDURE

POTENTIAL NURSING PROBLEMS:

Problem	Signs & Symptoms	Interventions
Blood glucose ***(related to sedentary lifestyle, circulating insulin deficiency secondary to pancreatic insufficiency; excessive dietary intake; insulin resistance; pregnancy)***	**Excess:** Fatigue; mild dehydration; elevated blood glucose; weight loss; weakness; polyuria; polydipsia; polyphagia; blurred vision; headache; paresthesia; poor skin turgor; dry mouth; nausea; vomiting; abdominal pain; Kussmaul respirations. **Deficit:** Tremor; decreased concentration; diaphoresis; elevated blood pressure; palpitations; headache; polyphagia; restlessness; lethargy; altered mental status; combativeness; altered speech; altered coordination	Check blood glucose before meals and at bedtime; administer prescribed insulin or oral drugs; educate and encourage the patient to participate in glucose self-check and record results; assess readiness to learn and barriers to learning; collaborate with the health-care provider (HCP) and dietitian to support medical nutritional therapy; collaborate with dietitian to assist the patient to select appropriate cultural foods; develop a plan of exercise commensurate with the patient's physical abilities; discuss lifestyle alterations necessary to support positive health management secondary to disease process; teach good hygiene and infection prevention; monitor laboratory studies that may be impacted by altered glucose and trend results (Hgb A_{1c}; blood urea nitrogen; creatinine; electrolytes; arterial pH; magnesium; urine ketones; urine microalbumin; white blood cell (WBC) count; amylase; Hgb/Hct; WBC; C-reactive protein; liver enzymes); facilitate oral hydration; correlate blood glucose with other laboratory values and medical condition(s); address the psychosocial aspects of the disease; monitor serum insulin levels

(table continues on page 880)

G

Problem	Signs & Symptoms	Interventions
Infection risk ***(related to altered blood glucose; exposure to opportunistic hosts; poor personal hygiene; broken skin; wound presence)***	Increased temperature; increased heart rate and respiratory rate; chills; change in mental status; fatigue; malaise; weakness; anorexia; headache; nausea; elevated blood glucose; hypotension; diminished oxygen saturation; elevated WBC; elevated C-reactive protein	Provide standard precautions in the provision of care; correlate symptoms with laboratory values and disease process; trend vital signs and laboratory values to monitor for improvement; administer prescribed antibiotics and medications for fever reduction; administer cooling measures; perform vigilant hand hygiene; educate patient and family regarding good hand hygiene; infuse ordered intravenous fluids to support adequate hydration; ensure implementation of infection prevention measures with consideration of age and culture such as adequate nutrition; provide aseptic wound care; ensure good skin care; ensure good oral care; ensure adequate rest; instruct patient to avoid exposure to opportunistic hosts; send cultures to the laboratory as ordered; correlate culture findings with selected antibiotics
Nutrition ***(related to excessive dietary intake more than body requirements, insulin deficiency, stress; anxiety; depression; cultural lifestyle; unhealthy food sources; financial restrictions)***	Increased thirst, increased urination, weight loss; fatigue; elevated blood glucose levels; inadequate glucose management; increased hunger	Monitor blood glucose results, refer to dietitian for evaluation, administer insulin or oral drugs; assess the cultural aspects of diet selection; correlate dietary intake with blood glucose and monitor trends; collaborate with a dietitian to develop a cultural- and age-appropriate diet plan; correlate nutritional intake and exercise; ensure that the patient understands the relationship between caloric intake and medication (insulin, oral drug); refer to social services, dietitian

Problem	Signs & Symptoms	Interventions
Noncompliance ***(related to refusal to accept new diagnosis; financial instability; cultural norms; complexity of the medical management; lack of knowledge)***	Insufficient disease management; alterations in blood glucose; poor self-management of medication administration; lack of supplies to support self-management; poor dietary control with inappropriate food selections	Assess the patient's ability to and prior efforts to manage the disease process; evaluate the ability to self-manage the disease including blood glucose screening, dietary management, exercise, and medication self-administration; assess for personal factors that may limit the patient's ability to self-perform such as visual, cognitive, and hearing; assess the financial ability to purchase the medication and supplies necessary to provide self-care; assess the level of family support; ensure the patient has the adequate knowledge to perform self-care and if not provide the necessary training; ensure the patient knows the signs and symptoms related to the disease process; teach correct dietary selections meeting cultural- and age-appropriate needs; refer to social services or home health; discuss how to manage diabetes during travel

PRETEST:

- Positively identify the patient using at least two person-specific identifiers before services, treatments, or procedures are performed.
- *Patient Teaching:* Inform the patient this test can assist in evaluating blood sugar control over approximately the past 3 mo.
- Obtain a history of the patient's health concerns, symptoms, surgical procedures, and results of previously performed laboratory and diagnostic studies. Include a list of known allergens, especially allergies or sensitivities to latex.
- Obtain a list of the patient's current medications, including over-the-counter medications and dietary supplements (see Effects of Natural Products on Laboratory Values online at Davis*Plus*).
- Review the procedure with the patient. Inform the patient that specimen collection takes approximately 5 to 10 min. Address concerns about pain and explain that there may be some discomfort during the venipuncture.
- ***Sensitivity to social and cultural issues,*** as well as concern for modesty, is important in providing psychological

support before, during, and after the procedure.

- Note that there are no food, fluid, or medication restrictions unless by medical direction.

INTRATEST:

Potential Complications: N/A

- Avoid the use of equipment containing latex if the patient has a history of allergic reaction to latex.
- Instruct the patient to cooperate fully and to follow directions. Direct the patient to breathe normally and to avoid unnecessary movement.
- Observe standard precautions, and follow the general guidelines in Patient Preparation and Specimen Collection online at Davis*Plus*. Positively identify the patient, and label the appropriate specimen container with the corresponding patient demographics, initials of the person collecting the specimen, date, and time of collection. Perform a venipuncture.
- Remove the needle and apply direct pressure with dry gauze to stop bleeding. Observe/assess venipuncture site for bleeding or hematoma formation and secure gauze with adhesive bandage.
- Promptly transport the specimen to the laboratory for processing and analysis.

G

POST-TEST:

- Inform the patient that a report of the results will be made available to the requesting HCP, who will discuss the results with the patient.
- ***Nutritional Considerations:*** Increased hemoglobin A_{1c} levels may be associated with diabetes. There is no "diabetic diet"; however, many meal-planning approaches with nutritional goals are endorsed by the ADA. 🍁 Patients who adhere to dietary recommendations report a better general feeling of health, better weight management, greater control of glucose and lipid values, and improved use of insulin. Instruct the patient, as appropriate, in nutritional management of diabetes. A variety of dietary patterns are beneficial for people with diabetes. The Mediterranean-style diet emphasizes inclusion of vegetables, whole grains, fruits, low-fat dairy, nuts, legumes, and nontropical vegetable oils (e.g., olive, canola, peanut, sunflower, flaxseed) along with fish and lean poultry. A similar dietary pattern known as the Dietary Approaches to Stop Hypertension (DASH) diet makes additional recommendations for the reduction of dietary sodium. Both dietary styles emphasize a reduction in consumption of red meats, which are high in saturated fats and cholesterol, and other foods containing sugar, saturated fats, trans fats, and sodium. A vegetarian diet as well as other potential weight loss diets such as Weight Watchers are also supported by the ADA. 🍁 If triglycerides also are elevated, the patient should be advised to eliminate or reduce alcohol. The nutritional needs of each patient with diabetic patient need to be determined individually (especially during pregnancy) with the appropriate HCPs, particularly professionals educated in nutrition.
- ***Social and Cultural Considerations:*** Numerous studies point to the prevalence of excess body weight in American children and adolescents. Experts estimate that obesity is present in 25% of the population aged 6 to 11 yr. The medical, social, and emotional consequences of excess body weight are significant. Special attention should be given to instructing the pediatric patient and caregiver regarding health risks and weight control education. 🍁
- ***Social and Cultural Considerations:*** Studies comparing risk for developing diabetes demonstrate that certain populations are disproportionately affected by type 2 diabetes and complications of type 2 diabetes as compared to the general population. Nonmodifiable risk factors include age, ethnicity, and family history of diabetes or metabolic syndrome. The risk of developing type 2 diabetes increases with age. In the United States, affected populations include

African Americans, Asian Americans, Hispanics, native Hawaiians and Pacific Islanders, American Indians, and Alaska natives. 🍁 Modifiable risk factors include lifestyle choices related to making healthy dietary choices, maintaining a healthy body weight, and meeting recommended levels of physical activity. The financial and emotional burdens of diabetes and related complications continue to grow at an alarming rate. A system for the prevention, management, and support of patients with type 2 diabetes should be provided through the coordinated efforts of multidisciplinary partners using strategies that are culturally appropriate.

- Recognize anxiety related to test results, and be supportive of perceived loss of independence and fear of shortened life expectancy. The ADA recommends A_{1C} testing four times a year for insulin-dependent type 1 or type 2 diabetes when glycemic targets are not being met or when therapy has changed and twice a year when treatment goals are being met for non–insulin-dependent type 2 diabetes. The ADA also recommends that testing for diabetes commence at age 45 for asymptomatic individuals, be considered for adults of any age who are overweight and have additional risk factors, and continue every 3 yr in the absence of symptoms. 🍁
- Depending on the results of this procedure, additional testing may be performed to evaluate or monitor progression of the disease process and determine the need for a change in therapy. Evaluate test results in relation to the patient's symptoms and other tests performed.

Patient Education:

- Instruct the patient and caregiver to report signs and symptoms of hypoglycemia (weakness, confusion, diaphoresis, rapid pulse) or hyperglycemia (thirst, polyuria, hunger, lethargy).
- Discuss the implications of abnormal test results on the patient's lifestyle.
- Provide teaching and information regarding the clinical implications of the test results, as appropriate.
- Emphasize, if indicated, that good glycemic control delays the onset and slows the progression of diabetic retinopathy, nephropathy, and neuropathy.
- Educate the patient regarding access to counseling services, as appropriate.
- Provide contact information, if desired, for the ADA (www.diabetes.org), American Heart Association (www.americanheart.org), National Heart, Lung, and Blood Institute (www.nhlbi.nih.gov), and USDA's resource for nutrition (www.choosemyplate.gov). 🍁
- Reinforce information given by the patient's HCP regarding further testing, treatment, or referral to another HCP.
- Instruct the patient in the use of home testing strips or meters approved for glucose, ketones, or A_{1C} by the U.S. Food and Drug Administration, if prescribed. 🍁
- Answer any questions or address any concerns voiced by the patient or family.

Expected Patient Outcomes:

Understanding

- The patient and family state that diabetes is a disease that can adversely affect multiple body systems if not accurately controlled.
- The patient and family state that this laboratory study is a way to assess blood glucose control over time.

Ability

- The patient demonstrates proficiency in the ability to perform a self-monitored glucose accurately.
- The patient demonstrates proficiency in the ability to perform insulin self-administration correctly or to take oral antihyperglycemic drugs.

Response

- The patient complies with the request for periodic A_{1C} laboratory studies to better manage the disease process over time.

G

- The patient complies with recommended diet and exercise to better control blood glucose.

RELATED STUDIES:

- Related tests include C-peptide, cholesterol (total and HDL), CT cardiac scoring, creatinine/eGFR, EMG, ENG, fluorescein angiography, fructosamine, fundoscopy, gastric emptying scan, glucagon, glucose, glucose tolerance tests, insulin, insulin antibodies, ketones, microalbumin, plethysmography, slit-lamp biomicroscopy, triglycerides, and visual fields test.
- Refer to the Endocrine System table online at Davis*Plus* for related tests by body system.

Gonioscopy

SYNONYM/ACRONYM: N/A

COMMON USE: To detect abnormalities in the structure of the anterior chamber of the eye such as in glaucoma.

AREA OF APPLICATION: Eyes.

DESCRIPTION: Gonioscopy is a technique used for examination of the anterior chamber structures of the eye (i.e., the trabecular meshwork and the anatomical relationship of the trabecular meshwork to the iris). The trabecular meshwork is the drainage system of the eye, and gonioscopy is performed to determine if the drainage angle is damaged, blocked, or clogged. Gonioscopy in combination with biomicroscopy is considered to be the most thorough basis to confirm a diagnosis of glaucoma and to differentiate between open-angle and angle-closure glaucoma. The angle structures of the anterior chamber are normally not visible because light entering the eye through the cornea is reflected back into the anterior chamber. Placement of a special contact lens (goniolens) over the cornea allows reflected light to pass back through the cornea and onto a reflective mirror in the contact lens. It is in this way that the angle structures can be visualized. There are two types of gonioscopy: indirect and direct. The more commonly used indirect technique employs a mirrored goniolens and biomicroscope. Direct gonioscopy is performed with a gonioscope containing a dome-shaped contact lens known as a gonioprism. The gonioprism eliminates internally reflected light, allowing direct visualization of the angle. Interpretation of visual examination is usually documented in a colored hand-drawn diagram. Scheie's classification is used to standardize definition of angles based on appearance by gonioscopy. Shaffer's classification is based on the angular width of the angle recess.

This procedure is contraindicated for: N/A

INDICATIONS

- Assess degenerative conditions of the anterior chamber.
- Assess for hyperpigmentation.
- Assess peripheral anterior synechiae (PAS).

- Assess for the presence of glaucoma (confirmation of normal structures and estimation of angle width).
- Assess for the presence of uveitis.
- Evaluate growth or tumor in the angle.
- Evaluate posttrauma evaluation for angle recession.
- Investigate conditions affecting the ciliary body.
- Investigate suspected neovascularization of the angle.

POTENTIAL MEDICAL DIAGNOSIS

Scheie's Classification Based on Visible Angle Structures

Classification	Appearance
Wide open	All angle structures seen
Grade I narrow	Difficult to see over the iris root
Grade II narrow	Ciliary band obscured
Grade III narrow	Posterior trabeculae hazy
Grade IV narrow	Only Schwalbe's line visible

Shaffer's Classification Based on Angle Width

Classification	Appearance
Wide open (20°–45°)	Closure improbable
Moderately narrow (10°–20°)	Closure possible
Extremely narrow (less than 10°)	Closure possible
Partially/totally closed	Closure present

Normal findings

- Normal appearance of anterior chamber structures and wide, unblocked, normal angle

Abnormal findings related to

- Corneal endothelial disorders (Fuchs' endothelial dystrophy, iridocorneal endothelial syndrome)
- Glaucoma
- Lens disorders (cataract, displaced lens)
- Malignant ocular neoplasm in angle
- Neovascularization in angle
- Ocular hemorrhage
- PAS
- Schwartz's syndrome
- Trauma
- Tumors
- Uveitis

CRITICAL FINDINGS: N/A

INTERFERING FACTORS

- Inability of the patient to cooperate or remain still during the test because of age, significant pain, or mental status may interfere with the test results.

NURSING IMPLICATIONS AND PROCEDURE

PRETEST:

- Positively identify the patient using at least two person-specific identifiers before services, treatments, or procedures are performed.
- *Patient Teaching:* Inform the patient this procedure can assist in evaluating the eye for disease.
- Obtain a history of the patient's health concerns (especially known or suspected vision loss; changes in visual acuity, including type and cause, use of glasses or contact lenses, eye

conditions with treatment regimens, and eye surgery), symptoms, surgical procedures, and results of previously performed laboratory and diagnostic studies. Include a list of known allergens, especially allergies or sensitivities to latex.

- Obtain a list of the patient's current medications, including over-the-counter medications and dietary supplements (see Effects of Natural Products on Laboratory Values online at Davis*Plus*).
- Instruct the patient to remove contact lenses or glasses, as appropriate. Instruct the patient regarding the importance of keeping the eyes open for the test.
- Review the procedure with the patient. Explain that the patient will be requested to fixate the eyes during the procedure. Address concerns about pain related to the procedure. Explain that no pain will be experienced during the test, but there may be moments of discomfort. Explain that some discomfort may be experienced after the test when the numbness wears off from anesthetic drops administered prior to the test. Inform the patient that the test is performed by a health-care provider (HCP) specially trained to perform this procedure and takes about 5 min to complete.
- ***Sensitivity to social and cultural issues,*** as well as concern for modesty, is important in providing psychological support before, during, and after the procedure.
- Note that there are no food, fluid, or medication restrictions unless by medical direction.

G

INTRATEST:

Potential Complications: N/A

- Observe standard precautions, and follow the general guidelines in Patient Preparation and Specimen Collection online at Davis*Plus*. Positively identify the patient.
- Instruct the patient to cooperate fully and to follow directions. Ask the patient to remain still during the procedure because movement produces unreliable results.
- Seat the patient comfortably. Instill topical anesthetic in each eye, as ordered, and allow time for it to work. Topical anesthetic drops are placed in the eye with the patient looking up and the solution directed at the six o'clock position of the sclera (white of the eye) near the limbus (gray, semitransparent area of the eyeball where the cornea and sclera meet). Neither the dropper nor the bottle should touch the eyelashes.
- Ask the patient to place the chin in the chin rest and gently press the forehead against the support bar. Ask the patient to open his or her eyes wide and look at desired target. Explain that the HCP or optometrist will place a lens on the eye while a narrow beam of light is focused on the eye.

POST-TEST:

- Inform the patient that a report of the results will be made available to the requesting HCP, who will discuss the results with the patient.
- Recognize anxiety related to test results, and be supportive of impaired activity related to vision loss or anticipated loss of driving privileges. Glaucoma is a leading cause of blindness in the United States. Additional information can be obtained from the American Optometric Association at (www.opto.ca). 🍁 Discuss the implications of abnormal test results on the patient's lifestyle. Provide teaching and information regarding the clinical implications of the test results, as appropriate.
- Reinforce information given by the patient's HCP regarding further testing, treatment, or referral to another HCP. Answer any questions or address any concerns voiced by the patient or family.
- Depending on the results of this procedure, additional testing may be performed to evaluate or monitor progression of the disease process and determine the need for a change in therapy. Evaluate test results in relation to the patient's symptoms and other tests performed.

RELATED STUDIES:

- Related tests include fundoscopy, pachymetry, slit-lamp biomicroscopy, and visual field testing.
- Refer to the Ocular System table online at Davis*Plus* for related tests by body system.

Gram Stain

SYNONYM/ACRONYM: N/A

COMMON USE: To provide a quick reference for gram-negative or gram-positive organisms to assist in medical management.

SPECIMEN: Blood, biopsy specimen, or body fluid as collected for culture.

NORMAL FINDINGS: N/A

DESCRIPTION: Gram stain is a technique commonly used to identify bacterial organisms on the basis of their specific staining characteristics. The method involves smearing a small amount of specimen on a slide, and then exposing it to gentian or crystal violet, iodine, alcohol, and safranin O. Gram-positive bacteria retain the gentian or crystal violet and iodine stain complex after a decolorization step and appear purple-blue in color. Gram-negative bacteria do not retain the stain after decolorization but can pick up the pink color of the safranin O counterstain. Gram stains provide information regarding the adequacy of a sample. For example, a sputum Gram stain showing greater than 25 squamous epithelial cells per low-power field, regardless of the number of polymorphonuclear white blood cells, indicates contamination of the specimen with saliva, and the specimen should be rejected for subsequent culture. Gram stains are reviewed over a number of fields for an impression of the quantity of organisms present, which reflects the extent of infection. For example, a Gram stain of unspun urine showing the occasional presence of bacteria per low-power field suggests a correlating colony count of 10,000 bacteria/mL, while the presence of bacteria in most fields is clinically significant and suggests greater than 100,000 bacteria/mL of urine. Gram stain results should be correlated with culture and sensitivity results to interpret the significance of isolated organisms and to select appropriate antibiotic therapy.

This procedure is contraindicated for: N/A

INDICATIONS

- Provide a rapid determination of the acceptability of the specimen for further analysis.
- Provide rapid, presumptive information about the type of potential pathogen present in the specimen (i.e., gram-positive bacteria, gram-negative bacteria, or yeast).

G

POTENTIAL MEDICAL DIAGNOSIS

Gram Positive				
Actinomadura	*Actinomyces*	*Bacillus*	*Clostridium*	*Corynebacterium*
Enterococcus	Erysipelothrix	*Lactobacillus*	*Listeria*	*Micrococcus*
Mycobacterium (gram variable)	*Peptostreptococcus*	*Propionibacterium*	*Rhodococcus*	*Staphylococcus*
Streptococcus				

Gram Negative				
Acinetobacter	*Aeromonas*	*Alcaligenes*	*Bacteroides*	*Bordetella*
Borrelia	*Brucella*	*Campylobacter*	*Citrobacter*	*Chlamydia*
Enterobacter	*Escherichia*	*Flavobacterium*	*Francisella*	*Fusobacterium*
Gardnerella	*Haemophilus*	*Helicobacter*	*Klebsiella*	*Legionella*
Leptospira	*Moraxella*	*Neisseria*	*Pasteurella*	*Plesiomonas*
Porphyromonas	*Prevotella*	*Proteus*	*Pseudomonas*	*Rickettsia*
Salmonella	*Serratia*	*Shigella*	*Vibrio*	*Xanthomonas*
Yersinia				

Acid Fast or Partial Acid Fast	
Nocardia	*Mycobacterium*

Note: Treponema species are classified as gram-negative spirochetes, but they are most often visualized using dark-field or silver-staining techniques.

CRITICAL FINDINGS:

- Any positive results in blood, cerebrospinal fluid, or any body cavity fluid.

Note and immediately report to the requesting health-care provider (HCP) any critical findings and related symptoms. A listing of these findings varies among facilities. Timely notification of a critical finding for laboratory or diagnostic studies is a role expectation of the professional nurse. The notification processes vary among facilities. Upon receipt of the critical finding, the information should be read back to the caller to verify accuracy.

INTERFERING FACTORS

- Very young, very old, or dead cultures may react atypically to the Gram stain technique.

NURSING IMPLICATIONS AND PROCEDURE

PRETEST:

- Positively identify the patient using at least two person-specific identifiers

before services, treatments, or procedures are performed.
- *Patient Teaching:* Inform the patient this test can assist in identifying the presence of pathogenic organisms.
- Obtain a history of the patient's health concerns, symptoms, surgical procedures, and results of previously performed laboratory and diagnostic studies. Include a list of known allergens, especially allergies or sensitivities to latex.
- Obtain a list of the patient's current medications, including over-the-counter medications and dietary supplements (see Effects of Natural Products on Laboratory Values online at Davis*Plus*).
- Review the procedure with the patient. Inform the patient that the time it takes to collect a proper specimen varies according to the patient's level of cooperation as well as the specimen collection site. Address concerns about pain and explain that there may be some discomfort during the procedure.
- *Sensitivity to social and cultural issues,* as well as concern for modesty, is important in providing psychological support before, during, and after the procedure.
- Note that there are no food, fluid, or medication restrictions unless by medical direction.

INTRATEST:

Potential Complications: N/A

- Instruct the patient to cooperate fully and to follow directions.
- Observe standard precautions, and follow the general guidelines in Patient Preparation and Specimen Collection online at Davis*Plus*. Positively identify the patient, and label the appropriate specimen container with the corresponding patient demographics, initials of the person collecting the specimen, date, and time of collection.
- Specific collection instructions are found in the associated culture studies.
- Promptly transport the specimen to the laboratory for processing and analysis.

POST-TEST:

- Inform the patient that a report of the results will be made available to the requesting HCP, who will discuss the results with the patient.
- Administer antibiotics as ordered, and instruct the patient in the importance of completing the entire course of antibiotic therapy even if no symptoms are present.
- Recognize anxiety related to test results. Discuss the implications of abnormal test results on the patient's lifestyle. Provide teaching and information regarding the clinical implications of the test results, as appropriate.
- Reinforce information given by the patient's HCP regarding further testing, treatment, or referral to another HCP. Answer any questions or address any concerns voiced by the patient or family.
- Depending on the results of this procedure, additional testing may be performed to evaluate or monitor progression of the disease process and determine the need for a change in therapy. Evaluate test results in relation to the patient's symptoms and other tests performed.

RELATED STUDIES:

- Related tests include amniotic fluid analysis, relevant biopsies, bronchoscopy, cultures bacterial and viral, CSF analysis, CBC, pericardial fluid analysis, peritoneal fluid analysis, pleural fluid analysis, procalcitonin, synovial fluid analysis, and UA.
- Refer to the Gastrointestinal, Genitourinary, Immune, Reproductive, and Respiratory systems tables online at Davis*Plus* for related tests by body system.

G

Group A Streptococcal Screen

SYNONYM/ACRONYM: Strep screen, rapid strep screen, direct strep screen.

COMMON USE: To detect a group A streptococcal infection such as strep throat.

SPECIMEN: Throat swab (two swabs should be submitted so that a culture can be performed if the screen is negative).

NORMAL FINDINGS: (Method: Enzyme immunoassay or latex agglutination) Negative.

DESCRIPTION: Rheumatic fever is a possible sequela to an untreated streptococcal infection. Early diagnosis and treatment appear to lessen the seriousness of symptoms during the acute phase and overall duration of the infection and sequelae. The onset of strep throat is sudden and includes symptoms such as chills, headache, sore throat, malaise, and exudative gray-white patches on the tonsils or pharynx. The group A streptococcal screen should not be ordered unless the results would be available within 1 to 2 hr of specimen collection to make rapid, effective therapeutic decisions. A positive result can be a reliable basis for the initiation of therapy. A negative result is presumptive for infection and should be backed up by culture results. In general, specimens showing growth of less than 10 colonies on culture yield negative results by the rapid screening method. Evidence of group A streptococci disappears rapidly after the initiation of antibiotic therapy. A nucleic acid probe method has also been developed for rapid detection of group A streptococci.

This procedure is contraindicated for: N/A

INDICATIONS

- Assist in the rapid determination of the presence of group A streptococci.

POTENTIAL MEDICAL DIAGNOSIS

Positive findings in

- Rheumatic fever
- Scarlet fever
- Strep throat
- Streptococcal glomerulonephritis
- Tonsillitis

CRITICAL FINDINGS: N/A

INTERFERING FACTORS

- Polyester (rayon or Dacron) swabs are favored over cotton for best chance of detection. Fatty acids are created on cotton fibers during the sterilization process. Detectable target antigens on the streptococcal cell wall are destroyed without killing the organism when there is contact between the specimen and the fatty acids on the cotton collection swab. False-negative test results can be obtained on specimens collected with cotton tip swabs. Negative strep screens should always be followed with a traditional culture.
- Sensitivity of the method varies among manufacturers.
- Adequate specimen collection in children may be difficult to achieve, which explains the higher percentage of false-negative results in this age group.

G

NURSING IMPLICATIONS AND PROCEDURE

POTENTIAL NURSING PROBLEMS:

Problem	Signs & Symptoms	Interventions
Infection ***(related to exposure to bacterial organisms secondary to inadequate defense mechanism; insufficient nutrition; chronic disease)***	Temperature; increased heart rate; increased blood pressure; shaking; chills; mottled skin; lethargy; fatigue; swelling; pain; night sweats; confusion; positive streptococcal throat swab; swollen tender lymph nodes in neck; headache; rash; vomiting; red, tender, pus-filled tonsils	Promote good hygiene; assist with hygiene as needed; administer prescribed antibiotics, antipyretics; provide cooling measures; monitor vital signs and trend temperatures; encourage oral fluids; adhere to standard or universal precautions; obtain cultures as ordered; assess nutritional status and provide supplements as needed
Airway ***(related to infection; inflammation)***	Difficulty swallowing; tonsils that are red, swollen, with pus or white patches; swollen tender lymph nodes in neck; dyspnea; tachypnea	Assess respiratory characteristics (rate, rhythm, depth, accessory muscle use); use pulse oximetry; administer prescribed oxygen; administer prescribed antibiotics; provide humidification of oxygen as appropriate
Fatigue ***(related to infection and inflammation)***	Report of tiredness; inability to maintain activities of daily living at current level; inability to restore energy after rest or sleep	Discuss the implementation of energy conservation activities (even pace when working, frequent rest periods, items in easy reach, push items instead of pulling); limit naps to increase nighttime sleeping; set priorities for energy expenditures; administer ordered antibiotics
Health management ***(related to inadequate access to care; low income;***	Unable to or fails to recognize or process information toward improving health and preventing illness with associated mental	Collaborate with health-care provider (HCP) to develop a plan of care that supports health; ensure patient adheres to recommended medication

(table continues on page 892)

Problem	Signs & Symptoms	Interventions
inadequate support systems; cultural influences)	and physical effects; fails to keep appointments; fails to comply with recommended therapeutic regime	regime; ensure patient complies with health-care follow-up appointments; assess diet and lifestyle choices; assess health history; identify specific questions and reservations related to health management

G

PRETEST:

- Positively identify the patient using at least two person-specific identifiers before services, treatments, or procedures are performed.
- *Patient Teaching:* Inform the patient this test can assist in identifying a streptococcal infection.
- Obtain a history of the patient's health concerns, symptoms, surgical procedures, and results of previously performed laboratory and diagnostic studies. Include a list of known allergens, especially allergies or sensitivities to latex.
- Obtain a history of prior antibiotic therapy.
- Obtain a list of the patient's current medications, including over-the-counter medications and dietary supplements (see Effects of Natural Products on Laboratory Values online at Davis*Plus*).
- Before specimen collection, verify with the laboratory whether wet or dry swabs are preferred for collection.
- Review the procedure with the patient. Inform the patient that specimen collection takes approximately 5 to 10 min. Address concerns about pain and explain that there may be some discomfort during the swabbing procedure.
- *Sensitivity to social and cultural issues,* as well as concern for modesty, is important in providing psychological support before, during, and after the procedure.
- Note that there are no food, fluid, or medication restrictions unless by medical direction.

INTRATEST:

Potential Complications: N/A

- Instruct the patient to cooperate fully and to follow directions. Direct the patient to breathe normally and to avoid unnecessary movement.
- Observe standard precautions, and follow the general guidelines in Patient Preparation and Specimen Collection online at Davis*Plus*. Positively identify the patient, and label the appropriate specimen container with the corresponding patient demographics, initials of the person collecting the specimen, date, and time of collection. Vigorous swabbing of both tonsillar pillars and the posterior throat enhances the probability of streptococcal antigen detection.
- Promptly transport the specimen to the laboratory for processing and analysis.

POST-TEST:

- Inform the patient that a report of the results will be made available to the requesting HCP, who will discuss the results with the patient.
- Administer antibiotics as ordered, and emphasize to the patient or caregiver the importance of completing the entire course of antibiotic therapy even if no symptoms are present.
- Depending on the results of this procedure, additional testing may be performed to evaluate or monitor progression of the disease process and determine the need for a change in therapy. Evaluate test results in relation to the patient's symptoms and other tests performed.

Patient Education:
- Reinforce information given by the patient's HCP regarding further testing, treatment, or referral to another HCP.
- Answer any questions or address any concerns voiced by the patient or family.

Expected Patient Outcomes:

Understanding
- The patient and family discuss the effects of noncompliance on overall health.
- The patient and family state the importance of completing antibiotic therapy to prevent infection recurrence.

Ability
- The patient demonstrates proficiency in self-administration of prescribed antibiotics.
- The patient and family relate symptoms of infection that should be reported to the HCP.

Response
- The patient and family recognize the importance of accepting financial assistance as necessary to maintain health.
- The patient exhibits willingness to break long-held habits to improve health.

RELATED STUDIES:
- Related laboratory tests include analgesic and antipyretic drugs, antimicrobial drugs, ASO, chest x-ray, CBC, culture (throat, viral), and Gram stain.
- Refer to the Immune and Respiratory systems tables online at Davis*Plus* for related tests by body system.

G

Growth Hormone, Stimulation and Suppression Tests

SYNONYM/ACRONYM: Somatotropic hormone, somatotropin, GH, hGH.

COMMON USE: To assess pituitary function and evaluate the amount of secreted growth hormone to assist in diagnosing diseases such as giantism and dwarfism.

SPECIMEN: Serum collected in a gold-, red-, or red/gray-top tube.

NORMAL FINDINGS: (Method: Immunoassay)

Growth Hormone

Age	Conventional Units	SI Units (Conventional Units × 1)
Cord blood	8–40 ng/mL	8–40 mcg/L
1 d	5–50 ng/mL	5–50 mcg/L
1 wk	5–25 ng/mL	5–25 mcg/L
Child	2–10 ng/mL	2–10 mcg/L
Adult		
Male	0–5 ng/mL	0–5 mcg/L
Female	0–10 ng/mL	0–10 mcg/L
Male older than 60 yr	0–10 ng/mL	0–10 mcg/L
Female older than 60 yr	0–14 ng/mL	0–14 mcg/L

(table continues on page 894)

Age	Conventional Units	SI Units (Conventional Units × 1)
Stimulation Tests		
Rise above baseline	Greater than 5 ng/mL	Greater than 5 mcg/L
Peak response	Greater than 10 ng/mL	Greater than 10 mcg/L
Suppression Tests	0–2 ng/mL	0–2 mcg/L

POTENTIAL MEDICAL DIAGNOSIS

Increased in:

Production of GH is modulated by numerous factors, including stress, exercise, sleep, nutrition, and response to circulating levels of GH.

- Acromegaly
- Anorexia nervosa
- Chronic kidney disease
- Cirrhosis
- Diabetes (uncontrolled)
- Ectopic GH secretion (neoplasms of stomach, lung)
- Exercise
- Gigantism (pituitary)
- Hyperpituitarism
- Laron dwarfism
- Malnutrition
- Stress

Decreased in:

- Adrenocortical hyperfunction ***(inhibits secretion of GH)***
- Dwarfism (pituitary) ***(related to GH deficiency)***
- Hypopituitarism ***(related to lack of production)***

CRITICAL FINDINGS: N/A

Find and print out the full study on Fast Find at davispl.us/vanleeuwen7.

Ham's Test for Paroxysmal Nocturnal Hemoglobinuria

SYNONYM/ACRONYM: Acid hemolysis test for PNH.

COMMON USE: To assist in diagnosing a rare condition called paroxysmal nocturnal hemoglobinuria (PNH), wherein red blood cells undergo lysis during and after sleep with hemoglobin excreted in the urine.

SPECIMEN: Whole blood collected in lavender-top (EDTA) tube and serum collected in red-top tube.

NORMAL FINDINGS: (Method: Acidified hemolysis) No hemolysis seen.

POTENTIAL MEDICAL DIAGNOSIS

Increased in:

- Congenital dyserythropoietic anemia, type II
- PNH

Decreased in: N/A

CRITICAL FINDINGS: N/A

Find and print out the full study on Fast Find at davispl.us/vanleeuwen7.

H

Haptoglobin

SYNONYM/ACRONYM: Hapto, HP, Hp.

COMMON USE: To assist in evaluating for intravascular hemolysis related to transfusion reactions, chronic liver disease, hemolytic anemias, and tissue inflammation or destruction.

SPECIMEN: Serum collected in a gold-, red-, or red/gray-top tube.

NORMAL FINDINGS: (Method: Immunoturbidimetric)

Age	Conventional Units	SI Units (Conventional Units × 0.01)
Newborn	5–48 mg/dL (levels may be undetectable at birth)	0.05–0.48 g/L (levels may be undetectable at birth)
6 mo–16 yr	25–138 mg/dL (adult levels are reached by 1 yr)	0.25–1.38 g/L (adult levels are reached by 1 yr)
Adult	15–200 mg/dL	0.15–2 g/L

DESCRIPTION: Haptoglobin is an α_2-globulin produced in the liver. It binds with the free hemoglobin released when red blood cells (RBCs) are lysed. The complexed hemoglobin is then removed from circulation by the spleen. Haptoglobin is used as a marker for intravascular hemolysis because the amount of free hemoglobin from a significant number of lysed RBCs will exceed the amount of haptoglobin normally available for binding. In conditions such as hemolytic anemia (e.g., drug induced, inherited, acute transfusion reaction) the liver is unable to compensate so consumption exceeds production, and haptoglobin levels are decreased.

This procedure is contraindicated for: N/A

INDICATIONS

- Assist in the investigation of suspected transfusion reaction.
- Evaluate known or suspected chronic liver disease, as indicated by decreased levels of haptoglobin.
- Evaluate known or suspected disorders characterized by excessive RBC hemolysis, as indicated by decreased levels of haptoglobin.
- Evaluate known or suspected disorders involving a diffuse inflammatory process or tissue destruction, as indicated by elevated levels of haptoglobin.

POTENTIAL MEDICAL DIAGNOSIS

Increased in:

Haptoglobin is an acute-phase reactant protein, and any condition that stimulates an acute-phase response will result in elevations of haptoglobin.

- Biliary obstruction
- Disorders involving tissue destruction, such as cancers, burns, and acute myocardial infarction
- Infection or inflammatory diseases, such as ulcerative colitis, arthritis, and pyelonephritis
- Neoplasms
- Steroid therapy

Decreased in:

- Autoimmune hemolysis ***(related to increased excretion rate of haptoglobin bound to free hemoglobin; rate of excretion exceeds the liver's immediate ability to replenish)***
- Hemolysis due to drug reaction ***(related to increased excretion rate of haptoglobin bound to free hemoglobin; rate of excretion exceeds the liver's immediate ability to replenish)***
- Hemolysis due to mechanical destruction (e.g., artificial heart valves, contact sports, subacute bacterial endocarditis) ***(related to increased excretion rate of haptoglobin bound to free hemoglobin; rate of excretion exceeds the liver's immediate ability to replenish)***
- Hemolysis due to RBC membrane or metabolic defects ***(related to increased excretion rate of haptoglobin bound to free hemoglobin; rate of excretion exceeds the liver's immediate ability to replenish)***
- Hemolysis due to transfusion reaction ***(related to increased excretion rate of haptoglobin bound to free hemoglobin; rate of excretion exceeds the liver's immediate ability to replenish)***
- Hypersplenism ***(related to increased excretion rate of haptoglobin bound to free hemoglobin due to increased RBC destruction; rate of excretion exceeds the liver's immediate ability to replenish)***
- Ineffective hematopoiesis due to conditions such as folate deficiency or hemoglobinopathies ***(related to decreased numbers of RBCs or dysfunctional binding in the presence of abnormal hemoglobins)***
- Liver disease ***(related to decreased production)***
- Pregnancy ***(related to effect of estrogen)***

CRITICAL FINDINGS: N/A

INTERFERING FACTORS

- Drugs and other substances that may increase haptoglobin levels include anabolic steroids and danazol.
- Drugs and other substances that may decrease haptoglobin levels include aminosalicylic acid, chlorpromazine, dapsone, dextran, diphenhydramine, furazolidone, isoniazid, nitrofurantoin, norethindrone, oral contraceptives, quinidine, resorcinol, stibophen, tamoxifen, and tripelennamine.

NURSING IMPLICATIONS AND PROCEDURE

PRETEST:

- Positively identify the patient using at least two person-specific identifiers before services, treatments, or procedures are performed.
- *Patient Teaching:* Inform the patient this test can assist with evaluating causes of red blood cell loss.
- Obtain a history of the patient's health concerns, symptoms, surgical procedures, and results of previously performed laboratory and diagnostic studies. Include a list of known allergens, especially allergies or sensitivities to latex.
- Obtain a list of the patient's current medications, including over-the-counter medications and dietary supplements (see Effects of Natural Products on Laboratory Values online at Davis*Plus*).
- Review the procedure with the patient. Inform the patient that specimen collection takes approximately 5 to 10 min. Address concerns about pain and explain that there may be some discomfort during the venipuncture.
- Note that there are no food, fluid, or medication restrictions unless by medical direction.

INTRATEST:

Potential Complications: N/A

- Avoid the use of equipment containing latex if the patient has a history of allergic reaction to latex.
- Instruct the patient to cooperate fully and to follow directions. Direct the patient to breathe normally and to avoid unnecessary movement.
- Observe standard precautions, and follow the general guidelines in Patient Preparation and Specimen Collection online at Davis*Plus*. Positively identify the patient, and label the appropriate specimen container with the corresponding patient demographics, initials of the person collecting the specimen, date, and time of collection. Perform a venipuncture.
- Remove the needle and apply direct pressure with dry gauze to stop bleeding. Observe/assess venipuncture site for bleeding or hematoma formation and secure gauze with adhesive bandage.
- Promptly transport the specimen to the laboratory for processing and analysis.

POST-TEST:

- Inform the patient that a report of the results will be made available to the requesting health-care provider (HCP), who will discuss the results with the patient.
- Instruct the patient to immediately report symptoms of hemolysis, including chills, fever, flushing, back pain, and fast heartbeat, to the HCP.
- Reinforce information given by the patient's HCP regarding further testing, treatment, or referral to another HCP. Answer any questions or address any concerns voiced by the patient or family.
- Depending on the results of this procedure, additional testing may be performed to evaluate or monitor progression of the disease process and determine the need for a change in therapy. Evaluate test results in relation to the patient's symptoms and other tests performed.

H

RELATED STUDIES:

- Related tests include ALT, AST, bilirubin, blood group and type, CBC, CBC RBC count, CBC RBC indices, CBC RBC morphology, Coombs' antiglobulin, folate, G6PD, GGT, Ham's test, hepatobiliary scan, and osmotic fragility.
- Refer to the Hematopoietic, Hepatobiliary, and Immune systems tables online at Davis*Plus* for related tests by body system.

Helicobacter Pylori Antibody

SYNONYM/ACRONYM: *H. pylori.*

COMMON USE: To test blood for findings that would indicate past or current *Helicobacter pylori* infection.

SPECIMEN: Serum collected in a plain gold-, red-, or red/gray-top tube. Place separated serum into a standard transport tube within 2 hr of collection.

NORMAL FINDINGS: (Method: Enzyme-linked immunosorbent assay [ELISA]) Negative.

DESCRIPTION: There is a strong association between *Helicobacter pylori* infection and gastric cancer, duodenal and gastric ulcer, and chronic gastritis. Immunoglobulin G (IgG) antibodies can be detected for up to 1 yr after treatment. The presence of *H. pylori* can also be demonstrated by a positive urea breath test, positive stool culture, or positive endoscopic biopsy. Patients with symptoms and evidence of *H. pylori* infection are considered to be infected with the organism; patients who demonstrate evidence of *H. pylori* but are without symptoms are said to be colonized.

The urea breath test is an accurate way to identify the presence of *H. pylori*. For the urea breath test, the patient swallows a capsule containing urea made from an isotope of carbon. If *H. pylori* is present in the stomach, the bacteria will metabolize the urea and isotope labelled carbon dioxide will be released. The carbon dioxide is absorbed by the stomach tissue, passes into the blood where it travels to the lungs, and is excreted during respiration. Samples of exhaled breath are collected 10 to 15 min after the capsule has been ingested, and the presence of isotope labelled carbon in the exhaled carbon dioxide is measured. If the isotope is present, *H. pylori* is present in the stomach. When the organism has been effectively treated with antibiotics, the test changes from positive to negative.

A stool antigen test may be used to identify the presence of *H. pylori*. This is an accurate test and may be requested for patients who are unable to cooperate for the urea breath test.

Examination of tissue biopsy, obtained by endoscopy, from the lining of the stomach is another way to identify the presence of *H. pylori*. The sample is tested for urease activity and is histologically examined for the presence of inflammatory epithelial cells in the presence of the characteristically curve shaped *H. pylori* bacteria.

This procedure is contraindicated for: N/A

INDICATIONS

- Assist in differentiating between *H. pylori* infection and NSAID use as the cause of gastritis or peptic or duodenal ulcer.
- Assist in establishing a diagnosis of gastritis, gastric carcinoma, or peptic or duodenal ulcer.

POTENTIAL MEDICAL DIAGNOSIS

Positive findings in

- *H. pylori* infection
- *H. pylori* colonization

Negative findings in: N/A

CRITICAL FINDINGS: N/A

INTERFERING FACTORS: N/A

NURSING IMPLICATIONS AND PROCEDURE

POTENTIAL NURSING PROBLEMS:

Problem	Signs & Symptoms	Interventions
Infection ***(related to fecal matter–contaminated food or water)***	Dark- or tar-colored stools; bloating; abdominal pain; feeling full after eating a small meal; lack of appetite; nausea and vomiting; development of stomach cancer	Administer prescribed proton pump inhibitors; administer prescribed antibiotics; avoid alcoholic beverages
Pain ***(related to gastric irritation; gastric inflammation)***	Abdominal cramping; abdominal distention; report of pain; emotional symptoms of distress; crying; agitation; facial grimace; moaning; verbalization of pain; irritability; disturbed sleep; altered blood pressure and heart rate; nausea; vomiting	Collaborate with the patient and health-care provider (HCP) to identify the best pain management modality to provide relief; refrain from activities that may aggravate pain; monitor pain severity; administer prescribed proton pump inhibitors; administer prescribed antibiotics; administer H_2 receptor antagonists; administer prescribed antacids

(table continues on page 900)

H

Problem	Signs & Symptoms	Interventions
Nutrition ***(related to nausea and vomiting; alcohol use; diarrhea; gastrointestinal bleed; abdominal pain)***	Known inadequate caloric intake; weight loss; muscle wasting in arms and legs; skin that is flaky with loss of elasticity; inadequate absorption of iron, vitamins, and minerals	Document food intake with possible calorie count; assess barriers to eating; consider using a food diary; monitor daily weight; arrange dietary consult with assessment of cultural food selections; encourage limitation of coffee and other caffeinated beverages; discuss refraining from excessive alcohol use
Fatigue ***(related to bleeding; pain; inadequate nutrition; nausea; vomiting)***	Decreased concentration; increased physical complaints; inability to restore energy with sleep; reports being tired; inability to maintain normal routine; decreasing hemoglobin (Hgb) and hematocrit (Hct); nausea; vomiting; inadequate dietary intake; self-report of abdominal pain	Assess for physical cause of fatigue; pace activities to preserve energy stores; rate fatigue on a numeric scale to trend degree of fatigue over time; identify what aggravates and decreases fatigue; assess for related emotional factors such as depression; evaluate current medications in relation to fatigue; assess for physiologic factors such as anemia; monitor for black tarry stools that are indicative of bleeding; administer prescribed blood or blood products; administer prescribed antiemetic and antidiarrheal medication; monitor and trend HgbB/Hct

PRETEST:

- Positively identify the patient using at least two person-specific identifiers before services, treatments, or procedures are performed.
- Inform the patient that the test is used to assist in the diagnosis of *H. pylori* infection in patients with duodenal and gastric disease.
- Obtain a history of the patient's health concerns, symptoms, surgical procedures, and results of previously performed laboratory and diagnostic studies. Include a list of known allergens, especially allergies or sensitivities to latex.
- Obtain a list of the patient's current medications, including over-the-counter medications, dietary supplements, anticoagulants, aspirin and other salicylates (see Effects of Natural Products on Laboratory Values online at Davis*Plus*). Such products should be discontinued by medical direction for the appropriate number of days prior to a surgical procedure. Note the last time and dose of medication taken.
- Review the procedure with the patient. Inform the patient that specimen collection takes approximately 5 to 10 min. Address concerns

about pain and explain that there may be some discomfort during the venipuncture.

- *Sensitivity to social and cultural issues,* as well as concern for modesty, is important in providing psychological support before, during, and after the procedure.
- Note that there are no food, fluid, or medication restrictions unless by medical direction.

INTRATEST:

Potential Complications: N/A

- Avoid the use of equipment containing latex if the patient has a history of allergic reaction to latex.
- Instruct the patient to cooperate fully and to follow directions. Direct the patient to breathe normally and to avoid unnecessary movement.
- Observe standard precautions, and follow the general guidelines in Patient Preparation and Specimen Collection online at Davis*Plus*. Positively identify the patient, and label the appropriate specimen container with the corresponding patient demographics, initials of the person collecting the specimen, date, and time of collection. Perform a venipuncture.
- Remove the needle and apply direct pressure with dry gauze to stop bleeding. Observe/assess venipuncture site for bleeding or hematoma formation and secure gauze with adhesive bandage.
- Promptly transport the specimen to the laboratory for processing and analysis.

POST-TEST:

- Inform the patient that a report of the results will be made available to the requesting HCP, who will discuss the results with the patient.
- Depending on the results of this procedure, additional testing may be performed to evaluate or monitor progression of the disease process and determine the need for a change in therapy. Evaluate test results in relation to the patient's symptoms and other tests performed.

Patient Education:

- Provide education regarding the disease, factors that can trigger symptoms, and possible treatment options that may include surgery.
- Stress the importance of adhering to requests for follow-up visits as ordered.
- Reinforce information given by the patient's HCP regarding further testing, treatment, or referral to another HCP.
- Inform the patient that a positive test result constitutes an independent risk factor for gastric cancer.
- Answer any questions or address any concerns voiced by the patient or family.

Expected Patient Outcomes:

Understanding

- The patient and family state the importance of taking prescribed antibiotics until completed to ensure infection is resolved.
- The patient and family state the importance of taking prescribed medications to manage infection and decrease pain

Ability

- The patient demonstrates proficient use of guided imagery and relaxation techniques to assist with pain management.
- The patient and family identify foods that cause gastric distress and develop a plan to avoid those foods.

Response

- The patient complies with the request to abstain from excessive alcohol use.
- The patient complies with the request to refrain from eating foods that cause gastric irritation.

RELATED STUDIES:

- Related tests include capsule endoscopy, EGD, gastric acid stimulation, gastric emptying scan, gastrin, and upper GI series.
- Refer to the Gastrointestinal System table online at Davis*Plus* for related test by body system.

H

Hemoglobin Electrophoresis

SYNONYM/ACRONYM: N/A

COMMON USE: To assist in evaluating hemolytic anemias and identifying hemoglobin variants, diagnose thalassemias, and sickle cell anemia.

SPECIMEN: Whole blood collected in a lavender-top (EDTA) tube.

NORMAL FINDINGS: (Method: Electrophoresis)

	Hgb A
Adult	Greater than 95%
	Hgb A_2
Adult	1.5%–3.7%
	Hgb F
Newborns and infants	
1 d–3 wk	70%–77%
6–9 wk	42%–64%
3–4 mo	7%–39%
6 mo	3%–7%
8–11 mo	0.6%–2.6%
Adult–older adult	Less than 2%

DESCRIPTION: Hemoglobin (Hgb) electrophoresis is a separation process used to identify normal and abnormal forms of Hgb. Electrophoresis and high-performance liquid chromatography as well as molecular genetics testing for mutations can also be used to identify abnormal forms of Hgb. Hgb A is the main form of Hgb in the normal adult. Hgb F is the main form of Hgb in the fetus, the remainder being composed of Hgb A_1 and A_2. Small amounts of Hgb F are normal in the adult. Hgb D, E, H, S, and C result from abnormal amino acid substitutions during the formation of Hgb and are inherited hemoglobinopathies.

Knowledge of genetics assists the nurse in identifying patients and family members who may benefit from additional education, risk assessment, and counseling. Genetics is the study and identification of genes, genetic mutations, and inheritance. For example, genetics provides some insight into the likelihood of inheriting a trait such as blue eyes or a medical condition such as a hemogloinopathy. Some conditions are the result of mutations involving a single gene, whereas other conditions may involve multiple genes and/or multiple chromosomes. Sickle cell disease is an example of an autosomal recessive disorder in which the offspring inherits a copy of the defective gene from each parent. Further information regarding inheritance of genes can be found in the study titled "Genetic Testing."

This procedure is contraindicated for: N/A

INDICATIONS

- Assist in the diagnosis of Hgb C disease.
- Assist in the diagnosis of thalassemia, especially in patients with a family history positive for the disorder.
- Differentiate among thalassemia types.
- Evaluate hemolytic anemia of unknown cause.
- Evaluate a positive sickle cell screening test to differentiate sickle cell trait from sickle cell disease.

POTENTIAL MEDICAL DIAGNOSIS

Increased in:

Hgb A_2

- Hyperthyroidism
- Megaloblastic anemia
- β-Thalassemias
- Sickle trait

Hgb F

- Anemia (aplastic, associated with chronic disease or due to blood loss)
- Erythropoietic porphyria
- Hereditary elliptocytosis or spherocytosis
- Hereditary persistence of fetal Hgb
- Hyperthyroidism
- Leakage of fetal blood into maternal circulation
- Leukemia (acute or chronic)
- Myeloproliferative disorders
- Paroxysmal nocturnal hemoglobinuria
- Pernicious anemia
- Sickle cell disease
- Thalassemias
- Unstable hemoglobins

Hgb C

- Hgb C disease (one of the most common structural variants in the human population; has a higher prevalence among people of African ancestry)

Hgb D

- Hgb D (rare hemoglobinopathy that may also be found in combination with Hgb S or thalassemia)

Hgb E

- Hgb E disease; thalassemia-like condition (second-most common hemoglobinopathy in the world; occurs with the highest frequency in people of South Asian [India, Bangladesh], Southeast Asian [Thailand, Laos, Cambodia], and African ancestry, where it is common for individuals to inherit alleles for both Hgb E and beta-thalassemia)

Hgb S

- Sickle cell trait or disease (most common variant in the United States; occurs with a frequency of about 8% among people of African ancestry) 🍁

Hgb H

- α-Thalassemias
- Hgb Bart's hydrops fetalis syndrome

Decreased in:

Hgb A_2

- Erythroleukemia
- Hgb H disease
- Iron-deficiency anemia (untreated)
- Sideroblastic anemia

CRITICAL FINDINGS: N/A

INTERFERING FACTORS

- High altitude ***related to a compensatory mechanism whereby red blood cell (RBC) production is increased to increase availability***

of oxygen binding to Hgb and dehydration ***related to hemoconcentration*** may increase values.
- Iron deficiency may decrease Hgb A_2, C, and S ***related to decreased amounts of Hgb in smaller, iron-deficient RBCs.***
- In patients less than 3 mo of age, false-negative results for Hgb S occur in coincidental polycythemia ***related to technical limitations of the procedure where increased total Hgb levels reflect a small, possibly undetectable percentage of Hgb S when compared to large amounts of Hgb F.***
- RBC transfusion within 4 mo of test can mask abnormal Hgb levels.

NURSING IMPLICATIONS AND PROCEDURE

POTENTIAL NURSING PROBLEMS:

Problem	Signs & Symptoms	Interventions
Health management ***(related to excessive demands; support deficit; conflicted decision making; limited resources; sense of powerlessness)***	Inability or failure to recognize or process information toward improving health and preventing illness with associated mental and physical effects	Assess health habits to obtain an interventional baseline; obtain a current health history; identify the patient's and family's learning styles; refrain from using medical jargon; observe for altered literacy cues; provide most important information first and reinforce with additional education; ensure the patient understands the ramifications of a lack of healthy behaviors on sickling events; identify number of emergency department visits for sickling crises; instruct the patient and family on situations that can precipitate a crisis; recommend genetic counseling
Pain ***(related to hypoxic vaso-occlusive crisis secondary to sickling disease)***	Emotional symptoms of distress; crying; agitation; facial grimace; moaning; verbalization of pain; rocking motions; irritability; disturbed sleep; diaphoresis; altered blood pressure and heart rate; nausea;	Collaborate with the patient and health-care provider (HCP) to identify the best pain management modality to provide relief; refrain from activities that may aggravate pain; use the application of heat or cold to the best effect in managing the pain; monitor pain severity; assess sickle pain characteristics, location, type, and duration; monitor pain severity (severe joint pain, abdominal, or back pain

Problem	Signs & Symptoms	Interventions
	vomiting; self-report of pain; limited mobility	may last for days); administer prescribed pain medication (typically intravenous morphine, hydromorphone, or fentanyl, NSAIDs); monitor Hgb and hematocrit (Hct) and transfuse with blood as ordered; use splinting of joints, joint support, moist heat to manage pain; consider distraction and rest periods
Coping ***(related to sense of powerlessness secondary to sickling event; feeling loss of control; poor support system; chronic nature of the disease process)***	Anxiety; demonstrated inability to cope; poor problem solving; inability to meet role expectations; fatigue; frequent illness; poor goal-directed behavior; fear; difficulty asking for help	Assess the ability to convey feelings clearly and appropriately; assess presence and stability of support structure; evaluate number of emergency department visits with sickling events; discuss concerns with the patient at a time that the pain is controlled; provide education related to the treatment of and chronic nature of the disease; consult with social services and case management for home support and community resources
Mobility ***(related to pain hypoxic vaso-occlusive crisis secondary to sickling disease)***	Difficulty in the performance of purposeful movement (walking, turning, transfers); pain with movement; reluctance or refusal to move; inability to perform directed movement	Assess baseline ability to move; assess need for assistive devices, encourage appropriate use; assess pain level; assess pain medication effectiveness; administer prescribed pain medication; assess emotional response to mobility deficits; ensure a safe environment with side rail up; ensure that room is not cluttered; facilitate ambulation as appropriate; monitor for skin breakdown and deep vein thrombosis

PRETEST:

- Positively identify the patient using at least two person-specific identifiers before services, treatments, or procedures are performed.
- ***Patient Teaching:*** Inform the patient this test can assist in diagnosing various types of anemias.
- Obtain a history of the patient's health concerns, symptoms, surgical

procedures, and results of previously performed laboratory and diagnostic studies. Include a list of known allergens, especially allergies or sensitivities to latex.
- Note any recent procedures that can interfere with test results.
- Obtain a list of the patient's current medications, including over-the-counter medications and dietary supplements (see Effects of Natural Products on Laboratory Values online at Davis*Plus*).
- Review the procedure with the patient. Inform the patient that specimen collection takes approximately 5 to 10 min. Address concerns about pain and explain that there may be some discomfort during the venipuncture.
- *Sensitivity to social and cultural issues,* as well as concern for modesty, is important in providing psychological support before, during, and after the procedure.
- Note that there are no food, fluid, or medication restrictions unless by medical direction.

H

INTRATEST:

Potential Complications: N/A

- Avoid the use of equipment containing latex if the patient has a history of allergic reaction to latex.
- Instruct the patient to cooperate fully and to follow directions. Direct the patient to breathe normally and to avoid unnecessary movement.
- Observe standard precautions, and follow the general guidelines in Patient Preparation and Specimen Collection online at Davis*Plus*. Positively identify the patient, and label the appropriate specimen container with the corresponding patient demographics, initials of the person collecting the specimen, date, and time of collection. Perform a venipuncture.
- Remove the needle and apply direct pressure with dry gauze to stop bleeding. Observe/assess venipuncture site for bleeding or hematoma formation and secure gauze with adhesive bandage.
- Promptly transport the specimen to the laboratory for processing and analysis.

POST-TEST:

- Inform the patient that a report of the results will be made available to the requesting HCP, who will discuss the results with the patient.
- Depending on the results of this procedure, additional testing may be performed to evaluate or monitor progression of the disease process and determine the need for a change in therapy. Evaluate test results in relation to the patient's symptoms and other tests performed.

Patient Education:

- Teach the patient that the frequency of sickling crises is reflective of disease control and need for review of therapeutic management.
- Reinforce information given by the patient's HCP regarding further testing, treatment, or referral to another HCP.
- Answer any questions or address any concerns voiced by the patient or family.
- Teach patient and family the pathophysiology of sickle cell disease in understandable terms. Provide contact information, if desired, for Sickle Cell Disease Association of America (www.sicklecelldisease.org). 🍁

Expected Patient Outcomes:

Understanding

- The patient and family state that the support of similar patients may assist with coping and disease management.
- The patient and family state that adherence to disease management recommendations can decrease sickling events.

Ability

- The patient and family describe lifestyle changes that can be made to decrease hypoxic episodes and the incidence of sickling crises.

- The patient and family identify symptoms of infection that should be reported to the HCP.

Response

- The patient and family comply with the request for genetic counseling.
- The patient and family comply with recommended therapeutic management for sickle cell disease.

RELATED STUDIES:

- Related tests include biopsy bone marrow, blood gases, CBC, CBC hematocrit, CBC hemoglobin, CBC RBC morphology, genetic testing methemoglobin, newborn screening, osmotic fragility, and sickle cell screen.
- Refer to the Hematopoietic System table online at Davis*Plus* for related tests by body system.

Hemosiderin

SYNONYM/ACRONYM: Hemosiderin stain, Pappenheimer body stain, iron stain.

COMMON USE: To assist in investigating recent intravascular hemolysis and to assist in the diagnosis of unexplained anemias, hemochromatosis, and renal tube damage.

SPECIMEN: Urine from a random first morning sample, collected in a clean plastic collection container.

NORMAL FINDINGS: (Method: Microscopic examination of Prussian blue–stained specimen) None seen.

POTENTIAL MEDICAL DIAGNOSIS

Increased in:

Any condition that involves hemolysis will release hemoglobin from RBCs into circulation. Hemoglobin is converted to hemosiderin in the renal tubular epithelial cells.

- Burns
- Cold hemagglutinin disease
- Hemochromatosis
- Hemolytic transfusion reactions
- Mechanical trauma to RBCs
- Megaloblastic anemia
- Microangiopathic hemolytic anemia
- Paroxysmal nocturnal hemoglobinuria
- Pernicious anemia
- Sickle cell anemia
- Thalassemia major

Decreased in: N/A

CRITICAL FINDINGS: N/A

Find and print out the full study on Fast Find at davispl.us/vanleeuwen7.

Hepatitis A Antibody

SYNONYM/ACRONYM: HAV serology.

COMMON USE: To test blood for the presence of antibodies that would indicate a past or current hepatitis A infection.

SPECIMEN: Serum collected in a gold-, red-, or red/gray-top tube. Place separated serum into a standard transport tube within 2 hr of collection.

NORMAL FINDINGS: (Method: Enzyme immunoassay) Negative.

DESCRIPTION: The hepatitis A virus (HAV) is classified as a picornavirus. Its primary mode of transmission is by the fecal-oral route under conditions of poor personal hygiene or inadequate sanitation. The incubation period is about 28 days, with a range of 15 to 50 days. Onset is usually abrupt, with the acute disease lasting about 1 wk. Therapy is supportive, and there is no development of chronic or carrier states. Assays for total (immunoglobulin G and immunoglobulin M [IgM]) hepatitis A antibody and IgM-specific hepatitis A antibody assist in differentiating recent infection from prior exposure. If results from the IgM-specific or from both assays are positive, recent infection is suspected. If the IgM-specific test results are negative and the total antibody test results are positive, past infection is indicated. The clinically significant assay—IgM-specific antibody—is often the only test requested. Jaundice occurs in 70% to 80% of adult cases of HAV infection and in 70% of pediatric cases.

This procedure is contraindicated for: N/A

INDICATIONS

- Screen individuals at high risk of exposure, such as those in long-term residential facilities or correctional facilities.
- Screen individuals with suspected HAV infection.

POTENTIAL MEDICAL DIAGNOSIS

Positive findings in

- Individuals with current HAV infection
- Individuals with past HAV infection

CRITICAL FINDINGS: N/A

INTERFERING FACTORS: N/A

H

NURSING IMPLICATIONS AND PROCEDURE

POTENTIAL NURSING PROBLEMS:

Problem	Signs & Symptoms	Interventions
Fatigue ***(related to decreased energy secondary to liver dysfunction associated with disease process and resulting inadequate absorption, metabolism and storage of nutrients)***	Decreased concentration; increased physical complaints; inability to restore energy with sleep; reports being tired; inability to maintain normal routine	Assess for physical cause of fatigue; pace activities to preserve energy stores; rate fatigue on a numeric scale to trend degree of fatigue over time; identify what aggravates and decreases fatigue; assess for related emotional factors such as depression; evaluate current medications in relation to fatigue; assess for physiologic factors such as anemia

Problem	Signs & Symptoms	Interventions
Knowledge ***(related to new condition or diagnosis; lack of familiarity or understanding with disease and treatment)***	Lack of interest or questions; multiple questions; anxiety in relation to disease process and management	Teach the patient that the disease is transmitted by fecal-oral route, crowded living conditions, poor personal hygiene, contaminated water, contaminated food, contaminated milk, and raw shellfish; assess patient's and family's knowledge regarding disease, transmission, and treatment; assess for cultural, literacy, or vision and hearing concerns that would interfere with learning; explain that adequate nutrition and rest can prevent disease complications; demonstrate proper hand-washing technique with re-demonstration; emphasize vigilant hand washing; explain that crowded living conditions and poor sanitation should be avoided; encourage family members to receive hepatitis vaccine; make patients aware that sexual partners should receive the hepatitis vaccine
Infection ***(related to crowded living conditions with poor sanitation; poor personal hygiene; fecal-oral exposure; exposure to contaminated water, milk, food; raw shellfish)***	Fever; fatigue; loss of appetite; jaundice; nausea and vomiting; dark-colored urine; abdominal pain; stool that is clay colored; joint pain; it is possible to be infected and have no symptoms	Explain that the best treatment is adequate rest, good nutrition, and adequate fluid intake; recommend that family and significant others receive the hepatitis vaccination; explain that alcohol should be avoided to decrease risk of liver damage; explain that over-the-counter medication should be checked with the health-care provider (HCP) before taking to ensure there is no risk to the liver; explain that jaundice can last several months

PRETEST:

- Positively identify the patient using at least two person-specific identifiers before services, treatments, or procedures are performed.
- *Patient Teaching:* Inform the patient this test can assist in evaluating for hepatitis infection.
- Obtain a history of the patient's health concerns, symptoms, surgical procedures, and results of previously performed laboratory and diagnostic studies. Include a list of known allergens, especially allergies or sensitivities to latex.
- Obtain a list of the patient's current medications, including over-the-counter medications and dietary supplements (see Effects of Natural Products on Laboratory Values online at Davis*Plus*).
- Review the procedure with the patient. Inform the patient that specimen collection takes approximately 5 to 10 min. Address concerns about pain and explain that there may be some discomfort during the venipuncture.
- Note that there are no food, fluid, or medication restrictions unless by medical direction.

INTRATEST:

Potential Complications: N/A

- Avoid the use of equipment containing latex if the patient has a history of allergic reaction to latex.
- Instruct the patient to cooperate fully and to follow directions. Direct the patient to breathe normally and to avoid unnecessary movement.
- Observe standard precautions, and follow the general guidelines in Patient Preparation and Specimen Collection online at Davis*Plus*. Positively identify the patient, and label the appropriate specimen container with the corresponding patient demographics, initials of the person collecting the specimen, date, and time of collection. Perform a venipuncture.
- Remove the needle and apply direct pressure with dry gauze to stop bleeding. Observe/assess venipuncture site for bleeding or hematoma formation and secure gauze with adhesive bandage.
- Promptly transport the specimen to the laboratory for processing and analysis.

POST-TEST:

- Inform the patient that a report of the results will be made available to the requesting HCP, who will discuss the results with the patient.
- Inform the patient that positive findings must be reported to local health department officials. 🍁
- *Nutritional Considerations:* Dietary recommendations may be indicated and will vary depending on the type and severity of the condition. Elimination of alcohol ingestion and a diet optimized for convalescence are commonly included in the treatment plan. Explain the importance of providing an adequate daily fluid intake of at least 4 L. Monitor the patient's weight, intake, and output each day and assess for development of ascites. Elimination of alcohol ingestion and a diet optimized for convalescence are commonly included in the treatment plan. As a general rule, small, frequent meals that are high in carbohydrates and low in fat will provide the required energy while not burdening the inflamed liver.
- *Social and Cultural Considerations:* Recognize anxiety related to test results, and offer support. Discuss the implications of abnormal test results on the patient's lifestyle. Provide teaching and information regarding the clinical implications of the test results, as appropriate. Counsel the patient, as appropriate, regarding risk of transmission and proper prophylaxis. Stress the importance of hand hygiene to prevent transmission of the virus. Immune globulin can be given before exposure (in the case of individuals who may be traveling to a location where the disease is endemic) or after exposure, during the incubation period. Prophylaxis is most effective when administered 2 wk after exposure.

- Depending on the results of this procedure, additional testing may be performed to evaluate or monitor progression of the disease process and determine the need for a change in therapy. Evaluate test results in relation to the patient's symptoms and other tests performed.

Patient Education:

- Reinforce information given by the patient's HCP regarding further testing, treatment, or referral to another HCP.
- Provide information regarding vaccine-preventable diseases where indicated (e.g., hepatitis A).
- Provide contact information, if desired, for the Centers for Disease Control and Prevention (www.cdc.gov/vaccines/vpd-vac and www.cdc.gov/DiseasesConditions) 🍁 for guidelines on vaccine-preventable diseases.
- Answer any questions or address any concerns voiced by the patient or family.

Expected Patient Outcomes:

Understanding

- The patient and family state the importance of washing hands after using the bathroom and prior to food preparation.
- The patient and family state that this disease is spread by contact with infected fecal matter.

Ability

- The patient and family demonstrate proficient hand washing.
- The patient and family verbalize the importance of using protective personal equipment, such as gloves if necessary, to prevent disease transmission.

Response

- The patient and family comply with the request to avoid drinking untreated water.
- The patient and family comply with the request to avoid washing food in untreated water.

RELATED STUDIES:

- Related tests include ALT, ALP, AST, bilirubin, GGT, and HBV, HBC, HBD, and HBE antigens and antibodies.
- Refer to the Hepatobiliary and Immune systems tables online at Davis*Plus* for related tests by body system.

Hepatitis B Antigen and Antibody

SYNONYM/ACRONYM: HBeAg, HBeAb, HBcAb, HBsAb, HBsAg.

COMMON USE: To test blood for the presence of antibodies that would indicate a past or current hepatitis B infection.

SPECIMEN: Serum collected in a gold-, red-, or red/gray-top tube. Place separated serum into a standard transport tube within 2 hr of collection.

NORMAL FINDINGS: (Method: Enzyme immunoassay) Negative.

DESCRIPTION: The hepatitis B virus (HBV) is classified as a double-stranded DNA retrovirus of the Hepadnaviridae family. Its primary modes of transmission are parenteral, perinatal, and sexual contact. Serological profiles vary with different scenarios (i.e., asymptomatic infection, acute/resolved infection, coinfection, and chronic carrier state). The formation and detectability of markers is also dose dependent. The following description refers to HBV infection that becomes resolved. The incubation period is generally 6 to 16 wk. The hepatitis B surface antigen (HBsAg) is the first marker to appear after infection. It is detectable 8 to 12 wk after exposure and often precedes symptoms. At about the time liver enzymes fall back to normal levels, the HBsAg titer has fallen to nondetectable levels. If the HBsAg remains detectable after 6 mo, the patient will likely become a chronic carrier who can transmit the virus. Hepatitis Be antigen (HBeAg) appears in the serum 10 to 12 wk after exposure. HBeAg can be found in the serum of patients with acute or chronic HBV infection and is a sign of active viral replication and infectivity. Levels of hepatitis Be antibody (HBeAb) appear about 14 wk after exposure, suggesting resolution of the infection and reduction of the patient's ability to transmit the disease. The more quickly HBeAg disappears, the shorter the acute phase of the infection. Immunoglobulin M–specific hepatitis B core antibody (HBcAb) appears 6 to 14 wk after exposure to HBsAg and continues to be detectable either until the infection is resolved or over the life span in patients who are in a chronic carrier state. In some cases, HBcAb may be the only detectable marker; hence, its lone appearance has sometimes been referred to as the *core window.* HBcAb is not an indicator of recovery or immunity; however, it does indicate current or previous infection. Hepatitis B surface antibody (HBsAb) appears 2 to 16 wk after HBsAg disappears. Appearance of HBsAb represents clinical recovery and immunity to the virus.

Onset of HBV infection is usually insidious. Most children and half of infected adults are asymptomatic. During the acute phase of infection, symptoms range from mild to severe. Chronicity decreases with age. HBsAg and HBcAb tests are used to screen donated blood before transfusion. HBsAg testing is often part of the routine prenatal screen. Vaccination of infants, children, and young adults is becoming a standard of care and in some cases a requirement.

This procedure is contraindicated for: N/A

INDICATIONS

- Detect exposure to HBV.
- Detect possible carrier status.
- Pre- and postvaccination testing.
- Routine prenatal testing.
- Screen donated blood before transfusion.
- Screen for individuals at high risk of exposure, such as patients on hemodialysis, persons with multiple sex partners, persons with a history of other sexually transmitted infections, individuals who misuse intravenous (IV) drugs, infants born to infected mothers, individuals residing in long-term residential facilities or correctional facilities, recipients of blood- or plasma-derived products, allied health-care workers, and public service employees who come in contact with blood and blood products.

POTENTIAL MEDICAL DIAGNOSIS

Positive findings in

- Patients currently infected with HBV
- Patients with a past HBV infection

CRITICAL FINDINGS: N/A

INTERFERING FACTORS

- Drugs that may decrease HBeAb and HBsAb include interferon alfa-2b.

NURSING IMPLICATIONS AND PROCEDURE

POTENTIAL NURSING PROBLEMS:

Problem	Signs & Symptoms	Interventions
Fatigue ***(related to decreased energy secondary to liver dysfunction associated with disease process and resulting inadequate absorption, metabolism and storage of nutrients)***	Decreased concentration; increased physical complaints; unable to restore energy with sleep; reports being tired; unable to maintain normal routine	Assess for physical cause of fatigue; pace activities to preserve energy stores; rate fatigue on a numeric scale to trend degree of fatigue over time; identify what aggravates and decreases fatigue; assess for related emotional factors such as depression; evaluate current medications in relation to fatigue; assess for physiologic factors such as anemia
Knowledge ***(related to new condition or diagnosis; lack of familiarity or understanding with disease and treatment)***	Lack of interest or questions; multiple questions; anxiety in relation to disease process and management	Teach the process of disease transmission: sharing needles with infected persons, unprotected sex with an infected person, sharing blood or body fluid with an infected person, blood products from an infected person; assess the patient's and family's knowledge of disease, transmission, and treatment; assess for cultural, literacy, or vision and hearing concerns that would interfere with learning; explain that adequate nutrition and rest can prevent disease complications; demonstrate proper hand-washing technique with re-demonstration; emphasize vigilant hand washing; discuss the implications of the disease as related to future blood donations (not possible); discuss safe sex; explain that razors, toothbrushes, and other personal care items should not be shared;

(table continues on page 914)

Problem	Signs & Symptoms	Interventions
		encourage family members to receive hepatitis vaccine; make patients aware that sexual partners should receive the hepatitis vaccine; explain that infected pregnant women can pass the disease to the child at birth
Infection ***(related to unprotected sex; exposure to blood and body fluids of an infected person; sharing needles with an infected person)***	Fever; fatigue; loss of appetite; jaundice; nausea and vomiting; dark-colored urine; abdominal pain; stool that is clay colored; joint pain; it is possible there will be no symptoms	Explain that the best treatment is adequate rest, good nutrition, and adequate fluid intake; recommend that family and significant others receive the hepatitis vaccination; explain that alcohol should be avoided to decrease risk of liver damage; explain that over-the-counter medication should be checked with the health-care provider (HCP) before taking to ensure there is no risk to the liver; explain that jaundice can last several months; administer prescribed medications
Activity ***(related to inadequate nutrient metabolism; increased basal metabolic rate associated with viral infection)***	Verbal report of weakness; inability to tolerate activity; shortness of breath with activity; altered heart rate, blood pressure, and respiratory rate with activity	Assess current level of physical activity; take baseline vital signs; trend vital signs with activity; assess response to activity; monitor for oxygen desaturation with activity; administer prescribed oxygen with activity; collaborate with physical therapy to support activity; monitor blood pressure for orthostatic changes; collaborate with the patient to establish activity goals and guidelines; pace activities to match energy stores; assist with self-care; monitor liver enzyme levels; encourage long, uninterrupted periods of rest; consider use of bedside commode; assist patient in setting realistic activity goals

H

PRETEST:

- Positively identify the patient using at least two person-specific identifiers before services, treatments, or procedures are performed.
- *Patient Teaching:* Inform the patient this test can assist in evaluating for hepatitis infection.
- Obtain a history of the patient's health concerns, symptoms, surgical procedures, and results of previously performed laboratory and diagnostic studies. Include a list of known allergens, especially allergies or sensitivities to latex.
- Obtain a history of IV drug use, high-risk sexual activity, or occupational exposure.
- Obtain a list of the patient's current medications, including over-the-counter medications and dietary supplements (see Effects of Natural Products on Laboratory Values online at Davis*Plus*).
- Review the procedure with the patient. Inform the patient that specimen collection takes approximately 5 to 10 min. Address concerns about pain and explain that there may be some discomfort during the venipuncture.
- *Sensitivity to social and cultural issues,* as well as concern for modesty, is important in providing psychological support before, during, and after the procedure.
- Note that there are no food, fluid, or medication restrictions unless by medical direction.

INTRATEST:

Potential Complications: N/A

- Avoid the use of equipment containing latex if the patient has a history of allergic reaction to latex.
- Instruct the patient to cooperate fully and to follow directions. Direct the patient to breathe normally and to avoid unnecessary movement.
- Observe standard precautions, and follow the general guidelines in Patient Preparation and Specimen Collection online at Davis*Plus*. Positively identify the patient, and label the appropriate specimen container with the corresponding patient demographics, initials of the person collecting the specimen, date, and time of collection. Perform a venipuncture.
- Remove the needle and apply direct pressure with dry gauze to stop bleeding. Observe/assess venipuncture site for bleeding or hematoma formation and secure gauze with adhesive bandage.
- Promptly transport the specimen to the laboratory for processing and analysis.

POST-TEST:

- Inform the patient that a report of the results will be made available to the requesting HCP, who will discuss the results with the patient.
- *Nutritional Considerations:* Dietary recommendations may be indicated and will vary depending on the type and severity of the condition. Explain the importance of providing an adequate daily fluid intake of at least 4 L. Monitor the patient's weight, intake, and output each day, and assess for development of ascites. Elimination of alcohol ingestion and a diet optimized for convalescence are commonly included in the treatment plan. As a general rule, small frequent meals that are high in carbohydrates and low in fat will provide the required energy while not burdening the inflamed liver.
- *Cultural and Social Considerations:* Recognize anxiety related to test results, and be supportive of impaired activity related to lack of neuromuscular control, perceived loss of independence, and fear of shortened life expectancy. Discuss the implications of abnormal test results on the patient's lifestyle. Provide teaching and information regarding the clinical implications of the test results, as appropriate. Educate the patient regarding access to counseling services. Counsel the patient, as appropriate, regarding risk of transmission and proper prophylaxis. Stress the importance

H

of hand hygiene to prevent transmission of the virus. Hepatitis B immune globulin (HBIG) vaccination should be given immediately after situations in which there is a potential for HBV exposure (e.g., accidental needle stick, perinatal period, sexual contact) for temporary, passive protection. Interferon alfa-2b may be useful in the treatment of hepatitis B. Antiviral drugs used to treat hepatitis B include lamivudine (Epivir), adefovir (Hepsera), telbivudine (Tyzeka) and entecavir (Baraclude). The specific course of treatment is decided through discussions between the patient and HCP.

- Counsel the patient and significant contacts, as appropriate, that HBIG immunization is available and has in fact become a requirement in many places as part of childhood immunization and employee health programs. Parents may choose to sign a waiver preventing their newborns from receiving the vaccine; they may choose not to vaccinate on the basis of philosophical, religious, or medical reasons. Vaccination regulations vary by state.
- Inform the patient that positive findings must be reported to local health department officials, who will question him or her regarding sexual partners. 🍁
- ***Cultural and Social Considerations:*** Offer support, as appropriate, to patients who may be the victims of sexual assault, including children and older adults. Educate the patient regarding access to counseling services. Provide a nonjudgmental, nonthreatening atmosphere for a discussion during which the risks of sexually transmitted infections are explained. It is also important to discuss the problems that the patient may experience (e.g., guilt, depression, anger).
- Depending on the results of this procedure, additional testing may be performed to evaluate or monitor progression of the disease process and determine the need for a change in therapy. Evaluate test results in relation to the patient's symptoms and other tests performed.

Patient Education:

- Reinforce information given by the patient's HCP regarding further testing, treatment, or referral to another HCP.
- Provide information regarding vaccine-preventable diseases where indicated (e.g., hepatitis B).
- Provide contact information, if desired, for the Centers for Disease Control and Prevention (www.cdc.gov/vaccines/vpd-vac and www.cdc.gov/DiseasesConditions). 🍁
- Answer any questions or address any concerns voiced by the patient or family.

Expected Patient Outcomes:

Understanding

- The patient and family state the importance of family members and sexual partners receiving hepatitis vaccine to protect against infection.
- The patient and family state the importance of family or significant other using personal protective equipment such as gloves to protect from infection and use good handwashing practices.

Ability

- Family and significant other demonstrate the proper technique in hand washing and in the application and removal of gloves as personal protective equipment.
- The patient and family relate the importance of hepatitis vaccine immunization to family members and significant others, as well as sexual partners.

Response

- The patient complies with the request to abstain from alcohol use.
- The patient complies with the request to rest prior to meals to increase appetite and calorie intake.

RELATED STUDIES:

- Related tests include ALT, ALP, antibodies, antimitochondrial, AST, bilirubin, biopsy liver, *Chlamydia* group antibody, cholangiography percutaneous transhepatic, culture anal, GGT, hepatitis C serology, HIV serology, liver and spleen scan, syphilis serology, and US liver.

- Refer to the Hepatobiliary and Immune systems tables online at Davis*Plus* for related tests by body system.

Hepatitis C Antibody

SYNONYM/ACRONYM: HCV serology, hepatitis non-A/non-B.

COMMON USE: To test blood for the presence of antibodies that would indicate a past or current hepatitis C infection.

SPECIMEN: Enzyme immunoassay and chemiluminescent immunoassay: Serum collected in a gold-, red-, or red/gray-top tube. Place separated serum into a standard transport tube within 2 hr of collection. Molecular testing for viral DNA or RNA: Serum, lavender-top (EDTA), or white-top (PPT EDTA) are acceptable.

NORMAL FINDINGS: (Method: Enzyme immunoassay, chemiluminescent immunoassay, branched chain DNA [bDNA], polymerase chain reaction [PCR], recombinant immunoblot assay [RIBA], viral RNA RT [reverse transcription] PCR). Negative.

DESCRIPTION: The hepatitis C virus (HCV) causes the majority of bloodborne non-A/non-B hepatitis cases. There are six main genotypes, or strains, of the virus, and 50 subtypes of the virus have been identified. It is possible to be infected with more than one genotype at a time. The virus is a flavivirus and contains a single-stranded RNA core. Its primary modes of transmission are parenteral, perinatal, and sexual contact. The incubation period varies widely, from 2 to 52 wk. Onset is insidious, and the risk of chronic liver disease after infection is high. On average, antibodies to hepatitis C are detectable in infected individuals within 4 to 10 wk of infection by enzyme immunoassay screening methods and as early as 2 to 3 wk of infection by PCR methods. Once infected with HCV, 75% to 85% of patients will become chronic carriers. Infected individuals and carriers have a high frequency of chronic liver diseases such as cirrhosis and chronic active hepatitis, and they have a higher risk of developing hepatocellular cancer. The transmission of hepatitis C by blood transfusion has decreased dramatically since it became part of the routine screening panel for blood donors. The possibility of prenatal transmission exists, especially in the presence of HIV coinfection. Therefore, this test is often included in prenatal testing packages. The test sequence begins with a qualitative immunoassay screening test for viral antibodies. Indeterminate or suspected false-positive results may be confirmed by the RIBA assay, which also detects viral antibodies. Nucleic acid amplification testing is the method used to document the presence of ongoing infection. Viral genotype testing is used to identify HCV RNA by RT PCR. Genotype and viral load testing (bDNA or RT PCR) are used to select and guide therapeutic interventions.

Genotype	Geographic Prevalence
Genotype 1	North America (found throughout the world)
Genotype 2	Worldwide
Genotype 3	Worldwide
Genotype 4	Northern Africa
Genotype 5	South Africa
Genotype 6	Asia

This procedure is contraindicated for: N/A

INDICATIONS

- Assist in the diagnosis of non-A/non-B viral hepatitis infection.
- Determine therapeutic approach based on identification of viral genotype.
- Monitor patients suspected of HCV infection but who have not yet produced antibody.
- Routine prenatal testing.
- Screen donated blood before transfusion.

POTENTIAL MEDICAL DIAGNOSIS

Positive findings in

- Patients currently infected with HCV
- Patients with a past HCV infection

Negative findings in: N/A

CRITICAL FINDINGS: N/A

INTERFERING FACTORS

- Drugs that may decrease hepatitis C antibody levels include interferon.

NURSING IMPLICATIONS AND PROCEDURE

POTENTIAL NURSING PROBLEMS:

Problem	Signs & Symptoms	Interventions
Knowledge ***(related to new condition or diagnosis; lack of familiarity or understanding with disease and treatment)***	Lack of interest or questions; multiple questions; anxiety in relation to disease process and management	Teach the process of disease transmission, sharing needles with infected persons, unprotected sex with an infected person, sharing blood or body fluid with an infected person, blood products from an infected person; assess the patient's and family's knowledge of the disease, transmission, and treatment; assess for cultural, literacy, or vision and hearing concerns that would interfere with learning; explain that adequate nutrition and rest can prevent disease complications; demonstrate

Problem	Signs & Symptoms	Interventions
		proper hand-washing technique with re-demonstration; emphasize vigilant hand washing; discuss the implications of the disease as related to future blood donations (not possible); discuss safe sex; explain that razors, toothbrushes, and other personal care items should not be shared
Infection ***(related to unprotected sex; exposure to blood and body fluids of an infected person; sharing needles with an infected person)***	Fever; fatigue; loss of appetite; jaundice; nausea and vomiting; dark-colored urine; abdominal pain; stool that is clay colored; joint pain; there may be no symptoms with chronic disease	Explain that the best treatment is adequate rest, good nutrition, and adequate fluid intake; administer prescribed interferon and ribavirin for chronic hepatitis
Fatigue ***(related to decreased energy secondary to liver dysfunction associated with disease process and resulting inadequate absorption, metabolism, and storage of nutrients)***	Decreased concentration; increased physical complaints; inability to restore energy with sleep; reports of being tired; inability to maintain normal routine	Assess for physical cause of fatigue; pace activities to preserve energy stores; rate fatigue on a numeric scale to trend degree of fatigue over time; identify what aggravates and decreases fatigue; assess for related emotional factors such as depression; evaluate current medications in relation to fatigue; assess for physiologic factors such as anemia
Nutrition ***(related to the inability to adequately store or metabolize foods; lack of appetite; refusal to eat; nausea and vomiting)***	Unintended weight loss; pale dry skin; dry mucous membranes; documented inadequate caloric intake; subcutaneous tissue loss; hair pulls out easily; paresthesias	Record accurate daily weight at the same time each day with the same scale; obtain an accurate nutritional history; assess for nausea and administer prescribed medication; assess attitude toward eating; promote a dietary consult to evaluate current eating habits and best method of nutritional

(table continues on page 920)

Problem	Signs & Symptoms	Interventions
		supplementation; develop short- and long-term eating strategies; monitor nutritional laboratory values such as albumin, transferrin, red blood cells (RBC), white blood cells (WBC), and serum electrolytes; encourage cultural home foods; provide a pleasant environment for eating; alter food seasoning to enhance flavor; provide parenteral or enteral nutrition as prescribed; encourage appropriate use of recommended vitamin supplements

H

PRETEST:

- Positively identify the patient using at least two person-specific identifiers before services, treatments, or procedures are performed.
- *Patient Teaching:* Inform the patient this test can assist in evaluating for hepatitis infection.
- Obtain a history of the patient's health concerns, symptoms, surgical procedures, and results of previously performed laboratory and diagnostic studies. Include a list of known allergens, especially allergies or sensitivities to latex.
- Obtain a history of intravenous drug use, high-risk sexual activity, and occupational exposure.
- Obtain a list of the patient's current medications, including over-the-counter medications and dietary supplements (see Effects of Natural Products on Laboratory Values online at Davis*Plus*).
- Review the procedure with the patient. Inform the patient that specimen collection takes approximately 5 to 10 min. Address concerns about pain and explain that there may be some discomfort during the venipuncture.
- *Sensitivity to social and cultural issues,* as well as concern for modesty, is important in providing psychological support before, during, and after the procedure.
- Note that there are no food, fluid, or medication restrictions unless by medical direction.

INTRATEST:

Potential Complications: N/A

- Avoid the use of equipment containing latex if the patient has a history of allergic reaction to latex.
- Instruct the patient to cooperate fully and to follow directions. Direct the patient to breathe normally and to avoid unnecessary movement.
- Observe standard precautions, and follow the general guidelines in Patient Preparation and Specimen Collection online at Davis*Plus*. Positively identify the patient, and label the appropriate specimen container with the corresponding patient demographics, initials of the person collecting the specimen, date, and time of collection. Perform a venipuncture.
- Remove the needle and apply direct pressure with dry gauze to stop

bleeding. Observe/assess venipuncture site for bleeding or hematoma formation and secure gauze with adhesive bandage.

- Promptly transport the specimen to the laboratory for processing and analysis.

POST-TEST:

- Inform the patient that a report of the results will be made available to the requesting health-care provider (HCP), who will discuss the results with the patient.
- *Nutritional Considerations:* Dietary recommendations may be indicated and will vary depending on the type and severity of the condition. Explain the importance of providing an adequate daily fluid intake of at least 4 L. Monitor the patient's weight, intake, and output each day, and assess for development of ascites. Elimination of alcohol ingestion and a diet optimized for convalescence are commonly included in the treatment plan. As a general rule, small, frequent meals that are high in carbohydrates and low in fat will provide the required energy while not burdening the inflamed liver.
- *Cultural and Social Considerations:* Recognize anxiety related to test results, and be supportive of impaired activity related to lack of neuromuscular control, perceived loss of independence, and fear of shortened life expectancy. Discuss the implications of abnormal test results on the patient's lifestyle. Provide teaching and information regarding the clinical implications of the test results, as appropriate. Educate the patient regarding access to counseling services. Counsel the patient, as appropriate, regarding the risk of transmission and proper prophylaxis. Stress the importance of hand hygiene to prevent transmission of the virus. Interferon alfa-2b may be useful in the treatment of hepatitis C. Antiviral drugs used to treat hepatitis C include boceprevir, daclatasvir, ledipasvir, peginterferon, ribavirin, simeprevir, sofosbuvir, and telaprevir. The specific course of treatment is decided through discussions between the patient and HCP. Therapeutic interventions are based on factors that include the type of virus identified, the patient's complete health history (including any history of liver disease, kidney disease, HIV coinfection, and previous treatment), and the patient's response to treatment. It should be noted that the average treatment is over a period of 12 wk but may extend over a period of a year and may be financially prohibitive for some patients.
- Inform the patient that positive findings must be reported to local health department officials, who will question him or her regarding sexual partners. ✱
- *Cultural and Social Considerations:* Offer support, as appropriate, to patients who may be the victims of sexual assault, including children and older adults. Educate the patient regarding access to counseling services. Provide a nonjudgmental, nonthreatening atmosphere for a discussion during which the risks of sexually transmitted infections are explained. It is also important to discuss the problems that the patient may experience (e.g., guilt, depression, anger).
- Depending on the results of this procedure, additional testing may be performed to evaluate or monitor progression of the disease process and determine the need for a change in therapy. Evaluate test results in relation to the patient's symptoms and other tests performed.

Patient Education:

- Reinforce information given by the patient's HCP regarding further testing, treatment, or referral to another HCP.
- There is no vaccine for hepatitis C. Provide contact information, if desired, for the Centers for Disease Control and Prevention (www.cdc.gov/DiseasesConditions) ✱ for information regarding hepatitis C.
- Answer any questions or address any concerns voiced by the patient or family.

Expected Patient Outcomes:

Understanding

- The patient and family state that this disease can lead to liver scarring and liver cancer.
- The patient and family state that this disease can last a lifetime and may result in liver transplant.

Ability

- The patient and family avoid situations where there can be exposure to infected blood.
- The patient takes precautions to avoid infecting others.

Response

- The patient and family accurately relate that it is possible that this disease may be present without significant symptoms.
- The patient complies with the recommendation to eat several small meals a day to support adequate nutrition.

RELATED STUDIES:

- Related tests include ALT, ALP, antibodies, antimitochondrial, AST, bilirubin, biopsy liver, *Chlamydia* group antibody, cholangiography percutaneous transhepatic, culture anal, GGT, hepatitis B serology, hepatobiliary scan, HIV serology, liver and spleen scan, syphilis serology, and US liver.
- Refer to the Hepatobiliary and Immune systems tables online at Davis*Plus* for related tests by body system.

H

Hepatitis D Antibody

SYNONYM/ACRONYM: Delta hepatitis.

COMMON USE: To test blood for the presence of antibodies that would indicate a past or current hepatitis D infections.

SPECIMEN: Serum collected in a gold-, red-, or red/gray-top tube. Place separated serum into a standard transport tube within 2 hr of collection.

NORMAL FINDINGS: (Method: Enzyme immunoassay [EIA]) Negative.

POTENTIAL MEDICAL DIAGNOSIS

Positive findings in

- Individuals currently infected with HDV
- Individuals with a past HDV infection

CRITICAL FINDINGS: N/A

Find and print out the full study on Fast Find at davispl.us/vanleeuwen7.

Hepatitis E Antibody

SYNONYM/ACRONYM: HEV.

COMMON USE: To test blood for the presence of antibodies that would indicate a past or current hepatitis E infection.

SPECIMEN: Serum collected in a gold-, red-, or red/gray-top tube. Place separated serum into a standard transport tube within 2 hr of collection.

NORMAL FINDINGS: (Method: Enzyme immunoassay) Negative.

POTENTIAL MEDICAL DIAGNOSIS

Positive findings in

- Individuals with current HEV infection
- Individuals with past HEV infection

CRITICAL FINDINGS: N/A

Find and print out the full study on Fast Find at davispl.us/vanleeuwen7.

Hepatobiliary Scan

SYNONYM/ACRONYM: Biliary tract radionuclide scan, cholescintigraphy, hepatobiliary imaging, hepatobiliary scintigraphy, gallbladder scan, HIDA or hepatobiliary iminodiacetic scan.

COMMON USE: To visualize and assess the cystic and common bile ducts of the gall bladder toward diagnosing obstructions, stones, inflammation, and tumor.

AREA OF APPLICATION: Bile ducts.

DESCRIPTION: The hepatobiliary scan is a nuclear medicine study of the hepatobiliary excretion system. It is primarily used to determine the patency of the cystic and common bile ducts, but it can also be used to determine overall hepatic function, gallbladder function, presence of gallstones (indirectly), and sphincter of Oddi dysfunction. A technetium (Tc-99m)–labelled iminodiacetic acid analogue (e.g., tribromoethyl) is administered by intravenous (IV) injection and excreted into the bile duct system. A gamma camera detects the radiation emitted from the injected contrast medium, and a representative image of the duct system is obtained. The results are correlated with other diagnostic studies, such as IV cholangiography, computed tomography (CT) scan of the gallbladder, and ultrasonography. Gallbladder emptying or ejection fraction can be determined by administering a fatty meal or cholecystokinin to the patient. This procedure can be used before and after surgery to determine the extent of bile reflux.

This procedure is contraindicated for

Patients who are pregnant or suspected of being pregnant, unless the potential benefits of a procedure using radiation far outweigh the risk of radiation exposure to the fetus and mother.

INDICATIONS

- Aid in the diagnosis of acute and chronic cholecystitis.
- Aid in the diagnosis of suspected gallbladder disorders, such as inflammation, perforation, or calculi.

- Assess enterogastric reflux.
- Assess obstructive jaundice when done in combination with radiography or ultrasonography.
- Determine common duct obstruction caused by tumors or choledocholithiasis.
- Evaluate biliary enteric bypass patency.
- Postoperatively evaluate gastric surgical procedures and abdominal trauma.

POTENTIAL MEDICAL DIAGNOSIS

Normal findings

- Normal shape, size, and function of the gallbladder with patent cystic and common bile ducts; radionuclide should pass through the biliary system, and a significant amount should be visualized in the gallbladder within 15 to 30 min.

Abnormal findings related to

Uneven distribution of the radionuclide, deposited in concentrated "hot spots," indicates areas where lesions, trauma, abnormal anatomy, or obstructions in the biliary system are located. Delayed visualization or absence of the radionuclide within 60 min or more is abnormal.

- Cholecystitis (acalculous, acute, chronic) ***evidenced by visualization of the biliary tree and lack of visualization of the gallbladder related to obstruction of the cystic duct by gallstones***
- Common bile duct obstruction secondary to gallstones, tumor, or stricture ***evidenced by visualization in the bile duct but absent visualization of the tracer in the small intestine, related to bile duct obstruction***
- Congenital biliary atresia or choledochal cyst ***evidenced by delayed visualization of the tracer and low ejection fracture (less than 35%)***
- Postoperative biliary leak, fistula, or obstruction
- Trauma-induced bile leak or cyst

CRITICAL FINDINGS: N/A

INTERFERING FACTORS

Factors that may alter the results of the study

- Inability of the patient to cooperate or remain still during the procedure because of age, significant pain, or mental status.
- Retained barium from a previous radiological procedure.
- Other nuclear scans done within the previous 24 to 48 hr.
- Metallic objects (e.g., jewelry, body rings) within the examination field, which may inhibit organ visualization and cause unclear images.
- Bilirubin levels greater than or equal to 30 mg/mL, 🍁 depending on the radionuclide used, indicate significant liver damage, which may decrease hepatic uptake.
- The use of opiate or morphine-based drugs 2 to 6 hr before the procedure may interfere with smooth muscle motility, affecting the passage of the radionuclide through the biliary system.
- Fasting for more than 24 hr before the procedure or receiving total parenteral nutrition may produce a false-positive result because ***the absence of the digestive process prevents the gallbladder from filling.***
- Ingestion of food or liquids within 2 to 4 hr before the scan.

Other considerations

- Failure to follow dietary restrictions before the procedure may cause the procedure to be canceled or repeated.
- Improper injection of the radionuclide that allows the tracer to seep

deep into the muscle tissue can produce erroneous hot spots.

- **Inaccurate timing of imaging after the radionuclide injection can affect the results.**

NURSING IMPLICATIONS AND PROCEDURE

See Potential Nursing Problems on Fast Find at davispl.us/vanleeuwen7.

PRETEST:

- Positively identify the patient using at least two person-specific identifiers before services, treatments, or procedures are performed.
- *Patient Teaching:* Inform the patient this procedure can assist in detecting inflammation or obstruction of the gallbladder or ducts.
- Obtain a history of the patient's health concerns, symptoms, surgical procedures, and results of previously performed laboratory and diagnostic studies. Include a list of known allergens, especially allergies or sensitivities to latex, anesthetics, sedatives, or radionuclides.
- Note any recent procedures that can interfere with test results, including examinations using iodine-based contrast medium.
- Record the date of the last menstrual period and determine the possibility of pregnancy in perimenopausal women.
- Obtain a list of the patient's current medications, including over-the-counter medications and dietary supplements (see Effects of Natural Products on Laboratory Values online at Davis*Plus*).
- Review the procedure with the patient. Address concerns about pain and explain that some pain may be experienced during the test, or there may be moments of discomfort. Reassure the patient that the radionuclide poses no radioactive hazard and rarely produces adverse effects. Inform the patient the procedure is performed in a nuclear medicine department by a health-care provider (HCP) specializing in this procedure, with support staff, and takes approximately 1 to 4 hr.
- Explain that an IV line may be inserted to allow infusion of fluids such as saline, anesthetics, sedatives, radionuclides, medications used in the procedure, or emergency medications.
- *Sensitivity to social and cultural issues,* as well as concern for modesty, is important in providing psychological support before, during, and after the procedure.
- Instruct the patient to remove jewelry and other metallic objects from the area to be examined prior to the procedure.
- Instruct the patient to restrict food and fluids for 4 to 6 hr prior to the procedure. Instruct the patient, as ordered, to discontinue use of opiate-based or morphine-based drugs 2 to 6 hr before the procedure. Protocols may vary among facilities.
- *Make sure a written and informed consent has been signed prior to the procedure and before administering any medications.*

INTRATEST:

Potential Complications:

Although it is rare, there is the possibility of allergic reaction to the radionuclide.

Establishing an IV site and injection of radionuclides is an invasive procedure. Complications are rare but do include bleeding from the puncture site ***related to a bleeding disorder or the effects of natural products and medications with known anticoagulant, antiplatelet, or thrombolytic properties;*** hematoma ***related to blood leakage into the tissue following needle insertion;*** infection ***that might occur if bacteria from the skin surface is introduced at the puncture site;*** or nerve injury ***that might occur if the needle strikes a nerve.***

- Observe standard precautions, and follow the general guidelines in

Patient Preparation and Specimen Collection online at Davis*Plus*. Positively identify the patient.

- Ensure that the patient has complied with dietary, fluids, and medication restrictions prior to the study, as instructed.
- Ensure that the patient has removed all external metallic objects prior to the procedure.
- Administer ordered prophylactic steroids or antihistamines before the procedure if the patient has a history of allergic reactions to radionuclides or medications.
- Instruct the patient to void prior to the procedure and to change into the gown, robe, and foot coverings provided.
- Record baseline vital signs and assess neurological status. Protocols may vary among facilities.
- Establish an IV fluid line for the injection of saline, anesthetics, sedatives, radionuclides, or emergency medications.
- Avoid the use of equipment containing latex if the patient has a history of allergic reaction to latex.
- Have emergency equipment readily available.
- Instruct the patient to cooperate fully and to follow directions. Instruct the patient to lie still during the procedure because movement produces unclear images.
- Administer sedative to a child or to an uncooperative adult, as ordered.
- Place the patient in a supine position on a flat table with foam wedges to help maintain position and immobilization.
- IV radionuclide is administered, and the upper right quadrant of the abdomen is scanned immediately, with images then taken every 5 min for the first 30 min and every 10 min for the next 30 min. If the gallbladder cannot be visualized, delayed views are taken in 2, 4, and 24 hr to differentiate acute from chronic cholecystitis or to detect the degree of obstruction.
- IV morphine may be administered during the study to initiate spasms of the sphincter of Oddi, forcing the radionuclide into the gallbladder, if the organ is not visualized within 1 hr of injection of the radionuclide. Imaging is then done 20 to 50 min later to determine delayed visualization or nonvisualization of the gallbladder.
- If gallbladder function or bile reflux is being assessed, the patient will be given a fatty meal or cholecystokinin 60 min after the injection.
- Remove the needle or catheter and apply a pressure dressing over the puncture site.
- Observe the needle/catheter insertion site for bleeding, inflammation, or hematoma formation.

POST-TEST:

- Inform the patient that a report of the results will be made available to the requesting HCP, who will discuss the results with the patient.
- Unless contraindicated, advise the patient to drink increased amounts of fluids for 24 to 48 hr to eliminate the radionuclide from the body. Inform the patient that radionuclide is eliminated from the body within 6 to 24 hr.
- Instruct the patient to resume usual diet, fluids, medications, and activity as directed by the HCP.
- Instruct the patient in the care and assessment of the injection site.
- If a woman who is breastfeeding must have a nuclear scan, she should not breastfeed the infant until the radionuclide has been eliminated. This could take as long as 3 days. She should be instructed to express the milk and discard it during the 3-day period to prevent cessation of milk production.
- Instruct the patient to immediately flush the toilet and to meticulously wash hands with soap and water after each voiding for 24 hr after the procedure.
- Instruct all caregivers to wear gloves when discarding urine for 24 hr after

the procedure. Wash gloved hands with soap and water before removing gloves, then wash ungloved hands.

- Recognize anxiety related to test results, and be supportive of perceived loss of independent function. Discuss the implications of abnormal test results on the patient's lifestyle. Provide teaching and information regarding the clinical implications of the test results, as appropriate.
- Reinforce information given by the patient's HCP regarding further testing, treatment, or referral to another HCP. Answer any questions or address any concerns voiced by the patient or family.
- Depending on the results of this procedure, additional testing may be needed to evaluate or monitor progression of the disease process and determine the need for a change in therapy. Evaluate test results in relation to the patient's symptoms and other tests performed.

Patient Education:

- Provide preoperative education for those requiring surgery.
- Provide education on how to use a pain scale appropriate to age, language, and culture.

Expected Patient Outcomes:

Understanding

- The patient and family state the importance of preoperative education and postoperative care.
- The patient and family state the importance of turning and deep breathing to prevent atelectasis.

Ability

- The patient demonstrates correct use of incentive spirometer.
- The patient demonstrates how to successfully turn and deep breathe.

Response

- The patient acknowledges the importance of taking timely pain medication to promote comfort.
- The patient agrees to progressive activity to decrease risk of postoperative complications.

RELATED STUDIES:

- Related tests include amylase, bilirubin, CT abdomen, lipase, liver and spleen scan, MRI abdomen, radiofrequency ablation liver, US abdomen, and US liver and bile ducts.
- Refer to the Hepatobiliary System table online at Davis*Plus* for related tests by body system.

Hexosaminidase A and B

SYNONYM/ACRONYM: TSD (Tay-Sachs disease) testing.

COMMON USE: To assist in diagnosing Tay-Sachs disease by identifying a hexosaminidase enzyme deficiency.

SPECIMEN: Serum collected in a yellow-top (acid-citrate-dextrose [ACD]) or a red-top tube for hexosaminidase enzyme assay; lavender-top (EDTA), pink-top (K_2 EDTA) or yellow-top tube (ACD) for molecular polymerase chain reaction (PCR) assay.

NORMAL FINDINGS: (Method: Fluorometry for enzyme assay, PCR/primer extension for molecular assay)

Enzyme Assay

Total Hexosaminidase	Conventional Units	SI Units (Conventional Units × 0.0167)
Noncarrier	589–955 nmol/hr/mL	9.83–15.95 units/L
Heterozygote	465–675 nmol/hr/mL	7.77–11.27 units/L
Tay-Sachs homozygote	Greater than 1,027 nmol/hr/mL	Greater than 17.15 units/L
Hexosaminidase A	**Conventional Units**	**SI Units (Conventional Units × 0.0167)**
Noncarrier	456–592 nmol/hr/mL or 55–76% of total hexosaminidase	7.62–9.88 units/L or 55–76% of total hexosaminidase
Heterozygote	197–323 nmol/hr/mL	3.29–5.39 units/L
Tay-Sachs homozygote	0 nmol/hr/mL	0 units/L
Hexosaminidase B	**Conventional Units**	**SI Units (Conventional Units × 0.0167)**
Noncarrier	12–32 nmol/hr/mL	0.2–0.54 units/L
Heterozygote	21–81 nmol/hr/mL	0.35–1.35 units/L
Tay-Sachs homozygote	Greater than 305 nmol/hr/mL	Greater than 5.09 units/L

Molecular assay: Negative for HEXA 7 mutations (samples are evaluated for seven specific HEXA gene mutations).

POTENTIAL MEDICAL DIAGNOSIS

Increased in:

Alterations in lysosomal enzymes metabolism are associated with various conditions.

- Total
  Gastric cancer
  Hepatic disease
  Myeloma
  Myocardial infarction
  Pregnancy
  Symptomatic porphyria
  Vascular complications of diabetes
- Hexosaminidase A
  Diabetes
  Pregnancy
- Hexosaminidase B
  Tay-Sachs disease

Decreased in:

- Total
  Sandhoff's disease ***(inherited disorder of enzyme metabolism lacking both essential enzymes for metabolizing gangliosides)***
- Hexosaminidase A
  Tay-Sachs disease ***(inherited disorder of enzyme metabolism lacking only the hexosaminidase A enzyme for metabolizing gangliosides)***
  Sandhoff's disease ***(inherited disorder of enzyme metabolism lacking both essential enzymes for metabolizing gangliosides)***
- Hexosaminidase B
  Sandhoff's disease

CRITICAL FINDINGS: N/A

Find and print out the full study on Fast Find at davispl.us/vanleeuwen7.

Holter Monitor

SYNONYM/ACRONYM: Ambulatory electrocardiography, ambulatory monitoring, event recorder, Holter electrocardiography.

COMMON USE: To evaluate cardiac symptoms associated with activity to assist with diagnosis of dysrhythmias and cardiomegaly.

AREA OF APPLICATION: Heart.

DESCRIPTION: The Holter monitor records electrical cardiac activity on a continuous basis for 24 to 72 hr. This noninvasive study includes the use of a portable device worn around the waist or over the shoulder that records cardiac electrical impulses on a magnetic tape. The recorder has a clock that allows accurate time markings on the tape and the patient is asked to keep a log or diary of daily activities and record any occurrence of cardiac symptoms. When the patient pushes a button indicating that symptoms (e.g., pain, palpitations, dyspnea, syncope) have occurred, an event marker is placed on the tape for later comparison with the cardiac activity recordings and the daily activity log. Some recorders allow the data to be transferred to the health-care provider's (HCP's) office by telephone, where the tape is interpreted by a computer to detect any significantly abnormal variations in the recorded waveform patterns.

This procedure is contraindicated for: N/A

INDICATIONS

- Detect dysrhythmias that occur during normal daily activities and correlate them with symptoms experienced by the patient.
- Evaluate activity intolerance related to oxygen supply and demand imbalance.
- Evaluate chest pain, dizziness, syncope, and palpitations.
- Evaluate the effectiveness of antidysrhythmic medications for dosage adjustment, if needed.
- Evaluate pacemaker function.
- Monitor for ischemia and dysrhythmias after myocardial infarction or cardiac surgery before changing rehabilitation and other therapy regimens.

POTENTIAL MEDICAL DIAGNOSIS

Normal findings

- Normal sinus rhythm

Abnormal findings related to

- Dysrhythmias such as premature ventricular contractions, bradycardias, tachycardias, conduction defects, and bradycardia
- Cardiomyopathy
- Hypoxic or ischemic changes
- Mitral valve abnormality
- Palpitations

CRITICAL FINDINGS: N/A

INTERFERING FACTORS

Factors that may impair the results of the examination

- Improper placement of the electrodes or movement of the electrodes.

- **Failure of the patient to maintain a daily log of symptoms or to push the button to produce a mark on the strip when experiencing a symptom.**

NURSING IMPLICATIONS AND PROCEDURE

PRETEST:

- Positively identify the patient using at least two person-specific identifiers before services, treatments, or procedures are performed.
- *Patient Teaching:* Inform the patient this procedure can assist in evaluating the heart's response to exercise or medication.
- Obtain a history of the patient's health concerns, symptoms, surgical procedures, and results of previously performed laboratory and diagnostic studies. Include a list of known allergens, especially allergies or sensitivities to latex.
- Obtain a list of the patient's current medications, including over-the-counter medications and dietary supplements (see Effects of Natural Products on Laboratory Values online at Davis*Plus*).
- Review the procedure with the patient. Inform the patient that it may be necessary to remove hair from the site before the procedure. Address concerns about pain related to the procedure and explain that no electricity is delivered to the body during this procedure and no discomfort is experienced during monitoring. Inform the patient that the electrocardiography (ECG) recorder is worn for 24 to 48 hr, at which time the patient is to return to the laboratory with an activity log to have the monitor and strip removed for interpretation.
- ***Sensitivity to social and cultural issues,*** as well as concern for modesty, is important in providing psychological support before, during, and after the procedure.
- Instruct the patient to wear loose-fitting clothing over the electrodes and not to disturb or disconnect the electrodes or wires.
- Advise the patient to avoid contact with magnetic or electrical devices that can affect the strip tracings (e.g., shavers, toothbrush, massager, blanket, microwave, metal detector) and to avoid showers and tub bathing.
- Instruct the patient to perform normal activities, such as walking, sleeping, climbing stairs, sexual activity, bowel or urinary elimination, cigarette smoking, emotional upsets, and medications, and to record them in an activity log.
- Instruct the patient regarding recording and pressing the button upon experiencing pain or discomfort.
- Advise the patient to report a light signal on the monitor, which indicates equipment malfunction or that an electrode has come off.
- Note that there are no food, fluid, or medication restrictions unless by medical direction.

INTRATEST:

Potential Complications: N/A

- Observe standard precautions, and follow the general guidelines in Patient Preparation and Specimen Collection online at Davis*Plus*. Positively identify the patient.
- Instruct the patient to void prior to the procedure and to change into the gown, robe, and foot coverings provided.
- Instruct the patient to cooperate fully and to follow directions.
- Place the patient in a supine position.
- Expose the chest. Prepare the skin surface with alcohol and remove excess hair. Use clippers to remove hair from the site if appropriate; cleanse thoroughly with alcohol and rub until red in color.
- Apply electropaste to the skin sites to provide conduction between the skin and electrodes, or apply prelubricated disposable disk electrodes.
- Apply two electrodes (negative electrodes) on the manubrium, one in the V_1 position (fourth intercostal space at the border of the right sternum), and

one at the V_5 position (level of the fifth intercostal space at the midclavicular line, horizontally and at the left axillary line). A ground electrode is also placed and secured to the skin of the chest or abdomen.
- After checking to ensure that the electrodes are secure, attach the electrode cable to the monitor and the lead wires to the electrodes.
- Check the monitor for paper supply and battery, insert the tape, and turn on the recorder. Tape all wires to the chest, and place the belt or shoulder strap in the proper position.

POST-TEST:

- After the patient has worn the monitor for the required 24 to 48 hr, gently remove the tape and other items securing the electrodes to him or her.
- Compare the activity log and tape recording for changes during the monitoring period.
- Inform the patient that a report of the results will be made available to the requesting HCP, who will discuss the results with the patient.
- Advise the patient to immediately report symptoms such as fast heart rate or difficulty breathing.
- Recognize anxiety related to test results, and be supportive of perceived loss of independence and fear of shortened life expectancy. Discuss the implications of abnormal test results on the patient's lifestyle. Provide teaching and information regarding the clinical implications of the test results, as appropriate. Educate the patient regarding access to counseling services.
- Reinforce information given by the patient's HCP regarding further testing, treatment, or referral to another HCP. Answer any questions or address any concerns voiced by the patient or family.
- Depending on the results of this procedure, additional testing may be needed to evaluate or monitor progression of the disease process and determine the need for a change in therapy. Evaluate test results in relation to the patient's symptoms and other tests performed.

RELATED STUDIES:

- Related tests include antidysrhythmic drugs, blood pool imaging, calcium, chest x-ray, echocardiography, echocardiography transesophageal, electrocardiogram, exercise stress test, magnesium, myocardial perfusion heart scan, PET heart, and potassium.
- Refer to the Cardiovascular System table online at Davis*Plus* for related tests by body system.

Homocysteine and Methylmalonic Acid

SYNONYM/ACRONYM: N/A

COMMON USE: To assist in evaluating increased risk for blood clots, plaque formation, and platelet aggregations associated with atherosclerosis and stroke risk.

SPECIMEN: Serum collected in a gold-, red-, or red/gray-top tube if methylmalonic acid and homocysteine are to be measured together. Alternatively, plasma collected in a lavender-top (EDTA) tube may be acceptable for the homocysteine measurement. The laboratory should be consulted before specimen collection because specimen type may be method dependent. Care must be taken to use the same type of collection container if serial measurements are to be taken.

NORMAL FINDINGS: (Method: Chromatography)

	Conventional & SI Units
Homocysteine	4.6–11.2 micromol/L
Methylmalonic Acid	70–270 nmol/L

POTENTIAL MEDICAL DIAGNOSIS

Increased in:

- Cerebrovascular disease ***(there is a relationship, but the pathophysiology is unclear)***
- Chronic kidney disease ***(pathophysiology is unclear)***
- Coronary artery disease (CAD) ***(there is a relationship, but the pathophysiology is unclear)***
- Folic acid deficiency ***(folate is required for completion of biochemical reactions involved in homocysteine metabolism)***
- Homocystinuria ***(inherited disorder of methionine metabolism that results in accumulation of homocysteine)***
- Peripheral vascular disease ***(related to vascular wall damage and formation of occlusive plaque)***
- Vitamin B_{12} deficiency ***(vitamin B_{12} is required for completion of biochemical reactions involved in homocysteine metabolism)***

Decreased in: N/A

CRITICAL FINDINGS: N/A

H

Find and print out the full study on Fast Find at davispl.us/vanleeuwen7.

Homovanillic Acid

SYNONYM/ACRONYM: HVA.

COMMON USE: To assist in diagnosis of neuroblastoma, pheochromocytoma, and ganglioblastoma and to monitor therapy.

SPECIMEN: Urine from a timed specimen collected in a clean plastic collection container with 6N HCl as a preservative.

NORMAL FINDINGS: (Method: Chromatography)

Age	Conventional Units	SI Units
Homovanillic Acid		*(Conventional Units × 5.49)*
3–6 yr	1.4–4.3 mg/24 hr	8–24 micromol/24 hr
7–10 yr	2.1–4.7 mg/24 hr	12–26 micromol/24 hr
11–16 yr	2.4–8.7 mg/24 hr	13–48 micromol/24 hr
Adult–older adult	1.4–8.8 mg/24 hr	8–48 micromol/24 hr
Vanillylmandelic Acid		*(Conventional Units × 5.05)*
3–6 yr	1–2.6 mg/24 hr	5–13 micromol/24 hr
7–10 yr	2–3.2 mg/24 hr	10–16 micromol/24 hr
11–16 yr	2.3–5.2 mg/24 hr	12–26 micromol/24 hr
Adult–older adult	1.4–6.5 mg/24 hr	7–33 micromol/24 hr

DESCRIPTION: Homovanillic acid (HVA) is the main terminal metabolite of dopamine. Vanillylmandelic acid is a major metabolite of epinephrine and norepinephrine. Both of these tests should be evaluated together for the diagnosis of neuroblastoma, one of the most common tumors affecting pediatric patients. Excretion may be intermittent; therefore, a 24-hr specimen is preferred. Creatinine is usually measured simultaneously to ensure adequate collection and to calculate an excretion ratio of metabolite to creatinine.

This procedure is contraindicated for: N/A

INDICATIONS

- Assist in the diagnosis of pheochromocytoma, neuroblastoma, and ganglioblastoma.
- Monitor the course of therapy.

POTENTIAL MEDICAL DIAGNOSIS

Increased in:

HVA is excreted in excessive amounts in the following conditions:

- Ganglioblastoma (tumor of the nervous system)
- Neuroblastoma (tumor usually originating in the adrenal gland)
- Pheochromocytoma (tumor usually originating in the adrenal gland)
- Riley-Day syndrome (inherited disorder of the nervous system; also known as familial dysautonomia)

Decreased in:

- Schizotypal personality disorders

CRITICAL FINDINGS: N/A

INTERFERING FACTORS

- Drugs and other substances that may increase HVA levels include acetylsalicylic acid, disulfiram, levodopa, pyridoxine, and reserpine.
- Drugs and other substances that may decrease HVA levels include moclobemide.
- All urine voided for the timed collection period must be included in the collection, or else falsely decreased values may be obtained. Compare output records with volume collected to verify that all voids were included in the collection.

NURSING IMPLICATIONS AND PROCEDURE

PRETEST:

- Positively identify the patient using at least two person-specific identifiers before services, treatments, or procedures are performed.
- *Patient Teaching:* Inform the patient this test can assist in screening for presence of a tumor.
- Obtain a history of the patient's health concerns, symptoms, surgical procedures, and results of previously performed laboratory and diagnostic studies. Include a list of known allergens, especially allergies or sensitivities to latex.
- Obtain a list of the patient's current medications, including over-the-counter medications and dietary supplements (see Effects of Natural Products on Laboratory Values online at Davis*Plus*).
- Review the procedure with the patient. Provide a nonmetallic urinal, bedpan, or toilet-mounted collection device. Address concerns about pain and explain that there should be no discomfort during the procedure.
- Usually a 24-hr time frame for urine collection is ordered. Inform the patient that all urine must be saved during that 24-hr period. Instruct the patient not to void directly into the laboratory collection container. Instruct the patient to avoid defecating in the collection device and to keep toilet tissue out of the collection

H

device to prevent contamination of the specimen. Place a sign in the bathroom to remind the patient to save all urine.

- Instruct the patient to void all urine into the collection device and then to pour the urine into the laboratory collection container. Alternatively, the specimen can be left in the collection device for a health-care staff member to add to the laboratory collection container.
- ***Sensitivity to social and cultural issues,*** as well as concern for modesty, is important in providing psychological support before, during, and after the procedure.
- If possible, and with medical direction, patients should withhold acetylsalicylic acid, disulfiram, pyridoxine, and reserpine for 2 days before specimen collection. Levodopa should be withheld for 2 wk before specimen collection.
- Note that there are no food or fluid restrictions unless by medical direction.

INTRATEST:

Potential Complications: N/A

- Ensure that the patient has complied with medication restrictions prior to the study, as instructed.
- Avoid the use of equipment containing latex if the patient has a history of allergic reaction to latex.
- Instruct the patient to cooperate fully and to follow directions.
- Observe standard precautions, and follow the general guidelines in Patient Preparation and Specimen Collection online at Davis*Plus*. Positively identify the patient, and label the appropriate specimen container with the corresponding patient demographics, initials of the person collecting the specimen, date, and time of collection.

Timed Specimen

- Obtain a clean 3-L urine specimen container, toilet-mounted collection device, and plastic bag (for transport of the specimen container). The specimen must be refrigerated or kept on ice throughout the entire collection period. If an indwelling urinary catheter is in place, the drainage bag must be kept on ice.
- Begin the test between 0600 and 0800 if possible. Collect first voiding and discard. Record the time the specimen was discarded as the beginning of the timed collection period. The next morning, ask the patient to void at the same time the collection was started and add this last voiding to the container. Urinary output should be recorded throughout the collection time.
- If an indwelling catheter is in place, replace the tubing and container system at the start of the collection time. Keep the container system on ice during the collection period, or empty the urine into a larger refrigerated container periodically during the collection period; monitor to ensure continued drainage, and conclude the test the next morning at the same hour the collection was begun.
- At the conclusion of the test, compare the quantity of urine with the urinary output record for the collection; if the specimen contains less than what was recorded as output, some urine may have been discarded, invalidating the test.
- Include on the collection container's label the amount of urine, test start and stop times, and ingestion of any foods or medications that can affect test results.
- Promptly transport the specimen to the laboratory for processing and analysis.

POST-TEST:

- Inform the patient that a report of the results will be made available to the requesting health-care provider (HCP), who will discuss the results with the patient.
- Instruct the patient to resume usual medications, as directed by the HCP.
- Recognize anxiety related to test results. Discuss the implications of abnormal test results on the patient's lifestyle. Provide teaching and

information regarding the clinical implications of the test results, as appropriate. Educate the patient regarding access to counseling services.

- Reinforce information given by the patient's HCP regarding further testing, treatment, or referral to another HCP. Answer any questions or address any concerns voiced by the patient or family.
- Depending on the results of this procedure, additional testing may be performed to evaluate or monitor progression of the disease process and determine the need for a change in therapy. Evaluate test results in relation to the patient's symptoms and other tests performed.

RELATED STUDIES:

- Related tests include angiography adrenal, CEA, catecholamines, CT kidneys, metanephrines, renin, and VMA.
- Refer to the Endocrine System table online at Davis*Plus* for related tests by body system.

Human Chorionic Gonadotropin

SYNONYM/ACRONYM: Chorionic gonadotropin, pregnancy test, HCG, hCG, α-HCG, β-subunit HCG.

COMMON USE: To assist in verification of pregnancy, screen for neural tube defects, and evaluate human chorionic gonadotropin (HCG)–secreting tumors.

SPECIMEN: Serum collected in a gold-, red-, or red/gray-top tube. Plasma collected in a green-top (heparin) tube is also acceptable.

NORMAL FINDINGS: (Method: Immunoassay)

	Conventional Units	SI Units (Conventional Units × 1)
Males and nonpregnant females	Less than 5 milli international units/mL	Less than 5 international units/L
Pregnant females by week of gestation:		
Less than 1 wk	5–50 milli international units/mL	5–50 international units/L
2 wk	5–100 milli international units/mL	5–100 international units/L
3 wk	200–3,000 milli international units/mL	200–3,000 international units/L
4 wk	10,000–80,000 milli international units/mL	10,000–80,000 international units/L
5–12 wk	10,000–200,000 milli international units/mL	10,000–200,000 international units/L
13–24 wk	5,000–80,000 milli international units/mL	5,000–80,000 international units/L
26–28 wk	3,000–15,000 milli international units/mL	3,000–15,000 international units/L

DESCRIPTION: Human chorionic gonadotropin (HCG) is a hormone secreted by the placenta beginning 8 to 10 days after conception, which coincides with implantation of the fertilized ovum. It stimulates secretion of progesterone by the corpus luteum. HCG levels peak at 8 to 12 wk of gestation and then fall to less than 10% of first trimester levels by the end of pregnancy. By postpartum week 2, levels are undetectable. HCG levels increase at a slower rate in ectopic pregnancy and spontaneous abortion than in normal pregnancy; a low rate of change between serial specimens is predictive of a nonviable fetus. As assays improve in sensitivity over time, ectopic pregnancies are increasingly being identified before rupture. HCG is used along with α-fetoprotein, dimeric inhibin-A, and estriol in prenatal screening for neural tube defects. These prenatal measurements are also known as *triple* or *quad markers,* depending on which tests are included. Serial measurements are needed for an accurate estimate of gestational stage and determination of fetal viability. Triple- and quad-marker testing has also been used to screen for trisomy 21 (Down syndrome). (To compare HCG to other tests in the triple- and quad-marker screening procedure, see study titled "α_1-Fetoprotein.") HCG is also produced by some germ cell tumors. Most assays measure both the intact and free β-HCG subunit, but if HCG is to be used as a tumor marker, the assay must be capable of detecting both intact and free β-HCG. Pregnancy testing is performed in many settings: at home using over-the-counter test kits, in the health-care provider (HCP)'s office using Clinical Laboratory Improvement Amendments (CLIA)-approved test kits or point-of-care instruments, and in full-service laboratories. HCG can be reliably measured using urine or blood specimens. Blood specimens are preferred because blood levels of HCG are detectable earlier than in urine specimens; urine specimens are susceptible to false-negative results if the specific gravity is too low, which is not a factor for blood specimens.

This procedure is contraindicated for: N/A

INDICATIONS

- Assist in the diagnosis of suspected HCG-producing tumors, such as choriocarcinoma, germ cell tumors of the ovary and testes, or hydatidiform moles.
- Confirm pregnancy, assist in the diagnosis of suspected ectopic pregnancy, or determine threatened or incomplete abortion.
- Determine adequacy of hormonal levels to maintain pregnancy.
- Monitor effects of surgery or chemotherapy.
- Monitor ovulation induction treatment.
- Prenatally detect neural tube defects and trisomy 21.

POTENTIAL MEDICAL DIAGNOSIS

Increased in:

- Choriocarcinoma ***(related to HCG-producing tumor)***
- Ectopic HCG-producing tumors (stomach, lung, colon, pancreas, liver, breast) ***(related to HCG-producing tumor)***
- Erythroblastosis fetalis ***(hemolytic anemia, as a result of fetal sensitization by incompatible***

maternal blood group antigens such as Rh, Kell, Kidd, and Duffy, is associated with increased HCG levels)

- Germ cell tumors (ovary and testes) ***(related to HCG-producing tumors)***
- Hydatidiform mole ***(related to HCG-secreting mole)***
- Islet cell tumors ***(related to HCG-producing tumors)***
- Multiple gestation pregnancy ***(related to increased levels produced by the presence of multiple fetuses)***
- Pregnancy ***(related to increased production by placenta)***

Decreased in:

Any condition associated with diminished viability of the placenta will reflect decreased levels.

- Ectopic pregnancy ***(HCG levels increase slower than in viable intrauterine pregnancies, plateau, and then decrease prior to rupture)***
- Incomplete abortion
- Intrauterine fetal demise
- Spontaneous abortion
- Threatened abortion

CRITICAL FINDINGS: N/A

INTERFERING FACTORS

- Drugs and other substances that may decrease HCG levels include epostane and mifepristone.
- Results may vary widely depending on the sensitivity and specificity of the assay. Performance of the test too early in pregnancy may cause false-negative results. HCG is composed of an α and a β subunit. The structure of the α subunit is essentially identical to the α subunit of follicle-stimulating hormone, luteinizing hormone, and thyroid-stimulating hormone. The structure of the β subunit differentiates HCG from the other hormones. False-positive results can therefore be obtained if the HCG assay does not detect β subunit.

H

NURSING IMPLICATIONS AND PROCEDURE

POTENTIAL NURSING PROBLEMS:

Problem	Signs & Symptoms	Interventions
Spirituality ***(related to potential or actual fetal death)***	Forgiveness; acceptance; anger at spiritual leaders; expressed feelings of hopeless, powerlessness; abandonment; refusals or inability to participate in spiritual activities (prayer); expresses feelings over lack of meaning with life or serenity	Encourage the verbalization of feelings in a safe, nonjudgmental environment; assess the desire for contact from associated spiritual advisor; foster a supportive relationship with the patient and family; encourage a display of objects (spiritual, religious) that provide emotional relief; assess for expressions of hope

(table continues on page 938)

Problem	Signs & Symptoms	Interventions
Fear ***(related to possible loss of potential child; ineffective coping; unfamiliar therapeutic regime; unknown)***	Expression of fear; preoccupation with fear; increased tension; increased blood pressure; increased heart rate; vomiting; diarrhea; nausea; fatigue; weakness; insomnia; shortness of breath; increased respiratory rate; withdrawal; panic attacks	Provide specific education related to pregnancy confirmation and identification of viability; provide specific information related to ongoing pregnancy; communicate with social services for needed support; ensure education is culturally appropriate; assist the patient and family to recognize effective coping strategies; assist the patient and family to acknowledge their fear; provide a safe environment to discuss fear; explore cultural influences that may enhance fear; utilize therapeutic touch as appropriate to decrease fear
Family process ***(related to failure to maintain a viable pregnancy)***	Stated feelings of failing to provide children; change in communication patterns between partners regarding having children; alterations in intimacy	Offer family counseling; facilitate opportunities for the patient and spouse to express their feelings and their perception of the problem; evaluate patient and family weaknesses, strengths, and coping strategies; help the family and patient break down concerns into manageable parts
Grief ***(related to fetal loss; inability to carry child to term)***	Apparent psychological and emotional distress; withdrawal; detachment; loss of appetite; refusal to participate in activities of daily living; anger; blame	Assess decision-making ability; encourage expression of grief; provide contact information for grief support group; assist to identify current support group; provide social services referral as appropriate; allow the patient and spouse to relive the loss and express feelings

PRETEST:

- Positively identify the patient using at least two person-specific identifiers before services, treatments, or procedures are performed.
- *Patient Teaching:* Inform the patient this test can assist in screening for pregnancy, identifying tumors, and evaluating fetal health.
- Obtain a history of the patient's health concerns, symptoms, surgical procedures, and results of previously performed laboratory and diagnostic studies. Include a list of known allergens, especially allergies or sensitivities to latex.
- Record the date of the last menstrual period and determine the possibility of pregnancy in perimenopausal women.
- Obtain a list of the patient's current medications, including over-the-counter medications and dietary supplements (see Effects of Natural Products on Laboratory Values online at Davis*Plus*).
- Review the procedure with the patient. Inform the patient that specimen collection takes approximately 5 to 10 min. Address concerns about pain and explain that there may be some discomfort during the venipuncture.
- *Sensitivity to social and cultural issues,* as well as concern for modesty, is important in providing psychological support before, during, and after the procedure.
- Note that there are no food, fluid, or medication restrictions unless by medical direction.

INTRATEST:

Potential Complications: N/A

- Avoid the use of equipment containing latex if the patient has a history of allergic reaction to latex.
- Instruct the patient to cooperate fully and to follow directions. Direct the patient to breathe normally and to avoid unnecessary movement.
- Observe standard precautions, and follow the general guidelines in Patient Preparation and Specimen Collection online at Davis*Plus*. Positively identify the patient, and label the appropriate specimen container with the corresponding patient demographics, initials of the person collecting the specimen, date, and time of collection. Perform a venipuncture.
- Remove the needle and apply direct pressure with dry gauze to stop bleeding. Observe/assess venipuncture site for bleeding or hematoma formation and secure gauze with adhesive bandage.
- Promptly transport the specimen to the laboratory for processing and analysis.

POST-TEST:

- Inform the patient that a report of the results will be made available to the requesting HCP, who will discuss the results with the patient.
- *Social and Cultural Considerations:* Recognize anxiety related to abnormal test results, and encourage the family to seek counseling if concerned with pregnancy termination or to seek genetic counseling if a chromosomal abnormality is determined. Provide teaching and information regarding the clinical implications of the test results, as appropriate. Decisions regarding elective abortion should take place in the presence of both parents. Provide a nonjudgmental, nonthreatening atmosphere for discussing the risks and difficulties of delivering and raising an infant who is developmentally challenged, as well as exploring other options (termination of pregnancy or adoption). It is also important to discuss feelings the mother and father may experience (e.g., guilt, depression, anger) if fetal abnormalities are detected.
- *Social and Cultural Considerations:* Offer support, as appropriate, to patients who may be the victims of rape or sexual assault. Educate the patient regarding access to counseling services. Provide a nonjudgmental, nonthreatening atmosphere for a discussion during which risks of

H

sexually transmitted infections are explained. It is also important to discuss problems the victim of sexual assault may experience (e.g., guilt, depression, anger) if there is possibility of pregnancy related to the assault.

- *Social and Cultural Considerations:* In patients with carcinoma, recognize anxiety related to test results and offer support. Provide teaching and information regarding the clinical implications of abnormal test results, as appropriate. Educate the patient regarding access to counseling services, as appropriate.
- Depending on the results of this procedure, additional testing may be performed to evaluate or monitor the patient's condition and determine the need for a change in therapy. Evaluate test results in relation to the patient's symptoms and other tests performed.

Patient Education:

- Reinforce information given by the patient's HCP regarding further testing, treatment, or referral to another HCP.
- Instruct the patient in the use of home test kits for pregnancy approved by the U.S. Food and Drug Administration, 🍁 as appropriate.
- Answer any questions or address any concerns voiced by the patient or family.

Expected Patient Outcomes:

Understanding

- The patient and family state that surgical intervention may be necessary in the event of fetal demise.
- The patient and family state that the purpose of surgical intervention post-miscarriage is to ensure all of the tissue is removed to prevent infection and facilitate future viable pregnancies.

Ability

- The patient and family accurately describe symptoms that may indicate a miscarriage and should be reported to the HCP.
- The patient and family accurately describe the purpose of future laboratory (HCG) studies to monitor and verify the continuation of the pregnancy.

Response

- The patient and family agree to attend a support group for those who have experienced fetal loss.
- The patient complies with scheduled follow-up laboratory studies to monitor pregnancy.

RELATED STUDIES:

- Related tests include biopsy chorionic villus, *Chlamydia* group antibody, chromosome analysis, CMV, estradiol, fetal fibronectin, α_1-fetoprotein, CBC, hematocrit, CBC hemoglobin, CBC WBC count and differential, progesterone, rubella antibody, rubeola antibody, syphilis serology, toxoplasma antibody, US abdomen, and US biophysical profile obstetric.
- Refer to the Endocrine, Immune, and Reproductive systems tables online at Davis*Plus* for related tests by body system.

Human Immunodeficiency Virus Type 1 and Type 2 Antibodies

SYNONYM/ACRONYM: HIV-1/HIV-2.

COMMON USE: Test blood for the presence of antibodies that would indicate a human immunodeficiency virus (HIV) infection.

SPECIMEN: Serum collected in a red-top tube. Place separated serum into a standard transport tube within 2 hr of collection.

NORMAL FINDINGS: (Method: Enzyme immunoassay) Negative.

DESCRIPTION: HIV is the etiological agent of AIDS and is transmitted through bodily secretions, especially by blood or sexual contact. The virus preferentially binds to the T4 helper lymphocytes and replicates within the cells using viral reverse transcriptase, integrase and protease enzymes. World Health Organization guidelines recommend that antiretroviral therapy (ART) should be offered to any person with HIV, regardless of CD4 test results or clinical stage, along with a discussion of the availability of daily oral pre-exposure prophylactic medications for patients considered to be at high risk for HIV infection. High-risk populations include gay and bisexual men, bisexual women, transgender people, sex workers, people who share intravenous (IV) needles contaminated with HIV-positive blood, people who receive HIV-positive blood products, and neonates who become infected in utero or during birth. Availability of postexposure prophylactic regimens should also be discussed as appropriate. The process for obtaining specimens and communicating test results has changed dramatically since the disease was first identified. However, confirmed positive HIV findings continue to have a significant medical, psychological, and social impact on affected individuals and their potentially infected contacts. Test methods and algorithms have been developed to include as many potentially infected people as possible. Testing is available in a variety of settings, including the traditional laboratory (generally from blood specimens), specialty laboratories by mail (generally oral, finger stick, or urine specimens collected at home and mailed to the testing facility), clinical settings (using approved rapid-test kits in labor and delivery for emergencies), and nonclinical community-based screening sites (using either approved rapid-test kits or mail-in test kits). Accuracy of test results varies depending on specimen type, quality of collection technique, and test method. In the traditional laboratory setting, initial HIV screening is generally performed using a combined immunoassay for HIV1 p24 antigen and antibodies to HIV1/HIV2. The antibody screening tests most commonly used do not distinguish between HIV1 and HIV2. A positive antigen/antibody screen may be followed by repeat testing by the same method, in duplicate, if recommended by the manufacturer. Otherwise, positive initial screens should be followed by an immunoassay that differentiates between HIV1 and HIV2 antibodies. A negative or indeterminate result for HIV1 obtained by HIV1/HIV2 differentiation testing could mean that the initial positive screen was related to the presence of HIV1 p24 antigen and the specimen was obtained after infection occurred but before the development of antibodies to the virus. Negative or indeterminate differentiation testing should be followed by a

H

nucleic acid amplification test (NAAT or NAT) to determine whether HIV1 viral RNA is present. Positive HIV1 NAT results indicate acute HIV infection. The HIV screening test is routinely recommended as part of a prenatal work-up, unless the patient declines, and is required for evaluating donated blood units before release for transfusion. The Centers for Disease Control and Prevention (CDC) has structured its recommendations to increase identification of patients who are infected with HIV as early as possible; early identification increases treatment options, increases frequency of successful treatment, and can decrease further spread of disease. The CDC recommends the following: 🍁

- Include HIV testing in routine medical care, and screen all patients between the ages of 13 and 64 years of age as part of routine medical care unless the patient requests to opt out.
- Implement new models to diagnose HIV infections outside medical settings; promote availability of rapid waived testing kits such as OraQuick.
- Prevent new infections by working with persons diagnosed with HIV and their partners; adapt a voluntary opt-out approach that includes elimination of pretest counseling and consent requirements specific for HIV. General consents should cover all aspects of care.
- Further decrease prenatal transmission of HIV by incorporating HIV testing as a routine part of prenatal medical care, and also perform third-trimester testing in areas with high rates of HIV infection among pregnant women. 🍁

HIV genotyping by polymerase chain reaction (PCR) methods may also be required to guide selection of medications for therapeutic regimens, assess potential for drug resistance, and monitor for transmission of drug resistant HIV. Genotyping is also useful to determine eligibility for new medications once resistance to conventional drugs has been identified.

This procedure is contraindicated for: N/A

INDICATIONS

- Evaluate donated blood units before transfusion.
- Perform as part of prenatal screening.
- Screen organ transplant donors.
- Test individuals who have documented and significant exposure to other infected individuals.
- Test exposed high-risk individuals for detection of antibody (e.g., persons with multiple sex partners, persons with a history of other sexually transmitted infections, people who use injection drugs, infants born to infected mothers, allied health-care workers, public service employees who have contact with blood and blood products).

POTENTIAL MEDICAL DIAGNOSIS

Positive findings in

- HIV1 or HIV2 infection

CRITICAL FINDINGS: N/A

INTERFERING FACTORS

- Drugs and other substances that may decrease HIV antibody levels include didanosine, dideoxycytidine, zalcitabine, and zidovudine.

- Negative HIV test results occur during the acute stage of the disease, when the virus is present but antibodies have not sufficiently developed to be detected. It may take up to 6 mo for the test to become positive. During this stage, the test for HIV antigen may not confirm an HIV infection.
- False-positive HIV test results can occur in patients who are immunocompromised due to conditions that include autoimmune disease, leukemias, and lymphomas.
- Test kits for HIV are very sensitive. As a result, nonspecific reactions may occur, leading to a false-positive result.

NURSING IMPLICATIONS AND PROCEDURE

POTENTIAL NURSING PROBLEMS:

Problem	Signs & Symptoms	Interventions
Knowledge ***(related to the emotional nature of the disease; new condition or diagnosis; lack of familiarity with or understanding of disease and treatment; treatment complexity; fear; misinterpretation of provided information)***	Lack of interest or questions; multiple questions; anxiety in relation to disease process and management; verbalization of inaccurate information; lack of follow-through with directions	Identify patient's, family's, and significant others' concerns about HIV infection; explain the importance of receiving pre- or postexposure HIV prophylaxis, hepatitis B vaccine, annual influenza vaccine, and pneumococcal vaccine to protect health; assist patient to identify at-risk behaviors (sexual activities and IV drug use); instruct to avoid raw foods that can cause infection from bacteria and protozoa in compromised individuals; avoid emptying cat litter boxes to avoid organism exposure; discuss safe sex practices, ways to express intimacy without infection exposure; discuss the importance of using safe needles for recreational drug use; encourage drug rehabilitation and provide contact information; explain the importance of refraining from blood donation

(table continues on page 944)

Problem	Signs & Symptoms	Interventions
Infection ***(related to decreased CD4 cells; detectable viral load; confirmed HIV antibody secondary to HIV infection)***	Fever; swollen lymph glands in the armpit, neck, and groin; sore throat; rash; unexplained fatigue; achy muscles and joints with pain; headache; weight loss; fever and night sweats; diarrhea lasting more than a week; mouth, anal, and genital sores; pneumonia; blotches (red, brown, pink, or purplish) on or under the skin located in the mouth, or nose; depression; memory loss; neurologic disorders	Monitor and trend vial load and CD4 laboratory results; explain the purpose of antiviral medication; administer prescribed antiviral medication (nucleoside and nonnucleoside reverse transcriptase inhibitors, protease inhibitors, integrase strand transfer inhibitors, fusion inhibitors); ensure legal regulations regarding testing are adhered to; reinforce the necessity of strict adherence to the designated treatment plan
Nutrition ***(related to fatigue; no appetite; oral candidiasis; nausea; vomiting; malabsorption; secondary to HIV infection)***	Weight loss; pale, dry skin; dry mucous membranes; documented inadequate caloric intake; loss of subcutaneous tissue, muscle, fat; hair pulls out easily; decreased body mass index	Record accurate daily weight at the same time each day with the same scale; obtain an accurate nutritional history; assess for nausea and administer prescribed medication; inspect the mouth and assess for oral candidiasis infection; administer prescribed medications antimonilial, anabolic steroids, testosterone supplements, human growth hormones, dronabinol; administer prescribed medications to enhance nutrient absorption within the gastrointestinal tract; discuss the patient use of total parenteral nutrition to support nutrition with the health-care provider (HCP);

H

Problem	Signs & Symptoms	Interventions
		assess attitude toward eating; promote a dietary consult to evaluate current eating habits and best method of nutritional supplementation; develop short- and long-term eating strategies; monitor nutritional laboratory values such as albumin, transferrin, red blood cells, white blood cells, and serum electrolytes; encourage cultural home foods; provide a pleasant environment for eating; alter food seasoning to enhance flavor; ensure appropriate use of recommended vitamin supplements

PRETEST:

- Positively identify the patient using at least two person-specific identifiers before services, treatments, or procedures are performed.
- *Patient Teaching:* Inform the patient that this laboratory test can assist in evaluating for HIV infection.
- Obtain a history of the patient's health concerns (especially a history of high risk behaviors, symptoms, surgical procedures, and results of previously performed laboratory and diagnostic studies. Include a list of known allergens, especially allergies or sensitivities to latex.
- Obtain a list of the patient's current medications, including over-the-counter medications and dietary supplements (see Effects of Natural Products on Laboratory Values online at Davis*Plus*).
- Review the procedure with the patient. Inform the patient that specimen collection takes approximately 5 to 10 min. Address concerns about pain and explain that there may be some discomfort during the venipuncture. Explain that a series of specimens may be required over time.
- Note that there are no food, fluid, or medication restrictions unless by medical direction.

INTRATEST:

Potential Complications: N/A

- Avoid the use of equipment containing latex if the patient has a history of allergic reaction to latex.
- Instruct the patient to cooperate fully and to follow directions. Direct the patient to breathe normally and to avoid unnecessary movement.
- Observe standard precautions, and follow the general guidelines in Patient Preparation and Specimen Collection online at Davis*Plus*. Positively identify the patient, and label the appropriate specimen container with the corresponding patient demographics, initials of the person collecting the specimen, date, and time of collection. Perform a venipuncture.

- Remove the needle and apply direct pressure with dry gauze to stop bleeding. Observe/assess venipuncture site for bleeding or hematoma formation and secure gauze with adhesive bandage.
- Promptly transport the specimen to the laboratory for processing and analysis.

POST-TEST:

- Inform the patient that a report of the results will be made available to the requesting HCP, who will discuss the results with the patient.
- Warn the patient that false-positive results occur and that the absence of antibody does not guarantee absence of infection, because the virus may be latent or may not have produced detectable antibody at the time of testing.
- *Social and Cultural Considerations:* Recognize anxiety related to test results, and be supportive of impaired activity related to weakness, perceived loss of independence, and fear of shortened life expectancy. Discuss the implications of abnormal test results on the patient's lifestyle. Provide teaching and information regarding the clinical implications of the test results, as appropriate. Educate the patient regarding access to counseling services. Provide contact information, if desired, for information related to HIV prevention, infection, and treatment provided by the National Institutes of Health (www.aidsinfo.nih.gov) or CDC (www.cdc.gov). 🍁
- *Social and Cultural Considerations:* Counsel the patient, as appropriate, regarding risk of transmission and proper prophylaxis, and reinforce the importance of strict adherence to the treatment regimen, including consultation with a pharmacist.
- *Social and Cultural Considerations:* Inform patient that positive findings must be reported to local health department officials, who will question him or her regarding sexual partners. 🍁
- *Social and Cultural Considerations:* Offer support, as appropriate, to patients who may be the victims of sexual assault. Educate the patient regarding access to counseling services. Provide a nonjudgmental, nonthreatening atmosphere for a discussion during which risks of sexually transmitted infections are explained. It is also important to discuss problems the patient may experience (e.g., guilt, depression, anger).
- Depending on the results of this procedure, additional testing may be performed to evaluate or monitor progression of the disease process and determine the need for a change in therapy. Evaluate test results in relation to the patient's symptoms and other tests performed.

Patient Education:

- Inform the patient that retesting may be necessary.
- Reinforce information given by the patient's HCP regarding further testing, treatment, or referral to another HCP.
- Provide information regarding pre- and postexposure HIV prophylaxis and vaccine-preventable diseases where indicated (e.g., hepatitis B, human papillomavirus). Provide contact information, if desired, for the CDC (www.cdc.gov/vaccines/vpd-vac) and (www.cdc.gov/DiseasesConditions). 🍁
- Instruct the patient in the use of home test kits approved by the U.S. Food and Drug Administration, if prescribed. Answer any questions or address any concerns voiced by the patient or family.

Expected Patient Outcomes:

Understanding

- The patient and family state the importance of avoiding activities that can cause exposure to infecting organisms.
- The patient and family state that donating infected blood can put others at risk, and that donation is prohibited.

Ability

- The patient and family accurately describe interventions that can prevent exposure to opportunistic infections.

- The patient proficiently self-administers prescribed medication to treat or prevent opportunistic infection.

Response

- The patient complies with the recommendation to take precautions during sexual activity to avoid placing others at risk.
- The patient complies with suggested dietary changes and takes the recommended medication designed to improve caloric intake.

RELATED STUDIES:

- Related tests include biopsy bone marrow, bronchoscopy, CD4/CD8 enumeration, *Chlamydia* group antibody, CBC, CBC platelet count, CBC WBC count and differential, culture and smear mycobacteria, culture viral, cytology sputum, CMV, culture skin, gallium scan, HBV antibody and antigen, HCV antibody, human T-cell lymphotropic virus types I and II, laparoscopy abdominal, LAP, lymphangiogram, MRI musculoskeletal, mediastinoscopy, β_2-microglobulin, newborn screening, and syphilis serology.
- Refer to the Immune System table online at Davis*Plus* for related tests by body system.

Human Leukocyte Antigen B27

H

SYNONYM/ACRONYM: HLA-B27.

COMMON USE: To assist in diagnosing juvenile rheumatoid arthritis, psoriatic arthritis, ankylosing spondylitis, and Reiter's syndrome.

SPECIMEN: Whole blood collected in a green-top (heparin) or a yellow-top (acid-citrate-dextrose [ACD]) tube.

NORMAL FINDINGS: (Method: Flow cytometry) Negative (indicating absence of the antigen).

POTENTIAL MEDICAL DIAGNOSIS

Positive findings in

- Ankylosing spondylitis
- Inflammatory bowel disease
- Juvenile rheumatoid arthritis
- Psoriatic arthritis
- Reiter's syndrome
- Sacroiliitis
- Uveitis

CRITICAL FINDINGS: N/A

Find and print out the full study on Fast Find at davispl.us/vanleeuwen7.

Human T-Lymphotropic Virus Type I and Type II Antibodies

SYNONYM/ACRONYM: HTLV-I/HTLV-II.

COMMON USE: To test the blood for the presence of antibodies that would indicate past or current human T-lymphocyte virus (HTLV) infection. Helpful in diagnosing certain types of leukemia.

SPECIMEN: Serum collected in a red-top tube. Place separated serum into a standard transport tube within 2 hr of collection.

NORMAL FINDINGS: (Method: Enzyme immunoassay) Negative.

POTENTIAL MEDICAL DIAGNOSIS

Positive findings in

- HTLV-I/HTLV-II infection

CRITICAL FINDINGS: N/A

Find and print out the full study on Fast Find at davispl.us/vanleeuwen7.

5-Hydroxyindoleacetic Acid

SYNONYM/ACRONYM: 5-HIAA.

COMMON USE: To assist in diagnosing carcinoid tumors.

H

SPECIMEN: Urine from a timed specimen collected in a clean plastic collection container with boric acid as a preservative.

NORMAL FINDINGS: (Method: High-pressure liquid chromatography)

Conventional Units	SI Units (Conventional Units × 5.23)
2–7 mg/24 hr	10.5–36.6 micromol/24 hr

POTENTIAL MEDICAL DIAGNOSIS

Increased in:

Serotonin is produced by the enterochromaffin cells of the small intestine and secreted ectopically by tumor cells. It is converted to 5-HIAA in the liver and excreted in the urine. Increased values are associated with malabsorption conditions, but the relationship is unclear.

- Celiac and tropical sprue
- Cystic fibrosis
- Foregut and midgut carcinoid tumors
- Oat cell carcinoma of the bronchus
- Ovarian carcinoid tumors
- Whipple's disease

Decreased in:

The documented relationship between decreased levels of serotonin, defective amino acid metabolism, and mental illness is not well understood.

- Chronic kidney disease ***(related to decreased renal excretion)***
- Depressive illnesses
- Hartnup's disease
- Mastocytosis
- Phenylketonuria
- Small intestine resection ***(related to a decrease in enterochromaffin-producing cells)***

CRITICAL FINDINGS: N/A

Find and print out the full study on Fast Find at davispl.us/vanleeuwen7.

Hypersensitivity Pneumonitis Serology

SYNONYM/ACRONYM: Farmer's lung disease serology, extrinsic allergic alveolitis.

COMMON USE: To assist in identification of pneumonia related to inhaled allergens containing *Aspergillus* or actinomycetes (dust, mold, or chronic exposure to moist organic materials).

SPECIMEN: Serum collected in a red-top tube. Place separated serum into a standard transport tube within 2 hr of collection.

NORMAL FINDINGS: (Method: Immunodiffusion) Negative.

POTENTIAL MEDICAL DIAGNOSIS

Increased in:

- Hypersensitivity pneumonitis

CRITICAL FINDINGS: N/A

Find and print out the full study on Fast Find at davispl.us/vanleeuwen7.

H

Hysterosalpingography

SYNONYM/ACRONYM: Hysterogram, uterography, uterosalpingography.

COMMON USE: To visualize and assess the uterus and fallopian tubes to assess for obstruction, adhesions, malformations, or injuries that may be related to infertility.

AREA OF APPLICATION: Uterus and fallopian tubes.

DESCRIPTION: Hysterosalpingography (HSG) is performed as part of an infertility study to identify anatomical abnormalities of the uterus or occlusion of the fallopian tubes. The procedure allows visualization of the uterine cavity, fallopian tubes, and peritubal area after the injection of iodinated contrast medium into the cervix. The contrast medium should flow through the uterine cavity, through the fallopian tubes, and into the peritoneal cavity, where it is absorbed if no obstruction exists. The procedure has therapeutic indications in that passage of the contrast medium through the tubes may clear mucous plugs, straighten kinked tubes, or break up adhesions, thus restoring fertility. This procedure is also used to evaluate the fallopian tubes after tubal ligation and to evaluate the results of reconstructive surgery.

This procedure is contraindicated for

Patients who are pregnant or suspected of being pregnant, unless the potential benefits of a procedure using radiation far outweigh the risk of radiation exposure to the fetus and mother.

- Conditions associated with adverse reactions to contrast medium (e.g., asthma, food allergies, or allergy to contrast medium).

Although patients are asked specifically if they have a known allergy to iodine or shellfish, it has been well established that the reaction is not to iodine; an actual iodine allergy would be problematic because iodine is required for the production of thyroid hormones. In the case of shellfish, the reaction is to a muscle protein called tropomyosin; in the case of iodinated contrast medium, the reaction is to the noniodinated part of the contrast molecule. Patients with a known hypersensitivity to the medium may benefit from premedication with corticosteroids and diphenhydramine; the use of nonionic contrast or an alternative noncontrast imaging study, if available, may be considered for patients who have severe asthma or who have experienced moderate to severe reactions to ionic contrast medium.

- Conditions associated with preexisting renal insufficiency (e.g., chronic kidney disease, single kidney transplant, nephrectomy, diabetes, multiple myeloma, treatment with aminoglycosides and NSAIDs) ***because iodinated contrast is nephrotoxic.***
- Patients who are chronically dehydrated before the test, especially older adults and patients whose health is already compromised ***because of their risk of contrast-induced acute kidney injury.***
- Patients with bleeding disorders ***because the puncture site may not stop bleeding.***
- Patients with menses, undiagnosed vaginal bleeding, or pelvic inflammatory disease.

INDICATIONS

- Assist in the investigation of abnormal uterine bleeding, amenorrhea, or recurrent abortion.
- Confirm the presence of fistulas, adhesions, polyps, or pelvic masses.
- Confirm tubal abnormalities such as adhesions and occlusions; evaluate the patency of the tubes.
- Confirm uterine abnormalities such as congenital malformation, traumatic injuries, missing or ectopic contraceptive devices, or indicate the presence of foreign bodies.
- Detect bicornate uterus.
- Evaluate adequacy of surgical tubal ligation and reconstructive surgery.

POTENTIAL MEDICAL DIAGNOSIS

Normal findings

- Contrast medium flowing freely into the fallopian tubes and from the uterus into the peritoneal cavity
- Normal position, shape, and size of the uterine cavity

Abnormal findings related to

- Bicornate uterus
- Developmental abnormalities
- Extrauterine pregnancy
- Internal scarring
- Kinking of the fallopian tubes due to adhesions
- Partial or complete blockage of fallopian tube(s)
- Tumors
- Uterine cavity anomalies
- Uterine fistulas
- Uterine masses or foreign body
- Uterine fibroid tumors (leiomyomas)

CRITICAL FINDINGS: N/A

INTERFERING FACTORS

Factors that may alter the results of the study

- Gas or feces in the gastrointestinal tract resulting from inadequate cleansing or failure to restrict food intake before the study.
- Retained barium from a previous radiological procedure.

- **Metallic objects (e.g., jewelry, body rings) within the examination field, which may inhibit organ visualization and cause unclear images.**
- **Inability of the patient to cooperate or remain still during the procedure because of age, significant pain, or mental status.**
- **Insufficient injection of contrast medium.**
- **Excessive traction during the test or tubal spasm, which may cause the appearance of a stricture in an otherwise normal fallopian tube.**

Other considerations

- **Excessive traction during the test may displace adhesions, making the fallopian tubes appear normal.**
- **Failure to follow pretesting preparations may cause the procedure to be canceled or repeated.**
- **The procedure may be terminated if chest pain or severe cardiac dysrhythmias occur.**

NURSING IMPLICATIONS AND PROCEDURE

PRETEST:

- Positively identify the patient using at least two person-specific identifiers before services, treatments, or procedures are performed.
- *Patient Teaching:* Inform the patient this procedure can assist in assessing the uterus and fallopian tubes.
- Obtain a history of the patient's health concerns, symptoms, surgical procedures, and results of previously performed laboratory and diagnostic studies. Include a list of known allergens, especially allergies or sensitivities to latex, anesthetics, sedatives, or contrast medium. Ensure results of coagulation testing are obtained and recorded prior to the procedure; a creatinine level is also needed before contrast medium is to be used.
- Obtain a history of the patient's reproductive system, symptoms, and results of previously performed laboratory tests and diagnostic and surgical procedures.
- Note any recent barium or other radiological contrast procedures. Ensure that barium studies were performed more than 4 days before the hysterosalpingography.
- Record the date of the last menstrual period and determine the possibility of pregnancy in perimenopausal women.
- Obtain a list of the patient's current medications, including over-the-counter medications, dietary supplements, anticoagulants, aspirin and other salicylates (see Effects of Natural Products on Laboratory Values online at Davis*Plus*). Such products should be discontinued by medical direction for the appropriate number of days prior to a surgical procedure. Note the last time and dose of medication taken.
- If iodinated contrast medium is scheduled to be used in patients receiving metformin for type 2 diabetes, the drug should be discontinued on the day of the test and continue to be withheld for 48 hr after the test. Iodinated contrast can temporarily impair kidney function, and failure to withhold metformin may indirectly result in drug-induced lactic acidosis, a dangerous and sometimes fatal adverse effect of metformin ***(related to renal impairment that does not support sufficient excretion of metformin).***
- Review the procedure with the patient. Address concerns about pain related to the procedure and explain that some pain may be experienced during the test, and there may be moments of discomfort. Explain to the patient that she may feel temporary sensations of nausea, dizziness, slow heartbeat, and menstrual-like cramping during the procedure, as well as shoulder pain from subphrenic irritation from the contrast medium as it spills into the peritoneal cavity. Inform the patient that the procedure is performed in a radiology department by a health-care provider (HCP), with support staff, and takes approximately 30 to 60 min.

H

- *Sensitivity to social and cultural issues,* as well as concern for modesty, is important in providing psychological support before, during and after the procedure.
- Instruct the patient to take a laxative or a cathartic, as ordered, on the evening before the examination.
- Instruct the patient to remove jewelry and other metallic objects from the area to be examined.
- Note that there are no food, fluid, or medication restrictions unless by medical direction or department protocol.
- *Make sure a written and informed consent has been signed prior to the procedure and before administering any medications.*

INTRATEST:

Potential Complications:

Risks from HSG can include uterine perforation, exposure to radiation, infection, allergic reaction to contrast medium, heavy vaginal bleeding, uterine perforation, severe abdominal pain or cramping, pelvic infection (uterine or of the fallopian tubes), and pulmonary embolism.

- Observe standard precautions, and follow the general guidelines in Patient Preparation and Specimen Collection online at Davis*Plus.* Positively identify the patient.
- Ensure the patient has complied with pretesting preparations prior to the study, as instructed.
- Ensure the patient has removed all external metallic objects from the area to be examined prior to the procedure.
- Assess for completion of bowel preparation according to the institution's procedure. Administer enemas or suppositories on the morning of the test, as ordered.
- Avoid the use of equipment containing latex if the patient has a history of allergic reaction to latex.
- Have emergency equipment readily available.
- Instruct the patient to void prior to the procedure and to change into the gown, robe, and foot coverings provided.
- Instruct the patient to cooperate fully and to follow directions. Instruct the patient to remain still throughout the procedure because movement produces unreliable results.
- Place the patient in a lithotomy position on the fluoroscopy table.
- A kidney, ureter, and bladder film is taken to ensure that no stool, gas, or barium will obscure visualization of the uterus and fallopian tubes.
- A speculum is inserted into the vagina, and contrast medium is introduced into the uterus through the cervix via a cannula, after which both fluoroscopic and radiographic images are taken.

POST-TEST:

- Inform the patient that a report of the results will be made available to the requesting HCP, who will discuss the results with the patient.
- Instruct the patient to resume usual medications and activity, as directed by the HCP. Kidney function should be assessed before metformin is resumed.
- Observe for delayed reaction to iodinated contrast medium, including rash, urticaria, tachycardia, hyperpnea, hypertension, palpitations, nausea, or vomiting.
- Instruct the patient to immediately report symptoms such as fast heart rate, difficulty breathing, skin rash, itching, chest pain, persistent right shoulder pain, or abdominal pain. Immediately report symptoms to the appropriate HCP.
- Inform the patient that a vaginal discharge is common and that it may be bloody, lasting 1 to 2 days after the test.
- Inform the patient that dizziness and cramping may follow this procedure, and that analgesia may be given if there is persistent cramping. Instruct the patient to contact the HCP in the event of severe cramping or profuse bleeding.

- Recognize anxiety related to test results. Discuss the implications of abnormal test results on the patient's lifestyle. Provide teaching and information regarding the clinical implications of the test results, as appropriate.
- Reinforce information given by the patient's HCP regarding further testing, treatment, or referral to another HCP. Answer any questions or address any concerns voiced by the patient or family.
- Depending on the results of this procedure, additional testing may be needed to evaluate or monitor progression of the disease process and determine the need for a change in therapy. Evaluate test results in relation to the patient's symptoms and other tests performed.

RELATED STUDIES:

- Related tests include CT abdomen, laparoscopy gynecological, MRI abdomen, US obstetric, US pelvis, and uterine fibroid embolization.
- Refer to the Reproductive System table online at Davis*Plus* for related tests by body system.

Hysteroscopy

SYNONYM/ACRONYM: N/A

COMMON USE: To visualize and assess the endometrial lining of the uterus to assist in diagnosing disorders such as fibroids, cancer, and polyps.

AREA OF APPLICATION: Uterus.

H

DESCRIPTION: Hysteroscopy is a diagnostic or minor surgical procedure of the uterus. It is done using a thin telescope (hysteroscope), which is inserted through the cervix with minimal or no dilation. Normal saline, glycine, or carbon dioxide is used to fill and distend the uterus. The inner surface of the uterus is examined, and laser beam or electrocautery can be accomplished during the procedure. Diagnostic hysteroscopy is used to diagnose uterine abnormalities and may be completed in conjunction with a dilatation and curettage (D & C). This procedure is usually done to assess abnormal uterine bleeding or repeated miscarriages. An operative hysteroscopy is done instead of abdominal surgery to treat many uterine conditions such as septums or fibroids (myomas). A resectoscope (a hysteroscope that uses high-frequency electrical current to cut or coagulate tissue) may be used to remove any localized myomas. Local, regional, or general anesthesia can be used, but usually general anesthesia is needed. The procedure may done in a health-care provider's (HCP) office, but if done as an outpatient surgical procedure, it is usually completed in a hospital setting.

This procedure is contraindicated for

Patients with bleeding disorders or receiving anticoagulant therapy ***related to the potential for continued bleeding as a result of the procedure.***

INDICATIONS

- Confirm the presence of uterine fibroids.
- Aid in the diagnosis and/or treatment of intrauterine adhesions.
- Investigate abnormal uterine bleeding.
- Assist in the removal of intrauterine devices.
- Assist in the removal of uterine polyps.

POTENTIAL MEDICAL DIAGNOSIS

Normal findings

- Normal uterine appearance

Abnormal findings related to

- Areas of active bleeding
- Adhesions
- Displaced intrauterine devices
- Fibroid tumors
- Polyps
- Uterine septum

H

CRITICAL FINDINGS: N/A

INTERFERING FACTORS

- Inability of the patient to cooperate or remain still during the test because of age, significant pain, or mental status may interfere with the test results.
- Failure to follow dietary restrictions and other pretesting preparations may cause the procedure to be canceled or repeated.

NURSING IMPLICATIONS AND PROCEDURE

PRETEST:

- Positively identify the patient using at least two person-specific identifiers before services, treatments, or procedures are performed.
- *Patient Teaching:* Inform the patient that this procedure can assist in assessing uterine health.
- Obtain a history of the patient's health concerns, symptoms, surgical procedures, and results of previously performed laboratory and diagnostic studies. Include a list of known allergens, especially allergies or sensitivities to latex.
- Record the date of last menstrual period and determine the possibility of pregnancy in perimenopausal women.
- Obtain a list of the patient's current medications, including over-the-counter medications and dietary supplements (see Effects of Natural Products on Laboratory Values online at Davis*Plus*).
- Review the procedure with the patient. Address concerns about pain and explain that a local anesthetic spray or liquid may be applied to the cervix to ease with insertion of the hysteroscope if general anesthesia is not used. Inform the patient that the procedure is usually performed in the office of a HCP or a surgery suite and takes about 30 to 45 min.
- *Sensitivity to social and cultural issues,* as well as concern for modesty, is important in providing psychological support before, during, and after the procedure.
- Explain that an intravenous (IV) line may be inserted to allow infusion of fluids such as saline, anesthetics, sedatives, or emergency medications.
- Instruct the patient that to reduce the risk of aspiration related to nausea and vomiting, solid food and milk or milk products are restricted for at least 6 hr, and clear liquids are restricted for at least 2 hr prior to general anesthesia, regional anesthesia, or sedation/analgesia (monitored anesthesia). The American Society of Anesthesiologists has fasting guidelines for risk levels according to patient status. More information can be located at www.asahq.org. 🍁 Patients on beta blockers before the surgical procedure should be instructed to take their medication as ordered during the perioperative period. Protocols may vary among facilities.
- Instruct the patient not to douche or use tampons or vaginal medications for 24 hr prior to the procedure.

- *Make sure a written and informed consent has been signed prior to the procedure and before administering any medications.*

INTRATEST:

Potential Complications:

Complications of the procedure may include bleeding.

- Observe standard precautions, and follow the general guidelines in Patient Preparation and Specimen Collection online at Davis*Plus*. Positively identify the patient.
- Ensure the patient has complied with dietary and fluid restrictions prior to the study, as instructed.
- Avoid the use of equipment containing latex if the patient has a history of allergic reaction to latex.
- Have emergency equipment readily available.
- Instruct the patient to void prior to the procedure and to change into the gown, robe, and foot coverings provided.
- Instruct the patient to cooperate fully and to follow directions.
- Record baseline vital signs, and continue to monitor throughout the procedure. Protocols may vary among facilities.
- Establish an IV fluid line for the injection of saline, sedatives, or emergency medications.
- Place the patient in the supine position on an examination table. Cleanse the vaginal area, and cover with a sterile drape.
- Monitor the patient for complications related to the procedure.

POST-TEST:

- Inform the patient that a report of the results will be made available to the requesting HCP, who will discuss the results with the patient.
- Instruct the patient to resume usual diet, fluids, medications, and activity as directed by the HCP.
- Instruct the patient to immediately report symptoms such as excessive uterine bleeding or fever.
- Recognize anxiety related to test results. Discuss the implications of abnormal test results on the patient's lifestyle. Provide teaching and information regarding the clinical implications of the test results, as appropriate.
- Reinforce information given by the patient's HCP regarding further testing, treatment, or referral to another HCP. Answer any questions or address any concerns voiced by the patient or family.
- Depending on the results of this procedure, additional testing may be needed to evaluate or monitor progression of the disease process and determine the need for a change in therapy. Evaluate test results in relation to the patient's symptoms and other tests performed.

RELATED STUDIES:

- Related tests include CBC hematocrit, CBC hemoglobin, CT abdomen, HCG, KUB, and US pelvis.
- Refer to the Reproductive System table online at Davis*Plus* for related tests by body system.

H

Immunofixation Electrophoresis, Blood and Urine

SYNONYM/ACRONYM: IFE.

COMMON USE: To identify the individual types of immunoglobulins, toward diagnosing diseases such as multiple myeloma, and to evaluate effectiveness of chemotherapy.

SPECIMEN: Serum collected in a gold-, red-, or red/gray-top tube. Place separated serum in a standard transport tube within 2 hr of collection. Urine from a random or timed collection in a clean plastic container.

NORMAL FINDINGS: (Method: Immunoprecipitation combined with electrophoresis) Test results are interpreted by a pathologist. Normal placement and intensity of staining provide information about the immunoglobulin bands.

DESCRIPTION: Immunofixation electrophoresis (IFE) is a qualitative technique that provides a detailed separation of individual immunoglobulins according to their electrical charges followed by the application of specific antiserum (anti-IgM, anti kappa, etc.) and a stain, to help visualize the patterns. It is usually requested when there is an abnormality in the gamma globulin fraction of a serum protein electrophoresis; either monoclonal or polyclonal. IFE is frequently used to identify the three main immunoglobulin groups (IgG, IgM, and IgA) and the light chain proteins (kappa and lambda). Antisera for IgE and IgD are available for use, if indicated. Abnormalities are revealed by changes produced in the individual bands, such as displacement compared to a normal pattern, intense color which reflects an increase, or absence of color which reflects a decrease. Urine IFE has replaced the Bence Jones screening test for light chains. IFE has replaced immunoelectrophoresis because it is more sensitive and easier to interpret. IFE is used to help detect, diagnose, and monitor the course and treatment of conditions like chronic kidney disease, multiple myeloma and Waldenström's macroglobulinemia.

This procedure is contraindicated for: N/A

INDICATIONS

- Assist in the diagnosis of multiple myeloma and amyloidosis.
- Assist in the diagnosis of suspected immunodeficiency.
- Assist in the diagnosis of suspected immunoproliferative disorders, such as multiple myeloma and Waldenström's macroglobulinemia.
- Identify biclonal or monoclonal gammopathies.
- Identify cryoglobulinemia.
- Monitor the effectiveness of chemotherapy or radiation therapy.

POTENTIAL MEDICAL DIAGNOSIS

See the "Immunoglobulins A, D, G, and M" and "Protein, total and fractions" studies.

CRITICAL FINDINGS: N/A

INTERFERING FACTORS

- Drugs and other substances that may increase immunoglobulin levels include asparaginase, cimetidine, and opioids.

- Drugs and other substances that may decrease immunoglobulin levels include dextran, oral contraceptives, methylprednisolone (high doses), and phenytoin.
- Chemotherapy and radiation treatments may alter the width of the bands and make interpretation difficult.

NURSING IMPLICATIONS AND PROCEDURE

POTENTIAL NURSING PROBLEMS:

Problem	Signs & Symptoms	Interventions
Powerlessness ***(related chronic illness; treatment for illness; loss of ability to provide self-care; progressive debilitation; terminal prognosis)***	Expression of loss of control over situation, self, outcome of disease; passive; apathetic; submissive; decreased participation in self-care; reluctant to express feelings	Assess need to be in control; assess feelings of hopelessness, depression, apathy; assist to identify situations that contribute to a feeling of powerlessness; assess the impact of the sense of powerlessness on the patient's sense of self; encourage verbalization of feelings; discuss therapeutic options offered by health-care provider (HCP); assist to identify strengths; identify coping strategies; encourage being responsible for self-care and personal environment to increase sense of control; give positive feedback
Hopelessness ***(related to chronic illness; impaired functionality; prolonged pain and discomfort)***	Decreased affect; decreased response to stimuli; feeling of emptiness; alterations in sleep patterns and appetite; expressions of apathy; withdrawn; states life has no meaning	Assess role of illness in relation to expressions of helplessness; assess grooming (energy to provide good personal hygiene); assess level of appetite; assess verbalization of helplessness; provide opportunities to express feelings in a safe environment; support development of a trusting relationship to decrease feelings of isolation; encourage verbalization of personal strengths and weaknesses; encourage realistic hope; assist in identification of coping skills

(table continues on page 958)

Problem	Signs & Symptoms	Interventions
Mobility ***(related to pain; weakness; depression; fatigue; decreased muscle strength; decreased coordination)***	Decreased purposeful movement; difficulty completing activities of daily living; limited range of motion; reluctance to move; pain	Assess the patient's ability to perform independent range-of-motion exercises; encourage performance of range-of-motion exercises; encourage and assist in moving every 2 hr to relieve tissue pressure; assist with activities of daily living; encourage use of assistive devices as needed to support mobility
Protection ***(related to failure of bone marrow; replacement of bone marrow by neoplastic cells; insufficient autoimmune response; chemotherapy; bone marrow transplant)***	Bleeding; infection; anemia	Monitor and trend hemoglobin and hematocrit; monitor and trend platelets and red blood cells (RBCs); monitor for symptoms of infection; take temperature every 4 hr; institute bleeding precautions, soft toothbrushes, avoid aspirin, avoid intramuscular and intravenous injections, coordinate laboratory draws to minimize venipuncture; administer prescribed steroids, erythropoietin; administer prescribed blood and blood products; avoid at-risk activities that could cause trauma; discuss exposure to microbes that could result in infection

PRETEST:

- Positively identify the patient using at least two person-specific identifiers before services, treatments, or procedures are performed.
- *Patient Teaching:* Inform the patient this test can assist in assessing the immune system.
- Obtain a history of the patient's health concerns, symptoms, surgical procedures, and results of previously performed laboratory and diagnostic studies. Include a list of known allergens, especially allergies or sensitivities to latex.
- Note any recent procedures that can interfere with test results. Assess whether the patient received any vaccinations or immunizations within the last 6 mo or any blood or blood components within the last 6 wk.
- Obtain a list of the patient's current medications, including over-the-counter medications and dietary supplements (see Effects of Natural Products on Laboratory Values online at Davis*Plus*).
- Review the procedure with the patient. Inform the patient that specimen collection takes approximately 5 to 10 min. Address concerns about pain and explain that there may be some discomfort during the venipuncture.

- Provide a nonmetallic urinal, bedpan, or toilet-mounted collection device.
- Note that usually a 24-hr time frame for urine collection is ordered. Inform the patient that all urine must be saved during that 24-hr period. Instruct the patient not to void directly into the laboratory collection container. Instruct the patient to avoid defecating in the collection device and to keep toilet tissue out of the collection device to prevent contamination of the specimen. Place a sign in the bathroom to remind the patient to save all urine.
- Instruct the patient to void all urine into the collection device and then to pour the urine into the laboratory collection container. Alternatively the specimen can be left in the collection device for a health-care staff member to add to the laboratory collection container.
- ***Sensitivity to social and cultural issues,*** as well as concern for modesty, is important in providing psychological support before, during, and after the procedure.
- Note that there are no food, fluid, or medication restrictions unless by medical direction.

INTRATEST:

Potential Complications: N/A

- Avoid the use of equipment containing latex if the patient has a history of allergic reaction to latex.
- Instruct the patient to cooperate fully and to follow directions. Direct the patient to breathe normally and to avoid unnecessary movement.
- Observe standard precautions, and follow the general guidelines in Patient Preparation and Specimen Collection online at Davis*Plus*. Positively identify the patient, and label the appropriate specimen container with the corresponding patient demographics, initials of the person collecting the specimen, date, and time of collection. Perform a venipuncture as appropriate.

Blood

- Perform a venipuncture.
- Remove the needle and apply direct pressure with dry gauze to stop bleeding. Observe/assess venipuncture site for bleeding or hematoma formation and secure gauze with adhesive bandage.

Urine

Clean-Catch Specimen

- Instruct the male patient to (1) thoroughly wash his hands, (2) cleanse the meatus, (3) void a small amount into the toilet, and (4) void directly into the specimen container.
- Instruct the female patient to (1) thoroughly wash her hands; (2) cleanse the labia from front to back; (3) while keeping the labia separated, void a small amount into the toilet; and (4) without interrupting the urine stream, void directly into the specimen container.

Blood or Urine

- Promptly transport the specimen to the laboratory for processing and analysis.

POST-TEST:

- Inform the patient that a report of the results will be made available to the requesting HCP, who will discuss the results with the patient.
- Depending on the results of this procedure, additional testing may be performed to evaluate or monitor progression of the disease process and determine the need for a change in therapy. Evaluate test results in relation to the patient's symptoms and other tests performed.

Patient Education:

- Reinforce information given by the patient's HCP regarding further testing, treatment, or referral to another HCP.
- Answer any questions or address any concerns voiced by the patient or family.
- Provide contact information for support groups.

Expected Patient Outcomes:

Understanding

- The patient and family state the importance of ambulation to prevent demineralization and support bone health.
- The patient and family state the importance of using assistive devices to support mobility and decrease injury risk.

Ability

- The patient strictly avoids at-risk activities that could result in trauma and bleeding.
- The patient makes dietary selections that include omitting fresh fruit to decrease exposure to bacteria.

Response

- The patient adheres to recommended therapeutic regime.
- The patient makes a positive effort to address feelings of hopelessness and powerlessness.

RELATED STUDIES:

- Related tests include anion gap, biopsy bone, biopsy bone marrow, biopsy liver, biopsy lymph node, cold agglutinin, CBC, CBC WBC count and differential, cryoglobulin, ESR, fibrinogen, quantitative immunoglobulin levels, LAP, liver and spleen scan, β-2-microglobulin, platelet antibodies, protein total and fractions, and UA.
- Refer to the Hematopoietic and Immune systems tables online at Davis*Plus* for related tests by body system.

Immunoglobulin E

I

SYNONYM/ACRONYM: IgE.

COMMON USE: To assess immunoglobulin E (IgE) levels in order to identify the presence of an allergic or inflammatory immune response.

SPECIMEN: Serum collected in a gold-, red-, or red/gray-top tube. Place separated serum into a standard transport tube within 2 hr of collection.

NORMAL FINDINGS: (Method: Immunoassay)

Age	Conventional & SI Units
Newborn	Less than 12 units/L
Less than 1 yr	Less than 50 units/L
2–4 yr	Less than 200 units/L
5–9 yr	Less than 300 units/L
10 yr and older	Less than 100 units/L

DESCRIPTION: Immunoglobulin E (IgE) is an antibody whose primary response is to allergic reactions and parasitic infections. Most of the body's IgE is bound to specialized tissue cells; little is available in the circulating blood. IgE binds to the membrane of special granulocytes called *basophils* in the circulating blood and *mast cells* in the tissues. Basophil and mast cell membranes have receptors for IgE. Mast cells are abundant in the skin and the tissues lining the respiratory and alimentary tracts. When IgE antibody becomes cross-linked with antigen/allergen, the release of histamine, heparin, and other chemicals from the granules in the cells is triggered. A sequence of events follows activation of IgE that affects smooth muscle contraction, vascular permeability, and inflammatory reactions. The inflammatory response allows proteins from the bloodstream to enter the tissues. Helminths (worm parasites) are especially susceptible to immunoglobulin-mediated cytotoxic chemicals. The inflammatory reaction proteins attract macrophages from the circulatory system and granulocytes, such as eosinophils, from circulation and bone marrow. Eosinophils also contain enzymes effective against the parasitic invaders.

A nasal smear can be examined for the presence of eosinophils to screen for allergic conditions. Either a single smear or smears of nasal secretions from each side of the nose should be submitted, at room temperature, for Hansel staining and evaluation. Normal findings vary by laboratory but generally, greater than 10% to 15% is considered eosinophilia or increased presence of eosonophils. Results may be invalid for patients already taking local or systemic corticosteroids.

This procedure is contraindicated for: N/A

INDICATIONS

Assist in the evaluation of allergy and parasitic infection.

POTENTIAL MEDICAL DIAGNOSIS

Increased in:

Conditions involving allergic reactions or infections that stimulate production of IgE.

- Alcoholism ***(alcohol may play a role in the development of environmentally instigated IgE-mediated hypersensitivity)***
- Allergy
- Asthma
- Bronchopulmonary aspergillosis
- Dermatitis
- Eczema
- Hay fever
- IgE myeloma
- Parasitic infestation
- Rhinitis
- Sinusitis
- Wiskott-Aldrich syndrome

Decreased in:

- Advanced carcinoma ***(related to generalized decrease in immune system response)***
- Agammaglobulinemia ***(related to decreased production)***
- Ataxia-telangiectasia ***(evidenced by familial immunodeficiency disorder)***
- IgE deficiency

CRITICAL FINDINGS: N/A

INTERFERING FACTORS

- Drugs and other substances that may cause a decrease in IgE levels include phenytoin and tryptophan.
- Penicillin G has been associated with increased IgE levels in some patients with drug-induced acute interstitial nephritis.
- Normal IgE levels do not eliminate allergic disorders as a possible diagnosis.

I

NURSING IMPLICATIONS AND PROCEDURE

POTENTIAL NURSING PROBLEMS:

Problem	Signs & Symptoms	Interventions
Powerlessness ***(related to chronic illness; treatment for illness; loss of ability to provide self-care; progressive debilitation; terminal prognosis)***	Expression of loss of control over situation, self, outcome of disease; passive; apathetic; submissive; decreased participation in self-care; reluctant to express feelings	Assess need to be in control; assess feelings of hopelessness, depression, apathy; assist to identify situations that contribute to a feeling of powerlessness; assess the impact of the sense of powerlessness on the patient's sense of self; encourage verbalization of feelings; discuss therapeutic options offered by health-care provider (HCP); assist to identify strengths; identify coping strategies; encourage being responsible for self-care and personal environment to increase sense of control; provide positive feedback
Mobility ***(related to pain; weakness; depression; fatigue; decreased muscle strength; decreased coordination)***	Decreased purposeful movement; difficulty completing activities of daily living; limited range of motion; reluctance to move; pain	Assess the patient's ability to perform independent range-of-motion exercises; encourage performance of range-of-motion exercises; encourage and assist in moving every 2 hr to relieve tissue pressure; assist with activities of daily living; encourage use of assistive devices as needed to support mobility
Knowledge ***(related to recent diagnosis; complexity of treatment; poor understanding of provided information; cultural or language barriers; anxiety;***	Lack of interest or questions; multiple questions; anxiety in relation to disease process and management; verbalizes inaccurate information; lack of follow-through with directions	Identify patient's, family's, and significant others' concerns about disease process; provide information about disease process, bone marrow analysis, and associated diagnostic studies that may be necessary (computed tomography, bone scan); facilitate and monitor ordered laboratory studies (complete blood count, immunoglobulin levels, C-reactive protein, protein

Problem	Signs & Symptoms	Interventions
emotional disturbance; unfamiliarity with medical management)		electrophoresis); discuss possible treatment modalities, chemotherapy, proteasome inhibitors, palliative radiation therapy, drug administration, stem cell transplant, pain management

PRETEST:

- Positively identify the patient using at least two person-specific identifiers before services, treatments, or procedures are performed.
- *Patient Teaching:* Inform the patient this test can assist in identification of an allergic or inflammatory response.
- Obtain a history of the patient's health concerns, symptoms, surgical procedures, and results of previously performed laboratory and diagnostic studies. Include a list of known allergens, especially allergies or sensitivities to latex.
- Obtain a list of the patient's current medications, including over-the-counter medications and dietary supplements (see Effects of Natural Products on Laboratory Values online at Davis*Plus*).
- Review the procedure with the patient. Inform the patient that specimen collection takes approximately 5 to 10 min. Address concerns about pain and explain that there may be some discomfort during the venipuncture.
- *Sensitivity to social and cultural issues,* as well as concern for modesty, is important in providing psychological support before, during, and after the procedure.
- Note that there are no food, fluid, or medication restrictions unless by medical direction.

INTRATEST:

Potential Complications: N/A

- Avoid the use of equipment containing latex if the patient has a history of allergic reaction to latex.
- Instruct the patient to cooperate fully and to follow directions. Direct the patient to breathe normally and to avoid unnecessary movement.
- Observe standard precautions, and follow the general guidelines in Patient Preparation and Specimen Collection online at Davis*Plus*. Positively identify the patient, and label the appropriate specimen container with the corresponding patient demographics, initials of the person collecting the specimen, date, and time of collection. Perform a venipuncture.
- Remove the needle and apply direct pressure with dry gauze to stop bleeding. Observe/assess venipuncture site for bleeding or hematoma formation and secure gauze with adhesive bandage.
- Promptly transport the specimen to the laboratory for processing and analysis.

POST-TEST:

- Inform the patient that a report of the results will be made available to the HCP, who will discuss the results with the patient.
- *Nutritional Considerations:* Increased IgE levels may be associated with allergy. Consideration should be given to diet if the patient has food allergies.
- Depending on the results of this procedure, additional testing may be performed to evaluate or monitor progression of the patient's condition and determine the need for a change in therapy. Evaluate test results in relation to the patient's symptoms and other tests performed.

I

Patient Education:
- Reinforce information given by the patient's HCP regarding further testing, treatment, or referral to another HCP.
- Answer any questions or address any concerns voiced by the patient or family.
- Explain that a negative result does not necessarily preclude the presence of a sensitivity to an allergen.

Expected Patient Outcomes:

Understanding
- The patient and family state the importance of maintaining an uncluttered home environment to decrease injury risk.
- The patient and family state the importance of conserving energy by including frequent rest periods during times of activity.

Ability
- The patient successfully changes position every 2 hr to decrease risk of skin breakdown.
- The patient demonstrates the ability to perform range-of-motion exercises proficiently.

Response
- The patient agrees to accept assistance with activities of daily living to enhance comfort and safety.
- The patient agrees to perform range-of-motion activities three times a day to decrease contracture risk.

RELATED STUDIES:
- Related tests include allergen-specific IgE, alveolar/arterial gradient, biopsy intestine, biopsy liver, biopsy muscle, blood gases, carbon dioxide, CBC, CBC platelet count, CBC WBC count and differential, eosinophil count, fecal analysis, hypersensitivity pneumonitis, lung perfusion scan, and PFT.
- Refer to the Immune and Respiratory systems tables online at Davis*Plus* for related tests by body system.

I

Immunoglobulins A, D, G, and M

SYNONYM/ACRONYM: IgA, IgD, IgG, and IgM.

COMMON USE: To quantitate immunoglobulins A, D, G, and M as indicators of immune system function, to assist in the diagnosis of conditions that result in deficient or excessive production of immunoglobulins; to investigate immune system disorders such as multiple myeloma.

SPECIMEN: Serum collected in a gold-, red-, or red/gray-top tube. Place separated serum in a standard transport tube within 2 hr of collection.

NORMAL FINDINGS: (Method: Nephelometry)

Age	Conventional Units	SI Units
Immunoglobulin A		*(Conventional Units × 0.01)*
Newborn	1–4 mg/dL	0.01–0.04 g/L
1–9 mo	2–80 mg/dL	0.02–0.8 g/L
10–12 mo	15–90 mg/dL	0.15–0.9 g/L
2–3 yr	18–150 mg/dL	0.18–1.5 g/L
4–5 yr	25–160 mg/dL	0.25–1.6 g/L
6–8 yr	35–200 mg/dL	0.35–2 g/L

Age	Conventional Units	SI Units
9–12 yr	45–250 mg/dL	0.45–2.5 g/L
Older than 12 yr	40–350 mg/dL	0.40–3.5 g/L
Immunoglobulin D		*(Conventional Units × 10)*
Newborn	Greater than 2 mg/dL	Greater than 20 g/L
Adult	Less than 15 mg/dL	Less than 150 g/L
Immunoglobulin G		*(Conventional Units × 0.01)*
Newborn	650–1,600 mg/dL	6.5–16 g/L
1–9 mo	250–900 mg/dL	2.5–9 g/L
10–12 mo	290–1,070 mg/dL	2.9–10.7 g/L
2–3 yr	420–1,200 mg/dL	4.2–12 g/L
4–6 yr	460–1,240 mg/dL	4.6–12.4 g/L
Greater than 6 yr	650–1,600 mg/dL	6.5–16 g/L
Immunoglobulin M		*(Conventional Units × 0.01)*
Newborn	Less than 25 mg/dL	Less than 0.25 g/L
1–9 mo	20–125 mg/dL	0.2–1.25 g/L
10–12 mo	40–150 mg/dL	0.4–1.5 g/L
2–8 yr	45–200 mg/dL	0.45–2 g/L
9–12 yr	50–250 mg/dL	0.5–2.5 g/L
Greater than 12 yr	50–300 mg/dL	0.5–3 g/L

DESCRIPTION: Immunoglobulins A, D, E, G, and M are made by plasma cells in response to foreign substances. Immunoglobulins neutralize toxic substances, support phagocytosis, and destroy invading microorganisms. They are made up of heavy and light chains. Immunoglobulins produced by the abnormal proliferation of a single plasma cell (clone) are called *monoclonal*. Polyclonal increases result when multiple cell lines produce excessive amounts of antibody. IgA is found mainly in secretions such as tears, saliva, and breast milk. It is believed to protect mucous membranes from viruses and bacteria. The function of IgD is not well understood, but it is believed to participate in the activation of B lymphocytes. For details on IgE, see the study titled "Immunoglobulin E." IgG is the predominant serum immunoglobulin and is important in long-term defense against disease. It is the only antibody that crosses the placenta. IgM is the largest immunoglobulin, and it is the first antibody to react to an antigenic stimulus. IgM also forms natural antibodies, such as ABO blood group antibodies. The presence of IgM in cord blood is an indication of congenital infection.

This procedure is contraindicated for: N/A

INDICATIONS

- Assist in the diagnosis of multiple myeloma.
- Evaluate humoral immunity status.
- Monitor therapy for multiple myeloma.
- IgA: Evaluate patients suspected of IgA deficiency prior to transfusion. Evaluate anaphylaxis associated with the transfusion of blood and blood products (anti-IgA antibodies may develop in patients with low

levels of IgA, possibly resulting in anaphylaxis when donated blood is transfused).

POTENTIAL MEDICAL DIAGNOSIS

Increased in:

IgA

Polyclonal

- Chronic liver disease ***(pathophysiology is unclear)***
- Immunodeficiency states, such as Wiskott-Aldrich syndrome ***(inherited condition of lymphocytes characterized by increased IgA and IgE)***
- Inflammatory bowel disease ***(IgG and/or IgA antibody positive for*** *Saccharomyces cerevisiae* ***with negative perinuclear-antineutrophil cytoplasmic antibody is indicative of Crohn's disease)***
- Lower gastrointestinal (GI) cancer ***(pathophysiology is unclear)***
- Rheumatoid arthritis ***(pathophysiology is unclear)***

Monoclonal

- IgA-type multiple myeloma ***(related to excessive production by a single clone of plasma cells)***

IgD

Polyclonal ***(pathophysiology is unclear, but increases are associated with increases in IgM)***

- Chronic infections
- Connective tissue disorders

Monoclonal

- IgD-type multiple myeloma ***(related to excessive production by a single clone of plasma cells)***

IgG

(Conditions that involve inflammation and/or development of an infection stimulate production of IgG.)

Polyclonal

- Autoimmune diseases, such as systemic lupus erythematosus, rheumatoid arthritis, and Sjögren's syndrome
- Chronic liver disease
- Chronic or recurrent infections
- Intrauterine devices ***(the IUD creates a localized inflammatory reaction that stimulates production of IgG)***
- Sarcoidosis

Monoclonal

- IgG-type multiple myeloma ***(related to excessive production by a single clone of plasma cells)***
- Leukemias
- Lymphomas

IgM

Polyclonal ***(humoral response to infections and inflammation; both acute and chronic)***

- Active sarcoidosis
- Chronic hepatocellular disease
- Collagen vascular disease
- Early response to bacterial or parasitic infection
- Hyper-IgM dysgammaglobulinemia
- Rheumatoid arthritis
- Variable in nephrotic syndrome
- Viral infection (hepatitis or mononucleosis)

Monoclonal

- Cold agglutinin hemolysis disease
- Malignant lymphoma
- Neoplasms (especially in GI tract)
- Reticulosis
- Waldenström's macroglobulinemia ***(related to excessive production by a single clone of plasma cells)***

Decreased in:

IgA

- Ataxia-telangiectasia
- Chronic sinopulmonary disease
- Genetic IgA deficiency

IgD
- Genetic IgD deficiency
- Malignant melanoma of the skin
- Pre-eclampsia

IgG
- Burns
- Genetic IgG deficiency
- Nephrotic syndrome
- Pregnancy

IgM
- Burns
- Secondary IgM deficiency associated with IgG or IgA gammopathies

CRITICAL FINDINGS: N/A

INTERFERING FACTORS
- Drugs and other substances that may increase immunoglobulin levels include asparaginase, cimetidine, and narcotics.
- Drugs and other substances that may decrease immunoglobulin levels include dextran, oral contraceptives, methylprednisolone (high doses), and phenytoin.
- Chemotherapy, immunosuppressive therapy, and radiation treatments decrease immunoglobulin levels.
- Specimens with macroglobulins, cryoglobulins, or cold agglutinins tested at cold temperatures may give falsely low values.

NURSING IMPLICATIONS AND PROCEDURE

POTENTIAL NURSING PROBLEMS:

Problem	Signs & Symptoms	Interventions
Hopelessness ***(related to chronic illness; impaired functionality; prolonged pain and discomfort)***	Decreased affect; decreased response to stimuli; feeling of emptiness; alterations in sleep patterns and appetite; expressions of apathy; withdrawn; states life has no meaning	Assess role of illness in relation to expressions of helplessness; assess grooming (energy to provide good personal hygiene); assess level of appetite; assess verbalization of helplessness; provide opportunities to express feelings in a safe environment; support development of a trusting relationship to decrease feelings of isolation; encourage verbalization of personal strengths and weaknesses; encourage realistic hope; assist in identification of coping skills
Protection ***(related to failure of bone marrow; replacement of bone marrow by neoplastic cells; insufficient***	Bleeding; infection; anemia	Monitor and trend hemoglobin and hematocrit; monitor and trend platelets and red blood cells (RBCs); monitor for symptoms of infection; take temperature every 4 hr; institute bleeding precautions, soft toothbrushes, avoid aspirin, avoid intramuscular and intravenous injections,

(table continues on page 968)

Problem	Signs & Symptoms	Interventions
autoimmune response; chemotherapy; bone marrow transplant)		coordinate laboratory draws to minimize venipuncture; administer prescribed steroids, erythropoietin; administer prescribed blood and blood products; avoid at-risk activities that could cause trauma; discuss exposure to microbes that could result in infection
Pain ***(related to invasion of bone marrow and pathological fractures secondary to medication diagnosis [multiple myeloma])***	Self-report of pain; guarding; crying; moaning; sleeplessness; restlessness; emotional symptoms of distress; agitation; facial grimace; rocking motions; irritability; diaphoresis; altered blood pressure and heart rate; nausea; vomiting	Assess pain characteristics, skeletal pain, low back, ribs; assess level of pain with movement; identify pain modalities that have relieved pain in the past; administer prescribed pain medication; monitor and trend vital signs; recommend use of nonpharmacologic pain management modalities, imagery, distraction, music, relaxation, correct body alignment

PRETEST:

- Positively identify the patient using at least two person-specific identifiers before services, treatments, or procedures are performed.
- *Patient Teaching:* Inform the patient this test can assess the immune system by evaluating the levels of immunoglobulins in the blood.
- Obtain a history of the patient's health concerns, symptoms, surgical procedures, and results of previously performed laboratory and diagnostic studies. Include a list of known allergens, especially allergies or sensitivities to latex.
- Obtain a list of the patient's current medications, including over-the-counter medications and dietary supplements (see Effects of Natural Products on Laboratory Values online at Davis*Plus*).
- Note any recent procedures that can interfere with test results.
- Review the procedure with the patient. Inform the patient that specimen collection takes approximately 5 to 10 min. Address concerns about pain and explain to the patient that there may be some discomfort during the venipuncture.
- *Sensitivity to social and cultural issues,* as well as concern for modesty, is important in providing psychological support before, during, and after the procedure.
- Note that there are no food, fluid, or medication restrictions unless by medical direction.

INTRATEST:

Potential Complications: N/A

- Avoid the use of equipment containing latex if the patient has a history of allergic reaction to latex.
- Instruct the patient to cooperate fully and to follow directions. Direct the

patient to breathe normally and to avoid unnecessary movement.
- Observe standard precautions, and follow the general guidelines in Patient Preparation and Specimen Collection online at Davis*Plus*. Positively identify the patient, and label the appropriate specimen container with the corresponding patient demographics, initials of the person collecting the specimen, date, and time of collection. Perform a venipuncture.
- Remove the needle and apply direct pressure with dry gauze to stop bleeding. Observe/assess venipuncture site for bleeding or hematoma formation and secure gauze with adhesive bandage.
- Promptly transport the specimen to the laboratory for processing and analysis.

POST-TEST:

- Inform the patient that a report of the results will be made available to the requesting health-care provider (HCP), who will discuss the results with the patient. A patient with IgA deficiency should not receive gamma globulin. Administration of gamma globulin may initiate sensitization of the immune system that could result in an anaphylactic shock during a subsequent RBC product transfusion, related to instigation by donor IgA in the product. IgA deficiency is a lifelong condition, if transfusion is necessary and products from an IgA-deficient donor are unavailable, washed RBCs can be used to decrease the risk of transfusion reaction.
- Depending on the results of this procedure, additional testing may be performed to evaluate or monitor progression of the disease process and determine the need for a change in therapy. Evaluate test results in relation to the patient's symptoms and other tests performed.

Patient Education:

- Reinforce information given by the patient's HCP regarding further testing, treatment, or referral to another HCP.
- Answer any questions or address any concerns voiced by the patient or family.
- Provide information on the disease process as it relates to altered laboratory results.

Expected Patient Outcomes:

Understanding

- The patient and family state the importance of notifying the HCP if the pain management regime is ineffective.
- The patient and family state that a combination of pain management modalities may be most effective in managing pain.

Ability

- The patient describes appropriate use of pain scale for quantifying the severity of pain experienced.
- The patient demonstrates proficiency in using a selected nonpharmacological pain management strategy to decrease pain intensity.

Response

- The patient complies with the recommendation to try using nonpharmacological measures to decrease pain.
- The patient complies with the recommendation to take pain medication around the clock to decrease the risk of peak pain periods.

RELATED STUDIES:

- Related tests include ALT, anion gap, ANA, bilirubin, biopsy bone, biopsy bone marrow, biopsy liver, biopsy lymph node, blood groups and antibodies, cold agglutinin, CBC, CBC WBC count and differential, Coomb's antiglobulin (direct and indirect), cryoglobulin, ESR, fibrinogen, IFE, GGT, LAP, liver and spleen scan, beta-2-microglobulin, platelet antibodies, protein total and fractions, RF, and uric acid.
- Refer to the Hematopoietic and Immune systems tables online at Davis*Plus* for related tests by body system.

Immunosuppressants: Cyclosporine, Methotrexate, Everolimus, Sirolimus, and Tacrolimus

SYNONYM/ACRONYM: *Cyclosporine* (Sandimmune), *methotrexate* (MTX, amethopterin, Folex, Metoject, Mexate, Rheumatrex), *everolimus* (Afinitor Disperz, Certican, Zortress), *sirolimus* (Rapamycin, Rapamune), *tacrolimus* (Advagraf, Prograf).

COMMON USE: To monitor appropriate drug dosage of immunosuppressant related to organ transplant maintenance.

SPECIMEN: Whole blood collected in lavender-top tube for cyclosporine, everolimus; sirolimus; tacrolimus. Serum collected in a red-top tube for methotrexate; specimen must be protected from light.

Immunosuppressant	Route of Administration	Recommended Collection Time
Cyclosporine	Oral or intravenous	12 hr after dose or immediately prior to next dose
Methotrexate	Oral	Varies according to dosing protocol
	Intramuscular	Varies according to dosing protocol
Everolimus	Oral	Immediately prior to next dose
Sirolimus	Oral	Immediately prior to next dose
Tacrolimus	Oral	Immediately prior to next dose

Leucovorin therapy, also called *leucovorin rescue,* is used in conjunction with administration of methotrexate. Leucovorin, a fast-acting form of folic acid, protects healthy cells from the toxic effects of methotrexate.

NORMAL FINDINGS: (Method: Immunoassay for cyclosporine and methotrexate; liquid chromatography with tandem mass spectrometry for everolimus, sirolimus, and tacrolimus)

	Therapeutic Dose		Half-Life (hr)	Volume of Distribution (L/kg)	Protein Binding (%)	Excretion
	Conventional Units	*SI Units (Conventional Units × 0.832)*				
Cyclosporine	100–300 ng/mL kidney transplant	83–250 nmol/L	8–24	4–6	90	Renal
	200–350 ng/mL cardiac, hepatic, pancreatic transplant	166–291 nmol/L	8–24	4–6	90	Renal
	100–300 ng/mL bone marrow transplant	83–250 nmol/L	8–24	4–6	90	Renal
	Conventional Units	*SI Units (Conventional Units × 1)*				
Methotrexate	Low dose: Less than 0.5 micromol/L after 48 hr High dose: Less than 5 micromol/L at 24 hr; less than 0.5 micromol/L at 48 hr; less than 0.1 micromol/L at 72 hr	Low dose: Less than 0.5 micromol/L after 48 hr High dose: Less than 5 micromol/L at 24 hr; less than 0.5 micromol/L at 48 hr; less than 0.1 micromol/L at 72 hr	5–9	0.4–1	50–70	Renal

(table continues on page 972)

	Therapeutic Dose		Half-Life (hr)	Volume of Distribution (L/kg)	Protein Binding (%)	Excretion
	Conventional Units	*SI Units (Conventional Units × 1.04)*				
Everolimus	Transplant: 3–8 ng/mL	Transplant: 3–8 nmol/L	18–35 (kidney); 30–35 (liver)	128–589	75	Biliary
	Oncology: 5–10 ng/mL	Oncology: 5–10 nmol/L	18–35	128–589	75	Biliary
	Conventional Units	*SI Units (Conventional Units × 1.1)*				
Sirolimus	Maintenance phase: kidney transplant: 4–12 ng/mL; liver transplant: 12–20 ng/mL	Kidney transplant: 4–13 nmol/L; liver transplant: 13–22 nmol/L	46–78	4–20	92	Biliary
	Conventional Units	*SI Units (Conventional Units × 1.24)*				
Tacrolimus	Maintenance phase: Kidney transplant: 6–12 ng/mL; liver transplant: 4–10 ng/mL; pancreas transplant: 10–18 ng/mL; bone marrow transplant: 10–20 ng/mL	Kidney transplant: 7–15 nmol/L; liver transplant: 5–12 nmol/L; pancreas transplant: 12–22 nmol/L; bone marrow transplant: 12–25 nmol/L	10–14	1.5	99	Biliary

Therapeutic targets for the initial phase post-transplantation are slightly higher than during the maintenance phase and are influenced by the specific therapy chosen for each patient with respect to coordination of treatment for other conditions and corresponding therapies. Therapeutic ranges for everolimus, sirolimus, and tacrolimus assume concomitant administration of cyclosporine and steroids.

DESCRIPTION: Cyclosporine is an immunosuppressive drug used in the management of organ rejection, especially rejection of heart, liver, pancreas, and kidney transplants. Its most serious adverse effect is renal impairment or chronic kidney disease. Cyclosporine is often administered in conjunction with corticosteroids (e.g., prednisone) for its anti-inflammatory or immune-suppressing properties and with other drugs (e.g., everolimus, sirolimus, tacrolimus) to reduce graft-versus-host disease. Methotrexate is a highly toxic drug that causes cell death by disrupting DNA synthesis. Methotrexate is also used in the treatment of rheumatoid arthritis, psoriasis, polymyositis, and Reiter's syndrome. Cyclosporine, sirolimus, and tacrolimus are metabolized by the cytochrome enzymes CYP3A4 and CYP3A5, which is essential to achieve the desired therapeutic effect. Testing for specific CYP450 genotype defects can be performed in some laboratories on blood and buccal specimens. Counseling and informed written consent are generally required for genetic testing. Test results can identify poor and ultrasensitive drug metabolizers. This allows for the possibility of personalized adjustments to their medication regimen or decisions to seek alternative drugs which in turn results in safer, more effective treatment.

Many factors must be considered in effective dosing and monitoring of therapeutic drugs, including patient age; weight; interacting medications; electrolyte balance; protein levels; water balance; conditions that affect absorption and excretion; as well as foods and dietary supplements that can either potentiate or inhibit the intended target concentration.

Important note: These medications are metabolized and excreted by the kidneys and are therefore contraindicated in patients with kidney disease and cautiously advised in patients with kidney impairment. Information regarding medications must be clearly and accurately communicated to avoid misunderstanding of the dose time in relation to the collection time. Miscommunication between the individual administering the medication and the individual collecting the specimen is the most frequent cause of subtherapeutic levels, toxic levels, and misleading information used in the calculation of future doses. Some pharmacies use a computerized pharmacokinetics approach to dosing that eliminates the need to be concerned about peak and trough collections; random specimens are adequate. If administration of the drug is delayed, notify the appropriate department(s) to reschedule the blood draw and notify the requesting health-care provider (HCP) if the delay has caused any real or perceived therapeutic harm.

This procedure is contraindicated for: N/A

INDICATIONS

Cyclosporine, Sirolimus, Tacrolimus

- Assist in the management of treatments to prevent organ rejection.
- Monitor for toxicity.

Everolimus

- Assist in the management of treatments to prevent organ rejection.
- Assist in the management of treatments for subependymal giant cell astrocytoma.
- Monitor effectiveness of treatment of renal cell carcinoma.
- Monitor for toxicity.

I

Methotrexate

- Monitor effectiveness of treatment of cancer and some autoimmune disorders.
- Monitor for toxicity.

POTENTIAL MEDICAL DIAGNOSIS

Level	Response
Normal levels	Therapeutic effect
Toxic levels	Adjust dose as indicated
Cyclosporine	Renal impairment
Methotrexate	Renal impairment
Everolimus, sirolimus, tacrolimus	Hepatic impairment

I

CRITICAL FINDINGS:

It is important to note the adverse effects of toxic and subtherapeutic levels. Care must be taken to investigate signs and symptoms of too little and too much medication.

Note and immediately report to the requesting HCP any critical findings and related symptoms. A listing of these findings varies among facilities. Timely notification of a critical finding for laboratory or diagnostic studies is a role expectation of the professional nurse. The notification processes vary among facilities. Upon receipt of the critical finding, the information should be read back to the caller to verify accuracy.

Cyclosporine Greater Than 500 ng/mL (SI: Greater Than 416 nmol/L)

Signs and symptoms of cyclosporine toxicity include increased severity of expected adverse effects, which include nausea, stomatitis, vomiting, anorexia, hypertension, infection, fluid retention, hypercalcemic metabolic acidosis, tremor, seizures, headache, and flushing. Possible interventions include close monitoring of blood levels to make dosing adjustments, inducing emesis (if orally ingested), performing gastric lavage (if orally ingested), withholding the drug, and initiating alternative therapy for a short time until the patient is stabilized.

Methotrexate: Greater Than 5 micromol/L

Signs and symptoms of methotrexate toxicity include increased severity of expected adverse effects, which include nausea, stomatitis, vomiting, anorexia, bleeding, infection, bone marrow depression, and, over a prolonged period of use, hepatotoxicity. The effect of methotrexate on normal cells can be reversed by administration of 5-formyltetrahydrofolate (citrovorum or leucovorin). 5-Formyltetrahydrofolate allows higher doses of methotrexate to be given.

Everolimus: Greater Than 15 ng/mL (SI: Greater Than 15 mcg/L)

Signs and symptoms of everolimus pulmonary toxicity include hypoxia, pleural effusion, cough, and dyspnea. Possible interventions include dosing adjustments, administration of corticosteroids, and monitoring of pulmonary function with chest x-ray. Use of everolimus is contraindicated in patients with severe hepatic impairment. Concomitant administration of strong CYP3A4 inhibitors may significantly increase everolimus levels.

Sirolimus: Greater Than 25 ng/mL (SI: Greater Than 28 mcg/L)

Signs and symptoms of sirolimus pulmonary toxicity include cough, shortness of breath, chest pain, and rapid heart rate. Possible interventions include dosing adjustments, administration of corticosteroids, and monitoring of pulmonary function with chest x-ray.

Tacrolimus: Greater Than 25 ng/mL (SI: Greater Than 31 mcg/L)
Signs and symptoms of tacrolimus toxicity include tremors, seizures, headache, high blood pressure, hyperkalemia, tinnitus, nausea, and vomiting. Possible interventions include treatment of hypertension, administration of antiemetics for nausea and vomiting, and dosing adjustments.

INTERFERING FACTORS

- Numerous drugs and other substances interact with cyclosporine and either increase cyclosporine levels or increase the risk of toxicity. These include acyclovir, aminoglycosides, amiodarone, amphotericin B, anabolic steroids, cephalosporins, cimetidine, danazol, erythromycin, furosemide, ketoconazole, melphalan, methylprednisolone, miconazole, NSAIDs, oral contraceptives, and trimethoprim-sulfamethoxazole.
- Drugs and other substances that may decrease cyclosporine levels include carbamazepine, ethotoin, phenobarbital, phenytoin, primidone, and rifampin.
- Drugs and other substances that may increase methotrexate levels or increase the risk of toxicity include NSAIDs, probenecid, salicylate, and sulfonamides.
- Antibiotics may decrease the absorption of methotrexate.
- Drugs and other substances that may increase everolimus levels include ketoconazole, amprenavir, aprepitant, atazanavir, clarithromycin, delavirdine, diltiazem, erythromycin, fluconazole, fosamprenavir, grapefruit juice, indinavir, itraconazole, nefazodone, nelfinavir, ritonavir, saquinavir, telithromycin, verapamil, and voriconazole.
- Drugs and other substances that may decrease everolimus levels include carbamazepine, dexamethasone, phenobarbital, phenytoin, rifabutin, rifampin, and St. John's Wort.
- Drugs and other substances that may increase sirolimus levels include bromocriptine, cimetidine, cisapride, clotrimazole, danazol, diltiazem, fluconazole, indinavir, metoclopramide, nicardipine, ritonavir, troleandomycin, and verapamil.
- Drugs and other substances that may increase sirolimus levels include carbamazepine, phenobarbital, phenytoin, rifapentine, and St. John's Wort.
- Drugs and other substances that may increase tacrolimus levels include bromocriptine, chloramphenicol, cimetidine, cisapride, clarithromycin, clotrimazole, cyclosporine, danazol, diltiazem, erythromycin, fluconazole, grapefruit juice, itraconazole, ketoconazole, methylprednisolone, metoclopramide, nelfinavir, nicardipine, nifedipine, troleandomycin, verapamil, and voriconazole.
- Drugs and other substances that may decrease tacrolimus levels include carbamazepine, ethotoin, octreotide, phenobarbital, primidone, rifabutin, rifampin, sirolimus, and St. John's Wort.

NURSING IMPLICATIONS AND PROCEDURE

PRETEST:

- Positively identify the patient using at least two person-specific identifiers before services, treatments, or procedures are performed.
- *Patient Teaching:* Inform the patient this test can assess in monitoring therapeutic and toxic drug levels.
- Obtain a history of the patient's health concerns, symptoms, surgical procedures, and results of previously performed laboratory and diagnostic

studies. Include a list of known allergens, especially allergies or sensitivities to latex.

- Obtain a history of the patient's genitourinary and immune systems, symptoms, and results of previously performed laboratory tests and diagnostic and surgical procedures. Some considerations prior to medication administration include documentation of adequate renal function with creatinine and BUN levels, documentation of adequate hepatic function with alanine aminotransferase (ALT) and bilirubin levels, and documentation of adequate hematological and immune function with platelet and white blood cell (WBC) count. Patients receiving methotrexate must be well hydrated and, depending on the therapy, may be treated with sodium bicarbonate for urinary alkalinization to enhance drug excretion. Leucovorin calcium rescue therapy may also be part of the protocol.
- Obtain a list of the patient's current medications, including over-the-counter medications and dietary supplements (see Effects of Natural Products on Laboratory Values online at DavisPlus online at Davis*Plus*).
- Review the procedure with the patient. Inform the patient that specimen collection takes approximately 5 to 10 min. Address concerns about pain and explain that there may be some discomfort during the venipuncture.
- ***Sensitivity to social and cultural issues,*** as well as concern for modesty, is important in providing psychological support before, during, and after the procedure.
- Note that there are no food, fluid, or medication restrictions unless by medical direction.

INTRATEST:

Potential Complications:

Note that lack of consideration for the proper collection time in relation to the dosing schedule can provide misleading information that may result in an erroneous interpretation of levels, creating the potential for a medication-error-related injury to the patient.

- Avoid the use of equipment containing latex if the patient has a history of allergic reaction to latex.
- Instruct the patient to cooperate fully and to follow directions. Direct the patient to breathe normally and to avoid unnecessary movement.
- Observe standard precautions, and follow the general guidelines in Patient Preparation and Specimen Collection online at Davis*Plus*. Consider recommended collection time in relation to the dosing schedule. Positively identify the patient, and label the appropriate specimen container with the corresponding patient demographics, initials of the person collecting the specimen, date, and time of collection, noting the last dose of medication taken. Perform a venipuncture.
- Remove the needle and apply direct pressure with dry gauze to stop bleeding. Observe/assess venipuncture site for bleeding or hematoma formation and secure gauze with adhesive bandage.
- Promptly transport the specimen to the laboratory for processing and analysis.

POST-TEST:

- Inform the patient that a report of the results will be made available to the requesting HCP, who will discuss the results with the patient.
- ***Nutritional Considerations:*** Patients taking immunosuppressant therapy tend to have decreased appetites due to the adverse effects of the medication. Instruct patients to consume a variety of foods within the basic food groups, maintain a healthy weight, be physically active, limit salt intake, limit alcohol intake, and be a nonsmoker.
- Recognize anxiety related to test results, and offer support. Patients receiving these drugs usually have conditions that can be intermittently moderately to severely debilitating, resulting in significant lifestyle changes. Educate the patient

regarding access to counseling services, as appropriate.

- Reinforce information given by the patient's HCP regarding further testing, treatment, or referral to another HCP. Explain to the patient the importance of following the medication regimen and give instructions regarding drug interactions. Answer any questions or address any concerns voiced by the patient or family.
- Instruct the patient to be prepared to provide the pharmacist with a list of other medications he or she is already taking in the event that the requesting HCP prescribes a medication.
- Depending on the results of this procedure, additional testing may be performed to evaluate or monitor progression of the disease process and determine the need for a change in therapy. Evaluate test results in relation to the patient's symptoms and other tests performed.

RELATED STUDIES:

- Related tests include ALT, AST, bilirubin, BUN, CBC platelet count, CBC WBC count and differential, and creatinine.
- Refer to the Genitourinary and Immune systems tables online at Davis*Plus* for related tests by body system.

Infectious Mononucleosis Screen

SYNONYM/ACRONYM: Monospot, heterophil antibody test, IM serology.

COMMON USE: To assess for Epstein-Barr virus and assist with diagnosis of infectious mononucleosis.

SPECIMEN: Serum collected in a gold-, red-, or red/gray-top tube. Place separated serum in a standard transport tube within 2 hr of collection.

NORMAL FINDINGS: (Method: Heterophile antibody test by agglutination; serological tests for EBV early antigen D antibody IgG, EBV nuclear antigen antibody IgG, EBV viral capsid antigen antibody IgG, EBV viral capsid antigen antibody IgM by immunoassay) Negative.

DESCRIPTION: Infectious mononucleosis is caused by the human herpesvirus 4, more commonly known as the *Epstein-Barr virus (EBV)*. The incubation period is 10 to 50 days, and the symptoms last 1 to 4 wk after the infection has fully developed. The hallmark of EBV infection is the presence of heterophil antibodies, also called *Paul-Bunnell-Davidsohn antibodies,* which are immunoglobulin M (IgM) antibodies that agglutinate sheep or horse red blood cells. The disease induces formation of abnormal lymphocytes in the lymph nodes; stimulates increased formation of heterophil antibodies; and is characterized by fever, cervical lymphadenopathy, tonsillopharyngitis, and hepatosplenomegaly. EBV is also thought to play a role in Burkitt's lymphoma, nasopharyngeal carcinoma, and chronic fatigue syndrome. If the results of the heterophil antibody screening test are negative and infectious mononucleosis is highly suspected, EBV-specific serology should be requested (EBV early antigen D antibody

IgG, EBV nuclear antigen antibody IgG, EBV viral capsid antigen antibody IgG, EBV viral capsid antigen antibody IgM). Molecular testing methods (e.g., polymerase chain reaction) are available to identify the presence of EBV viral DNA and to monitor viral load in patients being treated for other EBV-related diseases.

This procedure is contraindicated for: N/A

INDICATIONS

- Assist in confirming infectious mononucleosis.

POTENTIAL MEDICAL DIAGNOSIS

Positive findings in

- Infectious mononucleosis

Negative findings in: N/A

CRITICAL FINDINGS: N/A

INTERFERING FACTORS

- False-positive results may occur in the presence of narcotic addiction, serum sickness, lymphomas, hepatitis, leukemia, cancer of the pancreas, and phenytoin therapy.
- A false-negative result may occur if treatment was begun before antibodies developed or if the test was done less than 6 days after exposure to the virus.

NURSING IMPLICATIONS AND PROCEDURE

I

POTENTIAL NURSING PROBLEMS:

Problem	Signs & Symptoms	Interventions
Infection ***(related to Epstein-Barr viral infection secondary to exposure through kissing, cough, sneeze, sharing food utensils of an infected person)***	Fatigue, malaise, sore throat, fever, enlarged lymph nodes in the neck and armpits, swollen tonsils, headache, rash, swollen spleen	Rest, drink plenty of fluids (water and fruit juice), administer prescribed antibiotics to treat strep throat; administer prescribed steroids to treat swollen throat or tonsils; discuss gargling with warm saltwater to decrease pain of sore throat; discuss using over-the-counter ibuprofen or acetaminophen; discuss the importance of avoiding at-risk activities that may cause trauma and spleen rupture
Fatigue ***(related to Epstein-Barr viral infection secondary to exposure through kissing, cough,***	Decreased concentration; increased physical health concerns; unable to restore energy with sleep;	Monitor and trend mononucleosis screening results; pace activities to preserve energy stores; rate fatigue on a numeric scale to trend degree of

Problem	Signs & Symptoms	Interventions
sneeze, sharing food utensils of an infected person)	reports being tired; unable to maintain normal routine	fatigue over time; identify what aggravates and decreases fatigue; assess for related emotional factors such as depression; evaluate current medications in relation to fatigue; assess for physiologic factors such as anemia
Knowledge ***(related to recent diagnosis; complexity of treatment; poor understanding of provided information;*** cultural or language barriers; anxiety; emotional disturbance; unfamiliarity with medical management)	Lack of interest or questions; multiple questions; anxiety in relation to disease process and management; verbalizes inaccurate information; lack of follow-through with directions	Identify patient's, family's, and significant others' concerns about disease process; discuss the importance of fluids and rest for recovery; discuss the importance of avoiding vigorous activities, heavy lifting, roughhousing, or contact sports for at least 1 mo or as recommended by the health-care provider (HCP)

PRETEST:

- Positively identify the patient using at least two person-specific identifiers before services, treatments, or procedures are performed.
- *Patient Teaching:* Inform the patient this test can assist with diagnosing a mononucleosis infection.
- Obtain a history of the patient's health concerns, symptoms, surgical procedures, and results of previously performed laboratory and diagnostic studies. Include a list of known allergens, especially allergies or sensitivities to latex.
- Note any recent therapies that can interfere with test results.
- Obtain a list of the patient's current medications, including over-the-counter medications and dietary supplements (see Effects of Natural Products on Laboratory Values online at Davis*Plus*).
- Review the procedure with the patient. Inform the patient that specimen collection takes approximately 5 to 10 min. Address concerns about pain and explain that there may be some discomfort during the venipuncture.
- *Sensitivity to social and cultural issues,* as well as concern for modesty, is important in providing psychological support before, during, and after the procedure.
- Note that there are no food, fluid, or medication restrictions unless by medical direction.

INTRATEST:

Potential Complications: N/A

- Avoid the use of equipment containing latex if the patient has a history of allergic reaction to latex.
- Instruct the patient to cooperate fully and to follow directions. Direct the

patient to breathe normally and to avoid unnecessary movement.

- Observe standard precautions, and follow the general guidelines in Patient Preparation and Specimen Collection online at Davis*Plus*. Positively identify the patient, and label the appropriate specimen container with the corresponding patient demographics, initials of the person collecting the specimen, date, and time of collection. Perform a venipuncture.
- Remove the needle and apply direct pressure with dry gauze to stop bleeding. Observe/assess venipuncture site for bleeding or hematoma formation and secure gauze with adhesive bandage.
- Promptly transport the specimen to the laboratory for processing and analysis.

POST-TEST:

- Inform the patient that a report of the results will be made available to the requesting HCP, who will discuss the results with the patient.
- Recognize anxiety related to test results, and inform the patient that signs and symptoms of infection include fever, chills, sore throat, enlarged lymph nodes, and fatigue. Self-care while the disease runs its course include adequate fluid and nutritional intake along with sufficient rest. Activities that cause fatigue or stress should be avoided. Advise the patient to refrain from direct contact with others because the disease is transmitted through saliva.
- Reinforce information given by the patient's HCP regarding further testing, treatment, or referral to another HCP. Advise the patient to refrain from direct contact with others because the disease is transmitted through saliva. Answer any questions or address any concerns voiced by the patient or family.
- Depending on the results of this procedure, additional testing may be performed to evaluate or monitor progression of the disease process and determine the need for a change in therapy. Evaluate test results in relation to the patient's symptoms and other tests performed.

Patient Education:

- Inform the patient that approximately 10% of all results are false-negative or false-positive.
- Inform the patient that signs and symptoms of infection include fever, chills, sore throat, enlarged lymph nodes, and fatigue.
- Emphasize the importance of self-care while the disease runs its course, which includes adequate fluid and nutritional intake along with sufficient rest.

Expected Patient Outcomes:

Understanding

- The patient and family verbalize how to pace activities to conserve energy and manage fatigue in relation to activities of daily living.
- The patient and family state the importance of lengthy rest periods for recovery from mononucleosis.

Ability

- The patient follows the recommendation to increase fluid intake (water and juice).
- The patient follows the recommendation to take over-the-counter ibuprofen or acetaminophen for comfort as needed.

Response

- The patient complies with the request to get plenty of rest to facilitate the recovery process.
- The patient complies with the recommendation to avoid kissing to prevent infection of another individual with mononucleosis.

RELATED STUDIES:

- Related tests include CBC with peripheral blood smear evaluation and US abdomen.
- Refer to the Hepatobiliary and Immune systems tables online at Davis*Plus* for related tests by body system.

Insulin and Insulin Response to Glucose

SYNONYM/ACRONYM: N/A

COMMON USE: To assess the amount of insulin secreted in response to blood glucose to assist in diagnosis of types of hypoglycemia and insulin-resistant pathologies.

SPECIMEN: Serum collected in a red-top tube.

NORMAL FINDINGS: (Method: Immunoassay)

75-g Glucose Load	Insulin	SI Units (Conventional Units × 6.945)	Tolerance for Glucose (Hypoglycemia)
Fasting	Less than 17 micro international units/L	Less than 118.1 pmol/L	Less than 110 mg/dL
30 min	6–86 micro international units/L	41.7–597.3 pmol/L	Less than 200 mg/dL
1 hr	8–118 micro international units/L	55.6–819.5 pmol/L	Less than 200 mg/dL
2 hr	5–55 micro international units/L	34.7–382 pmol/L	Less than 140 mg/dL
3 hr	Less than 25 micro international units/L	Less than 174 pmol/L	65–120 mg/dL
4 hr	Less than 15 micro international units/L	Less than 104.2 pmol/L	65–120 mg/dL
5 hr	Less than 8 micro international units/L	Less than 55.6 pmol/L	65–115 mg/dL

DESCRIPTION: Insulin is a hormone secreted by the beta cells of the pancreatic islets of Langerhans in response to elevated blood glucose levels. Its overall effect is to help regulate the metabolism of glucose. Specifically, insulin decreases blood levels of glucose by promoting transport of glucose into the liver and muscles to be stored as glycogen. Insulin also participates in regulation of the processes required for metabolism of fats, carbohydrates, and proteins. The insulin response test measures insulin response to a standardized dose of glucose, administered over fixed period of time and is useful in evaluating patients with hypoglycemia and suspected insulin-resistance.

This procedure is contraindicated for: N/A

INDICATIONS

- Assist in the diagnosis of early or developing type 2 diabetes, as indicated by excessive production of insulin in relation to blood glucose levels (best shown with glucose tolerance tests or 2-hr postprandial tests).

- Assist in the diagnosis of insulinoma, as indicated by sustained high levels of insulin and absence of blood glucose–related variations.
- Confirm functional hypoglycemia, as indicated by circulating insulin levels appropriate to changing blood glucose levels.
- Differentiate between type 1 diabetes, in which insulin levels are high, and type 2 diabetes, in which insulin levels are low.
- Evaluate fasting hypoglycemia of unknown cause.
- Evaluate postprandial hypoglycemia of unknown cause.
- Evaluate uncontrolled type 1 diabetes.

POTENTIAL MEDICAL DIAGNOSIS

Increased in:

- Acromegaly ***(related to excess production of growth hormone, which increases insulin levels)***
- Alcohol use ***(related to stimulation of insulin production)***
- Cushing's syndrome ***(related to overproduction of cortisol, which increases insulin levels)***
- Excessive administration of insulin
- Insulin- and proinsulin-secreting tumors (insulinomas)
- Obesity ***(related to development of insulin resistance; body does not respond to insulin being produced)***
- Persistent hyperinsulinemic hypoglycemia ***(collection of hypoglycemic disorders of infants and children)***
- Reactive hypoglycemia in developing diabetes
- Severe liver disease

Decreased in:

- Beta cell failure ***(pancreatic beta cells produce insulin; therefore, damage to these cells will decrease insulin levels)***
- Type 1 diabetes or type 2 diabetes ***(related to lack of endogenous insulin)***

CRITICAL FINDINGS: N/A

INTERFERING FACTORS

- Drugs and other substances that may increase insulin levels include albuterol, amino acids, beclomethasone, betamethasone, broxaterol, calcium gluconate, cannabis, chlorpropamide, glibornuride, glipizide, glisoxepide, glucagon, glyburide, ibopamine, insulin, oral contraceptives, pancreozymin, prednisolone, prednisone, rifampin, terbutaline, tolazamide, tolbutamide, trichlormethiazide, and verapamil.
- Drugs and other substances that may decrease insulin levels include acarbose, calcitonin, cimetidine, clofibrate, diltiazem, doxazosin, enalapril, enprostil, ether, hydroxypropyl methylcellulose, metformin, niacin, nifedipine, nitrendipine, octreotide, phenytoin, propranolol, and psyllium.
- Administration of insulin or oral hypoglycemic drugs within 8 hr of the test can lead to falsely elevated levels.
- Hemodialysis destroys insulin and affects test results.

NURSING IMPLICATIONS AND PROCEDURE

PRETEST:

- Positively identify the patient using at least two person-specific identifiers before services, treatments, or procedures are performed.
- *Patient Teaching:* Inform the patient this test can assist in the evaluation of low blood sugar.
- Obtain a history of the patient's health concerns, symptoms, surgical procedures, and results of previously

performed laboratory and diagnostic studies. Include a list of known allergens, especially allergies or sensitivities to latex.

- Note any recent procedures that can interfere with test results.
- Obtain a list of the patient's current medications, including over-the-counter medications and dietary supplements (see Effects of Natural Products on Laboratory Values online at Davis*Plus*).
- Review the procedure with the patient. Inform the patient that multiple specimens may be required. Inform the patient that specimen collection takes approximately 5 to 10 min. Address concerns about pain and explain that there may be some discomfort during the venipuncture.
- ***Sensitivity to social and cultural issues,*** as well as concern for modesty, is important in providing psychological support before, during, and after the procedure.
- If a single sample is to be collected, the patient should have fasted and refrained, with medical direction, from taking insulin or other oral hypoglycemic drugs for at least 8 hr before specimen collection. Protocols may vary among facilities.
- ***Hypoglycemia:*** Serial specimens for insulin levels are collected in conjunction with glucose levels after administration of a 75-g glucose load. The patient should be prepared as for a standard oral glucose tolerance test over a 5-hr period. Protocols may vary among facilities.
- Note that there are no fluid restrictions unless by medical direction.

INTRATEST:

Potential Complications:

Note that the patient may have difficulty drinking the extremely sweet glucose beverage and become nauseous.

- Ensure that the patient has complied with dietary and medication restrictions and other pretesting preparations prior to the study, as instructed; assure that food or medications have been restricted as instructed prior to the specific procedure's protocol.
- Avoid the use of equipment containing latex if the patient has a history of allergic reaction to latex.
- Instruct the patient to cooperate fully and to follow directions. Direct the patient to breathe normally and to avoid unnecessary movement.
- Observe standard precautions, and follow the general guidelines in Patient Preparation and Specimen Collection online at Davis*Plus*. Positively identify the patient, and label the appropriate specimen container with the corresponding patient demographics, initials of the person collecting the specimen, date, and time of collection. Perform a venipuncture.
- Remove the needle and apply direct pressure with dry gauze to stop bleeding. Observe/assess venipuncture site for bleeding or hematoma formation and secure gauze with adhesive bandage.
- Promptly transport the specimen to the laboratory for processing and analysis.

POST-TEST:

- Inform the patient that a report of the results will be made available to the requesting health-care provider (HCP), who will discuss the results with the patient.
- Instruct the patient to resume usual diet and medication, as directed by the HCP.
- ***Nutritional Considerations:*** There is no "diabetic diet"; however, many meal-planning approaches with nutritional goals are endorsed by the American Diabetes Association (ADA). 🍁Patients who adhere to dietary recommendations report a better general feeling of health, better weight management, greater control of glucose and lipid values, and improved use of insulin. Instruct the patient, as appropriate, in nutritional management of diabetes. A variety of dietary patterns are beneficial for people with diabetes. The Mediterranean-style diet emphasizes

I

inclusion of vegetables, whole grains, fruits, low-fat dairy, nuts, legumes, and nontropical vegetable oils (e.g., olive, canola, peanut, sunflower, flaxseed) along with fish and lean poultry. A similar dietary pattern known as the Dietary Approaches to Stop Hypertension (DASH) diet makes additional recommendations for the reduction of dietary sodium. Both dietary styles emphasize a reduction in consumption of red meats, which are high in saturated fats and cholesterol, and other foods containing sugar, saturated fats, trans fats, and sodium. A vegetarian diet as well as other potential weight loss diets such as Weight Watchers are also supported by the ADA. 🍁 If triglycerides also are elevated, the patient should be advised to eliminate or reduce alcohol. The nutritional needs of each patient with diabetic patient need to be determined individually (especially during pregnancy) with the appropriate HCPs, particularly professionals educated in nutrition.

- Note that abnormal insulin response and impaired glucose tolerance may be associated with diabetes. Instruct the patient and caregiver to report signs and symptoms of hypoglycemia (weakness, confusion, diaphoresis, rapid pulse) or hyperglycemia (thirst, polyuria, hunger, lethargy).
- *Social and Cultural Considerations:* Numerous studies point to the prevalence of excess body weight in American children and adolescents. Experts estimate that obesity is present in 25% of the population aged 6 to 11 yr. The medical, social, and emotional consequences of excess body weight are significant. Special attention should be given to instructing the pediatric patient and caregiver regarding health risks and weight control education. 🍁
- Recognize anxiety related to test results, and be supportive of perceived loss of independence and fear of shortened life expectancy. Discuss the implications of abnormal test results on the patient's lifestyle. Provide teaching and information regarding the clinical implications of the test results, as appropriate. Emphasize, if indicated, that good glycemic control delays the onset and slows the progression of diabetic retinopathy, nephropathy, and neuropathy. Educate the patient regarding access to counseling services, as appropriate. Provide contact information, if desired, for the American Heart Association (www.americanheart.org), National Heart, Lung, and Blood Institute (www.nhlbi.nih.gov), Institute of Medicine of the National Academies (www.iom.edu), and USDA's resource for nutrition (www.choosemyplate.gov). 🍁
- Reinforce information given by the patient's HCP regarding further testing, treatment, or referral to another HCP. Instruct the patient in the use of home test kits approved by the U.S. Food and Drug Administration, if prescribed. Answer any questions or address any concerns voiced by the patient or family.
- Depending on the results of this procedure, additional testing may be performed to evaluate or monitor progression of the disease process and determine the need for a change in therapy. The ADA recommends A_{1C} testing four times a year for type 1 or type 2 diabetes when glycemic targets are not being met or when therapy has changed and twice a year when treatment goals are being met for non–insulin-dependent type 2 diabetes. The ADA also recommends that testing for diabetes commence at age 45 for asymptomatic individuals, be considered for adults of any age who are overweight and have additional risk factors, and continue every 3 yr in the absence of symptoms. 🍁

RELATED STUDIES:

- Related tests include ACTH, ALT, angiography adrenal, bilirubin, BUN, calcium, catecholamines, cholesterol (HDL, LDL, total), cortisol, C-peptide, DHEA, creatinine, fecal analysis, fecal fat, fructosamine, GGT, gastric emptying scan, glucagon, glucose, GTT, glycated hemoglobin, GH, HVA, insulin antibodies, ketones, lipoprotein electrophoresis, metanephrines, microalbumin, and myoglobin.

- Refer to the Endocrine System table online at Davis*Plus* for related tests by body system.

Insulin Antibodies

SYNONYM/ACRONYM: Islet cell antibody, glutamic acid decarboxylase antibody.

COMMON USE: To assist in the prediction, diagnosis, and management of type 1 diabetes as well as insulin resistance and insulin allergy.

SPECIMEN: Serum collected in a red-top tube.

NORMAL FINDINGS: (Method: Radioimmunoassay) Less than 0.4 Units/mL.

DESCRIPTION: The onset of type 1 diabetes has been shown to correspond to the development of a number of autoantibodies. The most common anti-insulin antibody is immunoglobulin (Ig) G, but IgA, IgM, IgD, and IgE antibodies also have anti-insulin properties. IgM is thought to participate in insulin resistance and IgE in insulin allergy. Increased use of human insulin instead of purified animal insulin has resulted in a significant decrease in the incidence of insulin antibody formation as a result of treatment for diabetics using insulin. The presence of insulin antibodies has been demonstrated to be a strong predictor for development of type 1 diabetes in individuals who do not have diabetes but are genetically predisposed.

This procedure is contraindicated for: N/A

INDICATIONS

- Assist in confirming insulin resistance.
- Assist in determining if hypoglycemia is caused by insulin abuse.
- Assist in determining insulin allergy.

POTENTIAL MEDICAL DIAGNOSIS

Increased in:

- Factitious hypoglycemia ***(assists in differentiating lack of response due to the presence of insulin antibodies from secretive self-administration of insulin)***
- Insulin allergy or resistance ***(antibodies bind to insulin and decrease amount of free insulin available for glucose metabolism)***
- Polyendocrine autoimmune syndromes
- Steroid-induced diabetes ***(an adverse effect of treatment for systemic lupus erythematosus)***

Decreased in: N/A

CRITICAL FINDINGS: N/A

INTERFERING FACTORS

Recent radioactive scans or radiation can interfere with test results when radioimmunoassay is the test method.

NURSING IMPLICATIONS AND PROCEDURE

PRETEST:

- Positively identify the patient using at least two person-specific identifiers before services, treatments, or procedures are performed.
- *Patient Teaching:* Inform the patient this test can assist in the diagnosis and management of type 1 diabetes.
- Obtain a history of the patient's health concerns, symptoms, surgical procedures, and results of previously performed laboratory and diagnostic studies. Include a list of known allergens, especially allergies or sensitivities to latex.
- Note any recent procedures that can interfere with test results.
- Obtain a list of the patient's current medications, including over-the-counter medications and dietary supplements (see Effects of Natural Products on Laboratory Values online at Davis*Plus*).
- Review the procedure with the patient. Inform the patient that specimen collection takes approximately 5 to 10 min. Address concerns about pain and explain that there may be some discomfort during the venipuncture.
- *Sensitivity to social and cultural issues,* as well as concern for modesty, is important in providing psychological support before, during, and after the procedure.
- Note that there are no food, fluid, or medication restrictions unless by medical direction.

INTRATEST:

Potential Complications: N/A

- Avoid the use of equipment containing latex if the patient has a history of allergic reaction to latex.
- Instruct the patient to cooperate fully and to follow directions. Direct the patient to breathe normally and to avoid unnecessary movement.
- Observe standard precautions, and follow the general guidelines in Patient Preparation and Specimen Collection online at Davis*Plus*. Positively identify the patient, and label the appropriate specimen container with the corresponding patient demographics, initials of the person collecting the specimen, date, and time of collection. Perform a venipuncture.
- Remove the needle and apply direct pressure with dry gauze to stop bleeding. Observe/assess venipuncture site for bleeding or hematoma formation and secure gauze with adhesive bandage.
- Promptly transport the specimen to the laboratory for processing and analysis.

POST-TEST:

- Inform the patient that a report of the results will be made available to the requesting health-care provider (HCP), who will discuss the results with the patient.
- Instruct the patient to resume usual diet and medication, as directed by the HCP.
- *Nutritional Considerations:* Abnormal findings may be associated with diabetes. There is no "diabetic diet"; however, many meal-planning approaches with nutritional goals are endorsed by the American Diabetes Association (ADA). 🍁 Patients who adhere to dietary recommendations report a better general feeling of health, better weight management, greater control of glucose and lipid values, and improved use of insulin. Instruct the patient, as appropriate, in nutritional management of diabetes. A variety of dietary patterns are beneficial for people with diabetes. The Mediterranean-style diet emphasizes inclusion of vegetables, whole grains, fruits, low-fat dairy, nuts, legumes, and nontropical vegetable oils (e.g., olive, canola, peanut, sunflower, flaxseed) along with fish and lean poultry. A similar dietary pattern known as the Dietary Approaches to Stop Hypertension (DASH) diet makes additional recommendations for the reduction of dietary sodium.

Both dietary styles emphasize a reduction in consumption of red meats, which are high in saturated fats and cholesterol, and other foods containing sugar, saturated fats, trans fats, and sodium. A vegetarian diet as well as other potential weight loss diets such as Weight Watchers are also supported by the ADA. ✦ If triglycerides also are elevated, the patient should be advised to eliminate or reduce alcohol. The nutritional needs of each patient with diabetic patient need to be determined individually (especially during pregnancy) with the appropriate HCPs, particularly professionals educated in nutrition.

- Note that the presence of insulin antibodies may be associated with diabetes. Instruct the patient and caregiver to report signs and symptoms of hypoglycemia (weakness, confusion, diaphoresis, rapid pulse) or hyperglycemia (thirst, polyuria, hunger, lethargy).
- Recognize anxiety related to test results, and be supportive of perceived loss of independence and fear of shortened life expectancy. Discuss the implications of abnormal test results on the patient's lifestyle. Provide teaching and information regarding the clinical implications of the test results, as appropriate. Emphasize, if indicated, that good glycemic control delays the onset and slows the progression of diabetic retinopathy, nephropathy, and neuropathy. Educate the patient regarding access to counseling services, as appropriate. Provide contact information, if desired, for the American Heart Association (www.americanheart.org), National Heart, Lung, and Blood Institute (www.nhlbi.nih.gov), Institute of Medicine of the National Academies (www.iom.edu), and USDA's resource for nutrition (www.choosemyplate.gov). ✦
- Reinforce information given by the patient's HCP regarding further testing, treatment, or referral to another HCP. Answer any questions or address any concerns voiced by the patient or family.
- Depending on the results of this procedure, additional testing may be performed to evaluate or monitor progression of the disease process and determine the need for a change in therapy. The ADA recommends A_{1C} testing four times a year for type 1 or type 2 diabetes when glycemic targets are not being met or when therapy has changed and twice a year when treatment goals are being met for non–insulin-dependent type 2 diabetes. The ADA also recommends that testing for diabetes commence at age 45 for asymptomatic individuals, be considered for adults of any age who are overweight and have additional risk factors, and continue every 3 yr in the absence of symptoms. ✦ Evaluate test results in relation to the patient's symptoms and other tests performed.

RELATED STUDIES:

- Related tests include C-peptide, glucose, GTT, glycated hemoglobin, and insulin.
- Refer to the Endocrine and Immune systems tables online at Davis*Plus* for related tests by body system.

Intraocular Muscle Function

SYNONYM/ACRONYM: IOM function.

COMMON USE: To assess the function of the extraocular muscle to assist with diagnosis of strabismus, amblyopia, and other ocular disorders.

AREA OF APPLICATION: Eyes.

DESCRIPTION: Evaluation of ocular motility is performed to detect and measure muscle imbalance in conditions classified as heterophorias or heterotropias. This evaluation is performed in a manner to assess fixation of each eye, alignment of both eyes in all directions, and the ability of both eyes to work together binocularly. Heterophorias are latent ocular deviations kept in check by the binocular power of fusion and made intermittent by disrupting fusion. Heterotropias are conditions that manifest constant ocular deviations. The prefixes *eso-* (tendency for the eye to turn in), *exo-* (tendency for the eye to turn out), and *hyper-* (tendency for one eye to turn up) indicate the direction in which the affected eye moves spontaneously. *Strabismus* is the failure of both eyes to spontaneously fixate on the same object because of a muscular imbalance (crossed eyes). *Amblyopia,* or lazy eye, is a term used for loss of vision in one or both eyes that cannot be attributed to an organic pathological condition of the eye or optic nerve. There are six extraocular muscles in each eye; their movement is controlled by three nerves. The actions of the muscles vary depending on the position of the eye when they become innervated. The cover test is commonly used because it is reliable, easy to perform, and does not require special equipment. The cover test method is described in this study. Another method for evaluation of ocular muscle function is the corneal light reflex test. It is useful with patients who cannot cooperate for prism cover testing or for patients who have poor fixation.

This procedure is contraindicated for: N/A

INDICATIONS

- Detection and evaluation of extraocular muscle imbalance.

POTENTIAL MEDICAL DIAGNOSIS

The examiner should determine the range of ocular movements in all gaze positions, usually to include up and out, in, down and out, up and in, down and in, and out. Limited movements in gaze position can be recorded semiquantitatively as −1 (minimal), −2 (moderate), −3 (severe), or −4 (total).

Normal findings

- Normal range of ocular movements in all gaze positions

Abnormal findings related to

- Amblyopia
- Heterophorias
- Heterotropias
- Strabismus

CRITICAL FINDINGS: N/A

INTERFERING FACTORS

Factors that may impair the results of the examination

- Inability of the patient to cooperate and remain still during the test because of age, significant pain, or mental status may interfere with the test results.
- Rubbing or squeezing the eyes may affect results.

NURSING IMPLICATIONS AND PROCEDURE

PRETEST:

- Positively identify the patient using at least two person-specific identifiers before services, treatments, or procedures are performed.
- *Patient Teaching:* Inform the patient this procedure can assist in evaluating eye muscle function.

- Obtain a history of the patient's health concerns (especially known or suspected vision loss, changes in visual acuity, including type and cause; use of glasses or contact lenses; eye conditions with treatment regimens, eye surgery), symptoms, surgical procedures, and results of previously performed laboratory and diagnostic studies. Include a list of known allergens, especially allergies or sensitivities to latex.
- Obtain a list of the patient's current medications, including over-the-counter medications and dietary supplements (see Effects of Natural Products on Laboratory Values online at Davis*Plus*).
- Review the procedure with the patient. Address concerns about pain and explain that no discomfort will be experienced during the test. Inform the patient that a health-care provider (HCP) performs the test in a quiet room and that to evaluate both eyes, the test can take 2 to 4 min.
- Instruct the patient to remove contact lenses or glasses, as appropriate. Instruct the patient regarding the importance of keeping the eyes open for the test.
- ***Sensitivity to social and cultural issues,*** as well as concern for modesty, is important in providing psychological support before, during, and after the procedure.
- Note that there are no food, fluid, or medication restrictions unless by medical direction.

INTRATEST:

Potential Complications: N/A

- Observe standard precautions, and follow the general guidelines in Patient Preparation and Specimen Collection online at Davis*Plus*. Positively identify the patient.
- Instruct the patient to cooperate fully and to follow directions. Ask the patient to remain still during the procedure because movement produces unreliable results.
- Note that one eye is tested at a time. The patient is given a fixation point, usually the testing personnel's index finger. An object, such as a small toy, can be used to ensure fixation in pediatric patients. The patient is asked to follow the fixation point with his or her gaze in the direction the fixation point moves. When testing is completed, the procedure is repeated using the other eye. The procedure is performed at a distance and near, first with and then without corrective lenses. The examiner should determine the range of ocular movements in all gaze positions, usually to include up and out, in, down and out, up and in, down and in, and out.

POST-TEST:

- Inform the patient that a report of the results will be made available to the requesting HCP, who will discuss the results with the patient.
- Recognize anxiety related to test results, and be supportive of impaired activity related to vision loss, anticipated loss of driving privileges, or the possibility of requiring corrective lenses (self-image).
- Reinforce information given by the patient's HCP regarding further testing, treatment, or referral to another HCP. Educate the patient, as appropriate, that he or she may be referred for special therapy to correct the anomaly, which may include glasses, prisms, eye exercises, eye patches, or chemical patching with drugs that modify the focusing power of the eye. The patient and family should be educated that the chosen therapy involves a process of mental retraining. The mode of therapy in itself does not correct vision. It is the process by which the brain becomes readapted to accept, receive, and store visual images received by the eye that results in vision correction. Therefore, the patient must be prepared to be alert, cooperative, and properly motivated. Answer any questions or address any concerns voiced by the patient or family.
- Depending on the results of this procedure, additional testing may

be performed to evaluate or monitor progression of the disease process and determine the need for a change in therapy. Evaluate test results in relation to the patient's symptoms and other tests performed.

RELATED STUDIES:

- Related tests include refraction and slit-lamp biomicroscopy.
- Refer to the Ocular System table online at Davis*Plus* for related tests by body system.

Intraocular Pressure

SYNONYM/ACRONYM: IOP.

COMMON USE: To evaluate changes in ocular pressure to assist in diagnosis of disorders such as glaucoma.

AREA OF APPLICATION: Eyes.

DESCRIPTION: The intraocular pressure (IOP) of the eye depends on a number of factors. The two most significant are the amount of aqueous humor present in the eye and the circumstances by which it leaves the eye. Other physiological variables that affect IOP include respiration, pulse, and the degree of hydration of the body. Individual eyes respond to IOP differently. Some can tolerate high pressures (20 to 30 mm Hg), and some will incur optic nerve damage at lower pressures. With respiration, variations of up to 4 mm Hg in IOP can occur, and changes of 1 to 2 mm Hg occur with every pulsation of the central retinal artery. IOP is measured with a tonometer; normal values indicate the pressure at which no damage is done to the intraocular contents. The rate of fluid leaving the eye, or its ability to leave the eye unimpeded, is the most important factor regulating IOP. There are three primary conditions that result in occlusion of the outflow channels for fluid. The most common condition is open-angle glaucoma, in which the diameter of the openings of the trabecular meshwork becomes narrowed, resulting in an increased IOP due to an increased resistance of fluid moving out of the eye. In secondary or angle closure glaucoma, the trabecular meshwork becomes occluded by tumor cells, pigment, red blood cells in hyphema, or other material. Additionally, the obstructing material may cover parts of the meshwork itself, as with scar tissue or other types of adhesions that form after severe iritis, an angle-closure glaucoma attack, or a central retinal vein occlusion. The third condition impeding fluid outflow in the trabecular channels occurs with pupillary block, most commonly associated with primary angle-closure glaucoma. In eyes predisposed to this condition, dilation of the pupil causes the iris to fold up like an accordion against the narrow-angle structures of the eye. Fluid in the posterior chamber has difficulty circulating into the anterior chamber; therefore, pressure in the posterior chamber increases, causing the iris to bow forward and obstruct the outflow channels even more. Angle-closure attacks occur quite suddenly and therefore do not give the eye a chance to adjust itself to the sudden increase in pressure. The eye becomes very red, the cornea edematous (patient may report seeing halos), and the pupil fixed and dilated, accompanied by a complaint of moderate pain. Pupil dilation can be initiated by emotional arousal or fear, conditions in which the eye must adapt to darkness (movie theaters), or mydriatics. Acute angle-closure glaucoma is an ocular emergency usually resolved by a peripheral iridotomy to allow movement of fluid between the anterior and posterior chambers. Iridotomy uses a laser to create a hole in the iris and is the preferred method of treatment. An iridectomy is a more invasive and less often used procedure that constitutes removal of a portion of the peripheral iris either by traditional surgery or by laser. Laser iridotomy is facilitated by the neodymium yttrium-aluminum-garnet laser, also known as the Nd:YAG laser. In some cases, an argon laser may be used alone or in combination with the YAG laser.

This procedure is contraindicated for: N/A

INDICATIONS

- Diagnosis or ongoing monitoring of glaucoma.
- Screening test included in a routine eye examination.

POTENTIAL MEDICAL DIAGNOSIS

Normal findings

- Normal IOP is between 10 and 20 mm Hg

Abnormal findings related to

- Open-angle glaucoma
- Primary angle-closure glaucoma
- Secondary glaucoma

CRITICAL FINDINGS:

Increased IOP in the presence of sudden pain, sudden change in vision, a partially dilated and nonreactive pupil, and firm globe implies acute angle-closure glaucoma, which is an ocular emergency requiring immediate attention to avoid permanent vision loss. This condition requires immediate examination by an ophthalmologist. Iridotomy is the most likely intervention.

Note and immediately report to the requesting health-care provider (HCP) any critical findings and related symptoms. A listing of these findings varies among facilities. Timely notification of a critical finding for laboratory or diagnostic studies is a role expectation of the professional nurse. The notification processes vary among facilities. Upon receipt of the critical finding, the information should be read back to the caller to verify accuracy.

INTERFERING FACTORS

- Inability of the patient to remain still and cooperative during the test may interfere with the test results.
- Rubbing or squeezing the eyes may affect results.

NURSING IMPLICATIONS AND PROCEDURE

PRETEST:

- Positively identify the patient using at least two person-specific identifiers before services, treatments, or procedures are performed.
- *Patient Teaching:* Inform the patient this procedure can assist in measuring eye pressure.
- Obtain a history of the patient's health concerns (especially known or suspected vision loss, changes

I

in visual acuity, including type and cause; use of glasses or contact lenses; eye conditions with treatment regimens, eye surgery), symptoms, surgical procedures, and results of previously performed laboratory and diagnostic studies. Include a list of known allergens, especially allergies or sensitivities to latex or topical anesthetics eyedrops.

- Obtain a list of the patient's current medications, including over-the-counter medications and dietary supplements (see Effects of Natural Products on Laboratory Values online at Davis*Plus*).
- Review the procedure with the patient. Explain that the patient will be requested to fixate the eyes during the procedure. Address concerns about pain and explain that he or she may feel coldness or a slight sting when the anesthetic/fluorescein drops are instilled at the beginning of the procedure but that no discomfort will be experienced during the test. Instruct the patient as to what should be expected with the use of the tonometer. The patient will experience less anxiety if he or she understands that the tonometer tip will touch the tear film and not the eye directly. Inform the patient that an HCP performs the test in a quiet, darkened room and that to evaluate both eyes, the test can take 1 to 3 min.
- Instruct the patient to remove contact lenses or glasses, as appropriate. Instruct the patient regarding the importance of keeping the eyes open for the test.
- ***Sensitivity to social and cultural issues,*** as well as concern for modesty, is important in providing psychological support before, during, and after the procedure.
- Note that there are no food, fluid, or medication restrictions unless by medical direction.

INTRATEST:

Potential Complications: N/A

- Observe standard precautions, and follow the general guidelines in Patient Preparation and Specimen Collection online at Davis*Plus*. Positively identify the patient.
- Instruct the patient to cooperate fully and to follow directions. Ask the patient to remain still during the procedure because any movement, such as coughing, breath-holding, or wandering eye movements, produces unreliable results.
- Seat the patient comfortably. Instruct the patient to look at directed target while the eyes are examined.
- Avoid the use of equipment containing latex if the patient has a history of allergic reaction to latex.
- Instill ordered topical anesthetic/ fluorescein drops in each eye, as ordered, and allow time for it to work. Topical anesthetic/fluorescein drops are placed in the eye with the patient looking up and the solution directed at the six o'clock position of the sclera (white of the eye) near the limbus (gray, semitransparent area of the eyeball where the cornea and sclera meet). Neither dropper nor bottle should touch the eyelashes.
- Instruct the patient to look straight ahead, keeping the eyes open and unblinking.
- A number of techniques are used to measure IOP. It can be measured by applanation at the slit lamp (Goldmann), with a handheld (Perkins) applanation tonometer, or with a non-touch airpuff tonometer.
- When the applanation tonometer is positioned on the patient's cornea, the instrument's headrest is placed against the patient's forehead. The tonometer should be held at an angle with the handle slanted away from the patient's nose. The tonometer tip should not touch the eyelids.
- When the tip is properly aligned and in contact with the fluorescein-stained tear film, force is applied to the tip using an adjustment control to the desired endpoint. The tonometer is removed from the eye. The reading is taken a second time, and if the pressure is elevated, a third reading is taken. The procedure is repeated on the other eye.

- With the airpuff tonometer, an air pump blows air onto the cornea, and the time it takes for the air puff to flatten the cornea is detected by infrared light and photoelectric cells. This time is directly related to the IOP.

POST-TEST:

- Inform the patient that a report of the results will be made available to the requesting HCP, who will discuss the results with the patient.
- Recognize anxiety related to test results, and be supportive of impaired activity related to vision loss or anticipated loss of driving privileges. Discuss the implications of abnormal test results on the patient's lifestyle. Provide teaching and information regarding the clinical implications of the test results, as appropriate. Provide contact information, if desired, for the Glaucoma Research Foundation (www.glaucoma.org). 🍁
- Reinforce information given by the patient's HCP regarding further testing, treatment, or referral to another HCP. Answer any questions or address any concerns voiced by the patient or family.
- Instruct the patient in the use of any ordered medications, usually eyedrops, that are intended to decrease IOP. Explain the importance of adhering to the therapy regimen, especially since increased IOP does not present symptoms. Instruct the patient in both the ocular adverse effects and systemic reactions associated with the prescribed medication. Encourage him or her to review corresponding literature provided by a pharmacist.
- Depending on the results of this procedure, additional testing may be performed to evaluate or monitor progression of the disease process and determine the need for a change in therapy. Evaluate test results in relation to the patient's symptoms and other tests performed.

RELATED STUDIES:

- Related tests include fundoscopy, gonioscopy, nerve fiber analysis, pachymetry, slit-lamp biomicroscopy, and visual field testing.
- Refer to the Ocular System table online at Davis*Plus* for related tests by body system.

I

Intravenous Pyelography

SYNONYM/ACRONYM: Antegrade pyelography, excretory urography (EUG), intravenous urography (IVU, IUG), IVP.

COMMON USE: To assess urinary tract dysfunction or evaluate progression of kidney disease such as stones, bleeding, and congenital anomalies.

AREA OF APPLICATION: Kidneys, ureters, bladder, and renal pelvis.

DESCRIPTION: Intravenous pyelography (IVP) is most commonly performed to determine urinary tract dysfunction or kidney disease. IVP uses intravenous (IV) radiopaque contrast medium to visualize the kidneys, ureters, bladder, and renal pelvis. The contrast medium concentrates in the blood and is filtered out by the glomeruli passing out through the renal tubules and concentrated in the urine. Renal function is reflected by the length of time it takes the contrast medium to appear and to be excreted by each kidney. A series of images is performed over a 30-min period to view passage of the contrast through the kidneys and ureters into the bladder. Tomography may be employed during the IVP to permit the examination of an individual layer or plane of the organ that may be obscured by surrounding overlying structures. Many facilities have replaced the IVP with computed tomography (CT) studies. CT provides detail of the anatomical structures in the urinary system and therefore greater sensitivity in the identification of renal pathology.

This procedure is contraindicated for

Patients who are pregnant or suspected of being pregnant, unless the potential benefits of a procedure using radiation far outweigh the risk of radiation exposure to the fetus and mother.

Patients with conditions associated with adverse reactions to contrast medium (e.g., asthma, food allergies, or allergy to contrast medium). Although patients are asked specifically if they have a known allergy to iodine or shellfish, it has been well established that the reaction is not to iodine; an actual iodine allergy would be problematic because iodine is required for the production of thyroid hormones. In the case of shellfish, the reaction is to a muscle protein called tropomyosin; in the case of iodinated contrast medium, the reaction is to the noniodinated part of the contrast molecule. Patients with a known hypersensitivity to the medium may benefit from premedication with corticosteroids and diphenhydramine; the use of nonionic contrast or an alternative noncontrast imaging study, if available, may be considered for patients who have severe asthma or who have experienced moderate to severe reactions to ionic contrast medium.

Conditions associated with preexisting renal insufficiency (e.g., chronic kidney disease, single kidney transplant, nephrectomy, diabetes, multiple myeloma, treatment with aminoglycosides and NSAIDs) ***because iodinated contrast is nephrotoxic.***

Patients who are chronically dehydrated before the test, especially older adults and patients whose health is already compromised, ***because of their risk of contrast-induced acute kidney injury.***

Patients with bleeding disorders or receiving anticoagulant therapy ***because the puncture site may not stop bleeding.***

INDICATIONS

- Aid in the diagnosis of renovascular hypertension.
- Evaluate the cause of blood in the urine.
- Evaluate the effects of urinary system trauma.
- Evaluate function of the kidneys, ureters, and bladder.
- Evaluate known or suspected ureteral obstruction.
- Evaluate the presence of kidney, ureter, or bladder calculi.
- Evaluate space-occupying lesions or congenital anomalies of the urinary system.

POTENTIAL MEDICAL DIAGNOSIS

Normal findings

- Normal size and shape of kidneys, ureters, and bladder
- Normal bladder and absence of masses or renal calculi, with prompt visualization of contrast medium through the urinary system

Abnormal findings related to

- Absence of a kidney (congenital malformation)
- Benign and malignant kidney tumors
- Bladder tumors

- Congenital kidney or urinary tract abnormalities
- Glomerulonephritis
- Hydronephrosis
- Prostatic enlargement
- Pyelonephritis
- Renal cysts
- Renal hematomas
- Renal or ureteral calculi
- Soft tissue masses
- Tumors of the collecting system

CRITICAL FINDINGS: N/A

INTERFERING FACTORS

Factors that may alter the results of the study

- Gas or feces in the gastrointestinal (GI) tract resulting from inadequate cleansing or failure to restrict food intake before the study.
- Retained barium from a previous radiological procedure.
- Metallic objects (e.g., jewelry, body rings) within the examination field, which may inhibit organ visualization and cause unclear images.
- Inability of the patient to cooperate or remain still during the procedure because of age, significant pain, or mental status.

Other considerations

- The procedure may be terminated if chest pain or severe cardiac dysrhythmias occur.
- Failure to follow dietary restrictions and other pretesting preparations may cause the procedure to be canceled or repeated.

NURSING IMPLICATIONS AND PROCEDURE

See Potential Nursing Problems on Fast Find at davispl.us/vanleeuwen7.

PRETEST:

- Positively identify the patient using at least two person-specific identifiers before services, treatments, or procedures are performed.
- *Patient Teaching:* Inform the patient this procedure can assist in assessing the kidneys, ureters, and bladder.
- Obtain a history of the patient's health concerns, symptoms, surgical procedures, and results of previously performed laboratory and diagnostic studies. Include a list of known allergens, especially allergies or sensitivities to latex, anesthetics, sedatives, or contrast medium. Ensure results of coagulation testing are obtained and recorded prior to the procedure; a creatinine level is also needed before contrast medium is to be used.
- Note any recent barium or other radiological contrast procedures. Ensure that barium studies were performed more than 4 days before the IVP.
- Record the date of the last menstrual period and determine the possibility of pregnancy in perimenopausal women.
- Obtain a list of the patient's current medications, including over-the-counter medications, dietary supplements, anticoagulants, aspirin and other salicylates (see Effects of Natural Products on Laboratory Values online at Davis*Plus*). Such products should be discontinued by medical direction for the appropriate number of days prior to a surgical procedure. Note the last time and dose of medication taken.
- If iodinated contrast medium is scheduled to be used in patients receiving metformin for type 2 diabetes, the drug should be discontinued on the day of the test and continue to be withheld for 48 hr after the test. Iodinated contrast can temporarily impair kidney function, and failure to withhold metformin may indirectly result in drug-induced lactic acidosis, a dangerous and sometimes fatal adverse effect of metformin ***(related to renal impairment that does not support sufficient excretion of metformin).***
- Review the procedure with the patient. Address concerns about pain related to the procedure and explain

that some pain may be experienced during the test, and there may be moments of discomfort. Inform the patient that the procedure is performed in a radiology department by a health-care provider (HCP)and takes approximately 30 to 60 min.

- ***Sensitivity to social and cultural issues,*** as well as concern for modesty, is important in providing psychological support before, during, and after the procedure.
- Instruct the patient to take a laxative or a cathartic, as ordered, on the evening before the examination; the bowel must be cleansed to achieve good visualization of the kidneys.
- Explain that an IV line may be inserted to allow infusion of fluids such as saline, anesthetics, sedatives, or emergency medications. Explain that the contrast medium will be injected, by catheter, at a separate site from the IV line.
- Inform the patient that a burning and flushing sensation may be felt throughout the body during injection of the contrast medium. After injection of the contrast medium, the patient may experience an urge to cough, flushing, nausea, or a salty or metallic taste.
- Instruct the patient to remove jewelry and other metallic objects from the area to be examined.
- Instruct the patient to fast and restrict fluids for 8 hr, as ordered, prior to the procedure. Fasting may be ordered as a precaution against aspiration related to possible nausea and vomiting during the administration of contrast. Protocols may vary among facilities. **Pediatric and Older Adult Considerations:** Special considerations regarding fluid restrictions may apply to patients experiencing chronic dehydration including older adult patients in whom dehydration is common; considerations may also be given to pediatric patients. Fluid restrictions for pediatric patients may be adjusted based on age and weight.
- *Make sure a written and informed consent has been signed prior to the procedure and before administering any medications.*

INTRATEST:

Potential Complications:

Allergic reaction to contrast media is a potential complication.

- Ensure the patient has removed all external metallic objects from the area to be examined prior to the procedure.
- Observe standard precautions, and follow the general guidelines in Patient Preparation and Specimen Collection online at Davis*Plus*. Positively identify the patient.
- Ensure the patient has complied with dietary, fluid, and medication restrictions prior to the procedure, as instructed. **Older Adult Considerations:** The combination of fluid restrictions and administration of laxatives may cause increased injury risk from falling for older adult patients, related to weakness. Additional monitoring and assistance while ambulating may be required.
- Assess for completion of bowel preparation according to the institution's procedure. Administer enemas or suppositories on the morning of the test, as ordered.
- Administer ordered prophylactic steroids or antihistamines before the procedure if the patient has a history of allergic reactions to any substance or drug. Use nonionic contrast medium for the procedure.
- Avoid the use of equipment containing latex if the patient has a history of allergic reaction to latex.
- Have emergency equipment readily available.
- Instruct the patient to void prior to the procedure and to change into the gown, robe, and foot coverings provided.
- Instruct the patient to cooperate fully and to follow directions. Instruct the patient to remain still throughout the procedure because movement produces unreliable results.
- Place the patient in the supine position on an examination table.

- A kidney, ureter, and bladder (KUB) or plain film is taken to ensure that no barium or stool obscures visualization of the urinary system.
- Insert an IV line, if one is not already in place, and inject the contrast medium.
- Instruct the patient to take slow, deep breaths if nausea occurs during the procedure.
- Monitor the patient for complications related to the procedure (e.g., allergic reaction, anaphylaxis, bronchospasm).
- Images are taken at 1, 5, 10, 15, 20, and 30 min following injection of the contrast medium into the urinary system. Instruct the patient to exhale deeply and to hold his or her breath while each image is taken.
- Remove the needle or catheter and apply a pressure dressing over the puncture site.
- Instruct the patient to void if a postvoiding exposure is required to visualize the empty bladder.

POST-TEST:

- Inform the patient that a report of the results will be made available to the requesting HCP, who will discuss the results with the patient.
- Instruct the patient to resume usual diet, fluids, medications, and activity, as directed by the HCP. Kidney function should be assessed before metformin is resumed if contrast was used.
- Observe for delayed reaction to iodinated contrast medium, including rash, urticaria, tachycardia, hyperpnea, hypertension, palpitations, nausea, or vomiting.
- Observe/assess the needle/catheter insertion site for bleeding, inflammation, or hematoma formation.
- Instruct the patient in the care and assessment of the injection site.
- Instruct the patient to apply cold compresses to the puncture site as needed, to reduce discomfort or edema.
- Monitor urinary output after the procedure. Decreased urine output may indicate impending renal failure.
- Recognize anxiety related to test results, and offer support. Discuss the implications of abnormal test results on the patient's lifestyle. Provide teaching and information regarding the clinical implications of the test results, as appropriate.
- Reinforce information given by the patient's HCP regarding further testing, treatment, or referral to another HCP. Answer any questions or address any concerns voiced by the patient or family.
- Depending on the results of this procedure, additional testing may be needed to evaluate or monitor progression of the disease process and determine the need for a change in therapy. Evaluate test results in relation to the patient's symptoms and other tests performed.

Patient Education:

- Teach the patient how to strain urine and to report any blood noted in the urine.
- Teach the patient the symptoms of infection that should be reported to the HCP.

Expected Patient Outcomes:

Understanding

- The patient and family state the importance of increasing oral fluid intake to facilitate stone removal.
- The patient and family state the importance of straining all urine to identify when a stone has passed.

Ability

- The patient successfully demonstrates the knees to chest position to decrease discomfort.
- The patient demonstrates relaxation techniques that successfully decrease pain.

Response

- The patient agrees to avoid high-calcium fluids (dairy, chocolate).
- The patient agrees to maintain in increased oral intake to mitigate stone reoccurrence.

RELATED STUDIES:

- Related tests include biopsy bladder, biopsy kidney, biopsy prostate, BUN, CT abdomen, CT kidneys, CT pelvis, creatinine, cystometry, cystoscopy, gallium scan, KUB, MRI abdomen, renogram, retrograde ureteropyelography, US abdomen, US bladder, US kidney, US prostate, urine markers of bladder cancer, urinalysis, urine cytology, and voiding cystourethrography.

- Refer to the Genitourinary System table online at Davis*Plus* for related tests by body system.

Intrinsic Factor Antibodies

SYNONYM/ACRONYM: IF antibodies, intrinsic factor blocking antibodies.

COMMON USE: To assist in the investigation of suspected pernicious anemia.

SPECIMEN: Serum collected in a gold-, red-, or red/gray-top tube. Place separated serum into a standard transport tube within 2 hr of collection.

NORMAL FINDINGS: (Method: Immunoassay) Negative.

POTENTIAL MEDICAL DIAGNOSIS

Increased in:

Conditions that involve the production of these blocking and binding autoantibodies

- Megaloblastic anemia
- Pernicious anemia
- Some patients with hyperthyroidism
- Some patients with type 1 diabetes

Decreased in: N/A

CRITICAL FINDINGS: N/A

Find and print out the full study on Fast Find at davispl.us/vanleeuwen7.

Iron

SYNONYM/ACRONYM: Fe.

COMMON USE: To monitor and assess blood iron levels related to treatment, blood loss, metabolism, anemia, and storage disorders.

SPECIMEN: Serum collected in a gold-, red-, or red/gray-top tube.

NORMAL FINDINGS: (Method: Spectrophotometry)

Age	Conventional Units	SI Units (Conventional Units × 0.179)
Newborn	100–250 mcg/dL	17.9–44.8 micromol/L
Infant–9 yr	20–105 mcg/dL	3.6–18.8 micromol/L
10–14 yr	20–145 mcg/dL	3.6–26 micromol/L
Adult		
Male	65–175 mcg/dL	11.6–31.3 micromol/L
Female	50–170 mcg/dL	9–30.4 micromol/L

Values tend to decrease in older adults.

DESCRIPTION: Iron plays a principal role in erythropoiesis, the formation and maturation of red blood cells (RBCs), and is required for hemoglobin (Hgb) synthesis. The human body contains between 4 and 5 grams of iron, about 65% of which is present in hemoglobin and 3% of which is present in myoglobin, the oxygen storage protein found in skeletal and cardiac muscle. A small amount is also found in cellular enzymes that catalyze the oxidation and reduction of iron. Excess iron is stored in the liver and spleen as ferritin and hemosiderin. Any iron present in the serum is in transit between the alimentary tract, the bone marrow, and available iron storage forms. Sixty to seventy percent of the body's iron is carried by its specific transport protein, transferrin. Normally, iron enters the body by oral ingestion; only 10% is absorbed, but as much as 20% to 30% can be absorbed in patients with iron-deficiency anemia. Unbound iron is highly toxic, but there is generally an excess of transferrin available to prevent the buildup of unbound iron in the circulation. Iron overload is as clinically significant as iron deficiency. An example of acute iron overload is the accidental poisoning of children caused by excessive intake of iron-containing multivitamins. Chronic iron overload can occur in patients receiving serial therapeutic transfusions of red blood cells over time for treatment of various cancers, hemoglobinopathies such as sickle cell anemia, the thalassemias, and other hemolytic anemias.

This procedure is contraindicated for: N/A

INDICATIONS

- Assist in the diagnosis of blood loss, as evidenced by decreased serum iron.
- Assist in the diagnosis of hemochromatosis or other disorders of iron metabolism and storage.
- Determine the differential diagnosis of anemia.
- Determine the presence of disorders that involve diminished protein synthesis or defects in iron absorption.
- Evaluate accidental iron poisoning.
- Evaluate iron overload in dialysis patients or patients with transfusion-dependent anemias.
- Evaluate thalassemia and sideroblastic anemia.
- Monitor hematological responses during pregnancy, when serum iron is usually decreased.
- Monitor response to treatment for anemia.

POTENTIAL MEDICAL DIAGNOSIS

Increased in:

- Acute iron poisoning (children) ***(related to excessive intake)***
- Acute leukemia
- Acute liver disease ***(possibly related to decrease in synthesis of iron storage proteins by damaged liver; iron accumulates and levels increase)***
- Aplastic anemia ***(related to repeated blood transfusions)***
- Excessive iron therapy ***(related to excessive intake)***
- Hemochromatosis ***(inherited disorder of iron overload; the iron is not excreted in proportion to the rate of accumulation)***
- Hemolytic anemias ***(related to release of iron from lysed RBCs)***
- Lead toxicity ***(lead can biologically mimic iron, displace it, and release it into circulation where its concentration increases)***

I

- Nephritis ***(related to decreased renal excretion; accumulation in blood)***
- Pernicious anemias (PA) ***(achlorhydria associated with PA prevents absorption of dietary iron, and it accumulates in the blood)***
- Sideroblastic anemias ***(enzyme disorder prevents iron from being incorporated into Hgb, and it accumulates in the blood)***
- Thalassemia ***(treatment for some types of thalassemia include blood transfusions, which can lead to iron overload)***
- Transfusions (repeated)
- Vitamin B_6 deficiency ***(this vitamin is essential to Hgb formation; deficiency prevents iron from being incorporated into Hgb, and it accumulates in the blood)***

Decreased in:

- Acute and chronic infection ***(iron is a nutrient for invading organisms)***
- Carcinoma ***(related to depletion of iron stores)***
- Chronic blood loss (gastrointestinal, uterine) ***(blood contains iron incorporated in Hgb)***
- Dietary deficiency
- Hypothyroidism ***(pathophysiology is unclear)***
- Intestinal malabsorption
- Iron-deficiency anemia ***(related to depletion of iron stores)***
- Nephrosis ***(anemia is common in people with kidney disease; fewer RBCs are made because of a deficiency of erythropoietin related to the damaged kidneys, blood can be lost in dialysis, and iron intake may be lower due to lack of appetite)***
- Postoperative state
- Pregnancy ***(related to depletion of iron stores by developing fetus)***
- Protein malnutrition (kwashiorkor) ***(protein is required to form transport proteins, RBCs, and Hgb)***

CRITICAL FINDINGS:

- Mild toxicity: Greater than 350 mcg/dL (SI: Greater than 62.6 micromol/L)
- Serious toxicity: Greater than 400 mcg/dL (SI: Greater than 71.6 micromol/L)
- Lethal: Greater than 1,000 mcg/dL (SI: Greater than 179 micromol/L)

Note and immediately report to the requesting health-care provider (HCP) any critical findings and related symptoms. A listing of these findings varies among facilities. Timely notification of a critical finding for laboratory or diagnostic studies is a role expectation of the professional nurse. The notification processes vary among facilities. Upon receipt of the critical finding, the information should be read back to the caller to verify accuracy.

Intervention may include chelation therapy by administration of deferoxamine mesylate (Desferal).

INTERFERING FACTORS

- Drugs and other substances that may increase iron levels include blood transfusion products, chemotherapy drugs, iron (intramuscular), iron dextran, iron-protein-succinylate, methimazole, methotrexate, oral contraceptives, and rifampin.
- Drugs and other substances that may decrease iron levels include acetylsalicylic acid, allopurinol, cholestyramine, corticotropin, cortisone, deferoxamine mesylate, and metformin.
- Gross hemolysis can interfere with test results.
- Failure to withhold iron-containing medications 24 hr before the test may falsely increase values.
- Failure to follow dietary restrictions before the procedure may cause the procedure to be canceled or repeated.

NURSING IMPLICATIONS AND PROCEDURE

POTENTIAL NURSING PROBLEMS:

Problem	Signs & Symptoms	Interventions
Fatigue ***(related to decreased oxygenation associated with unhealthy red blood cells secondary to inadequate iron)***	Verbalization of fatigue; altered ability to perform activities of daily living due to lack of energy; shortness of breath with exertion; increasingly frequent rest periods; presence of fatigue after sleep; inability to adhere to daily routine; altered level of concentration; complaints of tiredness	Monitor and trend CBC, Hgb, hematocrit (Hct), iron; monitor for shortness of breath; administer oxygen and use pulse oximetry as appropriate; assess ability to perform self-care; assess nutritional intake of iron-rich foods; encourage frequent rest periods; teach techniques for conserving energy expenditure; administer blood and blood products as ordered; administer prescribed iron supplements; monitor urine, stool, and sputum for bleeding; assess for medical or psychological factors contributing to fatigue; prioritize and bundle activities to conserve energy and decrease fatigue
Tissue perfusion (cerebral, peripheral, renal) ***(related to inadequate cellular oxygen associated with unhealthy red blood cells secondary to iron deficiency)***	Confusion; altered mental status; headaches; dizziness; visual disturbances; hypotension; dizziness; cool extremities; capillary refill greater than 3 sec; weak pedal pulses; altered level of consciousness; decreased urine output	Monitor blood pressure; assess for dizziness; check skin temperature for warmth; assess capillary refill; assess pedal pulses; monitor level of consciousness; monitor urine output to be in excess of 30 mL/hr; ensure adequate fluid intake or administer intravenous fluids as ordered; administer prescribed iron supplements
Nutrition ***(related to inability to digest foods, metabolize foods, ingest foods; refusal***	Unintended weight loss; current weight is 20% below ideal weight; pale dry skin; dry mucous membranes;	Record accurate daily weight at the same time each day with the same scale; obtain an accurate nutritional history; assess attitude toward eating; promote a dietary consult

(table continues on page 1002)

Problem	Signs & Symptoms	Interventions
to eat; increased metabolic needs associated with disease process; lack of understanding; unable to obtain healthy iron-rich foods)	documented inadequate caloric intake; subcutaneous tissue loss; hair pulls out easily; paresthesia	to evaluate current eating habits and best method of nutritional supplementation focusing on iron-rich foods; develop short- and long-term eating strategies; monitor serum iron; assess swallowing ability; encourage iron-rich cultural home foods; provide a pleasant environment for eating; alter food seasoning to enhance flavor; provide parenteral or enteral nutrition as prescribed
Bleeding loss ***(related to heavy menses; disease process with chronic blood loss [GI ulcer, malignancy]; overuse of NSAIDs)***	Altered level of consciousness; hypotension; increased heart rate; decreased Hgb and Hct; decreased serum iron; capillary refill greater than 3 sec; cool extremities; poor dietary selections	Monitor serum iron; increase frequency of vital sign assessment with variances in results; monitor for vital sign trends; administer blood or blood products as ordered; assess for disease process that may contribute to chronic blood loss; administer prescribed iron; assess stool for blood; consider dietary consult to support changed dietary selections; assess diet for iron-rich foods, and foods that inhibit absorption of iron

PRETEST:

- Positively identify the patient using at least two person-specific identifiers before services, treatments, or procedures are performed.
- *Patient Teaching:* Inform the patient this test can assist in evaluating the amount of iron in the blood.
- Obtain a history of the patient's health concerns, symptoms, surgical procedures, and results of previously performed laboratory and diagnostic studies. Include a list of known allergens, especially allergies or sensitivities to latex.
- Note any recent therapies that can interfere with test results. Specimen collection should be delayed for several days after blood transfusion.
- Obtain a list of the patient's current medications, including over-the-counter medications and dietary supplements (see Effects of Natural Products on Laboratory Values online at Davis*Plus*).
- Review the procedure with the patient. Inform the patient that specimen collection takes approximately 5 to 10 min. Address concerns about pain and explain that there may be some discomfort during the venipuncture.
- ***Sensitivity to social and cultural issues,*** as well as concern for modesty, is important in providing psychological support before, during, and after the procedure.
- Instruct the patient to fast for at least 12 hr before testing and, with medical

direction, to refrain from taking iron-containing medicines before specimen collection. Protocols may vary among facilities.

- Note that there are no fluid restrictions unless by medical direction.

INTRATEST:

Potential Complications: N/A

- Ensure that the patient has complied with dietary and medication restrictions prior to the procedure, as instructed.
- Avoid the use of equipment containing latex if the patient has a history of allergic reaction to latex.
- Instruct the patient to cooperate fully and to follow directions. Direct the patient to breathe normally and to avoid unnecessary movement.
- Observe standard precautions, and follow the general guidelines in Patient Preparation and Specimen Collection online at Davis*Plus*. Positively identify the patient, and label the appropriate specimen container with the corresponding patient demographics, initials of the person collecting the specimen, date, and time of collection. Perform a venipuncture.
- Remove the needle and apply direct pressure with dry gauze to stop bleeding. Observe/assess venipuncture site for bleeding or hematoma formation and secure gauze with adhesive bandage.
- Promptly transport the specimen to the laboratory for processing and analysis.

POST-TEST:

- Inform the patient that a report of the results will be made available to the requesting HCP, who will discuss the results with the patient.
- Instruct the patient to resume usual diet, fluids, medications, or activity, as directed by the HCP.
- *Nutritional Considerations:* Educate the patient with abnormally elevated iron values, as appropriate, on the importance of reading food labels. Foods high in iron include meats (especially liver), eggs, grains, and green leafy vegetables. It is also important to explain that iron levels in foods can be increased if foods are cooked in cookware containing iron.
- Depending on the results of this procedure, additional testing may be performed to evaluate or monitor progression of the disease process and determine the need for a change in therapy. Evaluate test results in relation to the patient's symptoms and other tests performed.

Patient Education:

- Patients must be educated to either increase or avoid intake of iron and iron-rich foods depending on their specific condition; for example, a patient with hemochromatosis or acute pernicious anemia should be educated to avoid foods rich in iron.
- Explain to the patient that the consumption of large amounts of alcohol damages the intestine and allows for the increased absorption of iron.
- Educate the patient that iron absorption is decreased by the absence (gastric resection) or diminished presence (use of antacids) of gastric acid.
- Teach the patient that phytic acids from cereals, tannins from tea and coffee, oxalic acid from vegetables, and minerals such as copper, zinc, and manganese interfere with iron absorption.
- Teach patient that iron absorption after a meal is also increased by factors in meat, fish, and poultry as well as by a high intake of calcium and ascorbic acid.
- Reinforce information given by the patient's HCP regarding further testing, treatment, or referral to another HCP.
- Answer any questions or address any concerns voiced by the patient or family. Educate the patient regarding access to nutritional counseling services.
- Provide contact information, if desired, for the the Institute of Medicine of the National Academies (www.iom.edu) or the USDA's resource for nutrition (www.choosemyplate.gov).

I

Expected Patient Outcomes:

Understanding

- The patient and family state factors that affect the absorption of iron, enhancing or decreasing absorption regardless of the original content of the iron-containing dietary source.

Ability

- The patient demonstrates proficiency in taking ordered iron supplements in a manner that enhances absorption.
- The patient demonstrates proficiency in selecting foods that are high in iron.

Response

- The patient complies with recommended lifestyle changes to increase or decrease iron intake based on laboratory results.
- The patient and family understand that a blood transfusion may be necessary to replace lost iron stores quickly to maintain health.

RELATED STUDIES:

- Related tests include biopsy bone marrow, biopsy liver, CBC, CBC RBC count, CBC RBC indices, CBC RBC morphology, CBC WBC count and differential, erythropoietin, ferritin, folate, FEP, gallium scan, hemosiderin, iron binding/transferrin, lead, porphyrins, reticulocyte count, and vitamin B_{12}.
- Refer to the Gastrointestinal and Hematopoietic systems tables online at Davis*Plus* for related tests by body system.

Iron-Binding Capacity (Total), Transferrin, and Iron Saturation

SYNONYM/ACRONYM: TIBC, Fe Sat.

COMMON USE: To monitor iron replacement therapy and assess blood iron levels to assist in diagnosing types of anemia such as iron deficiency.

SPECIMEN: Serum collected in a gold-, red-, or red/gray-top tube.

NORMAL FINDINGS: (Method: Spectrophotometry for TIBC and nephelometry for transferrin)

Test	Conventional Units	SI Units
		(Conventional Units × 0.179)
TIBC	250–450 mcg/dL	45–81 micromol/L
		(Conventional Units × 0.01)
Transferrin	215–380 mg/dL	2.15–3.8 g/L
Iron saturation		
Males	10%–50%	10%–50%
Females	15%–50%	15%–50%

TIBC = total iron-binding capacity.

DESCRIPTION: Iron plays a principal role in erythropoiesis, the formation and maturation of red blood cells (RBCs), and is required for hemoglobin (Hgb) synthesis. The human body contains between 4 and 5 grams of iron, about 65% of which is present in hemoglobin and 3% of which is present in myoglobin, the oxygen storage protein found in skeletal and cardiac muscle. A small amount is also found in cellular enzymes that catalyze the oxidation and reduction of iron. Excess iron is stored in the liver and spleen as ferritin and hemosiderin. Any iron present in the serum is in transit between the alimentary tract, the bone marrow, and available iron storage forms. Sixty to seventy percent of the body's iron is carried by its specific transport protein, transferrin. For this reason, total iron-binding capacity (TIBC) and transferrin are sometimes referred to interchangeably, even though other proteins carry iron and contribute to the TIBC. Unbound iron is highly toxic, but there is generally an excess of transferrin available to prevent the buildup of unbound iron in the circulation. The percentage of iron saturation is calculated by dividing the serum iron value by the TIBC value and multiplying by 100.

This procedure is contraindicated for: N/A

INDICATIONS

- Assist in the diagnosis of iron-deficiency anemia.
- Differentiate between iron-deficiency anemia and anemia secondary to chronic disease.
- Monitor hematological response to therapy during pregnancy and iron-deficiency anemias.
- Provide support for diagnosis of hemochromatosis or diseases of iron metabolism and storage.

POTENTIAL MEDICAL DIAGNOSIS

Increased in:

- Acute liver disease
- Hypochromic (iron-deficiency) anemias ***(insufficient circulating iron levels to saturate binding sites)***
- Late pregnancy

Decreased in:

- Chronic infections ***(transferrin is a negative acute-phase reactant protein that demonstrates decreased levels during periods of inflammation)***
- Cirrhosis ***(transferrin is a negative acute-phase reactant protein that demonstrates decreased levels during periods of inflammation)***
- Hemochromatosis ***(occurs early in the disease as intestinal absorption of iron available for binding increases)***
- Hemolytic anemias ***(transferrin becomes saturated, and the iron-binding capacity is significantly decreased)***
- Kidney disease ***(transferrin is a negative acute-phase reactant protein that demonstrates decreased levels during periods of inflammation)***
- Neoplastic diseases ***(transferrin is a negative acute-phase reactant protein that demonstrates decreased levels during periods of inflammation)***
- Protein depletion ***(transferrin contributes to the total protein concentration and will reflect a decrease in protein depletion)***
- Sideroblastic anemias ***(transferrin becomes saturated, and the iron-binding capacity is significantly decreased)***
- Thalassemia ***(transferrin becomes saturated, and the iron-binding capacity is significantly decreased)***

CRITICAL FINDINGS: N/A

INTERFERING FACTORS

- Drugs and other substances that may increase TIBC levels include mestranol and oral contraceptives.
- Drugs and other substances that may decrease TIBC levels include asparaginase, chloramphenicol, corticotropin, cortisone, and testosterone.

NURSING IMPLICATIONS AND PROCEDURE

PRETEST:

- Positively identify the patient using at least two person-specific identifiers before services, treatments, or procedures are performed.
- *Patient Teaching:* Inform the patient this test can assist in diagnosing anemia.
- Obtain a history of the patient's health concerns, symptoms, surgical procedures, and results of previously performed laboratory and diagnostic studies. Include a list of known allergens, especially allergies or sensitivities to latex.
- Obtain a list of the patient's current medications, including over-the-counter medications and dietary supplements (see Effects of Natural Products on Laboratory Values online at Davis*Plus*).
- Review the procedure with the patient. Inform the patient that specimen collection takes approximately 5 to 10 min. Address concerns about pain and explain that there may be some discomfort during the venipuncture.
- *Sensitivity to social and cultural issues,* as well as concern for modesty, is important in providing psychological support before, during, and after the procedure.
- Note that there are no food, fluid, or medication restrictions unless by medical direction.

INTRATEST:

Potential Complications: N/A

- Avoid the use of equipment containing latex if the patient has a history of allergic reaction to latex.
- Instruct the patient to cooperate fully and to follow directions. Direct the patient to breathe normally and to avoid unnecessary movement.
- Observe standard precautions, and follow the general guidelines in Patient Preparation and Specimen Collection online at Davis*Plus*. Positively identify the patient, and label the appropriate specimen container with the corresponding patient demographics, initials of the person collecting the specimen, date, and time of collection. Perform a venipuncture.
- Remove the needle and apply direct pressure with dry gauze to stop bleeding. Observe/assess venipuncture site for bleeding or hematoma formation and secure gauze with adhesive bandage.
- Promptly transport the specimen to the laboratory for processing and analysis.

POST-TEST:

- Inform the patient that a report of the results will be made available to the requesting health-care provider (HCP), who will discuss the results with the patient.
- Reinforce information given by the patient's HCP regarding further testing, treatment, or referral to another HCP. Answer any questions or address any concerns voiced by the patient or family.
- Depending on the results of this procedure, additional testing may be performed to evaluate or monitor progression of the disease process and determine the need for a change in therapy. Evaluate test results in relation to the patient's symptoms and other tests performed.

RELATED STUDIES:

- Related tests include biopsy bone marrow, biopsy liver, CBC, CBC RBC count, CBC RBC indices, CBC RBC morphology, CBC WBC count and differential, erythropoietin, ferritin, folate, FEP, gallium scan, hemosiderin, lead, porphyrins, reticulocyte count, and vitamin B_{12}.
- Refer to the Hematopoietic System table online at Davis*Plus* for related tests by body system.

Ketones, Blood and Urine

SYNONYM/ACRONYM: Ketone bodies, acetoacetate, acetone.

COMMON USE: To investigate diabetes as the cause of ketoacidosis and monitor therapeutic interventions.

SPECIMEN: Serum collected from gold-, red-, or red/gray-top tube. Urine, random or timed specimen, collected in a clean plastic collection container.

NORMAL FINDINGS: (Method: Colorimetric nitroprusside reaction) Negative.

DESCRIPTION: Ketone bodies refer to the three intermediate products of metabolism: acetone, acetoacetic acid, and β-hydroxybutyrate. Even though β-hydroxybutyrate is not a ketone, it is usually listed with the ketone bodies. In healthy individuals, ketones are produced and completely metabolized by the liver so that measurable amounts are not normally present in serum. Ketones appear in the urine before a significant serum level is detectable. If the patient has excessive fat metabolism, ketones are found in blood and urine. Excessive fat metabolism may occur if the patient has impaired ability to metabolize carbohydrates, inadequate carbohydrate intake, inadequate insulin levels, excessive carbohydrate loss, or increased carbohydrate demand. A strongly positive acetone result without severe acidosis, accompanied by normal glucose, electrolyte, and bicarbonate levels, is strongly suggestive of isopropyl alcohol poisoning. A low-carbohydrate or high-fat diet may cause a positive acetone test. Ketosis in people with diabetes is usually accompanied by increased glucose and decreased bicarbonate and pH. Extremely elevated levels of ketone bodies can result in coma. This situation is particularly life threatening in children younger than 10 yr.

This procedure is contraindicated for: N/A

INDICATIONS

- Assist in the diagnosis of starvation, stress, alcoholism, suspected isopropyl alcohol ingestion, glycogen storage disease, and other metabolic disorders.
- Detect and monitor treatment of diabetic ketoacidosis.
- Monitor the control of diabetes.
- Screen for ketonuria due to acute illness or stress in nondiabetic patients.
- Screen for ketonuria to assist in the assessment of inborn errors of metabolism.
- Screen for ketonuria to assist in the diagnosis of suspected isopropyl alcohol poisoning.

POTENTIAL MEDICAL DIAGNOSIS

Increased in:

Ketones are generated in conditions that involve the metabolism of carbohydrates, fatty acids, and protein.

- Acidosis
- Branched-chain ketonuria
- Carbohydrate deficiency
- Eclampsia
- Fasting or starvation
- Gestational diabetes
- Glycogen storage diseases
- High-fat or high-protein diet
- Hyperglycemia
- Ketoacidosis of alcoholism and diabetes
- Illnesses with marked vomiting and diarrhea

- Isopropyl alcohol ingestion
- Methylmalonic aciduria
- Postanesthesia period
- Propionyl coenzyme A carboxylase deficiency

Decreased in: N/A

CRITICAL FINDINGS:

- Strongly positive test results for glucose and ketones

Note and immediately report to the requesting health-care provider (HCP) any critical findings and related symptoms. A listing of these findings varies among facilities. Timely notification of a critical finding for laboratory or diagnostic studies is a role expectation of the professional nurse. The notification processes vary among facilities. Upon receipt of the critical finding, the information should be read back to the caller to verify accuracy.

Consideration may be given to verification of critical findings before action is taken. Policies vary among facilities and may include requesting immediate recollection and retesting by the laboratory or retesting using a rapid point-of-care testing instrument at the bedside, if available.

An elevated level of ketone bodies is evidenced by fruity-smelling breath, acidosis, ketonuria, and decreased level of consciousness. Administration of insulin and frequent blood glucose measurement may be indicated.

INTERFERING FACTORS

- Drugs and other substances that may cause an increase in serum ketone levels include acetylsalicylic acid (if therapy results in acidosis, especially in children), albuterol, nifedipine, and rimiterol. Increases have been shown in hyperthyroid patients receiving propranolol hydrochloride and propylthiouracil.
- Drugs and other substances that may cause a decrease in serum ketone levels include acetylsalicylic acid and valproic acid.
- Drugs and other substances that may increase urine ketone levels include acetylsalicylic acid (if therapy results in acidosis, especially in children), ether, metformin, and niacin.
- Drugs and other substances that may decrease urine ketone levels include acetylsalicylic acid.
- Urine should be checked within 60 min of collection.
- Bacterial contamination of urine can cause false-negative results.
- Failure to keep reagent strip container tightly closed can cause false-negative results. Light and moisture affect the ability of the chemicals in the strip to perform as expected.
- False-negative or weakly false-positive test results can be obtained when β-hydroxybutyrate is the predominating ketone body in cases of lactic acidosis.

NURSING IMPLICATIONS AND PROCEDURE

PRETEST:

- Positively identify the patient using at least two person-specific identifiers before services, treatments, or procedures are performed.
- ***Patient Teaching:*** Inform the patient this test can assist in diagnosing metabolic disorders such as diabetes.
- Obtain a history of the patient's health concerns, symptoms, surgical procedures, and results of previously performed laboratory and diagnostic studies. Include a list of known allergens, especially allergies or sensitivities to latex.
- Obtain a list of the patient's current medications, including over-the-counter medications and dietary supplements (see Effects of Natural

Products on Laboratory Values online at Davis*Plus*).

- Review the procedure with the patient. Inform the patient that blood specimen collection takes approximately 5 to 10 min. The amount of time required to collect a urine specimen depends on the level of cooperation from the patient. Address concerns about pain and explain that there may be some discomfort during the venipuncture.
- ***Sensitivity to social and cultural issues,*** as well as concern for modesty, is important in providing psychological support before, during, and after the procedure.
- Note that there are no food, fluid, or medication restrictions, unless by medical direction.

INTRATEST:

Potential Complications: N/A

- Observe standard precautions, and follow the general guidelines in Patient Preparation and Specimen Collection online at Davis*Plus*. Positively identify the patient, and label the appropriate specimen container with the corresponding patient demographics, initials of the person collecting the specimen, date, and time of collection. Perform a venipuncture as appropriate.

Blood

- Avoid the use of equipment containing latex if the patient has a history of allergic reaction to latex.
- Instruct the patient to cooperate fully and to follow directions. Direct the patient to breathe normally and to avoid unnecessary movement.
- Positively identify the patient, and label the appropriate specimen container with the corresponding patient demographics, initials of the person collecting the specimen, date, and time of collection. Perform a venipuncture. Alternatively, a fingerstick or heel stick method of specimen collection can be used.
- Remove the needle and apply direct pressure with dry gauze to stop bleeding. Observe/assess venipuncture site for bleeding or hematoma formation and secure gauze with adhesive bandage.

Urine

- Review the procedure with the patient. Explain to the patient how to collect a second-voided midstream void, then drink a glass of water, wait 30 min, and then try to void again.
- Instruct the patient to avoid excessive exercise and stress before specimen collection.

Clean-Catch Specimen

- Instruct the male patient to (1) thoroughly wash his hands, (2) cleanse the meatus, (3) void a small amount into the toilet, and (4) void directly into the specimen container.
- Instruct the female patient to (1) thoroughly wash her hands; (2) cleanse the labia from front to back; (3) while keeping the labia separated, void a small amount into the toilet; and (4) without interrupting the urine stream, void directly into the specimen container.

Blood or Urine

- Promptly transport the specimen to the laboratory for processing and analysis.

POST-TEST:

- Inform the patient that a report of the results will be made available to the requesting HCP, who will discuss the results with the patient.
- ***Nutritional Considerations:*** Increased levels of ketone bodies may be associated with diabetes. There is no "diabetic diet"; however, many meal-planning approaches with nutritional goals are endorsed by the American Diabetes Association (ADA). 🍁 Patients who adhere to dietary recommendations report a better general feeling of health, better weight management, greater control of glucose and lipid values, and improved use of insulin. Instruct the patient, as appropriate, in nutritional management of diabetes. A variety of dietary patterns are beneficial for people with diabetes. The Mediterranean-style diet emphasizes

inclusion of vegetables, whole grains, fruits, low-fat dairy, nuts, legumes, and nontropical vegetable oils (e.g., olive, canola, peanut, sunflower, flaxseed) along with fish and lean poultry. A similar dietary pattern known as the Dietary Approaches to Stop Hypertension (DASH) diet makes additional recommendations for the reduction of dietary sodium. Both dietary styles emphasize a reduction in consumption of red meats, which are high in saturated fats and cholesterol, and other foods containing sugar, saturated fats, trans fats, and sodium. A vegetarian diet as well as other potential weight loss diets such as Weight Watchers are also supported by the ADA. 🍁 If triglycerides also are elevated, the patient should be advised to eliminate or reduce alcohol. The nutritional needs of each patient with diabetic patient need to be determined individually (especially during pregnancy) with the appropriate HCPs, particularly professionals educated in nutrition.

K

- Impaired glucose tolerance may be associated with diabetes. Instruct the patient and caregiver to report signs and symptoms of hypoglycemia (weakness, confusion, diaphoresis, rapid pulse) or hyperglycemia (thirst, polyuria, hunger, lethargy).
- ***Nutritional Considerations:*** Increased levels of ketone bodies may be associated with poor carbohydrate intake in an unbalanced diet; therefore, the body breaks down fat instead of carbohydrate for energy. Increasing carbohydrate intake in the patient's diet reduces the levels of ketone bodies. Carbohydrates can be found in starches and sugars. Starch is a complex carbohydrate that can be found in foods such as grains (breads, cereals, pasta, rice) and starchy vegetables (corn, peas, potatoes). Sugar is a simple carbohydrate that can be found in natural foods (fruits and natural honey) and processed foods (desserts and candy).
- Recognize anxiety related to test results, and be supportive of perceived loss of independence and fear of shortened life expectancy. Discuss the implications of abnormal test results on the patient's lifestyle. Provide teaching and information regarding the clinical implications of the test results, as appropriate. Emphasize, if indicated, that good glycemic control delays the onset and slows the progression of diabetic retinopathy, nephropathy, and neuropathy. Educate the patient regarding access to counseling services, as appropriate. Provide contact information, if desired, for the American Heart Association (www.americanheart.org), National Heart, Lung, and Blood Institute (www.nhlbi.nih.gov), Institute of Medicine of the National Academies (www.iom.edu), and USDA's resource for nutrition (www.choosemyplate.gov). 🍁
- Reinforce information given by the patient's HCP regarding further testing, treatment, or referral to another HCP. Answer any questions or address any concerns voiced by the patient or family.
- Depending on the results of this procedure, additional testing may be performed to evaluate or monitor progression of the disease process and determine the need for a change in therapy. The ADA recommends A_{1C} testing four times a year for type 1 or type 2 diabetes when glycemic targets are not being met or when therapy has changed and twice a year when treatment goals are being met for type 2 diabetes. The ADA also recommends that testing for diabetes commence at age 45 for asymptomatic individuals, be considered for adults of any age who are overweight and have additional risk factors, and continue every 3 yr in the absence of symptoms. 🍁 Evaluate test results in relation to the patient's symptoms and other tests performed.

RELATED STUDIES:

- Related tests include ACTH, angiography adrenal, anion gap, blood gases, BUN, calcium, catecholamines, cholesterol (HDL, LDL, total), cortisol, C-peptide, DHEA, electrolytes, fecal analysis, fecal fat, fluorescein angiography, fructosamine, fundoscopy, gastric emptying scan, GTT, glycated hemoglobin A_{1C}, HVA, insulin, insulin antibodies, lactic acid, lipoprotein electrophoresis, metanephrines, microalbumin, osmolality, phosphorus, UA, and visual fields test.

- Refer to the Endocrine System table online at Davis*Plus* for related tests by body system.

Kidney, Ureter, and Bladder Study

SYNONYM/ACRONYM: Flat plate of the abdomen, kidney, urine, and bladder (KUB), plain film of the abdomen.

COMMON USE: To visualize and assess the abdominal organs for obstruction or abnormality related to mass, trauma, bleeding, stones, or congenital anomaly.

AREA OF APPLICATION: Kidneys, ureters, bladder, and abdomen.

DESCRIPTION: A KUB x-ray examination provides information regarding the structure, size, and position of the abdominal organs; it also indicates whether there is any obstruction or abnormality of the abdomen caused by disease or congenital malformation. Calcifications of the renal calyces, renal pelvis, and any radiopaque calculi present in the urinary tract or surrounding organs may be visualized in addition to normal air and gas patterns within the intestinal tract. Perforation of the intestinal tract or an intestinal obstruction can be visualized on erect KUB images. KUB x-rays are among the first examinations done to diagnose intra-abdominal diseases such as intestinal obstruction, masses, tumors, ruptured organs, abnormal gas accumulation, and ascites.

This procedure is contraindicated for

Patients who are pregnant or suspected of being pregnant, unless the potential benefits of a procedure using radiation far outweigh the risk of radiation exposure to the fetus and mother.

INDICATIONS

- Determine the cause of acute abdominal pain or palpable mass.
- Evaluate the effects of lower abdominal trauma, such as internal hemorrhage.
- Evaluate known or suspected intestinal obstructions.
- Evaluate the presence of renal, ureter, or other organ calculi.
- Evaluate the size, shape, and position of the liver, kidneys, and spleen.
- Evaluate suspected abnormal fluid, air, or metallic objects in the abdomen.

POTENTIAL MEDICAL DIAGNOSIS

Normal findings

- Normal size and shape of kidneys
- Normal bladder, absence of masses and renal calculi, and no abnormal accumulation of air or fluid

Abnormal findings related to

- Abnormal accumulation of bowel gas
- Ascites

- Bladder distention
- Congenital renal anomaly
- Foreign body
- Hydronephrosis
- Intestinal obstruction
- Organomegaly
- Renal calculi
- Renal hematomas
- Ruptured viscus
- Soft tissue masses
- Trauma to liver, spleen, kidneys, and bladder
- Vascular calcification

CRITICAL FINDINGS:

- Bowel obstruction
- Ischemic bowel
- Visceral injury

Note and immediately report to the requesting health-care provider (HCP) any critical findings and related symptoms. A listing of these findings varies among facilities. Timely notification of a critical finding for laboratory or diagnostic studies is a role expectation of the professional nurse. The notification processes vary among facilities. Upon receipt of the critical finding, the information should be read back to the caller to verify accuracy.

INTERFERING FACTORS:

Factors that may alter the results of the study

- Inability of the patient to cooperate or remain still during the procedure because of age, significant pain, or mental status.
- Metallic objects (e.g., jewelry, body rings) within the examination field, which may inhibit organ visualization and cause unclear images.
- Improper adjustment of the radiographic equipment to accommodate obese or thin patients, which can cause overexposure or underexposure and a poor-quality study.
- Incorrect positioning of the patient, which may produce poor visualization of the area to be examined, for images done by portable equipment.
- Retained barium from a previous radiological procedure.

Other considerations N/A

NURSING IMPLICATIONS AND PROCEDURE

See Potential Nursing Problems on Fast Find at davispl.us/vanleeuwen7.

PRETEST:

- Positively identify the patient using at least two person-specific identifiers before services, treatments, or procedures are performed.
- *Patient Teaching:* Inform the patient this procedure can assist in assessing the status of the abdomen.
- Obtain a history of the patient's health concerns, symptoms, surgical procedures, and results of previously performed laboratory and diagnostic studies. Include a list of known allergens, especially allergies or sensitivities to latex.
- Record the date of the last menstrual period and determine the possibility of pregnancy in perimenopausal women.
- Obtain a list of the patient's current medications, including over-the-counter medications and dietary supplements (see Effects of Natural Products on Laboratory Values online at Davis*Plus*).
- Review the procedure with the patient. Address concerns about pain and explain that little to no pain is expected during the test, but there may be moments of discomfort. Inform the patient that the procedure is performed in the radiology department or at the bedside by a registered radiologic technologist and takes approximately 5 to 15 min to complete.

- *Sensitivity to social and cultural issues,* as well as concern for modesty, is important in providing psychological support before, during, and after the procedure.
- Instruct the patient to remove all metallic objects from the area to be examined.
- Note that there are no food, fluid, or medication restrictions unless by medical direction.

INTRATEST:

Potential Complications: N/A

- Observe standard precautions, and follow the general guidelines in Patient Preparation and Specimen Collection online at Davis*Plus*. Positively identify the patient.
- Ensure the patient has removed all metallic objects from the area to be examined prior to the procedure.
- Instruct the patient to void prior to the procedure and to change into the gown, robe, and foot coverings provided.
- Instruct the patient to cooperate fully and follow directions. Instruct the patient to remain still throughout the procedure because movement produces unreliable results.
- Avoid the use of equipment containing latex if the patient has a history of allergic reaction to latex.
- Place the patient on the table in a supine position with hands relaxed at the side.
- Instruct the patient to inhale deeply and hold his or her breath while the x-ray images are taken, and then to exhale after the images are taken.

POST-TEST:

- Inform the patient that a report of the results will be made available to the requesting HCP, who will discuss the results with the patient.
- Reinforce information given by the patient's HCP regarding further testing, treatment, or referral to another HCP. Answer any questions or address any concerns voiced by the patient or family.
- Depending on the results of this procedure, additional testing may be performed to evaluate or monitor progression of the disease process and determine the need for a change in therapy. Evaluate test results in relation to the patient's symptoms and other tests performed.

Patient Education:

- Teach the patient to call for pain relief medication as soon as it is needed.
- Teach the patient how to measure intake and output.

Expected Patient Outcomes:

Understanding

- The patient describes pain management strategies that work and those that do not work.
- The patient describes the meaning of pain relief in relation to his or her personal health.

Ability

- The patient can anticipate pain needs and request medication in a timely manner.
- The patient demonstrates how to accurately measure urinary output and intake.

Response

- The patient describes the meaning of pain within the context of his or her personal health.
- The patient agrees to discuss concerns with identified support (family, friends, group, spiritual advisor).

RELATED STUDIES:

- Related tests include angiography kidneys, calculus kidney stone panel, CT abdomen, CT kidneys, CT pelvis, IVP, and MRI abdomen, retrograde ureteropyelography, US abdomen, US kidney, US pelvis, and UA.
- Refer to the Gastrointestinal and Genitourinary systems tables online at Davis*Plus* for related tests by body system.

Kleihauer-Betke Test

SYNONYM/ACRONYM: Fetal hemoglobin, hemoglobin F, acid elution slide test.

COMMON USE: To assist in assessing occurrence and extent of fetal maternal hemorrhage and calculate the amount of Rh immune globulin to be administered.

SPECIMEN: Whole blood collected in a lavender-top (EDTA) tube. Freshly prepared blood smears are also acceptable. Cord blood may be requested for use as a positive control.

NORMAL FINDINGS: (Method: Microscopic examination of treated and stained peripheral blood smear) Less than 1% fetal cells present.

POTENTIAL MEDICAL DIAGNOSIS

Positive findings in

- Fetal-maternal hemorrhage ***(related to leakage of fetal RBCs into maternal circulation)***
- Hereditary persistence of fetal hemoglobin ***(the test does not differentiate fetal hemoglobin from neonate and adult)***

Negative findings in: N/A

CRITICAL FINDINGS: N/A

Find and print out the full study on Fast Find at davispl.us/vanleeuwen7.

Lactate Dehydrogenase and Isoenzymes

SYNONYM/ACRONYM: LDH and isos, LD, and isos.

COMMON USE: To assess myocardial or skeletal muscle damage toward diagnosing disorders such as myocardial infarction or damage to brain, liver, kidneys, and skeletal muscle.

SPECIMEN: Serum collected in a gold-, red-, or red/gray-top tube.

NORMAL FINDINGS: (Method: Enzymatic [L to P] for lactate dehydrogenase, electrophoretic analysis for isoenzymes) Reference ranges are method dependent and may vary among laboratories.

Lactate Dehydrogenase

Age	Conventional & SI Units
0–2 yr	125–275 units/L
2–3 yr	166–232 units/L
4–6 yr	104–206 units/L
7–12 yr	90–203 units/L
13–14 yr	90–199 units/L
15–43 yr	90–156 units/L
Greater than 43 yr	90–176 units/L

LDH Fraction	% of Total	Fraction of Total
LDH_1	14–26	0.14–0.26
LDH_2	29–39	0.29–0.39
LDH_3	20–26	0.2–0.26
LDH_4	8–16	0.08–0.16
LDH_5	6–16	0.06–0.16

POTENTIAL MEDICAL DIAGNOSIS

Total LDH Increased In

LDH is released from any damaged cell in which it is stored so conditions that affect the heart, liver, kidneys, red blood cells, skeletal muscle, or other tissue source and cause cellular destruction demonstrate elevated LDH levels.

- Alcoholism
- Carcinoma of the liver
- Cirrhosis
- Heart failure
- HELLP (hemolysis, elevated liver enzymes, low platelet count) syndrome of pregnancy
- Hemolytic anemias
- Hypoxia
- Kidney disease (severe)
- Leukemias
- Megaloblastic and pernicious anemia
- MI or pulmonary infarction
- Musculoskeletal disease
- Obstructive jaundice
- Pancreatitis
- Shock
- Viral hepatitis

Total LDH Decreased In: N/A

LDH Isoenzymes

- LDH_1 fraction increased over LDH_2 can be seen in acute MI, anemias (pernicious, hemolytic, acute sickle cell, megaloblastic, hemolytic), and acute kidney injury due to any cause. The LDH_1 fraction in particular is elevated in cases of germ cell tumors.
- Increases in the middle fractions are associated with conditions in which massive platelet destruction has occurred (e.g., pulmonary embolism, posttransfusion period) and in lymphatic system disorders (e.g., infectious mononucleosis, lymphomas, lymphocytic leukemias).
- An increase in LDH_5 occurs with musculoskeletal damage and many types of liver damage (e.g., cirrhosis, cancer, hepatitis).

CRITICAL FINDINGS: N/A

Find and print out the full study on Fast Find at davispl.us/vanleeuwen7.

Lactic Acid

SYNONYM/ACRONYM: Lactate.

COMMON USE: To assess for lactic acid acidosis related to poor organ perfusion and liver failure. May also be used to differentiate between lactic acid acidosis and ketoacidosis by evaluating blood glucose levels.

SPECIMEN: Plasma collected in a gray-top (sodium fluoride) or a green-top (lithium heparin) tube. Specimen should be transported tightly capped and in an ice slurry.

NORMAL FINDINGS: (Method: Spectrophotometry/enzymatic analysis)

	Conventional Units	SI Units (Conventional Units × 0.111)
0–90 d	3–32 mg/dL	0.3–3.6 mmol/L
3–24 mo	3–30 mg/dL	0.3–3.3 mmol/L
2 yr–adult	3–23 mg/dL	0.3–2.6 mmol/L

DESCRIPTION: Lactic acid, also known as *lactate,* is a by-product of anaerobic carbohydrate metabolism. Pyruvate, the normal end product of glucose metabolism, is converted to lactate in situations when energy is needed but there is insufficient oxygen in the system to favor the aerobic and customary energy cycle. Lactic acid levels increase with strenuous exercise, heart failure, severe infection, sepsis, or shock. Lactic acid levels can also increase from liver disease or damage, because lactate is normally metabolized by the liver. Lactic acidosis can be differentiated from ketoacidosis by the absence of ketosis and grossly elevated glucose levels.

This procedure is contraindicated for: N/A

INDICATIONS

- Assess tissue oxygenation.
- Evaluate acidosis.

POTENTIAL MEDICAL DIAGNOSIS

Increased in:

The liver is the major organ responsible for the breakdown of lactic acid. Any condition affecting normal liver function may also reflect increased blood levels of lactic acid.

- Cardiac failure ***(decreased blood flow and insufficient oxygen in tissues result in accumulation of lactic acid from anaerobic glycolysis)***
- Diabetes ***(inefficient aerobic glycolysis and decreased blood flow caused by diabetes result in accumulation of lactic acid from anaerobic glycolysis)***
- Hemorrhage ***(decreased blood circulation and insufficient oxygen in tissues result in accumulation of lactic acid from anaerobic glycolysis)***
- Hepatic coma ***(related to liver damage and decreased tissue oxygenation)***
- Ingestion of large doses of alcohol or acetaminophen ***(related to liver damage)***
- Lactic acidosis ***(related to strenuous exercise that results in accumulations in metabolic byproducts of anaerobic breakdown of sugars for energy)***
- Pulmonary embolism ***(decreased blood flow and insufficient oxygen in tissues result in accumulation of lactic acid from anaerobic glycolysis)***
- Pulmonary failure ***(decreased blood flow and insufficient oxygen in tissues result in accumulation of lactic acid from anaerobic glycolysis)***
- Reye's syndrome ***(related to liver damage)***
- Shock ***(decreased blood flow and insufficient oxygen in tissues result in accumulation of lactic acid from anaerobic glycolysis)***
- Strenuous exercise ***(related to lactic acidosis)***

Decreased in: N/A

CRITICAL FINDINGS:

Adults

- Greater than 31 mg/dL (SI: Greater than 3.4 mmol/L)

Children

- Greater than 37 mg/dL (SI: Greater than 4.1 mmol/L)

Note and immediately report to the requesting health-care provider (HCP) any critical findings and related symptoms. A listing of these findings varies among facilities. Timely notification of a critical finding for laboratory or diagnostic studies is a role expectation of the professional nurse. The notification processes vary among facilities. Upon receipt of the critical finding, the information should be read back to the caller to verify accuracy.

Consideration may be given to verification of critical findings before action is taken. Policies vary among facilities and may include requesting immediate recollection and retesting by the laboratory or retesting using a rapid point-of-care testing instrument at the bedside, if available.

Observe the patient for signs and symptoms of elevated levels of lactate, such as Kussmaul's breathing and increased pulse rate. In general, there is an inverse relationship between critically elevated lactate levels and survival.

INTERFERING FACTORS

- Drugs and other substances that may increase lactate levels include albuterol, aspirin, anticonvulsants (long-term use), isoniazid, metformin (Glucophage), oral contraceptives, sodium bicarbonate, and sorbitol.

- Falsely low lactate levels are obtained in samples with elevated levels of the enzyme lactate dehydrogenase because this enzyme reacts with the available lactate substrate.
- Using a tourniquet or instructing the patient to clench his or her fist during a venipuncture can cause elevated levels.
- Engaging in strenuous physical activity (i.e., activity in which blood flow and oxygen distribution cannot keep pace with increased energy needs) before specimen collection can cause an elevated result.
- Delay in transport of the specimen to the laboratory must be avoided. Specimens not processed by centrifugation in a tightly stoppered collection container within 15 min of collection should be rejected for analysis. It is preferable to transport specimens to the laboratory in an ice slurry to further retard cellular metabolism that might shift lactate levels in the sample before analysis.
- Failure to follow dietary restrictions before the procedure may cause the procedure to be canceled or repeated.

NURSING IMPLICATIONS AND PROCEDURE

POTENTIAL NURSING PROBLEMS:

Problem	Signs & Symptoms	Interventions
Confusion ***(related to hepatic dysfunction; decreased tissue oxygenation)***	Disorganized thinking, restlessness, irritability, altered concentration and attention span, changeable mental function over the day, hallucinations	Treat the medical condition; correlate confusion with the need to reverse altered electrolytes; evaluate medications; prevent falls and injury through appropriate use of postural support, bed alarm, or restraints; consider pharmacological interventions; record accurate intake and output to assess fluid status
Fever ***(related to liver disease; infection)***	Continuous low-grade temperature that is unaltered by treatment with antibiotics; temperature variances secondary to cirrhosis and liver damage; elevated white blood cells (WBCs); positive sepsis screen	Take temperature every 4 hr and trend for continuous low-grade fever; administer prescribed antipyretics as appropriate; administer prescribed antibiotics as appropriate; provide clean linens to keep cool and comfortable (diaphoresis); provide cooling measures (light clothing)

Problem	Signs & Symptoms	Interventions
Electrolyte ***(related to altered metabolic process; decreased oxygenation; hepatic dysfunction; shock; sepsis; excessive alcohol intake)***	Altered EKG; decreased serum bicarbonate; elevated lactic acid; symptoms of shock (cool, clammy skin, deceased mental status, decreased urinary output, hypotension); diagnosis of liver failure; elevated WBC (sepsis, HIV infection); elevated blood glucose (DKA)	Correlate lactic acid imbalance with disease process (liver function, shock, DKA); collaborate with the pharmacist and health-care provider (HCP) for appropriate pharmacologic interventions; assess and trend serum lactic acid and bicarbonate levels; assess and monitor arterial blood gas bicarbonate results; monitor EKG; administer sodium bicarbonate therapy as clinically appropriate (use extreme caution because use is controversial); monitor and trend blood glucose; assess for alcoholism (causing hepatic dysfunction)
Gas exchange ***(related to obstruction secondary to embolism; shock)***	Decreased activity tolerance; increased shortness of breath with activity; weakness; orthopnea; cyanosis; cough; increased heart rate; weight gain; edema in the lower extremities; weakness; increased respiratory rate; use of respiratory accessory muscles	Auscultate and trend breath sounds; use pulse oximetry to monitor oxygenation; administer oxygen as ordered; collaborate with physician to consider intubation and/or mechanical ventilation; place the head of the bed in high Fowler's position; administer diuretics, vasodilators as ordered; monitor potassium levels

PRETEST:

- Positively identify the patient using at least two person-specific identifiers before services, treatments, or procedures are performed.
- *Patient Teaching:* Inform the patient this test can assist with assessing organ function.
- Obtain a history of the patient's health concerns, symptoms, surgical procedures, and results of previously performed laboratory and diagnostic studies. Include a list of known allergens, especially allergies or sensitivities to latex.
- Obtain a list of the patient's current medications, including over-the-counter medications and dietary supplements (see Effects of Natural Products on Laboratory Values online at Davis*Plus*).
- Review the procedure with the patient. Instruct the patient to rest for 1 hr before specimen collection. Inform the patient that specimen collection takes approximately 5 to

10 min. Address concerns about pain and explain that there may be some discomfort during the venipuncture.

- Instruct the patient to fast and to restrict fluids overnight. Instruct the patient not to ingest alcohol for 12 hr before the test. Protocols may vary among facilities.
- *Sensitivity to social and cultural issues,* as well as concern for modesty, is important in providing psychological support before, during, and after the procedure.
- Note that there are no medication restrictions unless by medical direction.
- Prepare an ice slurry in a cup or plastic bag to have on hand for immediate transport of the specimen to the laboratory.

INTRATEST:

Potential Complications: N/A

- Ensure that the patient has complied with dietary restrictions and other pretesting preparations prior to the study, as instructed.
- Avoid the use of equipment containing latex if the patient has a history of allergic reaction to latex.
- Instruct the patient to cooperate fully and to follow directions. Direct the patient to breathe normally and to avoid unnecessary movement.
- Observe standard precautions, and follow the general guidelines in Patient Preparation and Specimen Collection online at Davis*Plus*. Positively identify the patient, and label the appropriate specimen container with the corresponding patient demographics, initials of the person collecting the specimen, date, and time of collection. Instruct the patient *not* to clench and unclench fist immediately before or during specimen collection. Do not use a tourniquet. Perform a venipuncture. The tightly capped sample should be placed in an ice slurry immediately after collection. Information on the specimen label should be protected from water in the ice slurry by first placing the specimen in a protective plastic bag.
- Remove the needle and apply direct pressure with dry gauze to stop bleeding. Observe/assess venipuncture site for bleeding or hematoma formation and secure gauze with adhesive bandage.
- Promptly transport the specimen to the laboratory for processing and analysis.

POST-TEST:

- Inform the patient that a report of the results will be made available to the requesting HCP, who will discuss the results with the patient.
- Instruct the patient to resume usual diet and fluids, as directed by the HCP.
- *Nutritional Considerations:* Instruct patients to consume water when exercising. Dehydration may occur when the body loses water during exercise. Early signs of dehydration include dry mouth, thirst, and concentrated dark yellow urine. If replacement fluids are not consumed at this time, the patient may become moderately dehydrated and exhibit symptoms of extreme thirst, dry oral mucus membranes, inability to produce tears, decreased urinary output, and lightheadedness. Severe dehydration manifests as confusion, lethargy, vertigo, tachycardia, anuria, diaphoresis, and loss of consciousness.
- Note that depending on the results of this procedure, additional testing may be performed to evaluate or monitor progression of the disease process and determine the need for a change in therapy. Evaluate test results in relation to the patient's symptoms and other tests performed.

Patient Education:

- Reinforce information given by the patient's HCP regarding further testing, treatment, or referral to another HCP.

L

- Answer any questions or address any concerns voiced by the patient or family.

Expected Patient Outcomes:

Understanding

- The patient and family state that an untreated elevated lactic acid has the potential to be life threatening.
- The patient states the importance of abstaining from alcohol to protect liver function.

Skill

- The patient follows the recommendation to refrain from excessive physical activity that may cause increased lactic acid levels.
- The patient and family accurately describe symptoms of hypoxemia that should be reported to HCP.

Response

- The patient expresses willingness to make lifestyle changes that will improve overall health.
- The patient complies with the HCP therapeutic regimen to manage blood glucose.

RELATED STUDIES:

- Related laboratory tests include ALT, alveolar/arterial oxygen ratio, ammonia, analgesic and antipyretic drugs, anion gap, AST, biopsy liver, blood gases, CK, glucose, ketones, plethysmography, potassium, procalcitonin, pulse oximetry, and sodium.
- Refer to the Cardiovascular, Endocrine, Hepatobiliary, Musculoskeletal, and Respiratory systems tables online at Davis*Plus* for related tests by body system.

Lactose Tolerance Test

SYNONYM/ACRONYM: LTT.

COMMON USE: To assess for lactose intolerance or other metabolic disorders.

SPECIMEN: Plasma collected in a gray-top (fluoride/oxalate) tube.

NORMAL FINDINGS: (Method: Spectrophotometry)

Change in Glucose Value*	Conventional Units	SI Units (Conventional Units × 0.0555)
Normal	Greater than 30 mg/dL	Greater than 1.7 mmol/L
Inconclusive	20–30 mg/dL	1.1–1.7 mmol/L
Abnormal	Less than 20 mg/dL	Less than 1.1 mmol/L

*Compared to fasting sample for infants, children, adults, and older adults.

DESCRIPTION: Lactose is a disaccharide found in dairy products. When ingested, lactose is broken down in the intestine by the sugar-splitting enzyme lactase, into glucose and galactose. When sufficient lactase is not available, intestinal bacteria metabolize the lactose, resulting in abdominal bloating, pain, flatus, and diarrhea. The lactose tolerance test screens for lactose intolerance by monitoring glucose levels after ingestion of a dose of lactose.

There is also a noninvasive method to determine lactose intolerance using the hydrogen breath test. The breakdown of lactose by intestinal bacteria produces hydrogen gas. Before the administration of lactose, the patient breathes into a balloon. The concentration of hydrogen is measured from a sample of the gas in the balloon. After the administration of lactose, the patient breathes into a balloon at 15-min intervals over a period of 3 to 5 hr, and subsequent samples are measured for levels of hydrogen gas. The breath test is considered normal if the increase in hydrogen is less than 12 parts per million over the fasting or pretest level.

This procedure is contraindicated for: N/A

INDICATIONS

- Evaluate patients for suspected lactose intolerance.

POTENTIAL MEDICAL DIAGNOSIS

Glucose Levels Increased In

- Normal response

Glucose Levels Decreased In

- Lactose intolerance (lactase is insufficient to break down ingested lactose into glucose)

CRITICAL FINDINGS:

Glucose

Adults & Children

- Less than 40 mg/dL (SI: Less than 2.22 mmol/L)
- Greater than 400 mg/dL (SI: Greater than 22.2 mmol/L)

Note and immediately report to the requesting health-care provider (HCP) any critical findings and related symptoms. A listing of these findings varies among facilities. Timely notification of a critical finding for laboratory or diagnostic studies is a role expectation of the professional nurse. The notification processes vary among facilities. Upon receipt of the critical finding, the information should be read back to the caller to verify accuracy.

Consideration may be given to verification of critical findings before action is taken. Policies vary among facilities and may include requesting immediate recollection and retesting by the laboratory or retesting using a rapid point-of-care testing instrument at the bedside, if available.

Symptoms of decreased glucose levels include headache, confusion, polyphagia, irritability, nervousness, restlessness, diaphoresis, and weakness. Possible interventions include oral or intravenous (IV) administration of glucose, IV or intramuscular injection of glucagon, and continuous glucose monitoring.

Symptoms of elevated glucose levels include abdominal pain, fatigue, muscle cramps, nausea, vomiting, polyuria, polyphagia, and polydipsia. Possible interventions include fluid replacement in addition to subcutaneous or IV injection of insulin with continuous glucose monitoring.

INTERFERING FACTORS

- Numerous medications may alter glucose levels (see study titled "Glucose").
- Delayed gastric emptying may decrease glucose levels.
- Smoking may falsely increase glucose levels.
- Failure to follow dietary and activity restrictions before the procedure may cause the procedure to be canceled or repeated.

NURSING IMPLICATIONS AND PROCEDURE

POTENTIAL NURSING PROBLEMS:

Problem	Signs & Symptoms	Interventions
Pain ***(related to altered gastrointestinal motility secondary to lactase deficiency)***	Lower abdominal cramping; gas; bloating; diarrhea	Instruct patient to eliminate or reduce consumption of dairy products; instruct patient to self-administer oral enzyme medication to manage lactose when ingested
Nutrition ***(related to the inability to digest dairy products secondary to lactase deficiency)***	Intolerance to dairy products; a history of lower abdominal cramping, gas, bloating, and diarrhea with the ingestion of dairy products	Obtain a history of gastrointestinal (GI) upset with the ingestion of dairy products; trial a lactose-free diet to assess if the symptoms of GI upset resolve; instruct in self-administration of oral enzyme medication to manage lactose when ingested; instruct patient to eliminate or limit consumption of obvious sources of dairy, such as milk, ice cream, cheese; assess foods for hidden dairy ingredients such as found in sherbet, sauces, gravy, and desserts.
Diarrhea ***(related to gastric irritation secondary to bowel irritation from undigested lactose)***	Frequent diarrhea after ingesting dairy products with lower abdominal cramping; gas; bloating	Instruct patient to eliminate or reduce consumption of dairy products; instruct patient to self-administer oral enzyme medication to manage lactose when ingested
Socialization ***(related to fear of explosive diarrhea secondary to bowel irritation from undigested lactose)***	Lower abdominal cramping; gas; bloating; pain; explosive diarrhea; embarrassment; fear of the inability to locate a bathroom when needed	Assist the patient to map out restroom locations in areas where he or she commonly socializes; encourage the patient to follow a lactose-free or limited diet; instruct the patient to self-administer oral enzyme medication to manage lactose when ingested to prevent explosive diarrhea and urgency

PRETEST:

- Positively identify the patient using at least two person-specific identifiers before services, treatments, or procedures are performed.
- ***Patient Teaching:*** Inform the patient this test can assist with evaluating tolerance to dairy products which contain lactose.
- Obtain a history of the patient's health concerns, symptoms, surgical procedures, and results of previously performed laboratory and diagnostic studies. Include a list of known allergens, especially allergies or sensitivities to latex.
- Obtain a list of the patient's current medications, including over-the-counter medications and dietary supplements (see Effects of Natural Products on Laboratory Values online at Davis*Plus*).
- Review the procedure with the patient. Obtain the pediatric patient's weight to calculate dose of lactose to be administered. Inform the patient that multiple samples will be collected over a 90-min interval. Inform the patient that each specimen collection takes approximately 5 to 10 min. Address concerns about pain related to the procedure. Inform the patient that the test may produce symptoms such as cramps and diarrhea. Instruct the patient not to smoke cigarettes or chew gum during the test. Explain that there may be some discomfort during the venipuncture.
- ***Sensitivity to social and cultural issues,*** as well as concern for modesty, is important in providing psychological support before, during, and after the procedure.
- Inform the patient that fasting for at least 12 hr before the test is required and that strenuous activity should also be avoided for at least 12 hr before the test. Protocols may vary among facilities.
- Note that there are no medication restrictions unless by medical direction.

INTRATEST:

Potential Complications:
The test may produce symptoms such as cramps and diarrhea that may range in intensity from mild to severe.

- Ensure that the patient has complied with dietary and activity restrictions as well as other pretesting preparations prior to the study, as instructed.
- Avoid the use of equipment containing latex if the patient has a history of allergic reaction to latex.
- Administer lactose dissolved in a small amount of room temperature water (250 mL), over a 5- to 10-min period. Dosage is 2 g/kg body weight to a maximum of 50 g for patients of all ages. The requesting HCP may specify a lower challenge dose if severe lactose intolerance is suspected. One pound is equal to 0.45 kg; therefore, a weight of 50 lb is equal to 22 kg. The appropriate dosage of lactose in this example would be 45 g. Record body weight, dose administered, and time of ingestion. Encourage the patient to drink one to two glasses of water during the test.
- Instruct the patient to cooperate fully and to follow directions. Direct the patient to breathe normally and to avoid unnecessary movement.
- Observe standard precautions, and follow the general guidelines in Patient Preparation and Specimen Collection online at Davis*Plus*. Positively identify the patient, and label the appropriate specimen container with the corresponding patient demographics, initials of the person collecting the specimen, date, and time of collection. Perform a venipuncture. Samples should be collected at baseline, 15, 30, 60, 90, and 120 min. Record any symptoms the patient reports throughout the course of the test.
- Remove the needle and apply direct pressure with dry gauze to stop bleeding. Observe/assess

venipuncture site for bleeding or hematoma formation and secure gauze with adhesive bandage.
- Promptly transport the specimen to the laboratory for processing and analysis. Glucose values change rapidly in an unprocessed, unpreserved specimen; therefore, if a Microtainer is used, each sample should be transported immediately after collection.

POST-TEST:

- Inform the patient that a report of the results will be made available to the requesting HCP, who will discuss the results with the patient.
- ***Nutritional Considerations:*** Instruct the patient with lactose intolerance to avoid milk products and to carefully read labels on prepared products. Yogurt, which contains inactive lactase enzyme, may be ingested. The lactase in yogurt is activated by the temperature and pH of the duodenum and substitutes for the lack of endogenous lactase. Advise the patient that products such as Lactaid tablets or drops may allow ingestion of milk products without sequelae. Many lactose-free food products are now available in grocery stores.
- Recognize anxiety related to test results, and be supportive of concerns related to a perceived change in lifestyle.
- Depending on the results of this procedure, additional testing may be performed to evaluate or monitor progression of the disease process and determine the need for a change in therapy. Evaluate test results in relation to the patient's symptoms and other tests performed.

Patient Education:

- Instruct the patient that resuming his or her usual diet may not be possible if lactose intolerance is identified.
- Educate patients on the importance of following the dietary advice of a nutritionist to ensure proper nutritional balance.
- Discuss the implications of abnormal test results on the patient's lifestyle.
- Provide teaching and information regarding the clinical implications of the test results, as appropriate.
- Reinforce information given by the patient's HCP regarding further testing, treatment, or referral to another HCP.
- Answer any questions or address any concerns voiced by the patient or family.
- Teach the patient regarding lifestyle changes that will be necessary to manage lactose intolerance on a daily basis.
- Teach the patient about lactose intolerance support groups that may assist in making lifestyle adjustments.

Expected Patient Outcomes:

Understanding

- The patient and family state that calcium supplements may need to be taken with the elimination or reduction of dairy products in the diet.
- The patient and family compose a list of sources of dairy in the diet that may need to be eliminated.

Ability

- The patient and family select foods that exclude dietary lactose.
- The patient demonstrates proficiency in self-administration of medication to manage lactose intolerance symptoms.

Response

- The patient complies with the dietary limitation of dairy products to prevent lactose intolerance flares.
- The patient and family follow normal social activities.

RELATED STUDIES:

- Related tests include D-xylose absorption, fecal analysis, and glucose.
- Refer to the Gastrointestinal System table online at Davis*Plus* for related tests by body system.

L

Laparoscopy, Abdominal

SYNONYM/ACRONYM: Abdominal peritoneoscopy.

COMMON USE: To visualize and assess the liver, gallbladder, and spleen to assist with surgical interventions, staging tumor, and performing diagnostic biopsies.

AREA OF APPLICATION: Abdomen and pelvis.

DESCRIPTION: Abdominal or gastrointestinal (GI) laparoscopy provides direct visualization of the liver, gallbladder, spleen, and stomach after insufflation of carbon dioxide (CO_2). In this procedure, a rigid laparoscope is introduced into the body cavity through a 1- to 2-cm abdominal incision. The endoscope has a microscope to allow visualization of the organs, and it can be used to insert instruments for performing certain procedures, such as biopsy and tumor resection. Under general anesthesia, the peritoneal cavity is inflated with 2 to 3 L of CO_2. The gas distends the abdominal wall so that the instruments can be inserted safely. Advantages of this procedure compared to an open laparotomy include reduced pain, reduced length of stay at the hospital or surgical center, and reduced time off from work.

L

This procedure is contraindicated for

- Patients who are pregnant or suspected of being pregnant, unless the potential benefits of a procedure using radiation far outweigh the risk of radiation exposure to the fetus and mother.
- Patients with bleeding disorders, especially those associated with uremia and cytotoxic chemotherapy.
- Patients with cardiac conditions or dysrhythmias.
- Patients with advanced respiratory or cardiovascular disease.
- Patients with intestinal obstruction, abdominal mass, abdominal hernia, or suspected intra-abdominal hemorrhage.
- Patients with a history of peritonitis or multiple abdominal operations causing dense adhesions.

INDICATIONS

- Assist in performing surgical procedures such as cholecystectomy, appendectomy, hernia repair, hiatal hernia repair, and bowel resection.
- Detect cirrhosis of the liver.
- Detect pancreatic disorders.
- Evaluate abdominal pain or abdominal mass of unknown origin.
- Evaluate abdominal trauma in an emergency.
- Evaluate and treat appendicitis.
- Evaluate the extent of splenomegaly as a result of portal hypertension.
- Evaluate jaundice of unknown origin.
- Obtain biopsy specimens of benign or cancerous tumors.
- Stage neoplastic disorders such as lymphomas, Hodgkin's disease, and hepatic carcinoma.

POTENTIAL MEDICAL DIAGNOSIS

Normal findings

- Normal appearance of the liver, spleen, gallbladder, pancreas, and other abdominal contents

Abnormal findings related to
- Abdominal adhesions
- Appendicitis
- Ascites
- Cancer of any of the organs
- Cirrhosis of the liver
- Gangrenous gallbladder
- Intra-abdominal bleeding
- Portal hypertension
- Splenomegaly

CRITICAL FINDINGS:
- Appendicitis

Note and immediately report to the requesting health-care provider (HCP) any critical findings and related symptoms. A listing of these findings varies among facilities. Timely notification of a critical finding for laboratory or diagnostic studies is a role expectation of the professional nurse. The notification processes vary among facilities. Upon receipt of the critical finding, the information should be read back to the caller to verify accuracy.

INTERFERING FACTORS

Factors that may impair clear visualization
- Gas or feces in the GI tract resulting from inadequate cleansing or failure to restrict food intake before the study.
- Retained barium from a previous radiological procedure.
- Inability of the patient to cooperate or remain still during the procedure because of age, significant pain, or mental status.
- Metallic objects (e.g., jewelry, body rings) within the examination field, which may inhibit organ visualization and cause unclear images.

Other considerations
- The procedure may be terminated if chest pain or severe cardiac dysrhythmias occur.
- Failure to follow dietary restrictions and other pretesting preparations may cause the procedure to be canceled or repeated.
- Patients who are in a hypoxemic or hypercapnic state will require continuous oxygen administration.

NURSING IMPLICATIONS AND PROCEDURE

See Potential Nursing Problems on Fast Find at davispl.us/vanleeuwen7.

PRETEST:
- Positively identify the patient using at least two person-specific identifiers before services, treatments, or procedures are performed.
- *Patient Teaching:* Inform the patient this procedure can assist in assessing the abdominal organs.
- Obtain a history of the patient's health concerns, symptoms, surgical procedures, and results of previously performed laboratory and diagnostic studies. Include a list of known allergens, especially allergies or sensitivities to latex, anesthetics or sedatives.
- Ensure that this procedure is performed before any barium studies.
- Record the date of the last menstrual period and determine the possibility of pregnancy in perimenopausal women.
- Obtain a list of the patient's current medications, including over-the-counter medications, dietary supplements, anticoagulants, aspirin and other salicylates (see Effects of Natural Products on Laboratory Values online at Davis*Plus*). Such products should be discontinued by medical direction for the appropriate number of days prior to a surgical procedure. Note the last time and dose of medication taken.
- Review the procedure with the patient. Address concerns about pain related to the procedure and explain that some pain may be experienced during the test, and there may be moments of discomfort. Inform the patient that the procedure is performed in a surgery department, by

L

an HCP, with support staff, and takes approximately 30 to 60 min.

- ***Sensitivity to social and cultural issues,*** as well as concern for modesty, is important in providing psychological support before, during, and after the procedure.
- Explain that an intravenous (IV) line may be inserted to allow infusion of fluids such as saline, anesthetics, sedatives, or emergency medications.
- Inform the patient that a laxative and cleansing enema may be needed the day before the procedure, with cleansing enemas on the morning of the procedure, depending on the institution's policy.
- Instruct the patient to remove jewelry and other metallic objects from the area to be examined prior to the procedure.
- Instruct the patient that to reduce the risk of aspiration related to nausea and vomiting, solid food and milk or milk products have been restricted for at least 6 hr, and clear liquids have been restricted for at least 2 hr prior to general anesthesia, regional anesthesia, or sedation/analgesia (monitored anesthesia). The American Society of Anesthesiologists has fasting guidelines for risk levels according to patient status. More information can be located at www.asahq.org. 🍁 Patients on beta blockers before the surgical procedure should be instructed to take their medication as ordered during the perioperative period. Protocols may vary among facilities.
- *Make sure a written and informed consent has been signed prior to the procedure and before administering any medications.*

INTRATEST:

Potential Complications:

Complications of the procedure may include bleeding and cardiac dysrhythmias. Patients with acute infection or advanced malignancy involving the abdominal wall are at increased risk for infection because organisms may be introduced into the normally sterile peritoneal cavity.

- Observe standard precautions, and follow the general guidelines in Patient Preparation and Specimen Collection online at Davis*Plus*. Positively identify the patient.
- Ensure that the patient has complied with dietary, fluid, and medication restrictions prior to the study, as instructed.
- Ensure the patient has removed all external metallic objects from the area to be examined.
- Ensure that nonallergy to anesthesia is confirmed before the procedure is performed under general anesthesia.
- Assess for completion of bowel preparation according to the institution's procedure.
- Avoid the use of equipment containing latex if the patient has a history of allergic reaction to latex.
- Have emergency equipment readily available.
- Instruct the patient to void prior to the procedure and to change into the gown, robe, and foot coverings provided.
- Instruct the patient to cooperate fully and to follow directions. Instruct the patient to remain still throughout the procedure because movement produces unreliable results.
- Obtain and record baseline vital signs.
- Establish an IV fluid line for the injection of saline, sedatives, or emergency medications.
- Administer medications, as ordered, to reduce discomfort and to promote relaxation and sedation.
- Place the patient on the laparoscopy table. If general anesthesia is to be used, it is administered at this time. Place the patient in a modified lithotomy position with the head tilted downward. Cleanse the abdomen with an antiseptic solution, and drape and catheterize the patient, if ordered.
- The HCP identifies the site for the scope insertion and administers local anesthesia if that is to be used. After deeper layers are anesthetized, a pneumoperitoneum needle is placed between the visceral and parietal peritoneum.

L

- CO_2 is insufflated through the pneumoperitoneum needle to separate the abdominal wall from the viscera and to aid in visualization of the abdominal structures. The pneumoperitoneum needle is removed, and the trocar and laparoscope are inserted through the incision.
- After the examination, collection of tissue samples, and performance of therapeutic procedures, the scope is withdrawn. All possible CO_2 is evacuated via the trocar, which is then removed. The skin incision is closed with sutures, clips, or sterile strips, and a small dressing or adhesive strip is applied.
- Observe/assess the incision site for bleeding, inflammation, or hematoma formation.

POST-TEST:

- Inform the patient that a report of the results will be made available to the requesting HCP, who will discuss the results with the patient.
- Instruct the patient to resume usual diet, fluids, and medication, as directed by the HCP.
- Monitor vital signs and neurological status every 15 min for 1 hr, then every 2 hr for 4 hr, and as ordered. Take temperature every 4 hr for 24 hr. Monitor intake and output at least every 8 hr. Compare with baseline values. Notify the HCP if temperature is elevated. Protocols may vary among facilities.
- Instruct the patient to restrict activity for 2 to 7 days after the procedure.
- Instruct the patient in the care and assessment of the incision site.
- If indicated, inform the patient of a follow-up appointment for the removal of sutures.
- Inform the patient that shoulder discomfort may be experienced for 1 or 2 days after the procedure as a result of abdominal distention caused by insufflation of CO_2 into the abdomen and that mild analgesics and cold compresses, as ordered, can be used to relieve the discomfort.
- Emphasize that any persistent shoulder pain, abdominal pain, vaginal bleeding, fever, redness, or swelling of the incisional area must be reported to the HCP immediately.
- Recognize anxiety related to test results. Discuss the implications of abnormal test results on the patient's lifestyle. Provide teaching and information regarding the clinical implications of the test results, as appropriate.
- Reinforce information given by the patient's HCP regarding further testing, treatment, or referral to another HCP. Answer any questions or address any concerns voiced by the patient or family.
- Depending on the results of this procedure, additional testing may be needed to evaluate or monitor progression of the disease process and determine the need for a change in therapy. Evaluate test results in relation to the patient's symptoms and other tests performed.

Patient Education:

- Teach the signs and symptoms of infection that are associated with interrupted skin integrity.
- Teach the importance of good nutrition in wound healing (protein, vitamin C, iron).

Expected Patient Outcomes:

Understanding

- The patient and family state the importance of taking antibiotics as prescribed until completed.
- The patient and family state the importance of adequate food and fluid intake toward healing.

Ability

- The patient and family successfully demonstrate wound care of incision site or drains.
- The patient successfully demonstrates how to use incentive spirometry.

Response

- The patient recognizes the importance of taking pain medication to facilitate the ease of breathing.
- The patient and family agree to monitor diet to assure good nutrition,

L

RELATED STUDIES:

- Related tests include amylase, barium swallow, biopsy bone marrow, CBC, CBC WBC count and differential, CT abdomen, CT biliary tract and liver, CT pancreas, CRP, ESR, gallium scan, hepatobiliary scan, KUB, lipase, liver and spleen scan, lymphangiogram, MRI abdomen, MRI pelvis, peritoneal fluid analysis, US abdomen, and US pelvis.
- Refer to the Gastrointestinal and Hepatobiliary systems tables online at Davis*Plus* for related tests by body system.

Laparoscopy, Gynecologic

SYNONYM/ACRONYM: Gynecologic pelviscopy, gynecologic laparoscopy, pelvic endoscopy, peritoneoscopy.

COMMON USE: To visualize and assess the ovaries, fallopian tubes, and uterus toward diagnosing inflammation, malformations, cysts, and fibroids and to evaluate causes of infertility.

AREA OF APPLICATION: Pelvis.

DESCRIPTION: Gynecologic laparoscopy provides direct visualization of the internal pelvic contents, including the ovaries, fallopian tubes, and uterus, after insufflation of carbon dioxide (CO_2). It is done to diagnose and treat pelvic organ disorders as well as to perform surgical procedures on the organs. In this procedure, a rigid laparoscope is introduced into the body cavity through a 1- to 2-cm periumbilical incision. The endoscope has a microscope to allow visualization of the organs, and it can be used to insert instruments for performing procedures such as biopsy (e.g., biopsy of suspected endometrial lesions) and tumor resection. Under general or local anesthesia, the peritoneal cavity is inflated with 2 to 3 L of CO_2. The gas distends the abdominal wall so that the instruments can be inserted safely. Advantages of this procedure compared to an open laparotomy include reduced pain, reduced length of stay at the hospital or surgical center, and reduced time off from work.

This procedure is contraindicated for

- Patients who are pregnant or suspected of being pregnant, unless the potential benefits of a procedure using radiation far outweigh the risk of radiation exposure to the fetus and mother.
- Patients with bleeding disorders, especially those associated with uremia and cytotoxic chemotherapy.
- Patients with cardiac conditions or dysrhythmias.
- Patients with advanced respiratory or cardiovascular disease.
- Patients with intestinal obstruction, abdominal mass, abdominal hernia, or suspected intra-abdominal hemorrhage.

INDICATIONS

- Detect ectopic pregnancy and determine the need for surgery.

- Detect pelvic inflammatory disease or abscess.
- Detect uterine fibroids, ovarian cysts, and uterine malformations (ovarian cysts may be aspirated during the procedure).
- Evaluate amenorrhea and infertility.
- Evaluate fallopian tubes and anatomic defects to determine the cause of infertility.
- Evaluate known or suspected endometriosis, salpingitis, and hydrosalpinx.
- Evaluate pelvic pain or masses of unknown cause.
- Evaluate reproductive organs after therapy for infertility.
- Obtain biopsy specimens to confirm suspected pelvic malignancies or metastasis.
- Perform tubal sterilization and ovarian biopsy.
- Perform vaginal hysterectomy.
- Remove adhesions or foreign bodies such as intrauterine devices.
- Treat endometriosis through electrocautery or laser vaporization.

POTENTIAL MEDICAL DIAGNOSIS

Normal findings

- Normal appearance of uterus, ovaries, fallopian tubes, and other pelvic contents

Abnormal findings related to

- Abscesses
- Adhesions or scar tissue
- Ascites
- Cancer staging
- Ectopic pregnancy
- Endometriosis
- Enlarged fallopian tubes
- Infection
- Ovarian cyst
- Ovarian tumor
- Pelvic adhesions
- Pelvic inflammatory disease
- Pelvic tumor
- Salpingitis
- Uterine fibroids

CRITICAL FINDINGS:

- Ectopic pregnancy
- Foreign body
- Tumor with significant mass effect

Note and immediately report to the requesting health-care provider (HCP) any critical findings and related symptoms. A listing of these findings varies among facilities. Timely notification of a critical finding for laboratory or diagnostic studies is a role expectation of the professional nurse. The notification processes vary among facilities. Upon receipt of the critical finding, the information should be read back to the caller to verify accuracy.

INTERFERING FACTORS

Factors that may impair clear visualization

- Gas or feces in the gastrointestinal (GI) tract resulting from inadequate cleansing or failure to restrict food intake before the study.
- Retained barium from a previous radiological procedure.
- Inability of the patient to cooperate or remain still during the procedure because of age, significant pain, or mental status.
- Metallic objects (e.g., jewelry, body rings) within the examination field, which may inhibit organ visualization and cause unclear images.

Other considerations

- The procedure may be terminated if chest pain or severe cardiac dysrhythmias occur.
- Failure to follow dietary restrictions and other pretesting preparations may cause the procedure to be canceled or repeated.
- Patients who are in a hypoxemic or hypercapnic state will require continuous oxygen administration.

L

NURSING IMPLICATIONS AND PROCEDURE

See Potential Nursing Problems on Fast Find at davispl.us/vanleeuwen7.

PRETEST:

- Positively identify the patient using at least two person-specific identifiers before services, treatments, or procedures are performed.
- *Patient Teaching:* Inform the patient this procedure can assist in assessing the abdominal and pelvic organs.
- Obtain a history of the patient's health concerns, symptoms, surgical procedures, and results of previously performed laboratory and diagnostic studies. Include a list of known allergens, especially allergies or sensitivities to latex, anesthetics or sedatives.
- Ensure that this procedure is performed before any barium studies.
- Record the date of the last menstrual period and determine the possibility of pregnancy in perimenopausal women.
- Obtain a list of the patient's current medications, including over-the-counter medications, dietary supplements, anticoagulants, aspirin and other salicylates (see Effects of Natural Products on Laboratory Values online at Davis*Plus*). Such products should be discontinued by medical direction for the appropriate number of days prior to a surgical procedure. Note the last time and dose of medication taken.
- Review the procedure with the patient. Address concerns about pain related to the procedure and explain that some pain may be experienced during the test, and there may be moments of discomfort. Inform the patient that the procedure is performed in a surgery department by an HCP and support staff and takes approximately 30 to 60 min.
- *Sensitivity to social and cultural issues,* as well as concern for modesty, is important in providing psychological support before, during, and after the procedure.
- Explain that an intravenous (IV) line may be inserted to allow infusion of fluids such as saline, anesthetics, sedatives, or emergency medications.
- Inform the patient that a laxative and cleansing enema may be needed the day before the procedure, with cleansing enemas on the morning of the procedure, depending on the institution's policy.
- Instruct the patient to remove jewelry and other metallic objects from the area to be examined prior to the procedure.
- Instruct the patient that to reduce the risk of aspiration related to nausea and vomiting, solid food and milk or milk products have been restricted for at least 6 hr, and clear liquids have been restricted for at least 2 hr prior to general anesthesia, regional anesthesia, or sedation/analgesia (monitored anesthesia). The American Society of Anesthesiologists has fasting guidelines for risk levels according to patient status. More information can be located at www.asahq.org. 🍁 Patients on beta blockers before the surgical procedure should be instructed to take their medication as ordered during the perioperative period. Protocols may vary among facilities.
- *Make sure a written and informed consent has been signed prior to the procedure and before administering any medications.*

INTRATEST:

Potential Complications:

Complications of the procedure may include bleeding and cardiac dysrhythmias. Patients with acute infection or advanced malignancy involving the abdominal wall are at increased risk for infection because organisms may be introduced into the normally sterile peritoneal cavity.

- Observe standard precautions, and follow the general guidelines in Patient Preparation and Specimen Collection online at Davis*Plus*. Positively identify the patient.
- Ensure that the patient has complied with dietary, fluid, and medication

restrictions prior to the study, as instructed.

- Ensure the patient has removed all external metallic objects from the area to be examined.
- Ensure that nonallergy to anesthesia is confirmed before the procedure is performed under general anesthesia.
- Assess for completion of bowel preparation according to the institution's procedure.
- Avoid the use of equipment containing latex if the patient has a history of allergic reaction to latex.
- Have emergency equipment readily available.
- Instruct the patient to void prior to the procedure and to change into the gown, robe, and foot coverings provided.
- Instruct the patient to cooperate fully and to follow directions. Instruct the patient to remain still throughout the procedure because movement produces unreliable results.
- Obtain and record baseline vital signs.
- Establish an IV fluid line for the injection of saline, sedatives, or emergency medications.
- Administer medications, as ordered, to reduce discomfort and to promote relaxation and sedation.
- Place the patient on the laparoscopy table. If general anesthesia is to be used, it is administered at this time. Place the patient in a modified lithotomy position with the head tilted downward. Cleanse the abdomen with an antiseptic solution, and drape and catheterize the patient, if ordered.
- The HCP identifies the site for the scope insertion and administers local anesthesia if that is to be used. After deeper layers are anesthetized, a pneumoperitoneum needle is placed between the visceral and parietal peritoneum.
- CO_2 is insufflated through the pneumoperitoneum needle to separate the abdominal wall from the viscera and to aid in visualization of the abdominal structures. The pneumoperitoneum needle is removed, and the trocar and laparoscope are inserted through the incision.
- The HCP inserts a uterine manipulator through the vagina and cervix and into the uterus so that the uterus, fallopian tubes, and ovaries can be moved to permit better visualization.
- After the examination, collection of tissue samples, and performance of therapeutic procedures (e.g., tubal ligation), the scope is withdrawn. All possible CO_2 is evacuated via the trocar, which is then removed. The skin incision is closed with sutures, clips, or sterile strips and a small dressing or adhesive strip is applied. After the perineum is cleansed, the uterine manipulator is removed and a sterile pad applied.
- Observe/assess the incision site for bleeding, inflammation, or hematoma formation.

POST-TEST:

- Inform the patient that a report of the results will be made available to the requesting HCP, who will discuss the results with the patient.
- Instruct the patient to resume usual diet, fluids, and medication, as directed by the HCP.
- Monitor vital signs and neurological status every 15 min for 1 hr, then every 2 hr for 4 hr, and as ordered. Take temperature every 4 hr for 24 hr. Monitor intake and output at least every 8 hr. Compare with baseline values. Notify the HCP if temperature is elevated. Protocols may vary among facilities.
- Instruct the patient to restrict activity for 2 to 7 days after the procedure.
- Instruct the patient in the care and assessment of the incision site.
- If indicated, inform the patient of a follow-up appointment for the removal of sutures.
- Inform the patient that shoulder discomfort may be experienced for 1 or 2 days after the procedure as a result of abdominal distention caused by insufflation of CO_2 into the abdomen and that mild analgesics and cold compresses, as ordered, can be used to relieve the discomfort.

L

- Emphasize that any persistent shoulder pain, abdominal pain, vaginal bleeding, fever, redness, or swelling of the incisional area must be reported to the HCP immediately.
- Recognize anxiety related to test results. Discuss the implications of abnormal test results on the patient's lifestyle. Provide teaching and information regarding the clinical implications of the test results, as appropriate.
- Reinforce information given by the patient's HCP regarding further testing, treatment, or referral to another HCP. Answer any questions or address any concerns voiced by the patient or family.
- Depending on the results of this procedure, additional testing may be needed to evaluate or monitor progression of the disease process and determine the need for a change in therapy. Evaluate test results in relation to the patient's symptoms and other tests performed.

Patient Education:
- Teach the patient to refrain from sexual activity and tampon use until infection is resolved.
- Teach the patient the signs and symptoms of pelvic inflammatory disease and to seek medical attention as soon as possible if they occur.

Expected Patient Outcomes:

Understanding
- The patient and family state the importance of good personal hygiene, perineal care, after bowel movement to minimize bacteria.
- The patient and family state the importance of family counseling to assist with concerns related to reproductive challenges.

Ability
- The patient demonstrates how to correctly apply a heating pad to the abdomen.
- The patient identifies pain strategies that work best and uses them competently.

Response
- The patient agrees to abstain from sexual relations until the infection, cause of inflammation is resolved.
- The patient agrees to attend classes on safe sex and how to avoid pelvic disease.

RELATED STUDIES:
- Related tests include cancer antigens, *Chlamydia* group antibody, CT abdomen, CT pelvis, HCG, MRI pelvis, Pap smear, progesterone, US pelvis, and uterine fibroid embolization.
- Refer to the Reproductive System table online at Davis*Plus* for related tests by body system.

L

Latex Allergy

SYNONYM/ACRONYM: N/A

COMMON USE: To assess for allergic reaction to products containing latex.

SPECIMEN: Serum collected in a gold-, red-, or red/gray-top tube.

NORMAL FINDINGS: (Method: Immunoassay) Negative.

POTENTIAL MEDICAL DIAGNOSIS

Positive findings in

Latex allergy

Negative findings in: N/A

CRITICAL FINDINGS: N/A

Find and print out the full study on Fast Find at davispl.us/vanleeuwen7.

Access Canadian content on Fast Find: Lab and Dx at davispl.us/vanleeuwen7

Lead

SYNONYM/ACRONYM: Pb.

COMMON USE: To assess for lead toxicity and monitor exposure to lead to assist in diagnosing lead poisoning.

SPECIMEN: Whole blood collected in a special lead-free royal blue– or tan-top tube. Plasma collected in a lavender-top (EDTA) tube is also acceptable.

NORMAL FINDINGS: (Method: Atomic absorption spectrophotometry)

	Conventional Units	SI Units (Conventional Units × 0.0483)
Children and adults (WHO, CDC; environmental exposure)	Less than 10 mcg/dL	Less than 0.48 micromol/L
OSHA (occupational exposure standard)	Less than 40 mcg/dL	Less than 1.93 micromol/L

OSHA = Occupational Safety and Health Administration; WHO = World Health Organization; CDC = Centers for Disease Control and Prevention.

DESCRIPTION: Lead is a heavy metal and trace element found in the environment. It is absorbed through the respiratory and gastrointestinal systems. It can also be transported from mother to fetus through the placenta. When there is frequent exposure to lead-containing items (e.g., paint, batteries, gasoline, pottery, bullets, printing materials) or occupations (mining, automobile, printing, and welding industries), lead poisoning can cause severe behavioral and neurological effects. The blood test is considered the best indicator of lead poisoning.

This procedure is contraindicated for: N/A

INDICATIONS

Assist in the diagnosis and treatment of lead poisoning.

POTENTIAL MEDICAL DIAGNOSIS

Increased in:

Heme synthesis involves the conversion of* D*-amino levulinic acid to porphobilinogen. Lead interferes with the enzyme that is responsible for this critical step in heme synthesis, amino levulinic acid dehydrase.

- Anemia of lead intoxication
- Lead encephalopathy
- Metal poisoning

Decreased in: N/A

CRITICAL FINDINGS:

- Levels greater than 30 mcg/dL (SI: Greater than 1.4 micromol/L) indicate significant exposure.
- Levels greater than 60 mcg/dL (SI: Greater than 2.9 micromol/L) may require chelation therapy.
- Levels greater than 70 mcg/dL (SI: Greater than 3.3 micromol/L) may cause severe brain damage and result in death.

Note and immediately report to the requesting health-care provider (HCP) any critical findings and related symptoms. A listing of these findings varies among facilities. Timely notification of a critical finding for laboratory or diagnostic studies is a role expectation of the professional nurse. The notification processes vary among facilities. Upon receipt of the critical finding, the information should be read back to the caller to verify accuracy.

Observe the patient for signs and symptoms of elevated lead levels to include headache, impaired hearing, weight loss, disturbances of the nervous system, severe stomach cramps, and anemia. The pediatric patient may also demonstrate delayed learning and delayed growth.

INTERFERING FACTORS

Contamination of the collection site and/or specimen with lead in dust can be avoided by taking special care to have the surfaces surrounding the collection location cleaned. Extra care should also be used to avoid contamination during the actual venipuncture.

NURSING IMPLICATIONS AND PROCEDURE

PRETEST:

- Positively identify the patient using at least two person-specific identifiers before services, treatments, or procedures are performed.
- *Patient Teaching:* Inform the patient this test can assist in detecting lead exposure.
- Obtain a history of the patient's health concerns, symptoms, surgical procedures, and results of previously performed laboratory and diagnostic studies. Include a list of known allergens, especially allergies or sensitivities to latex.
- Obtain a history of the patient's exposure to lead.
- Obtain a list of the patient's current medications, including over-the-counter medications and dietary supplements (see Effects of Natural Products on Laboratory Values online at Davis*Plus*).
- Review the procedure with the patient. Inform the patient that specimen collection takes approximately 5 to 10 min. Address concerns about pain and explain that there may be some discomfort during the venipuncture.
- *Sensitivity to social and cultural issues,* as well as concern for modesty, is important in providing psychological support before, during, and after the procedure.
- Note that there are no food, fluid, or medication restrictions unless by medical direction.

INTRATEST:

Potential Complications: N/A

- Avoid the use of equipment containing latex if the patient has a history of allergic reaction to latex.
- Instruct the patient to cooperate fully and to follow directions. Direct the patient to breathe normally and to avoid unnecessary movement.
- Observe standard precautions, and follow the general guidelines in Patient Preparation and Specimen Collection online at Davis*Plus*. Positively identify the patient, and label the appropriate specimen container with the corresponding patient demographics, initials of the person collecting the specimen, date, and time of collection. Perform a venipuncture.
- Remove the needle and apply direct pressure with dry gauze to stop bleeding. Observe/assess venipuncture site for bleeding or hematoma formation and secure gauze with adhesive bandage.
- Promptly transport the specimen to the laboratory for processing and analysis.

POST-TEST:

- Inform the patient that a report of the results will be made available

to the requesting HCP, who will discuss the results with the patient.
- Reinforce information given by the patient's HCP regarding further testing, treatment, or referral to another HCP. Answer any questions or address any concerns voiced by the patient or family.
- Depending on the results of this procedure, additional testing may be performed to evaluate or monitor progression of the disease process and determine the need for a change in therapy. Evaluate test results in relation to the patient's symptoms and other tests performed.

RELATED STUDIES:

- Related tests include δ-aminolevulinic acid, CBC, CBC RBC morphology, erythrocyte protoporphyrin, and urine porphyrins.
- Refer to the Hematopoietic System table online at Davis*Plus* for related tests by body system.

Leukocyte Alkaline Phosphatase

SYNONYM/ACRONYM: LAP, LAP score, LAP smear.

COMMON USE: To monitor response to therapy in Hodgkin's disease and diagnose other disorders of the hematological system such as aplastic anemia.

SPECIMEN: Whole blood collected in a lavender-top (EDTA) tube.

NORMAL FINDINGS: (Method: Microscopic evaluation of specially stained blood smears) 25 to 130 (score based on 0 to 4+ rating of 100 neutrophils).

POTENTIAL MEDICAL DIAGNOSIS

Increased in:

Conditions that result in an increase in leukocytes in all stages of maturity will reflect a corresponding increase in LAP.

- Aplastic leukemia
- Chronic inflammation
- Down's syndrome
- Hairy cell leukemia
- Hodgkin's disease
- Leukemia (acute and chronic lymphoblastic)
- Myelofibrosis with myeloid metaplasia
- Multiple myeloma
- Polycythemia vera ***(increase in all blood cell lines, including leukocytes)***
- Pregnancy
- Stress
- Thrombocytopenia

Decreased in:

- Chronic myelogenous leukemia
- Hereditary hypophosphatemia ***(insufficient phosphorus levels)***
- Idiopathic thrombocytopenia purpura
- Nephrotic syndrome ***(excessive loss of phosphorus)***
- Paroxysmal nocturnal hemoglobinuria ***(possibly related to the absence of LAP and other proteins anchored to the red blood cell wall, resulting in complement-mediated hemolysis)***
- Sickle cell anemia
- Sideroblastic anemia

CRITICAL FINDINGS: N/A

Find and print out the full study on Fast Find at davispl.us/vanleeuwen7.

Lipase

SYNONYM/ACRONYM: Triacylglycerol acylhydrolase.

COMMON USE: To assess for pancreatic disease related to inflammation, tumor, or cyst, specific to the diagnosis of pancreatitis.

SPECIMEN: Serum collected in a gold-, red-, or red/gray-top tube. Plasma collected in a green-top (heparin) tube is also acceptable.

NORMAL FINDINGS: (Method: Enzymatic spectrophotometry)

	Conventional & SI Units
Newborn–older adult	0–60 units/L

DESCRIPTION: Lipases are digestive enzymes secreted mainly by the pancreas into the duodenum. There are different lipolytic enzymes with specific substrates, but they are collectively described as lipase. Other lipases produced by the body include sources such as the salivary glands, tongue, liver, intestines, and stomach. Lipase participates in fat digestion by breaking down triglycerides into fatty acids and glycerol so the fatty acids can be absorbed and either used for energy or stored for later use. Lipase is released into the bloodstream when damage occurs to the pancreatic acinar cells.

This procedure is contraindicated for: N/A

INDICATIONS

- Assist in the diagnosis of acute and chronic pancreatitis.
- Assist in the diagnosis of pancreatic carcinoma.

POTENTIAL MEDICAL DIAGNOSIS

Increased in:

Lipase is contained in pancreatic tissue and is released into the serum when cell damage or necrosis occurs.

- Acute cholecystitis
- Bowel obstruction
- Cystic fibrosis
- Chronic diseases of the pancreas that cause permanent damage to acinar cells
- Chronic kidney disease ***(related to decreased urinary excretion)***
- Obstruction of the pancreatic duct
- Pancreatic carcinoma (early)
- Pancreatic cyst or pseudocyst
- Pancreatic inflammation
- Pancreatitis (acute and chronic)

Decreased in: N/A

CRITICAL FINDINGS: N/A

INTERFERING FACTORS

- Drugs and other substances that may increase lipase levels include acetaminophen, asparaginase, azathioprine, calcitriol, cholinergics, codeine, diazoxide, didanosine, felbamate, glycocholate, hydrocortisone, indomethacin, meperidine, methacholine, methylprednisolone, metolazone, morphine, narcotics, nitrofurantoin, pancreozymin, pentazocine, and taurocholate.
- Drugs and other substances that may decrease lipase levels include protamine and saline intravenous (IV) infusions.

- Endoscopic retrograde cholangiopancreatography (ECRP) may increase lipase levels; specimens should be collected prior to ERCP.
- Serum lipase levels increase with hemodialysis. Therefore, predialysis specimens should be collected for lipase analysis.

NURSING IMPLICATIONS AND PROCEDURE

POTENTIAL NURSING PROBLEMS:

Problem	Signs & Symptoms	Interventions
Nutrition ***(related to altered pancreatic function; excess alcohol intake; insufficient eating habits; altered pancreatic and liver function)***	Known inadequate caloric intake; weight loss; muscle wasting in arms and legs; stool that is pale or gray colored; skin that is flaky with loss of elasticity	Document food intake with possible calorie count; assess barriers to eating; consider using a food diary; monitor continued alcohol use, as it is a barrier to adequate protein nutrition; monitor glucose levels; record daily weight; provide dietary consult with assessment of cultural food selections
Fluid volume ***(related to vomiting; decreased oral intake; diaphoresis; nothing by mouth with a nasogastric tube; overly aggressive fluid resuscitation; compromised renal function; overly aggressive diuresis)***	**Deficient:** Decreased urinary output, fatigue, and sunken eyes, dark urine, decreased blood pressure, increased heart rate, and altered mental status **Overload:** Edema, shortness of breath, increased weight, ascites, rales, rhonchi, and diluted laboratory values	Record daily weight and monitor trends; record accurate intake and output; collaborate with health-care provider (HCP) with administration of IV fluids to support hydration; monitor laboratory values that reflect alterations in fluid status (potassium, blood urea nitrogen, creatinine, calcium, hemoglobin, and hematocrit); manage underlying cause of fluid alteration; monitor urine characteristics and respiratory status; establish baseline assessment data; collaborate with physician to adjust oral and IV fluids to provide optimal hydration status; administer replacement electrolytes as ordered
Pain ***(related to organ inflammation and surrounding tissues;***	Emotional symptoms of distress; crying; agitation; facial grimace; moaning; verbalization of pain; rocking	Collaborate with the patient and HCP to identify the best pain management modality to provide relief; refrain from activities that may aggravate pain; use the application of

(table continues on page 1040)

Problem	Signs & Symptoms	Interventions
excessive alcohol intake; infection)	motions; irritability; disturbed sleep; diaphoresis; altered blood pressure and heart rate; nausea; vomiting; self-report of pain; upper abdominal and gastric pain after eating fatty foods or alcohol intake with acute pancreatic disease; pain may be decreased or absent in chronic pancreatic disease	heat or cold to the best effect in managing the pain; monitor pain severity
Breathing ***(related to abdominal distention; ascites; pleural effusion; respiratory failure)***	Dyspnea; shortness of breath; increased work of breathing; nasal flare; respiratory rate greater than 24 breaths per minute; tachypnea; use of accessory muscles for breathing; anxiety	Monitor for cyanosis and pallor; monitor effect of administered medication on respiratory effort; evaluate need for intubation or mechanical ventilation; monitor and trend vital signs and rate and effort; monitor for snoring when sleeping; auscultate and access for adventitious breath sounds

L

PRETEST:

- Positively identify the patient using at least two person-specific identifiers before services, treatments, or procedures are performed.
- *Patient Teaching:* Inform the patient this test can assist in diagnosing pancreatitis.
- Obtain a history of the patient's health concerns, symptoms, surgical procedures, and results of previously performed laboratory and diagnostic studies. Include a list of known allergens, especially allergies or sensitivities to latex.
- Note any recent procedures that can interfere with test results.
- Obtain a list of the patient's current medications, including over-the-counter medications and dietary supplements (see Effects of Natural Products on Laboratory Values online at Davis*Plus*).
- Review the procedure with the patient. Inform the patient that specimen collection takes approximately 5 to 10 min. Address concerns about pain and explain that there may be some discomfort during the venipuncture.
- *Sensitivity to social and cultural issues,* as well as concern for modesty, is important in providing psychological support before, during, and after the procedure.
- Note that there are no food, fluid, or medication restrictions unless by medical direction.

INTRATEST:

Potential Complications: N/A

- Avoid the use of equipment containing latex if the patient has a history of allergic reaction to latex.
- Instruct the patient to cooperate fully and to follow directions. Direct the patient to breathe normally and to avoid unnecessary movement.
- Observe standard precautions, and follow the general guidelines in Patient Preparation and Specimen Collection online at Davis*Plus*. Positively identify the patient, and label the appropriate specimen container with the corresponding patient demographics, initials of the person collecting the specimen, date, and time of collection. Perform a venipuncture.
- Remove the needle and apply direct pressure with dry gauze to stop bleeding. Observe/assess venipuncture site for bleeding or hematoma formation and secure gauze with adhesive bandage.
- Promptly transport the specimen to the laboratory for processing and analysis.

POST-TEST:

- Inform the patient that a report of the results will be made available to the requesting HCP, who will discuss the results with the patient.
- *Nutritional Considerations:* Instruct the patient to ingest small, frequent meals if he or she has a gastrointestinal disorder; advise the patient to consider other dietary alterations as well. After acute symptoms subside and bowel sounds return, patients are usually prescribed a clear liquid diet, progressing to a low-fat, high-carbohydrate diet.
- Administer vitamin B_{12}, as ordered, to the patient with decreased lipase levels, especially if his or her disease prevents adequate absorption of the vitamin.
- Depending on the results of this procedure, additional testing may be performed to evaluate or monitor progression of the disease process and determine the need for a change in therapy. Evaluate test results in relation to the patient's symptoms and other tests performed.

Patient Education:

- Encourage the patient who abuses alcohol to avoid alcohol and to seek appropriate counseling for substance abuse.
- Reinforce information given by the patient's HCP regarding further testing, treatment, or referral to another HCP.
- Recognize anxiety related to test results and answer any questions or address any concerns voiced by the patient or family.
- Teach the patient and the patient's family that they should report any difficulty of breathing or shortness of breath to the nurse for immediate intervention.
- Reinforce information provided by the HCP that intubation or mechanical ventilation may be necessary to support breathing if there is no improvement.

Expected Patient Outcomes:

Understanding

- The patient and family design a plan of care for home that supports improved breathing.
- The patient and family identify signs and symptoms that indicate compromised breathing.

Ability

- The patient proficiently demonstrates relaxation techniques that improve his or her breathing pattern.
- The patient follows the prescribed therapeutic interventions that improve lung ventilation.

Response

- The patient complies with prescribed pain management to improve breathing.
- The patient and family accept information about advance directive options.

RELATED STUDIES:

- Related tests include ALT, ALP, amylase, AST, bilirubin, calcitonin stimulation, calcium, cancer antigens,

L

cholangiography percutaneous transhepatic, cholesterol, CBC, CBC WCB count and diff, ERCP, fecal fat, GGT, hepatobiliary scan, magnesium, MRI pancreas, mumps serology, pleural fluid analysis, peritoneal fluid analysis, triglycerides, US abdomen, and US pancreas.

- Refer to the Gastrointestinal and Hepatobiliary systems tables online at Davis*Plus* for related tests by body system.

Lipoprotein Electrophoresis

SYNONYM/ACRONYM: Lipid fractionation; lipoprotein phenotyping; $3ga_1$-lipoprotein cholesterol, high-density lipoprotein (HDL); β-lipoprotein cholesterol, low-density lipoprotein (LDL); pre-β-lipoprotein cholesterol, very-low-density lipoprotein (VLDL).

COMMON USE: To assist in categorizing lipoprotein as an indicator of cardiac health.

SPECIMEN: Serum collected in a gold-, red-, or red/gray-top tube.

NORMAL FINDINGS: (Method: Electrophoresis and 4°C test for specimen appearance) There is no quantitative interpretation of this test. The specimen appearance and electrophoretic pattern is visually interpreted.

Hyperlipoproteinemia: Fredrickson Type	Specimen Appearance	Electrophoretic Pattern
Type I	Clear with creamy top layer	Heavy chylomicron band
Type IIa	Clear	Heavy β band
Type IIb	Clear or faintly turbid	Heavy β and pre-β bands
Type III	Slightly to moderately turbid	Heavy β band
Type IV	Slightly to moderately turbid	Heavy pre-β band
Type V	Slightly to moderately turbid with creamy top layer	Intense chylomicron band and heavy β and pre-β bands

POTENTIAL MEDICAL DIAGNOSIS

- *Type I:* Hyperlipoproteinemia, or increased chylomicrons, can be primary ***resulting from an inherited deficiency of lipoprotein lipase*** or secondary ***caused by uncontrolled diabetes, systemic lupus erythematosus, and dysgammaglobulinemia.*** Total cholesterol is normal to moderately elevated, and triglycerides (mostly exogenous chylomicrons) are grossly elevated. If the condition is inherited, symptoms will appear in childhood.
- *Type IIa:* Hyperlipoproteinemia can be primary ***resulting from***

inherited characteristics or secondary ***caused by uncontrolled hypothyroidism, nephrotic syndrome, and dysgammaglobulinemia.*** Total cholesterol is elevated, triglycerides are normal, and LDLC is elevated. If the condition is inherited, symptoms will appear in childhood.

- *Type IIb:* Hyperlipoproteinemia ***can occur for the same reasons as in type IIa.*** Total cholesterol, triglycerides, and LDLC are all elevated.
- *Type III:* Hyperlipoproteinemia can be primary ***resulting from inherited characteristics*** or secondary ***caused by hypothyroidism, uncontrolled diabetes, alcoholism, and dysgammaglobulinemia.*** Total cholesterol and triglycerides are elevated, whereas LDLC is normal.
- *Type IV:* Hyperlipoproteinemia can be primary ***resulting from inherited characteristics*** or secondary ***caused by poorly controlled diabetes, alcoholism, nephrotic syndrome, chronic renal failure, and dysgammaglobulinemia.*** Total cholesterol is normal to moderately elevated, triglycerides are moderately to grossly elevated, and LDLC is normal.
- *Type V:* Hyperlipoproteinemia can be primary ***resulting from inherited characteristics,*** or secondary ***caused by uncontrolled diabetes, alcoholism, nephrotic syndrome, and dysgammaglobulinemia.*** Total cholesterol is normal to moderately elevated, triglycerides are grossly elevated, and LDLC is normal.

CRITICAL FINDINGS: N/A

Find and print out the full study on Fast Find at davispl.us/vanleeuwen7.

L

Liver and Spleen Scan

SYNONYM/ACRONYM: Liver and spleen scintigraphy, radionuclide liver scan, spleen scan.

COMMON USE: To visualize and assess the liver and spleen related to tumors, inflammation, cysts, abscess, trauma, and portal hypertension.

AREA OF APPLICATION: Abdomen.

DESCRIPTION: The liver and spleen scan is performed to help diagnose abnormalities in the function and structure of the liver and spleen. It is often performed in combination with lung scanning to help diagnose masses or inflammation in the diaphragmatic area. This procedure is useful for evaluating right-upper-quadrant pain, metastatic disease, jaundice, cirrhosis, ascites, traumatic infarction, and radiation-induced organ cellular necrosis. Technetium-99m (Tc-99m) sulfur colloid is injected by intravenous (IV) access and rapidly taken up through phagocytosis by the reticuloendothelial cells, which normally function to remove particulate matter, including radioactive colloids in the liver and spleen. Radionuclide uptake in the spleen should always be less than uptake in the liver.

Access Canadian content on Fast Find: Lab and Dx at davispl.us/vanleeuwen7

False-negative results may occur in patients with space-occupying lesions that prevent normal hepatic filling (e.g., tumors, cysts, abscesses) smaller than 2 cm. For evaluation of a suspected hemangioma, the most common benign cause of a hepatic filling defect, the patient's red blood cells are combined with Tc-99m and images are recorded of the liver. This scan can detect portal hypertension, demonstrated by a greater uptake of the radionuclide in the spleen than in the liver. Liver and spleen scans are generally being ordered with less frequency and are in some cases being replaced by more advanced technology to include computed tomography (CT), magnetic resonance imaging (MRI), ultrasonography (US), and SPECT scans. Single-photon emission computed tomography (SPECT) has significantly improved the resolution and accuracy of liver scanning. SPECT enables images to be recorded from multiple angles around the body and reconstructed by a computer to produce images, or *slices,* representing the organ at different levels. Diagnostic test results are interpreted in light of the results of liver function tests (alanine aminotransferase, albumin, alkaline phosphatase, aspartate aminotransferase, bilirubin, total protein). Liver scans are also used to assist with tumor staging, monitor disease progress, and follow response to therapeutic interventions.

This procedure is contraindicated for

Patients who are pregnant or suspected of being pregnant, unless the potential benefits of a procedure using radiation far outweigh the risk of radiation exposure to the fetus and mother.

INDICATIONS

- Assess the condition of the liver and spleen after abdominal trauma.
- Detect a bacterial or amebic abscess.
- Detect and differentiate between primary and metastatic tumor focal disease.
- Detect benign tumors, such as adenoma and cavernous hemangioma.
- Detect cystic focal disease.
- Detect diffuse hepatocellular disease, such as hepatitis and cirrhosis.
- Detect infiltrative processes that affect the liver, such as sarcoidosis and amyloidosis.
- Determine superior vena cava obstruction or Budd-Chiari syndrome.
- Differentiate between splenomegaly and hepatomegaly.
- Evaluate the effects of lower abdominal trauma, such as internal hemorrhage.
- Evaluate jaundice.
- Evaluate liver and spleen damage caused by radiation therapy or toxic drug therapy.
- Evaluate palpable abdominal masses.
- Evaluate post–liver transplantation for indications of organ rejection.

POTENTIAL MEDICAL DIAGNOSIS

Normal findings

- Normal size, contour, position, and function of the liver and spleen

Abnormal findings related to

The radioactive tracer accumulates in abnormal tissue, and "hot spots" identify specific areas of concern. "Cold spots," or the absence of tracer in areas where uptake is expected, also can identify specific areas of concern. Images can identify abnormalities in anatomical structures with regard to size, shape, and function (e.g., unexpected cold spots may inform with regard to dysfunctional tissue, filling defects).

- Abscesses
- Cirrhosis
- Cysts
- Hemangiomas ***evidenced by immediate uptake of the radionuclide by the filling defect***
- Hematomas
- Hepatitis
- Hodgkin's disease
- Infarction
- Infection
- Infiltrative process (amyloidosis and sarcoidosis)
- Inflammation of the diaphragmatic area
- Metastatic tumors
- Nodular hyperplasia
- Portal hypertension ***related to a reversal in the radionuclide uptake ratio (liver to spleen), which indicates a reversal in blood flow (as a result of portal hypertension)***
- Primary benign or malignant tumors
- Traumatic lesions

CRITICAL FINDINGS:

- Visceral injury

Note and immediately report to the requesting health-care provider (HCP) any critical findings and related symptoms. A listing of these findings varies among facilities. Timely notification of a critical finding for laboratory or diagnostic studies is a role expectation of the professional nurse. The notification processes vary among facilities. Upon receipt of the critical finding, the information should be read back to the caller to verify accuracy.

INTERFERING FACTORS

Factors that may alter the results of the study

- Inability of the patient to cooperate or remain still during the procedure because of age, significant pain, or mental status.
- Metallic objects (e.g., jewelry, body rings) within the examination field, which may inhibit organ visualization and cause unclear images.
- Other nuclear scans done within the preceding 24 to 48 hr.

Other considerations

- The scan may fail to detect focal lesions smaller than 2 cm in diameter.
- Improper injection of the radionuclide may allow the tracer to seep deep into the muscle tissue, producing erroneous hot spots.

NURSING IMPLICATIONS AND PROCEDURE

See Potential Nursing Problems on Fast Find at davispl.us/vanleeuwen7.

PRETEST:

- Positively identify the patient using at least two person-specific identifiers before services, treatments, or procedures are performed.
- *Patient Teaching:* Inform the patient this procedure can assist in evaluating liver and spleen function.
- Obtain a history of the patient's health concerns, symptoms, surgical procedures, and results of previously performed laboratory and diagnostic studies. Include a list of known allergens, especially allergies or sensitivities to latex, anesthetics, sedatives, or radionuclides.
- Note any recent procedures that can interfere with test results, including examinations using iodine-based contrast medium.
- Record the date of the last menstrual period and determine the possibility of pregnancy in perimenopausal women.

- Obtain a list of the patient's current medications, including over-the-counter medications and dietary supplements (see Effects of Natural Products on Laboratory Values online at Davis*Plus*).
- Review the procedure with the patient. Address concerns about pain related to the procedure and explain that some pain may be experienced during the test, or there may be moments of discomfort. Reassure the patient that the radionuclide poses no radioactive hazard and rarely produces adverse effects. Inform the patient the procedure is performed in a nuclear medicine department by an HCP specializing in this procedure, with support staff, and takes approximately 30 to 60 min.
- *Sensitivity to social and cultural issues,* as well as concern for modesty, is important in providing psychological support before, during, and after the procedure.
- Explain that an IV line may be inserted to allow infusion of fluids such as saline, anesthetics, sedatives, radionuclides, medications used in the procedure, or emergency medications.
- Instruct the patient to remove jewelry and other metallic objects from the area to be examined.
- Note that there are no food, fluid, or medication restrictions unless by medical direction.
- *Make sure a written and informed consent has been signed prior to the procedure and before administering any medications.*

INTRATEST:

Potential Complications:

Although it is rare, there is the possibility of allergic reaction to the radionuclide. Have emergency equipment and medications readily available. If the patient has a history of allergic reactions to any substance or drug, administer ordered prophylactic steroids or antihistamines before the procedure.

Establishing an IV site and injection of radionuclides is an invasive procedure. Complications are rare but do include bleeding from the puncture site ***related to a bleeding disorder, or the effects of natural products and medications with known anticoagulant, antiplatelet, or thrombolytic properties,*** hematoma ***related to blood leakage into the tissue following needle insertion,*** infection ***that might occur if bacteria from the skin surface is introduced at the puncture site,*** or nerve injury ***that might occur if the needle strikes a nerve.***

- Observe standard precautions, and follow the general guidelines in Patient Preparation and Specimen Collection online at Davis*Plus*. Positively identify the patient.
- Ensure that the patient has removed all external metallic objects from the area to be examined prior to the procedure.
- Administer ordered prophylactic steroids or antihistamines before the procedure if the patient has a history of allergic reactions to any substance or drug.
- Avoid the use of equipment containing latex if the patient has a history of allergic reaction to latex.
- Have emergency equipment readily available.
- Instruct the patient to void prior to the procedure and to change into the gown, robe, and foot coverings provided.
- Record baseline vital signs and assess neurological status. Protocols may vary among facilities.
- Establish an IV fluid line for the injection of saline, anesthetics, sedatives, radionuclides, or emergency medications.
- Instruct the patient to cooperate fully and to follow directions. Instruct the patient to remain still throughout the procedure because movement produces unreliable results.
- Administer sedative to a child or to an uncooperative adult, as ordered.
- Place the patient in a supine position on a flat table with foam wedges,

which help maintain position and immobilization.
- IV radionuclide is administered, and the abdomen is scanned immediately to screen for vascular lesions with images taken in various positions.
- Monitor the patient for complications related to the procedure (e.g., allergic reaction, anaphylaxis, bronchospasm).
- Remove the needle or catheter and apply a pressure dressing over the puncture site.
- Observe/assess the needle/catheter insertion site for bleeding, inflammation, or hematoma formation.
- The patient may be imaged by SPECT techniques to further clarify areas of suspicious radionuclide localization.

POST-TEST:

- Inform the patient that a report of the results will be made available to the requesting HCP, who will discuss the results with the patient.
- Instruct the patient to resume usual medication and activity, as directed by the HCP.
- Unless contraindicated, advise patient to drink increased amounts of fluids for 24 to 48 hr to eliminate the radionuclide from the body. Inform the patient that radionuclide is eliminated from the body within 6 to 24 hr.
- No other radionuclide tests should be scheduled for 24 to 48 hr after this procedure.
- Instruct the patient in the care and assessment of the injection site.
- If a woman who is breastfeeding must have a nuclear scan, she should not breastfeed the infant until the radionuclide has been eliminated. This could take as long as 3 days. She should be instructed to express the milk and discard it during the 3-day period to prevent cessation of milk production.
- Instruct the patient to immediately flush the toilet and to meticulously wash hands with soap and water after each voiding for 24 hr after the procedure.
- Instruct all caregivers to wear gloves when discarding urine for 24 hr after the procedure. Wash gloved hands with soap and water before removing gloves; then wash ungloved hands.
- ***Nutritional Considerations:*** A low-fat, low-cholesterol, and low-sodium diet should be consumed to reduce current disease processes. High fat consumption increases the amount of bile acids in the colon and should be avoided.
- Recognize anxiety related to test results, and be supportive of perceived loss of independent function. Discuss the implications of abnormal test results on the patient's lifestyle. Provide teaching and information regarding the clinical implications of the test results, as appropriate.
- Reinforce information given by the patient's HCP regarding further testing, treatment, or referral to another HCP. Answer any questions or address any concerns voiced by the patient or family.
- Depending on the results of this procedure, additional testing may be needed to evaluate or monitor progression of the disease process and determine the need for a change in therapy. Evaluate test results in relation to the patient's symptoms and other tests performed.

Patient Education:

- Teach the patient that the purpose of measuring abdominal girth is to monitor for the presence and extent of ascites.
- Teach the patient how to keep a food diary to monitor caloric intake.

Expected Patient Outcomes:

Understanding

- The patient and family state the importance of an adequate caloric intake for positive health.
- The patient and family state the importance of taking dietary supplements.

Ability

- The patient and family demonstrate accurate recording of intake and output.
- The patient successfully demonstrates taking own daily weight.

Response

- The patient agrees to recommended follow-up appointments and diagnostic and laboratory studies.
- The patient agrees to restrict fluid intake as appropriate.

RELATED STUDIES:

- Related tests include ALT, antibodies antimitochondrial, AST, bilirubin, biopsy liver, CT abdomen, CT biliary tract and liver, GGT, HAV, HBV, HCV, hepatobiliary scan, MRI abdomen, and US liver.
- Refer to the Hematopoietic, Hepatobiliary, and Immune systems tables online at Davis*Plus* for related tests by body system.

Lung Perfusion Scan

SYNONYM/ACRONYM: Lung perfusion scintigraphy, lung scintiscan, pulmonary scan, radioactive perfusion scan, radionuclide lung scan, ventilation-perfusion scan, V/Q scan.

COMMON USE: To assess pulmonary blood flow to assist in diagnosis of pulmonary embolism.

AREA OF APPLICATION: Chest/thorax.

DESCRIPTION: The lung perfusion scan is a nuclear medicine study performed to evaluate a patient for pulmonary embolus (PE) or other pulmonary disorders. Technetium (Tc-99m) is injected by intravenous (IV) access and distributed throughout the pulmonary vasculature. The scan, which produces a visual image of pulmonary blood flow, is useful in diagnosing or confirming pulmonary vascular obstruction. The diameter of the IV-injected macroaggregated albumin (MAA) is larger than that of the pulmonary capillaries; therefore, the MAA temporarily becomes lodged in the pulmonary vasculature. A gamma camera detects the radiation emitted from the injected radioactive material, and a representative image of the lung is obtained. This procedure is often done in conjunction with the lung ventilation scan to obtain clinical information that assists in differentiating among the many possible pathological conditions revealed by the procedure; the combined study is a V/Q scan. The results are correlated with other diagnostic studies, such as thoracic computed tomography, pulmonary function, chest x-ray, pulmonary angiography, ECG, and arterial blood gases. A recent chest x-ray is essential for accurate interpretation of the lung perfusion scan. An area of nonperfusion seen in the same area as a pulmonary parenchymal abnormality on the chest x-ray indicates that a PE is not present; the defect may represent some other pathological condition, such as pneumonia.

This procedure is contraindicated for

- Patients who are pregnant or suspected of being pregnant, unless the potential benefits of a procedure using radiation far outweigh the risk of radiation exposure to the fetus and mother.
- Patients with atrial and ventricular septal defects ***because the MAA particles will not reach the lungs.***
- Patients with pulmonary hypertension.

INDICATIONS

- Aid in the diagnosis of PE in a patient with a normal chest x-ray.
- Detect malignant tumor.
- Differentiate between PE and other pulmonary diseases, such as pneumonia, pulmonary effusion, atelectasis, asthma, bronchitis, and tumors.
- Evaluate perfusion changes associated with congestive heart failure and pulmonary hypertension.
- Evaluate pulmonary function preoperatively in a patient with pulmonary disease.

POTENTIAL MEDICAL DIAGNOSIS

Normal findings

- Diffuse and homogeneous uptake of the radioactive material by the lungs

Abnormal findings related to

The radioactive tracer accumulates in abnormal tissue, and "hot spots" in areas that would otherwise be expected to demonstrate a diffusely uniform distribution of radionuclide identify specific areas of concern.

- Asthma
- Atelectasis
- Bronchitis
- Chronic obstructive pulmonary disease
- Left atrial or pulmonary hypertension
- Lung displacement by fluid or chest masses
- Pneumonia
- Pneumonitis
- PE
- Tuberculosis

CRITICAL FINDINGS:

- PE

Note and immediately report to the requesting health-care provider (HCP) any critical findings and related symptoms. A listing of these findings varies among facilities. Timely notification of a critical finding for laboratory or diagnostic studies is a role expectation of the professional nurse. The notification processes vary among facilities. Upon receipt of the critical finding, the information should be read back to the caller to verify accuracy.

INTERFERING FACTORS

Factors that may alter the results of the study

- Inability of the patient to cooperate or remain still during the procedure because of age, significant pain, or mental status.
- Metallic objects (e.g., jewelry, body rings) within the examination field, which may inhibit organ visualization and cause unclear images.
- Other nuclear scans done on the same day.

Other considerations

- Improper injection of the radionuclide may allow the tracer to seep deep into the muscle tissue, producing erroneous hot spots.

NURSING IMPLICATIONS AND PROCEDURE

See Potential Nursing Problems on Fast Find at davispl.us/vanleeuwen7.

PRETEST:

- Positively identify the patient using at least two person-specific identifiers before services, treatments, or procedures are performed.

- *Patient Teaching:* Inform the patient this procedure can assist in assessing blood flow to the lungs.
- Obtain a history of the patient's health concerns, symptoms, surgical procedures, and results of previously performed laboratory and diagnostic studies. Include a list of known allergens, especially allergies or sensitivities to latex, anesthetics, sedatives, or radionuclides.
- Note any recent procedures that can interfere with test results, including examinations using iodine-based contrast medium.
- Record the date of the last menstrual period and determine the possibility of pregnancy in perimenopausal women.
- Obtain a list of the patient's current medications, including over-the-counter medications and dietary supplements (see Effects of Natural Products on Laboratory Values online at Davis*Plus*).
- Review the procedure with the patient. Address concerns about pain related to the procedure and explain that some pain may be experienced during the test, or there may be moments of discomfort. Reassure the patient that the radionuclide poses no radioactive hazard and rarely produces adverse effects. Inform the patient that the procedure is performed in a nuclear medicine department, by a health-care provider (HCP) specializing in this procedure, with support staff, and takes approximately 60 min.
- ***Sensitivity to social and cultural issues,*** as well as concern for modesty, is important in providing psychological support before, during, and after the procedure.
- Explain that an IV line may be inserted to allow infusion of fluids such as saline, anesthetics, sedatives, radionuclides, medications used in the procedure, or emergency medications.
- Instruct the patient to remove jewelry and other metallic objects from the area to be examined prior to the procedure.
- Note that there are no food, fluid, or medication restrictions unless by medical direction.
- *Make sure a written and informed consent has been signed prior to the procedure and before administering any medications.*

INTRATEST:

Potential Complications:

Although it is rare, there is the possibility of allergic reaction to the radionuclide. Have emergency equipment and medications readily available. If the patient has a history of allergic reactions to any substance or drug, administer ordered prophylactic steroids or antihistamines before the procedure.

Establishing an IV site and injection of radionuclides is an invasive procedure. Complications are rare but do include bleeding from the puncture site ***related to a bleeding disorder, or the effects of natural products and medications with known anticoagulant, antiplatelet, or thrombolytic properties,*** hematoma ***related to blood leakage into the tissue following needle insertion,*** infection ***that might occur if bacteria from the skin surface is introduced at the puncture site,*** or nerve injury ***that might occur if the needle strikes a nerve.***

- Observe standard precautions, and follow the general guidelines in Patient Preparation and Specimen Collection online at Davis*Plus*. Positively identify the patient.
- Ensure that the patient has removed all external metallic objects from the area to be examined prior to the procedure.
- Administer ordered prophylactic steroids or antihistamines before the procedure if the patient has a history of allergic reactions to any substance or drug.
- Avoid the use of equipment containing latex if the patient has a history of allergic reaction to latex.
- Have emergency equipment readily available.

L

- Instruct the patient to void prior to the procedure and to change into the gown, robe, and foot coverings provided.
- Record baseline vital signs and assess neurological status. Protocols may vary among facilities.
- Establish an IV fluid line for the injection of saline, anesthetics, sedatives, radionuclides, or emergency medications.
- Instruct the patient to cooperate fully and to follow directions. Instruct the patient to remain still throughout the procedure because movement produces unreliable results.
- Administer a sedative to a child or to an uncooperative adult, as ordered.
- Place the patient in a supine position on a flat table with foam wedges, which help maintain position and immobilization.
- IV radionuclide is administered, and the abdomen is scanned immediately to screen for vascular lesions with images taken in various positions.
- Monitor the patient for complications related to the procedure (e.g., allergic reaction, anaphylaxis, bronchospasm).
- Remove the needle or catheter and apply a pressure dressing over the puncture site.
- Observe/assess the needle/catheter insertion site for bleeding, inflammation, or hematoma formation.

POST-TEST:

- Inform the patient that a report of the results will be made available to the requesting HCP, who will discuss the results with the patient.
- Unless contraindicated, advise patient to drink increased amounts of fluids for 24 to 48 hr to eliminate the radionuclide from the body. Inform the patient that radionuclide is eliminated from the body within 6 to 24 hr.
- No other radionuclide tests should be scheduled for 24 to 48 hr after this procedure.
- Monitor vital signs and neurological status every 15 min for 1 hr, then every 2 hr for 4 hr, and then as ordered by the HCP. Compare with baseline values. Protocols may vary among facilities.
- Instruct the patient to resume usual medication and activity, as directed by the HCP.
- Observe for delayed allergic reactions, such as rash, urticaria, tachycardia, hyperpnea, hypertension, palpitations, nausea, or vomiting.
- Instruct the patient to immediately report symptoms such as fast heart rate, difficulty breathing, skin rash, itching, chest pain, persistent right shoulder pain, or abdominal pain. Immediately report symptoms to the appropriate HCP.
- Observe/assess the needle/catheter insertion site for bleeding, inflammation, or hematoma formation.
- Instruct the patient in the care and assessment of the injection site.
- If a woman who is breastfeeding must have a nuclear scan, she should not breastfeed the infant until the radionuclide has been eliminated. This could take as long as 3 days. She should be instructed to express the milk and discard it during the 3-day period to prevent cessation of milk production.
- Instruct the patient to immediately flush the toilet and to meticulously wash hands with soap and water after each voiding for 24 hr after the procedure.
- Instruct all caregivers to wear gloves when discarding urine for 24 hr after the procedure. Wash gloved hands with soap and water before removing gloves; then wash ungloved hands.
- Recognize anxiety related to test results, and be supportive of perceived loss of independent function. Discuss the implications of abnormal test results on the patient's lifestyle. Provide teaching and information regarding the clinical implications of the test results, as appropriate.
- Reinforce information given by the patient's HCP regarding further testing, treatment, or referral to another HCP. Answer any questions or address any concerns voiced by the patient or family.

L

- Depending on the results of this procedure, additional testing may be needed to evaluate or monitor progression of the disease process and determine the need for a change in therapy. Evaluate test results in relation to the patient's symptoms and other tests performed.

Patient Education:

- Teach the patient to report signs of bleeding (bleeding gums, black tarry stools, blood in urine, hematoma).
- Teach the patient the symptoms of pulmonary embolism and the importance of timely reporting.

Expected Patient Outcomes:

Understanding

- The patient and family state the importance of remaining on bed rest to prevent movement of the embolus.
- The patient and family state the importance of keeping oxygen on at all times.

Ability

- The patient demonstrates effective coping mechanisms to decrease anxiety.
- The patient demonstrates how to use controlled breathing to improve breathing patterns.

Response

- The patient agrees to visit the HCP's office for follow-up coagulation studies.
- The patient agrees to take pain medication to decrease breathing discomfort and improve oxygenation.

RELATED STUDIES:

- Related tests include α-1 AT, eosinophil count, ACE, alveolar/arterial gradient, angiography pulmonary, biopsy lung, blood gases, blood pool imaging, bronchoscopy, carbon dioxide, chest x-ray, CBC, CBC WCB count and differential, CT thoracic, culture and smear mycobacteria, culture blood, culture throat, culture sputum, culture viral, cytology sputum, ESR, IgE, gallium scan, lung ventilation scan, MRI chest, MRI venography, mediastinoscopy, aPTT, plethysmography, pleural fluid analysis, PET heart, PFT, pulse oximetry, and TB skin tests.
- Refer to the Respiratory System table online at Davis*Plus* for related tests by body system.

L

Lung Ventilation Scan

SYNONYM/ACRONYM: Aerosol lung scan, radioactive ventilation scan, ventilation scan, VQ lung scan, xenon lung scan.

COMMON USE: To assess pulmonary ventilation to assist in diagnosis of pulmonary embolism.

AREA OF APPLICATION: Chest/thorax.

DESCRIPTION: The lung ventilation scan is a nuclear medicine study performed to evaluate a patient for pulmonary embolus (PE) or other pulmonary disorders. It can evaluate respiratory function (i.e., demonstrating areas of the lung that are patent and capable of ventilation) and dysfunction (e.g., parenchymal abnormalities affecting ventilation, such as pneumonia). The procedure is performed after the patient inhales air mixed with a radioactive gas (xenon gas or technetium-DTPA) through a face mask and mouthpiece. The radioactive gas delineates areas of the lung during ventilation. The distribution of the gas throughout the lung is measured in three phases:

- *Wash-in phase:* Phase during buildup of the radioactive gas
- *Equilibrium phase:* Phase after the patient rebreathes from a closed delivery system
- *Wash-out phase:* Phase after the radioactive gas has been removed

This procedure is usually performed along with a lung perfusion scan. When PE is present, ventilation scans display a normal wash-in and wash-out of radioactivity from the lung areas. Parenchymal disease responsible for perfusion abnormalities will produce abnormal wash-in and wash-out phases. This test can be used to quantify regional ventilation in patients with pulmonary disease.

This procedure is contraindicated for

Patients who are pregnant or suspected of being pregnant, unless the potential benefits of a procedure using radiation far outweigh the risk of radiation exposure to the fetus and mother.

INDICATIONS

- Aid in the diagnosis of PE.
- Differentiate between PE and other pulmonary diseases, such as pneumonia, pulmonary effusion, atelectasis, asthma, bronchitis, and tumors.
- Evaluate regional respiratory function.
- Identify areas of the lung that are capable of ventilation.
- Locate hypoventilation (regional), which can result from chronic obstructive pulmonary disease (COPD) or excessive smoking.

POTENTIAL MEDICAL DIAGNOSIS

Normal findings

- Equal distribution of radioactive gas throughout both lungs and a normal wash-out phase

Abnormal findings related to

The radioactive tracer accumulates in abnormal tissue, and "hot spots" identify specific areas of concern.

- AIDS-related respiratory conditions
- Airway obstruction
- Atelectasis
- Bronchitis
- Bronchogenic carcinoma
- COPD
- Cyanosis
- Cystic fibrosis
- PE
- Pneumonia
- Regional hypoventilation
- Sarcoidosis
- Tuberculosis
- Tumor

CRITICAL FINDINGS:

- PE

Note and immediately report to the requesting health-care provider (HCP) any critical findings and related symptoms. A listing of these findings varies among facilities. Timely notification of a critical finding for laboratory or diagnostic studies is a role expectation of the professional nurse. The notification processes vary among facilities. Upon receipt of the critical finding, the information should be read back to the caller to verify accuracy.

INTERFERING FACTORS

Factors that may alter the results of the study

- Inability of the patient to cooperate or remain still during the procedure because of age, significant pain, or mental status.
- Metallic objects (e.g., jewelry, body rings) within the examination field,

which may inhibit organ visualization and cause unclear images.

- Other nuclear scans done within the preceding 24 to 48 hr.

Other considerations

- The presence of conditions that affect perfusion or ventilation (e.g., tumors that obstruct the pulmonary artery, vasculitis, pulmonary edema, sickle cell disease, parasitic disease, emphysema, effusion, infection) can simulate a perfusion defect similar to PE.

NURSING IMPLICATIONS AND PROCEDURE

See Potential Nursing Problems on Fast Find at davispl.us/vanleeuwen7.

PRETEST:

- Positively identify the patient using at least two person-specific identifiers before services, treatments, or procedures are performed.
- *Patient Teaching:* Inform the patient this procedure can assist in assessing air flow to the lungs.
- Obtain a history of the patient's health concerns, symptoms, surgical procedures, and results of previously performed laboratory and diagnostic studies. Include a list of known allergens, especially allergies or sensitivities to latex, anesthetics, sedatives, or radionuclides.
- Note any recent procedures that can interfere with test results, including examinations using iodine-based contrast medium.
- Record the date of the last menstrual period and determine the possibility of pregnancy in perimenopausal women.
- Obtain a list of the patient's current medications, including over-the-counter medications and dietary supplements (see Effects of Natural Products on Laboratory Values online at Davis*Plus*).
- Review the procedure with the patient. Address concerns about pain related to the procedure and explain that some pain may be experienced during the test, and there may be moments of discomfort. Reassure the patient that the radionuclide poses no radioactive hazard and rarely produces adverse effects. Inform the patient that the procedure is performed in a nuclear medicine department, usually by an HCP who specializes in this procedure, with support staff, and takes approximately 30 to 60 min.
- *Sensitivity to social and cultural issues,* as well as concern for modesty, is important in providing psychological support before, during, and after the procedure.
- Instruct the patient to remove jewelry and other metallic objects from the area to be examined.
- Note that there are no food, fluid, or medication restrictions unless by medical direction.
- *Make sure a written and informed consent has been signed prior to the procedure and before administering any medications.*

INTRATEST:

Potential Complications:

Although it is rare, there is the possibility of allergic reaction to the radionuclide.

- Observe standard precautions, and follow the general guidelines in Patient Preparation and Specimen Collection online at Davis*Plus*. Positively identify the patient.
- Ensure that the patient has removed all external metallic objects from the area to be examined prior to the procedure.
- Administer ordered prophylactic steroids or antihistamines before the procedure if the patient has a history of allergic reactions to any substance or drug.
- Avoid the use of equipment containing latex if the patient has a history of allergic reaction to latex.
- Have emergency equipment readily available.
- Instruct the patient to void prior to the procedure and to change into

the gown, robe, and foot coverings provided.

- Record baseline vital signs and assess neurological status. Protocols may vary among facilities.
- Instruct the patient to cooperate fully and to follow directions. Direct the patient to remain still throughout the procedure because movement produces unreliable results.
- Administer sedative to a child or to an uncooperative adult, as ordered.
- Place the patient in a supine position on a flat table with foam wedges, which help maintain position and immobilization.
- The radionuclide is administered through a mask, which is placed over the patient's nose and mouth. The patient is asked to hold his or her breath for a short period of time while the scan is taken.
- Monitor the patient for complications related to the procedure (e.g., allergic reaction, anaphylaxis, bronchospasm).

POST-TEST:

- Inform the patient that a report of the results will be made available to the requesting HCP, who will discuss the results with the patient.
- Advise patient, unless contraindicated, to drink increased amounts of fluids for 24 to 48 hr to eliminate the radionuclide from the body. Inform the patient that radionuclide is eliminated from the body within 6 to 24 hr.
- No other radionuclide tests should be scheduled for 24 to 48 hr after this procedure.
- Evaluate the patient's vital signs. Monitor vital signs and neurological status every 15 min for 1 hr, then every 2 hr for 4 hr, and then as ordered by the HCP. Compare with baseline values. Protocols may vary among facilities.
- Instruct the patient to resume medication or activity, as directed by the HCP.
- If a woman who is breastfeeding must have a nuclear scan, she should not breastfeed the infant until the radionuclide has been eliminated. This could take as long as 3 days. She should be instructed to express the milk and discard it during the 3-day period to prevent cessation of milk production.
- Instruct the patient to immediately flush the toilet and to meticulously wash hands with soap and water after each voiding for 24 hr after the procedure.
- Instruct all caregivers to wear gloves when discarding urine for 24 hr after the procedure. Wash gloved hands with soap and water before removing gloves; then wash ungloved hands.
- *Nutritional Considerations:* A low-fat, low-cholesterol, and low-sodium diet should be consumed to reduce current disease processes and/or decrease risk of hypertension and coronary artery disease.
- Recognize anxiety related to test results, and be supportive of perceived loss of independent function. Discuss the implications of abnormal test results on the patient's lifestyle. Provide teaching and information regarding the clinical implications of the test results, as appropriate.
- Reinforce information given by the patient's HCP regarding further testing, treatment, or referral to another HCP. Answer any questions or address any concerns voiced by the patient or family.
- Depending on the results of this procedure, additional testing may be needed to evaluate or monitor progression of the disease process and determine the need for a change in therapy. Evaluate test results in relation to the patient's symptoms and other tests performed.

Patient Education:

- Teach the patient to report signs of bleeding (bleeding gums, black tarry stools, blood in urine, hematoma).
- Teach the patient the symptoms of PE and the importance of timely reporting.

Expected Patient Outcomes:

Understanding

- The patient and family state the importance of remaining on bed rest to prevent movement of the embolus.

L

- The patient and family state the importance of keeping oxygen on at all times.

Ability
- The patient demonstrates effective coping mechanisms to decrease anxiety.
- The patient demonstrates how to use controlled breathing to improve breathing patterns.

Response
- The patient agrees to visit the HCP's office for follow-up coagulation studies.
- The patient agrees to take pain medication to decrease breathing discomfort and improve oxygenation.

RELATED STUDIES:
- Related tests include α-1 antitrypsin, alveolar/arterial ratio, ACE, angiography pulmonary, biopsy lung, blood gases, blood pool imaging, bronchoscopy, carbon dioxide, chest x-ray, CBC, CBC WBC count and differential, CT thorax, culture and smear mycobacteria, culture blood, culture sputum, culture throat, culture viral, cytology sputum, D-dimer, gallium scan, lung perfusion scan, MRI chest, MRI venography, mediastinoscopy, aPTT, plethysmography, pleural fluid analysis, PET heart, PFT, TB skin tests, US venous Doppler extremity studies, and venography.
- Refer to the Respiratory System table online at Davis*Plus* for related tests by body system.

Lupus Anticoagulant Antibodies

L

SYNONYM/ACRONYM: Lupus inhibitor phospholipid type, lupus antiphospholipid antibodies, LA.

COMMON USE: To assess for systemic dysfunction related to anticoagulation and assist in diagnosing conditions such as lupus erythematosus and fetal loss.

SPECIMEN: Plasma collected in a completely filled blue-top (3.2% sodium citrate) tube. If the patient's hematocrit exceeds 55%, the volume of citrate in the collection tube must be adjusted.

NORMAL FINDINGS: (Method: Dilute Russell viper venom test time) Negative.

DESCRIPTION: Lupus anticoagulant (LA) antibodies are immunoglobulins, usually of the immunoglobulin G class. They are also called lupus antiphospholipid antibodies because they interfere with phospholipid-dependent coagulation tests such as activated partial thromboplastin time (aPTT) by reacting with the phospholipids in the test system. They are not associated with a bleeding disorder unless thrombocytopenia or antiprothrombin antibodies are already present. They are associated with an increased risk of thrombosis. The combination of noninflammatory thrombosis of blood vessels, low platelet count, and history of miscarriage is termed *antiphospholipid antibody syndrome* and is confirmed by the presence of at least one of the clinical criteria (vascular thrombosis confirmed by histopathology or imaging studies; pregnancy morbidity defined as either one or more unexplained deaths of a morphologically normal fetus at or beyond the 10th week of gestation, one or more premature births of a morphologically normal neonate before the 34th week of gestation due to eclampsia or severe pre-eclampsia, or three or more unexplained consecutive spontaneous abortions before the 10th week of gestation) and one of the laboratory criteria (ACA, IgG, or IgM, detectable at greater than 40 units on two or more occasions at least 12 wk apart; or LA detectable on two or more occasions at least 12 wk apart; or anti-β_2 glycoprotein 1 antibody, IgG, or IgM, detectable on two or more occasions at least 12 wk apart, all measured by a standardized ELISA, according to recommended procedures).

This procedure is contraindicated for: N/A

INDICATIONS

- Evaluate prolonged aPTT.
- Investigate reasons for fetal death.

POTENTIAL MEDICAL DIAGNOSIS

Positive findings in

- Antiphospholipid antibody syndrome ***(LA are nonspecific antibodies associated with this syndrome)***
- Fetal loss ***(thrombosis associated with LA can form clots that lodge in the placenta and disrupt nutrition to the fetus)***
- Raynaud's disease ***(LA can be detected with this condition and can cause vascular inflammation)***
- Rheumatoid arthritis ***(LA can be detected with this condition and can cause vascular inflammation)***
- Systemic lupus erythematosus ***(related to formation of thrombi as a result of LA binding to phospholipids on cell walls)***
- Thromboembolism ***(related to formation of thrombi as a result of LA binding to phospholipids on cell walls)***

Negative findings in: N/A

CRITICAL FINDINGS: N/A

INTERFERING FACTORS

- Drugs and other substances that may cause a positive LA test result include calcium channel blockers, chlorpromazine, heparin, hydralazine, hydantoins, isoniazid, methyldopa, phenytoin, phenothiazines, procainamide, quinine, and quinidine.
- Placement of a tourniquet for longer than 1 min can result in venous stasis and changes in the concentration of plasma proteins to be measured. Platelet activation may also occur under these conditions, causing erroneous results.
- Vascular injury during phlebotomy can activate platelets and coagulation factors, causing erroneous results.
- Hemolyzed specimens must be rejected because hemolysis is an indication of platelet and coagulation factor activation.
- Icteric or lipemic specimens interfere with optical testing methods, producing erroneous results.
- Hematocrit greater than 55% may cause falsely prolonged results because of anticoagulant excess relative to plasma volume.
- Incompletely filled collection tubes, specimens contaminated with heparin, clotted specimens, or unprocessed specimens not delivered to the laboratory within 1 to 2 hr of collection should be rejected.

L

NURSING IMPLICATIONS AND PROCEDURE

POTENTIAL NURSING PROBLEMS:

Problem	Signs & Symptoms	Interventions
Pain ***(related to joint inflammation and stiffness)***	Report of joint pain; emotional symptoms of distress; crying; agitation; facial grimace; moaning; rocking motions; irritability; disturbed sleep; diaphoresis; altered blood pressure and heart rate; nausea; vomiting	Collaborate with the patient and health-care provider (HCP) to identify the best pain management modality to provide relief; refrain from activities that may aggravate pain; use the application of heat or cold to the best effect in managing the pain; monitor pain severity; administer prescribed opioids; discuss with patient what has worked to relieve joint pain in the past; assess the effect of pain on personal, social, and professional obligations; take prescribed anti-inflammatory medication; consider using a bed cradle to keep weight of linens off of legs; collaborate with physical therapy to splint joints; discuss use of imagery or distraction to control pain; avoid prolonged periods of inactivity that could exacerbate joint pain and stiffness
Fatigue ***(related to associated anemia; disease progression; depression; pain; disturbed rest)***	Decreased concentration; increased physical complaints; inability to restore energy with sleep; reports being tired; inability to maintain normal routine; depression; excessive sleep; diminished performance	Assess for physical cause of fatigue; pace activities to preserve energy stores; rate fatigue on a numeric scale to trend degree of fatigue over time; identify what aggravates and decreases fatigue; assess for related emotional factors such as depression; evaluate current medications in relation to fatigue; assess for physiologic factors such as anemia; provide adequate rest periods; encourage warm shower or bath before bedtime; instruct patient to change position frequently while sleeping

L

Problem	Signs & Symptoms	Interventions
Grief ***(related to loss of relationship with potential child [fetal loss])***	Anger; blame; emotional distress; despair; helplessness; powerlessness; emotional pain; depression; detachment; crying; loud vocalization of grief; shock	Assess for behaviors that indicate grief; assess for shock, disbelief; identify stage of grieving; assess for cultural or spiritual aspects of grief; assess decision-making capacity that may be altered due to grief; collaborate with social services to support patient during time of grief; listen to and allow the patient to verbalize feelings; encourage self-care activities to support own health and healing; refer to community resources such as grief support groups; consider recommendation of pharmacological intervention as appropriate

PRETEST:

- Positively identify the patient using at least two person-specific identifiers before services, treatments, or procedures are performed.
- ***Patient Teaching:*** Inform the patient that this test can assist in evaluation of clotting disorders.
- Obtain a history of the patient's health concerns, symptoms, surgical procedures, and results of previously performed laboratory and diagnostic studies. Include a list of known allergens, especially allergies or sensitivities to latex.
- Obtain a list of the patient's current medications, including over-the-counter medications, dietary supplements, anticoagulants, aspirin and other salicylates (see Effects of Natural Products on Laboratory Values online at Davis*Plus*). Such products should be discontinued by medical direction for the appropriate number of days prior to a surgical procedure. Note the last time and dose of medication taken.
- Review the procedure with the patient. Inform the patient that specimen collection takes approximately 5 to 10 min. Address concerns about pain and explain that there may be some discomfort during the venipuncture.
- ***Sensitivity to social and cultural issues,*** as well as concern for modesty, is important in providing psychological support before, during, and after the procedure.
- Heparin therapy should be discontinued 2 days before specimen collection, with medical direction. Warfarin(Coumadin) therapy should be discontinued 2 wk before specimen collection, with medical direction.
- Note that there are no food or fluid restrictions unless by medical direction.

INTRATEST:

Potential Complications: N/A

- Ensure that the patient has complied with pretesting preparations prior to the study, as instructed.
- Avoid the use of equipment containing latex if the patient has a history of allergic reaction to latex.
- Instruct the patient to cooperate fully and to follow directions. Direct the

patient to breathe normally and to avoid unnecessary movement.

- Observe standard precautions, and follow the general guidelines in Patient Preparation and Specimen Collection online at Davis*Plus*. Positively identify the patient, and label the appropriate specimen container with the corresponding patient demographics, initials of the person collecting the specimen, date, and time of collection. Perform a venipuncture. Fill tube completely. *Important note:* When multiple specimens are drawn, the blue-top tube should be collected after sterile (i.e., blood culture) tubes. Otherwise, when using a standard vacutainer system, the blue-top tube is the first tube collected. When a butterfly is used, due to the added tubing, an extra red-top tube should be collected before the blue-top tube to ensure complete filling of the blue-top tube.
- Remove the needle and apply direct pressure with dry gauze to stop bleeding. Observe/assess venipuncture site for bleeding or hematoma formation and secure gauze with adhesive bandage.
- Promptly transport the specimen to the laboratory for processing and analysis. The recommendation for processed and unprocessed samples stored in unopened tubes is that testing should be completed within 1 to 4 hr of collection.

L

POST-TEST:

- Inform the patient that a report of the results will be made available to the requesting HCP, who will discuss the results with the patient.
- Recognize anxiety related to test results, and offer support.
- Depending on the results of this procedure, additional testing may be performed to evaluate or monitor progression of the disease process and determine the need for a change in therapy. Evaluate test results in relation to the patient's symptoms and other tests performed.

Patient Education:

- Instruct the patient to resume usual medications, as directed by the HCP.
- Provide teaching and information regarding the clinical implications of the test results, as appropriate.
- Take time to discuss feelings the mother and father may experience (e.g., guilt, depression, anger) if test results are abnormal.
- Teach patient to avoid caffeinated foods before bedtime.
- Educate the patient regarding access to counseling services. Provide contact information, if desired, for the Lupus Foundation of America (www.lupus.org). 🍁
- Reinforce information given by the patient's HCP regarding further testing, treatment, or referral to another HCP.
- Answer any questions or address any concerns voiced by the patient or family.

Expected Patient Outcomes:

Understanding

- The patient states that taking anti-inflammatory medication as early as possible in the morning will decrease joint stiffness sooner.
- The patient states that anti-inflammatory medication should not be taken on an empty stomach.

Ability

- The patient demonstrates effective use of alternative measures (imagery, distraction) to manage pain.
- The patient demonstrates proficiency for range-of-motion exercises that can be used to decrease joint stiffness.

Response

- The patient complies with recommendation to attend grief counseling to assist in managing grief process.
- The patient complies with recommendation to attend grief support group, as sharing grief experiences can assist emotional healing.

RELATED STUDIES:

- Related tests include antibody, anticardiolipin antibodies, anticyclic citrullinated peptide, ANA, arthroscopy, BMD, bone scan, CRP, ESR,

FDP, MRI musculoskeletal, aPTT, protein S, PT/INR and mixing studies, radiography bone, RF, synovial fluid analysis, and US obstetric.

Refer to the Hematopoietic, Immune, Musculoskeletal, and Reproductive systems tables online at Davis*Plus* for related tests by body system.

Luteinizing Hormone

SYNONYM/ACRONYM: LH, luteotropin, interstitial cell–stimulating hormone (ICSH).

COMMON USE: To assess gonadal function related to fertility issues and response to therapy.

SPECIMEN: Serum collected in a gold-, red-, or red/gray-top tube. Plasma collected in a green-top (heparin) tube is also acceptable.

NORMAL FINDINGS: (Method: Immunoassay)

Concentration by Gender and by Phase (in Females)	Conventional and SI Units
Male	
Less than 2 yr	0.5–1.9 international units/mL
2–10 yr	Less than 0.5 international units/mL
11–20 yr	0.5–5.3 international units/mL
Adult	1.2–7.8 international units/mL
Female	
Less than 2–10 yr	Less than 0.5 international units/mL
11–20 yr	0.5–9 international units/mL
Phase in Females	
Follicular	1.7–15 international units/mL
Ovulatory	21.9–80 international units/mL
Luteal	0.6–16.3 international units/mL
Postmenopausal	14.2–52.3 international units/mL

DESCRIPTION: The secretion and inhibition of human reproductive hormones is maintained by a fine balance of feedback mechanisms involving the hypothalmus, pituitary gland, ovaries, and testes. Gonadotropin-releasing hormone (Gn-RH), a peptide neurohormone produced and released by the hypothalamus, signals the anterior pituitary gland to release luteinizing hormone and follicle-stimulating hormone. GnRH is secreted during the neonatal period and gonadotropins are detectable in the blood at an early age. A negative feedback mechanism initiated by FSH and LH levels inhibits further secretion by suppressing the release of Gn-RH until puberty. During the prepubital period and following into adulthood, nocturnal pulses of Gn-RH induce nocturnal, pulsatile secretions of luteinizing hormone (LH). The mechanism by which increased release of Gn-RH permits increased secretion of gonadotropins is not well understood. LH affects gonadal function in both men and women. In women, a surge of LH normally occurs at the midpoint of the menstrual cycle (ovulatory phase) due to initiation of a positive feedback loop involving estrogen and which results in ovulation. As the corpus luteum develops progesterone levels rise, signaling the pituitary to stop secreting LH. In males, LH stimulates the interstitial cells of Leydig, located in the testes, to produce testosterone. For this reason, in reference to males, LH is sometimes called *interstitial cell-stimulating hormone.* Serial specimens may be required to accurately demonstrate blood levels.

This procedure is contraindicated for: N/A

L

INDICATIONS

- Distinguish between primary and secondary causes of gonadal failure.
- Evaluate children with precocious puberty.
- Evaluate male and female infertility, as indicated by decreased LH levels.
- Evaluate response to therapy to induce ovulation.
- Support diagnosis of infertility caused by anovulation, as evidenced by lack of LH surge at the midpoint of the menstrual cycle.

POTENTIAL MEDICAL DIAGNOSIS

Increased in:

Conditions of decreased gonadal function cause a feedback response that stimulates LH secretion.

- Anorchia
- Gonadal failure
- Menopause
- Primary gonadal dysfunction

Decreased in:

- Anorexia nervosa ***(pathophysiology is unclear)***
- Kallmann's syndrome ***(pathophysiology is unclear)***
- Malnutrition ***(pathophysiology is unclear)***
- Pituitary or hypothalamic dysfunction ***(these organs control production of LH; failure of the pituitary to produce LH or of the hypothalamus to produce gonadotropin-releasing hormone results in decreased LH levels)***
- Severe stress ***(pathophysiology is unclear)***

CRITICAL FINDINGS: N/A

INTERFERING FACTORS

- Drugs and other substances that may increase LH levels include clomiphene, gonadotropin-releasing hormone, goserelin, ketoconazole, leuprolide, mestranol, nafarelin, naloxone, nilutamide, spironolactone, and tamoxifen.
- Drugs and other substances that may decrease LH levels include anabolic steroids, anticonvulsants, conjugated estrogens, cyproterone, danazol, digoxin, D-Trp-6-LHRH, estradiol valerate, estrogen/progestin therapy, finasteride, ganirelix, goserelin, ketoconazole, leuprolide, desogestrel/ethinylestradiol (Marvelon), medroxyprogesterone, megestrol, metformin, octreotide, oral contraceptives, phenothiazine, pimozide, pravastatin, progesterone, and tamoxifen.
- In menstruating women, values vary in relation to the phase of the menstrual cycle.
- LH secretion follows a circadian rhythm, with higher levels occurring during sleep.

NURSING IMPLICATIONS AND PROCEDURE

POTENTIAL NURSING PROBLEMS:

Problem	Signs & Symptoms	Interventions
Self-esteem ***(related to altered self-view associated with infertility)***	Verbalizes feelings that express being a failure as a man or woman associated with inability to impregnate or become pregnant; dissatisfaction with present state of intimacy with significant other	Monitor for negative self-statements; assess for withdrawal; monitor for real or perceived rejection of others; encourage verbalization of self-worth; encourage discussion of perceived changes in family role; monitor for anxiety; recommend personal and family counseling; facilitate support group participation
Knowledge ***(related to recent diagnosis; complexity of treatment; poor understanding of provided information; cultural or language barriers; anxiety; emotional disturbance; unfamiliarity with medical management)***	Lack of interest or questions; multiple questions; anxiety in relation to disease process and management; verbalizes inaccurate information; lack of follow-through with directions	Identify patient's, family's, and significant other's concerns about disease process; provide information regarding fertility testing and treatment; encourage participation in a support group to decrease anxiety
Anxiety ***(related to failure versus desire to conceive)***	Stated feelings of inadequacy, helplessness; restlessness and irritability; altered sleep pattern; lack of appetite or overeating; difficulty concentrating and focusing	Assess the level of anxiety; assist the patient to identify coping strategies that decrease anxiety; administer prescribed medications to decrease anxiety; provide education that is culturally and age appropriate, and at an appropriate literacy level; encourage a discussion of fears and concerns causing the anxiety; refer to social services and a support group as applicable

(table continues on page 1064)

Problem	Signs & Symptoms	Interventions
Powerlessness ***(related inability to become pregnant secondary to failure to ovulate)***	Expression of loss of control over situation, self, outcome of disease; passive; apathetic; submissive; decreased participation in self-care; reluctant to express feelings	Assess need to be in control; assess feelings of hopelessness, depression, apathy; assess the impact of the sense of powerlessness on the patient's sense of self; encourage verbalization of feelings; discuss therapeutic options offered by health-care provider (HCP); assist to identify strengths; identify coping strategies

PRETEST:

- Positively identify the patient using at least two person-specific identifiers before services, treatments, or procedures are performed.
- ***Patient Teaching:*** Inform the patient this test can assist in assessing hormone and fertility disorders.
- Obtain a history of the patient's health concerns, symptoms, surgical procedures, and results of previously performed laboratory and diagnostic studies. Include a list of known allergens, especially allergies or sensitivities to latex.
- Record the date of the last menstrual period and determine the possibility of pregnancy in women who are perimenopausal.
- Obtain a list of the patient's current medications, including over-the-counter medications and dietary supplements (see Effects of Natural Products on Laboratory Values online at Davis*Plus*).
- Review the procedure with the patient. If the test is being performed to detect ovulation, inform the patient that it may be necessary to obtain a series of samples over a period of several days to detect peak LH levels. Inform the patient that specimen collection takes approximately 5 to 10 min. Address concerns about pain and explain that there may be some discomfort during the venipuncture.
- ***Sensitivity to social and cultural issues,*** as well as concern for modesty, is important in providing psychological support before, during, and after the procedure.
- Note that there are no food, fluid, or medication restrictions unless by medical direction.

INTRATEST:

Potential Complications: N/A

- Avoid the use of equipment containing latex if the patient has a history of allergic reaction to latex.
- Instruct the patient to cooperate fully and to follow directions. Direct the patient to breathe normally and to avoid unnecessary movement.
- Observe standard precautions, and follow the general guidelines in Patient Preparation and Specimen Collection online at Davis*Plus*. Positively identify the patient, and label the appropriate specimen container with the corresponding patient demographics, initials of the person collecting the specimen, date, and time of collection. Perform a venipuncture.
- Remove the needle and apply direct pressure with dry gauze to stop bleeding. Observe/assess venipuncture site for bleeding or hematoma formation and secure gauze with adhesive bandage.

- Promptly transport the specimen to the laboratory for processing and analysis.

POST-TEST:

- Inform the patient that a report of the results will be made available to the requesting HCP, who will discuss the results with the patient.
- Depending on the results of this procedure, additional testing may be performed to evaluate or monitor progression of the disease process and determine the need for a change in therapy. Evaluate test results in relation to the patient's symptoms and other tests performed.

Patient Education:

- Reinforce information given by the patient's HCP regarding further testing, treatment, or referral to another HCP.
- Instruct the patient in the use of home ovulation test kits approved by the U.S. Food and Drug Administration, as appropriate.
- Answer any questions or address any concerns voiced by the patient or family.

Expected Patient Outcomes:

Understanding

- The patient and family state the purpose of repeating laboratory studies to monitor and trend hormone levels.
- The patient states the efficacy of alternative methods to achieve pregnancy as described by HCP.

Ability

- The patient and family accurately describe the purpose of future laboratory studies to monitor hormone levels and evaluate response to therapy.
- The patient accurately self-administers medication to decrease anxiety.

Response

- The patient agrees to attend a support group for those who have infertility concerns.
- The patient identifies nonpharmacological coping strategies that help to decrease anxiety.

RELATED STUDIES:

- Related tests include ACTH, antisperm antibody, estradiol, FSH, progesterone, prolactin, and testosterone.
- Refer to the Endocrine and Reproductive systems tables online at Davis*Plus* for related tests by body system.

L

Lyme Antibody

SYNONYM/ACRONYM: N/A

COMMON USE: To detect antibodies to the organism that causes Lyme disease.

SPECIMEN: Serum collected in a gold-, red-, or red/gray-top tube.

NORMAL FINDINGS: (Method: Enzyme immunoassay) Less than 0.91 index; positives are confirmed by Western blot analysis.

DESCRIPTION: *Borrelia burgdorferi,* a deer tick–borne spirochete, is the organism that causes Lyme disease. Lyme disease affects multiple systems and is characterized by fever, arthralgia, and arthritis. The circular, red rash characterizing erythema migrans can appear 3 to 30 days after the tick bite. About one-half of patients in the early stage of Lyme disease (stage 1) and generally all of those in the advanced stage (stage 2—with cardiac, neurological, and rheumatoid manifestations) will have a positive test result. Patients in remission will also have a positive test response. The presence of immunoglobulin M (IgM) antibodies indicates acute infection. The presence of IgG antibodies indicates current or past infection. The Centers for Disease Control and Prevention (CDC) recommends a two-step testing process that begins with an immunofluorescence or enzyme-linked immunosorbent assay (ELISA) and is confirmed by using a Western blot test. 🍁

This procedure is contraindicated for: N/A

INDICATIONS

Assist in establishing a diagnosis of Lyme disease.

POTENTIAL MEDICAL DIAGNOSIS

Positive findings in

Lyme disease

Negative findings in: N/A

CRITICAL FINDINGS: N/A

INTERFERING FACTORS

- High rheumatoid-factor titers as well as cross-reactivity with Epstein-Barr virus and other spirochetes (e.g., *Rickettsia, Treponema*) may cause false-positive results.
- Positive test results should be confirmed by the Western blot method.

NURSING IMPLICATIONS AND PROCEDURE

POTENTIAL NURSING PROBLEMS:

Problem	Signs & Symptoms	Interventions
Infection ***(related to Borrelia burgdorferi bacteria; transmission of B. burgdorferi bacteria in utero from infected mother to baby)***	Macular flush; flu-like symptoms; headache; extreme fatigue; neck pain; joint pain; joint swelling; bone pain; classic bull's-eye rash; unexplained fever; difficulty swallowing; chest pain; shortness of breath; heart palpitations; nausea; vomiting; pain in feet; twitching; numbness; irritability; visual disturbance; mood swings; depression; paranoia	Administer prescribed antibiotics; administer prescribed medications to treat symptoms; minimize future exposure by following these recommendations: stay out of the woods in spring and summer, stay toward the center of the hiking trail, do not sit on the ground in leafy/grassy wooded areas, complete frequent self-check for ticks, wear long-sleeved shirts, tuck pants into socks, tuck shirt into pants, wear light-colored clothing to make attached ticks more visible, use bug repellant with DEET, strip down and do a full body check after being outdoors in endemic areas, check pets for ticks

Problem	Signs & Symptoms	Interventions
Fatigue ***(related to B. burgdorferi bacteria infection)***	Decreased concentration; increased physical health concerns; unable to restore energy with sleep; reports being tired; unable to maintain normal routine	Assess for physical cause of fatigue; pace activities to preserve energy stores; rate fatigue on a numeric scale to trend degree of fatigue over time; identify what aggravates and decreases fatigue; assess for related emotional factors such as depression; evaluate current medications in relation to fatigue; assess for physiologic factors such as anemia
Anxiety ***(related to physical and mental changes that may or may not be reversible secondary to bacterial infection with B. burgdorferi associated with tick bite)***	Consequences of *B. burgdorferi* infection to lifestyle and individual functionality; insomnia; restlessness; irritability; difficulty concentrating; anorexia; focus on self; expressions of concern; apprehension	Assess coping strategies used and their effectiveness; acknowledge the presence of anxiety; keep a calm presence while interacting with the patient; administer prescribed medications to decrease anxiety; use simple, straightforward language to increase understanding and decrease anxiety; support selected coping strategies; facilitate referral for psychiatric evaluation as needed; refer to Lyme disease support group

PRETEST:

- Positively identify the patient using at least two person-specific identifiers before services, treatments, or procedures are performed.
- *Patient Teaching:* Inform the patient this test can assist in diagnosing Lyme disease.
- Obtain a history of the patient's health concerns, symptoms, surgical procedures, and results of previously performed laboratory and diagnostic studies. Include a list of known allergens, especially allergies or sensitivities to latex. Discuss history of exposure; ask the patient if he or she lives in or visits wooded areas, wears long pants and long-sleeved shirts when in wooded areas or when doing yard work, or has ever been bitten by a tick.
- Obtain a list of the patient's current medications, including over-the-counter medications and dietary supplements (see Effects of Natural Products on Laboratory Values online at Davis*Plus*).
- Review the procedure with the patient. Inform the patient that several tests may be necessary to confirm diagnosis. Inform the patient that specimen collection takes approximately 5 to 10 min. Address concerns about pain and explain that there may be some discomfort during the venipuncture.
- ***Sensitivity to social and cultural issues,*** as well as concern for modesty, is important in providing psychological support before, during, and after the procedure.

- Note that there are no food, fluid, or medication restrictions unless by medical direction.

INTRATEST:

Potential Complications: N/A

- Avoid the use of equipment containing latex if the patient has a history of allergic reaction to latex.
- Instruct the patient to cooperate fully and to follow directions. Direct the patient to breathe normally and to avoid unnecessary movement.
- Observe standard precautions, and follow the general guidelines in Patient Preparation and Specimen Collection online at Davis*Plus*. Positively identify the patient, and label the appropriate specimen container with the corresponding patient demographics, initials of the person collecting the specimen, date, and time of collection. Perform a venipuncture.
- Remove the needle and apply direct pressure with dry gauze to stop bleeding. Observe/assess venipuncture site for bleeding or hematoma formation and secure gauze with adhesive bandage.
- Promptly transport the specimen to the laboratory for processing and analysis.

POST-TEST:

- Inform the patient that a report of the results will be made available to the requesting health-care provider (HCP), who will discuss the results with the patient.
- Recognize anxiety related to test results, and be supportive of impaired activity related to perceived loss of independence and fear of shortened life expectancy. Lyme disease can be debilitating and can result in significant changes in lifestyle. Discuss the implications of abnormal test results on the patient's lifestyle. Provide teaching and information regarding the clinical implications of the test results, as appropriate. Educate the patient regarding access to counseling services.
- Reinforce information given by the patient's HCP regarding further testing, treatment, or referral to another HCP. Warn the patient that false-positive test results can occur and that false-negative test results frequently occur. Answer any questions or address any concerns voiced by the patient or family.
- Depending on the results of this procedure, additional testing may be performed to evaluate or monitor progression of the disease process and determine the need for a change in therapy. Evaluate test results in relation to the patient's symptoms and other tests performed.

Patient Education:

- Advise the patient to wear light-colored clothing that covers extremities when in areas infested by deer ticks and to check body for ticks after returning from infested areas.
- Emphasize the importance of reporting continued signs and symptoms of the infection.
- Answer any questions or address any concerns voiced by the patient or family.

Expected Patient Outcomes:

Understanding

- The patient and family state that tick bite risk increases in specific designated geographical areas.
- The patient and family state the importance of taking prescribed antibiotic to treat infection, including that repeated antibiotic treatments may be necessary.

Ability

- The patient and family describe clothing that is appropriate to use in prevention of tick bites.
- The patient demonstrates proficiency in the self-administering of the prescribed antibiotic.

Response

- The patient follows recommendation to take measures to prevent future tick bites.
- The patient complies with recommendation to attend support group to decreased anxiety and increase understanding of disease process.

L

RELATED STUDIES:

- Related tests include ANA, CBC, ESR, rheumatoid factor, and synovial fluid analysis.
- Refer to the Immune and Musculoskeletal systems tables online at Davis*Plus* for related tests by body system.

Lymphangiography

SYNONYM/ACRONYM: Lymphangiogram.

COMMON USE: To visualize and assess the lymphatic system related to diagnosis of lymphomas such as Hodgkin's disease.

AREA OF APPLICATION: Lymphatic system.

DESCRIPTION: Lymphangiography involves visualization of the lymphatic system after the injection of an iodinated oil-based contrast medium into a lymphatic vessel in the hand or foot. The lymphatic system collects and filters lymph fluid; moving the fluid in one direction from the surrounding tissues to the neck where it re-enters the circulatory system. The lymphatic system consists of lymph vessels, lymph ducts, lymph nodes, tonsils, adenoids, spleen, and thymus. Lymph is a colorless to white fluid composed of lymphocytes (white blood cells produced by the bone marrow and thymus), excess plasma proteins, and chyle (emulsified fats) from the intestines. The filtration units of the lymphatic system are the lymph nodes and organs located in different parts of the body, such as the neck, armpit, groin, chest, and abdomen. The main function of the lymphatic system is to provide immunological defense for the body against injury from disease or toxic chemicals. Assessment of this system is important because cancer (e.g., lymphoma and Hodgkin's disease) often spreads via the lymphatic system. Painful edema of the extremities usually occurs when the flow of lymphatic fluid becomes obstructed by infection, injury, or cancer. Lymphangiography is performed for evaluating edema of unknown cause in an extremity, identification of lymph node involvement which may indicate metastases from a primary tumor, cancer staging in patients with an established diagnosis of lymphoma or metastatic tumor to assist in monitoring progression of the disease, to plan surgical intervention, and to monitor the effectiveness of therapeutic modalities such as chemotherapy or radiation treatment. Injection into the hand allows visualization of the axillary and supraclavicular nodes. Injection into the foot allows visualization of the lymphatics of the leg, inguinal and iliac regions, and retroperitoneum up to the thoracic duct. Less commonly, injection into the foot can be used to visualize the cervical region (retroauricular area).

This procedure is contraindicated for

Patients who are pregnant or suspected of being pregnant, unless the potential benefits of a procedure using radiation far outweigh the risk of radiation exposure to the fetus and mother.

Patients with conditions associated with adverse reactions to contrast medium (e.g., asthma, food allergies, or allergy to contrast medium).

Although patients are asked specifically if they have a known allergy to iodine or shellfish, it has been well established that the reaction is not to iodine; an actual iodine allergy would be problematic because iodine is required for the production of thyroid hormones. In the case of shellfish, the reaction is to a muscle protein called tropomyosin; in the case of iodinated contrast medium, the reaction is to the noniodinated part of the contrast molecule. Patients with a known hypersensitivity to the medium may benefit from premedication with corticosteroids and diphenhydramine; the use of nonionic contrast or an alternative noncontrast imaging study, if available, may be considered for patients who have severe asthma or who have experienced moderate to severe reactions to ionic contrast medium.

Patients with conditions associated with preexisting renal insufficiency (e.g., chronic kidney disease, single kidney transplant, nephrectomy, diabetes, multiple myeloma, treatment with aminoglycosides and NSAIDs) ***because iodinated contrast is nephrotoxic.***

Patients who are chronically dehydrated before the test, especially older adults and patients whose health is already compromised, ***because of their risk of contrast-induced acute kidney injury.***

Patients with bleeding disorders or receiving anticoagulant therapy ***because the puncture site may not stop bleeding.***

Patients with severe chronic lung disease, cardiac disease, or advanced liver disease.

INDICATIONS

- Determine the extent of adenopathy.
- Determine lymphatic cancer staging.
- Distinguish primary from secondary lymphedema.
- Evaluate edema of an extremity without known cause.
- Evaluate effects of chemotherapy or radiation therapy.
- Plan surgical treatment or evaluate effectiveness of chemotherapy or radiation therapy in controlling malignant tumors.

POTENTIAL MEDICAL DIAGNOSIS

Normal findings

- Normal lymphatic vessels and nodes that fill completely with contrast medium on the initial films. On 24-hr images, the lymph nodes are fully opacified and well circumscribed. The lymphatic channels are emptied a few hours after injection of the contrast medium.

Abnormal findings related to

- Abnormal lymphatic vessels
- Hodgkin's disease
- Metastatic tumor involving the lymph glands
- Nodal lymphoma
- Retroperitoneal lymphomas associated with Hodgkin's disease

CRITICAL FINDINGS: N/A

INTERFERING FACTORS

Factors that may alter the results of the study

- Gas or feces in the gastrointestinal tract resulting from inadequate cleansing or failure to restrict food intake before the study.
- Retained barium from a previous radiological procedure.

- Metallic objects (e.g., jewelry, body rings) within the examination field, which may inhibit organ visualization and cause unclear images.
- Inability of the patient to cooperate or remain still during the procedure because of age, significant pain, or mental status.
- Inability to cannulate the lymphatic vessels.

Other considerations

- Failure to follow dietary restrictions and other pretesting preparations may cause the procedure to be canceled or repeated.
- Be aware of risks associated with the contrast medium. The oil-based contrast medium may embolize into the lungs and will temporarily diminish pulmonary function. This can produce lipid pneumonia, which is a life-threatening complication.

NURSING IMPLICATIONS AND PROCEDURE

PRETEST:

- Positively identify the patient using at least two person-specific identifiers before services, treatments, or procedures are performed.
- *Patient Teaching:* Inform the patient this procedure can assist in assessing the lymphatic system.
- Obtain a history of the patient's health concerns, symptoms, surgical procedures, and results of previously performed laboratory and diagnostic studies. Include a list of known allergens, especially allergies or sensitivities to latex, anesthetics, sedatives, or contrast medium. Ensure results of coagulation testing are obtained and recorded prior to the procedure; a creatinine level is also needed before contrast medium is to be used.
- Note any recent procedures that can interfere with test results, including examinations using barium- or iodine-based contrast medium. Ensure that barium studies were performed more than 4 days before lymphangiography.
- Record the date of the last menstrual period and determine the possibility of pregnancy in perimenopausal women.
- Obtain a list of the patient's current medications, including over-the-counter medications and dietary supplements (see Effects of Natural Products on Laboratory Values online at Davis*Plus*).
- If iodinated contrast medium is scheduled to be used in patients receiving metformin for type 2 diabetes, the drug should be discontinued on the day of the test and continue to be withheld for 48 hr after the test. Iodinated contrast can temporarily impair kidney function, and failure to withhold metformin may indirectly result in drug-induced lactic acidosis, a dangerous and sometimes fatal adverse effect of metformin ***(related to renal impairment that does not support sufficient excretion of metformin).***
- Review the procedure with the patient. Address concerns about pain and explain there may be moments of discomfort and some pain experienced during the test. Inform the patient that the procedure is performed by a health-care provider (HCP), with support staff, and takes approximately 1 to 2 hr. Inform the patient that he or she will have to return the next day, and the set of images taken upon return will take only 30 min.
- *Sensitivity to social and cultural issues,* as well as concern for modesty, is important in providing psychological support before, during, and after the procedure.
- Instruct the patient to remove jewelry and other metallic objects from the area to be examined prior to the procedure.
- Instruct patient to withhold anticoagulant medication or to reduce dosage before the procedure, as ordered by the HCP.
- Note that there are no food or fluid restrictions unless by medical direction.

- *Make sure a written and informed consent has been signed prior to the procedure and before administering any medications.*

INTRATEST:

Potential Complications:

Injection of contrast medium is an invasive procedure. Complications are rare but do include risk for allergic reaction ***related to contrast reaction;*** bleeding from the puncture site ***related to a bleeding disorder, or the effects of natural products and medications with known anticoagulant, antiplatelet, or thrombolytic properties;*** hematoma ***related to blood leakage into the tissue following needle insertion;*** infection ***that might occur if bacteria from the skin surface is introduced at the puncture site,*** dyspnea, pain, or hypotension ***caused by micropulmonary emboli;*** and lipoid pneumonia ***caused by contrast flowing into the thoracic duct.***

- Observe standard precautions, and follow the general guidelines in Patient Preparation and Specimen Collection online at Davis*Plus*. Positively identify the patient.
- Ensure the patient has complied with medication restrictions and pretesting preparations prior to the study, as instructed.
- Ensure the patient has removed all external metallic objects from the area to be examined.
- Administer ordered prophylactic steroids or antihistamines before the procedure if the patient has a history of allergic reactions to any substance or drug.
- Avoid the use of equipment containing latex if the patient has a history of allergic reaction to latex.
- Have emergency equipment readily accessible.
- Instruct the patient to void prior to the procedure and to change into the gown, robe, and foot coverings provided.
- Instruct the patient to cooperate fully and to follow directions. Direct the patient to remain still throughout the procedure because movement produces unreliable results.
- Obtain and record baseline vital signs, and assess neurological status.
- Administer a mild sedative, as ordered.
- Place the patient in a supine position on an x-ray table. Cleanse the selected area and cover with a sterile drape.
- A local anesthetic is injected at the site, and a small incision is made or a needle inserted. A blue dye is injected intradermally into the area between the toes or fingers. The lymphatic vessels are identified as the dye moves. A local anesthetic is then injected into the dorsum of each foot or hand, and a small incision is made and cannulated for injection of the contrast medium.
- The contrast medium is then injected, and the flow of the contrast medium is followed by fluoroscopy or images. When the contrast medium reaches the upper lumbar level, the infusion of contrast medium is discontinued. X-ray images are taken of the chest, abdomen, and pelvis to determine the extent of filling of the lymphatic vessels. To examine the lymphatic nodes and to monitor the progress of delayed flow, 24-hr delayed images are taken.
- Monitor the patient for complications related to the contrast medium (e.g., allergic reaction, anaphylaxis, bronchospasm, lipid pneumonia).
- Remove the needle or catheter and apply a pressure dressing over the puncture site.
- Observe/assess the needle/catheter insertion site for bleeding, inflammation, or hematoma formation.
- When the cannula is removed the incision is sutured and bandaged.

POST-TEST:

- Inform the patient that a report of the results will be made available to the requesting HCP, who will discuss the results with the patient.
- Monitor vital signs and neurological status every 15 min for 30 min. Take

L

temperature every 4 hr for 24 hr. Monitor intake and output at least every 8 hr. Compare with baseline values. Notify the HCP if temperature is elevated. Protocols may vary among facilities.
- Observe/assess the cannula insertion site for bleeding, inflammation, or hematoma formation.
- Observe for a delayed allergic reaction to contrast medium or pulmonary embolus, which may include shortness of breath, increased heart rate, pleuritic pain, hypotension, low-grade fever, and cyanosis.
- Instruct the patient to immediately report symptoms such as fast heart rate, difficulty breathing, skin rash, itching, chest pain, persistent right shoulder pain, or abdominal pain. Immediately report symptoms to the appropriate HCP.
- Instruct the patient in the care and assessment of the site.
- Instruct the patient to apply cold compresses to the puncture site as needed to reduce discomfort or edema.
- Instruct the patient to maintain bedrest up to 24 hr to reduce extremity swelling after the procedure, or as ordered.
- Instruct the patient to resume usual medications, as directed by the HCP. Kidney function should be assessed before metformin is resumed, if contrast was used.
- Recognize anxiety related to test results, and be supportive of perceived loss of independent function. Discuss the implications of abnormal test results on the patient's lifestyle. Provide teaching and information regarding the clinical implications of the test results, as appropriate.
- Reinforce information given by the patient's HCP regarding further testing, treatment, or referral to another HCP. Answer any questions or address any concerns voiced by the patient or family.
- Depending on the results of this procedure, additional testing may be needed to evaluate or monitor progression of the disease process and determine the need for a change in therapy. Evaluate test results in relation to the patient's symptoms and other tests performed.

RELATED STUDIES:

- Related tests include biopsy bone marrow, biopsy lymph nodes, CBC, CBC WBC count and differential, CT abdomen, CT pelvis, CT thoracic, gallium scan, laparoscopy abdominal, liver and spleen scan, MRI abdomen, mediastinoscopy, and US lymph nodes.
- Refer to the Endocrine and Immune systems tables online at Davis*Plus* for tests by related body system.

L

Magnesium, Blood

SYNONYM/ACRONYM: Mg^{2+}.

COMMON USE: To assess electrolyte balance related to magnesium levels to assist in diagnosis, monitoring diseases, and therapeutic interventions such as hemodialysis.

SPECIMEN: Serum collected in a gold-, red-, or red/gray-top tube.

NORMAL FINDINGS: (Method: Spectrophotometry)

Age	Conventional Units	SI Units (Conventional Units × 0.4114)
Newborn	1.7–2.5 mg/dL	0.7–1 mmol/L
Child	1.7–2.3 mg/dL	0.7–0.95 mmol/L
Adult	1.6–2.2 mg/dL	0.66–0.91 mmol/L

DESCRIPTION: Magnesium is required as a cofactor in numerous crucial enzymatic processes, such as protein synthesis, nucleic acid synthesis, and muscle contraction. Magnesium is also required for the use of adenosine diphosphate as a source of energy. It is the fourth most abundant cation and the second most abundant intracellular ion. Magnesium is needed for the transmission of nerve impulses and muscle relaxation. It controls absorption of sodium, potassium, calcium, and phosphorus; utilization of carbohydrate, lipid, and protein; and activation of enzyme systems that enable the B vitamins to function. Magnesium is also essential for oxidative phosphorylation, nucleic acid synthesis, and blood clotting. Urine magnesium levels reflect magnesium deficiency before serum levels. Magnesium deficiency severe enough to cause hypocalcemia and cardiac dysrhythmias can exist despite normal serum magnesium levels.

This procedure is contraindicated for: N/A

INDICATIONS

- Determine electrolyte balance in chronic kidney disease and alcoholism.
- Evaluate cardiac dysrhythmias (decreased magnesium levels can lead to excessive ventricular irritability).
- Evaluate known or suspected disorders associated with altered magnesium levels.
- Monitor the effects of various drugs on magnesium levels.

POTENTIAL MEDICAL DIAGNOSIS

Increased in:

- Addison's disease ***(related to insufficient production of aldosterone; decreased renal excretion)***
- Adrenocortical insufficiency ***(related to decreased renal excretion)***
- Dehydration ***(related to hemoconcentration)***
- Diabetic acidosis (severe) ***(related to acid-base imbalance)***
- Hypothyroidism ***(pathophysiology is unclear)***

M

- Massive hemolysis ***(related to release of intracellular magnesium; intracellular concentration is three times higher than normal plasma levels)***
- Overuse of antacids ***(related to excessive intake of magnesium-containing antacids)***
- Renal insufficiency ***(related to decreased urinary excretion)***
- Tissue trauma

Decreased in:
- Alcoholism ***(related to increased renal excretion and possible insufficient dietary intake)***
- Diabetic acidosis ***(insulin treatment lowers blood glucose and appears to increase intracellular transport of magnesium)***
- Glomerulonephritis (chronic) ***(related to diminished renal function; magnesium is reabsorbed in the renal tubules)***
- Hemodialysis ***(related to loss of magnesium due to dialysis treatment)***
- Hyperaldosteronism ***(related to increased excretion)***
- Hypocalcemia ***(decreased magnesium is associated with decreased calcium and vitamin D levels)***
- Hypoparathyroidism ***(related to decreased calcium)***
- Inadequate intake
- Inappropriate secretion of antidiuretic hormone ***(related to fluid overload)***
- Long-term hyperalimentation
- Malabsorption ***(related to impaired absorption of calcium and vitamin D)***
- Pancreatitis ***(secondary to alcoholism)***
- Pregnancy
- Severe loss of body fluids ***(diarrhea, lactation, sweating, laxative abuse)***

CRITICAL FINDINGS:

Adults
- Less than 1.2 mg/dL (SI: Less than 0.5 mmol/L)
- Greater than 4.9 mg/dL (SI: Greater than 2 mmol/L)

Children
- Less than 1.2 mg/dL (SI: Less than 0.5 mmol/L)
- Greater than 4.3 mg/dL (SI: Greater than 1.8 mmol/L)

Note and immediately report to the requesting health-care provider (HCP) any critical findings and related symptoms. A listing of these findings varies among facilities. Timely notification of a critical finding for laboratory or diagnostic studies is a role expectation of the professional nurse. The notification processes vary among facilities. Upon receipt of the critical finding, the information should be read back to the caller to verify accuracy.

Consideration may be given to verification of critical findings before action is taken. Policies vary among facilities and may include requesting immediate recollection and retesting by the laboratory or retesting using a rapid point-of-care testing instrument at the bedside, if available.

Symptoms such as tetany, weakness, dizziness, tremors, hyperactivity, nausea, vomiting, and convulsions occur at decreased (Less than 1.2 mg/dL [SI: Less than 0.5 mmol/L]) concentrations. Electrocardiographic (ECG) changes (prolonged P-R and Q-T intervals; broad, flat T waves; and ventricular tachycardia) may also occur. Treatment may include intravenous (IV) or oral administration of magnesium salts, monitoring for respiratory depression and areflexia (IV administration of magnesium salts), and monitoring for diarrhea and metabolic alkalosis (oral administration to replace magnesium).

M

Respiratory paralysis, decreased reflexes, and cardiac arrest occur at grossly elevated (Greater than 15 mg/dL [SI: Greater than 6.2 mmol/L]) levels. ECG changes, such as prolonged P-R and Q-T intervals, and bradycardia may be seen. Toxic levels of magnesium may be reversed with the administration of calcium, dialysis treatments, and removal of the source of excessive intake.

INTERFERING FACTORS

- Drugs and other substances that may increase magnesium levels include acetylsalicylic acid and progesterone.
- Drugs and other substances that may decrease magnesium levels include albuterol, aminoglycosides, amphotericin B, bendroflumethiazide, chlorthalidone, cisplatin, citrates, cyclosporine, digoxin, glucagon, and oral contraceptives.
- Magnesium is present in higher intracellular concentrations; therefore, hemolysis will result in a false elevation in values and such specimens should be rejected for analysis.
- Specimens should never be collected above an IV line because of the potential for dilution when the specimen and the IV solution combine in the collection container, falsely decreasing the result. There is also the potential of contaminating the sample with the substance of interest, if it is present in the IV solution, falsely increasing the result.

NURSING IMPLICATIONS AND PROCEDURE

POTENTIAL NURSING PROBLEMS:

Problem	Signs & Symptoms	Interventions
Fluid volume (water) ***(related to metabolic imbalances associated with disease process)***	**Deficiency:** Decreased urinary output, fatigue, and sunken eyes, dark urine, decreased blood pressure, increased heart rate, and altered mental status **Overload:** Edema, shortness of breath, increased weight, ascites, rales, rhonchi, and diluted laboratory values	Record daily weight and monitor trends; record accurate intake and output; collaborate with HCP with administration of IV fluids to support hydration; monitor laboratory values that reflect alterations in fluid status (potassium, blood urea nitrogen, creatinine, calcium, hemoglobin, hematocrit); manage underlying cause of fluid alteration; monitor urine characteristics and respiratory status; establish baseline assessment data; collaborate with HCP to adjust oral and IV fluids to provide optimal hydration status; administer replacement electrolytes as ordered; monitor serum magnesium levels

Problem	Signs & Symptoms	Interventions
Nutrition ***(related to excess caloric intake with large amounts of dietary sodium and fat; cultural lifestyle; overeating associated with anxiety, depression, compulsive disorder; genetics; inadequate or unhealthy food resources)***	Observable obesity; high-fat or sodium food selections; high body mass index; high consumption of ethnic foods; sedentary lifestyle; dietary religious beliefs and food selections; binge eating; diet high in refined sugar; repetitive dieting and failure	Discuss ideal body weight and the purpose and relationship between ideal weight and caloric intake to support cardiac health; review ways to decrease intake of saturated fats and increase intake of polyunsaturated fats; discuss limiting cholesterol intake to less than 300 mg per day; discuss limiting the intake of refined processed sugar; teach limiting sodium intake to the restriction recommended by the HCP; encourage intake of fresh fruits and vegetables, unprocessed carbohydrates, poultry, and grains
Electrolyte imbalance ***(related to metabolic imbalance)***	**Excess:** Nausea; vomiting; diarrhea; diaphoresis; flushing; sensation of heat; decreased mental functioning; weakness; drowsiness; hypotension; bradycardia; respiratory depression; coma. **Deficit:** Nystagmus; fatigue; convulsions; weakness; numbness	Correlate magnesium imbalance with disease process, nutritional intake, renal function, medications; monitor ECG status; monitor for respiratory changes; monitor for gastrointestinal changes; minimize metabolic complications; provide a safe environment to prevent injury; collaborate with the pharmacist and HCP for appropriate pharmacologic interventions; adjust medication dosage to compensate for renal impairment; collaborate with dietitian for dietary modifications
Cardiac output ***(related to increased preload; increased afterload; impaired cardiac contractility;***	Decreased peripheral pulses; decreased urinary output; cool, clammy skin; tachypnea; dyspnea; edema; altered level of consciousness;	Assess peripheral pulses and capillary refill; monitor blood pressure and check for orthostatic changes; assess respiratory rate, breath sounds, and orthopnea; assess skin color and temperature; assess level of consciousness;

(table continues on page 1078)

Problem	Signs & Symptoms	Interventions
cardiac muscle disease; altered cardiac conduction)	abnormal heart sounds; crackles in lungs; decreased activity tolerance; weight gain; fatigue; hypoxia	monitor urinary output; use pulse oximetry to monitor oxygenation; monitor sodium and potassium levels; monitor B-type natriuretic peptide levels; administer ordered angiontensin-converting enzyme inhibitors, beta-blockers, diuretics, aldosterone antagonists, and vasodilators; provide oxygen administration

PRETEST:

- Positively identify the patient using at least two person-specific identifiers before services, treatments, or procedures are performed.
- ***Patient Teaching:*** Inform the patient this test can assist in the evaluation of electrolyte balance.
- Obtain a history of the patient's health concerns, symptoms, surgical procedures, and results of previously performed laboratory and diagnostic studies. Include a list of known allergens, especially allergies or sensitivities to latex.
- Obtain a list of the patient's current medications, including over-the-counter medications and dietary supplements (see Effects of Natural Products on Laboratory Values online at Davis*Plus*).
- Review the procedure with the patient. Inform the patient that specimen collection takes approximately 5 to 10 min. Address concerns about pain and explain that there may be some discomfort during the venipuncture.
- ***Sensitivity to social and cultural issues,*** as well as concern for modesty, is important in providing psychological support before, during, and after the procedure.
- Note that there are no food, fluid, or medication restrictions unless by medical direction.

INTRATEST:

Potential Complications: N/A

- Avoid the use of equipment containing latex if the patient has a history of allergic reaction to latex.
- Instruct the patient to cooperate fully and to follow directions. Direct the patient to breathe normally and to avoid unnecessary movement.
- Observe standard precautions, and follow the general guidelines in Patient Preparation and Specimen Collection online at Davis*Plus*. Positively identify the patient, and label the appropriate specimen container with the corresponding patient demographics, initials of the person collecting the specimen, date, and time of collection. Perform a venipuncture.
- Remove the needle and apply direct pressure with dry gauze to stop bleeding. Observe/assess venipuncture site for bleeding or hematoma formation and secure gauze with adhesive bandage.
- Promptly transport the specimen to the laboratory for processing and analysis.

POST-TEST:

- Inform the patient that a report of the results will be made available to the requesting HCP, who will discuss the results with the patient.

M

- *Nutritional Considerations:* Educate the magnesium-deficient patient regarding good dietary sources of magnesium, such as green vegetables, seeds, legumes, shrimp, and some bran cereals. Advise the patient that high intake of substances such as phosphorus, calcium, fat, and protein interferes with the absorption of magnesium.
- Depending on the results of this procedure, additional testing may be performed to evaluate or monitor progression of the disease process and determine the need for a change in therapy. Evaluate test results in relation to the patient's symptoms and other tests performed.

Patient Education:

- Instruct the patient to report any signs or symptoms of electrolyte imbalance, such as dehydration, diarrhea, vomiting, or prolonged anorexia.
- Reinforce information given by the patient's HCP regarding further testing, treatment, or referral to another HCP.
- Recognize anxiety related to test results and answer any questions or address any concerns voiced by the patient or family.
- Educate the patient regarding access to nutritional counseling services.
- Provide contact information, if desired, for the Institute of Medicine of the National Academies (www.iom.edu) or USDA's resource for nutrition (www.choosemyplate.gov). 🍁
- Teach the importance of maintaining an appropriate magnesium level to their overall health.
- Teach the patient that kidney disease can contribute to an elevated magnesium level.

Expected Patient Outcomes:

Understanding

- The patient and family state that dietary magnesium intake may need to be increased to prevent hypomagnesemia.
- The patient and family state that kidney disease can contribute to high serum magnesium levels.

Ability

- The patient and family accurately select a diet that is appropriate to support the patient's personal magnesium needs.
- The patient and family identify foods in the patient's diet that should be added or deleted to support an appropriate magnesium level.

Response

- The patient complies with the recommendation to take dietary supplements to improve low magnesium levels.
- The patient and family discuss the possibility of hemodialysis as needed to manage serum magnesium levels.

RELATED STUDIES:

- Related tests include ACTH, aldosterone, anion gap, antidysrhythmic drugs, BUN, calcium, calculus kidney stone panel, CBC WBC count and differential, cortisol, CRP, CK and isoenzymes, creatinine, glucose, homocysteine, LDH and isoenzymes, magnesium urine, myoglobin, osmolality, PTH, phosphorus, potassium, renin, sodium, troponin, US abdomen, and vitamin D.
- Refer to the Cardiovascular, Endocrine, Gastrointestinal, Genitourinary, and Reproductive systems tables online at Davis*Plus* for related tests by body system.

M

Magnesium, Urine

SYNONYM/ACRONYM: Urine Mg^{2+}.

COMMON USE: To assess magnesium levels related to renal function.

SPECIMEN: Urine from a random or timed specimen collected in a clean plastic collection container with 6N hydrochloride as a preservative.

NORMAL FINDINGS: (Method: Spectrophotometry)

Conventional Units	SI Units (Conventional Units × 0.4114)
20–200 mg/24 hr	8.2–82.3 mmol/24 hr

POTENTIAL MEDICAL DIAGNOSIS

Increased in:

- Alcoholism ***(related to impaired absorption and increased urinary excretion)***
- Bartter's syndrome ***(inherited defect in renal tubules that results in urinary wasting of potassium and magnesium)***
- Transplant recipients on cyclosporine and prednisone ***(related to increased excretion by the kidney)***
- Use of corticosteroids ***(related to increased excretion by the kidney)***
- Use of diuretics ***(related to increased urinary excretion)***

Decreased in:

- Abnormal kidney function ***(related to diminished ability of renal tubules to reabsorb magnesium)***
- Crohn's disease ***(related to inadequate intestinal absorption)***
- Inappropriate secretion of antidiuretic hormone ***(related to diminished renal absorption)***
- Salt-losing conditions ***(related to diminished renal absorption)***

CRITICAL FINDINGS: N/A

Find and print out the full study on Fast Find at davispl.us/vanleeuwen7.

M

Magnetic Resonance Angiography

SYNONYM/ACRONYM: MRA.

COMMON USE: To visualize and assess blood flow in diseased and normal vessels toward diagnosis of vascular disease and to monitor and evaluate therapeutic interventions.

AREA OF APPLICATION: Vascular.

DESCRIPTION: Magnetic resonance imaging (MRI) is useful when the area of interest is soft tissue. The study can be performed with or without intravenous (IV) contrast (gadolinium). The technology does not involve radiation exposure and is considered safer than other imaging methods such as radiographs and computed tomography (CT). MRI uses a magnet and radio waves to produce an energy field that can be displayed as an image of the anatomic area of interest based on the water content of the tissue. The magnetic field causes the hydrogen atoms in tissue to line up, and when radio waves are directed toward the magnetic field, the hydrogen atoms absorb the radio waves and change their position. This change in the energy field is detected by the equipment, and an image is generated by the equipment's computer system using assigned values that correspond to the strength of the signal produced; the anatomical images are represented in various shades of gray. MRI produces cross-sectional images of the vessels in multiple planes without the use of ionizing radiation or the interference of bone or surrounding tissue. Images can be obtained in two-dimensional (series of slices) or three-dimensional sequences. Standard or closed MRI equipment has the appearance of an open tube or tunnel; open MRI equipment has no sides and provides an alternative for people who suffer from claustrophobia, pediatric patients, or patients who are obese. Some open MRI units are designed to allow the patient to stand or sit while images are taken in various body positions. IV gadolinium-based contrast media may be used to better visualize the vessels and tissues in the area of interest. Clear, high-quality images of abnormalities and disease processes significantly improve the diagnostic value of the study.

Magnetic resonance angiography (MRA) is an application of MRI that provides images of blood flow and diseased and normal blood vessels. In patients who are allergic to iodinated contrast medium, MRA is used in place of angiography. MRA is particularly useful for visualizing vascular abnormalities, dissections, and other pathology. Special imaging sequences allow the visualization of moving blood within the vascular system, and two common techniques are used to obtain images of flowing blood: time-of-flight and phase-contrast MRA. In time-of-flight imaging, incoming blood makes the vessels appear bright and surrounding tissue is suppressed. Phase-contrast images are produced by subtracting the stationary tissue surrounding the vessels where the blood is moving through vessels during the imaging, producing high-contrast images. MRA is the most accurate technique for imaging blood flowing in veins and small arteries (*laminar flow*), but it does not accurately depict blood flow in tortuous sections of vessels and distal to bifurcations and stenosis. Swirling blood may cause a signal loss and result in inadequate images, and the degree of vessel stenosis may be overestimated.

This procedure is contraindicated for

- Patients who are pregnant or suspected of being pregnant, unless the potential benefits of MRI far outweigh the risks to the fetus and mother. ***In pregnancy, gadolinium-based contrast medium (GBCAs) cross the placental barrier, enter the fetal circulation, and pass via the kidneys into the amniotic fluid. Although no definite adverse effects of GBCA administration on the human fetus have been documented, the potential bioeffects of fetal GBCA exposure are not well understood. GBCA administration should therefore be avoided during pregnancy unless no suitable alternative imaging is possible and the benefits of contrast administration outweigh the potential risk to the fetus.***

- Conditions associated with adverse reactions to contrast medium (e.g., asthma, food allergies, or allergy to contrast medium).

Although patients are asked specifically if they have a known allergy to iodine or shellfish (shellfish contain high levels of iodine), it has been well established that the reaction is not to iodine; an actual iodine allergy would be problematic because iodine is required for the production of thyroid hormones. In the case of shellfish, the reaction is to a muscle protein called tropomyosin; in the case of iodinated contrast medium, the reaction is to the noniodinated part of the contrast molecule. Patients with a known hypersensitivity to the medium may benefit from premedication with corticosteroids and diphenhydramine; the use of nonionic contrast or an alternative noncontrast imaging study, if available, may be considered for patients who have severe asthma or who have experienced moderate to severe reactions to ionic contrast medium.

- Patients with moderate to marked renal impairment (glomerular filtration rate less than 30 mL/min/1.73 m^2). Patients should be screened for kidney dysfunction prior to administration. The use of GBCAs should be avoided in these patients unless the benefits of the studies outweigh the risks and essential diagnostic information is not available using non–contrast-enhanced diagnostic studies.
- Patients with cardiac pacemakers that can be deactivated by MRI.
- Patients with metal in their body, such as dental amalgams, metallic body piercing items, tattoo inks containing iron (including tattooed eyeliners), shrapnel, bullet, ferrous metal in the eye, certain ferrous metal prosthetics, valves, aneurysm clips, intrauterine device, inner ear prostheses, or other metallic objects; these items can impair image quality. Metallic objects are also a significant safety issue for patients and health-care staff in the examination room during performance of an MRI. The MRI equipment consists of an extremely powerful magnet that can inactivate, move, or shift metallic objects inside a patient. Many metallic objects currently used in health-care procedures are made of materials that do not interfere with MRI studies; it is important for patients to provide specific information regarding medical procedures they have undergone in order to identify whether their device is safe to undergo MRI. Required information includes the date of the procedure and identification of the device. Metallic objects are not allowed inside the room with the MRI equipment because items such as watches, credit cards, and car keys can become dangerous projectiles.
- Patients with transdermal patches containing metallic components. The patch's liner contains a metal that controls absorption of the substance from the patch (e.g., drugs, nicotine, steroids, hormones). The patch may cause burns to the skin ***related to energy conducted through the metal which is converted to heat during the MRI.*** Other metallic objects on the skin may also cause burns.
- Patients who are claustrophobic.

INDICATIONS

- Detect pericardial abnormalities.
- Detect peripheral arterial disease (PAD).
- Detect thoracic and abdominal vascular diseases.
- Determine renal artery stenosis.
- Differentiate aortic aneurysms from tumors near the aorta.
- Evaluate cardiac chambers and pulmonary vessels.
- Evaluate postoperative angioplasty sites and bypass grafts.
- Identify congenital vascular diseases.

- Monitor and evaluate the effectiveness of medical or surgical treatment.

POTENTIAL MEDICAL DIAGNOSIS

Normal findings

- Normal blood flow in the area being examined, including blood flow rate

Abnormal findings related to

- Aortic aneurysm
- Coarctations
- Dissections
- PAD
- Thrombosis within a vessel
- Tumor invasion of a vessel
- Vascular abnormalities
- Vessel occlusion
- Vessel stenosis

CRITICAL FINDINGS:

- Aortic aneurysm
- Aortic dissection
- Occlusion
- Tumor with significant mass effect
- Vertebral artery dissection

Note and immediately report to the requesting health-care provider (HCP) any critical findings and related symptoms. A listing of these findings varies among facilities. Timely notification of a critical finding for laboratory or diagnostic studies is a role expectation of the professional nurse. The notification processes vary among facilities. Upon receipt of the critical finding, the information should be read back to the caller to verify accuracy.

INTERFERING FACTORS

Factors that may alter the results of the study

- Metallic objects (e.g., jewelry, body rings, dental amalgams) within the examination field, which may inhibit organ visualization and cause unclear images.
- Inability of the patient to cooperate or remain still during the procedure because of age, significant pain, or mental status.
- Patients with extreme cases of claustrophobia, unless sedation is given before the study.
- Patients who are extremely obese may require more radiation to obtain a clear image.

Other considerations

- If contrast medium is allowed to seep deep into the muscle tissue, vascular visualization will be impossible.
- The procedure may be canceled if the patient's weight exceeds the safety limit for the equipment.

NURSING IMPLICATIONS AND PROCEDURE

See Potential Nursing Problems on Fast Find at davispl.us/vanleeuwen7.

PRETEST:

- Positively identify the patient using at least two person-specific identifiers before services, treatments, or procedures are performed.
- ***Patient Teaching:*** Inform the patient this procedure can assist in assessing the vascular system.
- Obtain a history of the patient's health concerns (especially kidney dysfunction if the use of GBCA is anticipated), symptoms, surgical procedures, and results of previously performed laboratory and diagnostic studies. Include a list of known allergens, especially allergies or sensitivities to latex, anesthetics, sedatives, or contrast medium. Patients with a known hypersensitivity to contrast medium may benefit from premedication with corticosteroids and diphenhydramine.
- Ensure the results of blood urea nitrogen, creatinine, and estimated glomerular filtration rate are obtained if GBCA is to be used.
- Determine if the patient has ever had any device implanted into his or her body, including copper intrauterine

M

devices, pacemakers, ear implants, and heart valves.

- Obtain occupational history to determine the presence of metal in the body, such as shrapnel or flecks of ferrous metal in the eye (which can cause retinal hemorrhage).
- Note any recent procedures that can interfere with test results.
- Record the date of the last menstrual period and determine the possibility of pregnancy in perimenopausal women.
- Obtain a list of the patient's current medications, including over-the-counter medications and dietary supplements (see Effects of Natural Products on Laboratory Values online at Davis*Plus*).
- Review the procedure with the patient. Address concerns about pain related to the procedure and explain that no pain will be experienced during the test, but there may be moments of discomfort. Reassure the patient that if contrast is used, it poses no radioactive hazard and rarely produces adverse effects. Inform the patient the procedure is performed in an MRI department by an HCP who specializes in this procedure, with support staff, and takes approximately 30 to 60 min.
- Inform the patient that the technologist will place him or her in a supine position on a flat table in a large cylindrical scanner.
- Tell the patient to expect to hear loud banging from the scanner and possibly to see magnetophosphenes (flickering lights in the visual field); these will stop when the procedure is over.
- Explain that an IV line may be inserted to allow infusion of fluids such as saline, anesthetics, contrast medium, or sedatives.
- ***Sensitivity to social and cultural issues,*** as well as concern for modesty, is important in providing psychological support before, during, and after the procedure.
- Instruct the patient to remove external metallic objects from the area to be examined prior to the procedure.
- Note that there are no food, fluid, or medication restrictions unless by medical direction. Some protocols may require the patient to restrict prescribed oral iron supplements prior to the study because the iron may interfere with the study results. Restriction of food, fluids, alcohol, nicotine, and caffeine for 1 to 2 hr before the procedure may also be required in order to avoid vasoconstriction or vasodilation as well as nausea and vomiting related to anxiety while in the MRI scanner.

INTRATEST:

Potential Complications:

Injection of the contrast is an invasive procedure. Complications are rare but do include risk for allergic reaction ***related to contrast reaction;*** cardiac dysrhythmias; hematoma ***related to blood leakage into the tissue following needle insertion;*** bleeding from the puncture site ***related to a bleeding disorder or the effects of natural products and medications with known anticoagulant, antiplatelet, or thrombolytic properties;*** vascular or nerve injury ***that might occur if the needle strikes a nerve or nearby blood vessel;*** or infection ***that might occur if bacteria from the skin surface is introduced at the puncture site.***

Some patients are at risk for developing nephrogenic systemic fibrosis as a result of the use of gadolinium-based contrast medium ***related to ineffective renal clearance in patients with impaired kidney function.***

- Observe standard precautions, and follow the general guidelines in Patient Preparation and Specimen Collection online at Davis*Plus*. Positively identify the patient.
- Ensure that the patient has complied with dietary, fluid, and other pretesting preparations prior to the study, as instructed.
- Ensure that the patient has removed external metallic objects from the area to be examined prior to the procedure.

M

- Administer ordered prophylactic steroids or antihistamines before the procedure if the patient has a history of allergic reactions to any substance or drug.
- Avoid the use of equipment containing latex if the patient has a history of allergic reaction to latex.
- Have emergency equipment readily available.
- Instruct the patient to void prior to the procedure and to change into the gown, robe, and foot coverings provided.
- Instruct the patient to cooperate fully and to follow directions. Instruct the patient to remain still throughout the procedure because movement produces unreliable results. ECG or respiratory gating may be performed in conjunction with the scan to reduce artifacts during data collection due to respiratory or cardiac movement; apply MRI-safe electrodes at the appropriate sites.
- Supply earplugs to the patient to block out the loud, banging sounds that occur during the test. Instruct the patient to communicate with the technologist during the examination via a microphone within the scanner.
- Apply MRI-safe electrodes to the appropriate sites if an electrocardiogram or respiratory gating is to be performed in conjunction with the scan.
- Establish IV fluid line for the injection of fluids such as saline, anesthetics, contrast medium, or sedatives. Avoid the use of IV equipment that contains metal.
- Administer an antianxiety drug, as ordered, if the patient has claustrophobia. Administer a sedative to a child or to an adult who is uncooperative, as ordered.
- Assist the patient onto the examination table and into the appropriate position for imaging to begin.
- Imaging can begin shortly after the injection, if contrast is used.
- Ask the patient to inhale deeply and hold his or her breath while the images are taken, and then to exhale after the images are taken.
- Instruct the patient to take slow, deep breaths if nausea occurs during the procedure.
- Monitor the patient for complications related to the procedure (e.g., allergic reaction, anaphylaxis, bronchospasm).
- Remove the needle or catheter and apply a pressure dressing over the puncture site.
- Observe/assess the needle/catheter insertion site for bleeding, inflammation, or hematoma formation.

POST-TEST:

- Inform the patient that a report of the results will be made available to the requesting HCP, who will discuss the results with the patient.
- Observe for delayed allergic reactions, such as rash, urticaria, tachycardia, hyperpnea, hypertension, palpitations, nausea, or vomiting.
- Instruct the patient to immediately report symptoms such as fast heart rate, difficulty breathing, skin rash, itching, chest pain, persistent right shoulder pain, or abdominal pain. Immediately report symptoms to the appropriate HCP.
- Instruct the patient in the care and assessment of the injection site.
- Instruct the patient to apply cold compresses to the puncture site as needed to reduce discomfort or edema.
- Recognize anxiety related to test results. Discuss the implications of abnormal test results on the patient's lifestyle. Provide teaching and information regarding the clinical implications of the test results, as appropriate. Provide contact information, if desired, for the American Heart Association (www.americanheart.org), National Heart, Lung, and Blood Institute (www.nhlbi.nih.gov), or Legs for Life (www.legsforlife.org). 🍁
- Reinforce information given by the patient's HCP regarding further testing, treatment, or referral to another HCP. Answer any questions or address any concerns voiced by the patient or family.

M

- Depending on the results of this procedure, additional testing may be performed to evaluate or monitor progression of the disease process and determine the need for a change in therapy. Evaluate test results in relation to the patient's symptoms and other tests performed.

Patient Education:

- Teach the patient the importance of managing hypertension to decrease bleeding risk.
- Teach the signs and symptoms of transfusion reaction.

Expected Patient Outcomes:

Understanding

- The patient and family discuss the medical versus surgical options for aneurysm management.
- The patient and family discuss the risks and benefits of blood transfusion and the types of transfusion available.

Ability

- The patient and family successfully create a quiet environment.
- The patient successfully demonstrates how to take own blood pressure using an approved medical device.

Response

- The patient and family agree to vigilant follow-up care to monitor the size of the aneurysm.
- The patient agrees to blood replacement therapy.

RELATED STUDIES:

- Related tests include angiography of the body area of interest, BUN, CT angiography, creatinine, US arterial Doppler carotid, and US venous Doppler.
- Refer to the Cardiovascular System table online at Davis*Plus* for related tests by body system.

Magnetic Resonance Imaging, Abdomen

M

SYNONYM/ACRONYM: Abdominal MRI.

COMMON USE: To visualize and assess abdominal and hepatic structures toward diagnosis of tumor, metastasis, aneurysm, and abscess. Also used to monitor medical and surgical therapeutic interventions.

AREA OF APPLICATION: Liver and abdominal area.

DESCRIPTION: Magnetic resonance imaging (MRI) is useful when the area of interest is soft tissue. The study can be performed with or without intravenous (IV) contrast (gadolinium). The technology does not involve radiation exposure and is considered safer than other imaging methods such as radiographs and computed tomography (CT). MRI uses a magnet and radio waves to produce an energy field that can be displayed as an image of the anatomic area of interest based on the water content of the tissue. The magnetic field causes the hydrogen atoms in tissue to line up, and when radio waves are directed toward the magnetic field, the hydrogen atoms absorb the radio waves and change their position; this change in the energy field is detected by the equipment, and an image is generated by the equipment's computer system using assigned values that correspond to the strength of the signal produced; the anatomical images are represented in various shades of gray. MRI produces cross-sectional images of the abdomen in multiple planes without the use of ionizing radiation or the interference of bone or surrounding tissue. Images can be obtained in two-dimensional (series of slices) or three-dimensional sequences. Standard or closed MRI equipment has the appearance of an open tube or tunnel; open MRI equipment has no sides and provides an alternative for people who suffer from claustrophobia, pediatric patients, or patients who are obese. Some open MRI units are designed to allow the patient to stand or sit while images are taken in various body positions. IV gadolinium-based contrast media may be used to better visualize the vessels and tissues in the area of interest. Clear, high-quality images of abnormalities and disease processes significantly improve the diagnostic value of the study.

Abdominal MRI is performed to assist in diagnosing abnormalities of abdominal and hepatic structures. Contrast-enhanced imaging is effective for distinguishing peritoneal metastases from primary tumors of the gastrointestinal (GI) tract. Primary tumors of the stomach, pancreas, colon, and appendix often spread by intraperitoneal tumor shedding and subsequent peritoneal carcinomatosis. MRI uses the noniodinated paramagnetic contrast medium gadopentetate dimeglumine (Magnevist), which is administered IV to enhance differences between normal and abnormal tissues.

Magnetic resonance cholangiopancreatography (MRCP) is an imaging technique used specifically to evaluate the hepatobiliary system that is comprised of the liver, gallbladder, bile ducts, pancreas, and pancreatic ducts. MRCP is a less invasive way than endoscopic retrograde cholangiopancreatography (ERCP) to investigate abdominal pain, suspected malignancy, gall stones, or pancreatitis.

This procedure is contraindicated for

- Patients who are pregnant or suspected of being pregnant, unless the potential benefits of the MRI far outweigh the risks to the fetus and mother. ***In pregnancy, gadolinium-based contrast medium (GBCAs) cross the placental barrier, enter the fetal circulation, and pass via the kidneys into the amniotic fluid. Although no definite adverse effects of GBCA administration on the human fetus have been documented, the potential bioeffects of fetal GBCA exposure are not well understood. GBCA administration should therefore be avoided during pregnancy unless no suitable alternative imaging is possible and the benefits of contrast administration outweigh the potential risk to the fetus.***
- Conditions associated with adverse reactions to contrast medium (e.g., asthma, food allergies, or allergy to contrast medium).

Although patients are asked specifically if they have a known allergy to iodine or shellfish (shellfish contain high levels of iodine), it has been well established that the reaction is not to iodine; an actual iodine allergy would be problematic because iodine is required for the production of thyroid hormones. In the case of shellfish, the reaction is to a muscle protein called tropomyosin; in the case of iodinated contrast medium, the reaction is to the

M

noniodinated part of the contrast molecule. Patients with a known hypersensitivity to the medium may benefit from premedication with corticosteroids and diphenhydramine; the use of nonionic contrast or an alternative noncontrast imaging study, if available, may be considered for patients who have severe asthma or who have experienced moderate to severe reactions to ionic contrast medium.

Patients with moderate to marked renal impairment (glomerular filtration rate less than 30 mL/min/1.73 m^2). Patients should be screened for kidney dysfunction prior to administration. The use of GBCAs should be avoided in these patients unless the benefits of the studies outweigh the risks and if essential diagnostic information is not available using noncontrast-enhanced diagnostic studies.

Patients with cardiac pacemakers that can be deactivated by MRI.

Patients with metal in their body, such as dental amalgams, metallic body piercing items, tattoo inks containing iron (including tattooed eyeliners), shrapnel, bullet, ferrous metal in the eye, certain ferrous metal prosthetics, valves, aneurysm clips, intrauterine device, inner ear prostheses, or other metallic objects; these items can impair image quality. Metallic objects are also a significant safety issue for patients and health-care staff in the examination room during performance of an MRI. The MRI equipment consists of an extremely powerful magnet that can inactivate, move, or shift metallic objects inside a patient. Many metallic objects currently used in health-care procedures are made of materials that do not interfere with MRI studies; it is important for patients to provide specific information regarding medical procedures they have undergone in order to identify whether their device is safe to undergo MRI. Required information includes the date of the procedure and identification of the device. Metallic objects are not allowed inside the room with the MRI equipment because items such as watches, credit cards, and car keys can become dangerous projectiles.

Patients with transdermal patches containing metallic components. The patch's liner contains a metal that controls absorption of the substance from the patch (e.g., drugs, nicotine, steroids, hormones). The patch may cause burns to the skin ***related to energy conducted through the metal, which is converted to heat during the MRI.*** Other metallic objects on the skin may also cause burns.

Patients who are claustrophobic.

INDICATIONS

- Detect abdominal aortic diseases.
- Detect and stage cancer (primary or metastatic tumors of liver, pancreas, prostate, uterus, and bladder).
- Detect chronic pancreatitis.
- Detect renal vein thrombosis.
- Detect soft tissue abnormalities.
- Determine and monitor tissue damage in renal transplant patients.
- Determine the presence of blood clots, cysts, fluid or fat accumulation in tissues, hemorrhage, and infarctions.
- Determine vascular complications of pancreatitis, venous thrombosis, or pseudoaneurysm.
- Differentiate aortic aneurysms from tumors near the aorta.
- Differentiate liver tumors from liver abnormalities, such as cysts, cavernous hemangiomas, and hepatic amebic abscesses.
- Evaluate postoperative angioplasty sites and bypass grafts.
- Monitor and evaluate the effectiveness of medical or surgical interventions and the course of the disease.

M

POTENTIAL MEDICAL DIAGNOSIS

Normal findings

- Normal anatomic structures, soft tissue density, and biochemical constituents of body tissues, including blood flow

Abnormal findings related to

- Acute tubular necrosis
- Aneurysm
- Cholangitis
- Glomerulonephritis
- Hydronephrosis
- Internal bleeding
- Masses, lesions, infections, or inflammations
- Renal vein thrombosis
- Vena cava obstruction

CRITICAL FINDINGS:

- Acute GI bleed
- Aortic aneurysm
- Infection
- Tumor with significant mass effect

Note and immediately report to the requesting health-care provider (HCP) any critical findings and related symptoms. A listing of these findings varies among facilities. Timely notification of a critical finding for laboratory or diagnostic studies is a role expectation of the professional nurse. The notification processes vary among facilities. Upon receipt of the critical finding, the information should be read back to the caller to verify accuracy.

INTERFERING FACTORS

Factors that may alter the results of the study

- Metallic objects (e.g., jewelry, body rings, dental amalgams) within the examination field, which may inhibit organ visualization and cause unclear images.
- Inability of the patient to cooperate or remain still during the procedure because of age, significant pain, or mental status.
- Patients with extreme cases of claustrophobia, unless sedation is given before the study or an open MRI is utilized.
- Patients who are extremely obese may require more radiation to obtain a clear image.

Other considerations

- If contrast medium is allowed to seep deep into the muscle tissue, vascular visualization will be impossible.
- The procedure may be canceled if the patient's weight exceeds the safety limit for the equipment.

NURSING IMPLICATIONS AND PROCEDURE

See Potential Nursing Problems on Fast Find at davispl.us/vanleeuwen7.

PRETEST:

- Positively identify the patient using at least two person-specific identifiers before services, treatments, or procedures are performed.
- ***Patient Teaching:*** Inform the patient this procedure can assist in assessing the abdominal organs and structures.
- Obtain a history of the patient's health concerns (especially kidney dysfunction if the use of GBCA is anticipated), symptoms, surgical procedures, and results of previously performed laboratory and diagnostic studies. Include a list of known allergens, especially allergies or sensitivities to latex, anesthetics, sedatives, or contrast medium. Patients with a known hypersensitivity to contrast medium may benefit from premedication with corticosteroids and diphenhydramine.
- Ensure the results of blood urea nitrogen, creatinine, and estimated glomerular filtration rate are obtained if GBCA is to be used.
- Determine if the patient has ever had any device implanted into his or her body, including copper intrauterine

M

devices, pacemakers, ear implants, and heart valves.

- Obtain occupational history to determine the presence of metal in the body, such as shrapnel or flecks of ferrous metal in the eye (which can cause retinal hemorrhage).
- Note any recent procedures that can interfere with test results, including examinations using barium- or iodine-based contrast medium.
- Record the date of the last menstrual period and determine the possibility of pregnancy in perimenopausal women.
- Obtain a list of the patient's current medications, including over-the-counter medications and dietary supplements (see Effects of Natural Products on Laboratory Values online at Davis*Plus*).
- Review the procedure with the patient. Address concerns about pain related to the procedure and explain that no pain will be experienced during the test, but there may be moments of discomfort. Reassure the patient that if contrast is used, it poses no radioactive hazard and rarely produces adverse effects. Inform the patient the procedure is performed in an MRI department by an HCP specializing in this procedure, with support staff, and takes approximately 30 to 60 min.
- Inform the patient that the technologist will place him or her in a supine position on a flat table in a large cylindrical scanner.
- Tell the patient to expect to hear loud banging from the scanner and possibly to see magnetophosphenes (flickering lights in the visual field); these will stop when the procedure is over.
- ***Sensitivity to social and cultural issues,*** as well as concern for modesty, is important in providing psychological support before, during, and after the procedure.
- Explain that an IV line may be inserted to allow infusion of fluids such as saline, anesthetics, contrast medium, or sedatives.
- Instruct the patient to remove jewelry and all other metallic objects from the area to be examined prior to the procedure.
- Note that there are no food, fluid, or medication restrictions unless by medical direction. Some protocols may require the patient to restrict prescribed oral iron supplements prior to the study because the iron may interfere with the study results; fasting for 1 to 2 hr before the procedure may also be required in order to avoid nausea and vomiting related to anxiety while in the MRI scanner.

INTRATEST:

Potential Complications:

Injection of the contrast is an invasive procedure. Complications are rare but do include risk for allergic reaction ***related to contrast reaction;*** cardiac dysrhythmias; hematoma ***related to blood leakage into the tissue following needle insertion;*** bleeding from the puncture site ***related to a bleeding disorder or the effects of natural products and medications with known anticoagulant, antiplatelet, or thrombolytic properties;*** vascular or nerve injury ***that might occur if the needle strikes a nerve or nearby blood vessel;*** or infection ***that might occur if bacteria from the skin surface is introduced at the puncture site.***

Some patients are at risk for developing nephrogenic systemic fibrosis as a result of the use of gadolinium-based contrast medium ***related to ineffective renal clearance in patients with impaired kidney function.***

- Observe standard precautions, and follow the general guidelines in Patient Preparation and Specimen Collection online at Davis*Plus*. Positively identify the patient.
- Ensure that the patient has complied with dietary, fluid, and other pretesting preparations prior to the study, as instructed.
- Ensure that the patient has removed all external metallic objects from the area to be examined prior to the procedure.

M

- Administer ordered prophylactic steroids or antihistamines before the procedure if the patient has a history of allergic reactions to any substance or drug.
- Avoid the use of equipment containing latex if the patient has a history of allergic reaction to latex.
- Have emergency equipment readily available.
- Instruct the patient to void prior to the procedure and to change into the gown, robe, and foot coverings provided.
- Instruct the patient to cooperate fully and to follow directions. Instruct the patient to remain still throughout the procedure because movement produces unreliable results. Electrocardiogram or respiratory gating may be performed in conjunction with the scan to reduce artifacts during data collection due to respiratory or cardiac movement; apply MRI-safe electrodes at the appropriate sites.
- Supply earplugs to the patient to block out the loud, banging sounds that occur during the test. Instruct the patient to communicate with the technologist during the examination via a microphone within the scanner.
- Establish IV fluid line for the injection of fluids such as saline, anesthetics, contrast medium, or sedatives. Avoid the use of IV equipment that contains metal.
- Administer an antianxiety drug, as ordered, if the patient has claustrophobia. Administer a sedative to a child or to an adult who is uncooperative, as ordered.
- Assist the patient onto the examination table and into the appropriate position for imaging to begin.
- Imaging can begin shortly after the injection, if contrast is used.
- Ask the patient to inhale deeply and hold his or her breath while the images are taken and then to exhale after the images are taken.
- Instruct the patient to take slow, deep breaths if nausea occurs during the procedure.
- Monitor the patient for complications related to the procedure (e.g., allergic reaction, anaphylaxis, bronchospasm).
- Remove the needle or catheter and apply a pressure dressing over the puncture site.
- Observe/assess the needle/catheter insertion site for bleeding, inflammation, or hematoma formation.

POST-TEST:

- Inform the patient that a report of the results will be made available to the requesting HCP, who will discuss the results with the patient.
- Observe for delayed allergic reactions, such as rash, urticaria, tachycardia, hyperpnea, hypertension, palpitations, nausea, or vomiting
- Instruct the patient to immediately report symptoms such as fast heart rate, difficulty breathing, skin rash, itching, chest pain, persistent right shoulder pain, or abdominal pain. Immediately report symptoms to the appropriate HCP.
- Instruct the patient in the care and assessment of the injection site.
- Instruct the patient to apply cold compresses to the puncture site as needed to reduce discomfort or edema.
- Recognize anxiety related to test results. Discuss the implications of abnormal test results on the patient's lifestyle. Provide teaching and information regarding the clinical implications of the test results, as appropriate.
- Reinforce information given by the patient's HCP regarding further testing, treatment, or referral to another HCP. Answer any questions or address any concerns voiced by the patient or family.
- Depending on the results of this procedure, additional testing may be performed to evaluate or monitor progression of the disease process and determine the need for a change in therapy. Evaluate test results in relation to the patient's symptoms and other tests performed.

M

Patient Education:

- Teach the patient to call for pain relief medication as soon as it is needed.
- Teach the patient how to realistically evaluate the amount of food eaten.

Expected Patient Outcomes:

Understanding

- The patient describes pain management strategies that work and those that don't work.
- The patient and family state the pathophysiology related to the patient's specific disease process.

Ability

- The patient demonstrates effective coping mechanisms to decrease anxiety.
- The patient makes lifestyle changes that will support health and wellness.

Response

- The patient agrees to discuss concerns with identified support (family, friends, group, spiritual advisor).
- The patient agrees to lifestyle modifications to control disease process and symptoms.

RELATED STUDIES:

- Related tests include angiography abdomen, BUN, CT abdomen, creatinine, GI blood loss scan, KUB study, US abdomen, and US liver and biliary system.
- Refer to the Gastrointestinal, Genitourinary, and Hepatobiliary systems tables online at Davis*Plus* for related tests by body system.

Magnetic Resonance Imaging, Brain

SYNONYM/ACRONYM: Brain MRI.

COMMON USE: To visualize and assess intracranial abnormalities related to tumor, bleeding, lesions, and infarct such as stroke.

AREA OF APPLICATION: Brain area.

M

DESCRIPTION: Magnetic resonance imaging (MRI) is useful when the area of interest is soft tissue. The study can be performed with or without intravenous (IV) contrast (gadolinium). The technology does not involve radiation exposure and is considered safer than other imaging methods such as radiographs and computed tomography (CT). MRI uses a magnet and radio waves to produce an energy field that can be displayed as an image of the anatomic area of interest based on the water content of the tissue. The magnetic field causes the hydrogen atoms in tissue to line up, and when radio waves are directed toward the magnetic field, the hydrogen atoms absorb the radio waves and change their position. This change in the energy field is detected by the equipment, and an image is generated by the equipment's computer system using assigned values that correspond to the strength of the signal produced; the anatomical images are represented in various shades of gray. MRI produces cross-sectional images of pathological lesions of the brain in multiple planes without the use of ionizing radiation or the interference of bone or surrounding tissue. Images can be obtained in two-dimensional (series of slices) or three-dimensional sequences. Standard or closed MRI equipment has the appearance of an open tube or tunnel; open MRI equipment has no sides and provides an alternative for people who suffer from claustrophobia, pediatric patients, or patients who are obese. Some open MRI units are designed to allow the patient to stand or sit while images are taken in various body positions. IV gadolinium-based contrast media may be used to better visualize the vessels and tissues in the area of interest. Clear, high-quality images of abnormalities and disease processes significantly improve the diagnostic value of the study.

Standard brain MRI can distinguish solid, cystic, and hemorrhagic components of lesions. This procedure is done to aid in the diagnosis of intracranial abnormalities, including tumors, ischemia, infection, and multiple sclerosis, and in assessment of brain maturation in pediatric patients. Rapidly flowing blood on spin-echo MRI appears as an absence of signal or a void in the vessel's lumen. Blood flow can be evaluated in the cavernous and carotid arteries. Contrast-enhanced imaging is effective for enhancing differences between normal and abnormal tissues. Aneurysms may be diagnosed without traditional iodine-based contrast angiography, and old clotted blood in the walls of the aneurysm appear white. MRI uses the noniodinated contrast medium gadopentetate dimeglumine (Magnevist), which is administered IV.

Functional MRI (fMRI) is a neuroimaging application of MRI used to study how the brain is working. It identifies changes in blood flow, reflected by changes in the level of blood oxygenation, in response to activity. fMRI can identify metabolic changes in normal, diseased, or injured brain tissue. It is also used in research to study which parts of the brain are responsible for speech, physical movement, thought, and sensations; this type of research is also called brain mapping that has significant implications in understanding and managing the effects of stroke, brain tumors, and diseases such as Alzheimer's. fMRI is based on the blood oxygen level–dependent contrast mechanism that takes advantage of the inherent paramagnetic quality of deoxyhemoglobin. In a properly performed study, the patient is asked to perform a task; the MRI scanner detects changes in the signal strength of brain water protons produced as blood oxygen levels change, and the corresponding strength of the natural paramagnetic signal of deoxyhemoglobin changes.

Magnetic resonance spectroscopy (MRS) is an application of MRI based on the same principles as MRI, but instead of as an anatomical image, the data is displayed graphically as a series of peaks. The peaks represent specific elements and compounds that provide physiological data regarding the tissue of interest. MRS can be performed using MRI equipment with software adapted for the collection and interpretation of spectral data. MRS may be used alone or in conjunction with MRI whereby anatomical images are first collected by MRI followed by focused MRS images that reflect specific active metabolic processes. The frequency information used in MRS identifies specific chemical compounds, such as amino acids, lipids, and lactate, that are commonly involved in or produced by cellular activity. The presence or absence of different metabolites in the spectral analysis can be used to identify metabolic activity associated with a suspected tumor, differentiate between tumor types, provide information about brain lesions (brain tumors, Alzheimer's disease), and monitor response to therapeutic interventions. Other applications of MRS provide information about the spine (e.g., tumor, demyelinating diseases) and conditions involving skeletal muscle disease (muscular dystrophies).

This procedure is contraindicated for

- Patients who are pregnant or suspected of being pregnant, unless the potential benefits of the MRI far outweigh the risks to the fetus and mother. ***In pregnancy, gadolinium-based contrast medium (GBCAs) cross the placental barrier, enter the fetal circulation, and pass via the kidneys into the amniotic fluid. Although no definite adverse effects of GBCA administration on the human fetus have been documented, the potential bioeffects of fetal GBCA exposure are not well understood. GBCA administration should therefore be avoided during pregnancy unless no suitable alternative imaging is possible and the benefits of contrast administration outweigh the potential risk to the fetus.***
- Conditions associated with adverse reactions to contrast medium (e.g., asthma, food allergies, or allergy to contrast medium).

Although patients are asked specifically if they have a known allergy to iodine or shellfish (shellfish contain high levels of iodine), it has been well established that the reaction is not to iodine; an actual iodine allergy would be problematic because iodine is required for the production of thyroid hormones. In the case of shellfish, the reaction is to a muscle protein called tropomyosin; in the case of iodinated contrast medium, the reaction is to the noniodinated part of the contrast molecule. Patients with a known hypersensitivity to the medium may benefit from premedication with corticosteroids and diphenhydramine; the use of nonionic contrast or an alternative noncontrast imaging study, if available, may be considered for patients who have severe asthma or who have experienced moderate to severe reactions to ionic contrast medium.

- Patients with moderate to marked renal impairment (glomerular filtration rate less than 30 mL/min/1.73 m^2). Patients should be screened for kidney dysfunction prior to administration. The use of GBCAs should be avoided in these patients unless the benefits of the studies outweigh the risks and if essential diagnostic information is not available using non-contrast-enhanced diagnostic studies.
- Patients with cardiac pacemakers that can be deactivated by MRI.
- Patients with metal in their body, such as dental amalgams, metallic body piercing items, tattoo inks containing iron (including tattooed eyeliners), shrapnel, bullet, ferrous metal in the eye, certain ferrous metal prosthetics, valves, aneurysm clips, intrauterine device, inner ear prostheses, or other metallic objects; these items can impair image quality. Metallic objects are also a significant safety issue for patients and health-care staff in the examination room during performance of an MRI. The MRI equipment consists of an extremely powerful magnet that can inactivate, move, or shift metallic objects inside a patient. Many metallic objects currently used in health-care

procedures are made of materials that do not interfere with MRI studies; it is important for patients to provide specific information regarding medical procedures they have undergone in order to identify whether their device is safe to undergo MRI. Required information includes the date of the procedure and identification of the device. Metallic objects are not allowed inside the room with the MRI equipment because items such as watches, credit cards, and car keys can become dangerous projectiles.

Patients with transdermal patches containing metallic components. The patch's liner contains a metal that controls absorption of the substance from the patch (e.g., drugs, nicotine, steroids, hormones). The patch may cause burns to the skin ***related to energy conducted through the metal, which is converted to heat during the MRI.*** Other metallic objects on the skin may also cause burns.

Patients who are claustrophobic.

INDICATIONS

- Detect and locate brain tumors.
- Detect cause of cerebrovascular accident, cerebral infarct, or hemorrhage.
- Detect cranial bone, face, throat, and neck soft tissue lesions.
- Evaluate the cause of seizures, such as intracranial infection, edema, or increased intracranial pressure.
- Evaluate cerebral changes associated with dementia.
- Evaluate demyelinating disorders.
- Evaluate intracranial infections.
- Evaluate optic and auditory nerves.
- Evaluate the potential causes of headache, visual loss, and vomiting.
- Evaluate shunt placement and function in patients with hydrocephalus.
- Evaluate the solid, cystic, and hemorrhagic components of lesions.
- Evaluate vascularity of the brain and vascular integrity.
- Monitor and evaluate the effectiveness of medical or surgical interventions, chemotherapy, radiation therapy, and the course of disease.

POTENTIAL MEDICAL DIAGNOSIS

Normal findings

- Normal anatomic structures, soft tissue density, blood flow rate, face, nasopharynx, neck, tongue, and brain

Abnormal findings related to

- Abscess
- Acoustic neuroma
- Alzheimer's disease
- Aneurysm
- Arteriovenous malformation
- Benign meningioma
- Cerebral aneurysm
- Cerebral infarction
- Craniopharyngioma or meningioma
- Granuloma
- Intraparenchymal hematoma or hemorrhage
- Lipoma
- Metastasis
- Multiple sclerosis
- Optic nerve tumor
- Parkinson's disease
- Pituitary microadenoma
- Subdural empyema
- Ventriculitis

CRITICAL FINDINGS:

- Abscess
- Cerebral aneurysm
- Cerebral infarct
- Hydrocephalus
- Skull fracture or contusion
- Tumor with significant mass effect

Note and immediately report to the requesting health-care provider (HCP) any critical findings and related symptoms. A listing of these findings varies among facilities. Timely notification of a critical finding for laboratory or diagnostic studies is a role expectation of the professional nurse. The notification processes vary among facilities. Upon receipt of the critical finding, the information should be read back to the caller to verify accuracy.

INTERFERING FACTORS

Factors that may alter the results of the study

- Metallic objects (e.g., jewelry, body rings, dental amalgams) within the examination field, which may inhibit organ visualization and cause unclear images.
- Inability of the patient to cooperate or remain still during the procedure because of age, significant pain, or mental status.
- Patients with extreme cases of claustrophobia, unless sedation is given before the study or an open MRI is utilized.
- Patients who are extremely obese may require more radiation to obtain a clear image.

Other considerations

- If contrast medium is allowed to seep deep into the muscle tissue, vascular visualization will be impossible.
- The procedure may be canceled if the patient's weight exceeds the safety limit for the equipment.

NURSING IMPLICATIONS AND PROCEDURE

See Potential Nursing Problems on Fast Find at davispl.us/vanleeuwen7.

PRETEST:

- Positively identify the patient using at least two person-specific identifiers before services, treatments, or procedures are performed.
- *Patient Teaching:* Inform the patient this procedure can assist in assessing the brain.
- Obtain a history of the patient's health concerns (especially kidney dysfunction if the use of GBCA is anticipated), symptoms, surgical procedures, and results of previously performed laboratory and diagnostic studies. Include a list of known allergens, especially allergies or sensitivities to latex, anesthetics, sedatives, or contrast medium. Patients with a known hypersensitivity to contrast medium may benefit from premedication with corticosteroids and diphenhydramine.
- Ensure the results of blood urea nitrogen, creatinine, and estimated glomerular filtration rate are obtained if GBCA is to be used.
- Determine if the patient has ever had any device implanted into his or her body, including copper intrauterine devices, pacemakers, ear implants, and heart valves.
- Obtain occupational history to determine the presence of metal in the body, such as shrapnel or flecks of ferrous metal in the eye (which can cause retinal hemorrhage).
- Note any recent procedures that can interfere with test results, including examinations using barium- or iodine-based contrast medium.
- Record the date of the last menstrual period and determine the possibility of pregnancy in perimenopausal women.
- Obtain a list of the patient's current medications, including over-the-counter medications and dietary supplements (see Effects of Natural Products on Laboratory Values online at Davis*Plus*).
- Review the procedure with the patient. Address concerns about pain related to the procedure and explain that no pain will be experienced during the test, but there may be moments of discomfort. Reassure the patient that if contrast is used, it poses no radioactive hazard and rarely produces adverse effects. Inform the patient the procedure is performed in an MRI department, usually by an HCP who specializes in this procedure, with support staff, and takes approximately 30 to 60 min.

- Inform the patient that the technologist will place him or her in a supine position on a flat table in a large cylindrical scanner.
- Tell the patient to expect to hear loud banging from the scanner and possibly to see magnetophosphenes (flickering lights in the visual field); these will stop when the procedure is over.
- *Sensitivity to social and cultural issues,* as well as concern for modesty, is important in providing psychological support before, during, and after the procedure.
- Explain that an IV line may be inserted to allow infusion of fluids such as saline, anesthetics, contrast medium, or sedatives.
- Instruct the patient to remove jewelry and all other metallic objects from the area to be examined prior to the procedure.
- Note that there are no food, fluid, or medication restrictions unless by medical direction. Some protocols may require the patient to restrict prescribed oral iron supplements prior to the study because the iron may interfere with the study results; fasting for 1 to 2 hr before the procedure may also be required in order to avoid nausea and vomiting related to anxiety while in the MRI scanner.

INTRATEST:

Potential Complications:

Injection of the contrast is an invasive procedure. Complications are rare but do include risk for allergic reaction ***related to contrast reaction;*** cardiac dysrhythmias; hematoma ***related to blood leakage into the tissue following needle insertion;*** bleeding from the puncture site ***related to a bleeding disorder or the effects of natural products and medications with known anticoagulant, antiplatelet, or thrombolytic properties;*** vascular or nerve injury ***that might occur if the needle strikes a nerve or nearby blood vessel;*** or infection ***that might occur if bacteria from the skin surface is introduced at the puncture site.***

Some patients are at risk for developing nephrogenic systemic fibrosis as a result of the use of gadolinium-based contrast medium ***related to ineffective renal clearance in patients with impaired kidney function.***

- Observe standard precautions, and follow the general guidelines in Patient Preparation and Specimen Collection online at Davis*Plus*. Positively identify the patient.
- Ensure that the patient has complied with dietary, fluid, and other pretesting preparations prior to the study, as instructed.
- Ensure that the patient has removed all external metallic objects from the area to be examined prior to the procedure.
- Administer ordered prophylactic steroids or antihistamines before the procedure if the patient has a history of allergic reactions to any substance or drug.
- Avoid the use of equipment containing latex if the patient has a history of allergic reaction to latex.
- Have emergency equipment readily available.
- Instruct the patient to void prior to the procedure and to change into the gown, robe, and foot coverings provided.
- Instruct the patient to cooperate fully and to follow directions. Instruct the patient to remain still throughout the procedure because movement produces unreliable results. Electrocardiogram or respiratory gating may be performed in conjunction with the scan to reduce artifacts during data collection due to respiratory or cardiac movement; apply MRI-safe electrodes at the appropriate sites.
- Supply earplugs to the patient to block out the loud, banging sounds that occur during the test. Instruct the patient to communicate with the technologist during the examination via a microphone within the scanner.
- Apply MRI-safe electrodes to the appropriate sites if an electrocardiogram or respiratory gating is to be performed in conjunction with the scan.

M

- Establish IV fluid line for the injection of fluids such as saline, anesthetics, contrast medium, or sedatives. Avoid the use of IV equipment that contains metal.
- Administer an antianxiety drug, as ordered, if the patient has claustrophobia. Administer a sedative to a child or to an adult who is uncooperative, as ordered.
- Assist the patient onto the examination table and into the appropriate position for imaging to begin.
- Imaging can begin shortly after the injection, if contrast is used.
- Ask the patient to inhale deeply and hold his or her breath while the images are taken and then to exhale after the images are taken.
- Instruct the patient to take slow, deep breaths if nausea occurs during the procedure.
- Monitor the patient for complications related to the procedure (e.g., allergic reaction, anaphylaxis, bronchospasm).
- Remove the needle or catheter and apply a pressure dressing over the puncture site.
- Observe/assess the needle/catheter insertion site for bleeding, inflammation, or hematoma formation.

M

POST-TEST:

- Inform the patient that a report of the results will be made available to the requesting HCP, who will discuss the results with the patient.
- Observe for delayed allergic reactions, such as rash, urticaria, tachycardia, hyperpnea, hypertension, palpitations, nausea, or vomiting, if contrast medium was used.
- Instruct the patient to immediately report symptoms such as fast heart rate, difficulty breathing, skin rash, itching, chest pain, persistent right shoulder pain, or abdominal pain. Immediately report symptoms to the appropriate HCP.
- Instruct the patient to apply cold compresses to the puncture site as needed to reduce discomfort or edema.
- Recognize anxiety related to test results. Discuss the implications of abnormal test results on the patient's lifestyle. Provide teaching and information regarding the clinical implications of the test results, as appropriate.
- Reinforce information given by the patient's HCP regarding further testing, treatment, or referral to another HCP. Answer any questions or address any concerns voiced by the patient or family.
- Depending on the results of this procedure, additional testing may be performed to evaluate or monitor progression of the disease process and determine the need for a change in therapy. Evaluate test results in relation to the patient's symptoms and other tests performed.

Patient Education:

- Teach the patient, parent, or significant other reportable symptoms related to bleeding due to medication use.
- Teach the patient, parent, or significant other bleeding precautions that should be used with specific medications.

Expected Patient Outcomes:

Understanding

- The patient and family state the importance of refraining from risky activity that would result in trauma and bleeding.
- The patient and family state the importance of frequent positioning to decrease risk of pressure ulcer development.

Ability

- The patient successfully demonstrates range-of-motion technique.
- The patient successfully demonstrates the use of assistive devices.

Response

- The patient agrees to follow-up laboratory studies to manage medications to prevent stroke.
- The patient agrees to call for assistance when getting out of bed to decrease fall risk.

RELATED STUDIES:

- Related tests include Alzheimer's disease markers, angiography of the carotids, BUN, CSF analysis, CT brain, creatinine, EMG, evoked brain potentials, and PET brain.
- Refer to the Cardiovascular and Musculoskeletal systems tables online at Davis*Plus* for related tests by body system.

Magnetic Resonance Imaging, Breast

SYNONYM/ACRONYM: Breast MRI.

COMMON USE: To visualize and assess abnormalities in breast tissue to assist in evaluating structural abnormalities related to diagnoses such as cancer, abscess, and cysts.

AREA OF APPLICATION: Breast area.

DESCRIPTION: Magnetic resonance imaging (MRI) is useful when the area of interest is soft tissue. The study can be performed with or without intravenous (IV) contrast (gadolinium). The technology does not involve radiation exposure and is considered safer than other imaging methods such as radiographs and computed tomography (CT). MRI uses a magnet and radio waves to produce an energy field that can be displayed as an image of the anatomic area of interest based on the water content of the tissue. The magnetic field causes the hydrogen atoms in tissue to line up, and when radio waves are directed toward the magnetic field, the hydrogen atoms absorb the radio waves and change their position. This change in the energy field is detected by the equipment, and an image is generated by the equipment's computer system using assigned values that correspond to the strength of the signal produced; the anatomical images are represented in various shades of gray. MRI produces cross-sectional images of the breast in multiple planes without the use of ionizing radiation or the interference of bone or surrounding tissue. Images can be obtained in two-dimensional (series of slices) or three-dimensional sequences. Standard or closed MRI equipment has the appearance of an open tube or tunnel; open MRI equipment has no sides and provides an alternative for people who suffer from claustrophobia, pediatric patients, or patients who are obese. Some open MRI units are designed to allow the patient to stand or sit while images are taken in various body positions. IV gadolinium-based contrast media may be used to better visualize the vessels and tissues in the area of interest. Clear, high-quality images of abnormalities and disease processes significantly improve the diagnostic value of the study.

MRI imaging of the breast is not a replacement for traditional mammography, ultrasound, or biopsy. This examination is

Access Canadian content on Fast Find: Lab and Dx at davispl.us/vanleeuwen7

extremely helpful in evaluating mammogram abnormalities and identifying early breast cancer in women at high risk. Women at high risk include those who have had breast cancer, have an abnormal mutated breast cancer gene (BRCA1 or BRCA2), or have a mother or sister who has been diagnosed with breast cancer. Breast MRI is used most commonly in women at high risk when findings of a mammogram or ultrasound are inconclusive because of dense breast tissue or there is a suspected abnormality that requires further evaluation. MRI is also an excellent examination in the augmented breast, including both the breast implant and the breast tissue surrounding the implant. This same examination is also useful for staging breast cancer and determining the most appropriate treatment. MRI uses the noniodinated paramagnetic contrast medium gadopentetate dimeglumine (Magnevist), which is administered IV to enhance contrast differences between normal and abnormal tissues.

This procedure is contraindicated for

- Patients who are pregnant or suspected of being pregnant, unless the potential benefits of the MRI far outweigh the risks to the fetus and mother. ***In pregnancy, gadolinium-based contrast medium (GBCAs) cross the placental barrier, enter the fetal circulation, and pass via the kidneys into the amniotic fluid. Although no definite adverse effects of GBCA administration on the human fetus have been documented, the potential bioeffects of fetal GBCA exposure are not well understood. GBCA administration should therefore be avoided during pregnancy unless no suitable alternative imaging is possible and the benefits of contrast administration outweigh the potential risk to the fetus.***
- Conditions associated with adverse reactions to contrast medium (e.g., asthma, food allergies, or allergy to contrast medium).

  Although patients are asked specifically if they have a known allergy to iodine or shellfish (shellfish contain high levels of iodine), it has been well established that the reaction is not to iodine; an actual iodine allergy would be problematic because iodine is required for the production of thyroid hormones. In the case of shellfish, the reaction is to a muscle protein called tropomyosin; in the case of iodinated contrast medium, the reaction is to the noniodinated part of the contrast molecule. Patients with a known hypersensitivity to the medium may benefit from premedication with corticosteroids and diphenhydramine; the use of nonionic contrast or an alternative noncontrast imaging study, if available, may be considered for patients who have severe asthma or who have experienced moderate to severe reactions to ionic contrast medium.
- Patients with moderate to marked renal impairment (glomerular filtration rate less than 30 mL/min/1.73 m^2) because use of GBCAs is contraindicated. Patients should be screened for kidney dysfunction prior to administration. The use of GBCAs should be avoided in these patients unless the benefits of the studies outweigh the risks and if essential diagnostic information is not available using non-contrast-enhanced diagnostic studies.
- Patients with cardiac pacemakers that can be deactivated by MRI.
- Patients with metal in their body, such as dental amalgams, metallic body piercing items, tattoo inks

containing iron (including tattooed eyeliners), shrapnel, bullet, ferrous metal in the eye, certain ferrous metal prosthetics, valves, aneurysm clips, intrauterine device, inner ear prostheses, or other metallic objects; these items can impair image quality. Metallic objects are also a significant safety issue for patients and health-care staff in the examination room during performance of an MRI. The MRI equipment consists of an extremely powerful magnet that can inactivate, move, or shift metallic objects inside a patient. Many metallic objects currently used in health-care procedures are made of materials that do not interfere with MRI studies; it is important for patients to provide specific information regarding medical procedures they have undergone in order to identify whether their device is safe to undergo MRI. Required information includes the date of the procedure and identification of the device. Metallic objects are not allowed inside the room with the MRI equipment because items such as watches, credit cards, and car keys can become dangerous projectiles.

Patients with transdermal patches containing metallic components. The patch's liner contains a metal that controls absorption of the substance from the patch (e.g., drugs, nicotine, steroids, hormones). The patch may cause burns to the skin ***related to energy conducted through the metal, which is converted to heat during the MRI.*** Other metallic objects on the skin may also cause burns.

Patients who are claustrophobic.

INDICATIONS

- Evaluate breast implants.
- Evaluate dense breasts.
- Evaluate for residual cancer after lumpectomy.
- Evaluate inverted nipples.
- Evaluate small abnormalities.
- Evaluate tissue after lumpectomy or mastectomy.
- Evaluate women at high risk for breast cancer.

POTENTIAL MEDICAL DIAGNOSIS

Normal findings

- Normal anatomic structures, soft tissue density, and blood flow rate

Abnormal findings related to

- Breast abscess or cyst
- Breast cancer
- Breast implant rupture
- Hematoma
- Soft tissue masses
- Vascular abnormalities

CRITICAL FINDINGS: N/A

INTERFERING FACTORS

Factors that may alter the results of the study

- Metallic objects (e.g., jewelry, body rings) within the examination field, which may inhibit organ visualization and cause unclear images.
- Inability of the patient to cooperate or remain still during the procedure because of age, significant pain, or mental status.
- Patients with extreme cases of claustrophobia, unless sedation is given before the study or an open MRI is utilized.
- Patients who are extremely obese may require more radiation to obtain a clear image.

Other considerations

- If contrast medium is allowed to seep deep into the muscle tissue, vascular visualization will be impossible.
- The procedure may be canceled if the patient's weight exceeds the safety limit for the equipment.
- The procedure can be nonspecific; the examination is unable to image calcifications that can indicate breast cancer, and there may be difficulty distinguishing between cancerous and noncancerous tumors.

M

NURSING IMPLICATIONS AND PROCEDURE

See Potential Nursing Problems on Fast Find at davispl.us/vanleeuwen7.

PRETEST:

- Positively identify the patient using at least two person-specific identifiers before services, treatments, or procedures are performed.
- ***Patient Teaching:*** Inform the patient this procedure can assist in assessing the breast.
- Obtain a history of the patient's health concerns (especially kidney dysfunction if the use of GBCA is anticipated), symptoms, surgical procedures, and results of previously performed laboratory and diagnostic studies. Include a list of known allergens, especially allergies or sensitivities to latex, anesthetics, sedatives, or contrast medium. Patients with a known hypersensitivity to contrast medium may benefit from premedication with corticosteroids and diphenhydramine.
- Ensure the results of blood urea nitrogen, creatinine, and estimated glomerular filtration rate are obtained if GBCA is to be used.
- Determine if the patient has ever had any device implanted into his or her body, including copper intrauterine devices, pacemakers, ear implants, and heart valves.
- Obtain occupational history to determine the presence of metal in the body, such as shrapnel or flecks of ferrous metal in the eye (which can cause retinal hemorrhage).
- Note any recent procedures that can interfere with test results, including examinations using barium- or iodine-based contrast medium.
- Record the date of the last menstrual period and determine the possibility of pregnancy in perimenopausal women.
- Obtain a list of the patient's current medications, including over-the-counter medications and dietary supplements (see Effects of Natural Products on Laboratory Values online at Davis*Plus*).
- Review the procedure with the patient. Address concerns about pain related to the procedure and explain that no pain will be experienced during the test, but there may be moments of discomfort. Reassure the patient that if contrast is used, it poses no radioactive hazard and rarely produces adverse effects. Inform the patient that the procedure is performed in an MRI department by a health-care provider (HCP) who specializes in this procedure, with support staff, and takes approximately 30 to 60 min.
- Inform the patient that the technologist will place him or her in a prone position on a special imaging table in a large cylindrical scanner.
- Tell the patient to expect to hear loud banging from the scanner and possibly to see magnetophosphenes (flickering lights in the visual field); these will stop when the procedure is over.
- ***Sensitivity to social and cultural issues,*** as well as concern for modesty, is important in providing psychological support before, during, and after the procedure.
- Explain that an IV line may be inserted to allow infusion of fluids such as saline, anesthetics, contrast medium, or sedatives.
- Instruct the patient to remove jewelry and all other metallic objects from the area to be examined prior to the procedure.
- Note that there are no food, fluid, or medication restrictions unless by medical direction. Some protocols may require the patient to restrict prescribed oral iron supplements prior to the study because the iron may interfere with the study results; fasting for 1 to 2 hr before the procedure may also be required in order to avoid nausea and vomiting related to anxiety while in the MRI scanner.

M

INTRATEST:

Potential Complications:
Injection of the contrast is an invasive procedure. Complications are rare but do include risk for allergic reaction ***related to contrast reaction;*** cardiac dysrhythmias; hematoma ***related to blood leakage into the tissue following needle insertion;*** bleeding from the puncture site ***related to a bleeding disorder or the effects of natural products and medications with known anticoagulant, antiplatelet, or thrombolytic properties;*** vascular or nerve injury ***that might occur if the needle strikes a nerve or nearby blood vessel;*** or infection ***that might occur if bacteria from the skin surface is introduced at the puncture site.***

Some patients are at risk for developing nephrogenic systemic fibrosis as a result of the use of gadolinium-based contrast medium ***related to ineffective renal clearance in patients with impaired kidney function.***

- Observe standard precautions, and follow the general guidelines in Patient Preparation and Specimen Collection online at Davis*Plus*. Positively identify the patient.
- Ensure that the patient has complied with dietary, fluid, and other pretesting preparations prior to the study, as instructed.
- Ensure that the patient has removed all external metallic objects from the area to be examined prior to the procedure.
- Administer ordered prophylactic steroids or antihistamines before the procedure if the patient has a history of allergic reactions to any substance or drug.
- Avoid the use of equipment containing latex if the patient has a history of allergic reaction to latex.
- Have emergency equipment readily available.
- Instruct the patient to void prior to the procedure and to change into the gown, robe, and foot coverings provided.
- Instruct the patient to cooperate fully and to follow directions. Instruct the patient to remain still throughout the procedure because movement produces unreliable results. Electrocardiogram or respiratory gating may be performed in conjunction with the scan to reduce artifacts during data collection due to respiratory or cardiac movement; apply MRI-safe electrodes at the appropriate sites.
- Supply earplugs to the patient to block out the loud, banging sounds that occur during the test. Instruct the patient to communicate with the technologist during the examination via a microphone within the scanner.
- Establish IV fluid line for the injection of fluids such as saline, anesthetics, contrast medium, or sedatives. Avoid the use of IV equipment that contains metal.
- Administer an antianxiety drug, as ordered, if the patient has claustrophobia. Administer a sedative to a child or to an adult who is uncooperative, as ordered.
- Assist the patient onto the examination table, designed for breast imaging, and into the appropriate position for imaging to begin.
- Imaging can begin shortly after the injection, if contrast is used.
- Ask the patient to inhale deeply and hold his or her breath while the images are taken and then to exhale after the images are taken.
- Instruct the patient to take slow, deep breaths if nausea occurs during the procedure.
- Monitor the patient for complications related to the procedure (e.g., allergic reaction, anaphylaxis, bronchospasm).
- Remove the needle or catheter and apply a pressure dressing over the puncture site.
- Observe/assess the needle/catheter insertion site for bleeding, inflammation, or hematoma formation.

POST-TEST:

- Inform the patient that a report of the results will be made available

M

to the requesting HCP, who will discuss the results with the patient.

- Observe for delayed allergic reactions, such as rash, urticaria, tachycardia, hyperpnea, hypertension, palpitations, nausea, or vomiting.
- Instruct the patient to immediately report symptoms such as fast heart rate, difficulty breathing, skin rash, itching, chest pain, persistent right shoulder pain, or abdominal pain. Immediately report symptoms to the appropriate HCP.
- Instruct the patient in the care and assessment of the injection site.
- Instruct the patient to apply cold compresses to the puncture site as needed to reduce discomfort or edema.
- Recognize anxiety related to test results. Discuss the implications of abnormal test results on the patient's lifestyle. Provide teaching and information regarding the clinical implications of the test results, as appropriate. Educate the patient regarding access to counseling services.
- Reinforce information given by the patient's HCP regarding further testing, treatment, or referral to another HCP. Decisions regarding the need for and frequency of breast self-examination, mammography, MRI breast, or other cancer screening procedures should be made after consultation between the patient and HCP. The most current guidelines for breast cancer screening of the general population as well as of individuals with increased risk are available from the American Cancer Society (ACS) (www.cancer.org), American College of Obstetricians and Gynecologists (ACOG) (www.acog.org), and American College of Radiology (www.acr.org). The ACS recommends breast examinations be performed every 3 yr for women between the ages of 20 and 39 yr and annually for women over 40 yr of age; annual mammograms should be performed on women 40 yr and older as long as they are in good health. The ACS also recommends annual MRI testing, in addition to an annual mammogram, for women at high risk of developing breast cancer. 🍁 Genetic testing for inherited mutations (BRCA1 and BRCA2) associated with increased risk of developing breast cancer may be ordered for women at risk. The test is performed on a blood specimen. Answer any questions or address any concerns voiced by the patient or family.
- Depending on the results of this procedure, additional testing may be performed to evaluate or monitor progression of the disease process and determine the need for a change in therapy. Evaluate test results in relation to the patient's symptoms and other tests performed.

Patient Education:

- Provide information on disease signs and symptoms and management.
- Provide information on possible diagnostic and laboratory studies associated with disease management.

Expected Patient Outcomes:

Understanding

- The patient describes pain management strategies that work and those that don't work.
- The patient describes the meaning of pain relief in relation to his or her personal health.

Ability

- The patient demonstrates positive coping strategies.
- The patient successfully demonstrates care of surgical site, as appropriate.

Response

- The patient agrees to attend cancer support group meetings.
- The patient agrees to seek psychological counseling to adjust to body changes and intimacy concerns.

RELATED STUDIES:

- Related tests include biopsy breast, bone scan, BUN, cancer antigens, CT thorax, creatinine, ductography, genetic testing, mammogram, stereotactic biopsy breast, and US breast.
- Refer to the Reproductive System table online at Davis*Plus* for related tests by body system.

M

Magnetic Resonance Imaging, Chest

SYNONYM/ACRONYM: Chest MRI.

COMMON USE: To visualize and assess pulmonary and cardiovascular structures toward diagnosing tumor, masses, aneurysm, infarct, air, fluid, and evaluate the effectiveness of medical, and surgical interventions.

AREA OF APPLICATION: Chest/thorax.

DESCRIPTION: Magnetic resonance imaging (MRI) is useful when the area of interest is soft tissue. The study can be performed with or without intravenous (IV) contrast (gadolinium). The technology does not involve radiation exposure and is considered safer than other imaging methods such as radiographs and computed tomography (CT). MRI uses a magnet and radio waves to produce an energy field that can be displayed as an image of the anatomic area of interest based on the water content of the tissue. The magnetic field causes the hydrogen atoms in tissue to line up, and when radio waves are directed toward the magnetic field, the hydrogen atoms absorb the radio waves and change their position. This change in the energy field is detected by the equipment, and an image is generated by the equipment's computer system using assigned values that correspond to the strength of the signal produced; the anatomical images are represented in various shades of gray. MRI produces cross-sectional images of the chest in multiple planes without the use of ionizing radiation or the interference of bone or surrounding tissue. Images can be obtained in two-dimensional (series of slices) or three-dimensional sequences. Standard or closed MRI equipment has the appearance of an open tube or tunnel; open MRI equipment has no sides and provides an alternative for people who suffer from claustrophobia, pediatric patients, or patients who are obese. Some open MRI units are designed to allow the patient to stand or sit while images are taken in various body positions. IV gadolinium-based contrast media may be used to better visualize the vessels and tissues in the area of interest. Clear, high-quality images of abnormalities and disease processes significantly improve the diagnostic value of the study.

Chest MRI scanning is performed to assist in diagnosing abnormalities of cardiovascular and pulmonary structures. Two special techniques are available for evaluation of cardiovascular structures. One is the electrocardiograph (ECG)–gated multislice spin-echo sequence, used to diagnose anatomic abnormalities of the heart and aorta, and the other is the ECG-referenced gradient refocused sequence used to diagnose heart function and analyze blood flow patterns.

This procedure is contraindicated for

- Patients who are pregnant or suspected of being pregnant, unless the potential benefits of the MRI far outweigh the risks to the fetus and mother. ***In pregnancy, gadolinium-based contrast medium (GBCAs) cross the placental barrier, enter the fetal circulation, and pass via the kidneys into the amniotic fluid. Although no definite adverse effects of GBCA administration on the human fetus have been documented, the potential bioeffects of fetal GBCA exposure are not well understood. GBCA administration should therefore be avoided during pregnancy unless no suitable alternative imaging is possible and the benefits of contrast administration outweigh the potential risk to the fetus.***

Conditions associated with adverse reactions to contrast medium (e.g., asthma, food allergies, or allergy to contrast medium).

Although patients are asked specifically if they have a known allergy to iodine or shellfish (shellfish contain high levels of iodine), it has been well established that the reaction is not to iodine; an actual iodine allergy would be problematic because iodine is required for the production of thyroid hormones. In the case of shellfish, the reaction is to a muscle protein called tropomyosin; in the case of iodinated contrast medium, the reaction is to the noniodinated part of the contrast molecule. Patients with a known hypersensitivity to the medium may benefit from premedication with corticosteroids and diphenhydramine; the use of nonionic contrast or an alternative noncontrast imaging study, if available, may be considered for patients who have severe asthma or who have experienced moderate to severe reactions to ionic contrast medium.

Patients with moderate to marked renal impairment (glomerular filtration rate less than 30 mL/min/1.73 m^2) because use of GBCAs is contraindicated. Patients should be screened for kidney dysfunction prior to administration. The use of GBCAs should be avoided in these patients unless the benefits of the studies outweigh the risks and if essential diagnostic information is not available using non-contrast-enhanced diagnostic studies.

Patients with cardiac pacemakers that can be deactivated by MRI.

Patients with metal in their body, such as dental amalgams, metallic body piercing items, tattoo inks containing iron (including tattooed eyeliners), shrapnel, bullet, ferrous metal in the eye, certain ferrous metal prosthetics, valves, aneurysm clips, intrauterine device, inner ear prostheses, or other metallic objects; these items can impair image quality. Metallic objects are also a significant safety issue for patients and health-care staff in the examination room during performance of an MRI. The MRI equipment consists of an extremely powerful magnet that can inactivate, move, or shift metallic objects inside a patient. Many metallic objects currently used in health-care procedures are made of materials that do not interfere with MRI studies; it is important for patients to provide specific information regarding medical procedures they have undergone in order to identify whether their device is safe to undergo MRI. Required information includes the date of the procedure and identification of the device. Metallic objects are not allowed inside the room with the MRI equipment because items such as watches, credit cards, and car keys can become dangerous projectiles.

Patients with transdermal patches containing metallic components. The patch's liner contains a metal that controls absorption of the substance from the patch (e.g., drugs, nicotine, steroids, hormones). The patch may cause burns to the skin ***related to energy conducted through the metal,***

M

which is converted to heat during the MRI. Other metallic objects on the skin may also cause burns.

- Patients who are claustrophobic.

INDICATIONS

- Confirm diagnosis of cardiac and pericardiac masses.
- Detect aortic aneurysms.
- Detect myocardial infarction and cardiac muscle ischemia.
- Detect pericardial abnormalities.
- Detect pleural effusion.
- Detect thoracic aortic diseases.
- Determine blood, fluid, or fat accumulation in tissues, pleuritic space, or vessels.
- Determine cardiac ventricular function.
- Differentiate aortic aneurysms from tumors near the aorta.
- Evaluate cardiac chambers and pulmonary vessels.
- Evaluate postoperative angioplasty sites and bypass grafts.
- Identify congenital heart diseases.
- Monitor and evaluate the effectiveness of medical or surgical therapeutic regimen.

POTENTIAL MEDICAL DIAGNOSIS

Normal findings

- Normal heart and lung structures, soft tissue, and function, including blood flow rate

Abnormal findings related to

- Aortic dissection
- Congenital heart diseases, including pulmonary atresia, aortic coarctation, agenesis of the pulmonary artery, and transposition of the great vessels
- Constrictive pericarditis
- Intramural and periaortic hematoma
- Myocardial infarction
- Pericardial hematoma or effusion
- Pleural effusion

CRITICAL FINDINGS:

- Aortic aneurysm
- Aortic dissection
- Tumor with significant mass effect

Note and immediately report to the requesting health-care provider (HCP) any critical findings and related symptoms. A listing of these findings varies among facilities. Timely notification of a critical finding for laboratory or diagnostic studies is a role expectation of the professional nurse. The notification processes vary among facilities. Upon receipt of the critical finding, the information should be read back to the caller to verify accuracy.

INTERFERING FACTORS

Factors that may alter the results of the study

- Metallic objects (e.g., jewelry, body rings, dental amalgams) within the examination field, which may inhibit organ visualization and cause unclear images.
- Inability of the patient to cooperate or remain still during the procedure because of age, significant pain, or mental status.
- Patients with extreme cases of claustrophobia, unless sedation is given before the study or an open MRI is utilized.
- Patients who are extremely obese may require more radiation to obtain a clear image.

Other considerations

- If contrast medium is allowed to seep deep into the muscle tissue, vascular visualization will be impossible.
- The procedure may be canceled if the patient's weight exceeds the safety limit for the equipment.

M

NURSING IMPLICATIONS AND PROCEDURE

See Potential Nursing Problems on Fast Find at davispl.us/vanleeuwen7.

PRETEST:

- Positively identify the patient using at least two person-specific identifiers before services, treatments, or procedures are performed.
- *Patient Teaching:* Inform the patient this procedure can assist in assessing organs and structures inside the chest.
- Obtain a history of the patient's health concerns (especially kidney dysfunction if the use of GBCA is anticipated), symptoms, surgical procedures, and results of previously performed laboratory and diagnostic studies. Include a list of known allergens, especially allergies or sensitivities to latex, anesthetics, sedatives, or contrast medium. Patients with a known hypersensitivity to contrast medium may benefit from premedication with corticosteroids and diphenhydramine.
- Ensure the results of blood urea nitrogen, creatinine, and estimated glomerular filtration rate are obtained if GBCA is to be used.
- Determine if the patient has ever had any device implanted into his or her body, including copper intrauterine devices, pacemakers, ear implants, and heart valves.
- Obtain occupational history to determine the presence of metal in the body, such as shrapnel or flecks of ferrous metal in the eye (which can cause retinal hemorrhage).
- Note any recent procedures that can interfere with test results, including examinations using barium- or iodine-based contrast medium.
- Record the date of the last menstrual period and determine possibility of pregnancy in perimenopausal women.
- Obtain a list of the patient's current medications, including over-the-counter medications and dietary supplements (see Effects of Natural Products on Laboratory Values online at Davis*Plus*).
- Review the procedure with the patient. Address concerns about pain related to the procedure and explain that no pain will be experienced during the test, but there may be moments of discomfort. Reassure the patient that if contrast is used, it poses no radioactive hazard and rarely produces adverse effects. Inform the patient the procedure is performed in an MRI department, usually by an HCP who specializes in these procedures, with support staff, and takes approximately 30 to 60 min.
- Inform the patient that the technologist will place him or her in a supine position on a flat table in a large cylindrical scanner.
- Tell the patient to expect to hear loud banging from the scanner and possibly to see magnetophosphenes (flickering lights in the visual field); these will stop when the procedure is over.
- ***Sensitivity to social and cultural issues,*** as well as concern for modesty, is important in providing psychological support before, during, and after the procedure.
- Explain that an IV line may be inserted to allow infusion of fluids such as saline, anesthetics, contrast medium, or sedatives.
- Instruct the patient to remove jewelry and all other metallic objects from the area to be examined prior to the procedure.
- Note that there are no food, fluid, or medication restrictions unless by medical direction. Some protocols may require the patient to restrict prescribed oral iron supplements prior to the study because the iron may interfere with the study results; fasting for 1 to 2 hr before the procedure may also be required in order to avoid nausea and vomiting related to anxiety while in the MRI scanner.

INTRATEST:

Potential Complications:

Injection of the contrast is an invasive procedure. Complications are rare but do include risk for allergic reaction ***related to contrast reaction;***

cardiac dysrhythmias; hematoma ***related to blood leakage into the tissue following needle insertion;*** bleeding from the puncture site ***related to a bleeding disorder or the effects of natural products and medications with known anticoagulant, antiplatelet, or thrombolytic properties;*** vascular or nerve injury ***that might occur if the needle strikes a nerve or nearby blood vessel;*** or infection ***that might occur if bacteria from the skin surface is introduced at the puncture site.***

Some patients are at risk for developing nephrogenic systemic fibrosis as a result of the use of gadolinium-based contrast medium ***related to ineffective renal clearance in patients with impaired kidney function.***

- Observe standard precautions, and follow the general guidelines in Patient Preparation and Specimen Collection online at Davis*Plus*. Positively identify the patient.
- Ensure that the patient has complied with dietary, fluid, and other pretesting preparations prior to the study, as instructed.
- Ensure that the patient has removed all external metallic objects from the area to be examined prior to the procedure.
- Administer ordered prophylactic steroids or antihistamines before the procedure if the patient has a history of allergic reactions to any substance or drug.
- Avoid the use of equipment containing latex if the patient has a history of allergic reaction to latex.
- Have emergency equipment readily available.
- Instruct the patient to void prior to the procedure and to change into the gown, robe, and foot coverings provided.
- Instruct the patient to cooperate fully and to follow directions. Instruct the patient to remain still throughout the procedure because movement produces unreliable results. Electrocardiogram or respiratory gating may be performed in conjunction with the scan to reduce artifacts during data collection due to respiratory or cardiac movement; apply MRI-safe electrodes at the appropriate sites.
- Supply earplugs to the patient to block out the loud, banging sounds that occur during the test. Instruct the patient to communicate with the technologist during the examination via a microphone within the scanner.
- Apply MRI-safe electrodes to the appropriate sites if an electrocardiogram or respiratory gating is to be performed in conjunction with the scan.
- Establish IV fluid line for the injection of fluids such as saline, anesthetics, contrast medium, or sedatives. Avoid the use of IV equipment that contains metal.
- Administer an antianxiety drug, as ordered, if the patient has claustrophobia. Administer a sedative to a child or to an adult who is uncooperative, as ordered.
- Assist the patient onto the examination table and into the appropriate position for imaging to begin.
- Imaging can begin shortly after the injection, if contrast is used.
- Ask the patient to inhale deeply and hold his or her breath while the images are taken and then to exhale after the images are taken.
- Instruct the patient to take slow, deep breaths if nausea occurs during the procedure.
- Monitor the patient for complications related to the procedure (e.g., allergic reaction, anaphylaxis, bronchospasm).
- Remove the needle or catheter and apply a pressure dressing over the puncture site.
- Observe/assess the needle/catheter insertion site for bleeding, inflammation, or hematoma formation.

POST-TEST:

- Inform the patient that a report of the results will be made available to the requesting HCP, who will discuss the results with the patient.
- Observe for delayed allergic reactions, such as rash, urticaria,

tachycardia, hyperpnea, hypertension, palpitations, nausea, or vomiting.

- Instruct the patient to immediately report symptoms such as fast heart rate, difficulty breathing, skin rash, itching, chest pain, persistent right shoulder pain, or abdominal pain. Immediately report symptoms to the appropriate HCP.
- Instruct the patient in the care and assessment of the injection site.
- Instruct the patient to apply cold compresses to the puncture site as needed to reduce discomfort or edema.
- Recognize anxiety related to test results. Discuss the implications of abnormal test results on the patient's lifestyle. Provide teaching and information regarding the clinical implications of the test results, as appropriate.
- Reinforce information given by the patient's HCP regarding further testing, treatment, or referral to another HCP. Answer any questions or address any concerns voiced by the patient or family.
- Depending on the results of this procedure, additional testing may be performed to evaluate or monitor progression of the disease process and determine the need for a change in therapy. Evaluate test results in relation to the patient's symptoms and other tests performed.

Patient Education:

- Teach the patient about the pathophysiology of myocardial infarction.
- Teach the patient the purpose of ordered medications (morphine, nitroglycerin, calcium channel blockers, beta blockers).

Expected Patient Outcomes:

Understanding

- The patient and family explain the link between activity and cardiac health.
- The patient and family explain how oxygen administration supports cardiac function.

Ability

- The patient and family create a quiet environment to reduce energy demands.
- The patient and family plan rest periods during the day to conserve oxygen.

Response

- The patient agrees to make lifestyle changes that will support positive cardiac health.
- The patient agrees to attend cardiac rehabilitation.

RELATED STUDIES:

- Related tests include BNP, blood gases, blood pool imaging, BUN, chest x-ray, CT cardiac scoring, CT thorax, CRP, CK and isoenzymes, creatinine, echocardiography, exercise stress test, Holter monitor, myocardial infarct scan, myocardial perfusion heart scan, myoglobin, pleural fluid analysis, PET scan of the heart, and troponins.
- Refer to the Cardiovascular and Respiratory systems tables online at Davis*Plus* for related tests by body system.

M

Magnetic Resonance Imaging, Musculoskeletal

SYNONYM/ACRONYM: Musculoskeletal (knee, shoulder, hand, wrist, foot, elbow, hip, spine) MRI.

COMMON USE: To visualize and assess bones, joints, and surrounding structures to assist in diagnosing defects, cysts, tumors, and fracture.

AREA OF APPLICATION: Bones, joints, soft tissues.

Access Canadian content on Fast Find: Lab and Dx at davispl.us/vanleeuwen7

DESCRIPTION: Magnetic resonance imaging (MRI) is useful when the area of interest is soft tissue. The study can be performed with or without intravenous (IV) contrast (gadolinium). The technology does not involve radiation exposure and is considered safer than other imaging methods such as radiographs and computed tomography (CT). MRI uses a magnet and radio waves to produce an energy field that can be displayed as an image of the anatomic area of interest based on the water content of the tissue. The magnetic field causes the hydrogen atoms in tissue to line up, and when radio waves are directed toward the magnetic field, the hydrogen atoms absorb the radio waves and change their position. This change in the energy field is detected by the equipment, and an image is generated by the equipment's computer system using assigned values that correspond to the strength of the signal produced; the anatomical images are represented in various shades of gray. MRI produces cross-sectional images of bones and joints in multiple planes without the use of ionizing radiation or the interference of bone or surrounding tissue. Images can be obtained in two-dimensional (series of slices) or three-dimensional sequences. Standard or closed MRI equipment has the appearance of an open tube or tunnel; open MRI equipment has no sides and provides an alternative for people who suffer from claustrophobia, pediatric patients, or patients who are obese. Some open MRI units are designed to allow the patient to stand or sit while images are taken in various body positions. IV gadolinium-based contrast media may be used to better visualize the vessels and tissues in the area of interest. Clear, high-quality images of abnormalities and disease processes significantly improve the diagnostic value of the study.

Musculoskeletal MRI is performed to assist in diagnosing abnormalities of bones and joints and surrounding soft tissue structures, including cartilage, synovium, ligaments, and tendons. MRI eliminates the risks associated with exposure to x-rays and causes no harm to cells. Contrast-enhanced imaging is effective for evaluating scarring from previous surgery, vascular abnormalities, and differentiation of metastases from primary tumors. MRI uses the noniodinated paramagnetic contrast medium gadopentetate dimeglumine (Magnevist), which is administered IV to enhance differences between normal and abnormal tissues.

Magnetic resonance spectroscopy (MRS) is an application of MRI based on the same principles as MRI, but instead of as an anatomical image, the data is displayed graphically as a series of peaks. The peaks represent specific elements and compounds that provide physiological data regarding the tissue of interest. MRS can be performed using MRI equipment with software adapted for the collection and interpretation of spectral data. MRS may be used alone or in conjunction with MRI whereby anatomical images are first collected by MRI followed by focused MRS images that reflect specific active metabolic processes. The frequency information used in MRS identifies specific chemical compounds, such as amino acids, lipids, and lactate,

M

that are commonly involved in or produced by cellular activity. The presence or absence of different metabolites in the spectral analysis can be used to identify metabolic activity associated with a suspected tumor, differentiate between tumor types, provide information about the spine (e.g., demyelinating diseases) or conditions involving skeletal muscle disease (muscular dystrophies), and monitor response to therapeutic interventions. Other applications of MRS include studies of brain lesions (brain tumors, Alzheimer's disease).

This procedure is contraindicated for

- Patients who are pregnant or suspected of being pregnant, unless the potential benefits of the MRI far outweigh the risks to the fetus and mother. ***In pregnancy, gadolinium-based contrast medium (GBCAs) cross the placental barrier, enter the fetal circulation, and pass via the kidneys into the amniotic fluid. Although no definite adverse effects of GBCA administration on the human fetus have been documented, the potential bioeffects of fetal GBCA exposure are not well understood. GBCA administration should therefore be avoided during pregnancy unless no suitable alternative imaging is possible and the benefits of contrast administration outweigh the potential risk to the fetus.***
- Conditions associated with adverse reactions to contrast medium (e.g., asthma, food allergies, or allergy to contrast medium).

Although patients are asked specifically if they have a known allergy to iodine or shellfish (shellfish contain high levels of iodine), it has been well established that the reaction is not to iodine; an actual iodine allergy would be problematic because iodine is required for the production of thyroid hormones. In the case of shellfish, the reaction is to a muscle protein called tropomyosin; in the case of iodinated contrast medium, the reaction is to the noniodinated part of the contrast molecule. Patients with a known hypersensitivity to the medium may benefit from premedication with corticosteroids and diphenhydramine; the use of nonionic contrast or an alternative noncontrast imaging study, if available, may be considered for patients who have severe asthma or who have experienced moderate to severe reactions to ionic contrast medium.

- Patients with moderate to marked renal impairment (glomerular filtration rate less than 30 mL/min/1.73 m^2). Patients should be screened for kidney dysfunction prior to administration. The use of GBCAs should be avoided in these patients unless the benefits of the studies outweigh the risks and if essential diagnostic information is not available using non-contrast-enhanced diagnostic studies.
- Patients with cardiac pacemakers that can be deactivated by MRI.
- Patients with metal in their body, such as dental amalgams, metallic body piercing items, tattoo inks containing iron (including tattooed eyeliners), shrapnel, bullet, ferrous metal in the eye, certain ferrous metal prosthetics, valves, aneurysm clips, intrauterine device, inner ear prostheses, or other metallic objects; these items can impair image quality. Metallic objects are also a significant safety issue for patients and health-care staff in the examination room during performance of an MRI. The MRI equipment consists of an extremely powerful magnet that can inactivate, move, or shift metallic objects inside a patient. Many metallic objects currently used in health-care procedures are made of

materials that do not interfere with MRI studies; it is important for patients to provide specific information regarding medical procedures they have undergone in order to identify whether their device is safe to undergo MRI. Required information includes the date of the procedure and identification of the device. Metallic objects are not allowed inside the room with the MRI equipment because items such as watches, credit cards, and car keys can become dangerous projectiles.

Patients with transdermal patches containing metallic components. The patch's liner contains a metal that controls absorption of the substance from the patch (e.g., drugs, nicotine, steroids, hormones). The patch may cause burns to the skin ***related to energy conducted through the metal, which is converted to heat during the MRI.*** Other metallic objects on the skin may also cause burns.

Patients who are claustrophobic.

INDICATIONS

- Confirm diagnosis of osteomyelitis.
- Detect avascular necrosis of the femoral head or knee.
- Detect benign and cancerous tumors and cysts of the bone or soft tissue.
- Detect bone infarcts in the epiphyseal or diaphyseal sites.
- Detect changes in bone marrow.
- Detect tears or degeneration of ligaments, tendons, and menisci resulting from trauma or pathology.
- Determine cause of low back pain, including herniated disk and spinal degenerative disease.
- Differentiate between primary and secondary malignant processes of the bone marrow.
- Differentiate between a stress fracture and a tumor.
- Evaluate meniscal detachment of the temporomandibular joint.

POTENTIAL MEDICAL DIAGNOSIS

Normal findings

- Normal bones, joints, and surrounding tissue structures; no articular disease, bone marrow disorders, tumors, infections, or trauma to the bones, joints, or muscles

Abnormal findings related to

- Avascular necrosis of femoral head or knee, as found in Legg-Calvé-Perthes disease
- Bone marrow disease, such as Gaucher's disease, aplastic anemia, sickle cell disease, or polycythemia
- Degenerative spinal disease, such as spondylosis or arthritis
- Fibrosarcoma
- Hemangioma (muscular or osseous)
- Herniated disk
- Infection
- Meniscal tears or degeneration
- Osteochondroma
- Osteogenic sarcoma
- Osteomyelitis
- Rotator cuff tears
- Spinal stenosis
- Stress fracture
- Synovitis
- Tumor

CRITICAL FINDINGS: N/A

INTERFERING FACTORS

Factors that may alter the results of the study

- Metallic objects (e.g., jewelry, body rings, dental amalgams) within the examination field, which may inhibit organ visualization and cause unclear images.
- Inability of the patient to cooperate or remain still during the procedure because of age, significant pain, or mental status.
- Patients with extreme cases of claustrophobia, unless sedation is given before the study or an open MRI is utilized.

- **Patients who are extremely obese may require more radiation to obtain a clear image.**

Other considerations

- **If contrast medium is allowed to seep deep into the muscle tissue, vascular visualization will be impossible.**
- **The procedure may be canceled if the patient's weight exceeds the safety limit for the equipment.**

NURSING IMPLICATIONS AND PROCEDURE

PRETEST:

- Positively identify the patient using at least two person-specific identifiers before services, treatments, or procedures are performed.
- ***Patient Teaching:*** Inform the patient this procedure can assist in assessing bones, muscles, and joints.
- Obtain a history of the patient's health concerns (especially kidney dysfunction if the use of GBCA is anticipated), symptoms, surgical procedures, and results of previously performed laboratory and diagnostic studies. Include a list of known allergens, especially allergies or sensitivities to latex, anesthetics, sedatives, or contrast medium. Patients with a known hypersensitivity to contrast medium may benefit from premedication with corticosteroids and diphenhydramine.
- Ensure the results of blood urea nitrogen, creatinine, and estimated glomerular filtration rate are obtained if GBCA is to be used.
- Determine if the patient has ever had any device implanted into his or her body, including copper intrauterine devices, pacemakers, ear implants, and heart valves.
- Obtain occupational history to determine the presence of metal in the body, such as shrapnel or flecks of ferrous metal in the eye (which can cause retinal hemorrhage).
- Note any recent procedures that can interfere with test results, including examinations using barium- or iodine-based contrast medium.
- Record the date of the last menstrual period and determine the possibility of pregnancy in perimenopausal women.
- Obtain a list of the patient's current medications, including over-the-counter medications and dietary supplements (see Effects of Natural Products on Laboratory Values online at Davis*Plus*).
- Review the procedure with the patient. Address concerns about pain related to the procedure and explain that no pain will be experienced during the test, but there may be moments of discomfort. Reassure the patient that if contrast is used, it poses no radioactive hazard and rarely produces adverse effects. Inform the patient the procedure is performed in an MRI department, usually by a health-care provider (HCP) specializing in this procedure, with support staff, and takes approximately 30 to 60 min.
- Inform the patient that the technologist will place him or her in a supine position on a flat table in a large cylindrical scanner.
- Tell the patient to expect to hear loud banging from the scanner and possibly to see magnetophosphenes (flickering lights in the visual field); these will stop when the procedure is over.
- ***Sensitivity to social and cultural issues,*** as well as concern for modesty, is important in providing psychological support before, during, and after the procedure.
- Explain that an IV line may be inserted to allow infusion of fluids such as saline, anesthetics, contrast medium, or sedatives.
- Instruct the patient to remove jewelry and all other metallic objects from the area to be examined prior to the procedure.
- Note that there are no food, fluid, or medication restrictions unless by medical direction. Some protocols

M

may require the patient to restrict prescribed oral iron supplements prior to the study because the iron may interfere with the study results; fasting for 1 to 2 hr before the procedure may also be required in order to avoid nausea and vomiting related to anxiety while in the MRI scanner.

INTRATEST:

Potential Complications:
Injection of the contrast is an invasive procedure. Complications are rare but do include risk for allergic reaction ***related to contrast reaction***; cardiac dysrhythmias; hematoma ***related to blood leakage into the tissue following needle insertion;*** bleeding from the puncture site ***related to a bleeding disorder or the effects of natural products and medications with known anticoagulant, antiplatelet, or thrombolytic properties;*** vascular or nerve injury ***that might occur if the needle strikes a nerve or nearby blood vessel;*** or infection ***that might occur if bacteria from the skin surface is introduced at the puncture site.***

Some patients are at risk for developing nephrogenic systemic fibrosis as a result of the use of gadolinium-based contrast medium ***related to ineffective renal clearance in patients with impaired kidney function.***

- Observe standard precautions, and follow the general guidelines in Patient Preparation and Specimen Collection online at Davis*Plus*. Positively identify the patient.
- Ensure that the patient has complied with dietary, fluid, and other pretesting preparations prior to the study, as instructed.
- Ensure that the patient has removed all external metallic objects from the area to be examined prior to the procedure.
- Administer ordered prophylactic steroids or antihistamines before the procedure if the patient has a history of allergic reactions to any substance or drug.
- Avoid the use of equipment containing latex if the patient has a history of allergic reaction to latex.
- Have emergency equipment readily available.
- Instruct the patient to void prior to the procedure and to change into the gown, robe, and foot coverings provided.
- Instruct the patient to cooperate fully and to follow directions. Instruct the patient to remain still throughout the procedure because movement produces unreliable results. Electrocardiogram or respiratory gating may be performed in conjunction with the scan to reduce artifacts during data collection due to respiratory or cardiac movement; apply MRI-safe electrodes at the appropriate sites.
- Supply earplugs to the patient to block out the loud, banging sounds that occur during the test. Instruct the patient to communicate with the technologist during the examination via a microphone within the scanner.
- Establish IV fluid line for the injection of fluids such as saline, anesthetics, contrast medium, or sedatives. Avoid the use of IV equipment that contains metal.
- Administer an antianxiety drug, as ordered, if the patient has claustrophobia. Administer a sedative to a child or to an adult who is uncooperative, as ordered.
- Assist the patient onto the examination table and into the appropriate position for imaging to begin.
- Imaging can begin shortly after the injection, if contrast is used.
- Ask the patient to inhale deeply and hold his or her breath while the images are taken and then to exhale after the images are taken.
- Instruct the patient to take slow, deep breaths if nausea occurs during the procedure.
- Monitor the patient for complications related to the procedure (e.g., allergic reaction, anaphylaxis, bronchospasm).
- Remove the needle or catheter and apply a pressure dressing over the puncture site.

M

- Observe/assess the needle/catheter insertion site for bleeding, inflammation, or hematoma formation.

POST-TEST:

- Inform the patient that a report of the results will be made available to the requesting HCP, who will discuss the results with the patient.
- Observe for delayed allergic reactions, such as rash, urticaria, tachycardia, hyperpnea, hypertension, palpitations, nausea, or vomiting, if contrast medium was used.
- Instruct the patient to immediately report symptoms such as fast heart rate, difficulty breathing, skin rash, itching, chest pain, persistent right shoulder pain, or abdominal pain. Immediately report symptoms to the appropriate HCP.
- Instruct the patient in the care and assessment of the injection site.
- Instruct the patient to apply cold compresses to the puncture site as needed, to reduce discomfort or edema.
- Recognize anxiety related to test results, and be supportive of impaired activity related to anticipated chronic pain resulting from joint inflammation, impairment in mobility, musculoskeletal deformity, and loss of independence. Discuss the implications of abnormal test results on the patient's lifestyle. Provide teaching and information regarding the clinical implications of the test results, as appropriate. Educate the patient regarding access to counseling services, as appropriate. Provide contact information, if desired, for the American College of Rheumatology (www.rheumatology.org) or for the Arthritis Foundation (www.arthritis.org). 🍁
- Reinforce information given by the patient's HCP regarding further testing, treatment, or referral to another HCP. Answer any questions or address any concerns voiced by the patient or family.
- Depending on the results of this procedure, additional testing may be performed to evaluate or monitor progression of the disease process and determine the need for a change in therapy. Evaluate test results in relation to the patient's symptoms and other tests performed.

RELATED STUDIES:

- Related tests include anticyclic citrullinated antibodies, ANA, arthrogram, arthroscopy, bone mineral densitometry, bone scan, BUN, CRP, CT spine, creatinine, ESR, radiography of the bone, synovial fluid analysis, RF, and vertebroplasty.
- Refer to the Musculoskeletal System table online at Davis*Plus* for related tests by body system.

M

Magnetic Resonance Imaging, Pancreas

SYNONYM/ACRONYM: Pancreatic MRI.

COMMON USE: To visualize and assess the pancreas for structural defects, tumor, masses, staging cancer, and evaluating the effectiveness of medical and surgical interventions.

AREA OF APPLICATION: Pancreatic/upper abdominal area.

DESCRIPTION: Magnetic resonance imaging (MRI) is very useful when the area of interest is soft tissue. The study can be performed with or without intravenous (IV) contrast (gadolinium). The technology does not involve radiation exposure and is considered safer than other imaging methods such as radiographs and computed tomography (CT). MRI uses a magnet and radio waves to produce an energy field that can be displayed as an image of the anatomic area of interest based on the water content of the tissue. The magnetic field causes the hydrogen atoms in tissue to line up, and when radio waves are directed toward the magnetic field, the hydrogen atoms absorb the radio waves and change their position. This change in the energy field is detected by the equipment, and an image is generated by the equipment's computer system using assigned values that correspond to the strength of the signal produced; the anatomical images are represented in various shades of gray. MRI produces cross-sectional images of the pancreas in multiple planes without the use of ionizing radiation or the interference of bone or surrounding tissue. Images can be obtained in two-dimensional (series of slices) or three-dimensional sequences. Standard or closed MRI equipment has the appearance of an open tube or tunnel; open MRI equipment has no sides and provides an alternative for people who suffer from claustrophobia, pediatric patients, or patients who are obese. Some open MRI units are designed to allow the patient to stand or sit while images are taken in various body positions. IV gadolinium-based contrast media may be used to better visualize the vessels and tissues in the area of interest. Clear, high-quality images of abnormalities and disease processes significantly improve the diagnostic value of the study.

MRI of the pancreas is employed to evaluate small pancreatic adenocarcinomas, islet cell tumors, ductal abnormalities and calculi, or parenchymal abnormalities. A T1-weighted, fat-saturation series of images is probably best for evaluating the pancreatic parenchyma. This sequence is ideal for showing fat planes between the pancreas and peripancreatic structures and for identifying abnormalities such as fatty infiltration of the pancreas, hemorrhage, adenopathy, and carcinomas. T2-weighted images are most useful for depicting intrapancreatic or peripancreatic fluid collections, pancreatic neoplasms, and calculi. Imaging sequences can be adjusted to display fluid in the biliary tree and pancreatic ducts. MRI uses the noniodinated paramagnetic contrast medium gadopentetate dimeglumine (Magnevist), which is administered IV to enhance contrast differences between normal and abnormal tissues.

This procedure is contraindicated for

Patients who are pregnant or suspected of being pregnant, unless the potential benefits of the MRI far outweigh the risks to the fetus and mother. ***In pregnancy, gadolinium-based contrast medium (GBCAs) cross the placental barrier, enter the fetal circulation, and pass via the kidneys into the amniotic fluid. Although no definite adverse effects of GBCA administration on the human fetus have been documented, the potential bioeffects of fetal GBCA exposure are not well understood. GBCA administration should therefore be avoided during pregnancy unless no suitable alternative imaging is possible and the benefits of contrast administration outweigh the potential risk to the fetus.***

Conditions associated with adverse reactions to contrast medium (e.g., asthma, food allergies, or allergy to contrast medium).

Although patients are asked specifically if they have a known allergy to iodine or shellfish (shellfish contain high levels of iodine), it has been well established that the reaction is not to iodine; an actual iodine allergy would be problematic because iodine is required for the production of thyroid hormones. In the case of shellfish, the reaction is to a muscle protein called tropomyosin; in the case of iodinated contrast medium, the reaction is to the noniodinated part of the contrast molecule. Patients with a known hypersensitivity to the medium may benefit from premedication with corticosteroids and diphenhydramine; the use of nonionic contrast or an alternative noncontrast imaging study, if available, may be considered for patients who have severe asthma or who have experienced moderate to severe reactions to ionic contrast medium.

Patients with moderate to marked renal impairment (glomerular filtration rate less than 30 mL/min/1.73 m^2). Patients should be screened for kidney dysfunction prior to administration. The use of GBCAs should be avoided in these patients unless the benefits of the studies outweigh the risks and if essential diagnostic information is not available using noncontrast-enhanced diagnostic studies.

Patients with cardiac pacemakers that can be deactivated by MRI.

Patients with metal in their body, such as dental amalgams, metallic body piercing items, tattoo inks containing iron (including tattooed eyeliners), shrapnel, bullet, ferrous metal in the eye, certain ferrous metal prosthetics, valves, aneurysm clips, intrauterine device, inner ear prostheses, or other metallic objects; these items can impair image quality. Metallic objects are also a significant safety issue for patients and health-care staff in the examination room during performance of an MRI. The MRI equipment consists of an extremely powerful magnet that can inactivate, move, or shift metallic objects inside a patient. Many metallic objects currently used in health-care procedures are made of materials that do not interfere with MRI studies; it is important for patients to provide specific information regarding medical procedures they have undergone in order to identify whether their device is safe to undergo MRI. Required information includes the date of the procedure and identification of the device. Metallic objects are not allowed inside the room with the MRI equipment because items such as watches, credit cards, and car keys, can become dangerous projectiles.

Patients with transdermal patches containing metallic components. The patch's liner contains a metal that controls absorption of the substance from the patch (e.g., drugs, nicotine, steroids, hormones). The patch may cause burns to the skin ***related to energy conducted through the metal, which is converted to heat during the MRI.*** Other metallic objects on the skin may also cause burns.

Patients who are claustrophobic.

INDICATIONS

- Detect pancreatic fatty infiltration, hemorrhage, and adenopathy.
- Detect a pancreatic mass.
- Detect pancreatitis.
- Detect primary or metastatic tumors of the pancreas and provide cancer staging.
- Detect soft tissue abnormalities.
- Determine vascular complications of pancreatitis, venous thrombosis, or pseudoaneurysm
- Differentiate tumors from other abnormalities, such as cysts,

cavernous hemangiomas, and pancreatic abscesses.

- Monitor and evaluate the effectiveness of medical or surgical interventions and course of disease.

POTENTIAL MEDICAL DIAGNOSIS

Normal findings

- Normal anatomic structures and soft tissue density and biochemical constituents of the pancreatic parenchyma, including blood flow

Abnormal findings related to

- Islet cell tumor
- Metastasis
- Pancreatic duct obstruction or calculi
- Pancreatic fatty infiltration, hemorrhage, and adenopathy
- Pancreatic mass
- Pancreatitis

CRITICAL FINDINGS: N/A

INTERFERING FACTORS

Factors that may alter the results of the study

- Metallic objects (e.g., jewelry, body rings, dental amalgams) within the examination field, which may inhibit organ visualization and cause unclear images.
- Inability of the patient to cooperate or remain still during the procedure because of age, significant pain, or mental status.
- Patients with extreme cases of claustrophobia, unless sedation is given before the study or an open MRI is utilized.
- Patients who are extremely obese may require more radiation to obtain a clear image.

Other considerations

- If contrast medium is allowed to seep deep into the muscle tissue, vascular visualization will be impossible.
- The procedure may be canceled if the patient's weight exceeds the safety limit for the equipment.

NURSING IMPLICATIONS AND PROCEDURE

See Potential Nursing Problems on Fast Find at davispl.us/vanleeuwen7.

PRETEST:

- Positively identify the patient using at least two person-specific identifiers before services, treatments, or procedures are performed.
- ***Patient Teaching:*** Inform the patient this procedure can assist in assessing the pancreas, organs, and structures inside the abdomen.
- Obtain a history of the patient's health concerns (especially kidney dysfunction if the use of GBCA is anticipated), symptoms, surgical procedures, and results of previously performed laboratory and diagnostic studies. Include a list of known allergens, especially allergies or sensitivities to latex, anesthetics, sedatives, or contrast medium. Patients with a known hypersensitivity to contrast medium may benefit from premedication with corticosteroids and diphenhydramine.
- Ensure the results of BUN, creatinine, and estimated glomerular filtration rate are obtained if GBCA is to be used.
- Determine if the patient has ever had any device implanted into his or her body, including copper intrauterine devices, pacemakers, ear implants, and heart valves.
- Obtain occupational history to determine the presence of metal in the body, such as shrapnel or flecks of ferrous metal in the eye (which can cause retinal hemorrhage).
- Note any recent procedures that can interfere with test results, including examinations using barium- or iodine-based contrast medium.
- Record the date of the last menstrual period and determine the possibility of pregnancy in perimenopausal women.

- Obtain a list of the patient's current medications, including over-the-counter medications and dietary supplements (see Effects of Natural Products on Laboratory Values online at Davis*Plus*).
- Review the procedure with the patient. Address concerns about pain related to the procedure and explain that no pain will be experienced during the test, but there may be moments of discomfort. Reassure the patient that if contrast is used, it poses no radioactive hazard and rarely produces adverse effects. Inform the patient that the procedure is performed in an MRI department by a health-care provider (HCP) specializing in this procedure, with support staff, and takes approximately 30 to 60 min.
- Inform the patient that the technologist will place him or her in a supine position on a flat table in a large cylindrical scanner.
- Tell the patient to expect to hear loud banging from the scanner and possibly to see magnetophosphenes (flickering lights in the visual field); these will stop when the procedure is over.
- ***Sensitivity to social and cultural issues,*** as well as concern for modesty, is important in providing psychological support before, during, and after the procedure.
- Explain that an IV line may be inserted to allow infusion of fluids such as saline, anesthetics, contrast medium, or sedatives.
- Instruct the patient to remove jewelry and all other metallic objects from the area to be examined prior to the procedure.
- Note that there are no food, fluid, or medication restrictions unless by medical direction. Some protocols may require the patient to restrict prescribed oral iron supplements prior to the study because the iron may interfere with the study results; fasting for 1 to 2 hr before the procedure may also be required in order to avoid nausea and vomiting related to anxiety while in the MRI scanner.

M

INTRATEST:

Potential Complications:

Injection of the contrast is an invasive procedure. Complications are rare but do include risk for allergic reaction ***related to contrast reaction***; cardiac dysrhythmias; hematoma ***related to blood leakage into the tissue following needle insertion;*** bleeding from the puncture site ***related to a bleeding disorder or the effects of natural products and medications with known anticoagulant, antiplatelet, or thrombolytic properties;*** vascular or nerve injury ***that might occur if the needle strikes a nerve or nearby blood vessel;*** or infection ***that might occur if bacteria from the skin surface is introduced at the puncture site.***

Some patients are at risk for developing nephrogenic systemic fibrosis as a result of the use of gadolinium-based contrast medium ***related to ineffective renal clearance in patients with impaired kidney function.***

- Observe standard precautions, and follow the general guidelines in Patient Preparation and Specimen Collection online at Davis*Plus*. Positively identify the patient.
- Ensure that the patient has complied with dietary, fluid, and other pretesting preparations prior to the study, as instructed.
- Ensure that the patient has removed all external metallic objects from the area to be examined prior to the procedure.
- Administer ordered prophylactic steroids or antihistamines before the procedure if the patient has a history of allergic reactions to any substance or drug.
- Avoid the use of equipment containing latex if the patient has a history of allergic reaction to latex.
- Have emergency equipment readily available.
- Instruct the patient to void prior to the procedure and to change into the gown, robe, and foot coverings provided.

- Instruct the patient to cooperate fully and to follow directions. Instruct the patient to remain still throughout the procedure because movement produces unreliable results. Electrocardiogram or respiratory gating may be performed in conjunction with the scan to reduce artifacts during data collection due to respiratory or cardiac movement; apply MRI-safe electrodes at the appropriate sites.
- Supply earplugs to the patient to block out the loud, banging sounds that occur during the test. Instruct the patient to communicate with the technologist during the examination via a microphone within the scanner.
- Establish IV fluid line for the injection of fluids such as saline, anesthetics, contrast medium, or sedatives. Avoid the use of IV equipment that contains metal.
- Administer an antianxiety drug, as ordered, if the patient has claustrophobia. Administer a sedative to a child or to an adult who is uncooperative, as ordered.
- Assist the patient onto the examination table and into the appropriate position for imaging to begin.
- Imaging can begin shortly after the injection, if contrast is used.
- Ask the patient to inhale deeply and hold his or her breath while the images are taken and then to exhale after the images are taken.
- Instruct the patient to take slow, deep breaths if nausea occurs during the procedure.
- Monitor the patient for complications related to the procedure (e.g., allergic reaction, anaphylaxis, bronchospasm).
- Remove the needle or catheter and apply a pressure dressing over the puncture site.
- Observe/assess the needle/catheter insertion site for bleeding, inflammation, or hematoma formation.

POST-TEST:

- Inform the patient that a report of the results will be made available to the requesting HCP, who will discuss the results with the patient.
- Observe for delayed allergic reactions, such as rash, urticaria, tachycardia, hyperpnea, hypertension, palpitations, nausea, or vomiting.
- Instruct the patient to immediately report symptoms such as fast heart rate, difficulty breathing, skin rash, itching, chest pain, persistent right shoulder pain, or abdominal pain. Immediately report symptoms to the appropriate HCP.
- Instruct the patient in the care and assessment of the injection site.
- Instruct the patient to apply cold compresses to the puncture site as needed, to reduce discomfort or edema.
- Recognize anxiety related to test results. Discuss the implications of abnormal test results on the patient's lifestyle. Provide teaching and information regarding the clinical implications of the test results, as appropriate.
- Reinforce information given by the patient's HCP regarding further testing, treatment, or referral to another HCP. Answer any questions or address any concerns voiced by the patient or family.
- Depending on the results of this procedure, additional testing may be performed to evaluate or monitor progression of the disease process and determine the need for a change in therapy. Evaluate test results in relation to the patient's symptoms and other tests performed.

Patient Education:

- Teach the patient that the consumption of alcohol can exacerbate the pain due to pancreatic stimulation.
- Arrange dietary consultation to assist the patient in managing his or her nutritional status.

Expected Patient Outcomes:

Understanding

- The patient and family acknowledge the importance of progressing the diet slowly to evaluate food tolerance and make adjustments as needed.

M

- The patient and family acknowledge the importance of taking dietary supplements to support positive nutrition.

Ability

- The patient and family demonstrate the ability to select low-fat foods to include in the diet plan.
- The patient and family demonstrate the ability to accurately record intake and output.

Response

- The patient agrees to avoid drinking alcoholic and caffeinated beverages.
- The patient participates in a pain management plan that provides an acceptable level of relief.

RELATED STUDIES:

- Related tests include amylase, angiography of the abdomen, BUN, calcitonin, cholangiopancreatography endoscopic retrograde, CT abdomen, creatinine, hepatobiliary scan, 5-hydroxyindoleacetic acid, lipase, peritoneal fluid analysis, US liver and biliary system, and US pancreas.
- Refer to the Endocrine and Hepatobiliary systems tables online at Davis*Plus* for related tests by body system.

Magnetic Resonance Imaging, Pelvis

SYNONYM/ACRONYM: Pelvis MRI.

COMMON USE: To visualize and assess the pelvis and surrounding structure for tumor, masses, staging cancer, and inflammation and to evaluate the effectiveness of medical and surgical interventions.

AREA OF APPLICATION: Pelvic area.

M

DESCRIPTION: Magnetic resonance imaging (MRI) is useful when the area of interest is soft tissue. The study can be performed with or without intravenous (IV) contrast (gadolinium). The technology does not involve radiation exposure and is considered safer than other imaging methods such as radiographs and computed tomography (CT). MRI uses a magnet and radio waves to produce an energy field that can be displayed as an image of the anatomic area of interest based on the water content of the tissue. The magnetic field causes the hydrogen atoms in tissue to line up, and when radio waves are directed toward the magnetic field, the hydrogen atoms absorb the radio waves and change their position. This change in the energy field is detected by the equipment, and an image is generated by the equipment's computer system using assigned values that correspond to the strength of the signal produced; the anatomical images are represented in various shades of gray. MRI produces cross-sectional images of the pelvic area in multiple planes without the use of ionizing radiation or the interference of bone or surrounding tissue. Images can be obtained in two-dimensional (series of slices) or three-dimensional sequences. Standard or closed MRI equipment has the appearance of an open tube or tunnel; open MRI equipment has no sides and provides an alternative for people who suffer from claustrophobia, pediatric patients, or patients who are obese. Some open MRI units are designed to allow the patient to stand or sit while images are taken in various body positions. IV gadolinium-based contrast media may be used to better visualize the vessels and tissues in the area of interest. Clear, high-quality images of abnormalities and disease processes significantly improve the diagnostic value of the study.

Pelvic MRI is performed to assist in diagnosing abnormalities of the pelvis and associated structures. Contrast-enhanced MRI is effective for evaluating metastases from primary tumors. MRI is highly effective for depicting small-volume peritoneal tumors, carcinomatosis, and peritonitis and for determining the response to surgical and chemical therapies. MRI uses the noniodinated paramagnetic contrast medium gadopentetate dimeglumine (Magnevist), which is administered IV to enhance differences between normal and abnormal tissues. Oral and rectal contrast administration may be used to isolate the bowel from adjacent pelvic organs and improve organ visualization.

This procedure is contraindicated for

- Patients who are pregnant or suspected of being pregnant, unless the potential benefits of the MRI far outweigh the risks to the fetus and mother. ***In pregnancy, gadolinium-based contrast medium (GBCAs) cross the placental barrier, enter the fetal circulation, and pass via the kidneys into the amniotic fluid. Although no definite adverse effects of GBCA administration on the human fetus have been documented, the potential bioeffects of fetal GBCA exposure are not well understood. GBCA administration should therefore be avoided during pregnancy unless no suitable alternative imaging is possible and the benefits of contrast administration outweigh the potential risk to the fetus.***
- Conditions associated with adverse reactions to contrast medium (e.g., asthma, food allergies, or allergy to contrast medium).

  Although patients are asked specifically if they have a known allergy to iodine or shellfish (shellfish contain high levels of iodine), it has been well established that the reaction is not to iodine; an actual iodine allergy would be problematic because iodine is required for the production of thyroid hormones. In the case of shellfish, the reaction is to a muscle protein called tropomyosin; in the case of iodinated contrast medium, the reaction is to the noniodinated part of the contrast molecule. Patients with a known hypersensitivity to the medium may benefit from premedication with corticosteroids and diphenhydramine; the use of nonionic contrast or an alternative noncontrast imaging study, if available, may be considered for patients who have severe asthma or who have experienced moderate to severe reactions to ionic contrast medium.
- Patients with moderate to marked renal impairment (glomerular filtration rate less than 30 mL/min/1.73 m^2). Patients should be screened for kidney dysfunction prior to administration. The use of GBCAs should be avoided in these patients unless the benefits of the studies outweigh the risks and if essential diagnostic information is not available using non–contrast-enhanced diagnostic studies.
- Patients with cardiac pacemakers that can be deactivated by MRI.
- Patients with metal in their body, such as dental amalgams, metallic

M

body piercing items, tattoo inks containing iron (including tattooed eyeliners), shrapnel, bullet, ferrous metal in the eye, certain ferrous metal prosthetics, valves, aneurysm clips, intrauterine device, inner ear prostheses, or other metallic objects; these items can impair image quality. Metallic objects are also a significant safety issue for patients and health-care staff in the examination room during performance of an MRI. The MRI equipment consists of an extremely powerful magnet that can inactivate, move, or shift metallic objects inside a patient. Many metallic objects currently used in health-care procedures are made of materials that do not interfere with MRI studies; it is important for patients to provide specific information regarding medical procedures they have undergone in order to identify whether their device is safe to undergo MRI. Required information includes the date of the procedure and identification of the device. Metallic objects are not allowed inside the room with the MRI equipment because items such as watches, credit cards, and car keys can become dangerous projectiles.

Patients with transdermal patches containing metallic components. The patch's liner contains a metal that controls absorption of the substance from the patch (e.g., drugs, nicotine, steroids, hormones). The patch may cause burns to the skin ***related to energy conducted through the metal, which is converted to heat during the MRI.*** Other metallic objects on the skin may also cause burns.

Patients who are claustrophobic.

INDICATIONS

- Detect cancer (primary or metastatic tumors of ovary, prostate, uterus, and bladder) and provide cancer staging.
- Detect pelvic vascular diseases.
- Detect peritonitis.
- Detect soft tissue abnormalities.
- Determine blood clots, cysts, fluid or fat accumulation in tissues, hemorrhage, and infarctions.
- Differentiate tumors from tissue abnormalities, such as cysts, cavernous hemangiomas, and abscesses.
- Monitor and evaluate the effectiveness of medical or surgical interventions and course of the disease.

POTENTIAL MEDICAL DIAGNOSIS

Normal findings

- Normal pelvic structures and soft tissue density and biochemical constituents of pelvic tissues, including blood flow

Abnormal findings related to

- Adenomyosis
- Ascites
- Fibroids
- Masses, lesions, infections, or inflammations
- Peritoneal tumor or carcinomatosis
- Peritonitis
- Pseudomyxoma peritonei

CRITICAL FINDINGS: N/A

INTERFERING FACTORS

Factors that may alter the results of the study

- Metallic objects (e.g., jewelry, body rings, dental amalgams) within the examination field, which may inhibit organ visualization and cause unclear images.
- Inability of the patient to cooperate or remain still during the procedure because of age, significant pain, or mental status.
- Patients with extreme cases of claustrophobia, unless sedation is given before the study or an open MRI is utilized.
- Patients who are extremely obese may require more radiation to obtain a clear image.

Other considerations

- If contrast medium is allowed to seep deep into the muscle tissue, vascular visualization will be impossible.
- The procedure may be canceled if the patient's weight exceeds the safety limit for the equipment.

NURSING IMPLICATIONS AND PROCEDURE

See Potential Nursing Problems on Fast Find at davispl.us/vanleeuwen7.

PRETEST:

- Positively identify the patient using at least two person-specific identifiers before services, treatments, or procedures are performed.
- ***Patient Teaching:*** Inform the patient this procedure can assist in assessing the pelvis and surrounding structures.
- Obtain a history of the patient's health concerns (especially kidney dysfunction if the use of GBCA is anticipated), symptoms, surgical procedures, and results of previously performed laboratory and diagnostic studies. Include a list of known allergens, especially allergies or sensitivities to latex, anesthetics, sedatives, or contrast medium. Patients with a known hypersensitivity to contrast medium may benefit from premedication with corticosteroids and diphenhydramine.
- Ensure the results of blood urea nitrogen, creatinine, and estimated glomerular filtration rate are obtained if GBCA is to be used.
- Determine if the patient has ever had any device implanted into his or her body, including copper intrauterine devices, pacemakers, ear implants, and heart valves.
- Obtain occupational history to determine the presence of metal in the body, such as shrapnel or flecks of ferrous metal in the eye (which can cause retinal hemorrhage).
- Note any recent procedures that can interfere with test results, including examinations using barium- or iodine-based contrast medium.
- Record the date of the last menstrual period and determine the possibility of pregnancy in perimenopausal women.
- Obtain a list of the patient's current medications, including over-the-counter medications and dietary supplements (see Effects of Natural Products on Laboratory Values online at Davis*Plus*).
- Review the procedure with the patient. Address concerns about pain related to the procedure and explain that no pain will be experienced during the test, but there may be moments of discomfort. Reassure the patient that if contrast is used, it poses no radioactive hazard and rarely produces adverse effects. Inform the patient the procedure is performed in an MRI department by a health-care provider (HCP) specializing in this procedure, with support staff, and takes approximately 30 to 60 min.
- Inform the patient that the technologist will place him or her in a supine position on a flat table in a large cylindrical scanner.
- Tell the patient to expect to hear loud banging from the scanner and possibly to see magnetophosphenes (flickering lights in the visual field); these will stop when the procedure is over.
- ***Sensitivity to social and cultural issues,*** as well as concern for modesty, is important in providing psychological support before, during, and after the procedure.
- Explain that an IV line may be inserted to allow infusion of fluids such as saline, anesthetics, contrast medium, or sedatives.
- Instruct the patient to remove jewelry and all other metallic objects from the area to be examined prior to the procedure.
- Note that there are no food, fluid, or medication restrictions unless by medical direction. Some protocols may require the patient to restrict prescribed oral iron supplements

M

prior to the study because the iron may interfere with the study results; fasting for 1 to 2 hr before the procedure may also be required in order to avoid nausea and vomiting related to anxiety while in the MRI scanner.

INTRATEST:

Potential Complications:

Injection of the contrast is an invasive procedure. Complications are rare but do include risk for allergic reaction ***related to contrast reaction;*** cardiac dysrhythmias; hematoma ***related to blood leakage into the tissue following needle insertion;*** bleeding from the puncture site ***related to a bleeding disorder or the effects of natural products and medications with known anticoagulant, antiplatelet, or thrombolytic properties;*** vascular or nerve injury ***that might occur if the needle strikes a nerve or nearby blood vessel;*** or infection ***that might occur if bacteria from the skin surface is introduced at the puncture site.***

Some patients are at risk for developing nephrogenic systemic fibrosis as a result of the use of gadolinium-based contrast medium ***related to ineffective renal clearance in patients with impaired kidney function.***

- Observe standard precautions, and follow the general guidelines in Patient Preparation and Specimen Collection online at Davis*Plus*. Positively identify the patient.
- Ensure that the patient has complied with dietary, fluid, and other pretesting preparations prior to the study, as instructed.
- Ensure that the patient has removed all external metallic objects from the area to be examined prior to the procedure.
- Administer ordered prophylactic steroids or antihistamines before the procedure if the patient has a history of allergic reactions to any substance or drug.
- Avoid the use of equipment containing latex if the patient has a history of allergic reaction to latex.
- Have emergency equipment readily available.
- Instruct the patient to void prior to the procedure and to change into the gown, robe, and foot coverings provided.
- Instruct the patient to cooperate fully and to follow directions. Instruct the patient to remain still throughout the procedure because movement produces unreliable results. Electrocardiogram or respiratory gating may be performed in conjunction with the scan to reduce artifacts during data collection due to respiratory or cardiac movement; apply MRI-safe electrodes at the appropriate sites.
- Supply earplugs to the patient to block out the loud, banging sounds that occur during the test. Instruct the patient to communicate with the technologist during the examination via a microphone within the scanner.
- Establish IV fluid line for the injection of fluids such as saline, anesthetics, contrast medium, or sedatives. Avoid the use of IV equipment that contains metal.
- Administer an antianxiety drug, as ordered, if the patient has claustrophobia. Administer a sedative to a child or to an adult who is uncooperative, as ordered.
- Assist the patient onto the examination table and into the appropriate position for imaging to begin.
- Imaging can begin shortly after the injection, if contrast is used.
- Ask the patient to inhale deeply and hold his or her breath while the images are taken and then to exhale after the images are taken.
- Instruct the patient to take slow, deep breaths if nausea occurs during the procedure.
- Monitor the patient for complications related to the procedure (e.g., allergic reaction, anaphylaxis, bronchospasm).
- Remove the needle or catheter and apply a pressure dressing over the puncture site.
- Observe/assess the needle/catheter insertion site for bleeding, inflammation, or hematoma formation.

M

POST-TEST:

- Inform the patient that a report of the results will be made available to the requesting HCP, who will discuss the results with the patient.
- Observe for delayed allergic reactions, such as rash, urticaria, tachycardia, hyperpnea, hypertension, palpitations, nausea, or vomiting.
- Instruct the patient to immediately report symptoms such as fast heart rate, difficulty breathing, skin rash, itching, chest pain, persistent right shoulder pain, or abdominal pain. Immediately report symptoms to the appropriate HCP.
- Instruct the patient in the care and assessment of the injection site.
- Instruct the patient to apply cold compresses to the puncture site as needed, to reduce discomfort or edema.
- Recognize anxiety related to test results. Discuss the implications of abnormal test results on the patient's lifestyle. Provide teaching and information regarding the clinical implications of the test results, as appropriate.
- Reinforce information given by the patient's HCP regarding further testing, treatment, or referral to another HCP. Answer any questions or address any concerns voiced by the patient or family.
- Depending on the results of this procedure, additional testing may be performed to evaluate or monitor progression of the disease process and determine the need for a change in therapy. Evaluate test results in relation to the patient's symptoms and other tests performed.

Patient Education:

- Teach the pathophysiology of the disease process.
- Teach the patient the importance of calling for pain medication as soon as it is needed for effective pain management.

Expected Patient Outcomes:

Understanding

- The patient and family correctly describe treatment options related to disease process.
- The patient and family acknowledge the importance of family or group counseling related to end-of-life issues.

Ability

- The patient and family demonstrate the ability to maintain a quiet environment for emotional and physical rest.
- The patient and family demonstrate successful coping strategies.

Response

- The patient and family agree to family or individual support group counseling related to prognosis and end-of-life issues.
- The patient and family agree to all follow-up diagnostic and laboratory studies needed to monitor health status and the effectiveness of treatment modalities.

RELATED STUDIES:

- Related tests include BUN, CT pelvis, creatinine, cystourethrography voiding, IVP, KUB study, renogram, and US pelvis.
- Refer to the Genitourinary System table online at Davis*Plus* for related tests by body system.

Magnetic Resonance Imaging, Pituitary

SYNONYM/ACRONYM: Pituitary MRI, MRI of the parasellar region.

COMMON USE: To visualize and assess the pituitary and surrounding structures of the brain for lesions, hemorrhage, cysts, abscess, tumors, cancer, and infection.

AREA OF APPLICATION: Brain/pituitary area.

DESCRIPTION: Magnetic resonance imaging (MRI) is very useful when the area of interest is soft tissue. The study can be performed with or without intravenous (IV) contrast (gadolinium). The technology does not involve radiation exposure and is considered safer than other imaging methods such as radiographs and computed tomography (CT). MRI uses a magnet and radio waves to produce an energy field that can be displayed as an image of the anatomic area of interest based on the water content of the tissue. The magnetic field causes the hydrogen atoms in tissue to line up, and when radio waves are directed toward the magnetic field, the hydrogen atoms absorb the radio waves and change their position. This change in the energy field is detected by the equipment, and an image is generated by the equipment's computer system using assigned values that correspond to the strength of the signal produced; the anatomical images are represented in various shades of gray. MRI produces cross-sectional images of the vessels in multiple planes without the use of ionizing radiation or the interference of bone or surrounding tissue. Images can be obtained in two-dimensional (series of slices) or three-dimensional sequences. Standard or closed MRI equipment has the appearance of an open tube or tunnel; open MRI equipment has no sides and provides an alternative for people who suffer from claustrophobia, pediatric patients, or patients who are obese. Some open MRI units are designed to allow the patient to stand or sit while images are taken in various body positions. IV gadolinium-based contrast media may be used to better visualize the pituitary gland and parasellar region in the area of interest. Clear, high-quality images of abnormalities and disease processes significantly improve the diagnostic value of the study.

Pituitary MRI shows the relationship of pituitary lesions to the optic chiasm and cavernous sinuses. MRI has the capability of distinguishing the solid, cystic, and hemorrhagic components of lesions. Rapidly flowing blood on spin-echo MRI appears as an absence of signal or a void in the vessel's lumen. Blood flow can be evaluated in the cavernous and carotid arteries. Suprasellar aneurysms may be diagnosed without angiography, and old clotted blood in the walls of the aneurysms appears white. MRI uses the non-iodinated paramagnetic contrast medium gadopentetate dimeglumine (Magnevist) that is administered IV to enhance contrast differences between normal and abnormal tissues.

M

This procedure is contraindicated for

◆ Patients who are pregnant or suspected of being pregnant, unless the potential benefits of the MRI far outweigh the risks to the fetus and mother. ***In pregnancy, gadolinium-based contrast medium (GBCAs) cross the placental barrier, enter the fetal circulation, and pass via the kidneys into the amniotic fluid. Although no definite adverse effects of GBCA administration on the human fetus have been documented, the potential bioeffects of fetal GBCA exposure are not well understood. GBCA administration should therefore be avoided during pregnancy unless no suitable alternative imaging is possible and***

the benefits of contrast administration outweigh the potential risk to the fetus.

- Conditions associated with adverse reactions to contrast medium (e.g., asthma, food allergies, or allergy to contrast medium).

Although patients are asked specifically if they have a known allergy to iodine or shellfish (shellfish contain high levels of iodine), it has been well established that the reaction is not to iodine; an actual iodine allergy would be problematic because iodine is required for the production of thyroid hormones. In the case of shellfish, the reaction is to a muscle protein called tropomyosin; in the case of iodinated contrast medium, the reaction is to the noniodinated part of the contrast molecule. Patients with a known hypersensitivity to the medium may benefit from premedication with corticosteroids and diphenhydramine; the use of nonionic contrast or an alternative noncontrast imaging study, if available, may be considered for patients who have severe asthma or who have experienced moderate to severe reactions to ionic contrast medium.

- Patients with moderate to marked renal impairment (glomerular filtration rate less than 30 mL/min/1.73 m^2). Patients should be screened for kidney dysfunction prior to administration. The use of GBCAs should be avoided in these patients unless the benefits of the studies outweigh the risks and if essential diagnostic information is not available using noncontrast-enhanced diagnostic studies.
- Patients with cardiac pacemakers that can be deactivated by MRI.
- Patients with metal in their body, such as dental amalgams, metallic body piercing items, tattoo inks containing iron (including tattooed eyeliners), shrapnel, bullet, ferrous metal in the eye, certain ferrous metal prosthetics, valves, aneurysm clips, intrauterine device, inner ear prostheses, or other metallic objects; these items can impair image quality. Metallic objects are also a significant safety issue for patients and health-care staff in the examination room during performance of an MRI. The MRI equipment consists of an extremely powerful magnet that can inactivate, move, or shift metallic objects inside a patient. Many metallic objects currently used in health-care procedures are made of materials that do not interfere with MRI studies; it is important for patients to provide specific information regarding medical procedures they have undergone in order to identify whether their device is safe to undergo MRI. Required information includes the date of the procedure and identification of the device. Metallic objects are not allowed inside the room with the MRI equipment because items such as watches, credit cards, and car keys can become dangerous projectiles.
- Patients with transdermal patches containing metallic components. The patch's liner contains a metal that controls absorption of the substance from the patch (e.g., drugs, nicotine, steroids, hormones). The patch may cause burns to the skin ***related to energy conducted through the metal, which is converted to heat during the MRI.*** Other metallic objects on the skin may also cause burns.
- Patients who are claustrophobic.

INDICATIONS

- Detect microadenoma or macroadenoma of the pituitary.
- Detect parasellar abnormalities.
- Detect tumors of the pituitary.
- Evaluate potential cause of headache, visual loss, and vomiting.
- Evaluate the solid, cystic, and hemorrhagic components of lesions.
- Evaluate vascularity of the pituitary.

- Monitor and evaluate the effectiveness of medical or surgical interventions and course of disease.

POTENTIAL MEDICAL DIAGNOSIS

Normal findings

- Normal anatomic structures, density, and biochemical constituents of the pituitary, including blood flow

Abnormal findings related to

- Abscess
- Aneurysm
- Choristoma
- Craniopharyngioma or meningioma
- Empty sella
- Granuloma
- Infarct or hemorrhage
- Macroadenoma or microadenoma
- Metastasis
- Parasitic infection

CRITICAL FINDINGS: N/A

INTERFERING FACTORS

Factors that may alter the results of the study

- Metallic objects (e.g., jewelry, body rings, dental amalgams) within the examination field, which may inhibit organ visualization and cause unclear images.
- Inability of the patient to cooperate or remain still during the procedure because of age, significant pain, or mental status.
- Patients with extreme cases of claustrophobia, unless sedation is given before the study or an open MRI is utilized.
- Patients who are extremely obese may require more radiation to obtain a clear image.

Other considerations

- If contrast medium is allowed to seep deep into the muscle tissue, vascular visualization will be impossible.
- The procedure may be canceled if the patient's weight exceeds the safety limit for the equipment.

NURSING IMPLICATIONS AND PROCEDURE

See Potential Nursing Problems on Fast Find at davispl.us/vanleeuwen7.

PRETEST:

- Positively identify the patient using at least two person-specific identifiers before services, treatments, or procedures are performed.
- *Patient Teaching:* Inform the patient this procedure can assist in assessing the pituitary gland and surrounding brain tissue.
- Obtain a history of the patient's health concerns (especially kidney dysfunction if the use of GBCA is anticipated), symptoms, surgical procedures, and results of previously performed laboratory and diagnostic studies. Include a list of known allergens, especially allergies or sensitivities to latex, anesthetics, sedatives, or contrast medium. Patients with a known hypersensitivity to contrast medium may benefit from premedication with corticosteroids and diphenhydramine.
- Ensure the results of blood urea nitrogen, creatinine, and estimated glomerular filtration rate are obtained if GBCA is to be used.
- Determine if the patient has ever had any device implanted into his or her body, including copper intrauterine devices, pacemakers, ear implants, and heart valves.
- Obtain occupational history to determine the presence of metal in the body, such as shrapnel or flecks of ferrous metal in the eye (which can cause retinal hemorrhage).
- Note any recent procedures that can interfere with test results, including examinations using barium- or iodine-based contrast medium.
- Record the date of the last menstrual period and determine the possibility of pregnancy in perimenopausal women.

- Obtain a list of the patient's current medications, including over-the-counter medications and dietary supplements (see Effects of Natural Products on Laboratory Values online at Davis*Plus*).
- Review the procedure with the patient. Address concerns about pain related to the procedure and explain that no pain will be experienced during the test, but there may be moments of discomfort. Reassure the patient that if contrast is used, it poses no radioactive hazard and rarely produces adverse effects. Inform the patient the procedure is performed in an MRI department by a health-care provider (HCP) specializing in this procedure, with support staff, and takes approximately 30 to 60 min.
- Inform the patient that the technologist will place him or her in a supine position on a flat table in a large cylindrical scanner.
- Tell the patient to expect to hear loud banging from the scanner and possibly to see magnetophosphenes (flickering lights in the visual field); these will stop when the procedure is over.
- ***Sensitivity to social and cultural issues,*** as well as concern for modesty, is important in providing psychological support before, during, and after the procedure.
- Explain that an IV line may be inserted to allow infusion of fluids such as saline, anesthetics, contrast medium, or sedatives.
- Instruct the patient to remove jewelry and all other metallic objects from the area to be examined prior to the procedure.
- Note that there are no food, fluid, or medication restrictions unless by medical direction. Some protocols may require the patient to restrict prescribed oral iron supplements prior to the study because the iron may interfere with the study results; fasting for 1 to 2 hr before the procedure may also be required in order to avoid nausea and vomiting related to anxiety while in the MRI scanner.

INTRATEST:

Potential Complications:

Injection of the contrast is an invasive procedure. Complications are rare but do include risk for allergic reaction ***related to contrast reaction;*** cardiac dysrhythmias; hematoma ***related to blood leakage into the tissue following needle insertion;*** bleeding from the puncture site ***related to a bleeding disorder or the effects of natural products and medications with known anticoagulant, antiplatelet, or thrombolytic properties;*** vascular or nerve injury ***that might occur if the needle strikes a nerve or nearby blood vessel;*** or infection ***that might occur if bacteria from the skin surface is introduced at the puncture site.***

Some patients are at risk for developing nephrogenic systemic fibrosis as a result of the use of gadolinium-based contrast medium ***related to ineffective renal clearance in patients with impaired kidney function.***

- Observe standard precautions, and follow the general guidelines in Patient Preparation and Specimen Collection online at Davis*Plus*. Positively identify the patient.
- Ensure that the patient has complied with dietary, fluid, and other pretesting preparations prior to the study, as instructed.
- Ensure that the patient has removed all external metallic objects from the area to be examined prior to the procedure.
- Administer ordered prophylactic steroids or antihistamines before the procedure if the patient has a history of allergic reactions to any substance or drug.
- Avoid the use of equipment containing latex if the patient has a history of allergic reaction to latex.
- Have emergency equipment readily available.
- Instruct the patient to void prior to the procedure and to change into the gown, robe, and foot coverings provided.

M

- Instruct the patient to cooperate fully and to follow directions. Instruct the patient to remain still throughout the procedure because movement produces unreliable results. Electrocardiogram or respiratory gating may be performed in conjunction with the scan to reduce artifacts during data collection due to respiratory or cardiac movement; apply MRI-safe electrodes at the appropriate sites.
- Supply earplugs to the patient to block out the loud, banging sounds that occur during the test. Instruct the patient to communicate with the technologist during the examination via a microphone within the scanner.
- Establish IV fluid line for the injection of fluids such as saline, anesthetics, contrast medium, or sedatives. Avoid the use of IV equipment that contains metal.
- Administer an antianxiety drug, as ordered, if the patient has claustrophobia. Administer a sedative to a child or to an adult who is uncooperative, as ordered.
- Assist the patient onto the examination table and into the appropriate position for imaging to begin.
- Imaging can begin shortly after the injection, if contrast is used.
- Ask the patient to inhale deeply and hold his or her breath while the images are taken and then to exhale after the images are taken.
- Instruct the patient to take slow, deep breaths if nausea occurs during the procedure.
- Monitor the patient for complications related to the procedure (e.g., allergic reaction, anaphylaxis, bronchospasm).
- Remove the needle or catheter and apply a pressure dressing over the puncture site.
- Observe/assess the needle/catheter insertion site for bleeding, inflammation, or hematoma formation.

POST-TEST:

- Inform the patient that a report of the results will be made available to the requesting HCP, who will discuss the results with the patient.
- Observe for delayed allergic reactions, such as rash, urticaria, tachycardia, hyperpnea, hypertension, palpitations, nausea, or vomiting.
- Instruct the patient to immediately report symptoms such as fast heart rate, difficulty breathing, skin rash, itching, chest pain, persistent right shoulder pain, or abdominal pain. Immediately report symptoms to the appropriate HCP.
- Instruct the patient in the care and assessment of the injection site.
- Instruct the patient to apply cold compresses to the puncture site as needed to reduce discomfort or edema.
- Recognize anxiety related to test results. Discuss the implications of abnormal test results on the patient's lifestyle. Provide teaching and information regarding the clinical implications of the test results, as appropriate.
- Reinforce information given by the patient's HCP regarding further testing, treatment, or referral to another HCP. Answer any questions or address any concerns voiced by the patient or family.
- Depending on the results of this procedure, additional testing may be performed to evaluate or monitor progression of the disease process and determine the need for a change in therapy. Evaluate test results in relation to the patient's symptoms and other tests performed.

Patient Education:

- Teach the pathophysiology of the disease process.
- Provide information on possible diagnostic and laboratory studies associated with disease management.

Expected Patient Outcomes:

Understanding

- The patient and family correctly describe treatment options related to disease process.
- The patient and family acknowledge the importance of family or group

counseling related to end-of-life issues.

Ability

- The patient demonstrates effective coping mechanisms to decrease anxiety.
- The patient and family create a quiet environment that will assist in their learning.

Response

- The patient agrees to discuss concerns with identified support (family, friends, group, spiritual advisor).
- The patient agrees to seek psychological counseling to adjust to body changes and intimacy concerns.

RELATED STUDIES:

- Related tests include ACTH and challenge tests, angiography brain, BUN, cortisol and challenge tests, CT brain, creatinine, EEG, MRI brain, and PET brain.
- Refer to the Endocrine system table online at Davis*Plus* for related tests by body system.

Magnetic Resonance Venography

SYNONYM/ACRONYM: MRV.

COMMON USE: To visualize and assess blood flow in diseased and normal veins toward diagnosis of vascular disease and to monitor and evaluate therapeutic interventions.

AREA OF APPLICATION: Vascular.

DESCRIPTION: Magnetic resonance imaging (MRI) is very useful when the area of interest is soft tissue. The study can be performed with or without intravenous (IV) contrast (gadolinium). The technology does not involve radiation exposure and is considered safer than other imaging methods such as radiographs and computed tomography (CT). MRI uses a magnet and radio waves to produce an energy field that can be displayed as an image of the anatomic area of interest based on the water content of the tissue. The magnetic field causes the hydrogen atoms in tissue to line up, and when radio waves are directed toward the magnetic field, the hydrogen atoms absorb the radio waves and change their position. This change in the energy field is detected by the equipment, and an image is generated by the equipment's computer system using assigned values that correspond to the strength of the signal produced; the anatomical images are represented in various shades of gray. MRI produces cross-sectional images of the vessels in multiple planes without the use of ionizing radiation or the interference of bone or surrounding tissue. Images can be obtained in two-dimensional (series of slices) or three-dimensional sequences. Standard or closed MRI equipment has the appearance of an open tube or tunnel; open MRI equipment has no sides and provides an alternative for people who suffer from claustrophobia, pediatric patients, or patients who are obese. Some open MRI units are designed to allow the patient to stand or sit while images are taken in various body positions. IV gadolinium-based contrast media may be used to better visualize the vessels and tissues in the area of interest. Clear, high-quality images of abnormalities and disease processes significantly improve the diagnostic value of the study.

Magnetic resonance venography (MRV) is an accurate, noninvasive technique used to detect deep vein thrombosis. This application of MRI provides images of blood flow in diseased and normal veins. In patients who are allergic to iodinated contrast medium, MRV is used in place of venography or CT venography. MRV is particularly useful for visualizing vascular abnormalities, thrombosis, and other pathology. MRV can be accomplished with a contrast-enhanced (CE) or non–contrast-enhanced method. Special imaging sequences allow the visualization of moving blood within the venous system. Two common techniques to obtain images of flowing blood are time-of-flight (TOF) and steady-state free precession (SSFP). In TOF imaging, incoming blood makes the vessels appear bright, and surrounding tissue is suppressed. SSFP is generally used for assessment of veins in the chest, abdomen, and pelvis. Although the initial evaluation of the iliac and lower extremity veins is usually accomplished with sonography, MRV is more efficient in detecting venous thrombus in the pelvic and calf veins, especially in obese patients and those with chronic asymptomatic thrombus.

This procedure is contraindicated for

- Patients who are pregnant or suspected of being pregnant, unless the potential benefits of MRI far outweigh the risks to the fetus and mother. ***In pregnancy, gadolinium-based contrast medium (GBCAs) cross the placental barrier, enter the fetal circulation, and pass via the kidneys into the amniotic fluid. Although no definite adverse effects of GBCA administration on the human fetus have been documented, the potential bioeffects of fetal GBCA exposure are not well understood. GBCA administration should therefore be avoided during pregnancy unless no suitable alternative imaging is possible and the benefits of contrast administration outweigh the potential risk to the fetus.***
- Conditions associated with adverse reactions to contrast medium (e.g., asthma, food allergies, or allergy to contrast medium).

Although patients are asked specifically if they have a known allergy to iodine or shellfish (shellfish contain high levels of iodine), it has been well established that the reaction is not to iodine; an actual iodine allergy would be problematic because iodine is required for the production of thyroid hormones. In the case of shellfish, the reaction is to a muscle protein called tropomyosin; in the case of iodinated contrast medium, the reaction is to the noniodinated part of the contrast molecule. Patients with a known hypersensitivity to the medium may benefit from premedication with corticosteroids and diphenhydramine; the use of nonionic contrast or an alternative noncontrast imaging study, if available, may be considered for patients who have severe asthma or who have experienced moderate to severe reactions to ionic contrast medium.

◈ Patients with moderate to marked renal impairment (glomerular filtration rate less than 30 mL/min/1.73 m^2). Patients should be screened for kidney dysfunction prior to administration. The use of GBCAs should be avoided in these patients unless the benefits of the studies outweigh the risks and if essential diagnostic information is not available using non-contrast-enhanced diagnostic studies.

◈ Patients with cardiac pacemakers that can be deactivated by MRI.

◈ Patients with metal in their body, such as dental amalgams, metallic body piercing items, tattoo inks containing iron (including tattooed eyeliners), shrapnel, bullet, ferrous metal in the eye, certain ferrous metal prosthetics, valves, aneurysm clips, intrauterine device, inner ear prostheses, or other metallic objects; these items can impair image quality. Metallic objects are also a significant safety issue for patients and health-care staff in the examination room during performance of an MRI. The MRI equipment consists of an extremely powerful magnet that can inactivate, move, or shift metallic objects inside a patient. Many metallic objects currently used in health-care procedures are made of materials that do not interfere with MRI studies; it is important for patients to provide specific information regarding medical procedures they have undergone in order to identify whether their device is safe to undergo MRI. Required information includes the date of the procedure and identification of the device. Metallic objects are not allowed inside the room with the MRI equipment because items such as watches, credit cards, and car keys, can become dangerous projectiles.

◈ Patients with transdermal patches containing metallic components. The patch's liner contains a metal that controls absorption of the substance from the patch (e.g., drugs, nicotine, steroids, hormones). The patch may cause burns to the skin ***related to energy conducted through the metal, which is converted to heat during the MRI.*** Other metallic objects on the skin may also cause burns.

◈ Patients who are claustrophobic.

INDICATIONS

- Detect peripheral vascular disease (PVD).
- Detect axillary subclavian deep vein thrombosis.
- Detect cerebral vein disease.
- Detect pulmonary vein disease.
- Evaluate iliac and lower-extremity vein disease.
- Evaluate postoperative venous sites and bypass grafts.
- Identify deep vein thrombus in postsurgical patients.
- Monitor and evaluate the effectiveness of medical or surgical treatment.

POTENTIAL MEDICAL DIAGNOSIS

Normal findings

- Normal blood flow in the area being examined

Abnormal findings related to

- Cerebral vein thrombosis
- Deep vein thrombosis (DVT)
- Pulmonary emboli
- PVD
- Tumor invasion of a vein
- Vascular abnormalities
- Vein occlusion
- Vein stenosis

CRITICAL FINDINGS:

- Cerebral emboli
- Occlusion
- Pulmonary emboli
- Tumor with significant mass effect

Note and immediately report to the requesting health-care provider (HCP) any critical findings and related symptoms. A listing of these findings varies

M

among facilities. Timely notification of a critical finding for laboratory or diagnostic studies is a role expectation of the professional nurse. The notification processes vary among facilities. Upon receipt of the critical finding, the information should be read back to the caller to verify accuracy.

INTERFERING FACTORS

Factors that may alter the results of the study

- Metallic objects (e.g., jewelry, body rings, dental amalgams) within the examination field, which may inhibit organ visualization and cause unclear images.
- Inability of the patient to cooperate or remain still during the procedure because of age, significant pain, or mental status.
- Patients with extreme cases of claustrophobia, unless sedation is given before the study.
- Patients who are extremely obese may require more radiation to obtain a clear image.

Other considerations

- If contrast medium is allowed to seep deep into the muscle tissue, vascular visualization will be impossible.
- The procedure may be canceled if the patient's weight exceeds the safety limit for the equipment.

NURSING IMPLICATIONS AND PROCEDURE

See Potential Nursing Problems on Fast Find at davispl.us/vanleeuwen7.

PRETEST:

- Positively identify the patient using at least two person-specific identifiers before services, treatments, or procedures are performed.
- ***Patient Teaching:*** Inform the patient this procedure can assist in assessing the vascular system.
- Obtain a history of the patient's health concerns (especially kidney dysfunction if the use of GBCA is anticipated), symptoms, surgical procedures, and results of previously performed laboratory and diagnostic studies. Include a list of known allergens, especially allergies or sensitivities to latex, anesthetics, sedatives, or contrast medium. Patients with a known hypersensitivity to contrast medium may benefit from premedication with corticosteroids and diphenhydramine.
- Ensure the results of blood urea nitrogen, creatinine, and estimated glomerular filtration rate are obtained if GBCA is to be used.
- Determine if the patient has ever had any device implanted into his or her body, including copper intrauterine devices, pacemakers, ear implants, and heart valves.
- Obtain occupational history to determine the presence of metal in the body, such as shrapnel or flecks of ferrous metal in the eye (which can cause retinal hemorrhage).
- Note any recent procedures that can interfere with test results.
- Record the date of the last menstrual period and determine the possibility of pregnancy in perimenopausal women.
- Obtain a list of the patient's current medications, including over-the-counter medications and dietary supplements (see Effects of Natural Products on Laboratory Values online at Davis*Plus*).
- Review the procedure with the patient. Address concerns about pain related to the procedure and explain that no pain will be experienced during the test, but there may be moments of discomfort. Reassure the patient that if contrast is used, it poses no radioactive hazard and rarely produces adverse effects. Inform the patient the procedure is performed in an MRI department by an HCP who specializes in this procedure, with support staff, and takes approximately 30 to 60 min.

- Inform the patient that the technologist will place him or her in a supine position on a flat table in a large cylindrical scanner.
- Tell the patient to expect to hear loud banging from the scanner and possibly to see magnetophosphenes (flickering lights in the visual field); these will stop when the procedure is over.
- Explain that an IV line may be inserted to allow infusion of fluids such as saline, anesthetics, contrast medium, or sedatives.
- ***Sensitivity to social and cultural issues,*** as well as concern for modesty, is important in providing psychological support before, during, and after the procedure.
- Instruct the patient to remove external metallic objects from the area to be examined prior to the procedure.
- Note that there are no food, fluid, or medication restrictions unless by medical direction. Some protocols may require the patient to restrict prescribed oral iron supplements prior to the study because the iron may interfere with the study results. Restriction of food, fluids, alcohol, nicotine, and caffeine for 1 to 2 hr before the procedure may also be required in order to avoid vasoconstriction or vasodilation as well as nausea and vomiting related to anxiety while in the MRI scanner.

INTRATEST:

Potential Complications:

Injection of the contrast is an invasive procedure. Complications are rare but do include risk for allergic reaction ***related to contrast reaction;*** cardiac dysrhythmias; hematoma ***related to blood leakage into the tissue following needle insertion;*** bleeding from the puncture site ***related to a bleeding disorder or the effects of natural products and medications known to act as anticoagulants;*** vascular or nerve injury ***that might occur if the needle strikes a nerve or nearby blood vessel;*** or infection ***that might occur if bacteria from the skin surface is introduced at the puncture site.***

Some patients are at risk for developing nephrogenic systemic fibrosis as a result of the use of gadolinium-based contrast medium ***related to ineffective renal clearance in patients with impaired kidney function.***

- Observe standard precautions, and follow the general guidelines in Patient Preparation and Specimen Collection online at Davis*Plus*. Positively identify the patient.
- Ensure that the patient has complied with dietary, fluid, and other pretesting preparations prior to the study, as instructed.
- Ensure that the patient has removed external metallic objects from the area to be examined prior to the procedure.
- Administer ordered prophylactic steroids or antihistamines before the procedure if the patient has a history of allergic reactions to any substance or drug.
- Avoid the use of equipment containing latex if the patient has a history of allergic reaction to latex.
- Have emergency equipment readily available.
- Instruct the patient to void prior to the procedure and to change into the gown, robe, and foot coverings provided.
- Instruct the patient to cooperate fully and to follow directions. Instruct the patient to remain still throughout the procedure because movement produces unreliable results. Electrocardiogram or respiratory gating may be performed in conjunction with the scan to reduce artifacts during data collection due to respiratory or cardiac movement; apply MRI-safe electrodes at the appropriate sites.
- Supply earplugs to the patient to block out the loud, banging sounds that occur during the test. Instruct the patient to communicate with the technologist during the examination via a microphone within the scanner.

M

- Apply MRI-safe electrodes to the appropriate sites if an electrocardiogram or respiratory gating is to be performed in conjunction with the scan.
- Establish IV fluid line for the injection of fluids such as saline, anesthetics, contrast medium, or sedatives. Avoid the use of IV equipment that contains metal.
- Administer an antianxiety drug, as ordered, if the patient has claustrophobia. Administer a sedative to a child or to an adult who is uncooperative, as ordered.
- Assist the patient onto the examination table and into the appropriate position for imaging to begin.
- Imaging can begin shortly after the injection, if contrast is used.
- Ask the patient to inhale deeply and hold his or her breath while the images are taken, and then to exhale after the images are taken.
- Instruct the patient to take slow, deep breaths if nausea occurs during the procedure.
- Monitor the patient for complications related to the procedure (e.g., allergic reaction, anaphylaxis, bronchospasm).
- Remove the needle or catheter and apply a pressure dressing over the puncture site.
- Observe/assess the needle/catheter insertion site for bleeding, inflammation, or hematoma formation.

M

POST-TEST:

- Inform the patient that a report of the results will be made available to the requesting HCP, who will discuss the results with the patient.
- Observe for delayed allergic reactions, such as rash, urticaria, tachycardia, hyperpnea, hypertension, palpitations, nausea, or vomiting.
- Instruct the patient to immediately report symptoms such as fast heart rate, difficulty breathing, skin rash, itching, chest pain, persistent right shoulder pain, or abdominal pain. Immediately report symptoms to the appropriate HCP.
- Instruct the patient in the care and assessment of the injection site.
- Instruct the patient to apply cold compresses to the puncture site as needed to reduce discomfort or edema.
- Recognize anxiety related to test results. Discuss the implications of abnormal test results on the patient's lifestyle. Provide teaching and information regarding the clinical implications of the test results, as appropriate. Provide contact information, if desired, for the American Heart Association (www.americanheart.org), National Heart, Lung, and Blood Institute (www.nhlbi.nih.gov), and the Legs for Life (www.legsforlife.org). ♣
- Reinforce information given by the patient's HCP regarding further testing, treatment, or referral to another HCP. Answer any questions or address any concerns voiced by the patient or family.
- Depending on the results of this procedure, additional testing may be performed to evaluate or monitor progression of the disease process and determine the need for a change in therapy. Evaluate test results in relation to the patient's symptoms and other tests performed.

Patient Education:

- Teach the patient bleeding precautions when taking anticoagulants.
- Teach the patient to report bleeding to the HCP for evaluation.

Expected Patient Outcomes:

Understanding

- The patient and family state the purpose of taking anticoagulants is to prevent continued vascular occlusion.
- The patient and family state the purpose of follow-up laboratory studies is to monitor the effectiveness of prescribed medications at a safe level.

Ability

- The patient demonstrates the ability to self-medicate competently.

- The patient and family describe lifestyle changes that will be necessary to decrease bleeding risk and prevent further clot formation.

Response

- The patient agrees to lifestyle changes that will decrease bleeding risk.
- The patient agrees to attend appointments with HCP for examination and medication adjustments.

RELATED STUDIES:

- Related tests include angiography of the body area of interest, BUN, CT angiography, creatinine, D-dimer, US arterial Doppler carotid, US venous Doppler extremity studies, and venography lower extremity studies.
- Refer to the Cardiovascular System table online at Davis*Plus* for related tests by body system.

Mammography

SYNONYM/ACRONYM: Breast x-ray, mammogram.

COMMON USE: To visualize and assess breast tissue and surrounding lymph nodes for cancer, inflammation, abscess, tumor, and cysts.

AREA OF APPLICATION: Breast.

DESCRIPTION: Mammography, an x-ray examination of the breast, is most commonly used to detect breast cancer; however, it can also be used to detect and evaluate symptomatic changes associated with other breast diseases, including mastitis, abscess, cystic changes, cysts, benign tumors, masses, and lymph nodes. In addition, mammography can be used to locate a nonpalpable lesion for breast biopsy studies. While mammography cannot detect breast cancer with 100% accuracy, only about 10% to 15% of breast cancer cases are not detected. Recent advances in mammography technologies include full-field digital mammography (FFDM), computer-aided detection (CAD) systems, and three-dimensional (3-D) breast imaging or breast tomosynthesis. FFDM is performed in the same manner as conventional screen film mammography (SFM). The difference is that FFDM images are created by digitized signals rather than from x-ray film as with SFM. The FFDM detectors convert x-rays into electrical signals that are digitalized. The digital images can be visualized on a computer screen or printed on special paper. CAD systems use software to search images from SFM or FFDM for abnormal areas of breast tissue evidenced by denseness, abnormal size, or calcifications that may indicate the presence of cancer. Abnormal areas are "marked" for further review by a radiologist. 3-D breast imaging is performed in the same manner as conventional 2-D SFM. However, 3-D imaging uses equipment that rotates in an arc over the breast instead of the stationary system used in conventional SFM. The 3-D equipment generates a series of thin slices believed to produce

M

clearer images, especially of dense breast tissue. The new technologies are becoming more frequently used in screening mammography programs across the United States. Preliminary studies have demonstrated some improvement in detection rates, especially for some types of invasive cancer, and a reduction in recalls for additional imaging.

When a mass is detected, additional studies are performed to help differentiate the nature of the mass, as follows:

- Magnification views of the area in question
- Focal or "spot" views of the area in question, done with a specialized paddle-style compression device
- Ultrasound images of the area in question, which help differentiate between a fluid-filled cystic lesion and a solid lesion indicative of cancer or fibroadenomas

---

This procedure is contraindicated for

Patients who are pregnant or suspected of being pregnant, unless the potential benefits of a procedure using radiation far outweigh the risks to the fetus and mother.

Patients younger than age 25 or patients with very dense breast tissue ***because the density of the breast tissue is such that diagnostic x-rays are of limited value.***

INDICATIONS

- Differentiate between benign and neoplastic breast disease.
- Evaluate breast pain, skin retraction, nipple erosion, or nipple discharge.
- Evaluate known or suspected breast cancer.
- Evaluate nonpalpable breast masses.
- Evaluate opposite breast after mastectomy.
- Monitor postoperative and post-radiation treatment status of the breast.
- Evaluate size, shape, and position of breast masses.

POTENTIAL MEDICAL DIAGNOSIS

Normal findings

- Normal breast tissue, with no cysts, tumors, or calcifications

Abnormal findings related to

- Breast calcifications
- Breast cysts or abscesses
- Breast tumors
- Hematoma resulting from trauma
- Mastitis
- Soft tissue masses
- Vascular calcification

CRITICAL FINDINGS: N/A

INTERFERING FACTORS

Factors that may alter the results of the study

- Inability of the patient to cooperate or remain still during the procedure because of age, significant pain, or mental status.
- Metallic objects (e.g., jewelry, body rings) within the examination field, which may inhibit organ visualization and cause unclear images.
- Application of substances such as talcum powder, deodorant, or creams to the skin of breasts or underarms, which may alter test results.
- Previous breast surgery, breast augmentation, or the presence of breast implants, which may decrease the readability of the examination.

Other considerations

NURSING IMPLICATIONS AND PROCEDURE

See Potential Nursing Problems on Fast Find at davispl.us/vanleeuwen7.

PRETEST:

- Positively identify the patient using at least two person-specific identifiers before services, treatments, or procedures are performed.
- ***Patient Teaching:*** Inform the patient this procedure can assist in assessing breast status.
- Obtain a history of the patient's health concerns (especially known or suspected breast disease, and family history of breast disease), symptoms, surgical procedures, and results of previously performed laboratory and diagnostic studies. Knowledge of genetics assists the nurse in identifying patients and family members who may benefit from additional education, risk assessment, and counseling. Genetics is the study and identification of genes, genetic mutations, and inheritance. For example, genetics provides some insight into the likelihood of inheriting a trait such as blue eyes or a medical condition such as breast cancer. Genomic studies evaluate the interaction of groups of genes. The combined activity or combined expression of groups of genes allows assumptions or predictions to be made. As an example, genomic studies measure the levels of activity in multiple genes to predict how they, along with environmental and lifestyle decisions, influence the development of breast cancer, type 2 diabetes, coronary artery disease, myocardial infarction, or ischemic stroke. Further information regarding inheritance of genes can be found in the study titled "Genetic Testing." Include a list of known allergens, especially allergies or sensitivities to latex.
- Record the date of the last menstrual period and determine the possibility of pregnancy in perimenopausal women.
- Obtain a list of the patient's current medications, including over-the-counter medications and dietary supplements (see Effects of Natural Products on Laboratory Values online at Davis*Plus*).
- Review the procedure with the patient. Address concerns about pain related to the procedure. Inform the patient there may be discomfort associated with the study while the breast is being compressed, but the compression allows for better visualization of the breast tissue. Explain to the patient that the radiation dose will be kept to an absolute minimum. Inform the patient that the procedure is performed in the mammography department by a registered mammographer and takes approximately 15 to 30 min to complete.
- Inform the patient that the best time to schedule the examination is 1 wk after menses, when breast tenderness is decreased.
- ***Sensitivity to social and cultural issues,*** as well as concern for modesty, is important in providing psychological support before, during, and after the procedure.
- Inform the patient not to apply deodorant, body creams, or powders on the day of the procedure.
- Instruct the patient to remove jewelry and other metallic objects from the area of examination.
- Note that there are no food, fluid, or medication restrictions unless by medical direction.

INTRATEST:

Potential Complications: N/A

- Observe standard precautions, and follow the general guidelines in Patient Preparation and Specimen Collection online at Davis*Plus*. Positively identify the patient.
- Ensure that the patient has removed all jewelry and other metallic objects from the chest area.
- Avoid the use of equipment containing latex if the patient has a history of allergic reaction to latex.

M

- Instruct the patient to void prior to the procedure and to change into the gown and robe provided.
- Instruct the patient to cooperate fully and to follow directions. Instruct the patient to remain still throughout the procedure because movement produces unreliable results.
- Assist the patient to a standing or sitting position in front of the x-ray machine, which is adjusted to the level of the breasts. Position the patient's arms out of the range of the area to be imaged.
- Place breasts, one at a time, between the compression apparatus. Two images or exposures are taken of each breast. Ask the patient to hold her breath during each exposure. Additional images may be taken as requested by the radiologist before the patient leaves the mammography room.

POST-TEST:

- Inform the patient that a report of the results will be made available to the requesting health-care provider (HCP), who will discuss the results with the patient.
- Determine if the patient has any further questions or concerns.
- Recognize anxiety related to test results, and be supportive of fear of shortened life expectancy. Discuss the implications of abnormal test results on the patient's lifestyle. Provide teaching and information regarding the clinical implications of the test results, as appropriate. Educate the patient regarding access to counseling services. Provide contact information, if desired, for the American Cancer Society (www.cancer.org).
- Reinforce information given by the patient's HCP regarding further testing, treatment, or referral to another HCP. Decisions regarding the need for and frequency of breast self-examination, mammography, MRI breast, or other cancer screening procedures should be made after consultation between the patient and HCP. The most current guidelines for breast cancer screening of the general population as well as of individuals with increased risk are available from the American Cancer Society (ACS) (www.cancer.org), American College of Obstetricians and Gynecologists (ACOG) (www.acog.org), and American College of Radiology (www.acr.org). The ACS recommends breast examinations be performed every 3 yr for women between the ages of 20 and 39 yr and annually for women over 40 yr of age; annual mammograms should be performed on women 40 yr and older as long as they are in good health. The ACS also recommends annual MRI testing, in addition to an annual mammogram, for women at high risk of developing breast cancer. 🍁 Genetic testing for inherited mutations (BRCA1 and BRCA2) associated with increased risk of developing breast cancer may be ordered for women at risk. The test is performed on a blood specimen.
- Depending on the results of this procedure, additional testing may be performed to evaluate or monitor progression of the disease process and determine the need for a change in therapy. Evaluate test results in relation to the patient's symptoms and other tests performed.

Patient Education:

- Provide information on disease signs and symptoms and management.
- Provide information on possible diagnostic and laboratory studies associated with disease management.

Expected Patient Outcomes:

Understanding

- The patient and family state information provided related to medical and surgical options.
- The patient and family acknowledge the information provided related to prognosis associated with disease process.

Ability

- The patient demonstrates positive coping strategies.

- The patient successfully demonstrates care of surgical site.

Response

- The patient agrees to attend cancer support group meetings.
- The patient agrees to seek psychological counseling to adjust to body changes and intimacy concerns.

RELATED STUDIES:

- Related tests include biopsy breast, cancer antigens, ductography, genetic testing, MRI breast, stereotactic biopsy breast, and US breast.
- Refer to the Reproductive System table online at Davis*Plus* for related tests by body system.

Meckel's Diverticulum Scan

SYNONYM/ACRONYM: Ectopic gastric mucosa scan, Meckel's scan, Meckel's scintigraphy.

COMMON USE: To assess, evaluate, and diagnose the cause of abdominal pain and gastrointestinal bleeding.

AREA OF APPLICATION: Abdomen.

DESCRIPTION: Meckel's diverticulum scan is a nuclear medicine study performed to assist in diagnosing the cause of abdominal pain or occult gastrointestinal (GI) bleeding and to assess the presence and size of a congenital anomaly of the GI tract (especially in pediatric or young adult patients). After intravenous (IV) injection of technetium-99m pertechnetate, immediate and delayed imaging is performed, with various views of the abdomen obtained. The radionuclide is taken up and concentrated by parietal cells of the gastric mucosa, whether located in the stomach or in a Meckel's diverticulum. Up to 25% of Meckel's diverticulum is lined internally with ectopic gastric mucosal tissue. This tissue is usually located in the ileum and right lower quadrant of the abdomen; it secretes acid that causes ulceration of intestinal tissue, which results in abdominal pain and occult blood in stools.

This procedure is contraindicated for

Patients who are pregnant or suspected of being pregnant, unless the potential benefits of a procedure using radiation far outweigh the risk of radiation exposure to the fetus and mother.

INDICATIONS

- Aid in the diagnosis of unexplained abdominal pain and GI bleeding caused by hydrochloric acid and pepsin secreted by ectopic gastric mucosa, which ulcerates nearby mucosa.
- Detect sites of ectopic gastric mucosa.

POTENTIAL MEDICAL DIAGNOSIS

Normal findings

- Normal distribution of radionuclide by gastric mucosa at normal sites

Abnormal findings related to

- Meckel's diverticulum, as evidenced by focally increased radioactive uptake in areas other than normal structures

CRITICAL FINDINGS: N/A

INTERFERING FACTORS

Factors that may alter the results of the study

- Inability of the patient to cooperate or remain still during the procedure because of age, significant pain, or mental status.
- Metallic objects (e.g., jewelry, body rings) within the examination field, which may inhibit organ visualization and cause unclear images.
- Retained barium from a previous radiological procedure.
- Other nuclear scans done within the preceding 24 hr.

Other considerations

- Improper injection of the radio nuclide may allow the tracer to seep deep into the muscle tissue, producing erroneous hot spots.
- False-positive results may occur from nondiverticular bleeding, intussusception, duplication cysts, inflammatory bowel disease, hemangioma of the bowel, and other organ infections.
- Inadequate amount of gastric mucosa within Meckel's diverticulum can affect the ability to visualize abnormalities.
- Inaccurate timing for imaging after the radionuclide injection can affect the results.
- Failure to follow dietary restrictions before the procedure may cause the procedure to be canceled or repeated.

M

NURSING IMPLICATIONS AND PROCEDURE

PRETEST:

- Positively identify the patient using at least two person-specific identifiers before services, treatments, or procedures are performed.
- Inform the patient this procedure can assist in assessing GI bleeding.
- Obtain a history of the patient's health concerns, symptoms, surgical procedures, and results of previously performed laboratory and diagnostic studies. Include a list of known allergens, especially allergies or sensitivities to latex.
- Note any recent procedures that can interfere with test results.
- Record the date of the last menstrual period and determine the possibility of pregnancy in perimenopausal women.
- Obtain a list of the patient's current medications, including over-the-counter medications, dietary supplements, anticoagulants, aspirin and other salicylates (see Effects of Natural Products on Laboratory Values online at Davis*Plus*). Such products should be discontinued by medical direction for the appropriate number of days prior to a surgical procedure. Note the last time and dose of medication taken.
- Review the procedure with the patient. Address concerns about pain and explain that some pain may be experienced during the test, but there may be moments of discomfort. Reassure the patient that the radionuclide poses no radioactive hazard and rarely produces adverse effects. Inform the patient that the procedure is performed in a nuclear medicine department by a health-care provider (HCP)specializing in this procedure, with support staff, and takes approximately 60 min. **Pediatric Considerations:** Preparing children for a Meckel's diverticulum scan depends on the age of the child. Encourage parents to be truthful about what the child may experience during the procedure (e.g., they may feel a pinch or minor discomfort when the IV needle is inserted) and to use words that they know their child will understand. Toddlers and preschool-age children have a very short attention span, so the best time to talk about the test is right before the procedure. The child

should be assured that he or she will be allowed to bring a favorite comfort item into the examination room, and if appropriate, that a parent will be with the child during the procedure. Explain the importance of remaining still while the images are taken.

- ***Sensitivity to social and cultural issues,*** as well as concern for modesty, is important in providing psychological support before, during, and after the procedure.
- Explain that an IV line may be inserted to allow infusion of fluids such as saline, anesthetics, sedatives, radionuclides, medications used in the procedure, or emergency medications.
- Instruct the patient to remove jewelry and other metallic objects from the area to be examined.
- Instruct the patient to take a histamine blocker, as ordered, 2 days before the study to block GI secretion.
- *Make sure a written and informed consent has been signed prior to the procedure and before administering any medications.*
- Instruct the patient to fast and refrain from fluids for 8 hr prior to the procedure. Protocols may vary among facilities.

INTRATEST:

Potential Complications:

Although it is rare, there is the possibility of allergic reaction to the radionuclide. Have emergency equipment and medications readily available. If the patient has a history of allergic reactions to any substance or drug, administer ordered prophylactic steroids or antihistamines before the procedure.

Establishing an IV site and injecting radionuclides is an invasive procedure. Complications are rare but do include bleeding from the puncture site ***related to a bleeding disorder or the effects of natural products and medications with known anticoagulant, antiplatelet, or thrombolytic properties;*** hematoma ***related to blood leakage into the tissue following needle insertion;*** infection ***that might occur if bacteria from the skin surface is introduced at the puncture site;*** or nerve injury ***that might occur if the needle strikes a nerve.***

- Observe standard precautions, and follow the general guidelines in Patient Preparation and Specimen Collection online at Davis*Plus.* Positively identify the patient.
- Ensure that the patient has complied with dietary, fluid, and medication restrictions prior to the study, as instructed.
- Ensure that the patient has removed all external metallic objects from the area to be examined prior to the procedure.
- Avoid the use of equipment containing latex if the patient has a history of allergic reaction to latex.
- Have emergency equipment readily available.
- Instruct the patient to void prior to the procedure and to change into the gown, robe, and foot coverings provided.
- Record baseline vital signs and assess neurological status. Protocols may vary among facilities.
- Establish an IV fluid line for the injection of saline, anesthetics, sedatives, radionuclides, or emergency medications.
- Instruct the patient to cooperate fully and to follow directions. Instruct the patient to remain still throughout the procedure because movement produces unreliable results.
- Place the patient in a supine position on a flat table with foam wedges, which help maintain position and immobilization.
- IV radionuclide is administered, and the abdomen is scanned immediately to screen for vascular lesions. Images are taken in various positions every 5 min for the next hour.
- Monitor the patient for complications related to the procedure (e.g., allergic reaction, anaphylaxis, bronchospasm).

M

- Remove the needle or catheter and apply a pressure dressing over the puncture site.
- Observe/assess the needle/catheter insertion site for bleeding, inflammation, or hematoma formation.

POST-TEST:

- Inform the patient that a report of the results will be made available to the requesting HCP, who will discuss the results with the patient.
- Unless contraindicated, advise the patient to drink increased amounts of fluids for 24 to 48 hr to eliminate the radionuclide from the body. Inform the patient that radionuclide is eliminated from the body within 6 to 24 hr.
- No other radionuclide tests should be scheduled for 24 to 48 hr after this procedure.
- Instruct the patient to resume usual diet, fluids, and medications, as directed by the HCP.
- Monitor vital signs and neurological status every 15 min for 1 hr, then every 2 hr for 4 hr, and then as ordered by the HCP. Take temperature every 4 hr for 24 hr. Monitor intake and output at least every 8 hr. Compare with baseline values. Notify the HCP if temperature is elevated. Protocols may vary among facilities.
- Observe for delayed allergic reactions, such as rash, urticaria, tachycardia, hyperpnea, hypertension, palpitations, nausea, or vomiting.
- Instruct the patient to immediately report symptoms such as fast heart rate, difficulty breathing, skin rash, itching, chest pain, persistent right shoulder pain, or abdominal pain. Immediately report symptoms to the appropriate HCP.
- Instruct the patient in the care and assessment of the injection site.
- If a woman who is breastfeeding must have a nuclear scan, she should not breastfeed the infant until the radionuclide has been eliminated. This could take as long as 3 days. She should be instructed to express the milk and discard it during the 3-day period to prevent cessation of milk production.
- Instruct the patient to immediately flush the toilet and to meticulously wash hands with soap and water after each voiding for 24 hr after the procedure.
- Instruct all caregivers to wear gloves when discarding urine for 24 hr after the procedure. Wash gloved hands with soap and water before removing gloves; then wash ungloved hands.
- ***Nutritional Considerations:*** A low-fat, low-cholesterol, and low-sodium diet should be consumed to reduce current disease processes. High fat consumption increases the amount of bile acids in the colon and should be avoided.
- Recognize anxiety related to test results, and be supportive of perceived loss of independent function. Discuss the implications of abnormal test results on the patient's lifestyle. Provide teaching and information regarding the clinical implications of the test results, as appropriate.
- Reinforce information given by the patient's HCP regarding further testing, treatment, or referral to another HCP. Answer any questions or address any concerns voiced by the patient or family.
- Depending on the results of this procedure, additional testing may be needed to evaluate or monitor progression of the disease process and determine the need for a change in therapy. Evaluate test results in relation to the patient's symptoms and other tests performed.

RELATED STUDIES:

- Related tests include barium swallow, colonoscopy, CT abdomen, CT pelvis, esophageal manometry, EGD, fecal analysis, gastric acid stimulation, gastric emptying scan, gastrin stimulation, GI blood loss, MRI abdomen, MRI pelvis, and upper GI series.
- Refer to the Gastrointestinal System table online at Davis*Plus* for related tests by body system.

M

Mediastinoscopy

SYNONYM/ACRONYM: N/A

COMMON USE: To visualize and assess structures under the mediastinum to assist in obtaining biopsies for diagnosing and staging cancer and to evaluate the effectiveness of therapeutic interventions.

AREA OF APPLICATION: Mediastinum.

DESCRIPTION: Mediastinoscopy provides direct visualization of the structures that lie beneath the mediastinum, which is the area behind the sternum and between the lungs. The test is performed under general anesthesia by means of a mediastinoscope inserted through a surgical incision at the suprasternal notch. Structures that can be viewed include the trachea, the esophagus, the heart and its major vessels, the thymus gland, and the lymph nodes that receive drainage from the lungs. The procedure is performed primarily to visualize and obtain biopsy specimens of the mediastinal lymph nodes and to determine the extent of metastasis into the mediastinum for the determination of treatment planning in cancer patients.

This procedure is contraindicated for

Patients who are pregnant or suspected of being pregnant, unless the potential benefits of a procedure using radiation far outweigh the risk of radiation exposure to the fetus and mother.

Patients who have had a previous mediastinoscopy ***because scarring can make insertion of the scope and biopsy of lymph nodes difficult.***

Patients who have superior vena cava obstruction ***because this condition causes increased venous collateral circulation in the mediastinum.***

INDICATIONS

- Confirm radiological evidence of a thoracic infectious process of an indeterminate nature, coccidioidomycosis, or histoplasmosis.
- Confirm radiological or cytological evidence of carcinoma or sarcoidosis.
- Detect Hodgkin's disease.
- Detect metastasis into the anterior mediastinum or extrapleurally into the chest.
- Determine stage of known bronchogenic carcinoma, as indicated by the extent of mediastinal lymph node involvement.
- Evaluate a patient with signs and symptoms of obstruction of mediastinal lymph flow and a history of head or neck cancer to determine recurrence or spread.

POTENTIAL MEDICAL DIAGNOSIS

Normal findings

- Normal appearance of mediastinal structures
- No abnormal lymph node tissue

Abnormal findings related to

- Bronchogenic carcinoma
- Coccidioidomycosis
- Granulomatous infections
- Histoplasmosis

- Hodgkin's disease
- *Pneumocystis jiroveci*
- Sarcoidosis
- Tuberculosis

CRITICAL FINDINGS: N/A

INTERFERING FACTORS

Other considerations

- Failure to follow dietary restrictions before the procedure may cause the procedure to be canceled or repeated.

NURSING IMPLICATIONS AND PROCEDURE

PRETEST:

- Positively identify the patient using at least two person-specific identifiers before services, treatments, or procedures are performed.
- *Patient Teaching:* Inform the patient this procedure can assist in assessing structure in the middle of the chest.
- Obtain a history of the patient's health concerns, symptoms, surgical procedures, and results of previously performed laboratory and diagnostic studies. Include a list of known allergens, especially allergies or sensitivities to latex, anesthetics or sedatives.
- Ensure that the results of blood typing and crossmatching are obtained and recorded before the procedure in the event that an emergency thoracotomy is required.
- Note any recent procedures that can interfere with test results. Ensure that this procedure is performed before an upper gastrointestinal study or barium swallow.
- Record the date of the last menstrual period and determine the possibility of pregnancy in perimenopausal women.
- Obtain a list of the patient's current medications, including over-the-counter medications and dietary supplements (see Effects of Natural Products on Laboratory Values online at Davis*Plus*).
- Review the procedure with the patient. Inform the patient that prophylactic antibiotics may be administered prior to the procedure. Address concerns about pain related to the procedure and explain that a general anesthesia will be administered to promote relaxation and reduce discomfort prior to the mediastinoscopy. Explain that some pain may be experienced after the test. Inform the patient that the procedure is performed in the operating room by a health-care provider (HCP) specializing in this procedure, with support staff, and usually takes 30 to 60 min to complete.
- *Sensitivity to social and cultural issues,* as well as concern for modesty, is important in providing psychological support before, during, and after the procedure.
- Explain that an intravenous (IV) line may be inserted to allow infusion of fluids such as saline, anesthetics, sedatives, or emergency medications.
- Instruct the patient to remove jewelry and external metallic objects from the area to be examined prior to the procedure.
- Instruct the patient that to reduce the risk of aspiration related to nausea and vomiting, solid food and milk or milk products have been restricted for at least 8 hr, and clear liquids have been restricted for at least 2 hr prior to general anesthesia, regional anesthesia, or sedation/analgesia (monitored anesthesia). The American Society of Anesthesiologists has fasting guidelines for risk levels according to patient status. More information can be located at www.asahq.org. 🍁 Patients on beta blockers before the surgical procedure should be instructed to take their medication as ordered during the perioperative period. Protocols may vary among facilities. Instruct the patient to avoid taking anticoagulant medication or to reduce dosage as ordered prior to the procedure. Number of days to withhold

medication is dependent on the type of anticoagulant.
- *Make sure a written and informed consent has been signed prior to the procedure and before administering any medications.*

INTRATEST:

Potential Complications:

Complications of the procedure may include bleeding and cardiac arrhythmias.
- Observe standard precautions, and follow the general guidelines in Patient Preparation and Specimen Collection online at Davis*Plus*. Positively identify the patient.
- Ensure that the patient has complied with food, fluids, and medication restrictions prior to the procedure, as instructed.
- Ensure that the patient has removed jewelry and external metallic objects from the area to be examined prior to the procedure.
- Avoid the use of equipment containing latex if the patient has a history of allergic reaction to latex.
- Have emergency equipment readily available.
- Instruct the patient to void prior to the procedure and change into the gown, robe, and foot coverings provided.
- Record baseline vital signs and assess neurological status. Protocols may vary among facilities.
- Establish an IV fluid line for the injection of saline, sedatives, or emergency medications.
- Place electrocardiographic electrodes on the patient for cardiac monitoring. Establish baseline rhythm; determine if the patient has ventricular dysrhythmias.
- Avoid using morphine sulfate in patients with asthma or other pulmonary disease. This drug can further exacerbate bronchospasms and respiratory impairment.
- Place the patient in the supine position. General anesthesia is administered via an endotracheal tube.
- An incision is made at the suprasternal notch, and a path for the mediastinoscope is made using finger dissection. The lymph nodes can be palpated at this time. The lymph nodes on the right side of the mediastinum are most accessible and safest to biopsy by mediastinoscopy; the lymph nodes on the left side are more difficult to explore and biopsy because of their proximity to the aorta. Biopsy specimens of nodes on the left side of the mediastinum may need to be obtained by mediastinotomy, which involves performing a left anterior thoracotomy.
- Place tissue samples in properly labelled specimen containers, and promptly transport the specimen to the laboratory for processing and analysis.
- The scope is removed, and the incision is closed.
- Observe/assess the incision site for bleeding, inflammation, or hematoma formation.
- If the patient is stable and if no further surgery is immediately indicated, the patient is extubated.

POST-TEST:

- Inform the patient that a report of the results will be made available to the requesting HCP, who will discuss the results with the patient.
- Do not allow the patient to eat or drink for 12 to 24 hr.
- Instruct the patient to resume normal activity, medication, and diet in 24 hr or as tolerated after the examination, unless otherwise indicated.
- The patient should remain in a semi-Fowler's position on either side until vital signs revert to preprocedure levels.
- Monitor vital signs and neurological status every 15 min for 1 hr, then every 2 hr for 4 hr, and then as ordered by the HCP. Take temperature every 4 hr for 24 hr. Monitor intake and output, at least every 8 hr. Compare with baseline values. Notify the HCP if temperature changes. Protocols may vary among facilities.
- Observe for delayed allergic reactions, such as rash, urticaria, tachycardia, hyperpnea, hypertension, palpitations, nausea, or vomiting.

M

- Instruct the patient to immediately report symptoms such as fast heart rate, difficulty breathing, skin rash, itching, chest pain, persistent right shoulder pain, or abdominal pain. Immediately report symptoms to the appropriate HCP.
- Instruct the patient in the care and assessment of the site.
- Emphasize that any excessive bleeding; difficulty breathing; excessive coughing after biopsy; fever; or redness, swelling, or pain of the incisional area must be reported to the HCP immediately.
- Recognize anxiety related to test results, and be supportive of perceived loss of independent function. Discuss the implications of abnormal test results on the patient's lifestyle. Provide teaching and information regarding the clinical implications of the test results, as appropriate.
- Reinforce information given by the patient's HCP regarding further testing, treatment, or referral to another HCP. Answer any questions or address any concerns voiced by the patient or family.
- Depending on the results of this procedure, additional testing may be needed to evaluate or monitor progression of the disease process and determine the need for a change in therapy. Evaluate test results in relation to the patient's symptoms and other tests performed.

RELATED STUDIES:

- Related tests include ACE, β_2-microglobulin, biopsy liver, biopsy lung, biopsy lymph node, blood gases, bronchoscopy, carbon dioxide, chest x-ray, CBC, CBC WBC count and differential, CT thoracic, culture and smear mycobacteria, gallium scan, Gram stain, laparoscopy abdominal, LAP, liver and spleen scan, lung perfusion scan, lung ventilation scan, lymphangiogram, MRI chest, platelet count, pleural fluid analysis, PFT, and TB skin tests.
- Refer to the Immune and Respiratory system tables online at Davis*Plus* for related tests by body system.

Metanephrines

M

SYNONYM/ACRONYM: N/A

COMMON USE: To assist in the diagnosis of cancer of the adrenal medulla or to assess for the cause of hypertension.

SPECIMEN: Urine from a timed specimen collected in a clean amber plastic collection container with 6N hydrochloride as a preservative.

NORMAL FINDINGS: (Method: High-pressure liquid chromatography)

Age	Conventional Units	SI Units
Normetanephrines		*(Conventional Units × 5.07)*
3 mo–4 yr	54–249 mcg/24 hr	274–1,262 micromol/day
5–9 yr	31–398 mcg/24 hr	157–2,018 micromol/day
10–17 yr	67–531 mcg/24 hr	340–2,692 micromol/day
18–39 yr	35–482 mcg/24 hr	177–2,444 micromol/day
Greater than 40 yr	88–676 mcg/24 hr	446–3,427 micromol/day

Age	Conventional Units	SI Units
Metanephrines, Total		*(Conventional Units × 5.07)*
3 mo–4 yr	79–345 mcg/24 hr	401–1,749 micromol/day
5–9 yr	49–409 mcg/24 hr	248–2,074 micromol/day
10–17 yr	107–741 mcg/24 hr	543–3,757 micromol/day
18–39 yr	94–695 mcg/24 hr	477–3,524 micromol/day
40–49 yr	182–739 mcg/24 hr	923–3,747 micromol/day
Greater than 50 yr	224–832 mcg/24 hr	1,136–4,218 micromol/day

DESCRIPTION: Metanephrines are the inactive metabolites of epinephrine and norepinephrine. Metanephrines are either excreted or further metabolized into vanillylmandelic acid. Release of metanephrines in the urine is indicative of disorders associated with excessive catecholamine production, particularly pheochromocytoma. Vanillylmandelic acid and catecholamines are normally measured with urinary metanephrines. Creatinine is usually measured simultaneously to ensure adequate collection and to calculate an excretion ratio of metabolite to creatinine.

This procedure is contraindicated for: N/A

INDICATIONS

- Assist in the diagnosis of suspected pheochromocytoma.
- Assist in identifying the cause of hypertension.
- Verify suspected tumors associated with excessive catecholamine secretion.

POTENTIAL MEDICAL DIAGNOSIS

Increased in:

- Ganglioneuroma
- Neuroblastoma
- Pheochromocytoma
- Severe stress

Decreased in: N/A

CRITICAL FINDINGS: N/A

INTERFERING FACTORS

- Drugs and other substances that may increase metanephrine levels include monoamine oxidase inhibitors and prochlorperazine.
- Methylglucamine in x-ray contrast medium may cause false-negative results.
- All urine voided for the timed collection period must be included in the collection or else falsely decreased values may be obtained. Compare output records with volume collected to verify that all voids were included in the collection.

NURSING IMPLICATIONS AND PROCEDURE

PRETEST:

- Positively identify the patient using at least two person-specific identifiers before services, treatments, or procedures are performed.
- *Patient Teaching:* Inform the patient this test can assist in diagnosing adrenal gland health and hypertension.
- Obtain a history of the patient's health concerns, symptoms, surgical procedures, and results of previously performed laboratory and diagnostic studies. Include a list of known allergens, especially allergies or sensitivities to latex.

- Note any recent procedures that can interfere with test results.
- Obtain a list of the patient's current medications, including over-the-counter medications and dietary supplements (see Effects of Natural Products on Laboratory Values online at Davis*Plus*).
- Review the procedure with the patient. Provide a nonmetallic urinal, bedpan, or toilet-mounted collection device. Address concerns about pain and explain that there should be no discomfort during the procedure.
- Usually a 24-hr time frame for urine collection is ordered. Inform the patient that all urine must be saved during that 24-hr period. Instruct the patient not to void directly into the laboratory collection container. Instruct the patient to avoid defecating in the collection device and to keep toilet tissue out of the collection device to prevent contamination of the specimen. Place a sign in the bathroom to remind the patient to save all urine.
- Instruct the patient to void all urine into the collection device and then to pour the urine into the laboratory collection container. Alternatively, the specimen can be left in the collection device for a health-care staff member to add to the laboratory collection container.
- At the conclusion of the test, compare the quantity of urine with the urinary output record for the collection; if the specimen contains less than what was recorded as output, some urine may have been discarded, thus invalidating the test.
- ***Sensitivity to social and cultural issues,*** as well as concern for modesty, is important in providing psychological support before, during, and after the procedure.
- Instruct the patient to avoid excessive exercise and stress during the 24-hr collection of urine.
- Note that there are no food, fluid, or medication restrictions unless by medical direction.

M

INTRATEST:

Potential Complications: N/A

- Ensure that the patient has complied with activity restrictions during the procedure, as instructed.
- Avoid the use of equipment containing latex if the patient has a history of allergic reaction to latex.
- Instruct the patient to cooperate fully and to follow directions.
- Observe standard precautions, and follow the general guidelines in Patient Preparation and Specimen Collection online at Davis*Plus*. Positively identify the patient, and label the appropriate specimen container with the corresponding patient demographics, initials of the person collecting the specimen, date, and time of collection.

Timed Specimen

- Obtain a clean 3-L urine specimen container, toilet-mounted collection device, and plastic bag (for transport of the specimen container). The specimen must be refrigerated or kept on ice throughout the entire collection period. If an indwelling urinary catheter is in place, the drainage bag must be kept on ice.
- Begin the test between 0600 and 0800 if possible. Collect first voiding and discard. Record the time the specimen was discarded as the beginning of the timed collection period. The next morning, ask the patient to void at the same time the collection was started and add this last voiding to the container. Urinary output should be recorded throughout the collection time.
- If an indwelling catheter is in place, replace the tubing and container system at the start of the collection time. Keep the container system on ice during the collection period, or empty the urine into a larger container periodically during the collection period; monitor to ensure continued drainage, and conclude the test the next morning at the same hour the collection was begun.

- At the conclusion of the test, compare the quantity of urine with the urinary output record for the collection; if the specimen contains less than what was recorded as output, some urine may have been discarded, invalidating the test.
- Include on the collection container's label the amount of urine and test start and stop times.
- Promptly transport the specimen to the laboratory for processing and analysis.

POST-TEST:

- Inform the patient that a report of the results will be made available to the requesting health-care provider (HCP), who will discuss the results with the patient.
- Instruct the patient to resume usual activity, as directed by the HCP.
- Recognize anxiety related to test results, and be supportive of fear of shortened life expectancy. Discuss the implications of abnormal test results on the patient's lifestyle. Provide teaching and information regarding the clinical implications of the test results, as appropriate. Educate the patient regarding access to counseling services.
- Reinforce information given by the patient's HCP regarding further testing, treatment, or referral to another HCP. Answer any questions or address any concerns voiced by the patient or family.
- Depending on the results of this procedure, additional testing may be performed to evaluate or monitor progression of the disease process and determine the need for a change in therapy. Evaluate test results in relation to the patient's symptoms and other tests performed.

RELATED STUDIES:

- Related tests include angiography adrenal, cancer antigens, catecholamines, CT kidneys, HVA, renin, and VMA.
- Refer to the Endocrine System table online at Davis*Plus* for related tests by body system.

Methemoglobin

M

SYNONYM/ACRONYM: Hemoglobin, hemoglobin M, MetHb, Hgb M.

COMMON USE: To assess for cyanosis and hypoxemia associated with polycythemia, pathologies affecting hemoglobin, and potential inhaled drug toxicity.

SPECIMEN: Whole blood collected in green-top (heparin) tube. Specimen should be transported tightly capped and in an ice slurry.

NORMAL FINDINGS: (Method: Spectrophotometry)

Conventional Units	SI Units (Conventional Units × 155)
0.06–0.24 g/dL	9.3–37.2 micromol/L

Percentage of total hemoglobin = 0.41–1.15%.
Note: The conversion factor of ×155 is based on the molecular weight of hemoglobin of 64,500 daltons (d), or 64.5 kd.

POTENTIAL MEDICAL DIAGNOSIS

Increased in:

- Acquired methemoglobinemia (drugs, tobacco smoking, or ionizing radiation)
- Carbon monoxide poisoning ***(carbon monoxide is a form of deoxygenated hemoglobin)***
- Hereditary methemoglobinemia ***(evidenced by a deficiency of NADH-methemoglobin reductase or related to the presence of a hemoglobinopathy)***

Decreased in: N/A

CRITICAL FINDINGS:

Cyanosis can occur at levels greater than 10%.

Dizziness, fatigue, headache, and tachycardia can occur at levels greater than 30%.

Signs of central nervous system depression can occur at levels greater than 45%.

Death may occur at levels greater than 70%.

Note and immediately report to the requesting health-care provider (HCP) any critical findings and related symptoms. A listing of these findings varies among facilities. Timely notification of a critical finding for laboratory or diagnostic studies is a role expectation of the professional nurse. The notification processes vary among facilities. Upon receipt of the critical finding, the information should be read back to the caller to verify accuracy.

Possible interventions include airway protection, administration of oxygen, monitoring neurological status every hour, continuous pulse oximetry, hyperbaric oxygen therapy, and exchange transfusion. Administration of activated charcoal or gastric lavage may be effective if performed soon after the toxic material is ingested. Emesis should never be induced in patients with no gag reflex because of the risk of aspiration. Methylene blue may be used to reverse the process of methemoglobin formation, but it should be used cautiously when methemoglobin levels are greater than 30%. Use of methylene blue is contraindicated in the presence of glucose-6-phosphate dehydrogenase deficiency.

M

Find and print out the full study on Fast Find at davispl.us/vanleeuwen7.

Microalbumin

SYNONYM/ACRONYM: Albumin, urine.

COMMON USE: To assist in the identification and management of early diabetes in order to avoid or delay onset of diabetic associated kidney disease.

SPECIMEN: Urine from a random or timed specimen collected in a clean plastic collection container.

NORMAL FINDINGS: (Method: Immunoassay)

Test	Conventional Units	SI Units (Conventional Units × .001)
24-hr microalbumin to creatinine ratio	Less than 30 mg/g creatinine/24 hr	Less than 0.03 mg/g creatinine/24 hr
24-hr microalbumin		
Normal	Less than 30 mg/24 hr	Less than 0.03 mg/24 hr
Microalbuminuria	30–299 mg/24 hr	0.03–0.3 mg/24 hr
Clinical albuminuria	300 mg or greater/24 hr	0.3 mg or greater/24 hr

Simultaneous measurement of urine creatinine (Cr) or Cr clearance is usually requested. The American Diabetes Association (ADA) recommends annual measurement of serum Cr and estimated glomerular filtration rate (eGFR) regardless of microalbumin levels; numerous factors such as hydration status, the presence of an infection, or significant hyperglycemia can produce falsely increased or decreased microalbumin levels. Therefore, the ADA recommends classification of microalbuminuria after two of three 24-hr samples collected in a 3- to 6-mo period reflect abnormal results. The National Kidney Foundation defines microalbuminuria as equal to or greater than 30 mg/g Cr/24 hr based on eGFR measurements.

DESCRIPTION: The term *microalbumin* describes concentrations of albumin in urine that are greater than normal but undetectable by dipstick or traditional spectrophotometry methods. Microalbuminuria precedes the nephropathy associated with diabetes and is often elevated years before Cr clearance shows abnormal values. Studies have shown that the median duration from onset of microalbuminuria to development of nephropathy is 5 to 7 yr.

This procedure is contraindicated for: N/A

INDICATIONS

- Evaluate kidney disease.
- Screen patients with diabetes for early signs of nephropathy.

POTENTIAL MEDICAL DIAGNOSIS

Increased in:

Conditions resulting in increased renal excretion or loss of protein.

- Cardiomyopathy
- Diabetic nephropathy
- Exercise
- Hypertension (uncontrolled)
- Kidney disease
- Pre-eclampsia
- Urinary tract infections

Decreased in: N/A

CRITICAL FINDINGS: N/A

INTERFERING FACTORS

- Drugs and other substances that may decrease microalbumin levels include captopril, dipyridamole, enalapril, furosemide, indapamide, perindopril, quinapril, ramipril, tolrestat, and simvastatin.
- All urine voided for the timed collection period must be included in the collection, or else falsely decreased values may be obtained. Compare output records with volume collected to verify that all voids were included in the collection.

NURSING IMPLICATIONS AND PROCEDURE

POTENTIAL NURSING PROBLEMS:

Problem	Signs & Symptoms	Interventions
Blood glucose ***(related to sedentary lifestyle, circulating insulin deficiency secondary to pancreatic insufficiency; excessive dietary intake; insulin resistance; pregnancy)***	**Excess:** Fatigue; mild dehydration; elevated blood glucose; weight loss; weakness; polyuria; polydipsia; polyphagia; blurred vision; headache; paresthesia; poor skin turgor; dry mouth; nausea; vomiting; abdominal pain; Kussmaul respirations **Deficit:** Tremor; diaphoresis; decreased concentration; elevated blood pressure; palpitations; headache; polyphagia; restlessness; lethargy; altered mental status; combativeness; altered speech; altered coordination	Check blood glucose before meals and at bedtime; administer prescribed insulin or oral drugs; educate and encourage the patient to participate in glucose self-check and record results; assess readiness to learn and barriers to learning; collaborate with the health-care provider (HCP) and dietitian to support medical nutritional therapy; work with dietitian to assist the patient to select appropriate cultural foods; develop a plan of exercise commensurate with the patient's physical abilities; discuss lifestyle alterations necessary to support positive health management secondary to disease process; teach good hygiene and infection prevention; monitor laboratory studies that may be impacted by altered glucose and trend results (hemoglobin [Hgb] A_{1C}; blood urea nitrogen [BUN]; Cr; electrolytes; arterial pH; magnesium; urine ketones; urine microalbumin; white blood cell count; amylase; Hgb/hematocrit; C-reactive protein; liver enzymes); facilitate oral hydration; correlate blood glucose with other laboratory values and medical condition(s); address the psychosocial aspects of the disease; monitor serum insulin levels

M

Problem	Signs & Symptoms	Interventions
Nutrition ***(related to excessive dietary intake more than body requirements; insulin deficiency, stress; anxiety; depression; cultural lifestyle; unhealthy food sources; financial restrictions)***	Increased thirst, increased urination, weight loss; fatigue; elevated blood glucose levels; inadequate glucose management; increased hunger	Monitor blood glucose results; refer to dietitian for evaluation; administer insulin or oral antihyperglycemic drugs; assess the cultural aspects of diet selection; correlate dietary intake with blood glucose, and monitor trends; collaborate with a dietitian to develop a cultural- and age-appropriate diet plan; correlate nutritional intake and exercise; ensure that the patient understands the relationship between caloric intake and medication (insulin, oral antihyperglycemic drug); provide social services, dietary referrals if necessary
Renal impairment ***(related to elevated blood glucose levels over time; decreased renal perfusion; prolonged hypotension; heart disease with altered cardiac output)***	Altered fluid, electrolyte, and acid base balance; decreasing urinary output; elevated blood glucose	Review and trend diagnostic tests (BUN, Cr, urine osmolality, Cr clearance, microalbumin, blood glucose); teach accurate self-administration of medication to control blood pressure and blood glucose; teach accurate monitoring of blood glucose; ensure compliance with recommended dietary and exercise regimes; monitor and trend eGFR
Health management ***(related to complexity of health-care system; complexity of therapeutic management; altered metabolic process resulting in increased***	Health choices are ineffective in making a difference on outcomes; increasing symptoms of illness; verbalizes that therapeutic regime is too difficult; patient and family do not support HCP's	Assess effort to follow recommended regime; assess family and cultural factors that impact the success of the therapeutic regime; assess the patient's self-assessment of his or her health status; include the patient and family in designing the plan of care; tailor the plan of care to the patient's lifestyle;

(table continues on page 1158)

M

Problem	Signs & Symptoms	Interventions
or decreased potassium; knowledge deficit; conflicted decision making; cultural family health patterns; barriers to healthy decisions; mistrust of HCP)	suggestions for health improvement; refusal to follow recommended therapeutic regime	collaborate with the patient and family to develop a system of managing own health; focus on behaviors that will make the biggest positive impact on improved health

PRETEST:

- Positively identify the patient using at least two person-specific identifiers before services, treatments, or procedures are performed.
- *Patient Teaching:* Inform the patient this test can assist in evaluating for early kidney disease.
- Obtain a history of the patient's health concerns, symptoms, surgical procedures, and results of previously performed laboratory and diagnostic studies. Include a list of known allergens, especially allergies or sensitivities to latex.
- Obtain a list of the patient's current medications, including over-the-counter medications and dietary supplements (see Effects of Natural Products on Laboratory Values online at Davis*Plus*).
- Review the procedure with the patient. Provide a nonmetallic urinal, bedpan, or toilet-mounted collection device. Address concerns about pain and explain that there should be no discomfort during the procedure.
- Usually a 24-hr time frame for urine collection is ordered. Inform the patient that all urine must be saved during that 24-hr period. Instruct the patient not to void directly into the laboratory collection container. Instruct the patient to avoid defecating in the collection device and to keep toilet tissue out of the collection device to prevent contamination of the specimen. Place a sign in the bathroom to remind the patient to save all urine.
- Instruct the patient to void all urine into the collection device and then to pour the urine into the laboratory collection container. Alternatively, the specimen can be left in the collection device for a health-care staff member to add to the laboratory collection container.
- ***Sensitivity to social and cultural issues,*** as well as concern for modesty, is important in providing psychological support before, during, and after the procedure.
- Instruct the patient to avoid excessive exercise and stress during the 24-hr collection of urine.
- Note that there are no food, fluid, or medication restrictions unless by medical direction.

INTRATEST:

Potential Complications: N/A

- Ensure that the patient has complied with activity restrictions during the procedure.
- Avoid the use of equipment containing latex if the patient has a history of allergic reaction to latex.
- Instruct the patient to cooperate fully and to follow directions.
- Observe standard precautions, and follow the general guidelines in Patient Preparation and Specimen Collection online at Davis*Plus*. Positively identify the patient, and label the appropriate specimen container with the corresponding patient demographics, initials of the person collecting the specimen, date, and time of collection.

M

Random Specimen (Collect in Early Morning)

Clean-Catch Specimen

- Instruct the male patient to (1) thoroughly wash his hands; (2) cleanse the meatus; (3) void a small amount into the toilet; and (4) void directly into the specimen container.
- Instruct the female patient to (1) thoroughly wash her hands; (2) cleanse the labia from front to back; (3) while keeping the labia separated, void a small amount into the toilet; and (4) without interrupting the urine stream, void directly into the specimen container.

Indwelling Catheter

- Put on gloves. Empty drainage tube of urine. It may be necessary to clamp off the catheter for 15 to 30 min before specimen collection. Cleanse specimen port with antiseptic swab, and then aspirate 5 mL of urine with a 21- to 25-gauge needle and syringe. Transfer urine to a sterile container.

Timed Specimen

- Obtain a clean 3-L urine specimen container, toilet-mounted collection device, and plastic bag (for transport of the specimen container). The specimen must be refrigerated or kept on ice throughout the entire collection period. If an indwelling urinary catheter is in place, the drainage bag must be kept on ice.
- Begin the test between 0600 and 0800 if possible. Collect first voiding and discard. Record the time the specimen was discarded as the beginning of the timed collection period. The next morning, ask the patient to void at the same time the collection was started and add this last voiding to the container. Urinary output should be recorded throughout the collection time.
- If an indwelling catheter is in place, replace the tubing and container system at the start of the collection time. Keep the container system on ice during the collection period, or empty the urine into a larger container periodically during the collection period; monitor to ensure continued drainage, and conclude the test the next morning at the same hour the collection was begun.
- At the conclusion of the test, compare the quantity of urine with the urinary output record for the collection; if the specimen contains less than what was recorded as output, some urine may have been discarded, invalidating the test.
- Include on the collection container's label the amount of urine and test start and stop times.

General

- Promptly transport the specimen to the laboratory for processing and analysis.

POST-TEST:

- Inform the patient that a report of the results will be made available to the requesting HCP, who will discuss the results with the patient.
- ***Nutritional Considerations:*** Increased levels of microalbumin may be associated with diabetes. There is no "diabetic diet"; however, many meal-planning approaches with nutritional goals are endorsed by the ADA. 🍁 Patients who adhere to dietary recommendations report a better general feeling of health, better weight management, greater control of glucose and lipid values, and improved use of insulin. Instruct the patient, as appropriate, in nutritional management of diabetes. A variety of dietary patterns are beneficial for people with diabetes. The Mediterranean-style diet emphasizes inclusion of vegetables, whole grains, fruits, low-fat dairy, nuts, legumes, and nontropical vegetable oils (e.g., olive, canola, peanut, sunflower, flaxseed) along with fish and lean poultry. A similar dietary pattern known as the Dietary Approaches to Stop Hypertension (DASH) diet makes additional recommendations for the reduction of dietary sodium. Both dietary styles emphasize a reduction in consumption of red meats, which are high

M

in saturated fats and cholesterol, and other foods containing sugar, saturated fats, trans fats, and sodium. A vegetarian diet as well as other potential weight loss diets such as Weight Watchers are also supported by the ADA. 🍁 If triglycerides also are elevated, the patient should be advised to eliminate or reduce alcohol. The nutritional needs of each patient with diabetic patient need to be determined individually (especially during pregnancy) with the appropriate HCPs, particularly professionals educated in nutrition.

- Recognize anxiety related to test results, and be supportive of perceived loss of independence and fear of shortened life expectancy.
- Depending on the results of this procedure, additional testing may be performed to evaluate or monitor progression of the disease process and determine the need for a change in therapy. The ADA recommends A_{1C} testing four times a year for insulin-dependent type 1 or type 2 diabetes when glycemic targets are not being met or when therapy has changed and twice a year when treatment goals are being met for non–insulin-dependent type 2 diabetes. The ADA also recommends that testing for diabetes commence at age 45 for asymptomatic individuals, be considered for adults of any age who are overweight and have additional risk factors, and continue every 3 yr in the absence of symptoms. 🍁 Evaluate test results in relation to the patient's symptoms and other tests performed.

Patient Education:

- Instruct the patient to resume usual activity, as directed by the HCP.
- Instruct the patient and caregiver to report signs and symptoms of hypoglycemia or hyperglycemia.
- Discuss the implications of abnormal test results on the patient's lifestyle.
- Provide teaching and information regarding the clinical implications of the test results, as appropriate.
- Emphasize, if indicated, that good glycemic management delays the onset and slows the progression of diabetic retinopathy, nephropathy, and neuropathy.
- Educate the patient regarding access to counseling services, as appropriate. Provide contact information, if desired, for the American Heart Association (www.americanheart.org), the NHLBI (www.nhlbi.nih.gov), Institute of Medicine of the National Academies (www.iom.edu), USDA's resource for nutrition (www.choosemyplate.gov). 🍁
- Reinforce information given by the patient's HCP regarding further testing, treatment, or referral to another HCP.
- Answer any questions or address any concerns voiced by the patient or family.
- Teach the patient that diabetes that is not controlled can cause multiple health issues including renal failure resulting in necessary dialysis to support life.

Expected Patient Outcomes:

Understanding

- The patient and family state that a urine test can assess for early renal failure associated with diabetes.
- The patient and family state that chronic kidney disease can lead to death.

Ability

- The patient demonstrates proficiency in the ability to perform a self-check glucose accurately.
- The patient demonstrates proficiency in the ability to perform insulin self-administration correctly or to take oral antihyperglycemic drugs.

Response

- The patient complies with the HCP-recommended therapeutic regime to manage diabetes.
- The patient complies with the recommendation to attend support groups to learn how to manage disease process.

RELATED STUDIES:

- Related tests include A/G ratio, angiography kidneys, blood pool imaging, BUN, CBC, cortisol, creatinine, creatinine clearance, culture urine, cystometry, cystoscopy, cytology urine, echocardiography, echocardiography transesophageal, EPO, fluorescein angiography, fundoscopy, glucose, GTT, glycated hemoglobin, gonioscopy, Holter monitor, insulin, insulin antibodies, magnesium, protein total and fractions, renogram, UA, visual fields test, and voiding cystourethrography.
- Refer to the Endocrine and Genitourinary systems tables online at Davis*Plus* for related tests by body system.

Mumps Serology

SYNONYM/ACRONYM: N/A

COMMON USE: To assist in diagnosing a present or past mumps infection.

SPECIMEN: Serum collected in a gold-, red-, or red/gray-top tube. Place separated serum into a standard transport tube within 2 hr of collection.

NORMAL FINDINGS: (Method: Indirect immunofluorescence)

	IgM	Interpretation	IgG	Interpretation
Negative	0.89 index or less	No significant level of detectable antibody	Less than 5 IU/mL	No significant level of detectable antibody; indicative of nonimmunity
Indeterminate	0.9–1 index	Equivocal results; retest in 10–14 d	6–9 IU/mL	Equivocal results; retest in 10–14 d
Positive	1.1 index or greater	Antibody detected; indicative of recent immunization, current or recent infection	10 IU/mL or greater	Antibody detected; indicative of immunization, current or past infection

POTENTIAL MEDICAL DIAGNOSIS

Past or current mumps infection.

CRITICAL FINDINGS: N/A

Find and print out the full study on Fast Find at davispl.us/vanleeuwen7.

Myocardial Infarct Scan

SYNONYM/ACRONYM: PYP cardiac scan, infarct scan, pyrophosphate cardiac scan, acute myocardial infarction scan.

COMMON USE: To differentiate between new and old myocardial infarcts and evaluate myocardial perfusion.

AREA OF APPLICATION: Heart, chest/thorax.

DESCRIPTION: Technetium-99m stannous pyrophosphate (PYP) scanning, also known as *myocardial infarct imaging,* can identify areas of infarct or necrosis due to insufficient myocardial perfusion and provide information about the extent of myocardial infarction (MI). This procedure can distinguish new from old infarcts when a patient has had abnormal electrocardiograms (ECGs) and cardiac enzymes have returned to normal.

PYP uptake by acutely infarcted tissue may be related to the influx of calcium through damaged cell membranes, which accompanies myocardial necrosis; that is, the radionuclide may be binding to calcium phosphate crystals (hydroxyapatite). The PYP in these damaged cells can be viewed as spots of increased radionuclide uptake that appear in 12 hr at the earliest. PYP uptake usually takes place 24 to 72 hr after MI, and the radionuclide remains detectable for approximately 10 to 14 days after the MI. PYP uptake is proportional to the blood flow to the affected area; with large areas of necrosis, PYP uptake may be maximal around the periphery of a necrotic area, with little uptake being detectable in the poorly perfused center. Most of the PYP is concentrated in regions that have 20% to 40% of the normal blood flow. Single-photon emission computed tomography (SPECT) can be used to visualize the heart from multiple angles and planes, enabling areas of MI to be viewed with greater accuracy and resolution. This technique removes overlying structures that may confuse interpretation of the results. Multigated (MUGA) blood pool imaging, also known as radionuclide ventriculogram may also be performed in conjunction with a PYP scan. MUGA provides information about cardiac function such as ejection fraction, ventricular wall motion, ventricular dilation, stroke volume, and cardiac output. With the availability of newer biomarkers such as troponin, myocardial infarct imaging has become less important in the diagnosis of acute MI.

This procedure is contraindicated for

Patients who are pregnant or suspected of being pregnant, unless the potential benefits of a procedure using radiation far outweigh the risk of radiation exposure to the fetus and mother.

INDICATIONS

- Aid in the diagnosis of (or confirm and locate) acute MI when ECG and enzyme testing do not provide a diagnosis.

- Aid in the diagnosis of perioperative MI.
- Differentiate between a new and old infarction.
- Evaluate possible reinfarction or extension of the infarct.
- Obtain baseline information about infarction before cardiac surgery.

POTENTIAL MEDICAL DIAGNOSIS

Normal findings

- Normal coronary blood flow and tissue perfusion, with no PYP localization in the myocardium
- No uptake above background activity in the myocardium (*Note:* When PYP uptake is present, it is graded in relation to adjacent rib activity.)

Abnormal findings related to

- MI, indicated by increased PYP uptake in the myocardium

CRITICAL FINDINGS: N/A

INTERFERING FACTORS

Factors that may alter the results of the study

- Inability of the patient to cooperate or remain still during the procedure because of age, significant pain, or mental status.
- Metallic objects (e.g., jewelry, body rings) within the examination field, which may inhibit organ visualization and cause unclear images.
- Other nuclear scans done within the previous 24 to 48 hr.
- Conditions such as chest wall trauma, cardiac trauma, or recent cardioversion procedure.
- Other conditions that may interfere include:
  - Aneurysms
  - Cardiac neoplasms
  - Left ventricular aneurysm
  - Metastasis
  - Myocarditis
  - Pericarditis
  - Valvular and coronary artery calcifications

Other considerations

- Improper injection of the radionuclide may allow the tracer to seep deep into the muscle tissue, producing erroneous hot spots.

NURSING IMPLICATIONS AND PROCEDURE

See Potential Nursing Problems on Fast Find at davispl.us/vanleeuwen7.

PRETEST:

- Positively identify the patient using at least two person-specific identifiers before services, treatments, or procedures are performed.
- ***Patient Teaching:*** Inform the patient this procedure can assess blood flow to the heart.
- Obtain a history of the patient's health concerns, symptoms, surgical procedures, and results of previously performed laboratory and diagnostic studies. Include a list of known allergens, especially allergies or sensitivities to latex, anesthetics, sedatives, or radionuclides. The presence of other risk factors, such as family history of heart disease, smoking, obesity, diet, lack of physical activity, hypertension, diabetes, previous myocardial infarction, and previous vascular disease, should be investigated. Knowledge of genetics assists the nurse in identifying patients and family members who may benefit from additional education, risk assessment, and counseling. Genetics is the study and identification of genes, genetic mutations, and inheritance. For example, genetics provides some insight into the likelihood of inheriting a trait such as blue eyes or a medical condition such as coronary artery disease (CAD). Genomic studies evaluate the interaction of groups of genes. The combined activity or combined expression of groups of genes allows assumptions or predictions to be made. As an example, genomic

M

studies measure the levels of activity in multiple genes to predict how they, along with environmental and lifestyle decisions, influence the development of type 2 diabetes, CAD, MI, or ischemic stroke. Further information regarding inheritance of genes can be found in the study titled "Genetic Testing."

- Note any recent procedures that can interfere with test results, including examinations using iodine-based contrast medium.
- Record the date of the last menstrual period and determine the possibility of pregnancy in perimenopausal women.
- Obtain a list of the patient's current medications, including over-the-counter medications and dietary supplements (see Effects of Natural Products on Laboratory Values online at Davis*Plus*).
- Review the procedure with the patient. Address concerns about pain related to the procedure and explain that some pain may be experienced during the test, and there may be moments of discomfort. Reassure the patient that the radionuclide poses no radioactive hazard and rarely produces adverse effects. Inform the patient that the procedure is performed in a nuclear medicine department by a health-care provider (HCP) specializing in this procedure, with support staff, and will take approximately 30 to 60 min. Inform the patient that the technologist will administer an intravenous (IV) injection of the radionuclide and that he or she will need to return 2 to 3 hr later for the scan.
- ***Sensitivity to social and cultural issues,*** as well as concern for modesty, is important in providing psychological support before, during, and after the procedure.
- Explain that an IV line may be inserted to allow infusion of fluids such as saline, anesthetics, sedatives, radionuclides, medications used in the procedure, or emergency medications.
- Instruct the patient to fast, restrict fluids, and refrain from smoking for 4 hr prior to the procedure. Instruct the patient to withhold medications for 24 hr before the procedure. Protocols may vary among facilities.
- *Make sure a written and informed consent has been signed prior to the procedure and before administering any medications.*
- Instruct the patient to remove jewelry and other metallic objects from the area to be examined.

INTRATEST:

Potential Complications:

Although it is rare, there is the possibility of allergic reaction to the radionuclide. Have emergency equipment and medications readily available. If the patient has a history of allergic reactions to any substance or drug, administer ordered prophylactic steroids or antihistamines before the procedure.

Establishing an IV site and injecting radionuclides is an invasive procedure. Complications are rare but do include bleeding from the puncture site ***related to a bleeding disorder or the effects of natural products and medications with known anticoagulant, antiplatelet, or thrombolytic properties;*** hematoma ***related to blood leakage into the tissue following needle insertion;*** infection ***that might occur if bacteria from the skin surface is introduced at the puncture site;*** or nerve injury ***that might occur if the needle strikes a nerve.***

- Observe standard precautions, and follow the general guidelines in Patient Preparation and Specimen Collection online at Davis*Plus*. Positively identify the patient.
- Ensure that the patient has complied with dietary and medication restrictions and other pretesting preparations prior to the procedure, as instructed.
- Ensure that the patient has removed all external metallic objects prior to the procedure.
- Avoid the use of equipment containing latex if the patient has a history of allergic reaction to latex.

M

- Have emergency equipment readily available.
- Instruct the patient to void prior to the procedure and to change into the gown, robe, and foot coverings provided.
- Record baseline vital signs and assess neurological status. Protocols may vary among facilities.
- Establish an IV fluid line for the injection of saline, anesthetics, sedatives, radionuclides, or emergency medications.
- Instruct the patient to cooperate fully and to follow directions. Instruct the patient to lie very still during the procedure because movement will produce unclear images.
- Place the patient in a supine position on a flat table with foam wedges to help maintain position and immobilization.
- IV radionuclide is administered. The heart is scanned 2 to 4 hr after injection in various positions. In most circumstances, however, SPECT is done so that the heart can be viewed from multiple angles and planes.
- Monitor the patient for complications related to the procedure (e.g., allergic reaction, anaphylaxis, bronchospasm).
- Remove the needle or catheter and apply a pressure dressing over the puncture site.
- Observe/assess the needle/catheter insertion site for bleeding, inflammation, or hematoma formation.

POST-TEST:

- Inform the patient that a report of the results will be made available to the requesting HCP, who will discuss the results with the patient.
- Instruct the patient to resume normal activity and diet as directed by the HCP.
- Unless contraindicated, advise the patient to drink increased amounts of fluids for 24 to 48 hr to eliminate the radionuclide from the body. Inform the patient that radionuclide is eliminated from the body within 6 to 24 hr.
- No other radionuclide tests should be scheduled for 24 to 48 hr after this procedure.
- Evaluate the patient's vital signs. Monitor vital signs and neurological status every 15 min for 1 hr, then every 2 hr for 4 hr, and then as ordered by HCP. Take temperature every 4 hr for 24 hr. Monitor intake and output at least every 8 hr. Compare with baseline values. Notify the HCP if temperature is elevated. Protocols may vary among facilities.
- Observe for delayed allergic reactions, such as rash, urticaria, tachycardia, hyperpnea, hypertension, palpitations, nausea, or vomiting.
- Instruct the patient to immediately report symptoms such as fast heart rate, difficulty breathing, skin rash, itching, chest pain, persistent right shoulder pain, or abdominal pain. Immediately report symptoms to the appropriate HCP.
- Instruct the patient in the care and assessment of the injection site.
- If the patient must return for additional imaging, advise the patient to rest in the interim and restrict diet to liquids before redistribution studies.
- If a woman who is breastfeeding must have a nuclear scan, she should not breastfeed the infant until the radionuclide has been eliminated. This could take as long as 3 days. She should be instructed to express the milk and discard it during the 3-day period to prevent cessation of milk production.
- Instruct the patient to flush the toilet immediately after each voiding following the procedure and to meticulously wash hands with soap and water after each voiding for 24 hr after the procedure.
- Instruct all caregivers to wear gloves when discarding urine for 24 hr after the procedure. Wash gloved hands with soap and water before removing gloves; then wash ungloved hands.
- ***Nutritional Considerations:*** Abnormal findings may be associated with cardiovascular disease. Nutritional therapy is recommended for the patient identified to be at risk for developing CAD

M

or for individuals who have specific risk factors and/or existing medical conditions (e.g., elevated LDL cholesterol levels, other lipid disorders, type 1 diabetes, type 2 diabetes, insulin resistance, or metabolic syndrome). Other changeable risk factors warranting patient education include strategies to encourage patients, especially those who are overweight and with high blood pressure, to safely decrease sodium intake, achieve a normal weight, ensure regular participation in moderate aerobic physical activity three to four times per week, eliminate tobacco use, and adhere to a heart-healthy diet. If triglycerides also are elevated, the patient should be advised to eliminate or reduce alcohol. A variety of dietary patterns are beneficial for people with CAD, and there are many meal-planning approaches with nutritional goals endorsed by the American Diabetes Association (ADA). The Guideline on Lifestyle Management to Reduce Cardiovascular Risk published by the American College of Cardiology (ACC) and the American Heart Association (AHA) in conjunction with the National Heart, Lung, and Blood Institute (NHLBI) recommends a Mediterranean-style diet rather than a low-fat diet. The guideline emphasizes inclusion of vegetables, whole grains, fruits, low-fat dairy, nuts, legumes, and nontropical vegetable oils (e.g., olive, canola, peanut, sunflower, flaxseed) along with fish and lean poultry. 🍁 A similar dietary pattern known as the Dietary Approaches to Stop Hypertension (DASH) diet makes additional recommendations for the reduction of dietary sodium. Both dietary styles emphasize a reduction in consumption of red meats, which are high in saturated fats and cholesterol, and other foods containing sugar, saturated fats, trans fats, and sodium. The ADA also includes a vegetarian diet as well as other potential weight loss diets such as Weight Watchers. 🍁 The nutritional needs of each patient need to be determined individually (especially during pregnancy) with the appropriate HCPs, particularly professionals educated in nutrition.

- Recognize anxiety related to test results, and be supportive of fear of shortened life expectancy. Discuss the implications of abnormal test results on the patient's lifestyle. Provide teaching and information regarding the clinical implications of the test results, as appropriate. Educate the patient regarding access to counseling services. Provide contact information, if desired, for the AHA (www.americanheart.org), NHLBI (www.nhlbi.nih.gov), Institute of Medicine of the National Academies (www.iom.edu), and USDA's resource for nutrition (www.choosemyplate.gov). 🍁
- Reinforce information given by the patient's HCP regarding further testing, treatment, or referral to another HCP. Answer any questions or address any concerns voiced by the patient or family.
- Depending on the results of this procedure, additional testing may be needed to evaluate or monitor progression of the disease process and determine the need for a change in therapy. Evaluate test results in relation to the patient's symptoms and other tests performed.

Patient Education:

- Teach the patient about the pathophysiology of myocardial infarction.
- Teach the patient the purpose of ordered medications (morphine, nitroglycerin, calcium channel blockers, beta blockers).

Expected Patient Outcomes:

Understanding

- The patient and family state the link between activity and cardiac health.
- The patient and family state how oxygen administration supports cardiac function.

Ability

- The patient and family create a quiet environment to reduce energy demands.
- The patient and family plan rest periods during the day to conserve oxygen.

Response

- The patient and family agree to make lifestyle changes that will support positive cardiac health.
- The patient agrees to attend cardiac rehabilitation.

RELATED STUDIES:

- Related tests include angiography abdominal, BNP, blood pool imaging, chest x-ray, CT abdominal, CT thoracic, CK and isoenzymes, culture viral, echocardiography, echocardiography transesophageal, ECG, genetic testing, Holter monitor, MRA, MRI chest, myocardial perfusion scan, pericardial fluid analysis, and PET heart.
- Refer to the Cardiovascular System table online at Davis*Plus* for related tests by body system.

Myocardial Perfusion Heart Scan

SYNONYM/ACRONYM: Cardiac stress scan, nuclear stress test, sestamibi scan, stress thallium, thallium scan.

COMMON USE: To assess cardiac blood flow to evaluate for and assist in diagnosing coronary artery disease and myocardial infarction.

AREA OF APPLICATION: Heart, chest/thorax.

DESCRIPTION: Cardiac scanning is a nuclear medicine study that reveals clinical information about coronary blood flow, ventricular size, and cardiac function. Thallium-201 chloride rest or stress studies are used to evaluate myocardial blood flow to assist in diagnosing or determining the risk for ischemic cardiac disease, coronary artery disease (CAD), and myocardial infarction (MI). This procedure is an alternative to angiography or cardiac catheterization in cases in which these procedures may pose a risk to the patient. Thallium-201 is a potassium analogue and is taken up by myocardial cells proportional to blood flow to the cell and cell viability. During stress studies, the radionuclide is injected at peak exercise, after which the patient continues to exercise for several minutes. During exercise, areas of heart muscle supplied by normal arteries increase their blood supply, as well as the supply of thallium-201 delivery to the heart muscle, to a greater extent than regions of the heart muscle supplied by stenosed coronary arteries. This discrepancy in blood flow becomes apparent and quantifiable in subsequent imaging. Comparison of early stress images with images taken after 3 to 4 hr redistribution (delayed images) enables differentiation between normally perfused, healthy myocardium (which is normal at rest but ischemic on stress) and infarcted myocardium. In most cases, the goal of the exercise stress test is to increase heart rate to a level just below (85%) a person's age-predicted maximum target heart rate. The target heart rate can be calculated in a number of ways. One way is by subtracting the patient's age from 220 (theoretical maximum heart rate) and multiplying by 0.85 (85%). For example, the study target heart rate for a patient age 50 years would be (220 – 50) × 0.85 = 144.

Technetium-99m radionuclides such as sestamibi (2-methoxyisobutylisonitrile) are delivered similarly to thallium-201 during myocardial perfusion imaging, but they are extracted to a lesser degree on the first pass through the heart and are taken up by the mitochondria. Over a short period, the radionuclide concentrates in the heart to the same degree as thallium-201. The advantage of technetium-99m radionuclide is that immediate imaging is unnecessary because the radionuclide remains fixed to the heart muscle for several hours. The examination requires two separate injections, one for the rest portion and one for the stress portion of the procedure. These injections can take place on the same day or preferably over a 2-day period. Examination quality is improved if the patient is given a light, fatty meal after the radionuclide is injected to facilitate hepatobiliary clearance of the radioactivity.

If stress testing cannot be performed by exercising, a vasodilator such as dipyridamole (Persantine) or adenosine, can be administered orally or by intravenous (IV) injection. The coronary vasodilator is administered before the thallium-201 or other radionuclide, and the scanning procedure is then performed. Vasodilators increase blood flow in normal coronary arteries twofold to threefold without exercise, and they reveal perfusion defects when blood flow is compromised by vessel pathology. Vasodilator-mediated myocardial perfusion scanning is reserved for patients who are unable to participate in treadmill, bicycle, or handgrip exercises for stress testing because of lung disease, neurological disorders (e.g., multiple sclerosis, spinal cord injury), morbid obesity, and orthopedic disorders (e.g., arthritis, limb amputation).

Single-photon emission computed tomography (SPECT) can be used to visualize the heart from multiple angles and planes, providing three-dimensional functional images that enable areas of ischemia to be viewed with greater accuracy and resolution. This technique removes overlying structures that may confuse interpretation of the results. SPECT also provides accurate, quantitative information regarding the degree of cardiac damage. Based on the study findings, multigated (MUGA) blood pool imaging, also known as ***radionuclide ventriculogram,*** may also be performed in conjunction with a myocardial perfusion scan. MUGA provides information about cardiac function such as ejection fraction, ventricular wall motion, ventricular dilation, stroke volume, and cardiac output.

This procedure is contraindicated for

- Patients who have taken sildenafil (Viagra) within the previous 48 hr ***because this test may require the use of nitrates (nitroglycerin) that can precipitate life-threatening low blood pressure.***
- Patients who are pregnant or suspected of being pregnant, unless the potential benefits of a procedure using radiation far outweigh the risk of radiation exposure to the fetus and mother.
- Patients with bleeding disorders.

M

◆ Patients with left ventricular hypertrophy, right and left bundle branch block, and hypokalemia, and patients receiving cardiotonic therapy.

◆ Patients with anginal pain at rest or patients with severe atherosclerotic coronary vessels ***in whom dipyridamole testing cannot be performed.***

◆ Patients with asthma ***because chemical stress with vasodilators can cause bronchospasms.***

INDICATIONS

Adult

- Aid in the diagnosis of CAD or risk for CAD.
- Determine rest defects and reperfusion with delayed imaging in unstable angina.
- Evaluate the extent of CAD and determine cardiac function.
- Assess the function of collateral coronary arteries.
- Evaluate bypass graft patency and general cardiac status after surgery.
- Evaluate the site of an old MI to determine obstruction to cardiac muscle perfusion.
- Evaluate the effectiveness of medication regimen and balloon angioplasty procedure on narrow coronary arteries.

Pediatric

- Assess athletic potential.
- Establish baseline prior to physical rehabilitation therapy.
- Evaluate for cardiac dysfunction related to diagnosed or undiagnosed congenital heart defects or other cardiac issues that manifest symptoms when individual engages in physical activity or exertion.

POTENTIAL MEDICAL DIAGNOSIS

Normal findings

- Normal wall motion, ejection fraction (55%–70%), coronary blood flow, tissue perfusion, and ventricular size and function. Mitochondria are responsible for generating the energy required for all cellular function; the amount of radionuclide visualization should reflect normal, active cardiac tissue.

Abnormal findings related to

Poor visualization or "cold spots" are seen in areas of poor perfusion and diminished cardiac muscle activity.

- Abnormal stress and resting images, indicating previous MI
- Abnormal stress images with normal resting images, indicating transient ischemia
- Cardiac hypertrophy, indicated by increased radionuclide uptake in the myocardium
- Enlarged left ventricle
- Heart chamber disorder
- Heart failure
- Ventricular septal defects

CRITICAL FINDINGS: N/A

INTERFERING FACTORS

Factors that may alter the results of the study

- Inability of the patient to cooperate or remain still during the procedure because of age, significant pain, or mental status.
- Medications such as digoxin and quinidine, which can alter cardiac contractility, and nitrates, which can affect cardiac performance.
- Single-vessel disease, which can produce false-negative thallium-201 scanning results.
- Conditions such as chest wall or cardiac trauma, angina that is difficult to control, significant cardiac dysrhythmias, and recent cardioversion procedure.
- Suboptimal cardiac stress or patient exhaustion preventing maximum heart rate testing.
- Excessive eating or exercising between initial and redistribution

imaging 4 hr later, which produces false-positive results.

- Improper adjustment of the radiological equipment to accommodate obese or thin patients, which can cause overexposure or underexposure and a poor-quality study.
- Patients who are extremely obese may require more radiation to obtain a clear image.
- Incorrect positioning of the patient, which may produce poor visualization of the area to be examined.
- Metallic objects (e.g., jewelry, body rings) within the examination field, which may inhibit organ visualization and cause unclear images.

Other considerations

- Failure to follow dietary restrictions before the procedure may cause the procedure to be canceled or repeated.
- Improper injection of the radionuclide that allows the tracer to seep deep into the muscle tissue produces erroneous hot spots.
- Inaccurate timing for imaging after radionuclide injection can affect the results.
- This procedure may be terminated if chest pain, severe cardiac dysrhythmias, or signs of a cerebrovascular accident occur.
- The procedure may be canceled if the patient's weight exceeds the safety limit for the equipment.

NURSING IMPLICATIONS AND PROCEDURE

See Potential Nursing Problems on Fast Find at davispl.us/vanleeuwen7.

PRETEST:

- Positively identify the patient using at least two person-specific identifiers before services, treatments, or procedures are performed.
- *Patient Teaching:* Inform the patient this procedure can assist in assessing blood flow to the heart.
- Obtain a history of the patient's health concerns, symptoms, surgical procedures, and results of previously performed laboratory and diagnostic studies. Include a list of known allergens, especially allergies or sensitivities to latex, anesthetics, sedatives, or radionuclides. The presence of other risk factors, such as family history of heart disease, smoking, obesity, diet, lack of physical activity, hypertension, diabetes, previous myocardial infarction, and previous vascular disease, should be investigated. Knowledge of genetics assists the nurse in identifying patients and family members who may benefit from additional education, risk assessment, and counseling. Genetics is the study and identification of genes, genetic mutations, and inheritance. For example, genetics provides some insight into the likelihood of inheriting a trait such as blue eyes or a medical condition such as CAD. Genomic studies evaluate the interaction of groups of genes. The combined activity or combined expression of groups of genes allows assumptions or predictions to be made. As an example, genomic studies measure the levels of activity in multiple genes to predict how they, along with environmental and lifestyle decisions, influence the development of type 2 diabetes, CAD, MI, or ischemic stroke. Further information regarding inheritance of genes can be found in the study titled "Genetic Testing."
- Record the date of the last menstrual period and determine the possibility of pregnancy in perimenopausal women.
- Obtain a list of the patient's current medications, including over-the-counter medications and dietary supplements (see Effects of Natural Products on Laboratory Values online at Davis*Plus*).
- Review the procedure with the patient. Address concerns about

pain and explain that some pain may be experienced during the test, or there may be moments of discomfort. Inform the patient that the procedure is performed in a special department, usually in a radiology or vascular suite, by a health-care provider (HCP) specializing in this procedure, with support staff, and takes approximately 30 to 60 min.

Pediatric Considerations: Preparing children for a perfusion heart scan depends on the age of the child. Encourage parents to be truthful about what the child may experience during the procedure and to use words that they know their child will understand. Toddlers and preschool-aged children have a short attention span, so the best time to talk about the test is right before the procedure. The child should be assured that he or she will be allowed to bring a favorite comfort item into the examination room, and if appropriate, that a parent will be with the child during the procedure. Provide older children with information about the test, and allow them to participate in as many decisions as possible (e.g., choice of clothes to wear to the appointment) in order to reduce anxiety and encourage cooperation. If the child will be asked to perform specific movements or exercises for the test, encourage the child to practice the required activities, provide a CD that demonstrates the procedure, and teach strategies to remain calm, such as deep breathing, humming, or counting to himself or herself.

- ***Sensitivity to social and cultural issues,*** as well as concern for modesty, is important in providing psychological support before, during, and after the procedure.
- Explain that an IV line may be inserted to allow infusion of fluids such as saline, anesthetics, sedatives, radionuclides, medications used in the procedure, or emergency medications.
- Instruct the patient to wear walking shoes (if treadmill exercise testing is to be performed), and emphasize the importance of reporting fatigue, pain, or shortness of breath. Explain that vital signs to monitor heart rate (electrocardiogram), oxygen level (pulse oximetry), and blood pressure (sphygmomanometer) will be measured before, during (peak), and after the study. Also explain the importance of describing any adverse symptoms that may develop during the test (e.g., chest pain, fatigue, dyspnea, dysrhythmias, or changes in blood pressure), which may require the procedure to be terminated.
- Instruct the patient to remove dentures, jewelry, and other metallic objects from the area to be examined prior to the procedure.
- Instruct the patient to fast and refrain from consuming caffeinated beverages for 4 hr, refrain from smoking for 4 to 6 hr, and withhold medications for 24 hr before the test. Instruct the patient to avoid taking anticoagulant medication or to reduce dosage as ordered prior to the procedure. Protocols may vary among facilities.
- *Make sure a written and informed consent has been signed prior to the procedure and before administering any medications.*

INTRATEST:

Potential Complications:

Although it is rare, there is the possibility of allergic reaction to the radionuclide. Have emergency equipment and medications readily available. If the patient has a history of allergic reactions to any substance or drug, administer ordered prophylactic steroids or antihistamines before the procedure.

Establishing an IV site and injecting radionuclides is an invasive procedure. Complications are rare but do include bleeding from the puncture site ***related to a bleeding disorder or the effects of natural products and medications with known anticoagulant, antiplatelet, or thrombolytic properties;*** hematoma ***related to blood leakage into the tissue following needle insertion;*** infection ***that***

might occur if bacteria from the skin surface is introduced at the puncture site; or nerve injury ***that might occur if the needle strikes a nerve.***

- Observe standard precautions, and follow the general guidelines in Patient Preparation and Specimen Collection online at Davis*Plus*. Positively identify the patient.
- Ensure that the patient has complied with dietary, tobacco, and medication restrictions and other pretesting preparations prior to the procedure, as instructed.
- Ensure that the patient has removed external metallic objects from the area to be examined prior to the procedure.
- Avoid the use of equipment containing latex if the patient has a history of allergic reaction to latex.
- Have emergency equipment readily available.
- Administer ordered prophylactic steroids or antihistamines before the procedure if the patient has a history of allergic reactions to any substance or drug. Use nonionic contrast medium for the procedure.
- Instruct the patient to void prior to the procedure and change into the gown, robe, and foot coverings provided.
- Record baseline vital signs and assess neurological status. Protocols may vary among facilities.
- Establish an IV fluid line for the injection of saline, anesthetics, sedatives, radionuclides, or emergency medications.
- Instruct the patient to cooperate fully and to follow directions.
- Place electrocardiographic electrodes on the patient for cardiac monitoring. Establish baseline rhythm; determine if the patient has ventricular dysrhythmias. Monitor the patient's blood pressure throughout the procedure by using an automated blood pressure machine.
- Assist the patient onto the treadmill or bicycle ergometer and ask the patient to exercise to a calculated 80% to 85% of the maximum heart rate, as determined by the protocol selected.
- Wear gloves during the radionuclide injection and while handling the patient's urine.
- Thallium-201 is injected 60 to 90 sec before exercise is terminated, and imaging is done immediately in the supine position and repeated in 4 hr.
- Patients who cannot exercise are given dipyridamole 4 min before thallium-201 is injected.
- Inform the patient that movement during the resting procedure affects the results and makes interpretation difficult.
- Monitor the patient for complications related to the procedure (e.g., allergic reaction, anaphylaxis, or bronchospasm).
- Remove the needle or catheter and apply a pressure dressing over the puncture site.
- Observe/assess the needle/catheter insertion site for bleeding, inflammation, or hematoma formation.
- The results are recorded on film or in a computerized system for recall and postprocedure interpretation by the appropriate HCP.

POST-TEST:

- Inform the patient that a report of the results will be made available to the requesting HCP, who will discuss the results with the patient.
- Instruct the patient to resume normal diet and activity, as directed by the HCP.
- Unless contraindicated, advise patient to drink increased amounts of fluids for 24 to 48 hr to eliminate the radionuclide from the body. Inform the patient that radionuclide is eliminated from the body within 6 to 24 hr.
- No other radionuclide tests should be scheduled for 24 to 48 hr after this procedure.
- Evaluate the patient's vital signs. Monitor vital signs and neurological status every 15 min for 1 hr, then every 2 hr for 4 hr, and then as ordered by HCP. Take temperature every 4 hr for 24 hr. Monitor intake and output at least every 8 hr. Compare with baseline values. Notify the

M

HCP if temperature is elevated. Protocols may vary among facilities.

- Observe for delayed allergic reactions, such as rash, urticaria, tachycardia, hyperpnea, hypertension, palpitations, nausea, or vomiting.
- Instruct the patient to immediately report symptoms such as fast heart rate, difficulty breathing, skin rash, itching, chest pain, persistent right shoulder pain, or abdominal pain. Immediately report symptoms to the appropriate HCP.
- Instruct the patient in the care and assessment of the injection site.
- If the patient must return for additional imaging, advise the patient to rest in the interim and restrict diet to liquids before redistribution studies.
- If a woman who is breastfeeding must have a nuclear scan, she should not breastfeed the infant until the radionuclide has been eliminated. This could take as long as 3 days. She should be instructed to express the milk and discard it during the 3-day period to prevent cessation of milk production.
- Instruct the patient to flush the toilet immediately after each voiding following the procedure and to meticulously wash hands with soap and water after each voiding for 24 hr after the procedure.
- Instruct all caregivers to wear gloves when discarding urine for 24 hr after the procedure. Wash gloved hands with soap and water before removing gloves; then wash ungloved hands.
- ***Nutritional Considerations:*** Abnormal findings may be associated with cardiovascular disease. Nutritional therapy is recommended for the patient identified to be at risk for developing CAD or for individuals who have specific risk factors and/or existing medical conditions (e.g., elevated LDL cholesterol levels, other lipid disorders, type 1 diabetes, type 2 diabetes, insulin resistance, or metabolic syndrome). Other changeable risk factors warranting patient education include strategies to encourage patients, especially those who are overweight and with high blood pressure, to safely decrease sodium intake, achieve a normal weight, ensure regular participation in moderate aerobic physical activity three to four times per week, eliminate tobacco use, and adhere to a heart-healthy diet. If triglycerides also are elevated, the patient should be advised to eliminate or reduce alcohol. A variety of dietary patterns are beneficial for people with CAD and there are many meal-planning approaches with nutritional goals endorsed by the American Diabetes Association (ADA). The Guideline on Lifestyle Management to Reduce Cardiovascular Risk published by the American College of Cardiology (ACC) and the American Heart Association (AHA) in conjunction with the National Heart, Lung, and Blood Institute (NHLBI) recommends a Mediterranean-style diet rather than a low-fat diet. The guideline emphasizes inclusion of vegetables, whole grains, fruits, low-fat dairy, nuts, legumes, and nontropical vegetable oils (e.g., olive, canola, peanut, sunflower, flaxseed) along with fish and lean poultry. 🍁 A similar dietary pattern known as the Dietary Approaches to Stop Hypertension (DASH) diet makes additional recommendations for the reduction of dietary sodium. Both dietary styles emphasize a reduction in consumption of red meats, which are high in saturated fats and cholesterol, and other foods containing sugar, saturated fats, trans fats, and sodium. The ADA also includes a vegetarian diet as well as other potential weight loss diets such as Weight Watchers. 🍁 The nutritional needs of each patient need to be determined individually (especially during pregnancy) with the appropriate HCPs, particularly professionals educated in nutrition.
- ***Sensitivity to social and cultural issues:*** Numerous studies point to the prevalence of excess body weight in American children and adolescents. Experts estimate that obesity is present in 25% of the population aged 6 to 11 yr. The medical, social, and

M

emotional consequences of excess body weight are significant. Special attention should be given to instructing the child and caregiver regarding health risks and weight control education. 🍁

- Recognize anxiety related to test results, and be supportive of fear of shortened life expectancy. Discuss the implications of abnormal test results on the patient's lifestyle. Provide teaching and information regarding the clinical implications of the test results, as appropriate. Educate the patient regarding access to counseling services. Provide contact information, if desired, for the AHA (www.americanheart.org), NHLBI (www.nhlbi.nih.gov), Institute of Medicine of the National Academies (www.iom.edu), and USDA's resource for nutrition (www.choosemyplate.gov). 🍁
- Reinforce information given by the patient's HCP regarding further testing, treatment, or referral to another HCP. Answer any questions or address any concerns voiced by the patient or family.
- Depending on the results of this procedure, additional testing may be needed to evaluate or monitor progression of the disease process and determine the need for a change in therapy. Evaluate test results in relation to the patient's symptoms and other tests performed.

Patient Education:

- Teach the patient about the pathophysiology of myocardial infarction.
- Teach the patient the purpose of ordered medications (morphine, nitroglycerin, calcium channel blockers, beta blockers).

Expected Patient Outcomes:

Understanding

- The patient and family state the link between activity and cardiac health.
- The patient and family state how oxygen administration supports cardiac function.

Ability

- The patient and family create a quiet environment to reduce energy demands.
- The patient and family plan rest periods during the day to conserve oxygen.

Response

- The patient and family agree to make lifestyle changes that will support positive cardiac health.
- The patient agrees to attend cardiac rehabilitation.

RELATED STUDIES:

- Related tests include antidysrhythmic drugs, apolipoproteins (A, B, and C), atrial natriuretic peptide, BNP, calcium, cholesterol (total, HDL, LDL), CT cardiac scoring, CRP, CK and isoenzymes, echocardiography, echocardiography transesophageal, ECG, exercise stress test, fundoscopy, genetic testing, glucose, glycated hemoglobin, Holter monitor, homocysteine, ketones, LDH and isos, lipoprotein electrophoresis, magnesium, MRI chest, MI infarct scan, myoglobin, PET heart, potassium, triglycerides, and troponin.
- Refer to the Cardiovascular System table online at Davis*Plus* for related tests by body system.

Myoglobin

SYNONYM/ACRONYM: MB.

COMMON USE: A general assessment of damage to skeletal or cardiac muscle from trauma or inflammation.

SPECIMEN: Serum collected in a red- or red/gray-top tube.

NORMAL FINDINGS: (Method: Electrochemiluminescent immunoassay)

	Conventional Units	SI Units (Conventional Units × 0.0571)
Male	28–72 ng/mL	1.6–4.1 nmol/L
Female	25–58 ng/mL	1.4–3.3 nmol/L

Values are higher in males.

DESCRIPTION: Myoglobin is an oxygen-binding muscle protein normally found in skeletal and cardiac muscle. It is released into the bloodstream after muscle damage from ischemia, trauma, or inflammation. Although myoglobin testing is more sensitive than creatinine kinase and isoenzymes, it does not indicate the specific site involved.

Timing for Appearance and Resolution of Serum/Plasma *Cardiac Markers in Acute Myocardial Infarction*

Cardiac Marker	*Appearance (Hr)*	*Peak (Hr)*	*Resolution (Days)*
CK (total)	4–6	24	2–3
CK-MB	4–6	15–20	2–3
LDH	12	24–48	10–14
Myoglobin	1–3	4–12	1
Troponin I	2–8	15–20	5–7

CK = creatine kinase; CK-MB = creatine kinase myocardial band; LDH = lactate dehydrogenase.

This procedure is contraindicated for: N/A

INDICATIONS

- Assist in predicting a flare-up of polymyositis.
- Estimate damage from skeletal muscle injury or myocardial infarction (MI).

POTENTIAL MEDICAL DIAGNOSIS

Increased in:

Conditions that cause muscle damage; damaged muscle cells release myoglobin into circulation.

- Cardiac surgery
- Chronic kidney disease
- Cocaine use ***(rhabdomyolysis is a complication of cocaine use or overdose)***
- Exercise
- Malignant hyperthermia
- MI
- Progressive muscular dystrophy
- Rhabdomyolysis
- Shock
- Thrombolytic therapy

Decreased in:

- Myasthenia gravis
- Presence of antibodies to myoglobin, as seen in patients with polymyositis
- Rheumatoid arthritis

CRITICAL FINDINGS: N/A

INTERFERING FACTORS: N/A

NURSING IMPLICATIONS AND PROCEDURE

POTENTIAL NURSING PROBLEMS:

Problem	Signs & Symptoms	Interventions
Mobility ***(related to progressive muscle wasting associated with muscular dystrophy)***	Weakness; waddling gait; lordosis; large calf muscles; difficulty moving from lying to sitting position; clumsiness; falling; difficulty running	Encourage use of appropriate assistive devices, including braces and wheelchairs; encourage active and passive range-of-motion exercises; promote independence; provide physical therapy as prescribed by the health-care provider (HCP)
Family process ***(related to altered role performance secondary to progressive skeletal muscle disease or cardiac disease progression)***	Inability to perform in supportive family role; alteration in family finances; change in communication patterns; change in assignment of family tasks and performance of those tasks; alterations in intimacy	Encourage family counseling; facilitate opportunities for the patient and family to express their feelings; assess patient's and family's perception of the problems; evaluate patient and family weaknesses, strengths, and coping strategies; help family and patient break down concerns into manageable parts
Cardiac output, decreased ***(related to altered cardiac muscle contractility secondary to muscle damage associated with myocardial infarction)***	Hypotension; dizziness; poor oxygenation; poor urine output; shortness of breath; fatigue; decreased activity; weakness; altered level of consciousness; peripheral edema	Monitor vital signs (heart rate, blood pressure); monitor oxygenation (saturation greater than 90%); assess for dizziness or altered level of consciousness; daily weight; assess for peripheral edema, weak peripheral pulses; monitor electrocardiogram results; administer prescribed medications appropriately (diuretics, procainamide, beta blockers, antidysrhythmics, atropine, calcium channel blockers, amiodarone); monitor for cool skin, cyanosis; prepare for cardioversion, pacemaker

PRETEST:

- Positively identify the patient using at least two person-specific identifiers before services, treatments, or procedures are performed.
- *Patient Teaching:* Inform the patient this test can assist in diagnosing cardiac or skeletal muscle damage.
- Obtain a history of the patient's health concerns, symptoms, surgical

procedures, and results of previously performed laboratory and diagnostic studies. Include a list of known allergens, especially allergies or sensitivities to latex.

- Obtain a list of the patient's current medications, including over-the-counter medications and dietary supplements (see Effects of Natural Products on Laboratory Values online at Davis*Plus*).
- Review the procedure with the patient. Inform the patient that specimen collection takes approximately 5 to 10 min. Address concerns about pain and explain that there may be some discomfort during the venipuncture.
- ***Sensitivity to social and cultural issues,*** as well as concern for modesty, is important in providing psychological support before, during, and after the procedure.
- Note that there are no food, fluid, or medication restrictions unless by medical direction.

INTRATEST:

Potential Complications: N/A

- Avoid the use of equipment containing latex if the patient has a history of allergic reaction to latex.
- Instruct the patient to cooperate fully and to follow directions. Direct the patient to breathe normally and to avoid unnecessary movement.
- Observe standard precautions, and follow the general guidelines in Patient Preparation and Specimen Collection online at Davis*Plus*. Positively identify the patient, and label the appropriate specimen container with the corresponding patient demographics, initials of the person collecting the specimen, date, and time of collection. Perform a venipuncture.
- Remove the needle and apply direct pressure with dry gauze to stop bleeding. Observe/assess venipuncture site for bleeding or hematoma formation and secure gauze with adhesive bandage.
- Promptly transport the specimen to the laboratory for processing and analysis.

POST-TEST:

- Inform the patient that a report of the results will be made available to the requesting HCP, who will discuss the results with the patient.
- ***Nutritional Considerations:*** Abnormal myoglobin levels may be associated with cardiovascular disease. Nutritional therapy is recommended for the patient identified to be at risk for developing coronary artery disease (CAD) or for individuals who have specific risk factors and/or existing medical conditions (e.g., elevated LDL cholesterol levels, other lipid disorders, type 1 diabetes, type 2 diabetes, insulin resistance, or metabolic syndrome). Other changeable risk factors warranting patient education include strategies to encourage patients, especially those who are overweight and with high blood pressure, to safely decrease sodium intake, achieve a normal weight, ensure regular participation in moderate aerobic physical activity three to four times per week, eliminate tobacco use, and adhere to a heart-healthy diet. If triglycerides also are elevated, the patient should be advised to eliminate or reduce alcohol. A variety of dietary patterns are beneficial for people with CAD, and there are many meal-planning approaches with nutritional goals endorsed by theAmerican Diabetes Association (ADA). The Guideline on Lifestyle Management to Reduce Cardiovascular Risk published by the American College of Cardiology (ACC) and the American Heart Association (AHA) in conjunction with the National Heart, Lung, and Blood Institute (NHLBI) recommends a Mediterranean-style diet rather than a low-fat diet. The guideline emphasizes inclusion of vegetables, whole grains, fruits, low-fat dairy, nuts, legumes, and nontropical vegetable oils (e.g., olive, canola, peanut, sunflower, flaxseed) along with fish and lean poultry. 🍁 A similar dietary pattern known as the Dietary Approaches to Stop Hypertension (DASH) diet makes additional

M

recommendations for the reduction of dietary sodium. Both dietary styles emphasize a reduction in consumption of red meats, which are high in saturated fats and cholesterol, and other foods containing sugar, saturated fats, trans fats, and sodium. The ADA also includes a vegetarian diet as well as other potential weight loss diets such as Weight Watchers. 🍁 The nutritional needs of each patient need to be determined individually (especially during pregnancy) with the appropriate HCPs, particularly professionals educated in nutrition.

- Recognize anxiety related to test results, and be supportive of fear of shortened life expectancy.
- Depending on the results of this procedure, additional testing may be performed to evaluate or monitor progression of the disease process and determine the need for a change in therapy. Evaluate test results in relation to the patient's symptoms and other tests performed.

Patient Education:

- Discuss the implications of abnormal test results on the patient's lifestyle.
- Provide teaching and information regarding the clinical implications of the test results, as appropriate.
- Educate the patient regarding access to counseling services.
- Provide contact information, if desired, for the AHA (www.americanheart.org), NHLBI (www.nhlbi.nih.gov), Institute of Medicine of the National Academies (www.iom.edu), and USDA's resource for nutrition (www.choosemyplate.gov). 🍁
- Reinforce information given by the patient's HCP regarding further testing, treatment, or referral to another HCP.
- Answer any questions or address any concerns voiced by the patient or family.
- Teach the patient and family, as appropriate, that muscular dystrophy is an inherited disease.
- Teach the family how to communicate concerns regarding cardiac health and skeletal muscle disease appropriately.

Expected Patient Outcomes:

Understanding

- The patient and family acquire knowledge regarding cardiac or skeletal muscle disease.
- The patient and family state that addressing disease concerns in small segments can assist in finding solutions.

Ability

- The patient and family identify resources available for supportive care when needed.
- The patient demonstrates proficient use of assistive devices as needed for skeletal muscle disease or cardiac disease with limited activity.

Response

- The patient and family comply with the HCP recommendation for family genetic testing to identify those female members at risk for passing the disease to male children.
- The patient complies with the recommendation to use assistive devices to support mobility and decrease fall injury risk.

RELATED STUDIES:

- Related tests include antidysrhythmic drugs, apolipoprotein A and B, ANP, blood gases, BNP, calcium, cholesterol (total, HDL, and LDL), CRP, CK and isoenzymes, CT cardiac scoring, echocardiography, echocardiography transesophageal, ECG, exercise stress test, fundoscopy, genetic testing, glucose, glycated hemoglobin, Holter monitor, homocysteine, ketones, LDH and isoenzymes, lipoprotein electrophoresis, magnesium, MRI chest, MI infarct scan, myoglobin, pericardial fluid analysis, PET heart, potassium, triglycerides, and troponin.
- Refer to the Cardiovascular and Musculoskeletal systems tables online at Davis*Plus* for related tests by body system.

M

Nerve Fiber Analysis

SYNONYM/ACRONYM: NFA.

COMMON USE: To assist in measuring the thickness of the retinal nerve fiber layer, to assist in diagnosing diseases of the eye such as glaucoma.

AREA OF APPLICATION: Eyes.

POTENTIAL MEDICAL DIAGNOSIS

Normal findings
- Normal nerve fiber layer thickness

Abnormal findings related to
- Glaucoma or suspicion of glaucoma
- Ocular hypertension
- Optic nerve disease

CRITICAL FINDINGS: N/A

Find and print out the full study on Fast Find at davispl.us/vanleeuwen7.

Newborn Screening

SYNONYM/ACRONYM: NBS, newborn metabolic screening, tests for inborn errors of metabolism, early hearing loss detection and intervention for newborns.

COMMON USE: To evaluate newborns for congenital abnormalities, which may include hearing loss; identification of hemoglobin variants such as thalassemias and sickle cell anemia; presence of antibodies that would indicate a HIV infection; or metabolic disorders such as homocystinuria, maple syrup urine disease (MSUD), phenylketonuria (PKU), tyrosinuria, and unexplained physical or intellectual disabilities.

AREA OF APPLICATION: Ears for hearing tests.

SPECIMEN: Whole blood for metabolic tests.

NORMAL FINDINGS: (Method: Thyroxine, TSH, and HIV—immunoassay; amino acids—tandem mass spectrometry; hemoglobin variants—electrophoresis)

Hearing Test	
Age	**Normal Findings**
Neonates–3 d	Normal pure tone average of −10 to 15 dB

Thyroid-Stimulating Hormone (TSH)		
Age	**Conventional Units**	**SI Units (Conventional Units × 1)**
Neonates–3 d	Less than 40 micro-international units/mL	Less than 40 milli-international units/L

Thyroxine, Total		
Age	**Conventional Units**	**SI Units (Conventional Units × 12.9)**
Neonates–30 d	5.4–22.6 mcg/dL	69.7–291.5 nmol/L

Hemoglobinopathies	Normal Hemoglobin Pattern
Blood spot amino acid analysis	Normal findings. Numerous amino acids are evaluated by blood spot testing, and values vary by method and laboratory. The testing laboratory should be consulted for corresponding reference ranges.
HIV antibodies	Negative

DESCRIPTION: Newborn screening is a process used to evaluate infants for disorders that are treatable but difficult to identify by direct observation of diagnosable symptoms. The testing is conducted shortly after birth through a collaborative effort between government agencies, local public health departments, hospitals, and parents. Knowledge of genetics assists the nurse in identifying patients and family members who may benefit from additional education, risk assessment, and counseling. Genetics is the study and identification of genes, genetic mutations, and inheritance. For example, genetics provides some insight into the likelihood of inheriting a trait such as blue eyes or a medical condition such as cystic fibrosis (CF), an aminoacidopathy or hemoglobinopathy. Some conditions are the result of mutations involving a single gene, whereas other conditions may involve multiple genes and/or multiple chromosomes. Sickle cell disease is an example of an autosomal recessive disorder in which the offspring inherits a copy of the defective gene from each parent. Further information regarding inheritance of genes can be found in the study titled "Genetic Testing."

Every state and territory in the United States has a newborn screening program that includes early hearing loss detection and intervention (EHDI). The goal of EHDI is to assure that permanent hearing loss is identified before 3 mo of age, appropriate and timely intervention services are provided before 6 mo of age, families of infants with hearing loss receive culturally competent support, and tracking and data management systems for newborn hearing screens are linked with other relevant public health information systems. 🍁 For more detailed information. refer to the study titled "Audiometry Hearing Loss." Testing of interest that is not included in the mandatory list can be requested by a health-care provider (HCP), as appropriate. Confirmatory testing is performed if abnormal findings are produced by screening methods.

Properly collected blood spot cards contain sufficient sample to perform both screening and confirmatory testing. Confirmatory testing varies depending on the initial screen and can include fatty acid oxidation probe tests on skin samples, enzyme uptake testing of skin or muscle tissue samples, enzyme assays of blood samples, DNA testing, gas chromatography/mass spectrometry, and tandem mass spectrometry. Testing for common genetically transferred conditions can be performed on either or both prospective parents by blood tests, skin tests, or DNA testing. DNA testing can also be performed on the fetus, in utero, through the collection of fetal cells by amniocentesis or chorionic villus sampling. Counseling and written, informed consent are recommended and sometimes required before genetic testing.

The adrenal glands are responsible for production of the hormones cortisol, aldosterone, and male sex androgens. Most infants born with congenital adrenal hyperplasia (CAH) make too much of the androgen hormones and not enough cortisol or aldosterone. The complex feedback loops in the body call for the adrenal glands to increase production of cortisol and aldosterone, and as the adrenal glands work harder to increase production, they increase in size, resulting in hyperplasia. CAH is a group of conditions. Most frequently, lack of or dysfunction of an enzyme called 21-hydroxylase results in one of two types of CAH. The first is a salt-wasting condition in which insufficient levels of aldosterone causes too much salt and water to be lost in the urine. Newborns with this condition are poor feeders and appear lethargic or sleepy. Other symptoms include vomiting, diarrhea, and dehydration, which can lead to weight loss, low blood pressure, and decreased electrolytes. If untreated, these symptoms can result in metabolic acidosis and shock, which in CAH infants is called an *adrenal crisis*. Signs of an adrenal crisis include confusion, irritability, tachycardia, and coma. The second most common type of CAH is a condition in which having too much of the androgen hormones in the blood causes female babies to develop masculinized or virilized genitals. High levels of androgens leads to precocious sexual development, well before the normal age of puberty, in both boys and girls.

Inadequate production of the thyroid hormone thyroxine can result in congenital hypothyroidism, which when untreated manifests in severely delayed physical and intellectual development. Inadequate production may be due to a defect such as a missing, misplaced, or malfunctioning thyroid gland. Inadequate production may also be due to the mother's thyroid condition or treatment during pregnancy or, less commonly encountered in developed nations, a maternal deficiency of iodine. Most newborns do not exhibit signs and symptoms of thyroxine deficiency during the first few weeks of life while they function on the hormone provided by their mother. As the maternal thyroxine is metabolized, some of the symptoms that ensue include coarse, swollen facial features; wide, short hands; respiratory problems; a hoarse-sounding cry; poor weight gain and small stature; delayed occurrence of developmental milestones such as sitting up, crawling, walking, and talking; goiter; anemia; bradycardia; myxedema (accumulation of fluid under the skin); and hearing loss. Children who remain untreated usually demonstrate physical and intellectual disabilities. They may have an unsteady gait and lack coordination. Most demonstrate delays in development of speech, and some have behavioral problems.

Hemoglobin (Hgb) A is the main form of Hgb in the healthy adult. Hgb F is the main form of Hgb in the fetus, the remainder being composed of Hgb A_1 and A_2. Hgb S and C result from abnormal amino acid substitutions during the formation of Hgb and are inherited hemoglobinopathies. Hgb S results from an amino acid substitution during Hgb synthesis whereby valine replaces glutamic acid. Hemoglobin C Harlem results from the substitution of lysine for glutamic acid. Hgb electrophoresis is a separation process used to identify normal and abnormal forms of Hgb. Electrophoresis and high-performance liquid chromatography as well as molecular genetics testing for mutations can also be used to identify abnormal forms of Hgb. Individuals with sickle cell disease have chronic anemia because the abnormal Hgb is unable to carry oxygen. The red blood cells of affected individuals are also abnormal in shape, resembling a crescent or sickle rather than the normal disk shape. This abnormality, combined with cell-wall rigidity, prevents the cells from passing through smaller blood vessels. Blockages in blood vessels result in hypoxia, damage, and pain. Individuals with the sickle cell trait do not have the clinical manifestations of the disease but may pass the disease on to children if the other parent has the trait (or the disease) as well.

Amino acids are required for the production of proteins, enzymes, coenzymes, hormones, nucleic acids used to form DNA, pigments such as hemoglobin, and neurotransmitters. Testing for specific aminoacidopathies is generally performed on infants after an initial screening test with abnormal results. Certain congenital enzyme deficiencies interfere with normal amino acid metabolism and cause excessive accumulation of or deficiencies in amino acid levels. The major genetic disorders include PKU, MSUD, and tyrosinuria. Enzyme disorders can also result in conditions of dysfunctional fatty acid or organic acid metabolism in which toxic substances accumulate in the body and, if untreated, can result in death. Infants with these conditions often appear normal and healthy at birth. Symptoms can appear soon after feeding begins or not until the first months of life, depending on the specific condition. Most of the signs and symptoms of amino acid disorders in infants include poor feeding, lethargy, vomiting, and irritability. Newborns with MSUD produce urine that smells like maple syrup or burned sugar. Accumulation of ammonia, a by-product of protein metabolism, and the corresponding amino

N

acids, results in progressive liver damage, hepatomegaly, jaundice, and tendency to bruise and bleed. If untreated, there may be delays in growth, lack of coordination, permanent learning and intellectual disabilities. Early diagnosis and treatment of certain aminoacidopathies can prevent intellectual disabilities, reduced growth rates, and various unexplained symptoms.

CF is a genetic disease that affects normal functioning of the exocrine glands, causing them to excrete large amounts of electrolytes. CF is characterized by abnormal exocrine secretions within the lungs, pancreas, small intestine, bile ducts, and skin. Some of the signs and symptoms that may be demonstrated by the newborn with CF include failure to thrive, salty sweat, chronic respiratory problems (constant coughing or wheezing, thick mucus, recurrent lung and sinus infections, nasal polyps), and chronic gastrointestinal problems (diarrhea, constipation, pain, gas, and greasy, malodorous stools that are bulky and pale colored). Patients with CF have sweat electrolyte levels two to five times normal. Sweat test values, with family history and signs and symptoms, are required to establish a diagnosis of CF. Clinical presentation may include chronic problems of the gastrointestinal and/or respiratory system. CF is more common in Caucasians than in other populations. Testing of stool samples for decreased trypsin activity has been used as a screen for CF in infants and children, but this is a much less reliable method than the sweat test. Sweat conductivity is a screening method that estimates chloride levels. Sweat conductivity values greater than or equal to 50 mEq/L should be referred for quantitative analysis of sweat chloride. The sweat electrolyte test is still considered the gold standard diagnostic for CF.

Biotin is an important water-soluble vitamin/cofactor that aids in the metabolism of fats, carbohydrates, and proteins. A congenital enzyme deficiency of biotinidase prevents biotin released during normal cellular turnover or via digested dietary proteins from being properly recycled and absorbed, resulting in biotin deficiency. Signs and symptoms of biotin deficiency appear within the first few months and can result in hypotonia, poor coordination, respiratory problems, delays in development, seizures, behavioral disorders, and learning disabilities. Untreated, the deficiency can lead to loss of vision and hearing, ataxia, skin rashes, and hair loss.

Lactose, the main sugar in milk and milk products, is composed of galactose and glucose. Galactosemia occurs when there is a deficiency of the enzyme galactose-1-phosphate uridyl transferase, which is responsible for the conversion of galactose into glucose. The inability of dietary galactose and lactose to be metabolized results in the accumulation of galactose-1-phosphate, which causes damage to the liver, central nervous system, and other body systems. Newborns with galactosemia usually have diarrhea and vomiting within a few days of drinking milk or formula containing lactose. Other early symptoms include poor suckling and feeding, failure to gain weight or grow in length, lethargy, and irritability. The accumulation of galactose-1-phosphate and ammonia is damaging to the liver, and symptoms likely to follow if untreated include hypoglycemia, seizures, coma, hepatomegaly, jaundice, bleeding, shock, and life-threatening bacteremia or septicemia. Early cataracts can occur in about 10% of children with galactosemia. Most untreated children eventually die of liver failure.

HIV is the cause of AIDS and is transmitted through bodily secretions, especially by blood or sexual contact. The virus preferentially binds to the T4 helper lymphocytes and replicates within the cells. Current assays detect several viral proteins. Positive results should be confirmed by Western blot assay. This test is routinely recommended as part of a prenatal work-up and is required for evaluating donated blood units before release for transfusion. The Centers for Disease Control and Prevention (CDC) has structured its recommendations to increase identification of HIV-infected patients as early as possible; early identification increases treatment options, increases frequency of successful treatment, and can decrease further spread of disease. 🍁

N

Core Conditions Evaluated

Condition	Affected Component	Marker for Disease	Incidence	Potential Therapeutic Interventions	Outcomes of Therapeutic Interventions
Hearing loss	Damage to or malformations of the inner ear	Abnormal audiogram	1 in 3,000 births	Surgery, medications for infections, removal of substances blocking the ear canal, hearing aids	A shorter period of auditory deprivation has a positive impact on normal development.
Congenital adrenal hyperplasia (CAH) (classical)	Multiple types of CAH; majority have a deficiency of or nonfunctioning enzyme: 21-hydroxylase	17-Hydroxyprogesterone (17-OHP)	1 in 15,000 births (75% have salt-wasting type; 25% have virilization type)	Oral cortisone administration, surgery for females with virilization	Patients who begin treatment soon after birth usually have normal growth and development.
Congenital hypothyroidism	Missing, misplaced, or malfunctioning thyroid gland resulting in insufficient thyroxine; insufficient thyroxine due to maternal	Thyroxine (total), thyroid-stimulating hormone	1 in 3,000–4,000 births	Administration of L-thyroxine	Patients who begin treatment soon after birth usually have normal growth and development.

(table continues on page 1186)

N

Core Conditions Evaluated

Condition	Affected Component	Marker for Disease	Incidence	Potential Therapeutic Interventions	Outcomes of Therapeutic Interventions
	thyroid condition or treatment with antithyroid medications during pregnancy				
Sickle cell disease (SCD) and thalassemia	Variant hemoglobin	Hgb S: amino acid substitution of valine for glutamic acid in the beta-globin chain; Hgb C: amino acid substitution of lysine for glutamic acid in the beta-globin chain; thalassemia: loss of two amino acids in the alpha globin chain or decreased production of the beta globin chain	Hgb S: 1 in 3,700 births; Hgb S/C: 1 in 7,400 births; Hgb S/beta-thalassemia 1 in 50,000 births ✱ (found more often in people of African, Mediterranean, Middle Eastern, and Asian descent and in parts of the world where malaria is endemic)	Care of patients with Hgb S is complex, and the main goal is to prevent complications from infection, blindness from damaged blood vessels in the eye, anemia, dehydration, and fatigue; some thalassemias may require iron supplementation	The goal with treatment is to lessen symptoms. Treatment cannot cure the condition. Symptoms may occur in spite of good treatment.

Inborn Errors of Amino Acid Metabolism					
Argininosuccinic aciduria (ASA)	Deficiency of or nonfunctioning enzyme: argininosuccinic acid lyase	Argininosuccinic acid lyase	1 in 70,000 births	Consultation with a dietitian; low-protein diet supplemented by special medical foods and formula	Patients who begin treatment soon after birth and continue treatment throughout life usually have normal growth and development. Early treatment can help prevent high ammonia levels. Accumulation of ammonia can cause brain damage, resulting in lifelong learning problems, intellectual disabilities, or lack of coordination.

(table continues on page 1188)

N

N

Core Conditions Evaluated					
Condition	**Affected Component**	**Marker for Disease**	**Incidence**	**Potential Therapeutic Interventions**	**Outcomes of Therapeutic Interventions**
Citrullinemia type I	Deficiency of or nonfunctioning enzyme: argininosuccinate synthetase	Citrulline	1 in 57,000 births ✤	Consultation with a dietitian; low-protein diet supplemented by special medical foods and formula	Patients who begin treatment soon after birth and continue treatment throughout life usually have normal growth and development. Early treatment can help prevent high ammonia levels. Accumulation of ammonia can cause brain damage, resulting in lifelong learning problems, intellectual disabilities, or lack of coordination.

Homocystinuria	Deficiency of or nonfunctioning enzyme: cystathionine beta-synthase	Methionine	Less than 1 in 50,000 births (found more often in white people from the New England region of the United States and in people of Irish ancestry)	Consultation with dietitian; diet low in methionine supplemented by special medical foods; administration of vitamin B_6, vitamin B_{12}, folic acid, betaine, and L-cystine	Patients who begin treatment soon after birth and continue treatment throughout life usually have normal growth and development. Treatment may lower the chance for blood clots, heart disease, and stroke. Treatment also lessens the chance of eye problems such as cataract or lens dislocation, which can often be corrected by surgery.

(table continues on page 1190)

N

N

Core Conditions Evaluated

Condition	Affected Component	Marker for Disease	Incidence	Potential Therapeutic Interventions	Outcomes of Therapeutic Interventions
Maple syrup urine disease (MSUD)	Deficiency of or nonfunctioning enzyme group: branched-chain ketoacid dehydrogenase	Leucine and isoleucine	Less than 1 in 100,000 🍁 births (found more often in Mennonite people: about 1 in 380 babies of Mennonite background is born with MSUD; also found more often in people of French-Canadian ancestry)	Consultation with a dietitian; diet low in branched-chain amino acids supplemented by special medical foods and formula, administration of thiamine; liver transplant	Patients who begin treatment soon after birth and continue treatment throughout life usually have normal growth and development. Untreated or delayed treatment results in brain damage and intellectual disabilities.
Phenylketonuria	Deficiency of or nonfunctioning enzyme: phenylalanine hydroxylase (PAH)	Phenylalanine	1 in 10,000 🍁 births (found more often in people of Irish, Northern European, Turkish, or Native American ancestry	Consultation with a dietitian; diet low in phenylalanine supplemented by special medical foods and formula; administration of BH4 (tetrahydrobiopterin),	Patients who begin treatment soon after birth and continue treatment throughout life usually have normal growth and

				which helps the PAH enzyme convert phenylalanine into tyrosine; patients with this condition should avoid foods and vitamins containing the sugar substitute aspartame, which increases blood levels of phenylalanine	development. Some patients may experience delays in learning even after treatment, but without treatment or if treatment is delayed until after 6 mo of age, intellectual disabilities usually result.
Tyrosinemia type 1	Deficiency of or nonfunctioning enzyme: fumarylacetoacetase	Tyrosine	1 in 100,000 births (found more often in people of French-Canadian ancestry)	Consultation with a dietitian; diet low in tyrosine and phenylalanine supplemented by special medical foods and formula; administration of nitisinone to prevent liver and kidney damage; liver transplant	Patients who begin treatment soon after birth and continue treatment throughout life usually have normal growth and development. Without treatment, liver and kidney damage will occur.

(table continues on page 1192)

N

N

Core Conditions Evaluated

Condition	Affected Component	Marker for Disease	Incidence	Potential Therapeutic Interventions	Outcomes of Therapeutic Interventions
		Inborn Errors of Fatty Acid Metabolism			
Carnitine uptake disorder	Deficiency of or nonfunctioning enzyme: carnitine transporter	Free and total carnitine	Less than 1 in 50,000 births	Consultation with a dietitian; diet low in tyrosine and phenylalanine supplemented by special medical foods and formula	Patients who begin treatment soon after birth and continue treatment throughout life usually have normal growth and development. Without treatment, infants may incur brain damage resulting in permanent learning or intellectual disabilities.

Long-chain L-3-hydroxyacyl-CoA dehydrogenase deficiency	Deficiency of or nonfunctioning enzyme: long-chain L-3-hydroxyacyl-CoA dehydrogenase	Acylcarnitines	Extremely rare; actual incidence is unknown (found more often in people of Finnish ancestry)	Consultation with a dietitian; low-fat, high-carbohydrate diet supplemented by special medical foods and formula consumed in small, frequent meals to avoid hypoglycemia; infants may need to be woken up to eat if they do not wake up on their own; administration of medium-chain triglyceride oil (MCT oil), L-carnitine, and DHA (docosahexanoic acid), which may help prevent loss of eyesight	Patients who begin treatment soon after birth and continue treatment throughout life usually have normal growth and development. Continued episodes of hypoglycemia can lead to learning or intellectual disabilities. With treatment, some people still develop vision, muscle, liver, or heart problems.
Medium-chain acyl-CoA dehydrogenase deficiency	Deficiency of or nonfunctioning enzyme: medium-chain acyl-CoA dehydrogenase	Octanoylcarnitine and acylcarnitine	1 in 15,000 ✱ births (found more often in white people from Northern Europe and the United States)	Consultation with a dietitian; low-fat, high-carbohydrate diet supplemented by special medical foods and formula consumed in small,	Patients who begin treatment soon after birth and continue treatment throughout life usually have

(table continues on page 1194)

N

Core Conditions Evaluated

Condition	Affected Component	Marker for Disease	Incidence	Potential Therapeutic Interventions	Outcomes of Therapeutic Interventions
				frequent meals to avoid hypoglycemia; infants may need to be woken up to eat if they do not wake up on their own; administration of MCT oil and L-carnitine	normal growth and development. Continued episodes of hypoglycemia can lead to lack of coordination, chronic muscle weakness, learning or intellectual disabilities.
Trifunctional protein (TFP) deficiency	Deficiency of or nonfunctioning enzyme group: mitochondrial trifunctional protein	3-Hydroxy-hexadecanoylcarnitine	Extremely rare; actual incidence is unknown	Consultation with a dietitian; low-fat, high-carbohydrate diet supplemented by special medical foods and formula consumed in small, frequent meals to avoid hypoglycemia; infants may need	Most newborns with early TFP deficiency die of cardiac or respiratory problems, even when treated. Patients with childhood TFP deficiency who begin treatment

to be woken up to eat if they do not wake up on their own; administration of MCT oil and L-carnitine	soon after birth and continue treatment throughout life usually have normal growth and development. Continued episodes of hypoglycemia can lead to lack of coordination, chronic muscle weakness, learning or intellectual disabilities. Patients with mild/muscle TFP deficiency who begin treatment soon after birth and continue treatment throughout life usually have normal

(table continues on page 1196)

N

Core Conditions Evaluated

Condition	Affected Component	Marker for Disease	Incidence	Potential Therapeutic Interventions	Outcomes of Therapeutic Interventions
					growth and development. This form does not affect intelligence.
Very-long-chain acyl-CoA dehydrogenase deficiency	Deficiency of or nonfunctioning enzyme: very-long-chain acyl-CoA dehydrogenase	Tetradecenoylcarnitine	1 in 30,000 to 100,000 births worldwide; incidence is not higher in any geographic area or ethnic group than in another	Consultation with a dietitian; low-fat, high-carbohydrate diet supplemented by special medical foods and formula consumed in small, frequent meals to avoid hypoglycemia; infants may need to be woken up to eat if they do not wake up on their own; administration of MCT oil and L-carnitine	Patients who begin treatment soon after birth and continue treatment throughout life usually have normal growth and development.

N

Inborn Errors of Organic Acid Metabolism					
• Glutaric acidemia type 1	Deficiency of or nonfunctioning enzyme: glutaryl-CoA dehydrogenase	Glutarylcarn tine	1 in 40,000 births (found more often in people of Amish background in the United States, the Ojibway Indian population in Canada, and people of Swedish ancestry)	Consultation with a dietitian; diet high in carbohydrates, low in protein, especially lysine and tryptophan, supplemented by special medical foods and formula consumed in small, frequent meals; administration of riboflavin, carnitine	Patients who begin treatment soon after birth and continue treatment throughout life usually have normal growth and development.
3-Hydroxy, 3-methylglutaric aciduria	Deficiency of or nonfunctioning enzyme: HMG CoA lyase	Acylcarnitines	Extremely rare; actual incidence is unknown (found more often in people of Saudi Arabian, Portuguese, and Spanish ancestry)	Consultation with a dietitian; diet high in carbohydrates, low in protein, especially leucine, supplemented by special medical foods and formula consumed in small, frequent meals; administration of carnitine	Patients who begin treatment soon after birth and continue treatment throughout life usually have normal growth and development.

(table continues on page 1198)

N

Core Conditions Evaluated

Condition	Affected Component	Marker for Disease	Incidence	Potential Therapeutic Interventions	Outcomes of Therapeutic Interventions
Isovaleric acidemia	Deficiency of or nonfunctioning enzyme: isovaleryl-CoA dehydrogenase	Isovaleryl carnitine	1 in 230,000 births ✤	Consultation with a dietitian; diet high in carbohydrates, low in protein, especially leucine, supplemented by special medical foods and formula consumed in small, frequent meals; administration of glycine, carnitine	Patients who begin treatment soon after birth and continue treatment throughout life usually have normal growth and development.
Methyl malonic acidemias (vitamin B_{12} disorders)	Deficiency of or nonfunctioning enzyme: methylmalonyl-CoA mutase combined with mutations causing defects in vitamin B_{12} metabolism	Propionylcarnitine	1 in 80,000 births ✤	Consultation with a dietitian; diet high in carbohydrates, low in protein, especially leucine, valine, methionine, and threonine, supplemented by special medical foods and formula consumed in small, frequent meals;	Treatment may help some patients but not others. Some infants die even with treatment. Patients who begin treatment soon after birth and continue treatment throughout life

				administration of betaine, carnitine, vitamin B_{12}	may have permanent learning or intellectual disabilities or psychiatric disorders.
Beta ketothiolase	Deficiency of or nonfunctioning enzyme: mitochondrial acetoacetyl-CoA thiolase	3-Methylcrotoryl carnitine	Extremely rare; actual incidence is unknown	Consultation with a dietitian; diet high in carbohydrates, low in protein, supplemented by special medical foods and formula consumed in small, frequent meals; administration of carnitine	Patients who begin treatment soon after birth and continue treatment throughout life usually have normal growth and development.
Propionic acidemia	Deficiency of or nonfunctioning enzyme: propionyl-CoA carboxylase	Acylcarnitines	1 in 100,000 births (found more often in people of Saudi Arabian ancestry and the Inuit Indian population of Greenland) 🍁	Consultation with a dietitian; diet high in carbohydrates, low in protein, especially leucine, valine, methionine, and threonine, supplemented by special medical foods and formula	Patients who begin treatment soon after birth and continue treatment throughout life usually have normal growth and development.

(table continues on page 1200)

N

N

Core Conditions Evaluated

Condition	Affected Component	Marker for Disease	Incidence	Potential Therapeutic Interventions	Outcomes of Therapeutic Interventions
				consumed in small, frequent meals; administration of biotin, carnitine	Some patients, even with treatment, may have seizures, involuntary movement disorders, chronic infections, permanent learning or intellectual disabilities.
Multiple carboxylase (holocarboxylase)	Deficiency of or nonfunctioning enzyme: 3-methylcrotonyl-CoA carboxylase, 2-methylbutyryl-CoA dehydrogenase	3-Hydroxy-isovaleryl carnitine	Less than 1 in 100,000 births	Consultation with a dietitian; diet high in carbohydrates, low in protein, supplemented by special medical foods and formula consumed in small, frequent meals; administration of carnitine	Patients who begin treatment soon after birth and continue treatment through out life usually have normal growth and development.

Other Multisystem Diseases					
Biotinidase deficiency	Deficiency of or nonfunctioning enzyme: biotinidase	Biotinidase	1 in 75,000 to 80,000 births	Consultation with a dietitian; diet supplemented by special medical foods and formula; administration of biotin	Patients who begin treatment soon after birth and continue treatment throughout life usually have normal growth and development.
Cystic fibrosis	Deficiency of or nonfunctioning protein: cystic fibrosis transmembrane conductance regulator protein	CF mutation analysis or immunoreactive trypsinogen	1 in 3,600 to 3,700 births	Consultation with a dietitian; higher calorie diet supplemented by special medical foods and formula, additional hydration, administration of pancreatic enzymes and vitamins; bronchodilators, antibiotics, mucus thinners; percussive therapy, ThAIRapy vest; gene therapy, lung transplant	Patients who begin treatment soon after birth and continue treatment throughout life usually have normal growth and development. The goal with treatment is to lessen symptoms. Treatment cannot cure the condition. Symptoms may occur in spite of good treatment.

(table continues on page 1202)

N

Core Conditions Evaluated					
Condition	**Affected Component**	**Marker for Disease**	**Incidence**	**Potential Therapeutic Interventions**	**Outcomes of Therapeutic Interventions**
Core Conditions Evaluated in Many states					
Galactosemia (classical)	Deficiency of or nonfunctioning enzyme: galactose-1-phosphate uridyl transferase	Galactose-1-phosphate	Greater than 1 in 50,000 births	Consultation with a dietitian; diet free of lactose and galactose supplemented by special medical foods and formula; administration of calcium, vitamin D, and vitamin K	Patients who begin treatment soon after birth and continue treatment throughout life usually have normal growth and development. Some patients may experience delays in learning even after treatment, but without treatment or if treatment is delayed until after 10 days of age, developmental delays and learning disabilities usually result.

This procedure is contraindicated for: N/A

INDICATIONS

Hearing Tests

- Screen for hearing loss in infants to determine the need for a referral to an audiologist.

Blood Spot testing

- Assist in the diagnosis of CAH.
- Assist in the diagnosis of congenital hypothyroidism.
- Assist in the diagnosis of abnormal hemoglobins as with Hgb C disease, sickle cell trait or sickle cell disease, and thalassemias, especially in patients with a family history positive for any the disorders.
- Assist in identifying the cause of hemolytic anemia resulting from G-6-PD enzyme deficiency.
- Detect congenital errors of amino acid, fatty acid, or organic acid metabolism.
- Detect congenital errors responsible for urea cycle disorders.
- Screen for multisystem disorders such as CF, biotinidase deficiency, or galactosemia.
- Test for HIV antibodies in infants who have documented and significant exposure to other infected individuals.

POTENTIAL MEDICAL DIAGNOSIS

Abnormal findings related to

Hearing Test

- Abnormal audiogram ***(related to congenital damage or malformations of the inner ear, infections, residual amniotic fluid or vernix in the ear canal)***

Endocrine Disorders

Increased in:

- Congenital hypothyroidism (TSH) ***(related to decrease in total thyroxine hormone levels, which activates the feedback loop to increase production of TSH)***
- CAH (adrenocorticotropic hormone [ACTH] and androgens) ***(related to an autosomal recessive inherited disorder that results in missing or malfunctioning enzymes responsible for the production of cortisol and which may result in a salt-wasting condition or virilization of female genitalia)***

Decreased in:

- Congenital hypothyroidism (total T4) ***(related to missing or malfunctioning thyroid gland resulting in absence or decrease in total thyroxine hormone levels)***
- CAH (21-hydroxylase) ***(related to an autosomal recessive inherited disorder that results in missing or malfunctioning enzymes responsible for the production of cortisol and which may result in one of several conditions, including a salt-wasting condition or virilization of female genitalia)***
- CAH (cortisol) ***(related to an autosomal recessive inherited disorder that results in missing or malfunctioning enzymes responsible for the production of cortisol and which may result in a salt-wasting condition or virilization of female genitalia)***
- CAH (aldosterone) ***(related to an autosomal recessive inherited disorder that results in missing or malfunctioning enzymes responsible for the production of cortisol and which may result in a salt-wasting condition)***

Abnormal findings related to

Hemoglobinopathies

- Hgb S: Sickle cell trait or sickle cell anemia ***(related to an autosomal recessive inherited disorder that results in a genetic variation in***

the β-chain of hemoglobin, causing a conformational change in the hemoglobin molecule and affecting the oxygen-binding properties of hemoglobin, which results in sickle-shaped red blood cells)

- Hgb SC disease ***(related to an autosomal recessive inherited disorder that results in the presence of an abnormal combination of Hgb S with Hgb C and presents a milder form of sickle cell anemia)***
- Hgb S/β-thalassemias ***(related to an autosomal recessive inherited disorder that results in the presence of abnormal hemoglobin S/β-thalassemia, which combines the effects of thalassemia, a genetic disorder that results in decreased production of hemoglobin and sickle cell anemia, where sickled red blood cells lack the ability to combine effectively with oxygen)***

RBC Enzyme Defect

Decreased in:

- G6PD deficiency ***(usually related to an X-linked recessive inherited disorder that results in a deficiency of glucose-6-phosphate dehydrogenase, which causes a hemolytic anemia)***

Inborn Errors of Amino Acid Metabolism/Disorders of the Urea Cycle

- Aminoacidopathies ***(usually related to an autosomal recessive inherited disorder that results in insufficient or nonfunctional enzyme levels; specific amino acids are implicated)***
- Disorders of the urea cycle; specifically argininemia, argininosuccinic acidemia, citrullinemia, and hyperammonemia/hyperornithinemia/homocitrullinemia ***(usually related to an autosomal recessive inherited disorder that results in insufficient or nonfunctional enzyme levels; specific amino acids are implicated)***

Inborn Errors of Organic Acid Metabolism

- Organic acid disorders ***(usually related to an autosomal recessive inherited disorder that results in insufficient or nonfunctional enzyme levels; specific organic acids are implicated)***

Inborn Errors of Fatty Acid Metabolism

- Fatty acid oxidation disorders ***(usually related to an autosomal recessive inherited disorder that results in insufficient or nonfunctional enzyme levels; specific fatty acids are implicated)***

Other Multisystem Diseases

- Biotinidase deficiency ***(related to an autosomal recessive inherited disorder that results in deficiency of the enzyme biotinidase, which prevents absorption or recycling of the essential vitamin biotin)***
- Cystic fibrosis ***(related to an autosomal recessive inherited disorder that results in insufficient or nonfunctional CF transmembrane conductance regulator protein, which results in poor transport of salts, especially sodium and chloride, and significantly impairs pulmonary and gastrointestinal function)***
- Galactosemia (classical) ***(usually related to an autosomal recessive inherited disorder that results in insufficient or nonfunctional***

N

galactose-1-phosphate uridyl transferase enzyme levels

Infectious Diseases

Positive findings in

- HIV-1 or HIV-2 infection

CRITICAL FINDINGS: N/A

INTERFERING FACTORS

- Specimens for newborn screening that are collected earlier than 24 hr after the first feeding ***(false-negative results related to insufficient time after feeding for the abnormal metabolites to accumulate)*** or from neonates receiving total parenteral nutrition ***(false-negative results if circulating levels of the amino acids are increased above the detectable limit of the test)*** may produce invalid results.
- Specimens for newborn screening that are improperly applied to the filter paper circles may produce invalid results.
- Touching blood spots after collection on the filter paper card may contaminate the sample and produce invalid results.
- Failure to let the filter paper sample dry may affect test results.
- Specimens for newborn screening collected after transfusion may produce invalid results.
- Nonreactive HIV test results occur during the acute stage of the disease, when the virus is present but antibodies have not sufficiently developed to be detected. It may take up to 6 mo for the test to become positive. During this stage, the test for HIV antigen may not confirm an HIV infection.

NURSING IMPLICATIONS AND PROCEDURE

POTENTIAL NURSING PROBLEMS:

Problem	Signs & Symptoms	Interventions
Fear ***(related to diagnosed congenital anomaly of newborn; newborn disease; possibility infant death [HIV, sickle cell, etc.])***	Expression of fear; expresses concern over caring for a disabled child; preoccupation with fear; increased tension; increased blood pressure; increased heart rate; vomiting; diarrhea; nausea; fatigue; weakness; insomnia; shortness of breath; increased respiratory rate; withdrawal; panic attacks	Provide access to social services; provide specific and culturally appropriate education; assist the patient and family to recognize effective coping strategies; assist the patient to acknowledge his or her fear; provide a safe environment to discuss fear; explore cultural influences that may enhance fear

(table continues on page 1206)

Problem	Signs & Symptoms	Interventions
Knowledge ***(related to diagnosis of childhood disability or disease; complexity of treatment; poor understating of provided information; cultural or language barriers; anxiety; emotional disturbance; unfamiliar with medical management)***	Lack of interest or questions; multiple questions; anxiety in relation to disease process and management, including management of disabled child; verbalizes inaccurate information; lack of follow through with directions	Identify patient's, family's, and significant others's concerns about child's diagnosed disease or disability; provide information and support group information on caring for a disabled child; provide information on treatment options related to disease or disability (hearing loss, sickle cell anemia, etc.); provide information related to genetic counseling
Nutrition ***(related to inability to metabolize galactose)***	Lethargy; weight loss; failure to thrive; jaundice; bleeding; developmental delays; speech delays; irritability; convulsions	Provide information for use of lactose-free formula, soy formula, or a protein-based hydrolysate formula; ensure strict avoidance of dairy products, organ meats, MSG, foods with sodium or calcium caseinate, any processed food that includes margarine as an ingredient, and any fermented soy sauce, once off of formula and on a regular diet
Infection ***(related to infant exposure in utero secondary to maternal HIV disease [maternal fetal transmission]; infected mother breastfeeding)***	Positive polymerase chain reaction testing in infants; delay in developmental milestones (walking, crawling, etc.) in toddlers; school-aged children perform poorly; possible neurologic problems with ongoing disease	Administer ordered antiretroviral medication or prescribed treatment modality; discuss family support for treatment of the child and mother; assess infection in other family members and children; educate about the importance of adhering to treatment modalities; consider individual cultures and socioeconomic strategies to foster positive outcomes

PRETEST:

General

- Positively identify the patient using at least two person-specific identifiers before services, treatments, or procedures are performed.
- *Patient Teaching:* Education regarding newborn screening should begin during the prenatal period and be reinforced at the time of preadmission testing. Many birthing facilities and hospitals provide educational brochures to the parents. Physicians and physician delegates are responsible to inform parents of the newborn screening process before discharge. Inform the patient these procedures can assist in evaluating a number of congenital conditions, including hearing loss, thyroid function, adrenal gland function, and other metabolic enzyme disorders. Evaluation may also include HIV antibody testing if not performed prenatally or if otherwise clinically indicated.
- Obtain a history of the patient's health concerns, symptoms, surgical procedures, and results of previously performed laboratory and diagnostic studies. Include a list of known allergens, especially allergies or sensitivities to latex.
- Obtain a list of the patient's current medications, including over-the-counter medications and dietary supplements (see Effects of Natural Products on Laboratory Values online at Davis*Plus*).

Blood Tests

- Review the procedure with the parents or caregiver. Explain that blood specimens from neonates are collected by heel stick and applied to filter paper spots on the birth state's specific screening program card.

Hearing Test

- Review the procedure with the parents or caregiver. Address concerns about pain and explain that no discomfort will be experienced during the test. Inform the parents or caregiver that an audiologist or HCP trained in this procedure performs the test in a quiet room and that the test can take up 20 min to evaluate both ears. Explain that each ear is tested separately by using earphones and/or a device placed behind the ear to deliver sounds of varying intensities.
- ***Sensitivity to social and cultural issues,*** as well as concern for modesty, is important in providing psychological support before, during, and after the procedure.
- Most regulations require screening specimens to be collected between 24 and 48 hr after birth to allow sufficient time after protein intake for abnormal metabolites to be detected, and preferably before blood product transfusion or physical transfer to another facility.

INTRATEST:

Potential Complications: N/A

Hearing Test

- Perform otoscopy examination to ensure that the external ear canal is free from any obstruction (see study titled "Otoscopy").
- Test for closure of the canal from the pressure of the earphones by compressing the tragus. Tendency for the canal to close (often the case in children and elderly patients) can be corrected by the careful insertion of a small, stiff plastic tube into the anterior canal.
- Start the test by providing a trial tone of 15 to 20 dB above the expected threshold to the ear for 1 to 2 sec to familiarize the patient with the sounds. If no response is indicated, the level is increased until a response is obtained, and then it is raised in 10-dB increments or until the audiometer's limit is reached for the test frequency. The test results are plotted on a graph called an audiogram using symbols that indicate the ear tested and responses using earphones (air conduction) or oscillator (bone conduction).

Air Conduction

- In the air conduction test, the tone is delivered to an infant through insert earphones or ear muffins, and the auditory response is measured

N

through electrodes placed on the infant's scalp. Air conduction is tested first by starting at 1,000 Hz and gradually decreasing the intensity 10 dB at a time until there is no response, indicating that the tone is no longer heard. The intensity is then increased 5 dB at a time until the tone is heard again. This is repeated until the same response is achieved at a 50% response rate at the same hertz level. The threshold is derived from the lowest decibel level at which the patient correctly responds to three out of six trials to a tone at that hertz level. The test is continued for each ear with tones delivered at 1,000 Hz, 2,000 Hz, 4,000 Hz, and 8,000 Hz, and then again at 1,000 Hz, 500 Hz, and 250 Hz to determine a second threshold. Results are recorded on a graph called an audiogram. Averaging the air conduction thresholds at the 500-Hz, 1,000-Hz, and 2,000-Hz levels reveals the degree of hearing loss and is called the pure tone average.

Bone Conduction

- Bone conduction testing is performed in a similar manner to air conduction testing; a vibrator placed on the skull is used to deliver tones to an infant instead of earphones as in the air conduction test. The raised and lowered tones are delivered as in air conduction using 250 Hz, 500 Hz, 1,000 Hz, 2,000 Hz, and 4,000 Hz to determine the thresholds. An analysis of thresholds for air and bone conduction tones is done to determine the type of hearing loss (conductive, sensorineural, or mixed).

Otoacoustic Emissions

- In otoacoustic testing, microphones are placed in the infant's ears. Nearby sounds should echo in the ear canal and be detected by the microphones if the infant's hearing is normal.

Filter Paper Test

- Obtain kit and cleanse heel with antiseptic. Observe standard precautions, and follow the general guidelines in Patient Preparation and Specimen Collection online at Davis*Plus*. Use gauze to dry the stick area completely. Perform heel stick, gently squeeze infant's heel, and touch filter paper to the puncture site. When collecting samples for newborn screening, it is important to apply each blood drop to the correct side of the filter paper card and fill each circle with a single application of blood. Overfilling or underfilling the circles will cause the specimen card to be rejected by the testing facility. Additional information is required on newborn screening cards and may vary by testing location. Newborn screening cards should be allowed to air dry for several hours on a level, nonabsorbent, unenclosed area. If multiple patients are tested, do not stack cards. Regulations usually require the specimen cards to be submitted within 24 hr of collection. Observe/assess puncture site for bleeding or hematoma formation, and secure gauze with adhesive bandage.

POST-TEST:

- Inform the parent or caregiver that a report of the results will be made available to the requesting HCP, who will discuss the results with the parents or caregiver.
- ***Nutritional Considerations:*** Instruct the parents or caregiver in special dietary modifications to treat deficiency, and refer parents or caregiver to a qualified nutritionist, as appropriate. Amino acids are classified as essential (i.e., must be present simultaneously in sufficient quantities), conditionally or acquired essential (i.e., under certain stressful conditions, they become essential), and nonessential (i.e., can be produced by the body, when needed, if diet does not provide them). Essential amino acids include lysine, threonine, histidine, isoleucine, methionine, phenylalanine, tryptophan, and valine. Conditionally essential amino acids include cysteine, tyrosine, arginine, citrulline, taurine, and carnitine. Nonessential amino acids include alanine, glutamic acid, aspartic acid, glycine, serine,

N

proline, glutamine, and asparagine. A high intake of specific amino acids can cause other amino acids to become essential.

- *Social and Cultural Considerations:* Recognize anxiety related to test results, and be supportive of parents' or caregiver's perceived loss of impaired activity or independence related to hearing loss or physical limitations and their fear of shortened life expectancy for the newborn. Discuss the implications of abnormal test results on the patient's lifestyle. Provide teaching and information regarding the clinical implications of the test results, as appropriate. Educate the parents or caregiver regarding access to genetic or other counseling services. Provide contact information, if desired, for the March of Dimes (www.marchofdimes.com), National Library of Medicine (www.nlm.nih.gov/medlineplus/newbornscreening.html), general information (newbornscreening.info/Parents/facts.html), and state department of health newborn screening program. There are numerous support groups and informational Web sites for specific conditions, including the National Center for Hearing Assessment and Management (www.infanthearing.org), American Speech-Language-Hearing Association (www.asha.org), ABLEDATA (for assistive technology, sponsored by the National Institute on Disability and Rehabilitation Research, at www.abledata.com), Sickle Cell Disease Association of America (www.sicklecelldisease.org), Fatty Oxidation Disorders (FOD) Family Support Group (www.fodsupport.org), Organic Acidemia Association (www.oaanews.org), United Mitochondrial Disease Foundation (www.umdf.org), Cystic Fibrosis Foundation (www.cff.org), and for AIDS information, the National Institutes of Health (www.aidsinfo.nih.gov) and the CDC (www.cdc.gov). 🍁
- *Social and Cultural Considerations:* Inform parents or caregiver that positive neonatal HIV findings must be reported to local health department officials.
- *Social and Cultural Considerations:* Offer support, as appropriate, to parents who may be the victims of sexual assault. Educate the parents regarding access to counseling services. Provide a nonjudgmental, nonthreatening atmosphere for a discussion during which risks of sexually transmitted infections to the newborn are explained. It is also important to discuss problems the parents may experience (e.g., guilt, depression, anger).
- Depending on the results of these procedures, additional testing may be performed to evaluate or monitor progression of the disease process and determine the need for a change in therapy. Evaluate test results in relation to the patient's symptoms and other tests performed.

Patient Education:

- Reinforce information given by the patient's HCP regarding further testing, treatment, or referral to another HCP.
- Answer any questions or address any concerns voiced by the parents, family, or caregiver.
- Provide information regarding vaccine-preventable diseases where indicated (e.g., diphtheria, hepatitis B, measles, mumps, pertussis, polio, rotavirus, rubella, varicella). Provide contact information, if desired, for the CDC (www.cdc.gov/vaccines/vpd-vac) 🍁 for guidelines on sexually transmitted infections and vaccine preventable diseases.

Expected Patient Outcomes:

Understanding

- The parent or caregiver states the importance of alternative language training (sign language) for an infant with hearing loss as soon as possible to enhance growth and development.
- The parent or caregiver states that failure to refrain from feeding the child foods that include galactose can result in severe disability and death.

Ability

- The parent or caregiver demonstrates proficiency in accessing online resources as a source of ongoing information.

- The parent or caregiver develops a diet free of dairy products to support the child's health maintenance.

Response

- The parent or caregiver agrees to genetic counseling prior to having another child to identify risk of future disability in additional children.
- The parent or caregiver agrees to adhere to HIV treatment plan for self and child.

RELATED STUDIES:

- Related tests include amino acid screen, amniotic fluid analysis, audiometry hearing loss, biopsy chorionic villus, chloride sweat, chromosome analysis, CBC, evoked brain potential studies for hearing loss, genetic testing, glucose-6–phosphate dehydrogenase, hemoglobin electrophoresis, human immunodeficiency virus type 1 and type 2 antibodies, otoscopy, sickle cell screen, TSH, thyroxine total, and US thyroid.
- Refer to the Auditory, Endocrine, Genitourinary, Hematopoietic, Hepatobiliary, and Reproductive systems tables online at Davis*Plus* for related tests by body system.

N

Osmolality, Blood and Urine

SYNONYM/ACRONYM: Osmo.

COMMON USE: To assess fluid and electrolyte balance related to hydration, acid-base balance, and screening for toxins.

SPECIMEN: Serum collected in a gold-, red-, or red/gray-top tube; urine from an unpreserved random specimen collected in a clean plastic collection container.

NORMAL FINDINGS: (Method: Freezing point depression)

	Conventional Units	SI Units (Conventional Units × 1)
Serum	275–295 mOsm/kg	275–295 mmol/kg
Urine (random)	50–1200 mOsm/kg	50–1200 mmol/kg
Urine (24-hr collection)		
Newborn	75–300 mOsm/kg	75–300 mmol/kg
Children and adults	250–900 mOsm/kg	250–900 mmol/kg

DESCRIPTION: Osmolality is a measure of the number of particles in a solution; it is independent of particle size, shape, and charge. Measurement of osmotic concentration in serum provides clinically useful information about water and dissolved-particle transport across fluid compartment membranes. Urine osmolality provides information about the ability of the kidneys to concentrate urine. Urine osmolality, like serum osmolality, can be used to evaluate, monitor, and treat imbalances in fluid and electrolyte concentrations. Osmolality is used to assist in the diagnosis of metabolic, renal, and endocrine disorders. The simultaneous determination of serum and urine osmolality provides the opportunity to compare values between the two fluids. A normal urine-to-serum ratio is approximately 0.2 to 4.7 for random samples and greater than 3 for first-morning samples (dehydration normally occurs overnight). The major dissolved particles that contribute to osmolality are sodium, chloride, bicarbonate, urea, and glucose. Some of these substances are used in the following calculated estimate:

$$\text{Serum osmolality} = (2 \times Na^+) + (\text{glucose}/18) + (\text{BUN}/2.8)$$

Measured osmolality in serum or urine is higher than the estimated value because of other unmeasured organic particles in solution contributing to the osmotic concentration. The osmolal gap is the difference between the measured and calculated values and is normally 5 to 10 mOsm/kg. If the difference is greater than 15 mOsm/kg, consider ethylene glycol, isopropanol, methanol, or ethanol toxicity. These substances behave like antifreeze, lowering the freezing point in the blood, and provide misleadingly high results.

This procedure is contraindicated for: N/A

INDICATIONS

Serum

- Assist in the evaluation of antidiuretic hormone (ADH) function.
- Assist in rapid screening for toxic substances, such as ethylene glycol, ethanol, isopropanol, and methanol.
- Evaluate electrolyte and acid-base balance.
- Evaluate state of hydration.

Urine

- Evaluate concentrating ability of the kidneys.
- Evaluate diabetes insipidus ***a condition related to a dysfunction of the kidneys (nephrogenic diabetes insipidus) or pituitary gland (central diabetes insipidus); unrelated to type 1 or type 2 diabetes.***
- Evaluate neonatal patients with protein or glucose in the urine.
- Perform work-up for kidney disease.

POTENTIAL MEDICAL DIAGNOSIS

Increased in:

- Serum
  - Azotemia ***(related to accumulation of nitrogen-containing waste products that contribute to osmolality)***
  - Dehydration ***(related to hemoconcentration)***
  - Diabetes insipidus ***(related to excessive loss of water through urination that results in hemoconcentration)***
  - Diabetic ketoacidosis ***(related to excessive loss of water through urination that results in hemoconcentration)***
  - Hypercalcemia ***(related to electrolyte imbalance that results in water loss and hemoconcentration)***
  - Hypernatremia ***(related to insufficient intake of water or excessive loss of water; sodium is a major cation in the determination of osmolality)***
- Urine
  - Amyloidosis
  - Azotemia ***(related to decrease in renal blood flow; decrease in water excreted by the kidneys results in a more concentrated urine)***
  - Heart failure ***(decrease in renal blood flow related to diminished cardiac output; decrease in water excreted by the kidneys results in a more concentrated urine)***
  - Dehydration ***(related to decrease in water excreted by the kidneys that results in a more concentrated urine)***
  - Hyponatremia
  - Syndrome of inappropriate antidiuretic hormone production (SIADH) ***(related to decrease in water excreted by the kidneys that results in a more concentrated urine)***

Decreased in:

- Serum
  - Adrenocorticoid insufficiency
  - Hyponatremia ***(sodium is a major influence on osmolality; decreased sodium contributes to decreased osmolality)***
  - SIADH ***(related to increase in water reabsorbed by the kidneys that results in a more dilute serum)***
  - Water intoxication ***(related to excessive water intake, which has a dilutional effect)***
- Urine
  - Diabetes insipidus ***(related to decreased ability of the kidneys to concentrate urine)***
  - Hypernatremia ***(related to increased water excreted by the kidneys that results in a more dilute urine)***
  - Hypokalemia ***(related to increased water excreted by the kidneys that results in a more dilute urine)***
  - Primary polydipsia ***(related to increase in water intake that results in dilute urine)***

CRITICAL FINDINGS:

Serum

- Less than 265 mOsm/kg (SI: Less than 265 mmol/kg)

- Greater than 320 mOsm/kg (SI: Greater than 320 mmol/kg)

Note and immediately report to the requesting health-care provider (HCP) any critical findings and related symptoms. A listing of these findings varies among facilities. Timely notification of a critical finding for laboratory or diagnostic studies is a role expectation of the professional nurse. The notification processes vary among facilities. Upon receipt of the critical finding, the information should be read back to the caller to verify accuracy.

Serious clinical conditions may be associated with elevated or decreased serum osmolality. The following conditions are associated with elevated serum osmolality:

- *Respiratory arrest:* 360 mOsm/kg (SI: 360 mmol/kg)
- *Stupor of hyperglycemia:* 385 mOsm/kg (SI: 385 mmol/kg)
- *Grand mal seizures:* 420 mOsm/kg (SI: 420 mmol/kg)
- *Death:* greater than 420 mOsm/kg (SI: greater than 420 mmol/kg)

Symptoms of critically high levels include poor skin turgor, listlessness, acidosis (decreased pH), shock, seizures, coma, and cardiopulmonary arrest. Intervention may include close monitoring of electrolytes, administering intravenous fluids with the appropriate composition to shift water either into or out of the intravascular space as needed, monitoring cardiac signs, continuing neurological checks, and taking seizure precautions.

INTERFERING FACTORS

- Drugs and other substances that may increase serum osmolality include corticosteroids, glycerin, inulin, ioxitalamic acid, and mannitol 🍁.
- Drugs and other substances that may decrease serum osmolality include bendroflumethiazide, carbamazepine, chlorpromazine, chlorthalidone, cyclophosphamide, cyclothiazide, doxepin, hydrochlorothiazide, lorcainide, methyclothiazide, and polythiazide.
- Drugs and other substances that may increase urine osmolality include anesthetic drugs, chlorpropamide, cyclophosphamide, furosemide, mannitol, metolazone, octreotide, and vincristine.
- Drugs and other substances that may decrease urine osmolality include captopril, demeclocycline, glyburide, lithium, octreotide, tolazamide, and verapamil.

NURSING IMPLICATIONS AND PROCEDURE

PRETEST:

- Positively identify the patient using at least two person-specific identifiers before services, treatments, or procedures are performed.
- ***Patient Teaching:*** Inform the patient that the test is used to evaluate electrolyte and water balance.
- Obtain a history of the patient's health concerns, symptoms, surgical procedures, and results of previously performed laboratory and diagnostic studies. Include a list of known allergens, especially allergies or sensitivities to latex.
- Obtain a list of the patient's current medications, including over-the-counter medications and dietary supplements (see Effects of Natural Products on Laboratory Values online at Davis*Plus*).
- Review the procedure with the patient. Inform the patient that blood specimen collection takes approximately 5 to 10 min; random urine collection takes approximately 5 min and depends on the cooperation of the patient. Urine specimen collection may also be timed. Address concerns about pain and explain that there may be some discomfort during

O

the venipuncture; there will be no discomfort during urine collection.

- *Sensitivity to social and cultural issues,* as well as concern for modesty, is important in providing psychological support before, during, and after the procedure.
- Note that there are no food, fluid, or medication restrictions unless by medical direction.

INTRATEST:

Potential Complications: N/A

- Direct the patient to breathe normally and to avoid unnecessary movement during the venipuncture.
- Observe standard precautions, and follow the general guidelines in Patient Preparation and Specimen Collection online at Davis*Plus*. Positively identify the patient, and label the appropriate specimen container with the corresponding patient demographics, initials of the person collecting the specimen, date, and time of collection. Perform a venipuncture as appropriate.

Blood

- Avoid the use of equipment containing latex if the patient has a history of allergic reaction to latex.
- Perform a venipuncture.
- Remove the needle and apply direct pressure with dry gauze to stop bleeding. Observe/assess venipuncture site for bleeding or hematoma formation and secure gauze with adhesive bandage.

Urine

- Either a random specimen or a timed collection may be requested.

Timed Specimen

- Obtain a clean 3-L urine specimen container, toilet-mounted collection device, and plastic bag (for transport of the specimen container). The specimen must be refrigerated or kept on ice throughout the entire collection period. If an indwelling urinary catheter is in place, the drainage bag must be kept on ice.
- Begin the test between 0600 and 0800 if possible. Collect first voiding and discard. Record the time the specimen was discarded as the beginning of the timed collection period. The next morning, ask the patient to void at the same time the collection was started and add this last voiding to the container. Urinary output should be recorded throughout the collection time.
- If an indwelling catheter is in place, replace the tubing and container system at the start of the collection time. Keep the container system on ice during the collection period, or empty the urine into a larger container periodically during the collection period; monitor to ensure continued drainage, and conclude the test the next morning at the same hour the collection was begun.
- At the conclusion of the test, compare the quantity of urine with the urinary output record for the collection; if the specimen contains less than what was recorded as output, some urine may have been discarded, invalidating the test.
- Include on the collection container's label the amount of urine and test start and stop times.

Clean-Catch Specimen

- Instruct the male patient to (1) thoroughly wash his hands; (2) cleanse the meatus; (3) void a small amount into the toilet; and (4) void directly into the specimen container.
- Instruct the female patient to (1) thoroughly wash her hands; (2) cleanse the labia from front to back; (3) while keeping the labia separated, void a small amount into the toilet; and (4) without interrupting the urine stream, void directly into the specimen container.

Indwelling Catheter

- Put on gloves. Empty drainage tube of urine. It may be necessary to clamp off the catheter for 15 to 30 min before specimen collection. Cleanse specimen port with antiseptic swab, and then aspirate 5 mL of urine with a 21- to 25-gauge needle and syringe. Transfer urine to a sterile container.

O

Blood or Urine

- Promptly transport the specimen to the laboratory for processing and analysis.

POST-TEST:

- Inform the patient that a report of the results will be made available to the requesting HCP, who will discuss the results with the patient.
- *Nutritional Considerations:* Decreased osmolality may be associated with overhydration. Observe the patient for signs and symptoms of fluid-volume excess related to excess electrolyte intake, fluid-volume deficit related to active body fluid loss, or risk of injury related to an alteration in body chemistry. (For electrolyte-specific dietary references, see studies titled "Chloride," "Potassium," and "Sodium.")
- Increased osmolality may be associated with dehydration. Evaluate the patient for signs and symptoms of dehydration. Dehydration is a significant and common finding in geriatric and other patients in whom renal function has deteriorated.
- Recognize anxiety related to test results. Discuss the implications of abnormal test results on the patient's lifestyle. Provide teaching and information regarding the clinical implications of the test results, as appropriate. Educate the patient regarding access to counseling services. Provide contact information, if desired, for the National Kidney Foundation (www.kidney.org). 🍁
- Reinforce information given by the patient's HCP regarding further testing, treatment, or referral to another HCP. Answer any questions or address any concerns voiced by the patient or family.
- Depending on the results of this procedure, additional testing may be performed to evaluate or monitor progression of the disease process and determine the need for a change in therapy. Evaluate test results in relation to the patient's symptoms and other tests performed.

RELATED STUDIES:

- Related tests include ACTH, anion gap, ammonia, ADH, ANP, BNP, BUN, calcium, carbon dioxide, chloride, CBC hematocrit, CBC hemoglobin, cortisol, creatinine, echocardiography, echocardiography transesophageal, ethanol, glucose, ketones, lung perfusion scan, magnesium, phosphorus, potassium, sodium, and UA.
- Refer to the Endocrine and Genitourinary systems tables online at Davis*Plus* for related tests by body system.

Osmotic Fragility

O

SYNONYM/ACRONYM: Red blood cell osmotic fragility, OF.

COMMON USE: To assess the fragility of erythrocytes related to red blood cell lysis toward diagnosing diseases such as hemolytic anemia.

SPECIMEN: Whole blood collected in a green-top (heparin) tube and two peripheral blood smears.

NORMAL FINDINGS: (Method: Spectrophotometry) Hemolysis (unincubated) begins at 0.5% sodium chloride (NaCl) solution and is complete at 0.3% NaCl solution. Results are compared to a normal curve.

POTENTIAL MEDICAL DIAGNOSIS

Increased in:

Conditions that produce RBCs with a small surface-to-volume ratio or RBCs that are rounder than normal will have increased osmotic fragility.

- Acquired immune hemolytic anemias ***(abnormal RBCs in size and shape; spherocytes)***
- Hemolytic disease of the newborn ***(abnormal RBCs in size and shape; spherocytes)***
- Hereditary spherocytosis ***(abnormal RBCs in size and shape; spherocytes)***
- Malaria ***(related to effect of parasite on RBC membrane integrity)***
- Pyruvate kinase deficiency ***(abnormal RBCs in size and shape; spherocytes)***

Decreased in:

Conditions that produce RBCs with a large surface-to-volume ratio or RBCs that are flatter than normal will have decreased osmotic fragility.

- Asplenia ***(abnormal cells are not removed from circulation due to absence of spleen; target cells)***
- Hemoglobinopathies ***(abnormal RBCs in size and shape; target cells, drepanocytes)***
- Iron-deficiency anemia ***(abnormal RBCs in size and shape; target cells)***
- Liver disease ***(abnormal RBCs in size and shape; target cells)***
- Thalassemias ***(abnormal RBCs in size and shape; target cells)***

CRITICAL FINDINGS: N/A

Find and print out the full study on Fast Find at davispl.us/vanleeuwen7.

Osteocalcin

SYNONYM/ACRONYM: Bone GLA protein, BGP.

COMMON USE: To assist in assessment of risk for osteoporosis and to evaluate effectiveness of therapeutic interventions.

SPECIMEN: Serum collected in a red-top tube. Serum from a gold-, red/gray-top tube; plasma from a lavender (EDTA)-pink (K2EDTA), or green (sodium or lithium heparin)-top tube is also acceptable.

NORMAL FINDINGS: (Method: Electrochemiluminescence)

Age and Sex	Conventional Units	SI Units (Conventional Units × 1)
6 mo–6 yr		
Male	39–121 ng/mL	39–121 mcg/L
Female	44–130 ng/mL	44–130 mcg/L
7–9 yr		
Male	66–182 ng/mL	66–182 mcg/L
Female	73–206 ng/mL	73–206 mcg/L
10–12 yr		
Male	85–232 ng/mL	85–232 mcg/L
Female	77–262 ng/mL	77–262 mcg/L

Age and Sex	Conventional Units	SI Units (Conventional Units × 1)
13–15 yr		
Male	70–336 ng/mL	70–336 mcg/L
Female	33–222 ng/mL	33–222 mcg/L
16–17 yr		
Male	43–237 ng/mL	43–237 mcg/L
Female	24–99 ng/mL	24–99 mcg/L
Adult		
Male	3–40 ng/mL	3–40 mcg/L
Female		
Premenopausal	5–30 ng/mL	5–30 mcg/L
Postmenopausal	9–50 ng/mL	9–50 mcg/L

POTENTIAL MEDICAL DIAGNOSIS

Increased in:

- Adolescents undergoing a growth spurt ***(levels in the blood increase as the rate of bone formation increases)***
- Chronic kidney disease ***(related to accumulation in circulation due to decreased renal excretion)***
- Hyperthyroidism (primary and secondary) ***(related to increased bone turnover)***
- Metastatic skeletal disease ***(levels in the blood increase as bone destruction releases it into circulation)***
- Paget's disease ***(levels in the blood increase as bone destruction releases it into circulation)***
- Renal osteodystrophy ***(related to bone degeneration secondary to hyperparathyroidism of chronic kidney disease)***
- Some patients with osteoporosis ***(levels in the blood increase as bone destruction releases it into circulation)***

Decreased in:

- Growth hormone deficiency ***(bone mineralization is stimulated by growth hormone)***
- Pregnancy ***(increased demand by developing fetus results in an increase in maternal bone resorption)***
- Primary biliary cirrhosis ***(related to increased bone loss)***

CRITICAL FINDINGS: N/A

Find and print out the full study on Fast Find at davispl.us/vanleeuwen7.

O

Otoscopy

SYNONYM/ACRONYM: N/A

COMMON USE: To visualize and assess internal and external structures of the ear to evaluate for pain or hearing loss.

AREA OF APPLICATION: Ears.

DESCRIPTION: This noninvasive procedure is used to inspect the external ear, auditory canal, and tympanic membrane. Otoscopy is an essential part of any general physical examination but is also done before any other audiological studies when symptoms of ear pain or hearing loss are present.

This procedure is contraindicated for: N/A

INDICATIONS

- Detect causes of deafness, obstruction, stenosis, or swelling of the pinna or canal causing a narrowing or closure that prevents sound from entering.
- Detect ear abnormalities during routine physical examination.
- Diagnose cause of ear pain.
- Remove impacted cerumen (with a dull ring curette) or foreign bodies (with a forceps) that are obstructing the entrance of sound waves into the ear.
- Evaluate acute or chronic otitis media and effectiveness of therapy in controlling infections.

POTENTIAL MEDICAL DIAGNOSIS

Normal findings

- Normal structure and appearance of the external ear, auditory canal, and tympanic membrane.

  Pinna: Funnel-shaped cartilaginous structure; no evidence of infection, pain, dermatitis with swelling, redness, or itching

  External auditory canal: S-shaped canal lined with fine hairs, sebaceous and ceruminous glands; no evidence of redness, lesions, edema, scaliness, pain, accumulation of cerumen, drainage, or presence of foreign bodies

  Tympanic membrane: Shallow, circular cone that is shiny and pearl gray in color, semitransparent whitish cord crossing from front to back just under the upper edge, cone of light on the right side at the 4 o'clock position; no evidence of bulging, retraction, lusterless membrane, or obliteration of the cone of light

Abnormal findings related to

- Cerumen accumulation
- Ear trauma
- Foreign bodies
- Otitis externa
- Otitis media
- Tympanic membrane perforation or rupture

CRITICAL FINDINGS: N/A

INTERFERING FACTORS

Factors that may impair the results of the examination

- Obstruction of the auditory canal with cerumen, dried drainage, or foreign bodies that prevent introduction of the otoscope.

NURSING IMPLICATIONS AND PROCEDURE

PRETEST:

- Positively identify the patient using at least two person-specific identifiers before services, treatments, or procedures are performed.
- *Patient Teaching:* Inform the patient this procedure can assist in investigating suspected ear disorders.
- Obtain a history of the patient's health concerns (especially known or suspected hearing loss, including type and cause; ear conditions with treatment regimens; ear surgery; and other tests and procedures to assess and diagnose auditory deficit; presence of tympanotomy tube), symptoms (especially pain, itching, drainage), surgical procedures, and results of previously performed laboratory and diagnostic studies. Include a list of known allergens, especially allergies or sensitivities to latex.
- Obtain a list of the patient's current medications (especially antibiotic

O

regimen), including over-the-counter medications and dietary supplements (see Effects of Natural Products on Laboratory Values online at Davis*Plus*).

- Review the procedure with the patient. Inform the caregiver that he or she may need to restrain a child in order to prevent damage to the ear if the child cannot remain still. Address concerns about pain and explain that no discomfort will be experienced during the test. Inform the patient that a health-care provider (HCP) performs the test and that to evaluate both ears, the test can take 5 to 10 min.
- ***Sensitivity to social and cultural issues,*** as well as concern for modesty, is important in providing psychological support before, during, and after the procedure.
- Note that there are no food, fluid, or medication restrictions unless by medical direction.
- Ensure that the external auditory canal is clear of impacted cerumen.

INTRATEST:

Potential Complications: N/A

- Observe standard precautions, and follow the general guidelines in Patient Preparation and Specimen Collection online at Davis*Plus*. Positively identify the patient.
- Instruct the patient to cooperate fully and to follow directions. Ask the patient to remain still during the procedure because movement produces unreliable results.
- Administer ear drops or irrigation to prepare for cerumen removal, if ordered.
- Place adult patient in a sitting position; place a child in a supine position on the caregiver's lap. Request that the patient remain still during the examination. If the patient is a child, the caregiver should be informed that he or she may need to restrain the child in order to prevent damage to the ear if the child cannot remain still.
- Administer ear drops or irrigation to prepare for cerumen removal, if ordered. Assemble the otoscope with the correct-size speculum to fit the size of the patient's ear, and check the light source. For the adult, tilt the head slightly away and, with the nondominant hand, pull the pinna upward and backward. For a child, hold the head steady or have the caregiver hold the child's head steady, depending on the age, and pull the pinna downward. The HCP performing the examination would gently and slowly insert the speculum into the ear canal downward and forward with the handle of the otoscope held downward. For the child, hold the handle upward while placing the edge of the hand holding the otoscope on the head to steady it during insertion. If the speculum resists insertion, withdraw and attach a smaller one.
- Place an eye to the lens of the otoscope, turn on the light source, and advance the speculum into the ear canal until the tympanic membrane is visible. Examine the posterior and anterior membrane, cone of light, outer rim (annulus), umbo, handle of the malleus, folds, and pars tensa.
- Culture any effusion with a sterile swab and culture tube (see "Culture, Bacterial, Ear" study); alternatively, an HCP will perform a needle aspiration from the middle ear through the tympanic membrane during the examination. Other procedures such as cerumen and foreign body removal can also be performed.
- Pneumatic otoscopy can be done to determine tympanic membrane flexibility. This test permits the introduction of air into the canal that reveals a reduction in movement of the membrane in otitis media and absence of movement in chronic otitis media.

POST-TEST:

- Inform the patient that a report of the results will be made available to the requesting HCP, who will discuss the results with the patient.
- Administer ear drops of a soothing oil, as ordered, if the canal is irritated

O

by removal of cerumen or foreign bodies.

- Recognize anxiety related to test results, and be supportive of impaired activity related to hearing loss. Discuss the implications of abnormal test results on the patient's lifestyle. Provide teaching and information regarding the clinical implications of the test results, as appropriate.
- Reinforce information given by the patient's HCP regarding further testing, treatment, or referral to another HCP. Answer any questions or address any concerns voiced by the patient or family.
- Depending on the results of this procedure, additional testing may be performed to evaluate or monitor progression of the disease process and determine the need for a change in therapy. Evaluate test results in relation to the patient's symptoms and other tests performed.

RELATED STUDIES:

- Related tests include antimicrobial drugs, audiometry hearing loss, culture bacterial (ear), and Gram stain.
- Refer to the Auditory System table online at Davis*Plus* for related tests by body system.

Ova and Parasites, Stool

SYNONYM/ACRONYM: O & P.

COMMON USE: To assess for the presence of parasites, larvae, or eggs in stool to assist in diagnosing a parasitic infection.

SPECIMEN: Stool collected in a clean plastic, tightly capped container.

NORMAL FINDINGS: (Method: Macroscopic and microscopic examination) No presence of parasites, ova, or larvae.

DESCRIPTION: This test evaluates stool for the presence of intestinal parasites and their eggs. Some parasites are nonpathogenic; others, such as protozoa and worms, can cause serious illness.

O

This procedure is contraindicated for: N/A

INDICATIONS

- Assist in the diagnosis of parasitic infestation.

POTENTIAL MEDICAL DIAGNOSIS

Positive findings in

- Amebiasis— *Entamoeba histolytica* infection
- Ascariasis— *Ascaris lumbricoides* infection
- Blastocystis— *Blastocystis hominis* infection
- Cryptosporidiosis— *Cryptosporidium parvum* infection
- Enterobiasis— *Enterobius vermicularis* (pinworm) infection
- Giardiasis— *Giardia lamblia* infection
- Hookworm disease— *Ancylostoma duodenale, Necator americanus* infection
- Isospora— *Isospora belli* infection
- Schistosomiasis— *Schistosoma haematobium, S. japonicum, S. mansoni* infection
- Strongyloidiasis— *Strongyloides stercoralis* infection
- Tapeworm disease— *Diphyllobothrium, Hymenolepiasis, Taenia saginata, T. solium* infection

- Trematode disease— *Clonorchis sinensis, Fasciola hepatica, Fasciolopsis buski* infection
- Trichuriasis— *Trichuris trichiura* infection

CRITICAL FINDINGS: N/A

INTERFERING FACTORS

- Failure to test a fresh specimen may yield a false-negative result.
- Antimicrobial or antiamebic therapy within 10 days of test may yield a false-negative result.
- Failure to wait 1 wk after a gastrointestinal study using barium or after laxative use can affect test results.
- Drugs and other substances such as antacids, antibiotics, antidiarrheal compounds, bismuth, castor oil, iron, magnesia, or psyllium fiber (Metamucil) may interfere with analysis.

NURSING IMPLICATIONS AND PROCEDURE

POTENTIAL NURSING PROBLEMS:

Problem	Signs & Symptoms	Interventions
Infection (tapeworm) ***(related to drinking contaminated water; eating food contaminated with fecal matter infested with larva; eating raw or uncooked meat from an infected animal)***	It is possible that there will be no symptoms; nausea; poor appetite; weakness; abdominal pain; diarrhea; weight loss secondary to inadequate nutrient absorption; fever; the presence of a cystic mass or lumps; allergic reactions to the larvae; bacterial infections; neurologic symptoms; seizures	Administer prescribed tapeworm medication (praziquantel (Biltricide), albendazole, nitazoxanide); provide education on how to prevent an infection reoccurrence; emphasize vigilant hand washing
Infection (Giardiasis) ***(related to contact with infected fecal contaminated food, water, or soil; swallowing infected water while swimming [lakes, rivers, streams]; eating uncooked food containing Giardiasis)***	Diarrhea; greasy stools; gas; nausea; abdominal pain/cramps; dehydration	Administer prescribed intravenous fluids and antibiotics; encourage drinking oral liquids; explain the symptoms of dehydration to be monitored for (especially in children); provide education on how to prevent an infection reoccurrence; teach the patient that family members should stay away from those infected with Giardiasis; emphasize vigilant hand washing

(table continues on page 1222)

Problem	Signs & Symptoms	Interventions
Pain ***(related to intestinal infection; inflammation; diarrhea)***	Self-report of abdominal pain; abdominal bloating; abdominal cramping; emotional symptoms of distress; crying; agitation; facial grimace; moaning; irritability; disturbed sleep; diaphoresis; altered blood pressure and heart rate; nausea; vomiting	Collaborate with the patient and health-care provider (HCP) to identify the best pain management modality to provide relief; ensure compliance with taking ordered antibiotic to clear parasitic infection; refrain from activities that may aggravate pain; use the application of heat or cold to the best effect in managing the pain; monitor pain severity
Nutrition ***(related to ingestion of parasitic contaminated food, water)***	Positive stool culture for parasitic infection	Teach the patient to abstain from eating raw food; teach the patient and family to use vigilant hand washing before meals; emphasize the importance of using clean water for food preparation and drinking

PRETEST:

- Positively identify the patient using at least two person-specific identifiers before services, treatments, or procedures are performed.
- *Patient Teaching:* Inform the patient this test can assist in diagnosing a parasitic infection.
- Obtain a history of the patient's health concerns, symptoms, surgical procedures, and results of previously performed laboratory and diagnostic studies. Include a list of known allergens, especially allergies or sensitivities to latex. Document any travel to foreign countries.
- Note any recent therapies that can interfere with test results.
- Obtain a list of the patient's current medications, including over-the-counter medications and dietary supplements (see Effects of Natural Products on Laboratory Values online at Davis*Plus*).
- Review the procedure with the patient. Instruct the patient on hand-washing procedures, and inform the patient that the infection may be contagious. Warn the patient not to contaminate the specimen with urine, toilet paper, or toilet water. Address concerns about pain and explain to the patient that there should be no discomfort during the procedure.
- ***Sensitivity to social and cultural issues,*** as well as concern for modesty, is important in providing psychological support before, during, and after the procedure.
- Instruct the patient to avoid medications that interfere with test results.
- Note that there are no food or fluid restrictions unless by medical direction.

O

INTRATEST:

Potential Complications: N/A

- Instruct the patient to cooperate fully and to follow directions.
- Observe standard precautions, and follow the general guidelines in Patient Preparation and Specimen Collection online at Davis*Plus*. Positively identify the patient, and label the appropriate specimen container with the corresponding patient demographics, initials of the person collecting the specimen, date, and time of collection.
- Collect a stool specimen directly into the container. If the patient is bedridden, use a clean bedpan and transfer the specimen into the container using a tongue depressor.
- Specimens to be examined for the presence of pinworms are collected by the "Scotch tape" method in the morning before bathing or defecation. A small paddle with a piece of cellophane tape (sticky side facing out) is pressed against the perianal area. The tape is placed in a collection container and submitted to determine if ova are present. Sometimes adult worms are observed protruding from the rectum.
- Promptly transport the specimen to the laboratory for processing and analysis.

POST-TEST:

- Inform the patient that a report of the results will be made available to the requesting HCP, who will discuss the results with the patient.
- Recognize anxiety related to test results. Discuss the implications of abnormal test results on the patient's lifestyle. Provide teaching and information regarding the clinical implications of the test results, as appropriate.
- Depending on the results of this procedure, additional testing may be performed to evaluate or monitor progression of the disease process and determine the need for a change in therapy. Evaluate test results in relation to the patient's symptoms and other tests performed.

Patient Education:

- Reinforce information given by the patient's HCP regarding further testing, treatment, or referral to another HCP.
- Educate the patient with positive findings on the transmission of the parasite, as indicated.
- Warn the patient that one negative result does not rule out parasitic infestation and that additional specimens may be required.
- Answer any questions or address any concerns voiced by the patient or family.

Expected Patient Outcomes:

Understanding

- The patient and family state the importance of good hand hygiene to decrease risk of parasitic infection.
- The patient and family state that anal itching during the nighttime could indicate a enterobiasis (pinworm) infection.

Ability

- The patient and family demonstrate proficient hand washing.
- The patient and family describe changes in food and water handling that will need to be taken to prevent parasitic infection.

Response

- The patient and family comply with the request to clean surfaces to help prevent an ova and parasite infection.
- The patient complies with the recommendation to take the entire amount of prescribed antibiotics as appropriate to treat infection.

RELATED STUDIES:

- Related tests include biopsy intestinal, biopsy liver, biopsy muscle, culture stool, fecal analysis, and IgE.
- Refer to the Gastrointestinal and Immune systems tables online at Davis*Plus* for related tests by body system.

O

Oxalate, Urine

SYNONYM/ACRONYM: N/A

COMMON USE: To identify patients who are at risk for renal calculus formation or hyperoxaluria related to malabsorption.

SPECIMEN: Urine from a timed specimen collected in a clean plastic collection container with hydrogen chloride (HCl) as a preservative.

NORMAL FINDINGS: (Method: Spectrophotometry)

	Conventional Units	SI Units (Conventional Units × 11.1)
Children and adults	0–40 mg/24 hr	0–444 micromol/24 hr

POTENTIAL MEDICAL DIAGNOSIS

Increased in:

Conditions that result in malabsorption for any reason can lead to increased levels. Chronic diarrhea results in excessive loss of calcium to bind oxalate. Increased oxalate is absorbed by the intestine and excreted by the kidneys.

- Bacterial overgrowth
- Biliary tract disease
- Bowel disease
- Celiac disease
- Cirrhosis
- Crohn's disease
- Diabetes
- Ethylene glycol poisoning ***(ethylene glycol is metabolized to oxalate and excreted by the kidneys; crystals are present in urine)***
- Ileal resection
- Jejunal shunt
- Pancreatic disease
- Primary hereditary hyperoxaluria (rare)
- Pyridoxine (vitamin B_6) deficiency ***(pyridoxine is a cofactor in an enzyme reaction that converts glyoxylic acid to glycine; deficiency results in an increase in oxalate)***
- Sarcoidosis

Decreased in:

- Hypercalciuria ***(related to formation of calcium oxalate crystals)***
- Kidney disease ***(related to oxalate kidney stone disease)***

CRITICAL FINDINGS: N/A

Find and print out the full study on Fast Find at davispl.us/vanleeuwen7.

Pachymetry

SYNONYM/ACRONYM: N/A

COMMON USE: To assess the thickness of the cornea prior to LASIK surgery and evaluate glaucoma risk.

AREA OF APPLICATION: Eyes.

POTENTIAL MEDICAL DIAGNOSIS

Normal findings

- Normal corneal thickness of 535 to 555 micron

Abnormal findings related to

- Bullous keratopathy
- Corneal rejection after penetrating keratoplasty
- Fuchs' endothelial dystrophy
- Glaucoma

CRITICAL FINDINGS: N/A

Find and print out the full study on Fast Find at davispl.us/vanleeuwen7.

Papanicolaou Smear

SYNONYM/ACRONYM: Pap smear, cervical smear.

COMMON USE: To establish a cytological diagnosis of cervical and vaginal disease and identify the presence of genital infections, such as human papillomavirus, herpes, and cytomegalovirus.

SPECIMEN: Cervical and endocervical cells.

NORMAL FINDINGS: Method: (Microscopic examination of fixed and stained smear) Reporting of Pap smear findings may follow one of several formats and may vary by laboratory. Simplified content of the two most common formats for interpretation are listed in the table.

Bethesda System

Specimen type:

Smear, liquid-based, or other.

Specimen adequacy:

- ***Satisfactory*** for evaluation—endocervical transformation zone component is described as present or absent, along with other quality indicators (e.g., partially obscuring blood, inflammation).
- ***Unsatisfactory*** for evaluation—either the specimen is rejected and the reason given or the specimen is processed and examined but not evaluated for epithelial abnormalities and the reason is given.

General categorization:

- ***Negative for intraepithelial lesion or malignancy.***
- ***Epithelial cell abnormality*** (abnormality is specified in the interpretation section of the report).
- ***Other comments***

P

Bethesda System

Interpretation/result:

1. Negative for intraepithelial lesion or malignancy
   A. ***List organisms causing infection:***
   - *Trichomonas vaginalis;* fungal organisms consistent with *Candida* spp.; shift in flora suggestive of bacterial vaginosis; bacteria morphologically consistent with *Actinomyces* spp.; cellular changes consistent with herpes simplex virus

   B. Other nonneoplastic findings:
   - Reactive cellular changes associated with inflammation, radiation, intrauterine device; glandular cell status post-hysterectomy; atrophy.
2. Epithelial cell abnormalities
   A. ***Squamous cell abnormalities***
   - ASC of undetermined significance (ASC-US) cannot exclude HSIL (ASC-H)
   - LSIL encompassing HPV, mild dysplasia, CIN 1
   - HSIL encompassing moderate and severe dysplasia, CIS/CIN 2 and CIN 3 with features suspicious for invasion (if invasion is suspected)
   - Squamous cell carcinoma

   B. ***Glandular cell***
   - Atypical glandular cells (NOS or specify otherwise)
   - Atypical glandular cells, favor neoplastic (NOS or specify otherwise)
   - Endocervical adenocarcinoma in situ
   - Adenocarcinoma
3. Other
   A. Endometrial cells (in a woman of 40 yr or greater)

Automated review:
Indicates the case was examined by an automated device and the results are listed along with the name of the device.

Ancillary testing:
Describes the test method and result.

Educational notes and suggestions:
Should be consistent with clinical follow-up guidelines published by professional organizations with references included.

P

ASC = atypical squamous cells; ASC-H = high-grade atypical squamous cells; ASC-US = atypical squamous cells undetermined significance; CIN = cervical intraepithelial neoplasia; CIS = carcinoma in situ; HSIL = high-grade squamous intraepithelial lesion; LSIL = low-grade squamous intraepithelial lesion.

DESCRIPTION: The Papanicolaou (Pap) smear is primarily used for the early detection of cervical cancer. The interpretation of Pap smears is as heavily dependent on the collection and fixation technique as it is on the completeness and accuracy of the clinical information provided with the specimen. The patient's age, date of last menstrual period, parity, surgical status, postmenopausal status, use of hormone therapy (including use of oral contraceptives), history of radiation or chemotherapy, history of abnormal vaginal bleeding, and history of previous Pap smears are essential for proper interpretation. Human papillomavirus (HPV) is the most common sexually transmitted virus and primary causal factor in the development of cervical cancer. Therefore, specimens for HPV are often collected simultaneously with the PAP smear. The laboratory should be consulted about the availability of this option prior to specimen collection because specific test kits are required to allow for simultaneous sample collection. HPV infection can be successfully treated once it has been identified. There are three HPV vaccines (Cervarix, Gardasil, and Gardasil 9), usually given as a series of three injections, at 2 and 6 mo after the initial injection. ✦ Vaccination is recommended in the preteen years because the vaccine's protection is most effective if the immune response to HPV develops prior to sexual activity. All three vaccines protect against the HPV strains that carry the highest infection risk (strains 16 and 18), which are associated with approximately 65% to 70% of cervical cancers and the majority of other HPV-related anal/genital cancers. Cervarix is a 2-valent vaccine that targets HPV types 16 and 18; Gardasil is a 4-valent vaccine that targets HPV types 6, 11, 16, and 18; and Gardasil 9 is a 9-valent vaccine that targets HPV types 6, 11, 16, 18, 31, 33, 45, 52, and 58. Gardasil and Gardasil 9 are effective against HPV types that account for another 15% to 20% of cervical cancers; they are also effective against HPV types 6 and 11, the types that cause genital warts. The Centers for Disease Control and Prevention recommends vaccination for males (4-v HPV or 9-v HPV) aged 11 or 12 yr through 21 yr who are not already vaccinated or who have not completed the entire three-dose series; vaccination of males through age 26 yr (4-v HPV or 9-v HPV) for immunocompromised men or men who have oral or anal intercourse with other men; and for females (2-v HPV, 4-v HPV, or 9-v HPV) aged 11 or 12 yr through 26 yr who are not already vaccinated or who have not completed the entire three-dose series. Vaccination can begin at age 9 yr for both males and females. FDA approval was recently received for administration of Gardasil 9 for females aged 9 to 25 yr and males aged 9 to 15 yr. Additional FDA approval has been requested for males aged 16 to 26 yr. The Advisory Committee on Immunization Practices has reviewed the preliminary data and recommended off-label use for males aged 16 to 26 yr. ✦

A wet prep can be prepared simultaneously from a cervical or vaginal sample. The swab is touched to a microscope slide, and a small amount of saline is dropped on the slide. The slide is examined by microscope to determine the presence of harmful bacteria or *Trichomonas*.

A Schiller's test entails applying an iodine solution to the cervix. Normal cells pick up the iodine and stain brown. Abnormal cells do not pick up any color.

Improvements in specimen preparation have added to the increased quality of screening procedures. Liquid-based Pap tests have largely replaced the traditional Pap smear. Cervical cells collected in the liquid media are applied in a very thin layer onto slides, using a method that clears away contaminants such as blood or vaginal discharge. Samples can be "split" so that questionable findings by cytological screening can be followed up with more specific molecular methods like nucleic acid hybridization probes, polymerase chain reaction, intracellular microRNA quantification, or immunocytochemistry to detect the presence of high-risk HPV, *Chlamydia trachomatis, and Neisseria gonorrhoeae*. Computerized scanning systems are also being used to reduce the number of smears that require manual review by a cytotechnologist or pathologist.

There are now some alternatives to cone biopsy and cryosurgery for the treatment of cervical dysplasia. Patients with abnormal Pap smear results may have a cervical loop electrosurgical excision procedure (LEEP) performed to remove or destroy abnormal cervical tissue. In the LEEP procedure, a speculum is inserted into the vagina, the cervix is numbed, and a special electrically charged wire loop is used to painlessly remove the suspicious area. Postprocedure cramping and bleeding can occur. Laser ablation is another technique that can be employed for the precise removal of abnormal cervical tissue.

This procedure is contraindicated for: N/A

INDICATIONS

- Assist in the diagnosis of cervical dysplasia.
- Assist in the diagnosis of endometriosis, condyloma, and vaginal adenosis.
- Assist in the diagnosis of genital infections (herpes, *Candida* spp., *Trichomonas vaginalis,* cytomegalovirus, *Chlamydia,* lymphogranuloma venereum, HPV, and *Actinomyces* spp.).
- Assist in the diagnosis of primary and metastatic neoplasms.
- Evaluate hormonal function.

POTENTIAL MEDICAL DIAGNOSIS

Positive findings in

(See table [Bethesda system])

Decreased in: N/A

CRITICAL FINDINGS: N/A

INTERFERING FACTORS

- The smear should not be allowed to air dry before fixation.
- Lubricating jelly should not be used on the speculum ***because the viability of some organisms is adversely affected by gels and disinfectants.***
- Improper collection site may result in specimen rejection. Samples for cancer screening are obtained from the posterior vaginal fornix and from the cervix. Samples for hormonal evaluation are obtained from the vagina.
- Douching, sexual intercourse, using tampons, or using vaginal medication within 24 hr prior to specimen collection can interfere with the specimen's results.
- Collection of other specimens prior to the collection of the Pap smear may be cause for specimen rejection.
- Contamination with blood from samples collected during the patient's menstrual period may be cause for specimen rejection.

NURSING IMPLICATIONS AND PROCEDURE

POTENTIAL NURSING PROBLEMS:

Problem	Signs & Symptoms	Interventions
Sexuality ***(related to alterations in sexual role secondary to sexually transmitted infection)***	Hesitancy to discuss sexual relationship with significant other	Facilitate a discussion of realistic changes to sexual intimacy associated with sexually transmitted infection; provide a relaxed atmosphere in which to discuss sexuality concerns; provide contact information for a support group
Infection ***(related to unprotected sexual activity; lack of knowledge to take precautions to prevent infection)***	Genital warts	Administer prescribed medication for wart removal (antimitotic gel, immune-enhancing cream); explain to the patient that sometimes the warts will clear on their own
Fear ***(related to potential terminal diagnosis secondary to development of cancer)***	Verbalization of fear; restlessness; increased tension; continuous questioning; increased blood pressure, heart rate, respiratory rate	Evaluate verbal and nonverbal indicators of fear; assess for the cause of fear; acknowledge the patient's awareness of his or her fear; explain all procedures with simple age- and culture-appropriate language; administer prescribed mild tranquilizer; maintain a confident, assured professional manner in all patient interactions
Knowledge ***(related to new condition or diagnosis; lack of familiarity or understanding with disease and treatment)***	Lack of interest or questions; multiple questions; anxiety in relation to disease process and management	Identify sexual orientation; teach the process of disease transmission; teach that infection risk increases with the number of sexual partners over time; identify the patient's sexual activity; discuss importance of notifying sexual partners of exposure to infection; assess for cultural, literacy, or vision and hearing concerns that would interfere with learning; administer

(table continues on page 1230)

P

Problem	Signs & Symptoms	Interventions
		prescribed medication; explore with the patient the value of monogamous relationship to support positive health; teach the importance of taking the prescribed medication in its entirety to resolve infection

PRETEST:

- Positively identify the patient using at least two person-specific identifiers before services, treatments, or procedures are performed.
- ***Patient Teaching:*** Inform the patient this procedure can assist in diagnosing infection or disease of the reproductive system.
- Obtain a history of the patient's health concerns, symptoms, surgical procedures, and results of previously performed laboratory and diagnostic studies. Include a list of known allergens, especially allergies or sensitivities to latex.
- Record the date of the last menstrual period and determine the possibility of pregnancy in perimenopausal women.
- Note any recent procedures that can interfere with test results.
- Obtain a list of the patient's current medications, including over-the-counter medications and dietary supplements (see Effects of Natural Products on Laboratory Values online at Davis*Plus*).
- Review the procedure with the patient. Instruct the patient to avoid douching or sexual intercourse for 24 hr before specimen collection. Verify that the patient is not menstruating. Address concerns about pain and explain that there may be some discomfort during the procedure. Inform the patient that specimen collection is performed by a health-care provider (HCP) specializing in this procedure and takes approximately 5 to 10 min.
- ***Sensitivity to social and cultural issues,*** as well as concern for modesty, is important in providing psychological support before, during, and after the procedure.
- Note that there are no food, fluid, or medication restrictions unless by medical direction.
- Note that if the patient is taking vaginal antibiotic medication, testing should be delayed for 1 mo after the treatment has been completed.
- *Make sure a written and informed consent has been signed prior to the procedure and before administering any medications.*

INTRATEST:

Potential Complications: N/A

- Have the patient void before the procedure.
- Have the patient remove clothes below the waist.
- Instruct the patient to cooperate fully and to follow directions. Ask the patient to breathe normally and to avoid unnecessary movement during the procedure.
- Observe standard precautions, and follow the general guidelines in Patient Preparation and Specimen Collection online at Davis*Plus*. Positively identify the patient, and label the appropriate specimen container with the corresponding patient demographics, initials of the person collecting the specimen, date, and time of collection.
- Assist the patient into a lithotomy position on a gynecological examination table (with feet in stirrups). Drape the patient's legs.
- A plastic or metal speculum is inserted into the vagina and is

P

opened to gently spread apart the vagina for inspection of the cervix. The speculum may be dipped in warm water to aid in comfortable insertion.

- After the speculum is properly positioned, the cervical and vaginal specimens are obtained. A synthetic fiber brush is inserted deep enough into the cervix to reach the endocervical canal. The brush is then rotated one turn and removed. A plastic or wooden spatula is used to lightly scrape the cervix and vaginal wall.

Conventional Collection

- Specimens from both the brush and the spatula are plated on the glass slide. The brush specimen is plated using a gentle rolling motion, whereas the spatula specimen is plated using a light gliding motion across the slide. The specimens are immediately fixed to the slide with a liquid or spray containing 95% ethanol. The speculum is removed from the vagina. A pelvic and/or rectal examination is usually performed after specimen collection is completed.

ThinPrep Collection

- The ThinPrep bottle lid is opened and removed, exposing the solution. The brush and spatula specimens are then gently swished in the ThinPrep solution to remove the adhering cells. The brush and spatula are then removed from the ThinPrep solution, and the bottle lid is replaced and secured.

Chlamydia Vaginal Swab Collection Followed by NAA

- *Care provider specimen:* Collect vaginal fluid sample using the vaginal swab kit by contacting the swab to the lower third of the vaginal wall, rotating the swab for 10 to 30 sec to absorb the fluid. Immediately place the swab into the transport tube, and carefully break the swab shaft against the side of the tube. Tightly screw on the cap.
- *Patient self-collection instructions:* Partially open the package. Do not touch the soft tip or lay the swab down. If the soft tip is touched, the swab is laid down, or the swab is dropped, use a new vaginal swab specimen collection kit. Remove the swab. Carefully insert the swab into the vagina about 2 in. past the introitus, and gently rotate the swab for 10 to 30 sec, making sure the swab touches the walls of the vagina so that moisture is absorbed by the swab. Withdraw the swab without touching the skin. Immediately place the swab into the transport tube, and carefully break the swab shaft against the side of the tube. Tightly screw on the cap.

Chlamydia Endocervical Swab

- Remove excess mucus from the cervical os and surrounding mucosa using the cleaning swab (white shaft swab in the package with red printing). Discard this swab. Insert the specimen collection swab (blue shaft swab in the package with green printing) into the endocervical canal. Gently rotate the swab clockwise for 10 to 30 sec in the endocervical canal to ensure adequate sampling. Withdraw the swab carefully; avoid contact with the vaginal mucosa. Remove the cap from the swab specimen transport tube, and immediately place the specimen collection swab into the transport tube. Carefully break the swab shaft at the scoreline using care to avoid splashing of the contents. Recap the swab specimen transport tube tightly.

Chlamydia Male Urethral Swab

- Note that the patient should not have urinated for at least 1 hr prior to specimen collection. Insert the specimen collection swab (blue shaft swab in the package with the green printing) 2 to 4 cm into the urethra. Gently rotate the swab clockwise for 2 to 3 sec in the urethra to ensure adequate sampling. Withdraw the swab carefully. Remove the cap from the swab specimen transport tube, and immediately place the specimen collection swab into the specimen transport tube. Carefully break the swab shaft at the scoreline using care to avoid splashing of contents. Recap the swab specimen transport tube tightly.

Urine Specimen

- Note that the patient should not have urinated for at least 1 hr prior to specimen collection. Direct patient to provide a first-catch urine (approximately 20 to 30 mL of the initial urine stream) into a urine collection cup free of any preservatives. Collection of larger volumes of urine may result in specimen dilution that may reduce test sensitivity; lesser volumes may not adequately rinse organisms into the specimen. Female patients should not cleanse the labial area prior to providing the specimen. Add urine to the urine collection device. The final volume must be between the two black lines on the device (about 2 mL).

General

- Place samples in properly labelled specimen container and promptly transport the specimen to the laboratory for processing and analysis.

POST-TEST:

- Inform the patient that a report of the results will be made available to the requesting HCP, who will discuss the results with the patient.
- Cleanse or allow the patient to cleanse secretions or excess lubricant (if a pelvic and/or rectal examination is also performed) from the perineal area. Provide a sanitary pad if cervical bleeding occurs.
- Recognize anxiety related to test results, and offer support. Discuss the implications of abnormal test results on the patient's lifestyle. Provide teaching and information regarding the clinical implications of the test results, as appropriate. Educate the patient regarding access to counseling services.
- Decisions regarding the need for and frequency of conventional or liquid-based Pap tests or other cancer screening procedures should be made after consultation between the patient and HCP. The American Cancer Society's (ACS) guidelines for preventing cervical cancer recommend cytological screening every 3 yr for women aged 21 to 29 yr and co-testing for HPV and cytological screening every 5 yr for women aged 30 to 65 yr; no screening is recommended for women who have had a hysterectomy. The most current guidelines for cervical cancer screening of the general population as well as of individuals with increased risk are available from the ACS (www.cancer.org) and the American College of Obstetricians and Gynecologists (www.acog.org). 🍁
- Depending on the results of this procedure, additional testing may be performed to evaluate or monitor progression of the disease process and determine the need for a change in therapy. Evaluate test results in relation to the patient's symptoms and other tests performed.

Patient Education:

- Reinforce information given by the patient's HCP regarding further testing, treatment, or referral to another HCP.
- Provide information regarding vaccine-preventable diseases where indicated (e.g., cervical cancer and sexually transmitted infections such as hepatitis B and human papillomavirus).
- Provide information regarding vaccine-preventable diseases where indicated (e.g., cervical cancer, hepatitis A and B, HPV). Provide contact information, if desired, for the CDC (www.cdc.gov/vaccines/vpd-vac) 🍁 for guidelines on vaccine preventable diseases.
- Answer any questions or address any concerns voiced by the patient or family.

Expected Patient Outcomes:

Understanding

- The patient acknowledges the prescribed medication to treat the infection should be completed in its entirety.

Ability

- The patient displays appropriate coping skills related to changes in future sexual activity.

P

- The patient demonstrates proficiency on applying prescribed medication to genital warts

Response

- The patient agrees to discuss concerns regarding the possibility of social stigma associated with diagnosis.
- The patient agrees to notify sexual partner regarding diagnosis of infection.

RELATED STUDIES:

- Related tests include biopsy cervical, cancer antigens, *Chlamydia* group antibody, colposcopy, culture anal/genital, culture throat, culture urine, culture viral, CMV, cytology urine, laparoscopy gynecologic, US pelvis, and UA.
- Refer to the Immune and Reproductive systems tables online at Davis*Plus* for related tests by body system.

Parathyroid Hormone

SYNONYM/ACRONYM: Parathormone, PTH, intact PTH, whole molecule PTH.

COMMON USE: To assist in the diagnosis of parathyroid disease and disorders of calcium balance. Also used to monitor patients receiving renal dialysis.

SPECIMEN: Serum collected in a gold-, red-, or red/gray-top tube. Specimen should be transported tightly capped and in an ice slurry.

NORMAL FINDINGS: (Method: Immunoassay)

Age	Conventional Units	SI Units (Conventional Units × 1)
Cord blood	Less than 3 pg/mL	Less than 3 ng/L
2–20 yr	9–52 pg/mL	9–52 ng/L
Adult	10–65 pg/mL	10–65 ng/L

DESCRIPTION: Parathyroid hormone (PTH) is secreted by the parathyroid glands in response to decreased levels of circulating calcium. PTH assists in raising serum calcium levels by:

- Stimulating the release of calcium from bone into the bloodstream
- Promoting renal tubular reabsorption of calcium and decreased reabsorption of phosphate
- Enhancing renal production of active vitamin D metabolites which increases calcium absorption in the small intestine

C-terminal and N-terminal assays were used prior to the development of reliable intact or whole molecule PTH assays. A rapid PTH assay has been developed specifically for intraoperative monitoring of PTH in the surgical treatment of primary hyperparathyroidism. Rapid PTH assays have proved valuable because the decision of whether the hyperparathyroidism involves one or multiple glands depends on measurement of circulating PTH levels. Surgical outcomes indicate that a 50% decrease or more in intraoperative PTH from baseline measurements

P

can predict successful treatment with up to 97% accuracy. An intraoperative decrease of less than 50% indicates the need to identify and remove additional malfunctioning parathyroid tissue. In healthy individuals, intact PTH has a circulating half-life of about 5 min. N-terminal PTH has a circulating half-life of about 2 min and is found in minute quantities. Intact and N-terminal PTH are the only biologically active forms of the hormone. Ninety percent of circulating PTH is composed of inactive C-terminal and midregion fragments. PTH is cleared from the body by the kidneys.

This procedure is contraindicated for: N/A

INDICATIONS

- Assist in the diagnosis of hyperparathyroidism.
- Assist in the diagnosis of suspected secondary hyperparathyroidism due to chronic kidney disease, malignant tumors that produce ectopic PTH, and malabsorption syndromes.
- Detect incidental damage or inadvertent removal of the parathyroid glands during thyroid or neck surgery.
- Differentiate parathyroid and nonparathyroid causes of hypercalcemia.
- Evaluate autoimmune destruction of the parathyroid glands.
- Evaluate parathyroid response to altered serum calcium levels, especially those that result from malignant processes, leading to decreased PTH production.
- Evaluate source of altered calcium metabolism.

POTENTIAL MEDICAL DIAGNOSIS

Increased in:

- Fluorosis ***(skeletal fluorosis can cause a condition resembling secondary hyperparathyroidism, disruption in calcium homeostasis, and excessive PTH production)***
- Hyperparathyroidism: primary, secondary, or tertiary ***(all result in excess PTH production)***
- Hypocalcemia ***(compensatory increase in PTH in response to low calcium levels)***
- Pseudogout ***(calcium is lost due to deposits in the joint; decrease in calcium stimulates PTH production)***
- Pseudohypoparathyroidism ***(related to a congenital defect of the kidney that prevents a normal response to PTH in the presence of low calcium levels, signaling the parathyroid glands to secrete additional PTH)***
- Zollinger-Ellison syndrome ***(related to poor intestinal absorption of calcium and vitamin D; decreased calcium stimulates PTH production)***

Decreased in:

- Autoimmune destruction of the parathyroids ***(related to decreased parathyroid function)***
- DiGeorge's syndrome ***(related to hypoparathyroidism)***
- Hypercalcemia for any reason (e.g., tumors of the bone, breast, lung, kidney, pancreas, ovary) ***(compensatory response to high calcium levels)***
- Hyperthyroidism ***(related to increased calcium from bone loss; increased calcium levels inhibit PTH production)***
- Hypomagnesemia ***(magnesium is a calcium channel blocker; low magnesium levels allow for***

P

increased calcium, which inhibits PTH production)

- Nonparathyroid hypercalcemia (in the absence of kidney disease) ***(increased calcium levels inhibit PTH production)***
- Sarcoidosis ***(related to increased calcium levels)***
- Secondary hypoparathyroidism due to surgery

CRITICAL FINDINGS: N/A

INTERFERING FACTORS

- Drugs and other substances that may increase PTH levels include anticonvulsants, clodronate, estrogen/progestin therapy, foscarnet, furosemide, hydrocortisone, isoniazid, lithium, nifedipine, octreotide, pamidronate, phosphates, prednisone, rifampin, steroids, tamoxifen, and verapamil.
- Drugs and other substances that may decrease PTH levels include alfacalcidol, aluminum hydroxide, calcitriol, cimetidine, diltiazem, magnesium sulfate, parathyroid hormone, pindolol, prednisone, propranolol, and vitamin D.
- PTH levels are subject to diurnal variation, with highest levels occurring in the morning.
- PTH levels should always be measured in conjunction with calcium for proper interpretation.

NURSING IMPLICATIONS AND PROCEDURE

POTENTIAL NURSING PROBLEMS:

Problem	Signs & Symptoms	Interventions
Pain ***(related to low circulating parathyroid hormone levels; elevated circulating parathyroid hormone secondary to hyperplasia or adenoma of the parathyroid gland)***	**Deficit:** Muscle spasms; carpopedal spasms; abdominal cramping; tetany; easy fracture risk. **Excess:** Abdominal pain; peptic ulcer formation; constipation	Monitor and trend serum calcium levels; monitor and trend serum phosphorus levels; collaborate with pharmacist and health-care provider (HCP) to pharmacologically manage calcium levels; monitor and trend serum parathyroid hormone levels
Sensory perception ***(related to low circulating parathyroid hormone levels)***	**Deficit:** paresthesia of lips, hands, and feet; hyperactive reflexes	Monitor and trend serum calcium levels; monitor and trend serum phosphorus levels; collaborate with pharmacist and HCP to pharmacologically manage calcium levels; monitor and trend serum parathyroid hormone levels

(table continues on page 1236)

P

Problem	Signs & Symptoms	Interventions
Nutrition ***(related to inability to digest foods, metabolize foods, ingest foods; refusal to eat; increased metabolic needs associated with disease process; lack of understanding; inability to obtain healthy foods)***	Unintended weight loss; current weight is 20% below ideal weight; pale, dry skin; dry mucous membranes; documented inadequate caloric intake; subcutaneous tissue loss; hair pulls out easily; paresthesia	Record accurate daily weight at the same time each day with the same scale; obtain an accurate nutritional history; assess attitude toward eating; promote a dietary consult to evaluate current eating habits and best method of nutritional supplementation; develop short-term and long-term eating strategies; monitor nutritional laboratory values such as albumin, transferrin, red blood cells, white blood cells, and serum electrolytes; discourage caffeinated and carbonated beverages; assess swallowing ability; encourage cultural home foods; provide a pleasant environment for eating; alter food seasoning to enhance flavor; administer parenteral or enteral nutrition as prescribed

PRETEST:

- Positively identify the patient using at least two person-specific identifiers before services, treatments, or procedures are performed.
- *Patient Teaching:* Inform the patient this test can assist in diagnosing parathyroid disease.
- Obtain a history of the patient's health concerns, symptoms, surgical procedures, and results of previously performed laboratory and diagnostic studies. Include a list of known allergens, especially allergies or sensitivities to latex.
- Obtain a list of the patient's current medications, including over-the-counter medications and dietary supplements (see Effects of Natural Products on Laboratory Values online at Davis*Plus*).
- Review the procedure with the patient. In most patients with primary hyperparathyroidism, it is usually a single gland, rather than multiple of the four glands present, that is abnormal. Removal of abnormal glands, combined with intraoperative PTH monitoring, has become the surgical treatment of choice. Inform the surgical patient that a baseline PTH level will be collected prior to resection of the abnormal parathyroid glands. Explain that additional specimens will be collected during the procedure to indicate that all abnormal parathyroid tissue has been removed and the procedure can be concluded. The protocol may vary among HCPs regarding when the baseline level should be drawn (i.e., prior to anesthesia or

P

prior to incision). The amount of change between the baseline and intraoperative values considered adequate for determining successful, complete resection of the abnormal tissue may also vary by HCP; a decrease of 50% is typically used as a cutoff. Early-morning specimen collection is recommended because of the diurnal variation in PTH levels. Inform the patient that specimen collection takes approximately 5 to 10 min. Address concerns about pain and explain that there may be some discomfort during the venipuncture.

- ***Sensitivity to social and cultural issues,*** as well as concern for modesty, is important in providing psychological support before, during, and after the procedure.
- Note that there are no food, fluid, or medication restrictions unless by medical direction.
- Prepare an ice slurry in a cup or plastic bag to have on hand for immediate transport of the specimen to the laboratory.

INTRATEST:

Potential Complications: N/A

- Avoid the use of equipment containing latex if the patient has a history of allergic reaction to latex.
- Instruct the patient to cooperate fully and to follow directions. Direct the patient to breathe normally and to avoid unnecessary movement.
- Observe standard precautions, and follow the general guidelines in Patient Preparation and Specimen Collection online at Davis*Plus*. Positively identify the patient, and label the appropriate specimen container with the corresponding patient demographics, initials of the person collecting the specimen, date, and time of collection. Perform a venipuncture.
- Remove the needle and apply direct pressure with dry gauze to stop bleeding. Observe/assess venipuncture site for bleeding or hematoma formation and secure gauze with adhesive bandage.
- Promptly transport the specimen to the laboratory for processing and analysis. The sample should be placed in an ice slurry immediately after collection. Information on the specimen label should be protected from water in the ice slurry by first placing the specimen in a protective plastic bag.

POST-TEST:

- Inform the patient that a report of the results will be made available to the requesting HCP, who will discuss the results with the patient.
- ***Nutritional Considerations:*** Patients with abnormal parathyroid levels are also likely to experience the effects of calcium-level imbalances. Instruct the patient to report signs and symptoms of hypocalcemia and hypercalcemia to the HCP. (For critical findings, signs, and symptoms of calcium imbalance and for nutritional information, see studies titled "Calcium, Blood, Total and Ionized" and "Calcium, Urine.")
- Depending on the results of this procedure, additional testing may be performed to evaluate or monitor progression of the disease process and determine the need for a change in therapy. Evaluate test results in relation to the patient's symptoms and other tests performed.

Patient Education:

- Instruct the patient to resume usual diet, as directed by the HCP.
- Reinforce information given by the patient's HCP regarding further testing, treatment, or referral to another HCP.
- Recognize anxiety related to test results and answer any questions or address any concerns voiced by the patient or family.
- Teach the patient and family about the health risks associated with elevated and deficit parathyroid levels.

P

Expected Patient Outcomes:

Understanding

- The patient and family state symptoms of parathyroid disease that should be reported to the HCP.
- The patient and family state the cause of sensory perception loss associated with a deficit of parathyroid hormone.

Ability

- The patient demonstrates proficiency in self-administration of prescribed dietary supplements.
- The patient and family demonstrate proficiency in selecting a diet that supports appropriate levels of circulating serum calcium.

Response

- The patient complies with recommended follow-up laboratory studies to trend the disease process and tailor therapeutic interventions.
- The patient complies with recommendation to attend support groups to assist in disease management and coping.

RELATED STUDIES:

- Related tests include ALP, arthroscopy, calcitonin, calcium, collagen cross-linked telopeptides, evoked brain potentials, fecal fat, gastric emptying scan, gastric acid stimulation, gastrin stimulation test, parathyroid scan, phosphorus, RAIU, synovial fluid analysis, TSH, thyroxine, US thyroid and parathyroid, uric acid, UA, and vitamin D.
- Refer to the Endocrine System table online at Davis*Plus* for related tests by body system.

Parathyroid Scan

SYNONYM/ACRONYM: Parathyroid scintiscan.

COMMON USE: To assess the parathyroid gland toward diagnosing cancer and to perform postoperative evaluation of the parathyroid gland.

AREA OF APPLICATION: Parathyroid.

DESCRIPTION: Parathyroid scanning is performed to assist in the preoperative identification and localization of the parathyroid glands. Parathyroid hyperplasia has the effect of enlarging all four glands; parathyroid adenoma results in enlargement of a single gland while suppressing growth of the unaffected glands. The scan is also performed after surgery to verify the presence of the parathyroid gland in children and adults after thyroidectomy.

The radionuclide (iodine-123, technetium-99m (Tc-99m) pertechnetate, Tc-99m sestamibi, or a combination of the three radionuclides) is administered either orally or by intravenous (IV) 10 to 20 min before the imaging is performed. There are two types of parathyroid scan: single-tracer double-phase (STDP) scan and double-tracer subtraction test (DTST). In STDP, images are taken at 15 min and 3 hr after the Tc-99m sestamibi is injected. The tracer is observed in both the thyroid and parathyroid tissue at 15 min but is only retained and observed in abnormal parathyroid tissue after 3 hr. In DTST, images are taken about 15 min after administration of either iodine-123 or technetium-99m

P

(Tc-99m) pertechnetate where it can be observed that the thyroid gland has taken up the radionuclide; Tc-99m sestamibi is then injected and is taken up by both the thyroid and the parathyroid tissue. A second set of images is taken, and the first image is "subtracted" from the second so that the image of the thyroid is removed and images of the parathyroid glands remain.

Fine-needle aspiration biopsy guided by ultrasound is occasionally necessary to differentiate thyroid pathology, as well as pathology of other tissues, from parathyroid neoplasia.

This procedure is contraindicated for

Patients who are pregnant or suspected of being pregnant, unless the potential benefits of a procedure using radiation far outweigh the risk of radiation exposure to the fetus and mother.

INDICATIONS

- Aid in the diagnosis of hyperparathyroidism.
- Differentiate between extrinsic and intrinsic parathyroid adenoma but not between benign and malignant conditions.
- Evaluate the parathyroid in patients with severe hypercalcemia or in patients before parathyroidectomy.

POTENTIAL MEDICAL DIAGNOSIS

Normal findings

- No areas of increased perfusion or uptake in the thyroid or parathyroid

Abnormal findings related to

- Intrinsic and extrinsic parathyroid adenomas

CRITICAL FINDINGS: N/A

INTERFERING FACTORS

Factors that may alter the results of the study

- Inability of the patient to cooperate or remain still during the procedure because of age, significant pain, or mental status.
- Ingestion of foods containing iodine (e.g., iodized salt) and medications containing iodine (e.g., cough syrup, potassium iodide, vitamins, Lugol's solution, thyroid replacement medications), which can decrease uptake of the radionuclide.
- Other nuclear scans or iodinated contrast medium radiographic studies done within the previous 24 to 48 hr.
- Metallic objects (e.g., jewelry, body rings) within the examination field, which may inhibit organ visualization and cause unclear images.

Other considerations

- Improper injection of the radionuclide that allows the tracer to seep deep into the muscle tissue produces erroneous hot spots.

NURSING IMPLICATIONS AND PROCEDURE

PRETEST:

- Positively identify the patient using at least two person-specific identifiers before services, treatments, or procedures are performed.
- ***Patient Teaching:*** Inform the patient this procedure can assist in diagnosing parathyroid disease.
- Obtain a history of the patient's health concerns, symptoms, surgical procedures, and results of previously performed laboratory and diagnostic studies. Include a list of known allergens, especially allergies or sensitivities to latex, anesthetics, sedatives, or radionuclides.
- Note any recent procedures that can interfere with test results, including examinations using iodinated contrast medium or radioactive nuclides.

P

- Obtain a history of the patient's endocrine system, symptoms, and results of previously performed laboratory tests and diagnostic and surgical procedures.
- Record the date of the last menstrual period and determine the possibility of pregnancy in perimenopausal women.
- Obtain a list of the patient's current medications, including over-the-counter medications and dietary supplements (see Effects of Natural Products on Laboratory Values online at Davis*Plus*).
- Review the procedure with the patient. Address concerns about pain related to the procedure and explain that some pain may be experienced during the test. Inform the patient that the procedure is performed in a nuclear medicine department, usually by a health-care provider (HCP) specializing in this procedure, with support staff, and takes approximately 30 to 60 min.
- ***Sensitivity to social and cultural issues,*** as well as concern for modesty, is important in providing psychological support before, during, and after the procedure.
- Explain that an IV line may be inserted to allow infusion of fluids such as saline, anesthetics, sedatives, radionuclides, medications used in the procedure, or emergency medications.
- Instruct the patient to remove jewelry and other metallic objects from the area to be examined.
- Note that there are no food, fluid, or medication restrictions unless by medical direction.
- *Make sure a written and informed consent has been signed prior to the procedure and before administering any medications.*

INTRATEST:

Potential Complications:

Although it is rare, there is the possibility of allergic reaction to the radionuclide. Have emergency equipment and medications readily available. If the patient has a history of allergic reactions to any substance or drug, administer ordered prophylactic steroids or antihistamines before the procedure.

Establishing an IV site and injection of radionuclides is an invasive procedure. Complications are rare but do include bleeding from the puncture site ***related to a bleeding disorder, or the effects of natural products and medications with known anticoagulant, antiplatelet, and thrombolytic properties;*** hematoma ***related to blood leakage into the tissue following needle insertion;*** infection ***that might occur if bacteria from the skin surface is introduced at the puncture site;*** or nerve injury ***that might occur if the needle strikes a nerve.***

- Observe standard precautions, and follow the general guidelines in Patient Preparation and Specimen Collection online at Davis*Plus*. Positively identify the patient.
- Ensure that the patient has removed all external metallic objects from the area to be examined prior to the procedure.
- Instruct the patient to void prior to the procedure and to change into the gown, robe, and foot coverings provided.
- Record baseline vital signs and assess neurological status. Protocols may vary among facilities.
- Establish an IV fluid line for the injection of saline, anesthetics, sedatives, radionuclides, or emergency medications.
- Avoid the use of equipment containing latex if the patient has a history of allergic reaction to latex.
- Have emergency equipment readily available.
- Instruct the patient to cooperate fully and to follow directions. Instruct the patient to remain still throughout the procedure because movement produces unreliable results.
- Observe that technetium-99m (Tc-99m) pertechnetate is injected IV before DTST scanning.

- Place the patient in a supine position under a radionuclide gamma camera. Images are preformed 15 min after the injection.
- With the patient in the same position, Tc-99m sestamibi is injected, and a second image is obtained after 10 min.
- Iodine-123 may be administered orally in place of Tc-99m pertechnetate; the imaging sequence is performed as described previously.
- Remove the needle or catheter and apply a pressure dressing over the puncture site.
- Observe/assess the needle/catheter insertion site for bleeding, inflammation, or hematoma formation.

POST-TEST:

- Inform the patient that a report of the results will be made available to the requesting HCP, who will discuss the results with the patient.
- Observe/assess the needle/catheter insertion site for bleeding, inflammation, or hematoma formation.
- Instruct the patient in the care and assessment of the injection site.
- Advise the patient to drink increased amounts of fluids for 24 to 48 hr to eliminate the radionuclide from the body, unless contraindicated. Tell the patient that radionuclide is eliminated from the body within 6 to 24 hr.
- If a woman who is breastfeeding must have a nuclear scan, she should not breastfeed the infant until the radionuclide has been eliminated. This could take as long as 3 days. She should be instructed to express the milk and discard it during the 3-day period to prevent cessation of milk production.
- Instruct the patient to flush the toilet immediately and to meticulously wash hands with soap and water after each voiding for 24 hr after the procedure.
- Instruct all caregivers to wear gloves when discarding urine for 24 hr after the procedure. Wash gloved hands with soap and water before removing gloves; then wash ungloved hands.
- Recognize anxiety related to test results, and be supportive of perceived loss of independent function. Discuss the implications of abnormal test results on the patient's lifestyle. Provide teaching and information regarding the clinical implications of the test results, as appropriate.
- Reinforce information given by the patient's HCP regarding further testing, treatment, or referral to another HCP. Answer any questions or address any concerns voiced by the patient or family.
- Depending on the results of this procedure, additional testing may be needed to evaluate or monitor progression of the disease process and determine the need for a change in therapy. Evaluate test results in relation to the patient's symptoms and other tests performed.

RELATED STUDIES:

- Related tests include calcitonin, calcium, CT thoracic and MRI chest, PTH, phosphorus, US thyroid and parathyroid, and vitamin D.
- Refer to the Endocrine System table online at Davis*Plus* for related tests by body system.

P

Partial Thromboplastin Time, Activated

SYNONYM/ACRONYM: aPTT, APTT.

COMMON USE: To assist in assessing coagulation disorders and monitor the effectiveness of therapeutic interventions.

SPECIMEN: Plasma collected in a completely filled blue-top (3.2% sodium citrate) tube. If the patient's hematocrit exceeds 55%, the volume of citrate in the collection tube must be adjusted.

NORMAL FINDINGS: (Method: Clot detection) 25 to 35 sec. The aPTT is slightly prolonged in infants and children and is slightly shortened in older adults. Reference ranges vary with respect to the equipment and reagents used to perform the assay. For the patient on anticoagulants, therapeutic levels of heparin are achieved by adjusting the dosage so the aPTT value is 1.5 to 2.5 times the normal.

DESCRIPTION: The activated partial thromboplastin time (aPTT) test evaluates the function of the contact activation pathway, formerly known as intrinsic pathway (factors XII, XI, IX, VIII, prekallikrein, and high molecular weight kininogen) and the common pathway (factors V, X, II, and I) of the coagulation sequence. The aPTT time represents the time required for formation of a firm fibrin clot after tissue thromboplastin reagents and calcium are added to a plasma specimen. The aPTT is abnormal in 90% of patients with coagulation disorders and is useful in monitoring effective inactivation of factor II (thrombin) by heparin therapy. The test is prolonged when there is a 30% to 40% deficiency in one of the factors required or when factor inhibitors (e.g., antithrombin III, protein C, or protein S) are present. The aPTT and prothrombin time (PT) tests assist in identifying the cause of or tendency for bleeding as related to coagulation defects. A comparison between the results of aPTT and PT tests can allow some inferences to be made that a factor deficiency exists. A normal aPTT with a prolonged PT can occur only with factor VII deficiency. A prolonged aPTT with a normal PT could indicate a deficiency in factors XII, XI, IX, VIII, and VIII:C (von Willebrand factor). Factor deficiencies can also be identified by correction or substitution studies using normal serum. These studies are easy to perform and are accomplished by adding plasma from a healthy patient to a sample from a patient suspected to be factor deficient. When the aPTT is repeated and is corrected, or is within the reference range, it can be assumed that the prolonged aPTT is caused by a factor deficiency. If the result remains uncorrected, the prolonged aPTT is most likely due to a circulating anticoagulant. (For more information on factor deficiencies, see the "Coagulation Factors" study.)

This procedure is contraindicated for: N/A

INDICATIONS

- Detect congenital deficiencies in clotting factors, as seen in diseases such as hemophilia A (factor VIII) and hemophilia B (factor IX).
- Evaluate response to anticoagulant therapy with heparin or warfarin derivatives.
- Identify individuals who may be prone to bleeding during surgical, obstetric, dental, or invasive diagnostic procedures.
- Identify the possible cause of abnormal bleeding, such as epistaxis, hematoma, gingival bleeding, hematuria, and menorrhagia.

P

- Monitor the hemostatic effects of conditions such as liver disease, protein deficiency, and fat malabsorption.

POTENTIAL MEDICAL DIAGNOSIS

Prolonged in

- Afibrinogenemia, dysfibrinoginemia, or hypofibrinogenemia ***(related to insufficient levels of fibrinogen, which is required for clotting)***
- Circulating anticoagulants ***(related to the presence of coagulation factor inhibitors, e.g., developed from long-term factor VIII therapy, or circulating anticoagulants associated with conditions like tuberculosis, systemic lupus erythematosus, rheumatoid arthritis, and chronic glomerulonephritis)***
- Circulating products of fibrin and fibrinogen degradation ***(related to the presence of circulating breakdown products of fibrin)***
- Disseminated intravascular coagulation ***(related to increased consumption of clotting factors)***
- Factor deficiencies ***(related to insufficient levels of coagulation factors)***
- Patients on hemodialysis ***(related to the anticoagulant effect of heparin)***
- Severe liver disease ***(insufficient production of clotting factors related to liver damage)***
- Vitamin K deficiency ***(related to insufficient vitamin K levels required for clotting)***
- Von Willebrand's disease ***(related to a congenital deficiency of clotting factors)***

CRITICAL FINDINGS:

- *Adults and children:* Greater than 70 sec

Note and immediately report to the requesting health-care provider (HCP) any critical findings and related symptoms. A listing of these findings varies among facilities. Timely notification of a critical finding for laboratory or diagnostic studies is a role expectation of the professional nurse. The notification processes vary among facilities. Upon receipt of the critical finding, the information should be read back to the caller to verify accuracy.

Consideration may be given to verification of critical findings before action is taken. Policies vary among facilities and may include requesting immediate recollection and retesting by the laboratory or retesting using a rapid point-of-care testing instrument at the bedside, if available.

Important signs to note are prolonged bleeding from cuts or gums, hematoma at a puncture site, bruising easily, blood in the stool, persistent epistaxis, heavy or prolonged menstrual flow, and shock. Monitor vital signs, aPTT levels, unusual ecchymosis, occult blood, severe headache, unusual dizziness, and neurological changes until aPTT is within normal range.

INTERFERING FACTORS

- Drugs and other substances such as antistreplase, antihistamines, chlorpromazine, salicylates, and ascorbic acid may cause prolonged aPTT.
- Anticoagulant therapy with heparin will prolong the aPTT.
- Copper is a component of factor V, and severe copper deficiencies may result in prolonged aPTT values.
- Traumatic venipunctures can activate the coagulation sequence by contamination of the sample with tissue thromboplastin and can produce falsely shortened results.
- Failure to fill the tube sufficiently to yield a proper blood-to-anticoagulant ratio invalidates the results and is reason for specimen rejection.

- Excessive agitation that causes sample hemolysis can falsely shorten the aPTT because the hemolyzed cells activate plasma-clotting factors.
- Inadequate mixing of the tube can produce erroneous results.
- Specimens left unprocessed for longer than 24 hr should be rejected for analysis.
- High platelet count or inadequate centrifugation will result in decreased values.
- Hematocrit greater than 55% may cause falsely prolonged results because of anticoagulant excess relative to plasma volume.
- Incompletely filled collection tubes, specimens contaminated with heparin, clotted specimens, or unprocessed specimens not delivered to the laboratory within 1 to 2 hr of collection should be rejected.

NURSING IMPLICATIONS AND PROCEDURE

POTENTIAL NURSING PROBLEMS:

Problem	Signs & Symptoms	Interventions
Bleeding ***(related to alerted clotting factors secondary to heparin use or depleted clotting factors)***	Altered level of consciousness; hypotension; increased heart rate; decreased hemoglobin (Hgb) and hematocrit (Hct); capillary refill greater than 3 sec; cool extremities; blood in urine, stool, sputum; bleeding gums; nosebleed; bruises easily; elevated PTT	Increase frequency of vital sign assessment with variances in results; monitor for vital sign trends; administer blood or blood products as ordered; administer prescribed vitamin K; monitor and trend Hgb/Hct; assess skin for petechiae, purpura, hematoma; monitor for blood in emesis, or sputum; institute bleeding precautions (prevent unnecessary venipuncture; avoid intramuscular [IM] injections; prevent trauma; be gentle with oral care, suctioning; avoid use of a sharp razor); administer prescribed stool softener
Gas exchange ***(related to deficient oxygen capacity of the blood secondary to blood loss)***	Irregular breathing pattern, use of accessory muscles; altered chest excursion; adventitious breath sounds (crackles, rhonchi, wheezes, diminished breath sounds); copious secretions; signs of hypoxia; altered	Monitor respiratory rate and effort based on assessment of patient condition; assess lung sounds frequently; monitor for secretions, bloody sputum; suction as necessary; use pulse oximetry to monitor oxygen saturation; collaborate with HCP to administer oxygen as needed; elevate the head of the bed 30 degrees or higher; monitor intravenous (IV) fluids

P

Problem	Signs & Symptoms	Interventions
	blood gas results; confusion; lethargy; cyanosis	and avoid aggressive fluid resuscitation; assess level of consciousness; anticipate the need for possible intubation
Tissue perfusion ***(related to decreased hemoglobin secondary to bleeding; altered clotting factors)***	Hypotension; dizziness; cool extremities; pallor; capillary refill greater than 3 sec in fingers and toes; weak pedal pulses; altered level of consciousness; altered sensation	Monitor blood pressure; assess for dizziness; assess extremities for skin temperature, color, warmth; assess capillary refill; assess pedal pulses; monitor for numbness, tingling, hyperesthesia, hypoesthesia; monitor and trend PT and international normalized ratio; administer blood or blood products as ordered; administer vitamin K as ordered; administer IV fluids as ordered; administer fluid bolus as appropriate; administer medication to support blood pressure as ordered; monitor and trend aPTT results
Health management ***(related to complexity of health-care system; complexity of therapeutic management; knowledge deficit; cultural family health patterns; mistrust of HCP)***	Inability or failure to recognize or process information toward improving health and preventing illness with associated mental and physical effects	Facilitate collaboration with HCP to develop a plan of care that supports health; ensure patient adheres to recommended medication regime; encourage patient to comply with health-care follow-up appointments

PRETEST:

- Positively identify the patient using at least two person-specific identifiers before services, treatments, or procedures are performed.
- *Patient Teaching:* Inform the patient this test can assist in evaluating the effectiveness of blood clotting.
- Obtain a history of the patient's health concerns (especially any bleeding disorders), symptoms, surgical procedures, and results of previously performed laboratory and diagnostic studies. Include a list of known allergens, especially allergies or sensitivities to latex.

- Obtain a list of the patient's current medications, including over-the-counter medications, dietary supplements, anticoagulants, aspirin and other salicylates (see Effects of Natural Products on Laboratory Values online at Davis*Plus*). Such products should be discontinued by medical direction for the appropriate number of days prior to a surgical procedure. Note the last time and dose of medication taken.
- Review the procedure with the patient. Inform the patient that specimen collection takes approximately 5 to 10 min. Address concerns about pain and explain there may be some discomfort during the venipuncture.
- ***Sensitivity to social and cultural issues,*** as well as concern for modesty, is important in providing psychological support before, during, and after the procedure.
- Note that there are no food, fluid, or medication restrictions unless by medical direction.

INTRATEST:

Potential Complications: N/A

- Avoid the use of equipment containing latex if the patient has a history of allergic reaction to latex.
- Instruct the patient to cooperate fully and to follow directions. Direct the patient to breathe normally and to avoid unnecessary movement.
- Observe standard precautions, and follow the general guidelines in Patient Preparation and Specimen Collection online at Davis*Plus*. Positively identify the patient, and label the appropriate specimen container with the corresponding patient demographics, initials of the person collecting the specimen, date, and time of collection. Perform a venipuncture. Fill tube completely. *Important note:* When multiple specimens are drawn, the blue-top tube should be collected after sterile (i.e., blood culture) tubes. Otherwise, when using a standard vacutainer system, the blue-top tube is the first tube collected. When a butterfly is used and due to the added tubing, an extra red-top tube should be collected before the blue-top tube to ensure complete filling of the blue-top tube.
- Remove the needle and apply direct pressure with dry gauze to stop bleeding. Observe/assess venipuncture site for bleeding or hematoma formation and secure gauze with adhesive bandage.
- Promptly transport the specimen to the laboratory for processing and analysis. If delays in specimen transport and processing occur, it is important to consult with the testing laboratory. Whole blood specimens are stable at room temperature for up to 24 hr. Specimen stability requirements may also vary if the patient is receiving heparin therapy. Some laboratories require frozen plasma if testing will not be performed within 1 hr of collection. Criteria for rejection of specimens based on collection time may vary among facilities.

POST-TEST:

- Inform the patient that a report of the results will be made available to the requesting HCP, who will discuss the results with the patient.
- Depending on the results of this procedure, additional testing may be performed to evaluate or monitor progression of the disease process and determine the need for a change in therapy. Evaluate test results in relation to the patient's symptoms and other tests performed.

Patient Education:

- Instruct the patient to report severe bruising or bleeding from any areas of the skin or mucous membranes.
- Inform the patient with prolonged aPTT values of the importance of taking precautions against bruising and bleeding, including the use of a soft-bristle toothbrush, use of an electric razor, avoidance of constipation, avoidance of acetylsalicylic acid and similar products, and avoidance of IM injections.

P

- Inform the patient of the importance of periodic laboratory testing while taking an anticoagulant.
- Reinforce information given by the patient's HCP regarding further testing, treatment, or referral to another HCP.
- Answer any questions or address any concerns voiced by the patient or family.

Expected Patient Outcomes:

Understanding

- The patient and family state signs and symptoms of bleeding that should be reported to the HCP.
- The patient and family state the purpose of heparin infusion in relation to medical diagnosis.

Ability

- The patient demonstrates the proficient use of nasal spray and lip balm to prevent cracked mucous membranes and associated bleeding.
- The patient demonstrates proficiency in the self-examination of skin for bruising and bleeding.

Response

- The patient complies with the request to refrain from at-risk behavior that would cause bleeding.
- The patient and family comply with the request to refrain from using herbal supplements unless approved by the HCP due to increased bleeding risk.

RELATED STUDIES:

- Related tests include antithrombin III, bleeding time, coagulation factors, CBC, CBC platelet count, copper, D-dimer, FDP, plasminogen, protein C, protein S, PT/INR, and vitamin K.
- Refer to the Hematopoietic and Hepatobiliary systems tables online at Davis*Plus* for related tests by body system.

Parvovirus B19 Immunoglobulin G and Immunoglobulin M Antibodies

SYNONYM/ACRONYM: N/A

COMMON USE: To assist in confirming a diagnosis of a present or past parvovirus infection.

SPECIMEN: Serum collected in a gold-, red-, or red/gray-top tube. Place separated serum into a standard transport tube within 2 hr of collection.

NORMAL FINDINGS: (Method: Immunoassay)

Negative	Less than 0.9 index
Equivocal	0.9–1 index

POTENTIAL MEDICAL DIAGNOSIS

Positive findings in:

Parvovirus infection can be evidenced in a variety of conditions.

- Arthritis
- Erythema infectiosum (fifth disease)
- Erythrocyte aplasia
- Hydrops fetalis

Negative findings in: N/A

CRITICAL FINDINGS: N/A

Find and print out the full study on Fast Find at davispl.us/vanleeuwen7.

Pericardial Fluid Analysis

SYNONYM/ACRONYM: N/A

COMMON USE: To evaluate and classify the type of fluid between the pericardium membranes to assist with diagnosis of infection or fluid balance disorder.

SPECIMEN: Pericardial fluid collected in a red- or green-top (heparin) tube for glucose, a lavender-top (EDTA) tube for cell count, and sterile containers for microbiology specimens; fluid in a clear container for cytology. Ensure that there is an equal amount of fixative and fluid in the container for cytology.

NORMAL FINDINGS: (Method: Spectrophotometry for glucose; automated or manual cell count, macroscopic examination of cultured organisms, and microscopic examination of specimen for microbiology and cytology; microscopic examination of cultured microorganisms)

Pericardial Fluid	Reference Value
Appearance	Clear
Color	Pale yellow
Glucose	Parallels serum values
Red blood cell count	None seen
White blood cell count	Less than 300 cells/microL
Culture	No growth
Gram stain	No organisms seen
Cytology	No abnormal cells seen

DESCRIPTION: The heart is located within a protective membrane called the *pericardium*. The fluid between the pericardial membranes is called *serous fluid*. Normally, only a small amount of fluid is present because the rates of fluid production and absorption are about the same. Many abnormal conditions can result in the buildup of fluid within the pericardium. Specific tests are usually ordered in addition to a common battery of tests used to distinguish a transudate from an exudate. *Transudates* are effusions that form as a result of a systemic disorder that disrupts the regulation of fluid balance, such as a suspected perforation. *Exudates* are caused by conditions involving the tissue of the membrane itself, such as an infection or malignancy. Fluid is withdrawn from the pericardium by needle aspiration and tested as listed in the previous and following tables.

Characteristic	Transudate	Exudate
Appearance	Clear	Cloudy or turbid
Specific gravity	Less than 1.015	Greater than 1.015
Total protein	Less than 2.5 g/dL	Greater than 3 g/dL

P

Characteristic	Transudate	Exudate
Fluid-to-serum protein ratio	Less than 0.5	Greater than 0.5
LDH	Parallels serum value	Less than 200 units/L
Fluid-to-serum LDH ratio	Less than 0.6	Greater than 0.6
Fluid cholesterol	Less than 55 mg/dL	Greater than 55 mg/dL
White blood cell count	Less than 100 cells/microL	Greater than 1,000 cells/microL

LDH = lactate dehydrogenase.

This procedure is contraindicated for: N/A

INDICATIONS

- Evaluate effusion of unknown etiology.
- Investigate suspected hemorrhage, immune disease, malignancy, or infection.

POTENTIAL MEDICAL DIAGNOSIS

Increased in:

Condition/Test Showing Increased Result

- Bacterial pericarditis (red blood cell [RBC] count, white blood cell [WBC] count with a predominance of neutrophils)
- Hemorrhagic pericarditis (RBC count, WBC count)
- Malignancy (RBC count, abnormal cytology)
- Post–myocardial infarction syndrome, also called Dressler's syndrome (RBC count, WBC count with a predominance of neutrophils)
- Rheumatoid disease or systemic lupus erythematosus (SLE) (RBC count, WBC count)
- Tuberculous or fungal pericarditis (RBC count, WBC count with a predominance of lymphocytes)
- Viral pericarditis (RBC count, WBC count with a predominance of neutrophils)

Decreased in:

Condition/Test Showing Decreased Result

- Bacterial pericarditis (glucose)
- Malignancy (glucose)
- Rheumatoid disease or SLE (glucose)

CRITICAL FINDINGS:

Positive culture findings in any sterile body fluid.

Note and immediately report to the requesting health-care provider (HCP) any critical findings and related symptoms. A listing of these findings varies among facilities. Timely notification of a critical finding for laboratory or diagnostic studies is a role expectation of the professional nurse. The notification processes vary among facilities. Upon receipt of the critical finding, the information should be read back to the caller to verify accuracy.

INTERFERING FACTORS

- Bloody fluid may be the result of a traumatic tap.
- Unknown hyperglycemia or hypoglycemia may be misleading in the comparison of fluid and serum glucose levels. Therefore, it is advisable to collect comparative serum samples a few hours before performing pericardiocentesis.
- Failure to follow dietary restrictions before the procedure may cause the procedure to be canceled or repeated.

NURSING IMPLICATIONS AND PROCEDURE

PRETEST:

- Positively identify the patient using at least two person-specific identifiers before services, treatments, or procedures are performed.
- *Patient Teaching:* Inform the patient this procedure can assist with evaluating fluid around the heart.
- Obtain a history of the patient's health concerns, symptoms, surgical procedures, and results of previously performed laboratory and diagnostic studies. Include a list of known allergens, especially allergies or sensitivities to latex.
- Note any recent procedures that can interfere with test results.
- Record the date of the last menstrual period and determine the possibility of pregnancy in perimenopausal women.
- Obtain a list of the patient's current medications, including over-the-counter medications, dietary supplements, anticoagulants, aspirin and other salicylates (see Effects of Natural Products on Laboratory Values online at Davis*Plus*). Such products should be discontinued by medical direction for the appropriate number of days prior to a surgical procedure. Note the last time and dose of medication taken.
- Review the procedure with the patient. Inform the patient that it may be necessary to remove hair from the site before the procedure. Address concerns about pain and explain that a sedative and/or analgesia will be administered to promote relaxation and reduce discomfort prior to needle insertion through the chest wall. Explain that any discomfort with the needle insertion will be minimized with local anesthetics and systemic analgesics. Explain that the anesthetic injection may cause a stinging sensation. Explain that after the skin has been anesthetized, a large needle will be inserted through the chest to obtain the fluid. Inform the patient that specimen collection is performed by an HCP specializing in this procedure and usually takes approximately 30 min to complete.
- Explain that an intravenous (IV) line will be inserted to allow infusion of fluids, antibiotics, anesthetics, and analgesics.
- *Sensitivity to social and cultural issues,* as well as concern for modesty, is important in providing psychological support before, during, and after the procedure.
- Note that food and fluids should be restricted for 6 to 8 hr before the procedure, as directed by the HCP, unless the procedure is performed in an emergency situation to correct pericarditis. The requesting HCP may request that anticoagulants and aspirin be withheld. The number of days to withhold medication is dependent on the type of anticoagulant. Protocols may vary among facilities.
- *Make sure a written and informed consent has been signed prior to the procedure and before administering any medications.*

INTRATEST:

Potential Complications:

Pain, bleeding, swelling, infection, injury to the surrounding organs

- Ensure that the patient has complied with dietary, fluid, and medication restrictions prior to the procedure, as instructed. Notify the HCP if patient anticoagulant therapy has not been withheld.
- Have emergency equipment readily available.
- Have the patient void before the procedure.
- Have the patient remove clothes above the waist and put on a gown.
- Avoid the use of equipment containing latex if the patient has a history of allergic reaction to latex.
- Instruct the patient to cooperate fully and to follow directions. Direct the patient to breathe normally and to avoid unnecessary movement during the local anesthetic and the procedure.

P

- Record baseline vital signs, and continue to monitor throughout the procedure. Protocols may vary among facilities.
- Observe standard precautions, and follow the general guidelines in Patient Preparation and Specimen Collection online at Davis*Plus*. Positively identify the patient, and label the appropriate specimen container with the corresponding patient demographics, initials of the person collecting the specimen, date and time of collection, and site location.
- Establish an IV line to allow infusion of fluids, anesthetics, analgesics, or sedation.
- Assist the patient into a comfortable supine position with the head elevated 45° to 60°.
- Clip hair from the site as needed, cleanse the site with an antiseptic solution, and drape the area with sterile towels prior to the administration of local anesthesia. The skin at the injection site is then anesthetized.
- The precordial (V) cardiac lead wire is attached to the cardiac needle with an alligator clip. The cardiac needle is inserted just below and to the left of the breastbone, and fluid is removed.
- Monitor vital signs every 15 min for signs of hypovolemia or shock. Monitor electrocardiogram for needle-tip positioning to indicate accidental puncture of the right atrium.
- The needle is withdrawn, and slight pressure is applied to the site. Apply a sterile dressing to the site.
- Monitor the patient for complications related to the procedure (e.g., allergic reaction, anaphylaxis).
- Place samples in properly labelled specimen containers, and promptly transport the specimens to the laboratory for processing and analysis.

POST-TEST:

- Inform the patient that a report of the results will be made available to the requesting HCP, who will discuss the results with the patient.
- Instruct the patient to resume usual diet and medications, as directed by the HCP.
- Monitor vital signs and cardiac status every 15 min for the first hour, every 30 min for the next 2 hr, every hr for the next 4 hr, and every 4 hr for the next 24 hr. Take the patient's temperature every 4 hr for 24 hr. Monitor intake and output for 24 hr. Notify the HCP if temperature is elevated. Protocols may vary among facilities.
- Observe/assess the patient for signs of respiratory and cardiac distress, such as shortness of breath, cyanosis, or rapid pulse.
- Continue IV fluids until vital signs are stable and the patient can resume fluid intake independently.
- Inform the patient that 1 hr or more of bed rest is required after the procedure.
- Observe/assess the puncture site for bleeding or drainage and signs of inflammation each time vital signs are taken and daily thereafter for several days. Report to HCP if bleeding is present.
- Observe/assess for nausea and pain. Administer antiemetic and analgesic medications as needed and as directed by the HCP.
- Administer antibiotics, as ordered, and instruct the patient in the importance of completing the entire course of antibiotic therapy even if no symptoms are present.
- Recognize anxiety related to test results, and offer support. Discuss the implications of abnormal test results on the patient's lifestyle. Provide teaching and information regarding the clinical implications of the test results, as appropriate. Educate the patient regarding access to counseling services, if appropriate.
- Reinforce information given by the patient's HCP regarding further testing, treatment, or referral to another HCP. Answer any questions or address any concerns voiced by the patient or family.
- Depending on the results of this procedure, additional testing may be performed to evaluate or monitor progression of the disease process and determine the need for a change

P

in therapy. Evaluate test results in relation to the patient's symptoms and other tests performed.

RELATED STUDIES:

- Related tests include atrial natriuretic peptide, blood gases, B-type natriuretic peptide, cancer antigens, chest x-ray, CBC WBC count and differential, CK and isoenzymes, culture and smear mycobacteria, culture blood, culture fungal, culture viral, ECG, echocardiography, α_1-fetoprotein, homocysteine, LDH and isoenzymes, magnesium, MRI chest, MI scan, myoglobin, and troponin.
- Refer to the Cardiovascular and Immune systems tables online at Davis*Plus* for related tests by body system.

Peritoneal Fluid Analysis

SYNONYM/ACRONYM: Ascites fluid analysis.

COMMON USE: To evaluate and classify the type of fluid within the peritoneal cavity to assist with diagnosis of cancer, infection, necrosis, and perforation.

SPECIMEN: Peritoneal fluid collected in a red- or green-top (heparin) tube for amylase, glucose, and alkaline phosphatase; lavender-top (EDTA) tube for cell count; sterile containers for microbiology specimens; fluid in a clear container with anticoagulant for cytology. Ensure that there is an equal amount of fixative and fluid in the container for cytology.

NORMAL FINDINGS: (Method: Spectrophotometry for glucose, amylase, and alkaline phosphatase; automated or manual cell count, macroscopic examination of cultured organisms, and microscopic examination of specimen for microbiology and cytology; microscopic examination of cultured microorganisms)

Peritoneal Fluid	Reference Value
Appearance	Clear
Color	Pale yellow
Amylase	Parallels serum values
Alkaline phosphatase	Parallels serum values
CEA	Parallels serum values
Glucose	Parallels serum values
Red blood cell count	None seen
White blood cell count	Less than 300 cells/microL
Culture	No growth
Acid-fast stain	No organisms seen
Gram stain	No organisms seen
Cytology	No abnormal cells seen

P

DESCRIPTION: The peritoneal cavity and organs within it are lined with a protective membrane. The fluid between the membranes is called *serous fluid*. Normally only a small amount of fluid is present because the rates of fluid production and absorption are about the same. Many abnormal conditions can result in the buildup of fluid within the peritoneal cavity. Specific tests are usually ordered in addition to a common battery of tests used to distinguish a transudate from an exudate. *Transudates* are effusions that form as a result of a systemic disorder that disrupts the regulation of fluid balance, such as a suspected perforation. *Exudates* are caused by conditions involving the tissue of the membrane itself, such as an infection or malignancy. Fluid is withdrawn from the peritoneal cavity by needle aspiration and tested as listed in the previous and following tables.

This procedure is contraindicated for: N/A

INDICATIONS

- Evaluate ascites of unknown cause.
- Investigate suspected peritoneal rupture, perforation, malignancy, or infection.

Characteristic	Transudate	Exudate
Appearance	Clear	Cloudy or turbid
Specific gravity	Less than 1.015	Greater than 1.015
Total protein	Less than 2.5 g/dL	Greater than 3 g/dL
Fluid-to-serum protein ratio	Less than 0.5	Greater than 0.5
LDH	Parallels serum value	Less than 200 units/L
Fluid-to-serum LDH ratio	Less than 0.6	Greater than 0.6
Fluid cholesterol	Less than 55 mg/dL	Greater than 55 mg/dL
White blood cell count	Less than 100 cells/microL	Greater than 1,000 cells/microL

LDH = lactate dehydrogenase.

POTENTIAL MEDICAL DIAGNOSIS

Increased in:

Condition/Test Showing Increased Result

- Abdominal malignancy (red blood cell [RBC] count, carcinoembryonic antigen, abnormal cytology)
- Abdominal trauma (RBC count)
- Ascites caused by cirrhosis (white blood cell [WBC] count, neutrophils greater than 25% but less than 50%)
- Bacterial peritonitis (WBC count, neutrophils greater than 50%)
- Peritoneal effusion due to gastric strangulation, perforation, or necrosis (amylase, ammonia, alkaline phosphatase)
- Peritoneal effusion due to pancreatitis, pancreatic trauma, or pancreatic pseudocyst (amylase)
- Rupture or perforation of urinary bladder (ammonia, creatinine, urea)
- Tuberculous effusion (elevated lymphocyte count, positive acid-fast bacillus smear and culture [25% to 50% of cases])

Decreased in:

Condition/Test Showing Decreased Result

- Abdominal malignancy (glucose)
- Tuberculous effusion (glucose)

CRITICAL FINDINGS:

Positive culture findings in any sterile body fluid.

Note and immediately report to the requesting health-care provider (HCP) any critical findings and related symptoms. A listing of these findings varies

among facilities. Timely notification of a critical finding for laboratory or diagnostic studies is a role expectation of the professional nurse. The notification processes vary among facilities. Upon receipt of the critical finding, the information should be read back to the caller to verify accuracy.

INTERFERING FACTORS

- Bloody fluids may result from a traumatic tap.
- Unknown hyperglycemia or hypoglycemia may be misleading in the comparison of fluid and serum glucose levels. Therefore, it is advisable to collect comparative serum samples a few hours before performing paracentesis.

NURSING IMPLICATIONS AND PROCEDURE

PRETEST:

- Positively identify the patient using at least two person-specific identifiers before services, treatments, or procedures are performed.
- ***Patient Teaching:*** Inform the patient this procedure can assist with evaluation of fluid surrounding the abdominal organs.
- Obtain a history of the patient's health concerns, symptoms, surgical procedures, and results of previously performed laboratory and diagnostic studies. Include a list of known allergens, especially allergies or sensitivities to latex.
- Note any recent procedures that can interfere with test results.
- Record the date of the last menstrual period and determine the possibility of pregnancy in perimenopausal women.
- Obtain a list of the patient's current medications, including over-the-counter medications, dietary supplements, anticoagulants, aspirin and other salicylates (see Effects of Natural Products on Laboratory Values online at Davis*Plus*). Such products should be discontinued by medical direction for the appropriate number of days prior to a surgical procedure. Note the last time and dose of medication taken.
- Review the procedure with the patient. If patient has ascites, obtain weight and measure abdominal girth. Inform the patient that it may be necessary to remove hair from the site before the procedure. Address concerns about pain and explain that a sedative and/or analgesia will be administered to promote relaxation and reduce discomfort prior to needle insertion through the abdomen wall. Explain that any discomfort with the needle insertion will be minimized with local anesthetics and systemic analgesics. Explain that the anesthetic injection may cause an initial stinging sensation. Explain that after the skin has been anesthetized, a large needle will be inserted through the abdominal wall and a "popping" sensation may be experienced as the needle penetrates the peritoneum. Inform the patient that specimen collection is performed under sterile conditions by an HCP specializing in this procedure and usually takes approximately 30 min to complete.
- Explain that an intravenous (IV) line will be inserted to allow infusion of fluids, antibiotics, anesthetics, and analgesics.
- ***Sensitivity to social and cultural issues,*** as well as concern for modesty, is important in providing psychological support before, during, and after the procedure.
- Note that there are no food or fluid restrictions unless by medical direction. The requesting HCP may request that anticoagulants and aspirin be withheld. The number of days to withhold medication is dependent on the type of anticoagulant.
- *Make sure a written and informed consent has been signed prior to the procedure and before administering any medications.*

P

INTRATEST:

Potential Complications:

Bleeding, infection, puncture of surrounding vessels or organs

- Ensure that anticoagulant therapy has been withheld for the appropriate number of days prior to the procedure, as instructed. Notify the HCP if patient anticoagulant therapy has not been withheld.
- Have emergency equipment readily available.
- Have the patient void, or catheterize the patient to avoid accidental puncture of the bladder if he or she is unable to void.
- Have the patient remove clothing and change into a gown for the procedure.
- Avoid the use of equipment containing latex if the patient has a history of allergic reaction to latex.
- Instruct the patient to cooperate fully and to follow directions. Direct the patient to breathe normally and to avoid unnecessary movement during the local anesthetic and the procedure.
- Observe standard precautions, and follow the general guidelines in Patient Preparation and Specimen Collection online at Davis*Plus*. Positively identify the patient, and label the appropriate specimen container with the corresponding patient demographics, initials of the person collecting the specimen, date and time of collection, and site location.
- Record baseline vital signs and continue to monitor throughout the procedure. Protocols may vary among facilities.
- Establish an IV line to allow infusion of fluids, anesthetics, analgesics, or sedation.
- Assist the patient to a comfortable seated position with feet and back supported or in high Fowler's position.
- Clip hair from the site as needed, cleanse the site with an antiseptic solution, and drape the area with sterile towels prior to the administration of local anesthesia. The skin at the injection site is then anesthetized.
- The paracentesis needle is inserted 1 to 2 in. below the umbilicus, and fluid is removed. If lavage fluid is required (helpful if malignancy is suspected), saline or Ringer's lactate can be infused via the needle over a 15- to 20-min period before the lavage fluid is removed. Monitor vital signs every 15 min for signs of hypovolemia or shock.
- No more than 1,500 to 2,000 mL of fluid should be removed at a time, even in the case of a therapeutic paracentesis, because of the risk of hypovolemia and shock.
- The needle is withdrawn, and slight pressure is applied to the site. Apply a sterile dressing to the site.
- Monitor the patient for complications related to the procedure (e.g., allergic reaction, anaphylaxis).
- Place samples in properly labelled specimen containers, and promptly transport the specimens to the laboratory for processing and analysis.

POST-TEST:

- Inform the patient that a report of the results will be made available to the requesting HCP, who will discuss the results with the patient.
- Instruct the patient to resume usual medications, as directed by the HCP.
- Monitor vital signs every 15 min for the first hr, every 30 min for the next 2 hr, every hour for the next 4 hr, and every 4 hr for the next 24 hr. Take the patient's temperature every 4 hr for 24 hr. Monitor intake and output for 24 hr. Notify the HCP if temperature is elevated. Protocols may vary among facilities.
- Observe/assess the puncture site for bleeding or drainage and signs of inflammation each time vital signs are taken and daily thereafter for several days. Report to the HCP if bleeding is present.
- Obtain weight and measure abdominal girth if a large amount of fluid was removed.

P

- Inform the patient that 1 hr or more of bed rest is required after the procedure.
- Instruct the patient to immediately report severe abdominal pain. (*Note:* Rigidity of abdominal muscles indicates developing peritonitis.) Report to HCP if abdominal rigidity or pain is present.
- Observe/assess for nausea and pain. Administer antiemetic and analgesic medications as needed and as directed by the HCP.
- Administer antibiotics, as ordered, and instruct the patient in the importance of completing the entire course of antibiotic therapy even if no symptoms are present.
- Recognize anxiety related to test results, and offer support. Discuss the implications of abnormal test results on the patient's lifestyle. Provide teaching and information regarding the clinical implications of the test results, as appropriate. Educate the patient regarding access to counseling services, if appropriate.
- Reinforce information given by the patient's HCP regarding further testing, treatment, or referral to another HCP. Answer any questions or address any concerns voiced by the patient or family.
- Depending on the results of this procedure, additional testing may be performed to evaluate or monitor progression of the disease process and determine the need for a change in therapy. Evaluate test results in relation to the patient's symptoms and other tests performed.

RELATED STUDIES:

- Related tests include cancer antigens, CBC, CBC WBC count and differential, CT abdomen, CT biliary tract and liver, culture and smear mycobacteria, culture blood, culture fungal, culture viral, KUB studies, laparoscopy abdominal, liver and spleen scan, MRI abdomen, US abdomen, and US spleen.
- Refer to the Gastrointestinal and Immune systems tables online at Davis*Plus* for related tests by body system.

Phosphorus, Blood

SYNONYM/ACRONYM: Inorganic phosphorus, phosphate, PO_4.

COMMON USE: To assist in evaluating multiple body system functions by monitoring phosphorus levels in relation to other electrolytes. Used specifically to evaluate renal function in at-risk patients.

P

SPECIMEN: Serum collected in a gold-, red-, or red/gray-top tube. Plasma collected in green-top (heparin) tube is also acceptable.

NORMAL FINDINGS: (Method: Spectrophotometry)

Age	Conventional Units	SI Units (Conventional Units × 0.323)
0–5 d	4.6–8 mg/dL	1.5–2.6 mmol/L
1–3 yr	3.9–6.5 mg/dL	1.3–2.1 mmol/L
4–6 yr	4–5.4 mg/dL	1.3–1.7 mmol/L
7–11 yr	3.7–5.6 mg/dL	1.2–1.8 mmol/L

Age	Conventional Units	SI Units (Conventional Units × 0.323)
12–13 yr	3.3–5.4 mg/dL	1.1–1.7 mmol/L
14–15 yr	2.9–5.4 mg/dL	0.9–1.7 mmol/L
16–19 yr	2.8–4.6 mg/dL	0.9–1.5 mmol/L
Adult	2.5–4.5 mg/dL	0.8–1.4 mmol/L

Values may be slightly decreased in older adults due to dietary insufficiency or the effects of medications and the presence of multiple chronic or acute diseases with or without muted symptoms.

DESCRIPTION: Phosphorus, in the form of phosphate, is distributed throughout the body. Approximately 85% of the body's phosphorus is stored in bones; the remainder is found in cells and body fluids. It is the major intracellular anion and plays a crucial role in cellular metabolism, maintenance of cellular membranes, and formation of bones and teeth. Phosphorus also indirectly affects the release of oxygen from hemoglobin by affecting the formation of 2,3-bisphosphoglycerate. The reabsorption and excretion of phosphorus is largely regulated by the parathyroid glands and the kidneys. Levels of phosphorus are also affected by dietary intake and are dependent on the presence of activated vitamin D for absorption by the intestines. Calcium and phosphorus are interrelated with respect to absorption and metabolic function. They have an inverse relationship with respect to concentration; serum phosphorus is increased when serum calcium is decreased.

Hyperphosphatemia can result in an infant fed only cow's milk during the first few weeks of life because of the combination of a high phosphorus content in cow's milk and the inability of infants' kidneys to clear the excess phosphorus.

This procedure is contraindicated for: N/A

INDICATIONS

- Assist in establishing a diagnosis of hyperparathyroidism.
- Assist in the evaluation of chronic kidney disease.

POTENTIAL MEDICAL DIAGNOSIS

Increased in:

- Acromegaly ***(related to increased renal absorption)***
- Bone metastases ***(related to release from bone stores)***
- Chronic kidney disease ***(related to decreased renal excretion)***
- Diabetic ketoacidosis ***(acid-base imbalance causes intracellular phosphorus to move into the extracellular fluid)***
- Excessive levels of vitamin D ***(vitamin D promotes intestinal absorption of phosphorus; excessive levels promote phosphorus release from bone stores)***
- Hyperthermia ***(tissue damage causes intracellular phosphorus to be released into circulation)***
- Hypocalcemia ***(calcium and phosphorus have an inverse relationship)***
- Hypoparathyroidism ***(related to increased renal absorption)***
- Lactic acidosis ***(acid-base imbalance causes intracellular phosphorus to move into the extracellular fluid)***

P

- Milk alkali syndrome ***(increased dietary intake)***
- Pseudohypoparathyroidism ***(related to increased renal absorption)***
- Pulmonary embolism ***(related to respiratory acid-base imbalance and compensatory mechanisms)***
- Respiratory acidosis ***(acid-base imbalance causes intracellular phosphorus to move into the extracellular fluid)***

Decreased in:

- Acute gout ***(related to decreased circulating calcium in calcium crystal–induced gout; calcium and phosphorus have an inverse relationship)***
- Alcohol withdrawal ***(related to malnutrition)***
- Gram-negative bacterial septicemia
- Growth hormone deficiency
- Hyperalimentation therapy
- Hypercalcemia ***(calcium and phosphorus have an inverse relationship)***
- Hyperinsulinism ***(insulin increases intracellular movement of phosphorus)***
- Hyperparathyroidism ***(parathyroid hormone [PTH] increases renal excretion)***
- Hypokalemia
- Impaired renal absorption ***(decreases return of phosphorus to general circulation)***
- Malabsorption syndromes ***(related to insufficient intestinal absorption of phosphorus)***
- Malnutrition ***(related to deficient intake)***
- Osteomalacia ***(evidenced by hypophosphatemia)***
- PTH-producing tumors ***(PTH increases renal excretion)***
- Primary hyperparathyroidism ***(PTH increases renal excretion)***
- Renal tubular acidosis
- Renal tubular defects ***(related to decreased renal absorption)***
- Respiratory alkalosis
- Respiratory infections
- Rickets ***(related to vitamin D deficiency)***
- Salicylate poisoning
- Severe burns
- Severe vomiting and diarrhea ***(related to excessive loss)***
- Vitamin D deficiency ***(related to vitamin D deficiency, which reduces intestinal and renal tubular absorption of phosphorus)***

CRITICAL FINDINGS:

Adults

- Less than 1 mg/dL (SI: Less than 0.3 mmol/L)
- Greater than 8.9 mg/dL (SI: Greater than 2.9 mmol/L)

Children

- Less than 1.3 mg/dL (SI: Less than 0.4 mmol/L)
- Greater than 8.9 mg/dL (SI: Greater than 2.9 mmol/L)

Note and immediately report to the requesting health-care provider (HCP) any critical findings and related symptoms. A listing of these findings varies among facilities. Timely notification of a critical finding for laboratory or diagnostic studies is a role expectation of the professional nurse. The notification processes vary among facilities. Upon receipt of the critical finding, the information should be read back to the caller to verify accuracy.

Interventions including intravenous (IV) replacement therapy with sodium or potassium phosphate may be necessary. Close monitoring of both phosphorus and calcium is important during replacement therapy.

INTERFERING FACTORS

- Drugs and other substances that may increase phosphorus levels include anabolic steroids, β-adrenergic blockers,

P

ergocalciferol, furosemide, hydrochlorothiazide, methicillin (occurs with nephrotoxicity), oral contraceptives, parathyroid extract, phosphates, sodium etidronate, tetracycline (occurs with nephrotoxicity), and vitamin D.

- Drugs and other substances that may decrease phosphorus levels include acetazolamide, albuterol, aluminum salts, amino acids (via IV hyperalimentation), anesthetic drugs, anticonvulsants, calcitonin, epinephrine, fibrin hydrolysate, fructose, glucocorticoids, glucose, insulin, mannitol, oral contraceptives, pamidronate, phenothiazine, phytate, and plicamycin.
- Serum phosphorus levels are subject to diurnal variation: They are highest in late morning and lowest in the evening; therefore, serial samples should be collected at the same time of day for consistency in interpretation.
- Hemolysis will falsely increase phosphorus values.
- Specimens should never be collected above an IV line because of the potential for dilution when the specimen and the IV solution combine in the collection container, thereby falsely decreasing the result. There is also the potential of contaminating the sample with the substance of interest if it is present in the IV solution, thereby falsely increasing the result.

NURSING IMPLICATIONS AND PROCEDURE

PRETEST:

- Positively identify the patient using at least two person-specific identifiers before services, treatments, or procedures are performed.
- ***Patient Teaching:*** Inform the patient this test can assist in a general evaluation of body systems.
- Obtain a history of the patient's health concerns, symptoms, surgical procedures, and results of previously performed laboratory and diagnostic studies. Include a list of known allergens, especially allergies or sensitivities to latex.
- Obtain a list of the patient's current medications, including over-the-counter medications and dietary supplements (see Effects of Natural Products on Laboratory Values online at Davis*Plus*).
- Review the procedure with the patient. Inform the patient that specimen collection takes approximately 5 to 10 min. Address concerns about pain and explain that there may be some discomfort during the venipuncture.
- ***Sensitivity to social and cultural issues,*** as well as concern for modesty, is important in providing psychological support before, during, and after the procedure.
- Note that there are no food, fluid, or medication restrictions unless by medical direction.

INTRATEST:

Potential Complications: N/A

- Avoid the use of equipment containing latex if the patient has a history of allergic reaction to latex.
- Instruct the patient to cooperate fully and to follow directions. Direct the patient to breathe normally and to avoid unnecessary movement.
- Observe standard precautions, and follow the general guidelines in Patient Preparation and Specimen Collection online at Davis*Plus*. Positively identify the patient, and label the appropriate specimen container with the corresponding patient demographics, initials of the person collecting the specimen, date, and time of collection. Perform a venipuncture.
- Remove the needle and apply direct pressure with dry gauze to stop bleeding. Observe/assess venipuncture site for bleeding or hematoma formation and secure gauze with adhesive bandage.

- Promptly transport the specimen to the laboratory for processing and analysis.

POST-TEST:

- Inform the patient that a report of the results will be made available to the requesting HCP, who will discuss the results with the patient.
- ***Nutritional Considerations:*** Severe hypophosphatemia is common in older adult patients or patients who have been hospitalized for long periods of time. Good dietary sources of phosphorus include meat, dairy products, nuts, and legumes. To decrease phosphorus levels to normal in the patient with hyperphosphatemia, dietary restriction may be recommended. Other interventions may include the administration of phosphate binders or calcitriol (the activated form of vitamin D).
- ***Nutritional Considerations:*** Vitamin D is necessary for the body to absorb phosphorus. Educate the patient with vitamin D deficiency, as appropriate, that the main dietary sources of vitamin D are cod liver oil and fortified dairy foods such as milk, cheese, and orange juice. Explain to the patient that vitamin D is also synthesized by the body, in the skin, and is activated by sunlight.
- Reinforce information given by the patient's HCP regarding further testing, treatment, or referral to another HCP. Answer any questions or address any concerns voiced by the patient or family. Educate the patient regarding access to nutritional counseling services. Provide contact information, if desired, for the Institute of Medicine of the National Academies (www.iom.edu) and USDA's resource for nutrition (http://www.choosemyplate.gov/). 🍁
- Depending on the results of this procedure, additional testing may be performed to evaluate or monitor progression of the disease process and determine the need for a change in therapy. Evaluate test results in relation to the patient's symptoms and other tests performed.

RELATED STUDIES:

- Related tests include biopsy bone, blood gases, BUN, calcitonin, calcium, calculus kidney stone panel, carbon dioxide, chloride, collagen cross-linked N-telopeptides, CBC WBC count and differential, creatinine, fecal analysis, fecal fat, FDP, glucagon, glucose, GH, insulin, lactic acid, lung perfusion scan, lung ventilation scan, osmolality, osteocalcin, PTH, parathyroid scan, phosphorus urine, potassium, US abdomen, and vitamin D.
- Refer to the Endocrine, Gastrointestinal, Genitourinary, and Musculoskeletal systems tables online at Davis*Plus* for related tests by body system.

P

Phosphorus, Urine

SYNONYM/ACRONYM: Urine phosphate.

COMMON USE: To assist in evaluating calcium and phosphorus levels related to use of diuretics in progression of kidney disease.

SPECIMEN: Urine from an unpreserved random or timed specimen collected in a clean plastic collection container.

NORMAL FINDINGS: (Method: Spectrophotometry) Reference values are dependent on phosphorus and calcium intake. Phosphate excretion exhibits diurnal variation and is significantly higher at night.

Conventional Units	SI Units (Conventional Units × 0.0323)
400–1,300 mg/24 hr	12.9–42 mmol/24 hr

POTENTIAL MEDICAL DIAGNOSIS

Increased in:

- Abuse of diuretics ***(related to increased renal excretion)***
- Primary hyperparathyroidism ***(parathyroid hormone [PTH] increases renal excretion)***
- Renal tubular acidosis
- Vitamin D deficiency ***(related to decreased renal reabsorption)***

Decreased in:

- Hypoparathyroidism ***(PTH enhances renal excretion; therefore, a lack of PTH will decrease urine phosphorus levels)***
- Pseudohypoparathyroidism ***(PTH enhances renal reabsorption; therefore, a lack of response to PTH, as in pseudohypoparathyroidism, will decrease urine phosphorus levels)***
- Vitamin D intoxication ***(vitamin D promotes renal excretion of phosphorus)***

CRITICAL FINDINGS: N/A

Find and print out the full study on Fast Find at davispl.us/vanleeuwen7.

Plasminogen

SYNONYM/ACRONYM: Profibrinolysin, PMG.

COMMON USE: To assess thrombolytic disorders such as disseminated intravascular coagulation (DIC) and monitor thrombolytic therapy.

SPECIMEN: Plasma collected in a completely filled blue-top (3.2% sodium citrate) tube. If the patient's hematocrit exceeds 55%, the volume of citrate in the collection tube must be adjusted.

NORMAL FINDINGS: (Method: Chromogenic substrate for plasminogen activity and nephelometric for plasminogen antigen)

Plasminogen activity	80%–100% of normal
Plasminogen antigen	7.5–15.5 mg/dL

Plasminogen activity in newborns is half of adult ranges.

POTENTIAL MEDICAL DIAGNOSIS

Increased in:

- Pregnancy (late) ***(pathophysiology is unclear)***

Decreased in:

- DIC ***(related to increased consumption during the hyperfibrinolytic state by conversion to plasmin)***
- Fibrinolytic therapy with tissue plasminogen activators such as streptokinase or urokinase ***(related to increased consumption by conversion to plasmin)***

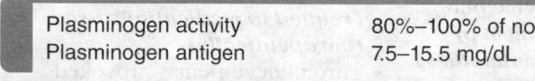

- Hereditary deficiency
- Liver disease ***(related to decreased production by damaged liver cells)***
- Neonatal hyaline membrane disease ***(possibly related to deficiency of plasminogen)***
- Postsurgical period ***(possibly related to trauma of surgery)***

CRITICAL FINDINGS: N/A

Find and print out the full study on Fast Find at davispl.us/vanleeuwen7.

Platelet Antibodies

SYNONYM/ACRONYM: Antiplatelet antibody; platelet-bound IgG/IgM, direct and indirect.

COMMON USE: To assess for the presence of platelet antibodies to assist in diagnosing thrombocytopenia related to autoimmune conditions and platelet transfusion compatibility issues.

SPECIMEN: Serum collected in a red-top tube for indirect immunoglobulin G (IgG) antibody. Whole blood collected in a lavender (EDTA)-, yellow (ACD)-, or pink (K2EDTA)-top tube for direct antibody.

NORMAL FINDINGS: (Method: Solid-phase enzyme-linked immunoassay) Negative.

POTENTIAL MEDICAL DIAGNOSIS

Increased in:

Development of platelet antibodies is associated with autoimmune conditions and medications.

- AIDS ***(related to medications used therapeutically)***
- Acute myeloid leukemia ***(related to medications used therapeutically)***
- Idiopathic thrombocytopenic purpura ***(related to development of platelet-associated IgG antibodies)***
- Immune complex diseases
- Multiple blood transfusions ***(related in most cases to sensitization to PLA1 antigens on donor red blood cells that will stimulate formation of antiplatelet antibodies)***
- Multiple myeloma ***(related to medications used therapeutically)***
- Neonatal immune thrombocytopenia ***(related to maternal platelet–associated antibodies directed against fetal platelets)***
- Paroxysmal hemoglobinuria
- Rheumatoid arthritis ***(related to medications used therapeutically)***
- Systemic lupus erythematosus ***(related to medications used therapeutically)***
- Thrombocytopenias provoked by drugs (see study titled "Complete Blood Count, Platelet Count")

Decreased in: N/A

CRITICAL FINDINGS: N/A

Find and print out the full study on Fast Find at davispl.us/vanleeuwen7.

P

Plethysmography

SYNONYM/ACRONYM: Impedance plethysmography, PVR.

COMMON USE: To measure changes in blood vessel size or changes in gas volume in the lungs to assist in diagnosing diseases such as deep vein thrombosis (DVT), chronic obstructive pulmonary disease (COPD), and some peripheral vascular disorders.

AREA OF APPLICATION: Veins, arteries, and lungs.

DESCRIPTION: Plethysmography is a noninvasive diagnostic manometric study used to measure changes in the size of blood vessels by determining volume changes in the blood vessels of the eye, extremities, and neck or to measure gas volume changes in the lungs.

Arterial plethysmography assesses arterial circulation in an upper or lower limb; it is used to diagnose extremity arteriosclerotic disease and to rule out occlusive disease. The test requires a normal extremity for comparison of results. The test is performed by applying a series of three blood pressure cuffs to the extremity. The amplitude of each pulse wave is then recorded.

Venous plethysmography, done with a series of cuffs, measures changes in venous capacity and outflow (volume and rate of outflow); it is used to diagnose a thrombotic condition that causes obstruction of the major veins of the extremity. When the cuffs are applied to an extremity in patients with venous obstruction, no initial increase in leg volume is recorded because the venous volume of the leg cannot dissipate quickly.

Body plethysmography measures the total amount (volume) of air within the thorax, whether or not the air is in ventilatory communication with the lung; the elasticity (compliance) of the lungs; and the resistance to airflow in the respiratory tree. It is used in conjunction with pulmonary stress testing and pulmonary function testing.

Impedance plethysmography is widely used to detect acute DVT of the leg, but it can also be used in the arm, abdomen, neck, or thorax. Doppler flow studies now are used to identify DVT, but ultrasound studies are less accurate in examinations below the knee.

This procedure is contraindicated for: N/A

INDICATIONS

Arterial Plethysmography

- Confirm suspected acute arterial embolization.
- Detect vascular changes associated with Raynaud's phenomenon and disease.
- Determine changes in toe or finger pressures when ankle pressures are elevated as a result of arterial calcifications.
- Determine the effect of trauma on the arteries in an extremity.

- Determine peripheral small-artery changes (ischemia) caused by diabetes, and differentiate these changes from neuropathy.
- Evaluate suspected arterial occlusive disease.
- Locate and determine the degree of arterial atherosclerotic obstruction and vessel patency in peripheral atherosclerotic disease, as well as inflammatory changes causing obliteration in the vessels in thromboangiitis obliterans.

Venous Plethysmography

- Detect partial or total venous thrombotic obstruction.
- Determine valve competency in conjunction with Doppler ultrasonography in the diagnosis of varicose veins.

Body Plethysmography

- Detect acute pulmonary disorders, such as atelectasis.
- Detect or determine the status of COPD, such as asthma or chronic bronchitis.
- Detect or determine the status of restrictive pulmonary disease, such as fibrosis.
- Detect infectious pulmonary diseases, such as pneumonia.
- Determine baseline pulmonary status before pulmonary rehabilitation to determine potential therapeutic benefit.
- Differentiate between obstructive and restrictive pulmonary pathology.

Impedance Plethysmography

- Act as a diagnostic screen for patients at risk for DVT.
- Detect and evaluate DVT.
- Evaluate degree of resolution of DVT after treatment.
- Evaluate patients with suspected pulmonary embolism (most pulmonary emboli are complications of DVT in the leg).

POTENTIAL MEDICAL DIAGNOSIS

Normal findings

- Arterial plethysmography:
  Normal arterial pulse waves: Steep upslope, more gradual downslope with narrow pointed peaks
  Normal pressure: Less than 20 mm Hg systolic difference between the lower and upper extremities; toe pressure greater than or equal to 80% of ankle pressure and finger pressure greater than or equal to 80% of wrist pressure
- Venous plethysmography:
  Normal venous blood flow in the extremities
  Venous filling times greater than 20 sec
- Body plethysmography:
  Thoracic gas volume: 2,400 mL
  Compliance: 0.2 L/cm H_2O
  Airway resistance: 0.6 to 2.5 cm H_2O/L per sec
- Impedance plethysmography:
  Sharp rise in volume with temporary occlusion
  Rapid venous outflow with release of the occlusion

Abnormal findings related to

- COPD, restrictive lung disease, lung infection, or atelectasis (body plethysmography)
- DVT (arterial, venous, or impedance plethysmography)
- Incompetent valves, thrombosis, or thrombotic obstruction in a major vein in an extremity
- Small-vessel diabetic changes
- Vascular disease (Raynaud's phenomenon)
- Vascular trauma

CRITICAL FINDINGS:

- DVT

Note and immediately report to the requesting health-care provider (HCP) any critical findings and related symptoms. A listing of these findings varies

among facilities. Timely notification of a critical finding for laboratory or diagnostic studies is a role expectation of the professional nurse. The notification processes vary among facilities. Upon receipt of the critical finding, the information should be read back to the caller to verify accuracy.

INTERFERING FACTORS

Arterial Plethysmography

Factors that may impair the results of the examination

- Cigarette smoking 2 hr before the study, which causes inaccurate results because the nicotine constricts the arteries
- Alcohol consumption
- Low cardiac output
- Shock
- Compression of pelvic veins (tumors or external compression by dressings)
- Environmental temperatures (hot or cold)
- Arterial occlusion proximal to the extremity to be examined, which can prevent blood flow to the limb

Venous Plethysmography

Factors that may impair the results of the examination

- Low environmental temperature or cold extremity, which constricts the vessels
- High anxiety level or muscle tenseness
- Venous thrombotic occlusion proximal to the extremity to be examined, which can affect blood flow to the limb

Body Plethysmography

Factors that may impair the results of the examination

- Inability of the patient to follow breathing instructions during the procedure

Impedance Plethysmography

Factors that may impair the results of the examination

- Movement of the extremity during electrical impedance recording, poor electrode contact, or nonlinear electrical output, which can cause false-positive results
- Constricting clothing or bandages

NURSING IMPLICATIONS AND PROCEDURE

See Potential Nursing Problems on Fast Find at davispl.us/vanleeuwen7.

PRETEST:

- Positively identify the patient using at least two person-specific identifiers before services, treatments, or procedures are performed.
- ***Patient Teaching:*** Inform the patient this procedure can assist in evaluating blood vessel size and lung ventilation.
- Obtain a history of the patient's health concerns, symptoms, surgical procedures, and results of previously performed laboratory and diagnostic studies. Include a list of known allergens, especially allergies or sensitivities to latex.
- Record the date of the last menstrual period and determine the possibility of pregnancy in perimenopausal women.
- Obtain a list of the patient's current medications, including over-the-counter medications and dietary supplements (see Effects of Natural Products on Laboratory Values online at Davis*Plus*).
- Review the procedure with the patient. Address concerns about pain related to the procedure and explain to the patient that no discomfort will be experienced during the test. Explain that there may be some discomfort during insertion of the naso-esophageal catheter if compliance testing is done. Inform the patient that the procedure is generally performed in a specialized area or at the

bedside by an HCP who specializes in this procedure, with support staff, and usually takes 30 to 60 min.

- Assess the patient's ability to comply with directions given for rest, positioning, and activity before and during the procedure.
- For body plethysmography, record the patient's weight, height, and gender. Determine whether the patient is claustrophobic.
- ***Sensitivity to social and cultural issues,*** as well as concern for modesty, is important in providing psychological support before, during, and after the procedure.
- Instruct the patient to refrain from smoking for 2 hr prior to the procedure.
- Note that there are no food, fluid, or medication restrictions unless by medical direction.

INTRATEST:

Potential Complications: N/A

- Observe standard precautions, and follow the general guidelines in Patient Preparation and Specimen Collection online at Davis*Plus*. Positively identify the patient.
- Ensure the patient has refrained from smoking for 2 hr before the procedure.
- Instruct the patient to void prior to the procedure and to change into the gown, robe, and foot coverings provided.
- Obtain and record baseline vital signs.
- Avoid the use of equipment containing latex if the patient has a history of allergic reaction to latex.
- Have emergency equipment readily available.
- Instruct the patient to report any unexpected symptoms that occur during the test.

Arterial Plethysmography

- Explain to the patient that cuffs are applied to the extremity to measure and compare blood flow.
- Place the patient in a semi-Fowler's position on an examination table or in bed.
- Ask the patient to notify medical personnel if he or she has unexpected symptoms during the test.
- Instruct the patient to remain still during the procedure.
- Apply three blood pressure cuffs to the extremity and attach a pulse volume recorder (plethysmograph), which records the amplitude of each pulse wave.
- Inflate the cuffs to 65 mm Hg to measure the pulse waves of each cuff. When compared with a normal limb, these measurements determine the presence of arterial occlusive disease.

Venous Plethysmography

- Explain to the patient that cuffs are applied to the extremity to measure and compare blood flow.
- Place the patient in a semi-Fowler's position on an examination table or in bed.
- Instruct the patient to remain still during the procedure.
- Apply two blood pressure cuffs to the extremity, one on the proximal part of the extremity (occlusion cuff) and the other on the distal part of the extremity (recorder cuff). Attach a third cuff to the pulse volume recorder.
- Inflate the recorder cuff to 10 mm Hg, and evaluate the effects of respiration on venous volume: Absence of changes during respirations indicates venous thrombotic occlusion.
- Inflate the occlusion cuff to 50 mm Hg, and record venous volume on the pulse monitor. Deflate the occlusion cuff after the highest volume is recorded in the recorder cuff. A delay in the return to preocclusion volume indicates venous thrombotic occlusion.

Body Plethysmography

- Place the patient in a sitting position on a chair in the body box. Explain to the patient that the cuffs are applied to the extremities to measure and compare blood flow.
- Position a nose clip to prevent breathing through the nose, and connect a mouthpiece to a measuring instrument.

P

- Ask the patient to breathe through the mouthpiece.
- Close the door to the box, and record the start time of the procedure. At the beginning of the study, instruct the patient to pant rapidly and shallowly, without allowing the glottis to close.
- For compliance testing, a double-lumen nasoesophageal catheter is inserted, and the bag is inflated with air. Intraesophageal pressure is recorded during normal breathing.

Impedance Plethysmography

- Explain to the patient that cuffs are applied to the extremity to measure and compare blood flow.
- Place the patient on his or her back with the leg being tested above the heart level.
- Flex the patient's knee slightly, and rotate the hips by shifting weight to the same side as the leg being tested.
- Apply conductive gel and electrodes to the legs, near the cuffs.
- Apply a blood pressure cuff to the thigh.
- Inflate the pressure cuff attached to the thigh temporarily to occlude venous return without interfering with arterial blood flow. Expect the blood volume in the other calf to increase.
- A tracing of changes in electrical impedance occurring during inflation and for 15 sec after cuff deflation is recorded.
- With DVT, blood volume increases less than expected because the veins are already at capacity.

POST-TEST:

- Inform the patient that a report of the results will be made available to the requesting HCP, who will discuss the results with the patient.
- Remove conductive gel and electrodes, as applied.
- Instruct the patient to resume usual activity and diet, as directed by the HCP.
- Monitor for severe ischemia, ulcers, and pain of the extremity after arterial, venous, or impedance plethysmography, and handle the extremity gently.
- Monitor respiratory pattern after body plethysmography, and allow the patient time to resume a normal breathing pattern.
- Monitor vital signs every 15 min until they return to baseline levels.
- Recognize anxiety related to test results, and be supportive of perceived loss of independent function. Discuss the implications of abnormal test results on the patient's lifestyle. Provide teaching and information regarding the clinical implications of the test results, as appropriate.
- Reinforce information given by the patient's HCP regarding further testing, treatment, or referral to another HCP. Answer any questions or address any concerns voiced by the patient or family.
- Depending on the results of this procedure, additional testing may be needed to evaluate or monitor progression of the disease process and determine the need for a change in therapy. Evaluate test results in relation to the patient's symptoms and other tests performed.

Patient Education:

- Teach the patient the purpose of ordered medications.
- Teach the patient the importance of calling for pain medication as soon as it is needed for effective pain management.

Expected Patient Outcomes:

Understanding

- The patient and family state the importance of keeping oxygen on at all times.
- The patient and family state the pathophysiology of the diagnosed disease process.

Ability

- The patient and family plan rest periods during the day to conserve oxygen.
- The patient demonstrates successful coping strategies.

Response

- The patient agrees to all follow-up diagnostic and laboratory studies

P

needed to monitor health status and the effectiveness of treatment modalities.

- The patient and family agree to family or individual support group counseling related to prognosis and end-of-life choices.

RELATED STUDIES:

- Related tests include α_1-AT, angiography pulmonary, anion gap, arterial/alveolar oxygen ratio, AT-III, biopsy lung, blood gases, bronchoscopy, carboxyhemoglobin, cardiolipin antibodies, chest x-ray, chloride sweat, cold agglutinin, CBC, CBC hemoglobin, CBC WBC count and differential, CT angiography, CT thoracic, culture and smear for mycobacteria, culture bacterial sputum, culture viral, cytology sputum, D-dimer, echocardiography, ECG, EMG, electroneurography, fibrinogen, Gram stain, IgE, lactic acid, lung perfusion scan, lung ventilation scan, lupus anticoagulant antibodies, MR angiography, MRI chest, MRI venography, osmolality, phosphorus, plasminogen, pleural fluid analysis, potassium, PFT, pulse oximetry, sodium, TB skin test, and US arterial and venous Doppler of the extremities.
- Refer to the Cardiovascular and Pulmonary systems tables online at Davis*Plus* for related tests by body system.

Pleural Fluid Analysis

SYNONYM/ACRONYM: Thoracentesis fluid analysis.

COMMON USE: To assess and categorize fluid obtained from within the pleural space for infection, cancer, and blood as well as identify the cause of its accumulation.

SPECIMEN: Pleural fluid collected in a green-top (heparin) tube for amylase, cholesterol, glucose, lactate dehydrogenase (LDH), pH, protein, and triglycerides; lavender-top (EDTA) tube for cell count; sterile containers for microbiology specimens; of fluid in a clear container with anticoagulant for cytology. Ensure that there is an equal amount of fixative and fluid in the container for cytology.

NORMAL FINDINGS: (Method: Spectrophotometry for amylase, cholesterol, glucose, LDH, protein, and triglycerides; ion-selective electrode for pH; automated or manual cell count; macroscopic and microscopic examination of cultured microorganisms; microscopic examination of specimen for microbiology and cytology)

Appearance	Clear
Color	Pale yellow
Amylase	Parallels serum values
Cholesterol	Parallels serum values
CEA	Parallels serum values
Glucose	Parallels serum values
LDH	Less than 200 units/L
Fluid LDH-to-serum LDH ratio	0.6 or less
Protein	3 g/dL

P

Appearance	Clear
Fluid protein-to-serum protein ratio	0.5 or less
Triglycerides	Parallel serum values
pH	7.37–7.43
RBC count	None seen
WBC count	Less than 1,000 cells/microL
Culture	No growth
Gram stain	No organisms seen
Cytology	No abnormal cells seen

CEA = carcinoembryonic antigen; LDH = lactate dehydrogenase; RBC = red blood cell; WBC = white blood cell.

DESCRIPTION: The pleural cavity and organs within it are lined with a protective membrane. The fluid between the membranes is called *serous fluid.* Normally, only a small amount of fluid is present because the rates of fluid production and absorption are about the same. Many abnormal conditions can result in the buildup of fluid within the pleural cavity. Specific tests are usually ordered in addition to a common battery of tests used to distinguish a transudate from an exudate. *Transudates* are effusions that form as a result of a systemic disorder that disrupts the regulation of fluid balance, such as a suspected perforation. *Exudates* are caused by conditions involving the tissue of the membrane itself, such as an infection or malignancy. Fluid is withdrawn from the pleural cavity by needle aspiration and tested as listed in the previous and following tables.

Characteristic	Transudate	Exudate
Appearance	Clear	Cloudy or turbid
Specific gravity	Less than 1.015	Greater than 1.015
Total protein	Less than 2.5 g/dL	Greater than 3 g/dL
Fluid protein-to-serum protein ratio	Less than 0.5	Greater than 0.5
LDH	Parallels serum value	Less than 200 units/L
Fluid LDH-to-serum LDH ratio	Less than 0.6	Greater than 0.6
Fluid cholesterol	Less than 55 mg/dL	Greater than 55 mg/dL
WBC count	Less than 100 cells/microL	Greater than 1,000 cells/microL

LDH = lactate dehydrogenase; WBC = white blood cell.

This procedure is contraindicated for: N/A

INDICATIONS

- Differentiate transudates from exudates.
- Evaluate effusion of unknown cause.
- Investigate suspected rupture, immune disease, malignancy, or infection.

POTENTIAL MEDICAL DIAGNOSIS

- *Bacterial or tuberculous empyema:* Elevated white blood cell (WBC) count with a predominance of neutrophils, increased fluid protein-to-serum protein ratio, increased fluid LDH-to-serum LDH ratio, decreased glucose, pH less than 7.3
- *Chylous pleural effusion:* Marked increase in both triglycerides (two to three times serum level) and chylomicrons
- *Effusion caused by pneumonia:* Elevated WBC count with a predominance of neutrophils and some eosinophils, increased fluid protein-to-serum protein ratio, increased fluid LDH-to-serum LDH ratio, pH less than 7.4 (and decreased glucose if bacterial pneumonia)
- *Esophageal rupture:* Significantly decreased pH (6) and elevated amylase
- *Hemothorax:* Bloody appearance, increased RBC count, elevated hematocrit
- *Malignancy:* Elevated WBC count with a predominance of lymphocytes, possible elevated RBC count, abnormal cytology, increased fluid protein-to-serum protein ratio, increased fluid LDH-to-serum LDH ratio, decreased glucose, pH less than 7.3
- *Pancreatitis:* Elevated WBC count with a predominance of neutrophils, elevated RBC count, pH greater than 7.3, increased fluid protein-to-serum protein ratio, increased fluid LDH-to-serum LDH ratio, increased amylase
- *Pulmonary infarction:* Elevated RBC count, elevated WBC count with a predominance of neutrophils, pH greater than 7.3, normal glucose, increased fluid protein-to-serum protein ratio, and increased fluid LDH-to-serum LDH ratio.
- *Pulmonary tuberculosis:* Elevated WBC count with a predominance of lymphocytes, positive acid-fast bacillus stain and culture, increased protein, decreased glucose, pH less than 7.3
- *Rheumatoid disease:* Elevated WBC count with a predominance of either lymphocytes or neutrophils, pH less than 7.3, decreased glucose, increased fluid protein-to-serum protein ratio, increased fluid LDH-to-serum LDH ratio, increased immunoglobulins
- *Systemic lupus erythematosus:* Similar findings as with rheumatoid disease, except that glucose is usually not decreased

CRITICAL FINDINGS:

Positive culture findings in any sterile body fluid.

Note and immediately report to the requesting health-care provider (HCP) any critical findings and related symptoms. A listing of these findings varies among facilities. Timely notification of a critical finding for laboratory or diagnostic studies is a role expectation of the professional nurse. The notification processes vary among facilities. Upon receipt of the critical finding, the information should be read back to the caller to verify accuracy.

INTERFERING FACTORS

- Bloody fluids may be the result of a traumatic tap.
- Unknown hyperglycemia or hypoglycemia may be misleading in the comparison of fluid and serum glucose levels. Therefore, it is advisable to collect comparative serum samples a few hours before performing thoracentesis.

P

NURSING IMPLICATIONS AND PROCEDURE

PRETEST:

- Positively identify the patient using at least two person-specific identifiers before services, treatments, or procedures are performed.
- *Patient Teaching:* Inform the patient this test can assist in identifying the type of fluid being produced within the body cavity.
- Obtain a history of the patient's health concerns, symptoms, surgical procedures, and results of previously performed laboratory and diagnostic studies. Include a list of known allergens, especially allergies or sensitivities to latex.
- Note any recent procedures that can interfere with test results.
- Record the date of the last menstrual period and determine the possibility of pregnancy in perimenopausal women.
- Obtain a list of the patient's current medications, including over-the-counter medications, dietary supplements, anticoagulants, aspirin and other salicylates (see Effects of Natural Products on Laboratory Values online at Davis*Plus*). Such products should be discontinued by medical direction for the appropriate number of days prior to a surgical procedure. Note the last time and dose of medication taken.
- Review the procedure with the patient. Inform the patient that it may be necessary to remove hair from the site before the procedure. Discuss with the patient that the requesting HCP may request that a cough suppressant be given before the thoracentesis. Address concerns about pain and explain that a sedative and/or analgesia will be administered to promote relaxation and reduce discomfort prior to needle insertion through the chest wall into the pleural space. Explain that any discomfort with the needle insertion will be minimized with local anesthetics and systemic analgesics. Explain that the local anesthetic injection may cause an initial stinging sensation. A sedative may be given to promote relaxation. Inform the patient that the needle insertion is performed under sterile conditions by an HCP specializing in this procedure. The procedure usually takes about 20 min to complete.
- Explain that an intravenous (IV) line will be inserted to allow infusion of fluids, antibiotics, anesthetics, and analgesics.
- ***Sensitivity to social and cultural issues,*** as well as concern for modesty, is important in providing psychological support before, during, and after the procedure.
- Note that there are no food or fluid restrictions unless by medical direction. The requesting HCP may request that anticoagulants and aspirin be withheld. The number of days to withhold medication is dependent on the type of anticoagulant.
- *Make sure a written and informed consent has been signed prior to the procedure and before administering any medications.*

INTRATEST:

Potential Complications:

Pneumothorax, bleeding, hemoptysis, and pulmonary edema.

- Ensure that anticoagulant therapy has been withheld for the appropriate number of days prior to the procedure. Notify the HCP if patient anticoagulant therapy has not been withheld.
- Have emergency equipment readily available. Keep resuscitation equipment on hand in the case of respiratory impairment or laryngospasm after the procedure.
- Avoid using morphine sulfate in those with asthma or other pulmonary disease. This drug can further exacerbate bronchospasms and respiratory impairment.
- Have the patient remove clothing and change into a gown for the procedure.

P

- Instruct the patient to cooperate fully and to follow directions. Direct the patient to breathe normally and to avoid unnecessary movement during the local anesthetic and the procedure.
- Observe standard precautions, and follow the general guidelines in Patient Preparation and Specimen Collection online at Davis*Plus*. Positively identify the patient, and label the appropriate specimen container with the corresponding patient demographics, initials of the person collecting the specimen, date and time of collection, and site location.
- Record baseline vital signs and continue to monitor throughout the procedure. Protocols may vary among facilities.
- Establish an IV line to allow infusion of fluids, anesthetics, analgesics, or sedation.
- Assist the patient into a comfortable sitting or side-lying position.
- Prior to the administration of local anesthesia, clip hair from the site as needed, cleanse the site with an antiseptic solution, and drape the area with sterile towels. The skin at the injection site is then anesthetized.
- The thoracentesis needle is inserted, and fluid is removed.
- The needle is withdrawn, and pressure is applied to the site with a petroleum jelly gauze. A pressure dressing is applied over the petroleum jelly gauze.
- Monitor the patient for complications related to the procedure (e.g., allergic reaction, anaphylaxis).
- Place samples in properly labelled specimen container, and promptly transport the specimen to the laboratory for processing and analysis.

POST-TEST:

- Inform the patient that a report of the results will be made available to the requesting HCP, who will discuss the results with the patient.
- Instruct the patient to resume usual medications, as directed by the HCP.
- Monitor vital signs every 15 min for the first hr, every 30 min for the next 2 hr, every hour for the next 4 hr, and every 4 hr for the next 24 hr. Take the patient's temperature every 4 hr for 24 hr. Monitor intake and output for 24 hr. Notify the HCP if temperature is elevated. Protocols may vary among facilities.
- Observe/assess the patient for signs of respiratory distress or skin color changes.
- Observe/assess the thoracentesis site for bleeding, inflammation, or hematoma formation each time vital signs are taken and daily thereafter for several days.
- Observe/assess the patient for hemoptysis, difficulty breathing, cough, air hunger, pain, or absent breathing sounds over the affected area. Report to HCP.
- Inform the patient that 1 hr or more of bed rest (lying on the unaffected side) is required after the procedure. Elevate the patient's head for comfort.
- Evaluate the patient for symptoms indicating the development of pneumothorax, such as dyspnea, tachypnea, anxiety, decreased breathing sounds, or restlessness. Prepare the patient for a chest x-ray, if ordered, to ensure that a pneumothorax has not occurred as a result of the procedure.
- Observe/assess for nausea and pain. Administer antiemetic and analgesic medications as needed and as directed by the HCP.
- Administer antibiotics, as ordered, and instruct the patient in the importance of completing the entire course of antibiotic therapy even if no symptoms are present.
- Recognize anxiety related to test results, and offer support. Discuss the implications of abnormal test results on the patient's lifestyle. Provide teaching and information regarding the clinical implications of the test results, as appropriate. Educate the patient regarding access to counseling services, if appropriate.

P

- Reinforce information given by the patient's HCP regarding further testing, treatment, or referral to another HCP. Answer any questions or address any concerns voiced by the patient or family.
- Depending on the results of this procedure, additional testing may be performed to evaluate or monitor progression of the disease process and determine the need for a change in therapy. Evaluate test results in relation to the patient's symptoms and other tests performed.

RELATED STUDIES:

- Related tests include antibodies anticyclic citrullinated peptide, ANA, biopsy lung, blood gases, cancer antigens, chest x-ray, CBC WBC count and differential, CT thoracic, CRP, culture and smear mycobacteria, culture blood, culture fungal, culture viral, ECG, ESR, Gram stain, MRI chest, and RF.
- Refer to the Immune and Respiratory systems tables online at Davis*Plus* for related tests by body system.

Porphyrins, Urine

SYNONYM/ACRONYM: Coproporphyrin, porphobilinogen, urobilinogen, and other porphyrins.

COMMON USE: To assess for porphyrins in the urine to assist with diagnosis of genetic disorders associated with porphyrin synthesis as well as heavy metal toxicity.

SPECIMEN: Urine from a random or timed specimen collected in a clean, amber-colored plastic collection container with sodium carbonate as a preservative.

NORMAL FINDINGS: (Method: High-performance liquid chromatography for porphyrins; spectrophotometry for δ-aminolevulinic acid and porphobilinogen)

Test	Conventional Units	SI Units
		(Conventional units × 1.53)
Coproporphyrin I	0–24 mcg/24 h	0–36.7 nmol/24 hr
Coproporphyrin III	0–74 mcg/24 hr	0–113.2 nmol/24 hr
		(Conventional units × 1.43)
Uroporphyrins	0–24 mcg/24 hr	0–34.3 nmol/24 hr
		(Conventional units × 1.34)
Hexacarboxylporphyrin	Less than 1 mcg/24 hr	Less than 1.34 nmol/24 hr
		(Conventional units × 1.27)
Heptacarboxylporphyrin	Less than 4 mcg/24 hr	Less than 5.1 nmol/24 hr
		(Conventional units × 4.42)
Porphobilinogen	Less than 2 mg/24 hr	Less than 8.8 micromol/24 hr
		(Conventional units × 7.626)
δ-Aminolevulinic acid	1.5–7.5 mg/24 hr	11.4–57.2 micromol/24 hr

POTENTIAL MEDICAL DIAGNOSIS

Increased in:

Accumulation of porphyrins or porphyrin precursors in the body is common to the various types of porphyrias. Excessive amounts of circulating porphyrins and precursors are excreted in the urine.

- Acute intermittent porphyria ***(related to an autosomal dominant disorder resulting in a deficiency of the enzyme porphobilinogen deaminase and increased excretion of porphobilinogen and delta-aminolevulinic acid [δ-ALA] in the urine)***
- Acquired or chemical porphyrias (heavy metal, benzene, or carbon tetrachloride toxicity; drug induced) ***(related to a disturbance in the heme biosynthetic pathway and increased excretion of delta-aminolevulinic acid in the urine)***
- ALAD deficiency porphyria ***(related to an autosomal recessive disorder resulting in a deficiency of the enzyme delta-aminolevulinic acid dehydratase and increased excretion of δ-ALA in the urine)***
- Hepatoerythropoietic porphyria ***(related to an autosomal recessive disorder resulting in a deficiency of the enzyme uroporphyrinogen decarboxylase and increased excretion of uroporphyrin and heptacarboxylporphyrin in the urine)***
- Hereditary coproporphyria ***(related to an autosomal dominant disorder resulting in a deficiency of the enzyme coproporphyrinogen oxidase and increased excretion of porphobilinogen, δ-ALA, and coproporphyrin in the urine)***
- Porphyria cutanea tarda ***(related to an acquired deficiency of the enzyme uroporphyrinogen decarboxylase activated by exposure to triggers such as iron, alcohol, hepatitis C virus, HIV, or estrogens and increased excretion of uroporphyrin, heptacarboxylporphyrin, and coproporphyrin in the urine)***
- Variegate porphyrias ***(related to an autosomal dominant disorder resulting in a deficiency of the enzyme protoporphyrinogen oxidase and increased excretion of porphobilinogen, coproporphyrin, and δ-ALA in the urine during attacks; excretion of normal levels may be found between attacks)***

Decreased in: N/A

CRITICAL FINDINGS: N/A

Find and print out the full study on Fast Find at davispl.us/vanleeuwen7.

P

Positron Emission Tomography, Brain

SYNONYM/ACRONYM: PET scan of the brain.

COMMON USE: To assess blood flow and metabolic processes of the brain to assist in diagnosis of disorders such as ischemic or hemorrhagic stroke or cancer and to evaluate head trauma.

AREA OF APPLICATION: Brain.

DESCRIPTION: Positron emission tomography (PET) combines the biochemical properties of nuclear medicine with the anatomic accuracy of computed tomography (CT). PET uses positron emissions from specific radionuclides. The positron radiopharmaceuticals generally have short half-lives, ranging from a few seconds to a few hours, and therefore they must be produced in a cyclotron located near where the test is being done. A radionuclide is basically composed of a measurable radioactive isotope and a biologically active molecule. The isotopes are derived from elements that are either naturally present in organic molecules (oxygen, nitrogen, and carbon) or can be substituted for naturally occurring elements (fluorine can be substituted for hydrogen). Selected molecules become biologically active radiolabelled analogs of their naturally occurring forms to create radionuclides that produce detailed functional images of the target organ's structure. Radionuclides are used to evaluate many aspects of organ function, including oxygen consumption and glucose metabolism; most PET studies are conducted in the areas of cardiology, neurology, and oncology. The studies are used to diagnose and stage diseases as well as to monitor the efficacy of therapeutic interventions. During the PET brain scan, the radiotracer is injected into the body where it migrates to the intended target organ, becomes involved in the physiological process of interest, and accumulates to the degree that radioactive emissions are detected by the PET scanner. The PET scanner translates the emissions from the radioactivity as the positron combines with the negative electrons from the tissues and forms gamma rays that can be detected by the scanner. This information is transmitted to the computer, which determines the location and its distribution and translates the emissions as color-coded images for viewing, quantitative measurements, activity changes in relation to time, and three-dimensional computer-aided analysis.

The brain uses oxygen and glucose almost exclusively to meet its energy needs, and therefore the brain's metabolism has been studied widely with PET. Each radionuclide tracer is designed to measure a specific body process, such as glucose metabolism, blood flow, or brain tissue perfusion. Fluorine-18, in the form of fluorodeoxyglucose (FDG), is one of the most versatile and commonly used radionuclides in PET. FDG is a glucose analogue. All cells use glucose, but diseases that involve increased metabolic activity will show a high level of radionuclide visualization, whereas those that are hypometabolic will show little to no radionuclide visualization. There is little localization of FDG in normal tissue with minimal amounts being evenly distributed, allowing rapid detection of abnormal disease states. The radionuclide can be administered by intravenous (IV) injection or inhaled as a gas. After the radionuclide becomes concentrated in the brain, PET images of blood flow or metabolic processes at the cellular level can be obtained. Oxygen-15 is used in circumstances that warrant the evaluation of blood flow in the brain to predict or identify areas affected by a stroke. PET scan

P

of the brain has had the greatest clinical impact in patients with epilepsy, dementia, neurodegenerative diseases, inflammation, cerebrovascular disease (indirectly), and brain tumors.

The expense of the study and the limited availability of radiopharmaceuticals limit the use of PET even though it is more sensitive than traditional nuclear scanning and single-photon emission computed tomography (SPECT). PET/CT and SPECT/CT are imaging applications that superimpose PET or SPECT and CT findings. The images are collected and produced by a single gantry system. The coregistered or image fusion of PET/CT or SPECT/CT findings can provide a detailed combination of anatomical and functional images. PET images can also be superimposed on MRI images.

This procedure is contraindicated for

Patients who are pregnant or suspected of being pregnant, unless the potential benefits of a procedure using radiation far outweigh the risk of radiation exposure to the fetus and mother.

INDICATIONS

- Detect Parkinson's disease and Huntington's disease, as evidenced by decreased metabolism.
- Determine the effectiveness of therapy, as evidenced by biochemical activity of normal and abnormal tissues.
- Determine physiological changes in psychosis and schizophrenia.
- Differentiate between tumor recurrence and radiation necrosis.
- Evaluate Alzheimer's disease and differentiate it from other causes of dementia, as evidenced by decreased cerebral flow and metabolism.
- Evaluate cranial tumors pre- and postoperatively and determine stage and appropriate treatment or procedure.
- Identify cerebrovascular accident or aneurysm, as evidenced by decreased blood flow and oxygen use.
- Identify focal seizures, as evidenced by decreased metabolism between seizures.

POTENTIAL MEDICAL DIAGNOSIS

Normal findings

- Normal patterns of tissue metabolism, blood flow, and homogeneous radionuclide distribution

Abnormal findings related to

- Alzheimer's disease ***(evidenced in later stages by areas lacking radionuclide visualization related to decreased cellular activity; cellular activity decreases as the disease progresses)***
- Aneurysm ***(evidenced by areas lacking radionuclide visualization related to decreased cellular activity; cellular activity decreases as the disease progresses)***
- Cerebral metastases ***(evidenced by areas of intense radionuclide visualization related to abnormally increased cellular activity)***
- Cerebrovascular accident ***(evidenced by areas lacking radionuclide visualization related to decreased cellular activity)***
- Creutzfeldt-Jakob disease
- Dementia ***(evidenced by areas lacking radionuclide visualization related to decreased cellular activity; cellular activity decreases as the disease progresses)***

P

- Head trauma ***(evidenced by areas lacking radionuclide visualization related to decreased cellular activity)***
- Huntington's disease ***(evidenced by focal areas of intense radionuclide visualization related to hyperactivity of the affected nerves and increased cellular metabolism; cellular activity decreases as the disease progresses)***
- Migraine
- Parkinson's disease ***(evidenced by focal areas of intense radionuclide visualization related to hyperactivity of the affected nerves and increased cellular metabolism; cellular activity decreases as the disease progresses)***
- Schizophrenia
- Seizure disorders ***(evidenced by focal areas of intense radionuclide visualization related to hyperactivity of the affected nerves and increased cellular metabolism)***
- Tumors ***(evidenced by areas of intense radionuclide visualization related to abnormally increased cellular activity)***

CRITICAL FINDINGS:

- Aneurysm
- Cerebrovascular accident
- Tumor with significant mass effect

Note and immediately report to the requesting health-care provider (HCP) any critical findings and related symptoms. A listing of these findings varies among facilities. Timely notification of a critical finding for laboratory or diagnostic studies is a role expectation of the professional nurse. The notification processes vary among facilities. Upon receipt of the critical finding, the information should be read back to the caller to verify accuracy.

INTERFERING FACTORS

Factors that may alter the results of the study

- Inability of the patient to cooperate or remain still during the procedure because of age, significant pain, or mental status.
- Drugs that alter glucose metabolism, such as tranquilizers or insulin, because hypoglycemia can alter PET results.
- The use of alcohol, tobacco, or caffeine-containing drinks at least 24 hr before the study, because the effects of these substances would make it difficult to evaluate the patient's true physiological state (e.g., alcohol is a vasoconstrictor and would decrease blood flow to the target organ).
- Metallic objects (e.g., jewelry, body rings) within the examination field, which may inhibit organ visualization and cause unclear images.

Other considerations

- Failure to follow dietary restrictions before the procedure may cause the procedure to be canceled or repeated.
- Improper injection of the radionuclide that allows the tracer to seep deep into the muscle tissue produces erroneous hot spots.
- False-positive findings may occur as a result of normal gastrointestinal tract uptake and uptake in areas of infection or inflammation.

P

NURSING IMPLICATIONS AND PROCEDURE

See Potential Nursing Problems on Fast Find at davispl.us/vanleeuwen7.

PRETEST:

- Positively identify the patient using at least two person-specific identifiers before services, treatments, or procedures are performed.

- ***Patient Teaching:*** Inform the patient that this procedure can assist in assessing blood flow to the brain and brain tissue metabolism.
- Obtain a history of the patient's health concerns, symptoms, surgical procedures, and results of previously performed laboratory and diagnostic studies. Include a list of known allergens, especially allergies or sensitivities to latex, anesthetics, sedatives, or radionuclides.
- Obtain a history of the patient's musculoskeletal system, symptoms, and results of previously performed laboratory tests and diagnostic and surgical procedures.
- Note any recent procedures that can interfere with test results, including examinations using barium- or iodine-based contrast medium.
- Record the date of the last menstrual period and determine the possibility of pregnancy in perimenopausal women.
- Obtain a list of the patient's current medications, including over-the-counter medications and dietary supplements (see Effects of Natural Products on Laboratory Values online at Davis*Plus*).
- Review the procedure with the patient. Address concerns about pain related to the procedure and explain that some pain may be experienced during the test, or there may be moments of discomfort. Reassure the patient that radioactive material poses minimal radioactive hazard because of its short half-life and rarely produces adverse effects. Inform the patient that the procedure is performed in a special department, usually in a radiology suite, by an HCP specializing in this procedure, with support staff, and takes approximately 60 to 120 min.
- ***Sensitivity to social and cultural issues,*** as well as concern for modesty, is important in providing psychological support before, during, and after the procedure.
- Explain that an IV line may be inserted to allow infusion of fluids such as saline, anesthetics, sedatives, radionuclides, medications used in the procedure, or emergency medications.
- Sometimes FDG examinations are done after blood has been drawn to determine circulating blood glucose levels. If blood glucose levels are high, insulin may be given.
- Instruct the patient to remove jewelry and other metallic objects from the area to be examined prior to the procedure.
- Instruct the patient to avoid taking anticoagulant medication or to reduce dosage as ordered prior to the procedure.
- Instruct the patient to restrict food for 4 hr; restrict alcohol, nicotine, or caffeine-containing drinks for 24 hr; and withhold medications for 24 hr before the test. Protocols may vary among facilities.
- *Make sure a written and informed consent has been signed prior to the procedure and before administering any medications.*

INTRATEST:

Potential Complications:

Although it is rare, there is the possibility of allergic reaction to the radionuclide. Have emergency equipment and medications readily available. If the patient has a history of allergic reactions to any substance or drug, administer ordered prophylactic steroids or antihistamines before the procedure.

Establishing an IV site and injecting radionuclides is an invasive procedure. Complications are rare but do include bleeding from the puncture site ***related to a bleeding disorder, or the effects of natural products and medications with known anticoagulant, antiplatelet, or thrombolytic properties;*** hematoma ***related to blood leakage into the tissue following needle insertion;*** infection ***that might occur if bacteria from the skin surface is introduced at the puncture site;*** or nerve injury ***that might occur if the needle strikes a nerve.***

- Observe standard precautions, and follow the general guidelines in Patient Preparation and Specimen Collection online at Davis*Plus*. Positively identify the patient.
- Ensure that the patient has complied with dietary, fluid, and medication restrictions and pretesting preparations prior to the procedure, as instructed.
- Ensure the patient has removed all jewelry and external metallic objects from the area to be examined prior to the procedure.
- Avoid the use of equipment containing latex if the patient has a history of allergic reaction to latex.
- Have emergency equipment readily available.
- Instruct the patient to void prior to the procedure and to change into the gown, robe, and foot coverings provided.
- Instruct the patient to cooperate fully and to follow directions. Ask the patient to remain still throughout the procedure because movement produces unreliable results.
- Record baseline vital signs and assess neurological status. Protocols may vary among facilities.
- Establish an IV fluid line for the injection of saline, anesthetics, sedatives, radionuclides, or emergency medications.
- Place the patient in the supine position on an examination table.
- The radionuclide is injected, and imaging is started after a 30-min delay. If comparative studies are indicated, additional injections may be needed.
- The patient may be asked to perform different cognitive activities (e.g., reading) to measure changes in brain activity during reasoning or remembering.
- The patient may be blindfolded or asked to use earplugs to decrease auditory and visual stimuli.
- Monitor the patient for complications related to the procedure (e.g., allergic reaction, anaphylaxis, bronchospasm).
- Remove the needle or catheter and apply a pressure dressing over the puncture site.
- Observe/assess the needle/catheter insertion site for bleeding, inflammation, or hematoma formation.

POST-TEST:

- Inform the patient that a report of the results will be made available to the requesting HCP, who will discuss the results with the patient.
- Instruct the patient to resume pretest diet, fluids, medications, or activity.
- Observe for delayed allergic reactions, such as rash, urticaria, tachycardia, hyperpnea, hypertension, palpitations, nausea, or vomiting.
- Instruct the patient to immediately report symptoms such as fast heart rate, difficulty breathing, skin rash, itching, chest pain, persistent right shoulder pain, or abdominal pain. Immediately report symptoms to the appropriate HCP.
- Observe/assess the needle/catheter insertion site for bleeding, inflammation, or hematoma formation.
- Instruct the patient in the care and assessment of the injection site.
- Instruct the patient to apply cold compresses to the puncture site as needed to reduce discomfort or edema.
- Instruct the patient to drink increased amounts of fluids for 24 to 48 hr to eliminate the radionuclide from the body, unless contraindicated. Educate the patient that radionuclide is eliminated from the body within 6 to 24 hr.
- Instruct the patient to flush the toilet immediately after each voiding and to meticulously wash hands with soap and water for 24 hr after the procedure.
- Instruct all caregivers to wear gloves when discarding urine for 24 hr after the procedure. Wash gloved hands with soap and water before removing gloves; then wash ungloved hands.
- If a woman who is breastfeeding must have a nuclear scan, she should not breastfeed the infant until the radionuclide has been eliminated, about

P

3 days. Instruct her to express the milk and discard it during the 3-day period to prevent cessation of milk production.

- No other radionuclide tests should be scheduled for 24 to 48 hr after this procedure.
- Recognize anxiety related to test results, and be supportive of perceived loss of independent function. Discuss the implications of abnormal test results on the patient's lifestyle. Provide teaching and information regarding the clinical implications of the test results, as appropriate.
- Reinforce information given by the patient's HCP regarding further testing, treatment, or referral to another HCP. Answer any questions or address any concerns voiced by the patient or family.
- Depending on the results of this procedure, additional testing may be needed to evaluate or monitor progression of the disease process and determine the need for a change in therapy. Evaluate test results in relation to the patient's symptoms and other tests performed.

Patient Education:

- Teach the patient, parent, or significant other reportable symptoms related to bleeding due to medication use.
- Teach the patient, parent, or significant other bleeding precautions that should be used with specific medications.

Expected Patient Outcomes:

Understanding

- The patient and family state the importance of refraining from risky activity that could result in trauma and bleeding.
- The patient and family state the importance of frequent positioning to decrease risk of pressure ulcer development.

Ability

- The patient and family successfully demonstrate range-of-motion technique.
- The patient and family successfully demonstrate the use of assistive devices.

Response

- The family agrees to psychological assistance to meet challenges of dementia, psychosis, Alzheimer's disease.
- The patient and family state the increased risk of falling, the patient agrees to call for assistance when getting out of bed to decrease fall risk, and appropriate restraint use is discussed.

RELATED STUDIES:

- Related tests include Alzheimer's disease markers, CT brain, EEG, MRI brain, and US arterial Doppler of the carotids.
- Refer to the Musculoskeletal System table online at Davis*Plus* for related tests by body system.

P

Positron Emission Tomography, Heart

SYNONYM/ACRONYM: PET scan of the heart.

COMMON USE: To assess blood flow and metabolic process of the heart to assist in diagnosis of disorders such as coronary artery disease, infarct, and aneurysm.

AREA OF APPLICATION: Heart, chest/thorax, vascular system.

DESCRIPTION: Positron emission tomography (PET) combines the biochemical properties of nuclear medicine with the anatomic accuracy of computed tomography (CT). PET uses positron emissions from specific radionuclides. The positron radiopharmaceuticals generally have short half-lives, ranging from a few seconds to a few hours, and therefore they must be produced in a cyclotron located near where the test is being done. A radionuclide is basically composed of a measurable radioactive isotope and a biologically active molecule. The isotopes are derived from elements that are either naturally present in organic molecules (oxygen, nitrogen, and carbon) or can be substituted for naturally occurring elements (fluorine can be substituted for hydrogen). Selected molecules become biologically active radiolabelled analogs of their naturally occurring forms to create radionuclides that produce detailed functional images of the target organ's structure. Radionuclides are used to evaluate many aspects of organ function, including oxy gen consumption and glucose metabolism; most PET studies are conducted in the areas of cardiology, neurology, and oncology. The studies are used to diagnose and stage diseases as well as to monitor the efficacy of therapeutic interventions. During the PET heart scan, the radiotracer is injected into the body where it migrates to the intended target organ, becomes involved in the physiological process of interest, and accumulates to the degree that radioactive emissions are detected by the PET scanner. The PET scanner translates the emissions from the radioactivity as the positron combines with the negative electrons from the tissues and forms gamma rays that can be detected by the scanner. This information is transmitted to the computer, which determines the location and its distribution and translates the emissions as color-coded images for viewing, quantitative measurements, activity changes in relation to time, and three-dimensional computer-aided analysis.

Cardiac muscle uses oxygen and glucose in many of its essential functions, and therefore the heart's metabolism has been studied widely with PET. Each radionuclide tracer is designed to measure a specific body process, such as glucose metabolism, blood flow, or cardiac tissue perfusion. Fluorine-18, in the form of fluorodeoxyglucose (FDG), is one of the most versatile and commonly used radionuclides in PET. FDG is a glucose analogue. All cells use glucose, but diseases that involve increased metabolic activity will show a high level of radionuclide visualization, whereas those that are hypometabolic will show little to no radionuclide visualization. There is little localization of FDG in normal tissue with minimal amounts being evenly distributed, allowing rapid detection of abnormal disease states. The radionuclide can be administered by intravenous (IV) injection or inhaled as a gas.

The expense of the study and the limited availability of radiopharmaceuticals limit the use of PET even though it is more sensitive than traditional nuclear scanning and single-photon emission computed tomography (SPECT). PET/CT and SPECT/CT are imaging applications that superimpose PET or SPECT and CT findings. The images are collected and produced by a single gantry system. The coregistered or image fusion of PET/CT or

SPECT/CT findings can provide a detailed combination of anatomical and functional images. PET images can also be superimposed on MRI images.

This procedure is contraindicated for

Patients who are pregnant or suspected of being pregnant, unless the potential benefits of a procedure using radiation far outweigh the risk of radiation exposure to the fetus and mother.

INDICATIONS

- Assess tissue permeability.
- Determine the effects of therapeutic drugs on malfunctioning or diseased tissue.
- Determine localization of areas of heart metabolism.
- Determine the presence of coronary artery disease (CAD), as evidenced by metabolic state during ischemia and after angina.
- Determine the size of heart infarcts.
- Identify cerebrovascular accident or aneurysm, as evidenced by decreasing blood flow and oxygen use.

POTENTIAL MEDICAL DIAGNOSIS

Normal findings

- Normal patterns of tissue metabolism, blood flow, and homogeneous radionuclide distribution

Abnormal findings related to

- Chronic obstructive pulmonary disease
- Areas of tissue necrosis and scar tissue ***(indicated by the lack of radionuclide visualization in areas of decreased blood flow and decreased glucose concentration)***
- Enlarged left ventricle
- Heart chamber disorder
- Ischemia and myocardial infarction ***(indicated by the lack of radionuclide visualization in areas of decreased blood flow and decreased glucose concentration)***
- Pulmonary edema

CRITICAL FINDINGS: N/A

INTERFERING FACTORS

Factors that may alter the results of the study

- Inability of the patient to cooperate or remain still during the procedure because of age, significant pain, or mental status.
- Drugs and other substances that alter glucose metabolism, such as tranquilizers or insulin, because hypoglycemia can alter PET results.
- The use of alcohol, tobacco, or caffeine-containing drinks at least 24 hr before the study, because the effects of these substances would make it difficult to evaluate the patient's true physiological state (e.g., alcohol is a vasoconstrictor and would decrease blood flow to the target organ).
- Metallic objects (e.g., jewelry, body rings) within the examination field, which may inhibit organ visualization and cause unclear images.

Other considerations

- Failure to follow dietary restrictions before the procedure may cause the procedure to be canceled or repeated.
- Improper injection of the radionuclide that allows the tracer to seep deep into the muscle tissue produces erroneous hot spots.
- False-positive findings may occur as a result of normal gastrointestinal tract uptake and uptake in areas of infection or inflammation.

NURSING IMPLICATIONS AND PROCEDURE

See Potential Nursing Problems on Fast Find at davispl.us/vanleeuwen7.

PRETEST:

- Positively identify the patient using at least two person-specific identifiers before services, treatments, or procedures are performed.
- *Patient Teaching:* Inform the patient this procedure can assist in assessing blood flow to the heart.
- Obtain a history of the patient's health concerns, symptoms, surgical procedures, and results of previously performed laboratory and diagnostic studies. Include a list of known allergens, especially allergies or sensitivities to latex, anesthetics, sedatives, or radionuclides.
- Obtain a history of the patient's cardiovascular and respiratory systems, symptoms, and results of previously performed laboratory tests and diagnostic and surgical procedures.
- Note any recent procedures that can interfere with test results, including examinations using barium- or iodine-based contrast medium.
- Record the date of the last menstrual period and determine the possibility of pregnancy in perimenopausal women.
- Obtain a list of the patient's current medications, including over-the-counter medications and dietary supplements (see Effects of Natural Products on Laboratory Values online at Davis*Plus*).
- Review the procedure with the patient. Address concerns about pain related to the procedure and explain that some pain may be experienced during the test, or there may be moments of discomfort. Reassure the patient that radioactive material poses minimal radioactive hazard because of its short half-life and rarely produces adverse effects. Inform the patient that the procedure is performed in a special department, usually in a radiology suite, by a health-care provider (HCP) specializing in this procedure, with support staff, and takes approximately 60 to 120 min.
- *Sensitivity to social and cultural issues,* as well as concern for modesty, is important in providing psychological support before, during, and after the procedure.
- Explain that an IV line may be inserted to allow infusion of fluids such as saline, anesthetics, sedatives, radionuclides, medications used in the procedure, or emergency medications.
- Sometimes FDG examinations are done after blood has been drawn to determine circulating blood glucose levels. If blood glucose levels are high, insulin may be given.
- Instruct the patient to remove jewelry and other metallic objects from the area to be examined prior to the procedure.
- Instruct the patient to avoid taking anticoagulant medication or to reduce dosage as ordered prior to the procedure.
- Instruct the patient to restrict food for 4 hr; restrict alcohol, nicotine, or caffeine-containing drinks for 24 hr; and withhold medications for 24 hr before the test. Protocols may vary among facilities.
- *Make sure a written and informed consent has been signed prior to the procedure and before administering any medications.*

INTRATEST:

Potential Complications:

Although it is rare, there is the possibility of allergic reaction to the radionuclide. Have emergency equipment and medications readily available. If the patient has a history of allergic reactions to any substance or drug, administer ordered prophylactic steroids or antihistamines before the procedure.

Establishing an IV site and injecting radionuclides is an invasive procedure. Complications are rare but do include bleeding from the

P

puncture site ***related to a bleeding disorder or the effects of natural products and medications with known anticoagulant, antiplatelet, or thrombolytic properties;*** hematoma ***related to blood leakage into the tissue following needle insertion;*** infection ***that might occur if bacteria from the skin surface is introduced at the puncture site;*** or nerve injury ***that might occur if the needle strikes a nerve.***

- Observe standard precautions, and follow the general guidelines in Patient Preparation and Specimen Collection online at Davis*Plus*. Positively identify the patient.
- Ensure that the patient has complied with dietary, fluid, and medication restrictions and pretesting preparations prior to the procedure, as instructed.
- Ensure the patient has removed all jewelry and external metallic objects from the area to be examined prior to the procedure.
- Administer ordered prophylactic steroids or antihistamines before the procedure if the patient has a history of allergic reactions to any substance or drug.
- Avoid the use of equipment containing latex if the patient has a history of allergic reaction to latex.
- Have emergency equipment readily available.
- Instruct the patient to void prior to the procedure and to change into the gown, robe, and foot coverings provided.
- Record baseline vital signs and assess neurological status. Protocols may vary among facilities.
- Establish an IV fluid line for the injection of saline, anesthetics, sedatives, radionuclides, or emergency medications.
- Instruct the patient to cooperate fully and to follow directions. Ask the patient to remain still throughout the procedure because movement produces unreliable results.
- Record baseline vital signs and assess neurological status. Protocols may vary among facilities.
- Place the patient in the supine position on an examination table.
- The radionuclide is injected and imaging is done at periodic intervals, with continuous scanning done for 1 hr. If comparative studies are indicated, additional injections may be needed.
- Monitor the patient for complications related to the procedure (e.g., allergic reaction, anaphylaxis, bronchospasm).
- Remove the needle or catheter and apply a pressure dressing over the puncture site.
- Observe/assess the needle site for bleeding, inflammation, or hematoma formation.

POST-TEST:

- Inform the patient that a report of the results will be made available to the requesting HCP, who will discuss the results with the patient.
- Instruct the patient to resume pretest diet, fluids, medications, and activity.
- Observe for delayed allergic reactions, such as rash, urticaria, tachycardia, hyperpnea, hypertension, palpitations, nausea, or vomiting.
- Instruct the patient to immediately report symptoms such as fast heart rate, difficulty breathing, skin rash, itching, chest pain, persistent right shoulder pain, or abdominal pain. Immediately report symptoms to the appropriate HCP.
- Observe/assess the needle/catheter insertion site for bleeding, inflammation, or hematoma formation.
- Instruct the patient to apply cold compresses to the puncture site as needed, to reduce discomfort or edema.
- Instruct the patient to drink increased amounts of fluids for 24 to 48 hr to eliminate the radionuclide from the body, unless contraindicated. Educate the patient that radionuclide is eliminated from the body within 6 to 24 hr.
- Instruct the patient to flush the toilet immediately after each voiding and to meticulously wash hands with soap and water for 24 hr after the procedure.

P

- Instruct all caregivers to wear gloves when discarding urine for 24 hr after the procedure. Wash gloved hands with soap and water before removing gloves; then wash ungloved hands.
- If a woman who is breastfeeding must have a nuclear scan, she should not breastfeed the infant until the radionuclide has been eliminated, about 3 days. Instruct her to express the milk and discard it during the 3-day period to prevent cessation of milk production.
- No other radionuclide tests should be scheduled for 24 to 48 hr after this procedure.
- ***Nutritional Considerations:*** Abnormal findings may be associated with cardiovascular disease. Nutritional therapy is recommended for the patient identified to be at risk for developing CAD or for individuals who have specific risk factors and/or existing medical conditions (e.g., elevated LDL cholesterol levels, other lipid disorders, type 1 diabetes, type 2 diabetes, insulin resistance, or metabolic syndrome). Other changeable risk factors warranting patient education include strategies to encourage patients, especially those who are overweight and with high blood pressure, to safely decrease sodium intake, achieve a normal weight, ensure regular participation in moderate aerobic physical activity three to four times per week, eliminate tobacco use, and adhere to a heart-healthy diet. If triglycerides also are elevated, the patient should be advised to eliminate or reduce alcohol. A variety of dietary patterns are beneficial for people with CAD, and there are many meal-planning approaches with nutritional goals endorsed by the American Diabetes Association (ADA). The Guideline on Lifestyle Management to Reduce Cardiovascular Risk published by the American College of Cardiology (ACC) and the American Heart Association (AHA) in conjunction with the National Heart, Lung, and Blood Institute (NHLBI) recommends a Mediterranean-style diet rather than a low-fat diet. The guideline emphasizes inclusion of vegetables, whole grains, fruits, low-fat dairy, nuts, legumes, and nontropical vegetable oils (e.g., olive, canola, peanut, sunflower, flaxseed) along with fish and lean poultry. 🍁 A similar dietary pattern known as the Dietary Approaches to Stop Hypertension (DASH) diet makes additional recommendations for the reduction of dietary sodium. Both dietary styles emphasize a reduction in consumption of red meats, which are high in saturated fats and cholesterol, and other foods containing sugar, saturated fats, trans fats, and sodium. The ADA also includes a vegetarian diet as well as other potential weight loss diets such as Weight Watchers. 🍁 The nutritional needs of each patient need to be determined individually (especially during pregnancy) with the appropriate HCPs, particularly professionals educated in nutrition.
- Recognize anxiety related to test results, and be supportive of perceived loss of independent function. Discuss the implications of abnormal test results on the patient's lifestyle. Provide teaching and information regarding the clinical implications of the test results, as appropriate.
- Provide contact information, if desired, for the AHA (www.americanheart.org), NHLBI (www.nhlbi.nih.gov), Institute of Medicine of the National Academies (www.iom.edu), and USDA's resource for nutrition (www.choosemyplate.gov). 🍁
- Reinforce information given by the patient's HCP regarding further testing, treatment, or referral to another HCP. Answer any questions or address any concerns voiced by the patient or family.
- Depending on the results of this procedure, additional testing may be needed to evaluate or monitor progression of the disease process and determine the need for a change in therapy. Evaluate test results in relation to the patient's symptoms and other tests performed.

P

Patient Education:

- Teach the patient about the pathophysiology of myocardial infarction.
- Teach the patient the purpose of ordered medications (morphine, nitroglycerin, calcium channel blockers, beta blockers).

Expected Patient Outcomes:

Understanding

- The patient and family acknowledge medical therapeutic management options.
- The patient and family acknowledge the importance of taking all prescribed medications to support cardiac health.

Ability

- The patient and family create a quiet environment to reduce energy demands.
- The patient and family plan rest periods during the day to conserve oxygen.

Response

- The patient and family agree to make lifestyle changes that will support positive cardiac health.
- The patient agrees to attend cardiac rehabilitation.

RELATED STUDIES:

- Related tests for cardiac indications include anion gap, antidysrhythmic drugs, apolipoproteins A, B, and C, arterial/alveolar oxygen ratio, ANP, α_1-AT, biopsy lung, blood gases, blood pool imaging, BNP, bronchoscopy, calcium, carboxyhemoglobin, chest x-ray, chloride sweat, cholesterol (total, HDL, and LDL), CRP, CBC, CT cardiac scoring, CT thoracic, CK and isoenzymes, culture and smear for mycobacteria, culture bacterial sputum, culture viral, cytology sputum, echocardiography, echocardiography transesophageal, ECG, electrolytes, exercise stress test, fundoscopy, glucose, glycated hemoglobin, Gram stain, Hgb, Holter monitor, homocysteine, ketones, LDH and isoenzymes, lipoprotein electrophoresis, magnesium, MRI chest, MI infarct scan, IgE, lactic acid, lung perfusion scan, lung ventilation scan, myocardial perfusion heart scan, myoglobin, osmolality, pericardial fluid analysis, phosphorus, plethysmography, pleural fluid analysis, PET heart, PFT, potassium, pulse oximetry, TB skin test, and triglycerides. Related tests for pulmonary indications include α_1-AT, anion gap, arterial/alveolar oxygen ratio, biopsy lung, blood gases, bronchoscopy, carboxyhemoglobin, chest x-ray, chloride sweat, CBC, CBC hemoglobin, CBC WBC count and differential, culture and smear for mycobacteria, culture bacterial sputum, culture viral, cytology sputum, electrolytes, Gram stain, IgE, lactic acid, lung perfusion scan, lung ventilation scan, osmolality, phosphorus, plethysmography, pleural fluid analysis, and pulse oximetry.
- Refer to the Cardiovascular and Respiratory systems tables online at Davis*Plus* for related tests by body system.

P

Positron Emission Tomography, Pelvis

SYNONYM/ACRONYM: PET scan of the pelvis.

COMMON USE: To assess blood flow and metabolism to the pelvis toward diagnosis of disorders such as colorectal tumor, assist in tumor staging, and monitor the effectiveness of therapeutic interventions.

AREA OF APPLICATION: Pelvis.

Access Canadian content on Fast Find: Lab and Dx at davispl.us/vanleeuwen7

DESCRIPTION: Positron emission tomography (PET) combines the biochemical properties of nuclear medicine with the anatomic accuracy of computed tomography (CT). PET uses positron emissions from specific radionuclides. The positron radiopharmaceuticals generally have short half-lives, ranging from a few seconds to a few hours, and therefore they must be produced in a cyclotron located near where the test is being done. A radionuclide is basically composed of a measurable radioactive isotope and a biologically active molecule. The isotopes are derived from elements that are either naturally present in organic molecules (oxygen, nitrogen, and carbon) or can be substituted for naturally occurring elements (fluorine can be substituted for hydrogen). Selected molecules become biologically active radiolabelled analogs of their naturally occurring forms to create radionuclides that produce detailed functional images of the target organ's structure. Radionuclides are used to evaluate many aspects of organ function, including oxygen consumption and glucose metabolism; most PET studies are conducted in the areas of cardiology, neurology, and oncology. The studies are used to diagnose and stage diseases as well as to monitor the efficacy of therapeutic interventions. During the PET pelvis scan, the radiotracer is injected into the body, and it migrates to the pelvis, becomes involved in the physiological process of interest, and accumulates to the degree that radioactive emissions are detected by the PET scanner. The PET scanner translates the emissions from the radioactivity as the positron combines with the negative electrons from the tissues and forms gamma rays that can be detected by the scanner. This information is transmitted to the computer, which determines the location and its distribution and translates the emissions as color-coded images for viewing, quantitative measurements, activity changes in relation to time, and three-dimensional computer-aided analysis. Colorectal tumor detection, tumor staging, evaluation of the effects of therapy, detection of recurrent disease, and detection of metastases are the main reasons to do a pelvic PET scan. Fluorine-18, in the form of fluorodeoxyglucose (FDG), is one of the more commonly used radionuclides. FDG is a glucose analogue, and because every cell uses glucose, the metabolic activity occurring in pelvic conditions such as colorectal cancer can be measured. There is little localization of FDG in normal tissue, allowing rapid detection of abnormal disease states.

The expense of the study and the limited availability of radiopharmaceuticals limit the use of PET even though it is more sensitive than traditional nuclear scanning and single-photon emission computed tomography (SPECT). PET/CT and SPECT/CT are imaging applications that superimpose PET or SPECT and CT findings. The images are collected and produced by a single gantry system. The coregistered or image fusion of PET/CT or SPECT/CT findings can provide a detailed combination of anatomical and functional images. PET images can also be superimposed on MRI images.

This procedure is contraindicated for

Patients who are pregnant or suspected of being pregnant, unless the potential benefits of a procedure using radiation far outweigh the risk of radiation exposure to the fetus and mother.

INDICATIONS

- Determine the effects of therapy.
- Determine the presence of colorectal cancer.
- Determine the presence of metastases of a cancerous tumor.
- Determine the recurrence of tumor or cancer.
- Identify the site for biopsy.

POTENTIAL MEDICAL DIAGNOSIS

Normal findings

- Normal patterns of tissue metabolism, blood flow, and radionuclide distribution
- No focal uptake of radionuclide

Abnormal findings related to

- Focal uptake of the radionuclide in pelvis
- Focal uptake in abnormal lymph nodes
- Focal uptake in tumor
- Focal uptake in metastases

CRITICAL FINDINGS: N/A

INTERFERING FACTORS

Factors that may alter the results of the study

- Inability of the patient to cooperate or remain still during the procedure because of age, significant pain, or mental status.
- Drugs that alter glucose metabolism, such as tranquilizers or insulin, because hypoglycemia can alter PET results.
- The use of alcohol, tobacco, or caffeine-containing drinks at least 24 hr before the study, because the effects of these substances would make it difficult to evaluate the patient's true physiological state (e.g., alcohol is a vasoconstrictor and would decrease blood flow to the target organ).
- Metallic objects within the examination field (e.g., jewelry, body rings), which may inhibit organ visualization and can produce unclear images.

Other considerations

- Failure to follow dietary restrictions before the procedure may cause the procedure to be canceled or repeated.
- Improper injection of the radionuclide that allows the tracer to seep deep into the muscle tissue produces erroneous hot spots.
- False-positive findings may occur as a result of normal gastrointestinal (GI) tract uptake and uptake in areas of infection or inflammation.

NURSING IMPLICATIONS AND PROCEDURE

See Potential Nursing Problems on Fast Find at davispl.us/vanleeuwen7.

PRETEST:

- Positively identify the patient using at least two person-specific identifiers before services, treatments, or procedures are performed.
- ***Patient Teaching:*** Inform the patient this procedure can assist in assessing the pelvis related to abnormal organ function.
- Obtain a history of the patient's health concerns, symptoms, surgical procedures, and results of previously performed laboratory and diagnostic studies. Include a list of known allergens, especially allergies or sensitivities to latex, anesthetics, sedatives, or radionuclides.

P

- Obtain a history of the patient's gastrointestinal system, symptoms, and results of previously performed laboratory tests and diagnostic and surgical procedures.
- Note any recent procedures that can interfere with test results, including examinations using barium- or iodine-based contrast medium.
- Record the date of the last menstrual period and determine the possibility of pregnancy in perimenopausal women.
- Obtain a list of the patient's current medications, including over-the-counter medications and dietary supplements (see Effects of Natural Products on Laboratory Values online at Davis*Plus*).
- Review the procedure with the patient. Address concerns about pain related to the procedure and explain that some pain may be experienced during the test, and there may be moments of discomfort. Reassure the patient that radioactive material poses minimal radioactive hazard because of its short half-life and rarely produces adverse effects. Inform the patient that the procedure is performed in a special department, usually in a radiology suite, by a health-care provider (HCP) specializing in this procedure, with support staff, and takes approximately 30 to 60 min.
- *Sensitivity to social and cultural issues,* as well as concern for modesty, is important in providing psychological support before, during, and after the procedure.
- Explain that an intravenous (IV) line may be inserted to allow infusion of fluids such as saline, anesthetics, sedatives, radionuclides, medications used in the procedure, or emergency medications.
- Sometimes FDG examinations are done after blood has been drawn to determine circulating blood glucose levels. If blood glucose levels are high, insulin may be given.
- Instruct the patient to remove jewelry and other metallic objects in the area to be examined.
- Instruct the patient to avoid taking anticoagulant medication or to reduce dosage as ordered prior to the procedure.
- Instruct the patient to restrict food for 4 hr; restrict alcohol, nicotine, or caffeine-containing drinks for 24 hr; and withhold medications for 24 hr before the test. Protocols may vary among facilities.
- *Make sure a written and informed consent has been signed prior to the procedure and before administering any medications.*

INTRATEST:

Potential Complications:

Although it is rare, there is the possibility of allergic reaction to the radionuclide. Have emergency equipment and medications readily available. If the patient has a history of allergic reactions to any substance or drug, administer ordered prophylactic steroids or antihistamines before the procedure.

Establishing an IV site and injecting radionuclides is an invasive procedure. Complications are rare but do include bleeding from the puncture site ***related to a bleeding disorder or the effects of natural products and medications with known anticoagulant, antiplatelet, or thrombolytic properties;*** hematoma ***related to blood leakage into the tissue following needle insertion;*** infection ***that might occur if bacteria from the skin surface is introduced at the puncture site;*** nerve injury ***that might occur if the needle strikes a nerve;*** or urinary trace infection ***related to use of a catheter.***

- Observe standard precautions, and follow the general guidelines in Patient Preparation and Specimen Collection online at Davis*Plus*. Positively identify the patient.
- Ensure that the patient has complied with dietary, fluid, and medication restrictions and pretesting preparations prior to the procedure, as instructed.

P

- Ensure the patient has removed all jewelry and external metallic objects from the area to be examined prior to the procedure.
- Administer ordered prophylactic steroids or antihistamines before the procedure if the patient has a history of allergic reactions to any substance or drug.
- Avoid the use of equipment containing latex if the patient has a history of allergic reaction to latex.
- Have emergency equipment readily available.
- Instruct the patient to void prior to the procedure and to change into the gown, robe, and foot coverings provided.
- Record baseline vital signs and assess neurological status. Protocols may vary among facilities.
- Establish an IV fluid line for the injection of saline, anesthetics, sedatives, radionuclides, or emergency medications.
- Instruct the patient to cooperate fully and to follow directions. Ask the patient to remain still throughout the procedure because movement produces unreliable results.
- Record baseline vital signs and assess neurological status. Protocols may vary among facilities.
- Place the patient in the supine position on an examination table.
- The radionuclide is injected, and imaging is started after a 45-min delay. Continuous scanning may be done for 1 hr. If comparative studies are indicated, additional injections of radionuclide may be needed.
- If required, the bladder may need to be lavaged via a urinary catheter with 2 L of 0.9% saline solution to remove concentrated radionuclide.
- Monitor the patient for complications related to the procedure (e.g., allergic reaction, anaphylaxis, bronchospasm).
- Remove the needle or catheter and apply a pressure dressing over the puncture site.
- Observe/assess the needle/catheter insertion site for bleeding, inflammation, or hematoma formation.

POST-TEST:

- Inform the patient that a report of the results will be made available to the requesting HCP, who will discuss the results with the patient.
- Instruct the patient to resume pretest diet, fluids, medications, and activity.
- Observe for delayed allergic reactions, such as rash, urticaria, tachycardia, hyperpnea, hypertension, palpitations, nausea, or vomiting.
- Instruct the patient to immediately report symptoms such as fast heart rate, difficulty breathing, skin rash, itching, chest pain, persistent right shoulder pain, or abdominal pain. Immediately report symptoms to the appropriate HCP.
- Observe/assess the needle/catheter insertion site for bleeding, inflammation, or hematoma formation.
- Instruct the patient to apply cold compresses to the puncture site as needed, to reduce discomfort or edema.
- Instruct the patient to drink increased amounts of fluids for 24 to 48 hr to eliminate the radionuclide from the body, unless contraindicated. Tell the patient that radionuclide is eliminated from the body within 6 to 24 hr.
- Instruct the patient to flush the toilet immediately after each voiding and to meticulously wash hands with soap and water for 24 hr after the procedure.
- Tell all caregivers to wear gloves when discarding urine for 24 hr after the procedure. Wash gloved hands with soap and water before removing gloves; then wash ungloved hands.
- If a woman who is breastfeeding must have a nuclear scan, she should not breastfeed the infant until the radionuclide has been eliminated, about 3 days. Instruct her to express the milk and discard it during the 3-day period to prevent cessation of milk production.

P

- No other radionuclide tests should be scheduled for 24 to 48 hr after this procedure.
- Recognize anxiety related to test results, and be supportive of perceived loss of independent function. Discuss the implications of abnormal test results on the patient's lifestyle. Provide teaching and information regarding the clinical implications of the test results, as appropriate.
- The American Cancer Society (ACS) recommends regular screening for colon cancer, beginning at age 50 yr for individuals without identified risk factors and sooner for those with identified risk factors. Its recommendations for frequency of screening are as follows: annually for occult blood testing (fecal occult blood testing or fecal immunochemical testing); every 5 yr for flexible sigmoidoscopy, double contrast barium enema, or computed tomography colonography; every 10 yr for colonoscopy; or every 3 yr for stool DNA testing. 🍁 Abnormal findings should be followed up by colonoscopy. There are both advantages and disadvantages to the screening tests that are available. Methods to use DNA testing of stool are being investigated and are designed to identify abnormal changes in DNA from the cells in the lining of the colon that are normally shed and excreted in stool. The DNA tests under development use multiple markers to identify colon cancers that demonstrate different, abnormal DNA changes. Unlike some of the current screening methods, the DNA tests would be able to detect precancerous polyps. The most current guidelines for colon cancer screening of the general population as well as of individuals with increased risk are available from the ACS (www.cancer.org), U.S. Preventive Services Task Force (www.uspreventiveservicestaskforce.org), and American College of Gastroenterology (www.gi.org). 🍁 Answer any questions or address any concerns voiced by the patient or family.
- Depending on the results of this procedure, additional testing may be needed to evaluate or monitor progression of the disease process and determine the need for a change in therapy. Evaluate test results in relation to the patient's symptoms and other tests performed.

Patient Education:

- Reinforce information given by the patient's HCP regarding further testing, treatment, or referral to another HCP.
- Provide information on disease signs and symptoms and management.
- Provide information on possible diagnostic and laboratory studies associated with disease management.

Expected Patient Outcomes:

Understanding

- The patient and family correctly describe treatment options related to disease process.
- The patient and family acknowledge the importance of family or group counseling related to end-of-life issues.

Ability

- The patient and family demonstrates positive coping strategies.
- The patient and family successfully demonstrate care of surgical site.

Response

- The patient and family agree to seek psychological counseling to adjust to body changes and intimacy concerns.
- The patient and family agree to attend cancer support group meetings.

RELATED STUDIES:

- Related tests include barium enema, biopsy intestinal, capsule endoscopy, cancer antigens, CT abdomen, CT colonoscopy, fecal analysis, KUB, MRI abdomen, and proctosigmoidoscopy.
- Refer to the Gastrointestinal System table online at Davis*Plus* for related tests by body system.

P

Potassium, Blood

SYNONYM/ACRONYM: Serum K^+.

COMMON USE: To evaluate fluid and electrolyte balance related to potassium levels toward diagnosing disorders such as acidosis, renal failure, dehydration, and monitor the effectiveness of therapeutic interventions.

SPECIMEN: Serum collected in a gold-, red-, or red/gray-top tube. Plasma collected in green-top (heparin) tube is also acceptable.

NORMAL FINDINGS: (Method: Ion-selective electrode)

Serum	Conventional & SI Units
Birth–7 d	3.2–5.5 mEq/L or mmol/L
8 d–1 mo	3.4–6 mEq/L or mmol/L
1–5 mo	3.5–5.6 mEq/L or mmol/L
6 mo–1 yr	3.5–6.1 mEq/L or mmol/L
2–19 yr	3.8–5.1 mEq/L or mmol/L
Adult–older adult	3.5–5.3 mEq/L or mmol/L

Note: Value ranges may vary depending on the laboratory. Serum values are 0.1 mmol/L higher than plasma values, and reference ranges should be adjusted accordingly. It is important that serial measurements be collected using the same type of collection container to reduce variability of results from collection to collection.

Older adults are at risk for hyperkalemia due to the decline in aldosterone levels, decline in kidney function, and effects of commonly prescribed medications that inhibit the renin-angiotensin-aldosterone system.

DESCRIPTION: Electrolytes dissociate into electrically charged ions when dissolved. Cations, including potassium, carry a positive charge. Body fluids contain approximately equal numbers of anions and cations, although the nature of the ions and their mobility differs between the intracellular and extracellular compartments. Both types of ions affect the electrical and osmolar functions of the body. Electrolyte quantities and the balance among them are controlled by oxygen and carbon dioxide exchange in the lungs; absorption, secretion, and excretion of many substances by the kidneys; and secretion of regulatory hormones by the endocrine glands. Potassium is the most abundant intracellular cation with a number of essential functions to include transmission of electrical impulses in cardiac and skeletal muscle and participation in enzyme reactions that transform glucose into energy and amino acids into proteins. Potassium also helps maintain acid-base equilibrium, and it has a significant and inverse relationship to pH: A decrease in pH of 0.1 increases the potassium level by 0.6 mmol/L.

P

Abnormal potassium levels can be caused by a number of contributing factors, which can be categorized as follows:

Altered renal excretion: Normally, 80% to 90% of the body's potassium is filtered out through the kidneys each day (the remainder is excreted in sweat and stool); kidney disease can result in abnormally high potassium levels.

Altered dietary intake: A severe potassium deficiency can be caused by an inadequate intake of dietary potassium.

Altered cellular metabolism: Damaged red blood cells (RBCs) release potassium into the circulating fluid, resulting in increased potassium levels.

This procedure is contraindicated for: N/A

INDICATIONS

- Assess a known or suspected disorder associated with kidney disease, glucose metabolism, trauma, or burns.
- Assist in the evaluation of electrolyte imbalances; this test is especially indicated in older adult patients, patients receiving hyperalimentation supplements, patients on hemodialysis, and patients with hypertension.
- Evaluate cardiac dysrhythmia to determine whether altered potassium levels are contributing to the problem, especially during digoxin therapy, which leads to ventricular irritability.
- Evaluate the effects of drug therapy, especially diuretics.
- Evaluate the response to treatment for abnormal potassium levels.
- Monitor known or suspected acidosis, because potassium moves from RBCs into the extracellular fluid in acidotic states.
- Routine screen of electrolytes in acute and chronic illness.

POTENTIAL MEDICAL DIAGNOSIS

Increased in:

- Acidosis ***(intracellular potassium ions are expelled in exchange for hydrogen ions in order to achieve electrical neutrality)***
- Acute kidney injury ***(potassium excretion is diminished, and it accumulates in the blood)***
- Addison's disease ***(due to lack of aldosterone, potassium excretion is diminished, and it accumulates in the blood)***
- Asthma ***(related to chronic inflammation and damage to lung tissue)***
- Burns ***(related to tissue damage and release by damaged cells)***
- Chronic interstitial nephritis ***(potassium excretion is diminished, and it accumulates in the blood)***
- Dehydration ***(related to hemoconcentration)***
- Dialysis ***(dialysis treatments simulate kidney function, but potassium builds up between treatments)***
- Diet ***(related to excessive intake of salt substitutes or of potassium salts in medications)***
- Exercise ***(related to tissue damage and release by damaged cells)***
- Hemolysis (massive) ***(potassium is the major intracellular cation)***
- Hyperventilation ***(in response to respiratory alkalosis, blood levels of potassium are increased in order to achieve electrical neutrality)***
- Hypoaldosteronism ***(due to lack of aldosterone, potassium excretion is diminished, and it accumulates in the blood)***
- Insulin deficiency ***(insulin deficiency results in movement of***

potassium from the cell into the extracellular fluid)
- Ketoacidosis ***(insulin deficiency results in movement of potassium from the cell into the extracellular fluid)***
- Leukocytosis
- Muscle necrosis ***(related to tissue damage and release by damaged cells)***
- Near drowning
- Pregnancy
- Prolonged periods of standing
- Tissue trauma ***(related to release by damaged cells)***
- Transfusion of old banked blood ***(aged cells hemolyze and release intracellular potassium)***
- Tubular unresponsiveness to aldosterone
- Uremia

Decreased in:
- Alcoholism ***(related to insufficient dietary intake)***
- Alkalosis ***(potassium uptake by cells is increased in response to release of hydrogen ions from cells)***
- Anorexia nervosa ***(related to significant changes in renal function that result in hypokalemia)***
- Bradycardia ***(hypokalemia can cause bradycardia)***
- Chronic, excessive licorice ingestion ***(from licorice root. Licorice inhibits short-chain dehydrogenase/reductase enzymes. These enzymes normally prevent cortisol from binding to aldosterone receptor sites in the kidney. In the absence of these enzymes, cortisol acts on the kidney and triggers the same effects as aldosterone, which include increased potassium excretion, sodium retention, and water retention.)***
- Crohn's disease ***(insufficient intestinal absorption)***
- Cushing's syndrome ***(aldosterone facilitates the excretion of potassium by the kidneys)***
- Diet deficient in meat and vegetables ***(insufficient dietary intake)***
- Excess insulin ***(insulin causes glucose and potassium to move into cells)***
- Familial periodic paralysis ***(related to fluid retention)***
- Gastrointestinal (GI) loss due to vomiting, diarrhea, nasogastric suction, or intestinal fistula
- Heart failure ***(related to fluid retention and hemodilution)***
- Hyperaldosteronism ***(aldosterone facilitates the excretion of potassium by the kidneys)***
- Hypertension ***(medications used to treat hypertension may result in loss of potassium; hypertension is often related to diabetes and kidney disease, which affect cellular retention and renal excretion of potassium, respectively)***
- Hypomagnesemia ***(magnesium levels tend to parallel potassium levels)***
- Intravenous (IV) therapy with inadequate potassium supplementation
- Laxative misuse ***(related to medications that cause potassium wasting)***
- Malabsorption ***(related to insufficient intestinal absorption)***
- Pica (eating substances of no nutritional value, e.g., clay)
- Renal tubular acidosis ***(condition results in excessive loss of potassium)***
- Sweating ***(related to increased loss)***
- Theophylline administration, excessive ***(theophylline drives potassium into cells, reducing circulating levels)***
- Thyrotoxicosis ***(related to changes in kidney function)***

P

CRITICAL FINDINGS:

Adults & children

- Less than 2.5 mEq/L or mmol/L (SI: Less than 2.5 mmol/L)
- Greater than 6.2 mEq/L or mmol/L (SI: Greater than 6.2 or mmol/L)

Newborns

- Less than 2.8 mEq/L or mmol/L (SI: Less than 2.8 mmol/L)
- Greater than 7.6 mEq/L or mmol/L (SI: Greater than 7.6 mmol/L)

Note and immediately report to the requesting health-care provider (HCP) any critical findings and related symptoms. A listing of these findings varies among facilities. Timely notification of a critical finding for laboratory or diagnostic studies is a role expectation of the professional nurse. The notification processes vary among facilities. Upon receipt of the critical finding, the information should be read back to the caller to verify accuracy.

Consideration may be given to verification of critical findings before action is taken. Policies vary among facilities and may include requesting immediate recollection and retesting by the laboratory or retesting using a rapid point-of-care testing instrument at the bedside, if available.

Symptoms of hyperkalemia include irritability, diarrhea, cramps, oliguria, difficulty speaking, and cardiac dysrhythmias (peaked T waves and ventricular fibrillation). Continuous cardiac monitoring is indicated. Administration of sodium bicarbonate or calcium chloride may be requested. If the patient is receiving an IV supplement, verify that the patient is voiding.

Symptoms of hypokalemia include malaise, thirst, polyuria, anorexia, weak pulse, low blood pressure, vomiting, decreased reflexes, and electrocardiographic changes (depressed T waves and ventricular ectopy). Replacement therapy is indicated.

INTERFERING FACTORS

- Drugs and other substances that can cause an increase in potassium levels include ACE inhibitors, atenolol, basiliximab, captopril, clofibrate in association with kidney disease, cyclosporine, dexamethasone, enalapril, etretinate, lisinopril in association with heart failure or hypertension, NSAIDs, some drugs with potassium salts (e.g., antibiotics such as penicillin), spironolactone, succinylcholine, and tacrolimus.
- Drugs and other substances that can cause a decrease in potassium levels include acetazolamide, acetylsalicylic acid, aldosterone, ammonium chloride, amphotericin B, bendroflumethiazide, benzthiazide, bicarbonate, captopril, cathartics, chlorothiazide, chlorthalidone, cisplatin, clorexolone, corticosteroids, cyclothiazide, dichlorphenamide, digoxin, diuretics, enalapril, foscarnet, fosphenytoin, furosemide, insulin, laxatives, metolazone, moxalactam (common when coadministered with amikacin), large doses of any IV penicillin, phenolphthalein (with chronic laxative misuse), polythiazide, quinethazone, sodium bicarbonate, tacrolimus, IV theophylline, thiazides, triamterene, and trichlormethiazide. A number of these medications initially increase the serum potassium level, but they also have a diuretic effect, which promotes potassium loss in the urine except in cases of renal insufficiency.
- Leukocytosis, as seen in leukemia, causes elevated potassium levels.
- False elevations can occur with vigorous pumping of the hand during venipuncture. Hemolysis of the sample and high platelet counts also increase potassium levels, as follows: (1) Because potassium is

P

an intracellular ion and concentrations are approximately 150 times extracellular concentrations, even a slight amount of hemolysis can cause a significant increase in levels. (2) Platelets release potassium during the clotting process, and therefore serum samples collected from patients with elevated platelet counts may produce spuriously high potassium levels. Plasma is the specimen of choice in patients known to have elevated platelet counts.

- False increases are seen in unprocessed samples left at room temperature because a significant amount of potassium leaks out of the cells within a few hours. Plasma or serum should be separated from cells within 4 hr of collection.
- Specimens should never be collected above an IV line because of the potential for dilution when the specimen and the IV solution combine in the collection container, falsely decreasing the result. There is also the potential of contaminating the sample with the substance of interest, if it is present in the IV solution, falsely increasing the result.

NURSING IMPLICATIONS AND PROCEDURE

POTENTIAL NURSING PROBLEMS:

Problem	Signs & Symptoms	Interventions
Electrolyte imbalance ***(related to metabolic imbalance associated with disease process)***	**Excess:** Nausea, weak or irregular pulse; sudden collapse, cardiac arrest **Deficit:** Thirst; tetany; weakness; constipation; arrhythmias; hypotension; nausea; vomiting; anorexia; polyuria; mental depression; cardiac arrest	Correlate potassium imbalance with disease process, nutritional intake, renal function, medications; monitor electrocardiogram status; monitor for respiratory changes; minimize metabolic complications; provide a safe environment to prevent injury; collaborate with the pharmacist and HCP for appropriate pharmacologic interventions; adjust medication dosage to compensate for renal impairment; collaborate with dietitian for dietary modifications; begin dialysis treatments if necessary (hemodialysis or peritoneal dialysis); reduce intake of high-potassium foods and dietary supplements

P

Problem	Signs & Symptoms	Interventions
Health management ***(related to complexity of health-care system; complexity of therapeutic management; altered metabolic process resulting in increased or decreased potassium; knowledge deficit; conflicted decision making; cultural family health patterns; barriers to healthy decisions; mistrust of HCP)***	Health choices are ineffective in making a difference on outcomes; increasing symptoms of illness; verbalizes that therapeutic regime is too difficult; patient and family do not support HCP's suggestions for health improvement; refuses to follow recommended therapeutic regime	Assess effort to follow recommended regime; assess family or cultural factors that impact the success of the therapeutic regime; assess the patient's self-assessment of his or her health status; include the patient and family in designing the plan of care; tailor the plan of care to the patient's lifestyle; collaborate with the patient and family to develop a system of managing own health; focus on behaviors that will make the biggest positive impact on improved health
Fluid volume (water) ***(related to metabolic imbalances associated with disease process)***	**Deficient:** Decreased urinary output; fatigue, sunken eyes; dark urine; decreased blood pressure; increased heart rate; altered mental status **Overload:** Edema; shortness of breath; increased weight; ascites; rales; rhonchi; diluted laboratory values	Record daily weight and monitor trends; record accurate intake and output; collaborate with HCP with administration of IV fluids to support hydration; monitor laboratory values that reflect alterations in fluid status (potassium, blood urea nitrogen, creatinine, calcium, hemoglobin, and hematocrit); manage underlying cause of fluid alteration; monitor urine characteristics and respiratory status; establish baseline assessment data; collaborate with HCP to adjust oral and IV fluids to provide optimal hydration status; administer replacement electrolytes as ordered; monitor serum potassium levels

(table continues on page 1298)

Problem	Signs & Symptoms	Interventions
Activity ***(related to compromised cardiac status; compromised renal status; weakness; lack of motivation; oxygen supply and demand imbalance)***	Verbal report of weakness; inability to tolerate activity; shortness of breath with activity; altered heart rate, blood pressure, and respiratory rate with activity	Assess current level of physical activity; take baseline vital signs; trend vital signs with activity; assess response to activity; monitor for oxygen desaturation with activity; administer prescribed oxygen with activity; collaborate with physical therapy to support activity; monitor blood pressure for orthostatic changes; collaborate with the patient to establish activity goals and guidelines; pace activities to match energy stores; assist with self-care

PRETEST:

- Positively identify the patient using at least two person-specific identifiers before services, treatments, or procedures are performed.
- ***Patient Teaching:*** Inform the patient this test can assist in evaluating electrolyte balance.
- Obtain a history of the patient's health concerns, symptoms, surgical procedures, and results of previously performed laboratory and diagnostic studies. Include a list of known allergens, especially allergies or sensitivities to latex.
- Obtain a list of the patient's current medications, including over-the-counter medications and dietary supplements (see Effects of Natural Products on Laboratory Values online at Davis*Plus*).
- Review the procedure with the patient. Inform the patient that specimen collection takes approximately 5 to 10 min. Address concerns about pain and explain that there may be some discomfort during the venipuncture.
- ***Sensitivity to social and cultural issues,*** as well as concern for modesty, is important in providing psychological support before, during, and after the procedure.
- Note that there are no food, fluid, or medication restrictions unless by medical direction.

INTRATEST:

Potential Complications: N/A

- Avoid the use of equipment containing latex if the patient has a history of allergic reaction to latex.
- Instruct the patient to cooperate fully and to follow directions. Direct the patient to breathe normally and to avoid unnecessary movement. Instruct the patient not to clench and unclench the fist immediately before or during specimen collection.
- Observe standard precautions, and follow the general guidelines in Patient Preparation and Specimen Collection online at Davis*Plus*. Positively identify the patient, and label the appropriate specimen container with the corresponding patient demographics, initials of the person collecting the specimen, date, and time of collection. Perform a venipuncture.

P

- Remove the needle and apply direct pressure with dry gauze to stop bleeding. Observe/assess venipuncture site for bleeding or hematoma formation and secure gauze with adhesive bandage.
- Promptly transport the specimen to the laboratory for processing and analysis.

POST-TEST:

- Inform the patient that a report of the results will be made available to the requesting HCP, who will discuss the results with the patient.
- *Nutritional Considerations:* Potassium is present in all plant and animal cells, making dietary replacement simple to achieve in the potassium-deficient patient. Fruits and vegetables (artichokes, avocados, bananas, cantaloupe, dried fruits, kiwi, mango, dried beans, nuts, oranges, peaches, pears, pomegranates, potatoes, prunes, pumpkin, spinach, sunflower seeds, swiss chard, tomatoes, and winter squash), dairy products (especially milk and milk products such as ice cream, yogurt, cream, buttermilk, half & half) and meats are rich in potassium.
- Observe the patient for signs and symptoms of fluid volume excess related to excess potassium intake (hyperkalemia), fluid volume deficit related to active loss (hypokalemia), or risk of injury related to an alteration in body chemistry. Symptoms of hypokalemia and hyperkalemia include dehydration, diarrhea, vomiting, or prolonged anorexia.
- Increased potassium levels may be associated with dehydration. Evaluate the patient for signs and symptoms of dehydration. Dehydration is a significant and common finding in older adult patients and other patients in whom kidney function has deteriorated.
- Decreased potassium levels may occur in patients receiving digoxin or potassium-wasting diuretics. Potassium levels should be monitored carefully because cardiac dysrhythmias can occur. Instruct the patient in electrolyte replacement therapy and changes in dietary intake that affect electrolyte levels, as ordered.
- Depending on the results of this procedure, additional testing may be performed to evaluate or monitor progression of the disease process and determine the need for a change in therapy. Evaluate test results in relation to the patient's symptoms and other tests performed.

Patient Education:

- Reinforce information given by the patient's HCP regarding further testing, treatment, or referral to another HCP.
- Recognize anxiety related to test results and answer any questions or address any concerns voiced by the patient or family.
- Educate the patient regarding access to nutritional counseling services. Provide contact information, if desired, for the Institute of Medicine of the National Academies (www.iom.edu) and USDA's resource for nutrition (www.choosemyplate.gov). 🍁
- Teach energy conservation techniques.
- Teach the appropriate use of assistive devices.

Expected Patient Outcomes:

Understanding

- The patient and family describe the signs and symptoms of physical overactivity.
- The patient and family state that monitoring of serum potassium levels will be necessary to maintain health.

Ability

- The patient demonstrates how to pace activities and conserve energy in the performance of the activities of daily living.
- The patient and family identify and list foods that can increase potassium levels.

Response

- The patient and family identify concerns about activity tolerance.

- The patient and family comply with the recommendation to access community resources to support a structured activity plan.

RELATED STUDIES:

- Related tests include ACTH, aldosterone, anion gap, antidysrhythmic drugs, alveolar/arterial gradient, ANP, BNP, blood gases, BUN, calcium, carbon dioxide, chloride, complement, CBC hematocrit, CBC hemoglobin, CBC WBC count and differential, Coomb's antiglobulin (direct and indirect), cortisol, CK and isoenzymes, creatinine, DHEAS, echocardiography, echocardiography transesophageal, fecal fat, glucose, G6PD, Ham's test, haptoglobin, hemosiderin, insulin, ketones, lactic acid, lung perfusion scan, magnesium, osmolality, osmotic fragility, plethysmography, urine potassium, PFT, PK, renin, sickle cell screen, sodium, and US abdomen.
- Refer to the Cardiovascular, Endocrine, Gastrointestinal, Genitourinary, Immune, and Respiratory systems tables online at Davis*Plus* for related tests by body system.

Potassium, Urine

SYNONYM/ACRONYM: Urine K^+.

COMMON USE: To evaluate electrolyte balance, acid-base balance, and hypokalemia.

SPECIMEN: Urine from an unpreserved random or timed specimen collected in a clean plastic collection container.

NORMAL FINDINGS: (Method: Ion-selective electrode)

Age	Conventional Units	SI Units (Conventional Units × 1)
6–10 yr		
Male	17–54 mEq/24 hr or mmol/24 hr	17–54 mmol/24 hr
Female	8–37 mEq/24 hr or mmol/24 hr	8–37 mmol/24 hr
10–14 yr		
Male	22–57 mEq/24 hr or mmol/24 hr	22–57 mmol/24 hr
Female	18–58 mEq/24 hr or mmol/24 hr	18–58 mmol/24 hr
Adult–older adult	26–123 mEq/24 hr or mmol/24 hr	26–123 mmol/24 hr

Note: Reference values depend on potassium intake and diurnal variation. Excretion is significantly higher at night.

Potassium excretion declines in older adults due to the decline in aldosterone levels, decline in kidney function, and effects of commonly prescribed medications that inhibit the renin-angiotensin-aldosterone system.

DESCRIPTION: Electrolytes dissociate into electrically charged ions when dissolved. Cations, including potassium, carry a positive charge. Body fluids contain approximately equal numbers of anions and cations, although the nature of the ions and their mobility differs between the intracellular and extracellular compartments. Both types of ions affect the electrical and osmolar functions of the body.

P

Electrolyte quantities and the balance among them are controlled by oxygen and carbon dioxide exchange in the lungs; absorption, secretion, and excretion of many substances by the kidneys; and secretion of regulatory hormones by the endocrine glands. Potassium is the most abundant intracellular cation. It is essential for the transmission of electrical impulses in cardiac and skeletal muscle. It also functions in enzyme reactions that transform glucose into energy and amino acids into proteins. Potassium helps maintain acid-base equilibrium, and it has a significant and inverse relationship to pH: A decrease in pH of 0.1 increases the potassium level by 0.6 mEq/L.

Abnormal potassium levels can be caused by a number of contributing factors, which can be categorized as follows:

Altered renal excretion: Normally, 80% to 90% of the body's potassium is filtered out through the kidneys each day (the remainder is excreted in sweat and stool); renal disease can result in abnormally high potassium levels.

Altered dietary intake: A severe potassium deficiency can be caused by an inadequate intake of dietary potassium.

Altered cellular metabolism: Damaged red blood cells (RBCs) release potassium into the circulating fluid, resulting in increased potassium levels.

Regulating electrolyte balance is one of the major functions of the kidneys. In normally functioning kidneys, urine potassium levels increase when serum levels are high and decrease when serum levels are low to maintain homeostasis. The kidneys respond to alkalosis by excreting potassium to retain hydrogen ions and increase acidity. In acidosis, the body excretes hydrogen ions and retains potassium. Analyzing these urinary levels can provide important clues to the functioning of the kidneys and other major organs. Urine potassium tests usually involve timed urine collections over a 12- or 24-hr period. Measurement of random specimens also may be requested.

This procedure is contraindicated for: N/A

INDICATIONS

- Determine the potential cause of renal calculi.
- Evaluate known or suspected endocrine disorder.
- Evaluate known or suspected kidney disease.
- Evaluate malabsorption disorders.

POTENTIAL MEDICAL DIAGNOSIS

Increased in:

- Albright-type kidney disease ***(related to excessive production of cortisol)***
- Cushing's syndrome ***(excessive corticosteroids, especially aldosterone levels, will increase urinary excretion of potassium)***
- Diabetic ketoacidosis ***(insulin deficiency forces potassium into the extracellular fluid; excess potassium is excreted in the urine)***
- Diuretic therapy ***(related to potassium-wasting effects of the medications)***
- Hyperaldosteronism ***(excessive aldosterone levels will increase urinary excretion of potassium)***
- Starvation (onset) ***(cells involved in providing energy through tissue breakdown release potassium into circulation)***
- Vomiting ***(elevated urine potassium is a hallmark of bulimia)***

P

Decreased in:

- Addison's disease ***(reduced aldosterone levels will diminish excretion of potassium by the kidneys)***
- Chronic kidney disease with decreased urine flow
- Potassium deficiency (chronic)

CRITICAL FINDINGS: N/A

INTERFERING FACTORS

- Drugs and other substances that can cause an increase in urine potassium levels include acetazolamide, acetylsalicylic acid, ammonium chloride, bendroflumethiazide, chlorthalidone, clopamide, corticosteroids, cortisone, diapamide, dichlorphenamide, diuretics, ethacrynic acid, fludrocortisone, furosemide, hydrochlorothiazide, hydrocortisone, intra-amniotic saline, mefruside, niacinamide, some oral contraceptives, thiazides, torsemide, triflocin, and viomycin.
- Drugs and other substances that can cause a decrease in urine potassium levels include anesthetic drugs, felodipine, and levarterenol.
- A dietary deficiency or excess of potassium can lead to spurious results.
- Diuretic therapy with excessive loss of electrolytes into the urine may falsely elevate results.
- All urine voided for the timed collection period must be included in the collection, or else falsely decreased values may be obtained. Compare output records with volume collected to verify that all voids were included in the collection.
- Potassium levels are subject to diurnal variation (output being highest at night), which is why 24-hr collections are recommended.

NURSING IMPLICATIONS AND PROCEDURE

PRETEST:

- Positively identify the patient using at least two person-specific identifiers before services, treatments, or procedures are performed.
- ***Patient Teaching:*** Inform the patient this test can assist in evaluating electrolyte balance.
- Obtain a history of the patient's health concerns, symptoms, surgical procedures, and results of previously performed laboratory and diagnostic studies. Include a list of known allergens, especially allergies or sensitivities to latex.
- Obtain a list of the patient's current medications, including over-the-counter medications and dietary supplements (see Effects of Natural Products on Laboratory Values online at Davis*Plus*).
- Review the procedure with the patient. Provide a nonmetallic urinal, bedpan, or toilet-mounted collection device. Address concerns about pain and explain that there should be no discomfort during the procedure.
- ***Sensitivity to social and cultural issues,*** as well as concern for modesty, is important in providing psychological support before, during, and after the procedure.
- Usually a 24-hr time frame for urine collection is ordered. Inform the patient that all urine must be saved during that 24-hr period. Instruct the patient not to void directly into the laboratory collection container. Instruct the patient to avoid defecating in the collection device and to keep toilet tissue out of the collection device to prevent contamination of the specimen. Place a sign in the bathroom to remind the patient to save all urine.
- Instruct the patient to void all urine into the collection device and then to pour the urine into the laboratory collection container. Alternatively, the specimen can be left in the collection device for a health-care staff member to add to the laboratory collection container.

- Note that there are no food, fluid, or medication restrictions unless by medical direction.

INTRATEST:

Potential Complications: N/A

- Avoid the use of equipment containing latex if the patient has a history of allergic reaction to latex.
- Instruct the patient to cooperate fully and to follow directions.
- Observe standard precautions, and follow the general guidelines in Patient Preparation and Specimen Collection online at Davis*Plus*. Positively identify the patient, and label the appropriate specimen container with the corresponding patient demographics, initials of the person collecting the specimen, date, and time of collection.

Random Specimen (Collect in Early Morning)

Clean-Catch Specimen

- Instruct the male patient to (1) thoroughly wash his hands, (2) cleanse the meatus, (3) void a small amount into the toilet, and (4) void directly into the specimen container.
- Instruct the female patient to (1) thoroughly wash her hands; (2) cleanse the labia from front to back; (3) while keeping the labia separated, void a small amount into the toilet; and (4) without interrupting the urine stream, void directly into the specimen container.

Indwelling Catheter

- Put on gloves. Empty drainage tube of urine. It may be necessary to clamp off the catheter for 15 to 30 min before specimen collection. Cleanse specimen port with antiseptic swab, and then aspirate 5 mL of urine with a 21- to 25-gauge needle and syringe. Transfer urine to a sterile container.

Timed Specimen

- Obtain a clean 3-L urine specimen container, toilet-mounted collection device, and plastic bag (for transport of the specimen container). The specimen must be refrigerated or kept on ice throughout the entire collection period. If an indwelling urinary catheter is in place, the drainage bag must be kept on ice.
- Begin the test between 0600 and 0800 if possible. Collect first voiding and discard. Record the time the specimen was discarded as the beginning of the timed collection period. The next morning, ask the patient to void at the same time the collection was started and add this last voiding to the container. Urinary output should be recorded throughout the collection time.
- If an indwelling catheter is in place, replace the tubing and container system at the start of the collection time. Keep the container system on ice during the collection period, or empty the urine into a larger container periodically during the collection period; monitor to ensure continued drainage, and conclude the test the next morning at the same hour the collection was begun.
- At the conclusion of the test, compare the quantity of urine with the urinary output record for the collection; if the specimen contains less than what was recorded as output, some urine may have been discarded, invalidating the test.
- Include on the collection container's label the amount of urine, test start and stop times, and ingestion of any foods or medications that can affect test results.

General

- Promptly transport the specimen to the laboratory for processing and analysis.

POST-TEST:

- Inform the patient that a report of the results will be made available to the requesting health-care provider (HCP), who will discuss the results with the patient.
- ***Nutritional Considerations:*** Potassium is present in all plant and animal cells, making dietary replacement simple to achieve in the potassium-deficient patient.
- Observe the patient for signs and symptoms of fluid volume excess

P

related to excess potassium intake, fluid volume deficit related to active loss, or risk of injury related to an alteration in body chemistry. Symptoms include dehydration, diarrhea, vomiting, or prolonged anorexia. Instruct the patient in electrolyte replacement therapy and changes in dietary intake that affect electrolyte levels, as ordered.

- Increased potassium levels may be associated with dehydration. Evaluate the patient for signs and symptoms of dehydration. Dehydration is a significant and common finding in older adult patients and other patients in whom renal function has deteriorated.
- Patients receiving digoxin or diuretics should have potassium levels monitored carefully because cardiac dysrhythmias can occur.
- Increased urine potassium levels may be associated with the formation of kidney stones. Educate the patient, if appropriate, on the importance of drinking a sufficient amount of water when kidney stones are suspected.
- Recognize anxiety related to test results. Discuss the implications of abnormal test results on the patient's lifestyle. Provide teaching and information regarding the clinical implications of the test results, as appropriate.
- Reinforce information given by the patient's HCP regarding further testing, treatment, or referral to another HCP. Answer any questions or address any concerns voiced by the patient or family.
- Depending on the results of this procedure, additional testing may be performed to evaluate or monitor progression of the disease process and determine the need for a change in therapy. Evaluate test results in relation to the patient's symptoms and other tests performed.

RELATED STUDIES:

- Related tests include ACTH, aldosterone, anion gap, BUN, calcium, calculus kidney stone panel, carbon dioxide, chloride, cortisol, creatinine, DHEAS, glucose, insulin, ketones, lactic acid, magnesium, osmolality, phosphorus, potassium, renin, sodium, and UA.
- Refer to the Endocrine, Gastrointestinal, and Genitourinary systems tables online at Davis*Plus* for related tests by body system.

Prealbumin

SYNONYM/ACRONYM: Transthyretin.

COMMON USE: To assess nutritional status and evaluate liver function toward diagnosing disorders such as malnutrition and chronic kidney disease.

P

SPECIMEN: Serum collected in a gold-, red-, or red/gray-top tube.

NORMAL FINDINGS: (Method: Nephelometry)

Age	Conventional Units	SI Units (Conventional Units × 10)
Newborn–1 mo	7–39 mg/dL	70–390 mg/L
1–6 mo	8–34 mg/dL	80–340 mg/L
6 mo–4 yr	2–36 mg/dL	20–360 mg/L
5–6 yr	12–30 mg/dL	120–300 mg/L
7 yr–adult/older adult	12–42 mg/dL	120–420 mg/L

DESCRIPTION: Prealbumin is a protein primarily produced by the liver. It is the major transport protein for triiodothyronine and thyroxine. It is also important in the metabolism of retinol-binding protein, which is needed for transporting vitamin A (retinol). Prealbumin has a short biological half-life of 2 days. It is used as an indicator of protein status and a marker for malnutrition. Prealbumin is often measured simultaneously with transferrin and albumin. The role of prealbumin in nutritional management has come into question by some health care providers (HCP) because it is a negative acute-phase protein. Prealbumin levels decrease during the acute phase of an inflammatory process such as in burns, infection, neoplasms, strenuous exercise, surgery, tissue infarction, and trauma, making the use of prealbumin less reliable as a predictor of malnutrition in certain clinical situations. Prealbumin may also be measured with C-reactive protein to assess for the coexistence of an inflammatory process and provide a more complete interpretation of the results.

This procedure is contraindicated for: N/A

INDICATIONS

Evaluate nutritional status.

POTENTIAL MEDICAL DIAGNOSIS

Increased in:

- Alcoholism ***(related to leakage of prealbumin from damaged hepatocytes and/or poor nutrition)***
- Chronic kidney disease ***(related to rapid turnover of prealbumin, which reflects a perceived elevation in the presence of overall loss of other proteins that take longer to produce)***
- Patients receiving steroids ***(these drugs stimulate production of prealbumin)***

Decreased in:

- Acute-phase inflammatory response ***(prealbumin is a negative acute-phase reactant protein; levels decrease in the presence of inflammation)***
- Diseases of the liver ***(related to decreased ability of the damaged liver to synthesize protein)***
- Hepatic damage ***(related to decreased ability of the damaged liver to synthesize protein)***
- Malnutrition ***(synthesis is decreased due to lack of proper diet)***
- Tissue necrosis ***(prealbumin is a negative acute-phase reactant protein; levels decrease in the presence of inflammation)***

CRITICAL FINDINGS: N/A

INTERFERING FACTORS

- Drugs and other substances that may increase prealbumin levels include anabolic steroids, anticonvulsants, danazol, oral contraceptives, prednisolone, prednisone, and propranolol.
- Drugs and other substances that may decrease prealbumin levels include amiodarone and diethylstilbestrol.
- Reference ranges are often based on fasting populations to provide some level of standardization for comparison. The presence of lipids in the blood may also interfere with the test method; fasting eliminates this potential source of error, especially if the patient has elevated lipid levels. The patient may be instructed to fast prior to the test; protocols vary among facilities.

NURSING IMPLICATIONS AND PROCEDURE

PRETEST:

- Positively identify the patient using at least two person-specific identifiers before services, treatments, or procedures are performed.
- ***Patient Teaching:*** Inform the patient this test can assist in assessing nutritional status.
- Obtain a history of the patient's health concerns, symptoms, surgical procedures, and results of previously performed laboratory and diagnostic studies. Include a list of known allergens, especially allergies or sensitivities to latex.
- Obtain a list of the patient's current medications, including over-the-counter medications and dietary supplements (see Effects of Natural Products on Laboratory Values online at Davis*Plus*).
- Review the procedure with the patient. Inform the patient that specimen collection takes approximately 5 to 10 min. Address concerns about pain and explain that there may be some discomfort during the venipuncture.
- ***Sensitivity to social and cultural issues,*** as well as concern for modesty, is important in providing psychological support before, during, and after the procedure.
- Instruct the patient to fast for 8 hr before specimen collection, if required.
- Note that there are no fluid or medication restrictions, unless by medical direction.

P

INTRATEST:

Potential Complications: N/A

- Ensure that the patient has complied with dietary restrictions prior to the study, as instructed.
- Avoid the use of equipment containing latex if the patient has a history of allergic reaction to latex.
- Instruct the patient to cooperate fully and to follow directions. Direct the patient to breathe normally and to avoid unnecessary movement.
- Observe standard precautions, and follow the general guidelines in Patient Preparation and Specimen Collection online at Davis*Plus*. Positively identify the patient, and label the appropriate specimen container with the corresponding patient demographics, initials of the person collecting the specimen, date, and time of collection. Perform a venipuncture.
- Remove the needle and apply direct pressure with dry gauze to stop bleeding. Observe/assess venipuncture site for bleeding or hematoma formation and secure gauze with adhesive bandage.
- Promptly transport the specimen to the laboratory for processing and analysis.

POST-TEST:

- Inform the patient that a report of the results will be made available to the requesting HCP, who will discuss the results with the patient.
- Instruct the patient to resume usual diet, as directed by the HCP.
- ***Nutritional Considerations:*** Nutritional therapy may be indicated for patients with decreased prealbumin levels. Educate the patient, as appropriate, that good dietary sources of complete protein (containing all eight essential amino acids) include meat, fish, eggs, and dairy products and that good sources of incomplete protein (lacking one or more of the eight essential amino acids) include grains, nuts, legumes, vegetables, and seeds.
- Reinforce information given by the patient's HCP regarding further testing, treatment, or referral to another HCP. Answer any questions or address any concerns voiced by the patient or family.
- Depending on the results of this procedure, additional testing may be performed to evaluate or monitor progression of the disease process and determine the need for a change in therapy. Evaluate test results in relation to the patient's symptoms and other tests performed.

RELATED STUDIES:

- Related tests include albumin, chloride, ferritin, iron/TIBC, potassium, protein, sodium, T_4, T_3, transferrin, and vitamin A.
- Refer to the Endocrine, Gastrointestinal, and Hepatobiliary systems tables online at Davis*Plus* for related tests by body system.

Prion Disease Testing

SYNONYM/ACRONYM: Transmissible spongiform encephalopathies, TSEs.

COMMON USE: Testing for prion diseases may be considered for patients with undiagnosed, rapidly progressive dementia.

SPECIMEN: Information is collected from a variety of sources that may include brain or tonsillar biopsy, cerebrospinal fluid (CSF). Analysis for the presence of 14-3-3 type protein, electroencephalogram (EEG), brain magnetic resonance imaging (MRI), neurologic exams, and patient history.

NORMAL FINDINGS: (Negative biopsy, normal CSF protein levels, normal EEG, normal MRI, normal neurologic examination.

DESCRIPTION: Prion diseases have been identified in humans and animals throughout the world. They are classified in a general category of brain diseases called proteinopathies. Prion diseases are rare, fatal (no known cure), and very difficult to diagnose. Prion diseases are caused by abnormal protein molecules called *scrapie prion proteins* (PrPSc) that cause irreversible damage to brain tissue. The protein molecules themselves appear to be capable of initiating the disease process, do not stimulate an immune response, and are extraordinarily resistant to destruction. Records describing the first prion disease date back to the 1700s, and the pathophysiology of transmissible spongiform encephalopathy (TSE) continues to elude scientists, as there is no known test that can reliably detect either the disease or its cause by conventional methods.

The term **prion** is derived from a combination of the words "protein" and "infectious" and was given to the protein in the 1980s by its Nobel Prize–winning discoverer, Stanley Prusiner. Cellular prion protein (PrPC) exists normally in humans and all other mammals; the highest concentration of PrPC is found in brain tissue, but it is also present in other tissue types (e.g., tonsil, appendix, spleen, intestinal, lymphatic). The trigger that leads to the aberrant conformational changes in the PrPC remains unknown, but the aberrant PrPSc protein will serve as a template to produce more abnormal protein once it has been transmitted into its host. There is significant scientific evidence that as the structurally abnormal PrPSc protein molecules develop, they gather in clusters and accumulate in affected tissue, especially brain tissue. The resulting damage leaves spongelike holes in the tissue that are evident upon microscopic examination of brain tissue; hence, the condition is termed *spongiform encephalopathy.* Difficulty in diagnosis is due to a number of factors that include latency (the infection can be developing for years before signs and symptoms appear) and the lack of specific, minimally invasive, rapid disease markers. Brain biopsy and neuropathologic examination at autopsy are the only methods that can positively confirm a diagnosis of prion disease. It is hoped that a growing understanding of molecular science will open doors that have thus far prevented our discovery of the cause, treatment, and cure for prion diseases. Current research projects are investigating the possibility of a connection between prion disease and the progressive loss of neuromuscular abilities associated with Alzheimer's disease, another familiar proteinopathy. Other diseases classified as proteinopathies include Parkinson's disease and amyotrophic lateral sclerosis.

Specific prion diseases are known to affect humans and animals. Scrapie, the first prion disease identified, affects sheep and goats. The scrapie-infected animals "scrape" off their wool or hair and exhibit signs and symptoms of a central nervous system disorder.

Prion diseases associated with animals:

- Bovine spongiform encephalopathy (BSE)—affects cattle; also known as mad cow disease
- Chronic wasting disease—affects deer, elk, and moose
- Feline spongiform encephalopathy
- Scrapie—affects sheep and goats
- Transmissible mink encephalopathy
- Ungulate spongiform encephalopathy—affects exotic animals such as kudu, nyala, and oryx

Human prion diseases can be acquired or inherited, or they can occur sporadically, unassociated with any cause. Even though the diseases are rare, there is cause for public health concern because transmission of tiny amounts of prion-contaminated material can initiate the conversion of normal to abnormal protein production in a healthy individual, and the disease that develops is always fatal. Some infections occur strictly within an animal species (e.g., sheep-to-sheep transmission), and some occur across animal species (e.g., animal-to-human transmission). Infection of animals is believed to occur as a result of direct transmission from animal to animal or by consumption of feed processed with infected animal parts; infection of humans is believed to occur as a result of the consumption of infected flesh (human or animal), blood transfusion, administration of human-derived pituitary growth hormones (production of genetically engineered hormones began in the 1980s), implantation of infected tissue (corneas and skin) or infected grafts (during spinal cord or brain surgery), and exposure to contaminated objects (e.g., surgical instruments used in neurosurgery). Blood product services have developed strict deferral policies regarding Creutzfeldt-Jakob disease (CJD), a human prion disease.

P

Three types of human prion diseases:

1. Acquired and iatrogenic prion diseases are very rare, accounting for less than 1% of reported cases. Kuru and variant CJD (vCJD) are types of acquired prion diseases caused by exposure to exogenous sources of PrPSc. Kuru is a disease that was originally identified in a New Guinea tribe that practiced cannibalism as part of the funeral ritual. Kuru is rarely encountered today because education regarding the mechanism of its transmission has resulted in its virtual eradication. vCJD is linked to exposure to BSE through consumption of contaminated beef, although there have been some cases of vCJD linked to blood transfusion. Unlike classic CJD, vCJD appears to affect younger patients (average age of 28 yr) and has a longer duration of illness (average of 12 to 14 mo). Iatrogenic prion disease occurs accidentally during a medical procedure (e.g., as a result of receiving prion-contaminated tissue implants or grafts, by injections of human derived hormones, or through exposure during a surgical procedure using contaminated instruments).
2. Inherited or familial prion diseases have a low incidence, accounting for 10% to 15% of reported cases. Familial prion diseases are defined by the presence of a mutation in the PrPC gene as determined by genetic testing. There are three distinct types of familial prion disease: familial Creutzfeldt-Jakob disease (fCJD), fatal familial insomnia (FFI), and Gerstmann-Sträussler-Scheinker disease (GSS).
3. Sporadic prion diseases are the most common, have no known cause, and comprise 85% to 90% of reported cases. There are also three types of sporadic diseases: sporadic Creutzfeldt-Jakob disease (sCJD), sporadic fatal insomnia (sFI), and variably protease-sensitive prionopathy (VPSPr). sCJD, or classical CJD, is the most common of all prion diseases. The average age of onset ranges between ages 45 and 75 yr and has a relatively short duration of illness; 70% of patients diagnosed with sCJD die in 6 mo or less. The period between production of the abnormal PrPSc protein and the onset of symptoms (latency period) can be anywhere between 1 and 30 yr. Once the abnormal protein begins accumulating, symptoms appear suddenly. Cognitive changes include memory lapses, moodiness, lack of interest in normal activities, and withdrawal from social contacts. Motor changes include unsteady gait, slurred speech, and difficulty swallowing. Blurred vision and hallucinations sometimes occur in the later phase of the disease. Mental and physical deterioration rapidly progress until, eventually, movement and speech are lost. Death is usually a complication of heart failure or respiratory failure.

This procedure is contraindicated for: N/A

INDICATIONS

- Identify family history of prion disease.
- Identify undiagnosed, rapidly progressive dementia.

POTENTIAL MEDICAL DIAGNOSIS

Normal findings

- No evidence of prion disease
- Negative tonsillar biopsy (if vCJD is being considered), ***as vCJD is the only type known to involve the lymph nodes, spleen, tonsil, and appendix.*** Note: A negative biopsy does not rule out vCJD.

Abnormal findings related to

Testing for sCJD, the most common type of prion disease, may include noninvasive testing such as brain MRI and EEG. Two types of MRI studies may be used to identify abnormalities in the cerebral cortex, striatum, and/or thalamus of the brain: fluid attenuated inversion recovery and diffusion weighted imaging. EEG studies of people with sCJD show the characteristic abnormal findings associated with CJD (periodic, sharp brain waves) at some stage of the disease in 65% of cases. The problem is that the abnormal patterns may be only intermittently manifested or they may not be demonstrated at all until the later stages of the disease. CSF analysis is a more invasive procedure and is used to identify an increase in CSF protein levels. Protein 14-3-3, brain-specific enolase, and tau protein have been associated with proteinopathies but are not specific for CJD. Two newer methods to detect prion proteins have been developed with good promise for detecting tiny amounts of PrPSc in human specimens. The real-time quaking-induced conversion (RT-QUIC) method utilizes a CSF specimen to detect CJD-associated prions. The protein misfolding cyclic amplification (PMCA) urine test detects evidence of vCJD-associated prions. More studies need to be done to determine whether these assays can be used diagnostically, but the hope is that reliable antemortem testing for TSEs, prior to the development of symptoms, may become a possibility.

- CJD ***evidenced by abnormal brain biopsy and neuropathologic findings at autopsy***

P

CRITICAL FINDINGS: N/A

INTERFERING FACTORS: N/A

NURSING IMPLICATIONS AND PROCEDURE

PRETEST:

- Positively identify the patient using at least two person-specific identifiers before services, treatments, or procedures are performed.
- *Patient Teaching:* Inform the patient that the testing ordered by the health-care provider (HCP) can assist in the differential diagnosis of types of conditions that affect the brain and nervous system.
- Obtain a history of the patient's health concerns, symptoms, surgical procedures, and results of previously performed laboratory and diagnostic studies. Include a list of known allergens, especially allergies or sensitivities to latex.
- Obtain a list of the patient's current medications, including over-the-counter medications and dietary supplements (see Effects of Natural Products on Laboratory Values online at Davis*Plus*).
- Review the procedure with the patient. Inform the patient that several tests may be necessary to establish a presumptive diagnosis. Inform the patient that CSF specimens are collected by lumbar puncture, as described in the cerebrospinal fluid analysis study. Address concerns about pain, and explain that there may be some discomfort during CSF specimen collection.
- ***Sensitivity to social and cultural issues,*** as well as concern for modesty, is important in providing psychological support before, during, and after the procedure.

- Follow the food, fluid, or medication instructions indicated in the individual studies.

INTRATEST:

Potential Complications: N/A

- Avoid the use of equipment containing latex if the patient has a history of allergic reaction to latex.
- Instruct the patient to cooperate fully and to follow directions. Direct the patient to breathe normally and to avoid unnecessary movement.
- Observe standard precautions, and follow the general guidelines in Patient Preparation and Specimen Collection online at Davis*Plus*. Positively identify the patient, and label the appropriate specimen container with the corresponding patient demographics, initials of the person collecting the specimen, date, and time of collection. Perform required specimen collection (see individual studies) and promptly transport the specimen to the laboratory for processing and analysis.
- CJD-specific infection-control guidelines have been developed to assist those involved in the care of CJD patients and disposal or cleaning of contaminated materials and equipment. Methods include steam autoclaving materials or immersing them in sodium hydroxide solution. Additional information can be obtained from the Centers for Disease Control and Prevention (CDC) (www.cdc.gov/prions/cjd/infection-control.html) and the World Health Organization (www.who.int/csr/resources/publications/bse/whocdscsraph2003.pdf?ua=1). 🍁
- CJD-specific infection control guidelines have been developed to assist funeral directors and their employees who are involved in funeral preparations. Information can be accessed at the websites provided for health-care workers.

POST-TEST:

- Inform the patient that a report of the results will be made available to the requesting HCP, who will discuss the results with the patient.
- Recognize anxiety related to test results, and provide emotional support if results are indicative of CJD. Encourage the family to seek counseling if concerned with providing care to the patient at home or for assistance to address fears about disease transmission during home care. Inform the patient and family that prion diseases are not on the list of nationally notifiable diseases. 🍁 Provide teaching and information regarding the clinical implications of the test results, as appropriate. Educate the patient regarding access to counseling services, as appropriate, especially regarding considerations for end-of-life preparations, including special funeral arrangements and the possibility of a postmortem autopsy.
- Reinforce information given by the patient's HCP regarding further testing, treatment, or referral to another HCP. Provide contact information, if desired, for the Creutzfeldt-Jacob Disease Foundation (www.cjdfoundation.org) and CDC (www.cdc.gov/DiseasesConditions). 🍁 Answer any questions or address any concerns voiced by the patient or family.
- Teach the patient and family about the disease progression. Explain that fear, anxiety, and grief are normal reactions. The patient may experience visual hallucinations, myoclonus, and dysesthesia, which can be very distressing for patients and their caregivers. Explain that as the disease progresses, the patient will lose awareness of his or her surroundings, of the disease, and of the symptoms. Inform the patient and family that there are drugs that can help alleviate the discomfort associated with some of the symptoms.
- Depending on the results of this procedure, additional testing may be performed to evaluate or monitor progression of the disease process and determine the need for a change in therapy. Evaluate test results in relation to the patient's symptoms and other tests performed.

P

Patient Education:

- Teach the pathophysiology associated with the disease process, including mode of transmission if known.
- Provide advance directive options to the patient and family with a discussion on end-of-life care.

Expected Patient Outcomes:

Understanding

- The patient and family state that the prognosis of the disease process is terminal.
- The patient and family state that treatment options focus on supportive measures.

Ability

- Family demonstrates adherence to safety measures that are necessary for those cognitively altered.
- Family demonstrates how to assist in performing basic care procedures (bathing, assistance with feeding, toileting).

Response

- Family agrees to attend support group for those with family members terminally ill.
- Family agrees to consider social services that may assist in the provision of home care.

RELATED STUDIES:

- Related tests include CSF analysis, EEG, MRI brain.
- Refer to the Musculoskeletal System table online at Davis*Plus* for related tests by body system.

Procalcitonin

SYNONYM/ACRONYM: PCT.

COMMON USE: To assist in diagnosing bacterial infection and risk for developing sepsis.

SPECIMEN: Serum collected in a gold-, red-, or red/gray-top tube. Plasma collected in a lavender-top (EDTA) or a green-top (lithium or sodium heparin) tube is also acceptable.

NORMAL FINDINGS: (Method: Fluorescence immunoassay)

Age	Conventional Units	SI Units (Conventional Units × 1)
Newborn	Less than 2 ng/mL	Less than 2 mcg/L
18–20 hr	Less than 20 ng/mL	Less than 20 mcg/L
48 hr	Less than 5 ng/mL	Less than 5 mcg/L
3 d–adult	Less than 0.1 ng/mL	Less than 0.1 mcg/L
	Interpretive Guidelines	
Interpretation	**Conventional Units**	**SI Units**
Bacterial infection absent or very unlikely	Less than 0.1 ng/mL	Less than 0.1 mcg/L
Bacterial infection possible; low risk for development of sepsis	Less than 0.5 ng/mL	Less than 0.5 mcg/L

P

Interpretive Guidelines		
Interpretation	**Conventional Units**	**SI Units**
Bacterial infection likely; development of sepsis is possible	0.5–2 ng/mL	0.5–2 mcg/L
Bacterial infection very likely; high risk for development of sepsis	2.1–9.9 ng/mL or greater	2.1–9.9 mcg/L or greater
Bacterial infection severe; septic shock is probable	10 ng/mL or greater	10 mcg/L or greater

DESCRIPTION: Sepsis is a very serious, potentially life-threatening systemic inflammatory response to infection. The host inflammatory reaction was termed *systemic inflammatory response syndrome* (SIRS) by the American College of Chest Physicians and the Society of Critical Care Medicine in 1992. SIRS is defined by documented clinical evidence of bacterial infection (e.g., culture results) in the presence of two of four other criteria: temperature greater than 100.4°F ✱ or less than 96.8°F, ✱ heart rate greater than 90 beats/min, hyperventilation (greater than 20 breaths/minute or $Paco_2$ less than 32 mm Hg), or white blood cell (WBC) count greater than 12 × 10^3/microL or less than 4 × 10^3/microL. The development of sepsis is initiated by the activation of circulating macrophages resulting from binding to receptors on the outer membrane of gram-negative or gram-positive bacteria. Other organisms, such as fungi, parasites, and viruses, are also capable of initiating SIRS, which can develop into sepsis. Severe sepsis involves a systemic inflammatory response that suppresses the immune system, activation of the coagulation process (reflected by prolonged prothrombin time and activated partial thromboplastin time, elevated D-dimer, and deficiency of protein C), cardiovascular insufficiency, and multiple organ failure. The incidence of sepsis in hospitals is especially high in noncardiac intensive care units. Early-onset neonatal sepsis occurs in the first 72 hours of life with 85% of cases presenting in the first 24 hours. Early-onset neonatal sepsis is the result of colonization of the neonate from the mother as it moved through the birth canal before delivery. The Centers for Disease Control and Prevention recommends universal screening for group B *Streptococcus* for all pregnant women at 35 to 37 weeks' gestation. Other organisms associated with early-onset neonatal sepsis include coagulase-negative *Staphylococcus*, *Escherichia coli*, *Haemophilus influenzae*, and *Listeria monocytogenes*.

Late-onset neonatal sepsis, during days 4 to 90, is acquired from the environment and has been associated with infection by *Acinetobacter*, *Candida*, coagulase-negative *Staphylococci*, *Enterobacter*, *E. coli*, group B *Streptococcus*, *Klebsiella*, *Pseudomonas*, *Serratia*, and *Staphylococcus aureus*, as well as some anaerobes. Normally procalcitonin, the precursor of the hormone calcitonin, is produced by the C cells of the thyroid. In SIRS, microbial toxins and inflammatory mediator proteins, including cytokines, tumor necrosis factor α, interleukin 1, prostaglandins, and platelet activating factor, may trigger the production of large amounts of procalcitonin by nonthyroidal, non-neuroendocrine cells throughout the body. Each phase of the inflammatory response creates another cascade of events that may conclude with septic shock and death. Procalcitonin is detectable within 2 to 4 hr after an SIRS-initiating event and peaks within 12 to 24 hr. Serial measurements are useful to monitor patients at risk of developing sepsis or to monitor response to therapy.

This procedure is contraindicated for: N/A

INDICATIONS

- Assist in the diagnosis of bacteremia and septicemia.
- Assist in the differential diagnosis of bacterial versus viral meningitis.
- Assist in the differential diagnosis of community-acquired bacterial versus viral pneumonia.
- Monitor response to antibacterial therapy.

P

POTENTIAL MEDICAL DIAGNOSIS

Increased in:

- Bacteremia or septicemia ***(related to SIRS induced overproduction of procalcitonin)***
- Major surgery ***(related to inflammation in the absence of sepsis)***
- Multiorgan failure ***(related to inflammation in the absence of sepsis)***
- Neuroendocrine tumors (medullary thyroid cancer, small-cell lung cancer, and carcinoid tumors) ***(related to procalcitonin-secreting tumor cells)***
- Severe burns ***(related to inflammation in the absence of sepsis)***
- Severe trauma ***(related to inflammation in the absence of sepsis)***
- Treatment with OKT3 antibodies (antibody used to protect a transplanted organ or graft from attack by T cells and subsequent rejection) and other drugs that stimulate the release of cytokines ***(related to inflammatory response in the absence of sepsis)***

Decreased in: N/A

CRITICAL FINDINGS: N/A

INTERFERING FACTORS: N/A

NURSING IMPLICATIONS AND PROCEDURE

PRETEST:

- Positively identify the patient using at least two person-specific identifiers before services, treatments, or procedures are performed.
- *Patient Teaching:* Inform the patient this test can assist in assessing for infection and response to antibiotic treatment.
- Obtain a history of the patient's health concerns (especially pain related to the inflammatory process in connective or other tissues), symptoms, surgical procedures, and results of previously performed laboratory and diagnostic studies. Include a list of known allergens, especially allergies or sensitivities to latex.
- Obtain a list of the patient's current medications, including over-the-counter medications and dietary supplements (see Effects of Natural Products on Laboratory Values online at Davis*Plus*).

- Review the procedure with the patient. Inform the patient that specimen collection takes approximately 5 to 10 min. Address concerns about pain and explain that there may be some discomfort during the venipuncture.
- *Sensitivity to social and cultural issues,* as well as concern for modesty, is important in providing psychological support before, during, and after the procedure.
- Note that there are no food, fluid, or medication restrictions unless by medical direction.

INTRATEST:

Potential Complications: N/A

- Avoid the use of equipment containing latex if the patient has a history of allergic reaction to latex.
- Instruct the patient to cooperate fully and to follow directions. Direct the patient to breathe normally and to avoid unnecessary movement.
- Observe standard precautions, and follow the general guidelines in Patient Preparation and Specimen Collection online at Davis*Plus*. Positively identify the patient, and label the appropriate specimen container with the corresponding patient demographics, initials of the person collecting the specimen, date, and time of collection. Perform a venipuncture.
- Remove the needle and apply direct pressure with dry gauze to stop bleeding. Observe/assess venipuncture site for bleeding or hematoma formation and secure gauze with adhesive bandage.
- Promptly transport the specimen to the laboratory for processing and analysis.

POST-TEST:

- Inform the patient that a report of the results will be made available to the requesting health-care provider (HCP), who will discuss the results with the patient.
- Answer any questions or address any concerns voiced by the patient or family.
- Depending on the results of this procedure, additional testing may be performed to evaluate or monitor progression of the disease process and determine the need for a change in therapy. Evaluate test results in relation to the patient's symptoms and other tests performed.

RELATED STUDIES:

- Related tests include ALKP, ALT, AST, antimicrobial drugs, bilirubin total and fractions, coagulation factors, CBC, CBC platelet count, CBC WBC count and differential, creatinine, CRP, culture bacterial blood, culture bacterial anal/genital, culture bacterial urine, ESR, Gram stain, lactic acid, aPTT, PT, and Protein C.
- Refer to the Immune System table online at Davis*Plus* for related tests by body system.

P

Proctosigmoidoscopy

SYNONYM/ACRONYM: Anoscopy (anal canal), proctoscopy (rectum), flexible fiberoptic sigmoidoscopy, flexible proctosigmoidoscopy, sigmoidoscopy (sigmoid colon).

COMMON USE: To visualize and assess the colon, rectum, and anus to assist in diagnosing disorders such as cancer, inflammation, prolapse, and evaluate the effectiveness of medical and surgical therapeutic interventions.

AREA OF APPLICATION: Anus, rectum, colon.

DESCRIPTION: Proctosigmoidoscopy allows direct visualization of the mucosa of the anal canal (anoscopy), rectum (proctoscopy), and distal sigmoid colon (sigmoidoscopy). The procedure can be performed using a rigid or flexible fiberoptic endoscope, but the flexible instrument is generally preferred. The endoscope is a multichannel device allowing visualization of the mucosal lining of the colon, instillation of air, removal of fluid and foreign objects, obtainment of tissue biopsy specimens, and use of a laser for the destruction of tissue and control of bleeding. The endoscope is advanced approximately 60 cm into the colon. This procedure is commonly used in patients with lower abdominal and perineal pain; changes in bowel habits; rectal prolapse during defecation; or passage of blood, mucus, or pus in the stool. Proctosigmoidoscopy can also be a therapeutic procedure, allowing removal of polyps or hemorrhoids or reduction of a volvulus. Biopsy specimens of suspicious sites may be obtained during the procedure.

This procedure is contraindicated for

- Patients with bleeding disorders, especially disorders associated with uremia and cytotoxic chemotherapy.
- Patients with cardiac conditions or dysrhythmias.
- Patients with bowel perforation, acute peritonitis, ischemic bowel necrosis, toxic megacolon, diverticulitis, recent bowel surgery, advanced pregnancy, severe cardiac or pulmonary disease, recent myocardial infarction, known or suspected pulmonary embolus, large abdominal aortic or iliac aneurysm, or coagulation abnormality.

INDICATIONS
- Confirm the diagnosis of diverticular disease.
- Confirm the diagnosis of Hirschsprung's disease and colitis in children.
- Determine the cause of pain and rectal prolapse during defecation.
- Determine the cause of rectal itching, pain, or burning.
- Evaluate the cause of blood, pus, or mucus in the stool.
- Evaluate postoperative anastomosis of the colon.
- Examine the distal colon before barium enema (BE) x-ray to obtain improved visualization of the area, and after a BE when x-ray findings are inconclusive.
- Reduce volvulus of the sigmoid colon.
- Remove hemorrhoids by laser therapy.
- Screen for and excise polyps.
- Screen for colon cancer.

POTENTIAL MEDICAL DIAGNOSIS

Normal findings
- Normal mucosa of the anal canal, rectum, and sigmoid colon

Abnormal findings related to
- Anal fissure or fistula
- Anorectal abscess
- Benign lesions
- Bleeding sites
- Bowel infection or inflammation
- Crohn's disease
- Diverticula
- Hypertrophic anal papillae
- Internal and external hemorrhoids
- Polyps
- Rectal prolapse
- Tumors
- Ulcerative colitis
- Vascular abnormalities

CRITICAL FINDINGS: N/A

INTERFERING FACTORS

Factors that may alter the results of the study

- Inability of the patient to cooperate or remain still during the procedure because of age, significant pain, or mental status.
- Strictures or other abnormalities preventing passage of the scope.
- Barium swallow or upper gastrointestinal (GI) series within the preceding 48 hr.
- Severe lower GI bleeding or the presence of feces, barium, blood, or blood clots.

Other considerations

- Failure to follow dietary restrictions before the procedure may cause the procedure to be canceled or repeated.
- Use of bowel preparations that include laxatives or enemas should be avoided in pregnant patients or patients with inflammatory bowel disease unless specifically directed by a health-care provider (HCP).

NURSING IMPLICATIONS AND PROCEDURE

See Potential Nursing Problems on Fast Find at davispl.us/vanleeuwen7.

PRETEST:

- Positively identify the patient using at least two person-specific identifiers before services, treatments, or procedures are performed.
- ***Patient Teaching:*** Inform the patient this procedure can assist in evaluating the rectum and lower colon for disease.
- Obtain a history of the patient's health concerns, symptoms, surgical procedures, and results of previously performed laboratory and diagnostic studies. Include a list of known allergens, especially allergies or sensitivities to latex, anesthetics, or sedatives.
- Note any recent procedures that can interfere with test results. Ensure that this procedure is performed before an upper GI study or barium swallow.
- Record the date of the last menstrual period and determine the possibility of pregnancy in perimenopausal women.
- Obtain a list of the patient's current medications, including over-the-counter medications, dietary supplements, anticoagulants, aspirin and other salicylates (see Effects of Natural Products on Laboratory Values online at Davis*Plus*). Such products should be discontinued by medical direction for the appropriate number of days prior to a surgical procedure. Note the last time and dose of medication taken.
- Note intake of oral iron preparations within 1 wk before the procedure because these cause black, sticky feces that are difficult to remove with bowel preparation.
- Review the procedure with the patient. Address concerns about pain related to the procedure and explain that some pain may be experienced during the test, and there may be moments of discomfort. Explain that a sedative and/or analgesia will be administered to promote relaxation and reduce discomfort prior to insertion of the anoscope. Inform the patient that the procedure is performed in a GI lab by an HCP specializing in this procedure, with support staff, and takes approximately 30 to 60 min.
- ***Sensitivity to social and cultural issues,*** as well as concern for modesty, is important in providing psychological support before, during, and after the procedure.
- Instruct the patient that a laxative may be needed the day before the procedure, with cleansing enemas on the morning of the procedure, depending on the institution's policy.
- Inform the patient that the urge to defecate may be experienced when the scope is passed. Encourage slow, deep breathing through the mouth to help alleviate the feeling.

P

- Inform the patient that flatus may be expelled during and after the procedure owing to air that is injected into the scope to improve visualization.
- Instruct the patient to eat a low-residue diet for 3 days prior to the procedure. Consume clear liquids only the evening before, and restrict food and fluids for 8 hr prior to the procedure. Protocols may vary among facilities.
- *Make sure a written and informed consent has been signed prior to the procedure and before administering any medications.*

INTRATEST:

Potential Complications:

Complications of the procedure may include bleeding and cardiac dysrhythmias.

- Observe standard precautions, and follow the general guidelines in Patient Preparation and Specimen Collection online at Davis*Plus*. Positively identify the patient.
- Ensure that the patient has complied with food, fluid, and medication restrictions and pretesting preparations prior to the procedure, as instructed.
- Administer two small-volume enemas 1 hr before the procedure.
- Avoid the use of equipment containing latex if the patient has a history of allergic reaction to latex.
- Have emergency equipment readily available.
- Instruct the patient to void prior to the procedure and change into the gown, robe, and foot coverings provided.
- Record baseline vital signs and continue to monitor throughout the procedure. Protocols may vary among facilities.
- Place the patient on an examination table in the left lateral decubitus position or the knee-chest position and drape with the buttocks exposed. The buttocks are placed at or extending slightly beyond the edge of the examination table or bed, preferably on a special examining table that tilts the patient into the desired position.
- The HCP visually inspects the perianal area and then performs a digital rectal examination with a well-lubricated, gloved finger. A fecal specimen may be obtained from the glove when the finger is removed from the rectum.
- A lubricated anoscope (7 cm in length) is inserted, and the anal canal is inspected (anoscopy). The anoscope is removed, and a lubricated proctoscope (27 cm in length) or flexible sigmoidoscope (35 to 60 cm in length) is inserted.
- The scope is manipulated gently to facilitate passage, and air may be insufflated through the scope to improve visualization. Suction and cotton swabs also are used to remove materials that hinder visualization.
- The patient is instructed to take deep breaths to aid in movement of the scope downward through the ascending colon to the cecum and into the terminal portion of the ileum.
- Examination is done as the scope is gradually withdrawn. Photographs are obtained for future reference.
- At the end of the procedure, the scope is completely withdrawn, and residual lubricant is cleansed from the anal area.
- Place fecal or tissue samples and polyps in properly labelled specimen containers, and promptly transport the specimen to the laboratory for processing and analysis.

POST-TEST:

- Inform the patient that a report of the results will be made available to the requesting HCP, who will discuss the results with the patient.
- Monitor vital signs and neurological status every 15 min for 1 hr, then every 2 hr for 4 hr, and then as ordered by the HCP. Monitor temperature every 4 hr for 24 hr. Monitor intake and output at least every 8 hr. Compare with baseline values. Notify the HCP if temperature changes. Protocols may vary among facilities.
- Monitor for any rectal bleeding.

- Instruct the patient to resume diet, medication, and activity, as directed by the HCP.
- Instruct the patient to expect slight rectal bleeding for 2 days after removal of polyps or biopsy specimens, but heavy rectal bleeding must be immediately reported to the HCP.
- Instruct the patient that any abdominal pain, tenderness, or distention; pain on defecation; or fever must be reported to the HCP immediately.
- Inform the patient that any bloating or flatulence is the result of air insufflation.
- Encourage the patient to drink several glasses of water to help replace fluid lost during test preparation.
- Recognize anxiety related to test results, and be supportive of perceived loss of independence and fear of shortened life expectancy. Discuss the implications of abnormal test results on the patient's lifestyle. Provide teaching and information regarding the clinical implications of the test results, as appropriate. Educate the patient regarding access to counseling services.
- Reinforce information given by the patient's HCP regarding further testing, treatment, or referral to another HCP. Decisions regarding the need for and frequency of occult blood testing, colonoscopy, or other cancer screening procedures should be made after consultation between the patient and HCP. The American Cancer Society (ACS) recommends regular screening for colon cancer, beginning at age 50 yr for individuals without identified risk factors and sooner for those with identified risk factors. Its recommendations for frequency of screening are as follows: annually for occult blood testing (fecal occult blood testing or fecal immunochemical testing); every 5 yr for flexible sigmoidoscopy, double contrast barium enema, or computed tomography colonography; every 10 yr for colonoscopy; or every 3 yr for stool DNA testing. 🍁 Abnormal findings should be followed up by colonoscopy. There are both advantages and disadvantages to the screening tests that are available today. Methods to use DNA testing of stool are being investigated and are designed to identify abnormal changes in DNA from the cells in the lining of the colon that are normally shed and excreted in stool. The DNA tests under development use multiple markers to identify colon cancers that demonstrate different, abnormal DNA changes. Unlike some of the current screening methods, the DNA tests would be able to detect precancerous polyps. The most current guidelines for colon cancer screening of the general population as well as of individuals with increased risk are available from the ACS (www.cancer.org), U.S. Preventive Services Task Force (www.uspreventiveservicestaskforce.org), and American College of Gastroenterology (www.gi.org). 🍁 Answer any questions or address any concerns voiced by the patient or family.
- Depending on the results of this procedure, additional testing may be needed to evaluate or monitor progression of the disease process and determine the need for a change in therapy. Evaluate test results in relation to the patient's symptoms and other tests performed.

Patient Education:
- Teach the patient and family disease specific-pathophysiology.
- Teach ostomy care as appropriate.

Expected Patient Outcomes:

Understanding
- The patient and family work with the health-care team to discuss treatment options and expected outcomes.
- The patient and family recognize that an HCP specialist (e.g., urology or oncology) may need to be consulted to manage the disease.

Ability
- The patient successfully demonstrates the ability to rate the degree of anxiety on a 1 to 10 scale.

- The patient and family successfully demonstrate how to manage the postoperative stool collection bag.

Response

- The patient and family agree to seek spiritual support as needed.
- The patient and family agree to review the process for completing an advance directive.

RELATED STUDIES:

- Related tests include barium enema, capsule endoscopy, colonoscopy, CBC, CT abdomen, fecal analysis, fecal fat, GI blood loss scan, MRI abdomen, and US prostate transrectal.
- Refer to the Gastrointestinal System table online at Davis*Plus* for related tests by body system.

Progesterone

SYNONYM/ACRONYM: N/A

COMMON USE: To assess ovarian function, assist in fertility work-ups, and monitor placental function during pregnancy related to disorders such as tumor, cysts, and threatened abortion.

SPECIMEN: Serum collected in a gold-, red-, or red/gray-top tube.

NORMAL FINDINGS: (Method: Immunochemiluminometric assay [ICMA])

Hormonal State	Conventional Units	SI Units (Conventional Units × 3.18)
Prepubertal	Less than 1 ng/mL	Less than 3 nmol/L
Adult male	Less than 1 ng/mL	Less than 3 nmol/L
Adult female		
Follicular phase	Less than 1 ng/mL	Less than 3 nmol/L
Luteal phase	2–25 ng/mL	6.4–79.5 nmol/L
Pregnancy, first trimester	10–44 ng/mL	31.8–140 nmol/L
Pregnancy, second trimester	19.5–82.5 ng/mL	62–262.4 nmol/L
Pregnancy, third trimester	65–229 ng/mL	206.7–728.2 nmol/L
Postmenopausal period	Less than 1 ng/mL	Less than 3 nmol/L

P

DESCRIPTION: Progesterone is a female sex hormone. Its function is to prepare the uterus for pregnancy and the breasts for lactation. Progesterone testing can be used to confirm that ovulation has occurred and to assess the functioning of the corpus luteum. Serial measurements can be performed to help determine the day of ovulation.

This procedure is contraindicated for: N/A

INDICATIONS

- Assist in the diagnosis of luteal-phase defects (performed in conjunction with endometrial biopsy).
- Evaluate patients at risk for early or spontaneous abortion.
- Identify patients at risk for ectopic pregnancy and assessment of corpus luteum function.

- Monitor patients ovulating during the induction of human chorionic gonadotropin (HCG), human menopausal gonadotropin, follicle-stimulating hormone/luteinizing hormone–releasing hormone, or clomiphene (serial measurements can assist in pinpointing the day of ovulation).
- Monitor patients receiving progesterone replacement therapy.

POTENTIAL MEDICAL DIAGNOSIS

Increased in:

- Chorioepithelioma of the ovary ***(related to progesterone-secreting tumor)***
- Congenital adrenal hyperplasia ***(related to excessive production of progesterone precursors)***
- Hydatidiform mole ***(related to progesterone-secreting tumor)***
- Lipoid ovarian tumor ***(related to progesterone-secreting tumor)***
- Ovulation ***(related to normal production of progesterone)***
- Pregnancy ***(related to normal production of progesterone)***
- Theca lutein cyst ***(related to progesterone-secreting cyst)***

Decreased in:

- Galactorrhea-amenorrhea syndrome ***(progesterone is not produced in the absence of ovulation)***
- Primary or secondary hypogonadism ***(related to diminished production of progesterone)***
- Short luteal-phase syndrome ***(related to diminished time frame for production and secretion)***
- Threatened abortion, fetal demise, toxemia of pregnancy, pre-eclampsia, placental failure ***(related to decreased production by threatened placenta)***

CRITICAL FINDINGS: N/A

INTERFERING FACTORS

- Drugs and other substances that may increase progesterone levels include clomiphene, corticotropin, hydroxyprogesterone, ketoconazole, mifepristone, progesterone, tamoxifen, and valproic acid.
- Drugs and other substances that may decrease progesterone levels include ampicillin, danazol, epostane, goserelin, and leuprolide.

NURSING IMPLICATIONS AND PROCEDURE

PRETEST:

- Positively identify the patient using at least two person-specific identifiers before services, treatments, or procedures are performed.
- *Patient Teaching:* Inform the patient this test can assist in evaluating hormone level during pregnancy.
- Obtain a history of the patient's health concerns, symptoms, surgical procedures, and results of previously performed laboratory and diagnostic studies. Include a list of known allergens, especially allergies or sensitivities to latex.
- Record the date of the last menstrual period and determine the possibility of pregnancy in perimenopausal women.
- Obtain a list of the patient's current medications, including over-the-counter medications and dietary supplements (see Effects of Natural Products on Laboratory Values online at Davis*Plus*).
- Review the procedure with the patient. Inform the patient that specimen collection takes approximately 5 to 10 min. Address concerns about pain and explain that there may be some discomfort during the venipuncture.
- *Sensitivity to social and cultural issues,* as well as concern for modesty, is important in providing psychological support before, during, and after the procedure.

P

- Note that there are no food, fluid, or medication restrictions unless by medical direction.

INTRATEST:

Potential Complications: N/A

- Avoid the use of equipment containing latex if the patient has a history of allergic reaction to latex.
- Instruct the patient to cooperate fully and to follow directions. Direct the patient to breathe normally and to avoid unnecessary movement.
- Observe standard precautions, and follow the general guidelines in Patient Preparation and Specimen Collection online at Davis*Plus*. Positively identify the patient, and label the appropriate specimen container with the corresponding patient demographics, initials of the person collecting the specimen, date, and time of collection. Perform a venipuncture.
- Remove the needle and apply direct pressure with dry gauze to stop bleeding. Observe/assess venipuncture site for bleeding or hematoma formation and secure gauze with adhesive bandage.
- Promptly transport the specimen to the laboratory for processing and analysis.

POST-TEST:

- Inform the patient that a report of the results will be made available to the requesting health-care provider (HCP), who will discuss the results with the patient.
- Recognize anxiety related to test results, and provide support. Provide teaching and information regarding the clinical implications of the test results, as appropriate. Provide a nonjudgmental, nonthreatening atmosphere for exploring other options (e.g., adoption). Educate the patient regarding access to counseling services, as appropriate.
- Reinforce information given by the patient's HCP regarding further testing, treatment, or referral to another HCP. Instruct the patient in the use of home pregnancy test kits approved by the U.S. Food and Drug Administration. Answer any questions or address any concerns voiced by the patient or family.
- Depending on the results of this procedure, additional testing may be performed to evaluate or monitor progression of the disease process and determine the need for a change in therapy. Evaluate test results in relation to the patient's symptoms and other tests performed.

RELATED STUDIES:

- Related tests include ACTH, AFP, amniotic fluid analysis, antibodies cardiolipin, biopsy chorionic villus, estradiol, fetal fibronectin, FSH, HCG, LH, prolactin, testosterone, and US BPP obstetric.
- Refer to the Endocrine and Reproductive systems tables online at Davis*Plus* for related tests by body system.

P

Prolactin

SYNONYM/ACRONYM: Luteotropic hormone, lactogenic hormone, lactogen, HPRL, PRL.

COMMON USE: To assess for lactation disorders and identify the presence of prolactin-secreting tumors to assist in diagnosing disorders such as lactation failure.

SPECIMEN: Serum collected in a gold-, red-, or red/gray-top tube. Specimen should be transported tightly capped and in an ice slurry.

NORMAL FINDINGS: (Method: Immunoassay)

Age	Conventional Units	SI Units (Conventional Units × 1)
Prepubertal males and females	3.2–20 ng/mL	3.2–20 mcg/L
Adult males	4–23 ng/mL	4–23 mcg/L
Adult females	4–30 ng/mL	4–30 mcg/L
Pregnant	5.3–215.3 ng/mL	5.3–215.3 mcg/L
Postmenopausal	2.4–24 ng/mL	2.4–24 mcg/L

DESCRIPTION: Prolactin is a hormone secreted by the pituitary gland. It is normally elevated in pregnant and lactating females. The main function of prolactin is to induce and sustain milk production in lactating females. Prolactin levels rise late in pregnancy, peak with the initiation of lactation, and surge each time a woman breastfeeds. Prolactin levels are highest at night during sleep and shortly after awakening. Levels are known to increase during periods of physical and emotional stress. Elevated prolactin levels are also known to affect fertility by inhibiting secretion of gonadotropin-releasing hormone from the hypothalamus; thereby also inhibiting secretion of luteinizing hormone and follicle-stimulating hormone from the pituitary gland and suppressing ovulation. Reduced fertility during lactation offers some natural protection against pregnancy. The function of prolactin in males and nonpregnant females is unknown but there is an association between high levels and infertility.

This procedure is contraindicated for: N/A

INDICATIONS

- Assist in the diagnosis of primary hypothyroidism, as indicated by elevated levels.
- Assist in the diagnosis of suspected tumor involving the lungs or kidneys (elevated levels indicating ectopic prolactin production).
- Evaluate failure of lactation in the postpartum period.
- Evaluate sexual dysfunction of unknown cause in men and women.
- Evaluate suspected postpartum hypophyseal infarction (Sheehan's syndrome), as indicated by decreased levels.

POTENTIAL MEDICAL DIAGNOSIS

Increased in:

- Adrenal insufficiency ***(secondary to hypopituitarism)***
- Amenorrhea ***(pathophysiology is unclear)***
- Anorexia nervosa ***(pathophysiology is unclear)***
- Breastfeeding ***(stimulates secretion of prolactin)***
- Chiari-Frommel and Argonz-Del Castillo syndromes ***(endocrine disorders in which pituitary or hypothalamic tumors secrete excessive amounts of prolactin)***

P

- Chest wall injury ***(trauma in this location can stimulate production of prolactin)***
- Chronic kidney disease ***(related to decreased renal excretion)***
- Ectopic prolactin-secreting tumors (e.g., lung, kidney)
- Galactorrhea ***(production of breast milk related to prolactin-secreting tumor)***
- Hypothalamic and pituitary disorders
- Hypothyroidism (primary) ***(related to pituitary gland dysfunction)***
- Pituitary tumor
- Polycystic ovary (Stein-Leventhal) syndrome
- Pregnancy
- Shingles
- Stress ***(stimulates secretion of prolactin)***
- Surgery (pituitary stalk section)

Decreased in:

- Sheehan's syndrome ***(severe hemorrhage after obstetric delivery that causes pituitary infarct; secretion of all pituitary hormones is diminished)***

CRITICAL FINDINGS: N/A

INTERFERING FACTORS

- Drugs and other substances that may increase prolactin levels include amitriptyline, amoxapine, azosemide, benserazide, butaperazine, butorphanol, carbidopa, chlorpromazine, cimetidine, clomipramine, desipramine, diethylstilbestrol, enalapril, enflurane, fenoldopam, flunarizine, fluphenazine, fluvoxamine, furosemide, growth hormone–releasing hormone, haloperidol, hexarelin, imipramine, insulin, interferon, labetalol, loxapine, megestrol, mestranol, methyldopa, metoclopramide, molindone, morphine, nitrous oxide, oral contraceptives, oxcarbazepine, parathyroid hormone, pentagastrin, perphenazine, phenytoin, pimozide, prochlorperazine, ranitidine, remoxipride, reserpine, sulpiride, sultopride, thiethylperazine, thioridazine, thiothixene, thyrotropin-releasing hormone, trifluoperazine, trimipramine, tumor necrosis factor, veralipride, verapamil, and zometapine.
- Drugs and other substances that may decrease prolactin levels include anticonvulsants, apomorphine, bromocriptine, cabergoline, calcitonin, cyclosporine, dexamethasone, D-Trp-6-LHRH, levodopa, metoclopramide, morphine, nifedipine, octreotide, pergolide, ranitidine, rifampin, ritanserin, ropinirole, secretin, and tamoxifen.
- Episodic elevations can occur in response to sleep, stress, exercise, hypoglycemia, and breastfeeding.
- Prolactin secretion is subject to diurnal variation with highest levels occurring in the morning.
- Failure to follow dietary restrictions before the procedure may cause the procedure to be canceled or repeated.

NURSING IMPLICATIONS AND PROCEDURE

PRETEST:

- Positively identify the patient using at least two person-specific identifiers before services, treatments, or procedures are performed.
- ***Patient Teaching:*** Inform the patient that test can assist in evaluating breast feeding hormone level.
- Obtain a history of the patient's health concerns, symptoms, surgical procedures, and results of previously performed laboratory and diagnostic studies. Include a list of known

allergens, especially allergies or sensitivities to latex.

- Obtain a list of the patient's current medications, including over-the-counter medications and dietary supplements (see Effects of Natural Products on Laboratory Values online at Davis*Plus*).
- Review the procedure with the patient. Specimen collection should occur between 0800 and 1000 Inform the patient that specimen collection takes approximately 5 to 10 min. Address concerns about pain and explain there may be some discomfort during the venipuncture.
- ***Sensitivity to social and cultural issues,*** as well as concern for modesty, is important in providing psychological support before, during, and after the procedure.
- Instruct the patient to fast for 12 hr before specimen collection because hyperglycemia can cause a short-term increase in prolactin levels.
- Note that there are no fluid or medication restrictions unless by medical direction.
- Prepare an ice slurry in a cup or plastic bag to have on hand for immediate transport of the specimen to the laboratory.

INTRATEST:

Potential Complications: N/A

- Ensure that the patient has complied with dietary restrictions prior to the procedure, as instructed.
- Avoid the use of equipment containing latex if the patient has a history of allergic reaction to latex.
- Instruct the patient to cooperate fully and to follow directions. Direct the patient to breathe normally and to avoid unnecessary movement.
- Observe standard precautions, and follow the general guidelines in Patient Preparation and Specimen Collection online at Davis*Plus*. Positively identify the patient, and label the appropriate specimen container with the corresponding patient demographics, initials of the person collecting the specimen, date, and time of collection. Perform a venipuncture.
- Remove the needle and apply direct pressure with dry gauze to stop bleeding. Observe/assess venipuncture site for bleeding or hematoma formation and secure gauze with adhesive bandage.
- Promptly transport the specimen to the laboratory for processing and analysis. The specimen should be placed in an ice slurry immediately after collection. Information on the specimen label should be protected from water in the ice slurry by first placing the specimen in a protective plastic bag.

POST-TEST:

- Inform the patient that a report of the results will be made available to the requesting health-care provider (HCP), who will discuss the results with the patient.
- Instruct the patient to resume usual diet, as directed by the HCP.
- Reinforce information given by the patient's HCP regarding further testing, treatment, or referral to another HCP. Answer any questions or address any concerns voiced by the patient or family.
- Depending on the results of this procedure, additional testing may be performed to evaluate or monitor progression of the disease process and determine the need for a change in therapy. Evaluate test results in relation to the patient's symptoms and other tests performed.

RELATED STUDIES:

- Related tests include ACE, BMD, CT pituitary, DHEAS, estradiol, FSH, GH, HCG, insulin, laparoscopy gynecologic, LH, MRI pituitary, progesterone, RAIU, TSH, and thyroxine.
- Refer to the Endocrine and Reproductive systems tables online at Davis*Plus* for related tests by body system.

P

Prostate-Specific Antigen

SYNONYM/ACRONYM: PSA.

COMMON USE: To assess prostate health and assist in diagnosis of disorders such as prostate cancer, inflammation, and benign tumor and to evaluate effectiveness of medical and surgical therapeutic interventions.

SPECIMEN: Serum collected in a gold-, red-, or red/gray-top tube.

NORMAL FINDINGS: (Method: Immunoassay)

Gender	Free PSA ng/mL	Total PSA Conventional Units ng/mL (SI Units mcg/L [Conventional Units × 1])		
Male (Ages)		Caucasians	African Americans	Individuals of Asian descent
40–49 yr	0–0.5	0–2.5	0–2	0–2
50–59 yr	0–0.7	0–3.5	0–4	0–3
60–69 yr	0–1	0-4.5	0–4.5	0–4
70 yr and older	0–1.2	0–6.5	0–5.5	0–5
Post–radical prostatectomy (30–60 d)		Less than 0.1		

DESCRIPTION: Prostate-specific antigen (PSA) is produced exclusively by the epithelial cells of the prostate, periurethral, and perirectal glands. Used in conjunction with the digital rectal examination (DRE), PSA is a useful screening test for early detection and monitoring cancer of the prostate. Risk of diagnosis is higher in African American men, who are 61% more likely than Caucasian men to develop prostate cancer. Family history and age at diagnosis are other strong correlating factors. PSA circulates in both free and bound (complexed) forms. A low ratio of free to complexed PSA (i.e., less than 10%) is suggestive of prostate cancer; a ratio of greater than 30% is rarely associated with prostate cancer. PSA velocity, the rate of PSA increase over time, is being used to indicate the potential aggressiveness of the cancer in order to identify the appropriate interventions and to monitor the effectiveness of treatment.

P

Estimated Risk for Developing Prostate Cancer in Men With a Slightly Elevated Total PSA (Between 4 and 10 ng/mL ✱)

Free PSA (%)	Probability of Developing Prostate Cancer
Greater than 30%	8%–20%
21%–30%	16%–19%
11%–20%	20%–25%
1%–10%	40%–50%
PSA velocity ng/mL	
Change of less than 0.75/yr	Low
Change of greater than 0.75/yr	Suspicious

Approximately 15% to 40% of patients who have had their prostate removed will encounter an increase in PSA. Patients treated for prostate cancer and who have had a PSA recurrence can still develop a metastasis for as long as 8 years after the postsurgical PSA level increased. The majority of prostate tumors develop slowly and require minimal intervention, but patients with an increase in PSA greater than 2 ng/mL in a year are more likely to have an aggressive form of prostate cancer with a greater risk of death.

The Prostate Health Index (PHI) is another multi-marker strategy being used to improve the positive prediction rate of prostate cancer, especially when PSA levels are considered to be moderately increased (between 4–10 ng/mL). The PHI applies information provided by the results of prostate marker blood tests to a mathematical formula and offers additional information for clinical decision making. The 3 tests used in the formula are the total PSA, free PSA, and p2PSA (an isoform of PSA) where:

PHI = p2PSA/(free PSA × total PSA)

PHI less than 27% have a relatively low probability for prostate cancer, PHI between 27% and 55% predict a moderate probability for prostate cancer, and PHI greater than 55% have an increased risk for prostate cancer.

Personalized medicine provides a technology to predict the progression of prostate cancer, likelihood of recurrence, or development of related metastatic disease. New technology makes it possible to combine data such as analysis of molecular biomarkers and cellular structure specific to the individual's biopsy tissue, standard tissue biopsy results, Gleason score, number of positive tumor cores, tumor stage, presurgical and postsurgical PSA levels, and postsurgical margin status with computerized mathematical programs to create a personalized report that predicts the likelihood of post-prostatectomy disease progression. Serial measurements of PSA in the blood are often performed before and after surgery.

P

PSA is also produced in females, most notably in breast tissue. There is some evidence that elevated PSA levels in breast cancer patients are associated with positive estrogen and progesterone status.

Important note: When following patients using serial testing, the same method of measurement should be consistently used.

This procedure is contraindicated for: N/A

INDICATIONS

- Evaluate the effectiveness of treatment for prostate cancer (prostatectomy): Levels decrease if treatment is effective; rising levels are associated with recurrence and a poor prognosis.
- Investigate or evaluate an enlarged prostate gland, especially if prostate cancer is suspected.
- Stage prostate cancer.

POTENTIAL MEDICAL DIAGNOSIS

Increased in:

A breach in the protective barrier between the prostatic lumen and the bloodstream due to significant disease will allow measurable levels of circulating PSA.

- Benign prostatic hyperplasia
- Prostate cancer
- Prostatic infarct
- Prostatitis
- Urinary retention

Decreased in: N/A

CRITICAL FINDINGS: N/A

INTERFERING FACTORS

- Drugs and other substances that decrease PSA levels include buserelin, dutasteride, finasteride, and flutamide.
- Increases may occur if ejaculation occurs within 24 hr prior to specimen collection. Increases can occur due to prostatic needle biopsy, cystoscopy, or prostatic infarction either by undergoing catheterization or the presence of an indwelling catheter; therefore, specimens should be collected prior to or 6 wk after the procedure. There is conflicting information regarding the effect of DRE on PSA values, and some health-care providers (HCPs) may specifically request specimen collection prior to DRE.

NURSING IMPLICATIONS AND PROCEDURE

P

POTENTIAL NURSING PROBLEMS:

Problem	Signs & Symptoms	Interventions
Knowledge ***(related to postoperative care and treatment secondary to prostate cancer)***	Lack of interest or questions; multiple questions; anxiety in relation to disease process and management; verbalization of inaccurate information	Assess the patient's understanding of the need for further treatment, radiation therapy, chemotherapy; discuss postoperative infection risk and the associated signs and symptoms; discuss the possibility of postoperative incontinence and erectile dysfunction

Problem	Signs & Symptoms	Interventions
Fear ***(related to lack of understanding about diagnosis; treatment; potential death)***	Anxiety; apprehension; verbalization of fear; restlessness; increased tension; continuous questioning; increased blood pressure, heart rate, respiratory rate	Evaluate verbal and nonverbal indicators of fear; assess for the cause of fear; acknowledge the patient's awareness of his fear; explain all procedures with simple age- and culturally appropriate language; administer prescribed mild tranquilizer; maintain a confident, assured, professional manner in all patient interactions
Hopelessness ***(related to chronic illness; impaired functionality; prolonged pain and discomfort)***	Decreased affect; decreased response to stimuli; feeling of emptiness; alterations in sleep patterns and appetite; expressions of apathy; withdrawn; states life has no meaning	Assess role of illness in relation to expressions of helplessness; assess level of appetite; assess verbalization of helplessness; provide opportunities to express feelings in a safe environment; support development of a trusting relationship to decrease feelings of isolation; encourage verbalization of personal strengths and weaknesses; encourage realistic hope; assist in identification of coping skills
Powerlessness ***(related to chronic illness; treatment for illness; loss of ability to provide self-care; progressive debilitation; terminal prognosis; changes in sexuality)***	Expression of loss of control over situation, self, outcome of disease; passive; apathetic; submissive; decreased participation in self-care; reluctant to express feelings	Assess need to be in control; assess feelings of hopelessness, depression, apathy; assist to identify situations that contribute to a feeling of powerlessness; assess the impact of the sense of powerlessness on the patient's sense of self; encourage verbalization of feelings; discuss therapeutic options offered by HCP; assist to identify strengths; identify coping strategies; encourage being responsible for self-care and personal environment to increase sense of control; receive positive feedback

P

PRETEST:

- Positively identify the patient using at least two person-specific identifiers before services, treatments, or procedures are performed.
- ***Patient Teaching:*** Inform the patient this test can assist in assessing prostate health.
- Obtain a history of the patient's health concerns, symptoms, surgical procedures, and results of previously performed laboratory and diagnostic studies. Include a list of known allergens, especially allergies or sensitivities to latex.
- Note any recent procedures that can interfere with test results.
- Obtain a list of the patient's current medications, including over-the-counter medications and dietary supplements (see Effects of Natural Products on Laboratory Values online at Davis*Plus*).
- Review the procedure with the patient. Inform the patient that specimen collection takes approximately 5 to 10 min. Address concerns about pain and explain that there may be some discomfort during the venipuncture.
- ***Sensitivity to social and cultural issues,*** as well as concern for modesty, is important in providing psychological support before, during, and after the procedure.
- Note that there are no food, fluid, or medication restrictions unless by medical direction.

INTRATEST:

Potential Complications: N/A

- Avoid the use of equipment containing latex if the patient has a history of allergic reaction to latex.
- Instruct the patient to cooperate fully and to follow directions. Direct the patient to breathe normally and to avoid unnecessary movement.
- Observe standard precautions, and follow the general guidelines in Patient Preparation and Specimen Collection online at Davis*Plus*. Positively identify the patient, and label the appropriate specimen container with the corresponding patient demographics, initials of the person collecting the specimen, date, and time of collection. Perform a venipuncture.
- Remove the needle and apply direct pressure with dry gauze to stop bleeding. Observe/assess venipuncture site for bleeding or hematoma formation and secure gauze with adhesive bandage.
- Promptly transport the specimen to the laboratory for processing and analysis.

POST-TEST:

- Inform the patient that a report of the results will be made available to the requesting HCP, who will discuss the results with the patient.
- ***Nutritional Considerations:*** There is growing evidence that inflammation and oxidation play key roles in the development of numerous diseases, including prostate cancer. Research also indicates that diets containing dried beans, fresh fruits and vegetables, nuts, spices, whole grains, and smaller amounts of red meats can increase the amount of protective antioxidants. Regular exercise, especially in combination with a healthy diet, can bring about changes in the body's metabolism that decrease inflammation and oxidation.
- Recognize anxiety related to test results, and offer support. Counsel the patient, as appropriate, that sexual dysfunction related to altered body function, drugs, or radiation may occur. Discuss the implications of abnormal test results on the patient's lifestyle. Provide teaching and information regarding the clinical implications of the test results, as appropriate. Recommendations made by various medical associations and national health organizations regarding prostate cancer screening are moving away from routine PSA screening and toward informed decision making. The American Cancer Society (ACS) recommends that discussions about screening

should begin at age 50 yr for men at average risk, 45 yr for men at high risk, and 40 yr for men at the highest risk of developing prostate cancer. Educate the patient regarding access to counseling services. Provide contact information, if desired, for the Prostate Cancer Foundation (www.prostatecancerfoundation.org).

- Depending on the results of this procedure, additional testing may be performed to evaluate or monitor progression of the disease process and determine the need for a change in therapy. Evaluate test results in relation to the patient's symptoms and other tests performed.

Patient Education:

- Reinforce information given by the patient's HCP regarding further testing, treatment, or referral to another HCP.
- Answer any questions or address any concerns voiced by the patient or family.
- Note that decisions regarding the need for and frequency of routine PSA testing or other cancer screening procedures should be made after consultation between the patient and HCP.
- Consult the most current guidelines for prostate cancer screening of the general population as well as of individuals with increased risk which are available from the ACS (www.cancer.org) and American Urological Association (www.aua.org).

Expected Patient Outcomes:

Understanding

- The patient and family state that postoperative urinary incontinence may occur and take up to a year to resolve.
- The patient and family state that erectile dysfunction may occur as a postoperative complication.

Ability

- The patient describes the correct technique for the self-administration of a sitz bath.
- The patient accurately describes how to perform Kegel exercises to improve control over urination.

Response

- The patient complies with the request to perform sitz baths to facilitate wound healing and prevent infection.
- The patient complies with the recommended follow-up appointments.

RELATED STUDIES:

- Related tests include biopsy prostate, cystoscopy, cystourethrography voiding, retrograde ureteropyelography, semen analysis, and US prostate.
- Refer to the Genitourinary System table online at Davis*Plus* for related tests by body system.

Protein, Blood, Total and Fractions

P

SYNONYM/ACRONYM: TP, SPEP (fractions include albumin, α_1-globulin, α_2-globulin, β-globulin, and γ-globulin).

COMMON USE: To assess nutritional status related to various disease and conditions such as dehydration, burns, and malabsorption.

SPECIMEN: Serum collected in a gold-, red-, or red/gray-top tube.

NORMAL FINDINGS: (Method: Spectrophotometry for total protein, electrophoresis for protein fractions)

Total Protein

Age	Conventional Units	SI Units (Conventional Units × 10)
Newborn–5 d	3.8–6.2 g/dL	38–62 g/L
1–3 yr	5.9–7 g/dL	59–70 g/L
4–6 yr	5.9–7.8 g/dL	59–78 g/L
7–9 yr	6.2–8.1 g/dL	62–81 g/L
10–19 yr	6.3–8.6 g/dL	63–86 g/L
Adult	6–8 g/dL	60–80 g/L

Values may be slightly decreased in older adults due to insufficient intake or the effects of medications and the presence of multiple chronic or acute diseases with or without muted symptoms.

Protein Fractions

	Conventional Units	SI Units (Conventional Units × 10)
Albumin	3.4–4.8 g/dL	34–48 g/L
α_1-Globulin	0.2–0.4 g/dL	2–4 g/L
α_2-Globulin	0.4–0.8 g/dL	4–8 g/L
β-Globulin	0.5–1 g/dL	5–10 g/L
γ-Globulin	0.6–1.2 g/dL	6–12 g/L

Values may be slightly decreased in older adults due to insufficient intake or the effects of medications and the presence of multiple chronic or acute diseases with or without muted symptoms.

DESCRIPTION: Protein is essential to all physiological functions. Proteins consist of amino acids, the building blocks of blood and body tissues. Protein is also required for the regulation of metabolic processes, immunity, and proper water balance. Total protein includes albumin and globulins. Albumin, the protein present in the highest concentrations, is the main transport protein in the body. Albumin also significantly affects plasma oncotic pressure, which regulates the distribution of body fluid between blood vessels, tissues, and cells. α_1-Globulin includes α_1-antitrypsin, α_1-fetoprotein, α_1-acidglycoprotein, α_1-antichymotrypsin, inter-α_1-trypsin inhibitor, high-density lipoproteins, and group-specific component (vitamin D–binding protein). α_2-Globulin includes haptoglobin, ceruloplasmin, and α_2-macroglobulin. β-Globulin includes transferrin, hemopexin, very-low-density lipoproteins, low-density lipoproteins, β_2-microglobulin, fibrinogen, complement, and C-reactive protein. γ-Globulin includes immunoglobulin (Ig) G, IgA, IgM, IgD, and IgE. After an acute infection or trauma, levels of many of the liver-derived proteins increase, whereas albumin level decreases; these conditions may not reflect an abnormal total protein determination.

P

This procedure is contraindicated for: N/A

INDICATIONS

- Evaluation of edema, as seen in patients with low total protein and low albumin levels.
- Evaluation of nutritional status.

POTENTIAL MEDICAL DIAGNOSIS

Increased in:

- α_1-Globulin proteins in acute and chronic inflammatory diseases
- α_2-Globulin proteins occasionally in diabetes, pancreatitis, and hemolysis
- β-Globulin proteins in hyperlipoproteinemias and monoclonal gammopathies
- γ-Globulin proteins in chronic liver diseases, chronic infections, autoimmune disorders, hepatitis, cirrhosis, and lymphoproliferative disorders
- Total protein:
  Dehydration ***(related to hemoconcentration)***
  Monoclonal and polyclonal gammopathies ***(related to excessive γ-globulin protein synthesis)***
  Myeloma ***(related to excessive γ-globulin protein synthesis)***
  Sarcoidosis ***(related to excessive γ-globulin protein synthesis)***
  Some types of chronic liver disease
  Tropical diseases (e.g., leprosy) ***(related to inflammatory reaction)***
  Waldenström's macroglobulinemia ***(related to excessive γ-globulin protein synthesis)***

Decreased in:

- α_1-Globulin proteins in hereditary deficiency
- α_2-Globulin proteins in nephrotic syndrome, malignancies, numerous subacute and chronic inflammatory disorders, and recovery stage of severe burns
- β-Globulin proteins in hypo-β-lipoproteinemias and IgA deficiency
- γ-Globulin proteins in immune deficiency or suppression
- Total protein:
  Administration of intravenous (IV) fluids ***(related to hemodilution)***
  Burns ***(related to fluid retention, loss of albumin from chronic open burns)***
  Chronic alcoholism ***(related to insufficient dietary intake; diminished protein synthesis by damaged liver)***
  Chronic ulcerative colitis ***(related to poor intestinal absorption)***
  Cirrhosis ***(related to damaged liver, which cannot synthesize adequate amount of protein)***
  Crohn's disease ***(related to poor intestinal absorption)***
  Glomerulonephritis ***(related to alteration in permeability that results in excessive loss by kidneys)***
  Heart failure ***(related to fluid retention)***
  Hyperthyroidism ***(possibly related to increased metabolism and corresponding protein synthesis)***
  Malabsorption ***(related to insufficient intestinal absorption)***
  Malnutrition ***(related to insufficient intake)***
  Neoplasms
  Nephrotic syndrome ***(related to alteration in permeability that results in excessive loss by kidneys)***
  Pregnancy ***(related to fluid retention, dietary insufficiency, increased demands of growing fetus)***
  Prolonged immobilization ***(related to fluid retention)***
  Protein-losing enteropathies ***(related to excessive loss)***
  Severe skin disease
  Starvation ***(related to insufficient intake)***

CRITICAL FINDINGS: N/A

INTERFERING FACTORS

- Drugs and other substances that may increase protein levels include amino acids (if given by IV), anabolic steroids, angiotensin, anticonvulsants, corticosteroids, corticotropin, furosemide, insulin, isotretinoin, levonorgestrel, oral

P

contraceptives, progesterone, radiographic medium, and thyroid drugs.

- Drugs and other substances that may decrease protein levels include acetylsalicylic acid, arginine, benzene, carvedilol, citrates, floxuridine, laxatives, mercury compounds, oral contraceptives, pyrazinamide, rifampin, trimethadione, and valproic acid.
- Values are significantly lower (5% to 10%) in recumbent patients.
- Hemolysis can falsely elevate results.
- Venous stasis can falsely elevate results; the tourniquet should not be left on the arm for longer than 60 sec.

NURSING IMPLICATIONS AND PROCEDURE

PRETEST:

- Positively identify the patient using at least two person-specific identifiers before services, treatments, or procedures are performed.
- ***Patient Teaching:*** Inform the patient this test can assist in assessing nutritional status related to disease process.
- Obtain a history of the patient's health concerns, symptoms, surgical procedures, and results of previously performed laboratory and diagnostic studies. Include a list of known allergens, especially allergies or sensitivities to latex.
- Obtain a list of the patient's current medications, including over-the-counter medications and dietary supplements (see Effects of Natural Products on Laboratory Values online at Davis*Plus*).
- Review the procedure with the patient. Inform the patient that specimen collection takes approximately 5 to 10 min. Address concerns about pain and explain that there may be some discomfort during the venipuncture.
- ***Sensitivity to social and cultural issues,*** as well as concern for modesty, is important in providing psychological support before, during, and after the procedure.
- Note that there are no food, fluid, or medication restrictions unless by medical direction.

INTRATEST:

Potential Complications: N/A

- Avoid the use of equipment containing latex if the patient has a history of allergic reaction to latex.
- Instruct the patient to cooperate fully and to follow directions. Direct the patient to breathe normally and to avoid unnecessary movement.
- Observe standard precautions, and follow the general guidelines in Patient Preparation and Specimen Collection online at Davis*Plus*. Positively identify the patient, and label the appropriate specimen container with the corresponding patient demographics, initials of the person collecting the specimen, date, and time of collection. Perform a venipuncture.
- Remove the needle and apply direct pressure with dry gauze to stop bleeding. Observe venipuncture site for bleeding or hematoma formation and secure gauze with adhesive bandage.
- Promptly transport the specimen to the laboratory for processing and analysis.

POST-TEST:

- Inform the patient that a report of the results will be made available to the requesting health-care provider (HCP), who will discuss the results with the patient.
- ***Nutritional Considerations:*** Educate the patient, as appropriate, that good dietary sources of complete protein (containing all eight essential amino acids) include meat, fish, eggs, and dairy products and that good sources of incomplete protein (lacking one or more of the eight essential amino acids) include

P

grains, nuts, legumes, vegetables, and seeds.

- Reinforce information given by the patient's HCP regarding further testing, treatment, or referral to another HCP. Answer any questions or address any concerns voiced by the patient or family.
- Depending on the results of this procedure, additional testing may be performed to evaluate or monitor progression of the disease process and determine the need for a change in therapy. Evaluate test results in relation to the patient's symptoms and other tests performed.

RELATED STUDIES:

- Related tests include albumin, ALP, ACE, anion gap, AST, biopsy liver, biopsy lung, calcium, carbon dioxide, chloride, CBC WBC count and differential, cryoglobulin, fecal analysis, fecal fat, gallium scan, GGT, IgA, IgG, IgM, IFE, liver and spleen scan, magnesium, mediastinoscopy, β_2-microglobulin, osmolality, protein urine total and fractions, PFT, radiography bone, RF, sodium, TSH, thyroxine, and UA.
- Refer to the Gastrointestinal, Hepatobiliary, and Immune systems tables online at Davis*Plus* for related tests by body system.

Protein C

SYNONYM/ACRONYM: Protein C antigen, protein C functional.

COMMON USE: To assess coagulation function and assist in diagnosis of disorders such as thrombosis and protein C deficiency.

SPECIMEN: Plasma collected in a completely filled blue-top (3.2% sodium citrate) tube. If the patient's hematocrit exceeds 55%, the volume of citrate in the collection tube must be adjusted.

NORMAL FINDINGS: (Method: Clot detection) 70% to 140% activity. Values are significantly reduced in children because of liver immaturity. Levels rise to approximately 50% of adult levels by age 5 yr and reach adult levels by age 16 yr.

POTENTIAL MEDICAL DIAGNOSIS

Increased in: N/A

Decreased in:

- Congenital deficiency
- Disseminated intravascular coagulation ***(related to increased consumption)***
- Liver disease ***(related to decreased synthesis by the liver)***
- Oral anticoagulant therapy ***(patients deficient in protein C may be at risk of developing warfarin-induced skin necrosis unless an immediate-acting anticoagulant like heparin is administered until therapeutic warfarin levels are achieved)***
- Septic shock ***(related to increased consumption and decreased synthesis due to hepatic impairment)***
- Vitamin K deficiency ***(related to production of dysfunctional protein in the absence of vitamin K)***

CRITICAL FINDINGS: N/A

Find and print out the full study on Fast Find at davispl.us/vanleeuwen7.

Protein S

SYNONYM/ACRONYM: Protein S antigen, protein S functional.

COMMON USE: To assess coagulation function, assist in the diagnosis of disorders such as disseminated intravascular coagulation (DIC), and evaluate oral anticoagulation therapy.

SPECIMEN: Plasma collected in a completely filled blue-top (3.2% sodium citrate) tube. If the patient's hematocrit exceeds 55%, the volume of citrate in the collection tube must be adjusted.

NORMAL FINDINGS: (Method: Clot detection)

	Conventional Units
Adult	70%–140% activity
Pediatric	12%–60% activity

Note: The low end of "normal" is lower in patients younger than age 16 because of the immaturity of the liver.

POTENTIAL MEDICAL DIAGNOSIS

Increased in: N/A

Decreased in:
- Acute phase reactions ***(related to increased levels of C4b-binding protein in response to inflammation, which decrease levels of available functional protein)***
- Congenital deficiency
- DIC ***(related to increased consumption)***
- Estrogen (replacement therapy, oral contraceptives, and pregnancy) ***(elevated estrogen levels are associated with decreased protein levels; estrogen does not stimulate hypercoagulable states)***
- Liver disease ***(related to decreased synthesis by the liver)***
- Oral anticoagulant therapy
- Vitamin K deficiency ***(related to production of dysfunctional protein in the absence of vitamin K)***

CRITICAL FINDINGS: N/A

Find and print out the full study on Fast Find at davispl.us/vanleeuwen7.

P

Protein, Urine: Total Quantitative and Fractions

SYNONYM/ACRONYM: N/A

COMMON USE: To assess for the presence of protein in the urine toward diagnosing disorders affecting the kidneys and urinary tract, such as cancer, infection, and pre-eclampsia.

SPECIMEN: Urine from an unpreserved random or timed specimen collected in a clean plastic collection container.

NORMAL FINDINGS: (Method: Spectrophotometry for total protein, electrophoresis for protein fractions)

Normal 24-Hour Urine Volume

The ranges are very general averages and were not calculated on the basis of normal average body weights. Literature shows that the expected urinary output can be estimated by formula where the expected output is as follows:

Infants: 1–2 mL/kg/hr
Children and adolescents: 0.5–1 mL/kg/hr
Adults: 1 mL/kg/hr

Newborns	15–60 mL
Infants	
3–10 d	100–300 mL
11–59 d	250–450 mL
2–12 mo	400–500 mL
Children and adolescents	
13 mo–4 yr	500–700 mL
5–7 yr	650–1,000 mL
8–14 yr	800–1,400 mL
Adults and older adults	800–2,500 mL (average 1,200 mL)

Normally, more urine is produced during the day than at night. With advancing age, the reverse will often occur. The total expected outcome for adults appears to remain the same regardless of age.

	Conventional Units	SI Units (Conventional Units × 0.001)
Total protein	30–150 mg/24 hr	0.03–0.15 g/24 hr
Second and third trimesters of pregnancy	45–185 mg/24 hr	0.045–0.185 g/24 hr

The 24-hr urine volume is recorded and provided with the results of the protein measurement. Electrophoresis for fractionation is qualitative: No monoclonal gammopathy detected. (Urine protein electrophoresis should be ordered along with serum protein electrophoresis.)

DESCRIPTION: Most proteins, with the exception of the immunoglobulins, are synthesized and catabolized in the liver, where they are broken down into amino acids. The amino acids are converted to ammonia and ketoacids. Ammonia is converted to urea via the urea cycle. Urea is excreted in the urine. Normally, proteins do not pass from the blood through the kidneys' filtration process into the urine. The presence of protein in the urine is a significant indication of kidney disease. The predominant causes of proteinuria are (1) lack of filtration due to damaged glomeruli and (2) a breakdown in the kidneys' tubular reabsorption process. Chronic conditions such as diabetes, hypertension, and sickle cell anemia cause incremental and potentially irreversible kidney damage. Acute conditions such as urinary tract infections and kidney stones can also damage the kidneys. Proteinuria can also be the result of extremely elevated serum protein levels, as seen with immunoglobulin-secreting malignancies such as multiple myeloma. The kappa and lambda light chain portions of the immunoglobulins, also known as *Bence Jones proteins,* are detected using electrophoresis techniques and are classic findings in conditions such as myeloma, Waldenström's macroglobulinemia, and lymphoma.

This procedure is contraindicated for: N/A

INDICATIONS

- Assist in the detection of Bence Jones proteins (light chains).
- Assist in the diagnosis of myeloma, Waldenström's macroglobulinemia, lymphoma, and amyloidosis.
- Evaluate kidney function.

POTENTIAL MEDICAL DIAGNOSIS

Increased in:

- Diabetic nephropathy ***(related to disease involving renal glomeruli, which increases permeability of protein)***
- Fanconi's syndrome ***(related to abnormal protein deposits in the kidney, which can cause Fanconi's syndrome)***
- Heavy metal poisoning ***(related to disease involving renal glomeruli, which increases permeability of protein)***
- Malignancies of the urinary tract ***(tumors secrete protein into the urine)***
- Monoclonal gammopathies ***(evidenced by large amounts of Bence Jones protein light chains excreted in the urine)***
- Multiple myeloma ***(evidenced by large amounts of Bence Jones protein light chains excreted in the urine)***
- Nephrotic syndrome ***(related to disease involving renal glomeruli, which increases permeability of protein)***
- Postexercise period ***(related to muscle exertion)***
- Pre-eclampsia ***(numerous factors contribute to increased permeability of the kidneys to protein)***
- Sickle cell disease ***(related to increased destruction of red blood cells and excretion of hemoglobin protein)***
- Urinary tract infections ***(related to disease involving renal glomeruli, which increases permeability of protein)***

Decreased in: N/A

CRITICAL FINDINGS: N/A

INTERFERING FACTORS

- Drugs and other substances that may increase urine protein levels include acetaminophen, aminosalicylic acid, amphotericin B, ampicillin, antimony compounds, antipyrine, arsenicals, ascorbic acid, bacitracin, bismuth subsalicylate, bromate, capreomycin, captopril, carbamazepine, carbarsone, cephaloglycin, cephaloridine, chlorpromazine, chlorpropamide, chlorthalidone, chrysarobin, colistimethate, colistin, corticosteroids, cyclosporine, demeclocycline, diatrizoic acid, dihydrotachysterol, doxycycline, enalapril, gentamicin, gold, hydrogen sulfide, iodopyracet, iopanoic acid, iophenoxic acid, ipodate, kanamycin, corn oil (Lipomul), lithium, mefenamic acid, melarsoprol, mercury compounds, methicillin, methylbromide, mezlocillin, mitomycin, nafcillin, naphthalene,

P

neomycin, NSAIDs, oxacillin, paraldehyde, penicillamine, penicillin, phenolphthalein, phenols, phensuximide, piperacillin, plicamycin, polymyxin, probenecid, pyrazolones, radiographic medium, rifampin, sodium bicarbonate, streptokinase, sulfisoxazole, suramin, tetracyclines, thallium, thiosemicarbazones, tolbutamide, tolmetin, triethylenemelamine, and vitamin D.

- Drugs and other substances that may decrease urine protein levels include benazepril, captopril, cyclosporine, diltiazem, enalapril, fosinopril, interferon, lisinopril, losartan, lovastatin, prednisolone, prednisone, and quinapril.
- All urine voided for the timed collection period must be included in the collection, or else falsely decreased values may be obtained. Compare output records with volume collected to verify that all voids were included in the collection.

NURSING IMPLICATIONS AND PROCEDURE

PRETEST:

- Positively identify the patient using at least two person-specific identifiers before services, treatments, or procedures are performed.
- *Patient Teaching:* Inform the patient this test can assist in assessing the cause of protein in the urine.
- Obtain a history of the patient's health concerns, symptoms, surgical procedures, and results of previously performed laboratory and diagnostic studies. Include a list of known allergens, especially allergies or sensitivities to latex.
- Obtain a list of the patient's current medications, including over-the-counter medications and dietary supplements (see Effects of Natural Products on Laboratory Values online at Davis*Plus*).
- Review the procedure with the patient. Provide a nonmetallic urinal, bedpan, or toilet-mounted collection device. Address concerns about pain and explain that there should be no discomfort during the procedure.
- Usually a 24-hr time frame for urine collection is ordered. Inform the patient that all urine must be saved during that 24-hr period. Instruct the patient not to void directly into the laboratory collection container. Instruct the patient to avoid defecating in the collection device and to keep toilet tissue out of the collection device to prevent contamination of the specimen. Place a sign in the bathroom to remind the patient to save all urine.
- Instruct the patient to void all urine into the collection device and then to pour the urine into the laboratory collection container. Alternatively, the specimen can be left in the collection device for a health-care staff member to add to the laboratory collection container.
- *Sensitivity to social and cultural issues,* as well as concern for modesty, is important in providing psychological support before, during, and after the procedure.
- Note that there are no food, fluid, or medication restrictions unless by medical direction.

INTRATEST:

Potential Complications: N/A

- Avoid the use of equipment containing latex if the patient has a history of allergic reaction to latex.
- Instruct the patient to cooperate fully and to follow directions.
- Observe standard precautions, and follow the general guidelines in Patient Preparation and Specimen Collection online at Davis*Plus*. Positively identify the patient, and label the appropriate specimen container with the corresponding patient demographics, initials of the person collecting the specimen, date, and time of collection.

P

Random Specimen (Collect in Early Morning)

Clean-Catch Specimen

- Instruct the male patient to (1) thoroughly wash his hands, (2) cleanse the meatus, (3) void a small amount into the toilet, and (4) void directly into the specimen container.
- Instruct the female patient to (1) thoroughly wash her hands; (2) cleanse the labia from front to back; (3) while keeping the labia separated, void a small amount into the toilet; and (4) without interrupting the urine stream, void directly into the specimen container.

Indwelling Catheter

- Put on gloves. Empty drainage tube of urine. It may be necessary to clamp off the catheter for 15 to 30 min before specimen collection. Cleanse specimen port with antiseptic swab, and then aspirate 5 mL of urine with a 21- to 25-gauge needle and syringe. Transfer urine to a sterile container.

Timed Specimen

- Obtain a clean 3-L urine specimen container, toilet-mounted collection device, and plastic bag (for transport of the specimen container). The specimen must be refrigerated or kept on ice throughout the entire collection period. If an indwelling urinary catheter is in place, the drainage bag must be kept on ice.
- Begin the test between 0600 and 0800 if possible. Collect first voiding and discard. Record the time the specimen was discarded as the beginning of the timed collection period. The next morning, ask the patient to void at the same time the collection was started and add this last voiding to the container. Urinary output should be recorded throughout the collection time.
- If an indwelling catheter is in place, replace the tubing and container system at the start of the collection time. Keep the container system on ice during the collection period, or empty the urine into a larger container periodically during the collection period; monitor to ensure continued drainage, and conclude the test the next morning at the same hour the collection was begun.
- At the conclusion of the test, compare the quantity of urine with the urinary output record for the collection; if the specimen contains less than the recorded output, some urine may have been discarded, invalidating the test.
- Include on the collection container's label the amount of urine collected and test start and stop times.

General

- Promptly transport the specimen to the laboratory for processing and analysis.

POST-TEST:

- Inform the patient that a report of the results will be made available to the requesting health-care provider (HCP), who will discuss the results with the patient.
- Recognize anxiety related to test results. Discuss the implications of abnormal test results on the patient's lifestyle. Provide teaching and information regarding the clinical implications of the test results, as appropriate.
- Reinforce information given by the patient's HCP regarding further testing, treatment, or referral to another HCP. Answer any questions or address any concerns voiced by the patient or family.
- Depending on the results of this procedure, additional testing may be performed to evaluate or monitor progression of the disease process and determine the need for a change in therapy. Evaluate test results in relation to the patient's symptoms and other tests performed.

RELATED STUDIES:

- Related tests include amino acid screen, ACE, β_2-microglobulin, biopsy bladder, biopsy bone marrow, bladder cancer markers, BUN, calcium, CBC, CT kidneys, CT pelvis, creatinine, cryoglobulin, culture urine, cytology urine, cystometry, cystoscopy, glucose, glycated hemoglobin, Hgb electrophoresis, IgA, IgG, IgM, IFE, IVP, lead, LAP, MRI musculoskeletal, microalbumin, osmolality, porphyrins, protein blood total and fractions, renogram, sickle cell screen, US bladder, US spleen, UA, and voiding cystourethrography.

- Refer to the Genitourinary and Immune systems tables online at Davis*Plus* for related tests by body system.

Prothrombin Time and International Normalized Ratio

SYNONYM/ACRONYM: Protime, PT, and INR.

COMMON USE: To assess and monitor coagulation status related to therapeutic interventions and disorders such as vitamin K deficiency.

SPECIMEN: Plasma collected in a completely filled blue-top (sodium citrate) tube. If the patient's hematocrit exceeds 55%, the volume of citrate in the collection tube must be adjusted.

NORMAL FINDINGS: (Method: Clot detection) 10 to 13 sec.

- International normalized ratio (INR) = 0.9 to 1.1 for patients not receiving anticoagulation therapy; 2 to 3 for patients receiving treatment for venous thrombosis, pulmonary embolism, and valvular heart disease.
- INR = 2.5 to 3.5 for patients with mechanical heart valves and/or receiving treatment for recurrent systemic embolism.
- For patients receiving anticoagulants, therapeutic levels of warfarin are achieved by adjusting the dosage so the prothrombin time (PT) value is 1.5 to 2.5 times longer than normal or so the INR is between 2 and 3.

DESCRIPTION: PT is a coagulation test performed to measure the time it takes for a firm fibrin clot to form after tissue thromboplastin (factor III) and calcium are added to a sample of plasma. Coagulation factors in the patient's sample, including prothrombin (factor II) react with the reagents and complete the process of coagulation in proportion to the amount of available coagulation factors. The PT is used to evaluate the tissue factor pathway, formerly called the extrinsic pathway of the coagulation sequence in patients receiving oral warfarin anticoagulants. Prothrombin is a vitamin K–dependent protein produced by the liver; measurement is reported as time in seconds or percentage of normal activity.

The goal of long-term anticoagulation therapy is to achieve a balance between in vivo thrombus formation and hemorrhage. It is a delicate clinical balance, and because of differences in instruments and reagents, there is a wide variation in PT results among laboratories. Worldwide concern for the need to provide more consistency in monitoring patients receiving anticoagulant therapy led to the development of an international committee. In the early 1980s, manufacturers of instruments and reagents began comparing their measurement systems with a single reference material provided by the World Health Organization (WHO). The international effort successfully developed an algorithm to provide comparable PT values regardless of differences in laboratory methodology. Reagent and instrument manufacturers compare their results to the WHO reference and derive a factor called an international sensitivity index (ISI) that is applied to a mathematical formula to standardize the results. Laboratories convert their PT values into an INR by using the following formula:

$$INR = (\text{patient PT result/normal patient average})^{(ISI)}$$

PT evaluation can now be based on an INR using a standardized thromboplastin reagent to assist in making decisions regarding oral anticoagulation therapy.

The metabolism of many commonly prescribed medications is driven by the cytochrome P450 (CYP450) family of enzymes. Genetic variants can alter enzymatic activity that results in a spectrum of effects ranging from the total absence of drug metabolism to ultrafast metabolism. Impaired drug metabolism can prevent the intended therapeutic effect or even lead to serious adverse drug reactions. Poor metabolizers are at increased risk for drug-induced adverse effects due to accumulation of drug in the blood, whereas ultra-rapid metabolizers require a higher-than-normal dosage because the drug is metabolized over a shorter duration than intended. In the case of prodrugs that require activation before metabolism, the opposite occurs: Poor metabolizers may require a higher dose because the activated drug is becoming available more slowly than intended, and ultra-rapid metabolizers may require less because the activated drug is becoming available sooner than intended. Other genetic phenotypes used to report CYP450 results are intermediate metabolizer and extensive metabolizer. Genetic testing can be performed on blood samples submitted to a laboratory. Test method commonly used is polymerase chain reaction. Counseling and informed written consent are generally required for genetic testing. CYP2C9 is a gene in the CYP450 family that metabolizes prodrugs like the anticoagulant warfarin. Three major gene mutations, CYP2CP*2, CYP2C9*3, and VKORC1, are associated with warfarin response and are estimated to account for up to 45% of variations in warfarin dose response. CYP450 testing is available and should be used in conjunction with other factors, including all prescription and over-the-counter medications being used; mode of drug administration; use of tobacco products, foods, and supplements; age, weight, environment, activity level, and diseases with which the patient may be dealing.

Some inferences of factor deficiency can be made by comparison of results obtained from the activated partial thromboplastin time (aPTT) and PT tests. A normal aPTT with a prolonged PT can occur only with factor

P

VII deficiency. A prolonged aPTT with a normal PT could indicate a deficiency in factors XII, XI, IX, and VIII as well as VIII:C (von Willebrand factor). Factor deficiencies can also be identified by correction or substitution studies using normal serum. These studies are easy to perform and are accomplished by adding plasma from a healthy patient to a sample from a suspected factor-deficient patient. When the PT is repeated and corrected, or within the reference range, it can be assumed that the prolonged PT is due to a factor deficiency (see study titled "Coagulation Factors"). If the result remains uncorrected, the prolonged PT is most likely due to a circulating anticoagulant.

This procedure is contraindicated for: N/A

INDICATIONS

- Differentiate between deficiencies of clotting factors II, V, VII, and X, which prolong the PT, and congenital coagulation disorders such as hemophilia A (factor VIII) and hemophilia B (factor IX), which do not alter the PT.
- Evaluate the response to anticoagulant therapy with warfarin derivatives and determine dosage required to achieve therapeutic results.
- Identify individuals who may be prone to bleeding during surgical, obstetric, dental, or invasive diagnostic procedures.
- Identify the possible cause of abnormal bleeding, such as epistaxis, hematoma, gingival bleeding, hematuria, and menorrhagia.
- Monitor the effects of conditions such as liver disease, protein deficiency, and fat malabsorption on hemostasis.
- Screen for prothrombin deficiency.
- Screen for vitamin K deficiency.

POTENTIAL MEDICAL DIAGNOSIS

Increased in:

- Afibrinogenemia, dysfibrinogenemia, or hypofibrinogenemia ***(related to insufficient levels of fibrinogen, which is required for clotting; its absence prolongs PT)***
- Alcohol use ***(related to decreased liver function, which results in decreased production of clotting factors and prolonged PT)***
- Biliary obstruction ***(related to poor absorption of fat-soluble vitamin K; vitamin K is required for clotting and its absence prolongs PT)***
- Disseminated intravascular coagulation ***(related to increased consumption of clotting factors; PT is increased)***
- Hereditary deficiencies of factors II, V, VII, and X ***(related to deficiency of factors required for clotting; their absence prolongs PT)***
- Liver disease (cirrhosis) ***(related to decreased liver function, which results in decreased production of clotting factors and prolonged PT)***
- Massive transfusion of packed red blood cells (RBCs) ***(related to dilutional effect of replacing a significant fraction of the total blood volume; there are insufficient clotting factors in plasma-poor, packed RBC products. Blood products contain anticoagulants, which compound the lack of adequate clotting factors in the case of massive transfusion)***
- Poor fat absorption ***(tropical sprue, celiac disease, and chronic diarrhea are conditions that prevent absorption of fat-soluble vitamins, including vitamin K, which is required for clotting; its absence prolongs PT)***

- Presence of circulating anticoagulant ***(related to the production of inhibitors of specific factors, e.g., developed from long-term factor VIII therapy or circulating anticoagulants associated with conditions like tuberculosis, systemic lupus erythematosus, rheumatoid arthritis, and chronic glomerulonephritis)***
- Salicylate intoxication ***(related to decreased liver function)***
- Vitamin K deficiency ***(related to dietary deficiency or disorders of malabsorption; vitamin K is required for clotting; its absence prolongs PT)***

Decreased in:

- Increased absorption of vitamin K ***(related to dietary increases in fat, which enhances absorption of vitamin K, or increases of green leafy vegetables that contain large amounts of vitamin K)***
- Ovarian hyperfunction
- Regional enteritis or ileitis

CRITICAL FINDINGS:

INR

- Greater than 5

Prothrombin Time

- Greater than 27 sec

Note and immediately report to the requesting health-care provider (HCP) any critical findings and related symptoms. A listing of these findings varies among facilities. Timely notification of a critical finding for laboratory or diagnostic studies is a role expectation of the professional nurse. The notification processes vary among facilities. Upon receipt of the critical finding, the information should be read back to the caller to verify accuracy.

Consideration may be given to verification of critical findings before action is taken. Policies vary among facilities and may include requesting immediate recollection and retesting by the laboratory or retesting using a rapid point-of-care testing instrument at the bedside, if available.

Important signs to note relate to bleeding in specific areas of the body and include prolonged bleeding from cuts or gums, hematoma at a puncture site, hemorrhage, blood in the stool, backache or flank pain, dark-colored urine, joint pain, persistent epistaxis, heavy or prolonged menstrual flow, and shock. Monitor vital signs, unusual ecchymosis, occult blood, severe headache, unusual dizziness, and neurological changes until PT is within normal range. Intramuscular (IM) administration of vitamin K, an anticoagulant reversal drug, may be requested by the HCP.

INTERFERING FACTORS

- Drugs and other substances that may increase the PT in patients receiving anticoagulation therapy include acetaminophen, acetylsalicylic acid, amiodarone, anabolic steroids, anisindione, anistreplase, antibiotics, antipyrine, carbenicillin, cathartics, chloral hydrate, chlorthalidone, cholestyramine, clofibrate, corticotropin, demeclocycline, diazoxide, diflunisal, disulfiram, diuretics, doxycycline, erythromycin, ethyl alcohol, hydroxyzine, laxatives, mercaptopurine, miconazole, nalidixic acid, neomycin, niacin, oxyphenbutazone, phenytoin, quinidine, quinine, thyroxine, and tosylate bretylium.
- Drugs and other substances that may decrease the PT in patients receiving anticoagulation therapy include amobarbital, anabolic steroids, antacids, antihistamines, barbiturates, carbamazepine, chloral hydrate, chlordane, chlordiazepoxide, cholestyramine, clofibrate,

P

colchicine, corticosteroids, diuretics, oral contraceptives, penicillin, primidone, raloxifene, rifabutin, rifampin, simethicone, spironolactone, tacrolimus, tolbutamide, and vitamin K.

- Traumatic venipunctures can activate the coagulation sequence by contaminating the sample with tissue thromboplastin and producing falsely shortened PT.
- Hematocrit greater than 55% may cause falsely prolonged results because of anticoagulant excess relative to plasma volume.
- Incompletely filled collection tubes, specimens contaminated with heparin, clotted or hemolyzed specimens, or unprocessed specimens not delivered to the laboratory within 24 hr of collection should be rejected.
- Excessive agitation causing sample hemolysis can falsely shorten the PT because the hemolyzed cells activate plasma-clotting factors.

NURSING IMPLICATIONS AND PROCEDURE

POTENTIAL NURSING PROBLEMS:

Problem	Signs & Symptoms	Interventions
Bleeding ***(related to altered clotting factors secondary to warfarin use or depleted clotting factors)***	Altered level of consciousness; hypotension; increased heart rate; decreased hemoglobin (Hgb) and hematocrit (Hct); capillary refill greater than 3 sec; cool extremities; blood in urine, stool, sputum; bleeding gums; nosebleed; bruises easily	Increase frequency of vital sign assessment with variances in results; monitor for vital sign trends; administer blood or blood products as ordered; administer prescribed vitamin K; monitor and trend Hgb/Hct; assess skin for petechiae, purpura, hematoma; monitor for blood in emesis, or sputum; institute bleeding precautions (prevent unnecessary venipuncture; avoid IM injections; prevent trauma; be gentle with oral care, suctioning; avoid use of a sharp razor); administer prescribed stool softener; monitor and trend PT/INR in relation to warfarin dosage
Gas exchange ***(related to deficient oxygen capacity of the blood secondary to blood loss)***	Irregular breathing pattern, use of accessory muscles; altered chest excursion; adventitious breath sounds (crackles,	Monitor respiratory rate and effort based on assessment of patient condition; assess lung sounds frequently; monitor for secretions, bloody sputum; suction as necessary; use pulse

(table continues on page 1346)

Problem	Signs & Symptoms	Interventions
	rhonchi, wheezes, diminished breath sounds); copious secretions; signs of hypoxia; altered blood gas results; confusion; lethargy; cyanosis	oximetry to monitor oxygen saturation; collaborate with HCP to administer oxygen as needed; elevate the head of the bed 30 degrees or higher; monitor intravenous (IV) fluids and avoid aggressive fluid resuscitation; assess level of consciousness; anticipate the need for possible intubation
Tissue perfusion ***(related to decreased Hgb secondary to bleeding; altered clotting factors)***	Hypotension; dizziness; cool extremities; pallor; capillary refill greater than 3 sec in fingers and toes; weak pedal pulses; altered level of consciousness; altered sensation	Monitor blood pressure; assess for dizziness; assess extremities for skin temperature, color, warmth; assess capillary refill; assess pedal pulses; monitor for numbness, tingling, hyperesthesia, hypoesthesia; monitor and trend PT and INR; administer blood or blood products as ordered; administer vitamin K as ordered; administer IV fluids as ordered; use fluid bolus as appropriate; administer medication to support blood pressure as ordered
Health management ***(related to inaccurate self-medication of warfarin; complexity of health-care system; complexity of therapeutic management; knowledge deficit; cultural family health patterns; mistrust of HCP)***	Inability or failure to recognize or process information toward improving health and preventing illness with associated mental and physical effects	Collaborate with HCP to develop a plan of care that supports health; ensure patient adheres to recommended medication regime; encourage patient to comply with health-care follow-up appointments

P

PRETEST:

- Positively identify the patient using at least two person-specific identifiers before services, treatments, or procedures are performed.
- ***Patient Teaching:*** Inform the patient this test can assist in evaluating coagulation and monitor therapy.
- Obtain a history of the patient's health concerns (especially any bleeding disorders), symptoms, surgical procedures, and results of previously performed laboratory and diagnostic studies. Include a list of known allergens, especially allergies or sensitivities to latex.
- Obtain a list of the patient's current medications, including over-the-counter medications, dietary supplements, anticoagulants, aspirin and other salicylates (see Effects of Natural Products on Laboratory Values online at Davis*Plus*). Such products should be discontinued by medical direction for the appropriate number of days prior to a surgical procedure. Note the last time and dose of medication taken.
- Review the procedure with the patient. Inform the patient that specimen collection takes approximately 5 to 10 min. Address concerns about pain and explain that there may be some discomfort during the venipuncture.
- ***Sensitivity to social and cultural issues,*** as well as concern for modesty, is important in providing psychological support before, during, and after the procedure.
- Note that there are no food, fluid, or medication restrictions unless by medical direction.

INTRATEST:

Potential Complications: N/A

- Avoid the use of equipment containing latex if the patient has a history of allergic reaction to latex.
- Instruct the patient to cooperate fully and to follow directions. Direct the patient to breathe normally and to avoid unnecessary movement.
- Observe standard precautions, and follow the general guidelines in Patient Preparation and Specimen Collection online at Davis*Plus*. Positively identify the patient, and label the appropriate specimen container with the corresponding patient demographics, initials of the person collecting the specimen, date, and time of collection. Perform a venipuncture. Fill tube completely. *Important note:* When multiple specimens are drawn, the blue-top tube should be collected after sterile (i.e., blood culture) tubes. Otherwise, when using a standard vacutainer system, the blue-top tube is the first tube collected. When a butterfly is used and due to the added tubing, an extra red-top tube should be collected before the blue-top tube to ensure complete filling of the blue-top tube.
- Remove the needle and apply direct pressure with dry gauze to stop bleeding. Observe/assess venipuncture site for bleeding or hematoma formation and secure gauze with adhesive bandage.
- Promptly transport the specimen to the laboratory for processing and analysis. If delays in specimen transport and processing occur, it is important to consult with the testing laboratory. Whole blood specimens are stable at room temperature for up to 24 hr. Some laboratories will accept refrigerated whole blood samples up to 48 hr from the time of collection. Criteria for rejection of specimens based on collection time may vary among facilities.

POST-TEST:

- Inform the patient that a report of the results will be made available to the requesting HCP, who will discuss the results with the patient.
- Frequent monitoring of the PT/INR is important. Concern with monitoring is mostly involved with elevated values. However, decreased PT results can indicate a risk for thrombosis. There are three factors, known as Virchow's

P

triad, that increase the risk of developing a venous thrombus:

- Hypercoagulability, or a tendency for blood to coagulate at an abnormally rapid rate
- Venous stasis, or an impaired rate of blood flow through a vessel
- Vessel wall trauma or injury

Possible nursing interventions to decrease risk of thrombus include education for the patient regarding leg exercises, avoidance of constrictive clothing (e.g., stockings or tight socks), or avoidance of behaviors that might constrict blood flow, such as crossing of the legs or maintaining a dependent position for long periods of time.

- ***Nutritional Considerations:*** Foods high in vitamin K may alter PT/INR findings for patients on anticoagulant therapy if consumed in quantities that differ significantly (either more or less) from the normal dietary intake. Foods that contain vitamin K include asparagus, beans, cabbage, cauliflower, chickpeas, egg yolks, green tea, pork, liver, milk, soybean products, tomatoes, mayonnaise, vegetable oils, and green leafy vegetables such as leaf lettuce, watercress, parsley, broccoli, brussels sprouts, kale, spinach, swiss chard, and collard, mustard, and turnip greens.
- ***Nutritional Considerations:*** Avoid alcohol and alcohol products while taking warfarin because the combination of the two increases the risk of gastrointestinal bleeding.
- Depending on the results of this procedure, additional testing may be performed to evaluate or monitor progression of the disease process and determine the need for a change in therapy. Evaluate test results in relation to the patient's symptoms and other tests performed.

Patient Education:

- Instruct the patient to report bleeding from any areas of the skin or mucous membranes.
- Inform the patient with prolonged PT/INR of the importance of taking precautions against bruising and bleeding, including the use of a soft bristle toothbrush, use of an electric razor, avoidance of constipation, avoidance of aspirin products, and avoidance of IM injections.
- Inform the patient of the importance of periodic laboratory testing while taking an anticoagulant.
- Reinforce the importance of refraining from alcohol use while on warfarin.
- Reinforce information given by the patient's HCP regarding further testing, treatment, or referral to another HCP.
- Instruct the patient in the use of home test kits for PT/INR approved by the U.S. Food and Drug Administration, as appropriate.
- Answer any questions or address any concerns voiced by the patient or family.

Expected Patient Outcomes:

Understanding

- The patient and family state signs and symptoms of bleeding that should be reported to the HCP.
- The patient and family state the benefit of taking warfarin to the patient's overall health.

Ability

- The patient demonstrates proficiency and accuracy in the self-administration of warfarin.
- The patient and family identify foods high in vitamin K and include balanced quantities in the diet (relative to the patient's diet prior to warfarin therapy).

Response

- The patient and family discuss barriers to compliance with therapeutic management and make efforts to adhere to recommendations.
- The patient complies with recommended follow-up appointments for PT and INR evaluation.

RELATED STUDIES:

- Related tests include, ALP, ALT, ANA, AT-III, AST, bilirubin, biopsy liver, bleeding time, calcium, coagulation factors, CBC, CBC platelet count, CT liver and biliary tract,

P

cryoglobulin, D-dimer, fecal analysis, fecal fat, FDP, fibrinogen, GGT, gastric acid emptying scan, genetic testing, hepatitis antibodies (A, B, C, D), liver and spleen scan, lupus anticoagulant, aPTT, plasminogen, protein C, protein S, US abdomen, US liver, and vitamin K.

- Refer to the Cardiovascular, Hematopoietic, and Hepatobiliary systems tables online at Davis*Plus* for related tests by body system.

Pseudocholinesterase and Dibucaine Number

SYNONYM/ACRONYM: CHS, PCHE, AcCHS.

COMMON USE: To assess for pseudocholinesterase deficiency to assist in diagnosing a congenital deficiency. Special attention must be given to results for preoperative patients because positive results indicate risk for apnea with use of succinylcholine as an anesthetic drug.

SPECIMEN: Plasma collected in a lavender-top (EDTA) tube. Serum collected in a red-top tube is also acceptable.

NORMAL FINDINGS: (Method: Spectrophotometry, kinetic)

Test	Conventional Units
Pseudocholinesterase	
Males	3,334–7,031 units/L
Females	2,504–6,297 inits/L

Dibucaine Number	Fraction (%) of Activity Inhibited
Normal homozygote	79%–84%
Heterozygote	55%–70%
Abnormal homozygote	16%–28%

POTENTIAL MEDICAL DIAGNOSIS

Increased in:

Increased levels are observed in a number of conditions without specific cause.

- Diabetes
- Hyperthyroidism
- Nephrotic syndrome
- Obesity

Decreased in:

The enzyme is produced in the liver, and any condition affecting liver function may result in decreased production of circulating enzyme.

- Acute infection
- Anemia (severe)
- Carcinomatosis
- Cirrhosis
- Congenital deficiency
- Hepatic carcinoma
- Hepatocellular disease
- Infectious hepatitis
- Insecticide exposure ***(organic phosphate exposure decreases enzyme activity)***

- Malnutrition ***(possibly related to decreased availability of transport proteins; condition associated with decreased enzyme activity)***
- Muscular dystrophy
- Myocardial infarction
- Plasmapheresis ***(iatrogenic cause)***
- Succinylcholine hypersensitivity ***(this chemical is a trigger in susceptible individuals)***
- Tuberculosis ***(chronic infection is known to decrease enzyme activity)***
- Uremia ***(pathological condition known to decrease enzyme activity)***

CRITICAL FINDINGS:

A positive result indicates that the patient is at risk for prolonged or unrecoverable apnea related to the inability to metabolize succinylcholine. Notify the anesthesiologist if the test result is positive and surgery is scheduled.

Note and immediately report to the requesting health-care provider (HCP) any critical findings and related symptoms. A listing of these findings varies among facilities. Timely notification of a critical finding for laboratory or diagnostic studies is a role expectation of the professional nurse. The notification processes vary among facilities. Upon receipt of the critical finding, the information should be read back to the caller to verify accuracy.

Find and print out the full study on Fast Find at davispl.us/vanleeuwen7.

Pulmonary Function Studies

SYNONYM/ACRONYM: Pulmonary function tests (PFTs).

COMMON USE: To assess respiratory function to assist in evaluating obstructive versus restrictive lung disease and to monitor and assess the effectiveness of therapeutic interventions.

AREA OF APPLICATION: Lungs, respiratory system.

DESCRIPTION: Pulmonary function studies provide information about the volume, pattern, and rates of airflow involved in respiratory function. These studies may also include tests involving the diffusing capabilities of the lungs (i.e., volume of gases diffusing across a membrane). A complete pulmonary function study includes the determination of all lung volumes, spirometry, diffusing capacity, maximum voluntary ventilation, flow-volume loop, and maximum expiratory and inspiratory pressures. (See Figure 1 showing lung volumes measured during PFT.) Other studies include small airway volumes.

The studies are conducted using a mechanical device called a *spirometer*. The amount of gas breathed in and out by the patient is measured and converted into a series of electrical signals that are displayed in a *spirogram*.

Pulmonary function studies are classified according to lung volumes and capacities, rates

P

of flow, and gas exchange. The exception is the diffusion test, which records the movement of a gas during inspiration and expiration. Lung volumes and capacities constitute the amount of air inhaled or exhaled from the lungs; this value is compared to normal reference values specific for the patient's age, height, and gender. The following are volumes and capacities measured by spirometry that do not require timed testing.

Tidal volume (TV)	Total amount of air inhaled and exhaled with one breath
Residual volume (RV)	Amount of air remaining in the lungs after a maximum expiration effort; this indirect type of measurement can be done by body plethysmography (see study titled "Plethysmography")
Inspiratory reserve volume (IRV)	Maximum amount of air inhaled at the point of maximum expiration
Expiratory reserve volume (ERV)	Maximum amount of air exhaled after a resting expiration; can be calculated by the VC minus the IC
Vital capacity (VC)	Maximum amount of air exhaled after a maximum inspiration (can be calculated by adding the IC and the ERV)
Total lung capacity (TLC)	Total amount of air that the lungs can hold after maximum inspiration; can be calculated by adding the VC and the RV
Inspiratory capacity (IC)	Maximum amount of air inspired after normal expiration; can be calculated by adding the IRV and the TV
Functional residual capacity (FRC)	Volume of air that remains in the lungs after normal expiration can be calculated by adding the RV and ERV

The volumes, capacities, and rates of flow measured by spirometry that do require timed testing include the following:

Forced vital capacity (FVC)	Maximum amount of air that can be forcefully exhaled after a full inspiration
Forced expiratory volume (FEV1)	Amount of air that can be forcefully exhaled in the first second after a full inspiration (can also be determined at 2 or 3 sec)
Maximal midexpiratory flow (MMEF)	Also known as *forced expiratory flow rate* (FEF_{25-75}), or the maximal rate of airflow during a forced expiration

(table continues on page 1352)

Forced inspiratory flow rate (FIF)	Volume inspired from the RV at a point of measurement (can be expressed as a percentage to identify the corresponding volume pressure and inspired volume)
Peak inspiratory flow rate (PIFR)	Maximum airflow during a forced maximal inspiration
Peak expiratory flow rate (PEFR)	Maximum airflow expired during FVC
Flow-volume loops (F-V)	Flows and volumes recorded during forced expiratory volume and forced inspiratory VC procedures
Maximal inspiratory-expiratory pressures	Strengths of the respiratory muscles in neuromuscular disorders
Maximal voluntary ventilation (MVV)	Maximal volume of air inspired and expired in 1 min (may be done for shorter periods and multiplied to equal 1 min)

Other studies for gas-exchange capacity, small airway abnormalities, and allergic responses in hyperactive airway disorders can be performed during the conventional pulmonary function study. These include the following:

Diffusing capacity of the lungs (DL)	Rate of transfer of carbon monoxide through the alveolar and capillary membrane in 1 min
Closing volume (CV)	Measure of the closure of small airways in the lower alveoli by monitoring volume and percentage of alveolar nitrogen after inhalation of 100% oxygen
Isoflow volume (isoV)	Flow-volume loop test followed by inhalation of a mixture of helium and oxygen to determine small airway disease
Body plethysmography	Measure of thoracic gas volume and airway resistance
Bronchial provocation	Quantification of airway response after inhalation of methacholine
Arterial blood gases (ABGs)	Measure of oxygen, pH, and carbon dioxide in arterial blood

Values are expressed in units of mL, %, L, L/sec, and L/min, depending on the test performed.

Note: See Figure 1 showing some examples of PFT results presented in graphic form; the graphs assist in interpreting the findings and establishing the diagnosis of respiratory conditions.

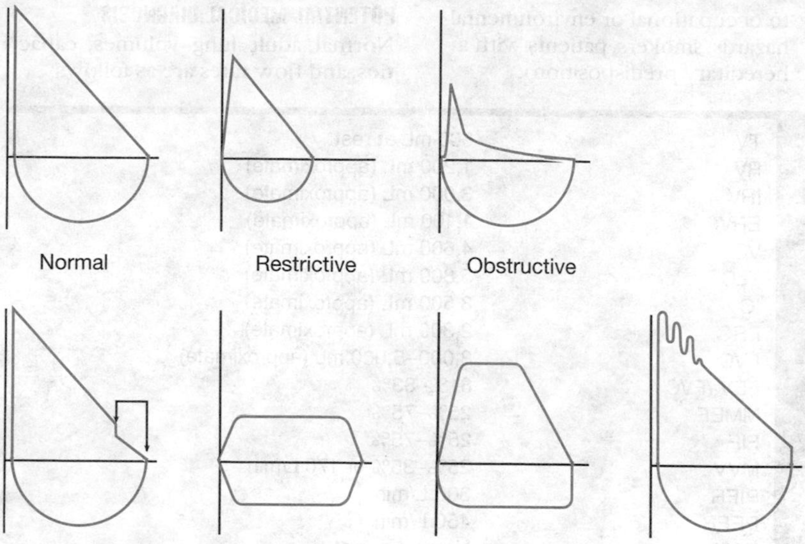

Figure 1 Examples of PFT results presented in graphic form.

This procedure is contraindicated for

Patients with cardiac insufficiency, recent myocardial infarction, and presence of chest pain that affects inspiration or expiration ability.

INDICATIONS

- Detect chronic obstructive pulmonary disease (COPD) and/or restrictive pulmonary diseases that affect the chest wall (e.g., neuromuscular disorders, kyphosis, scoliosis) and lungs, as evidenced by abnormal airflows and volumes.
- Determine airway response to inhalants in patients with an airway-reactive disorder.
- Determine the diffusing capacity of the lungs (DCOL).
- Determine the effectiveness of therapy regimens, such as bronchodilators, for pulmonary disorders.
- Determine the presence of lung disease when other studies, such as x-rays, do not provide a definitive diagnosis, or determine the progression and severity of known COPD and restrictive pulmonary disease.
- Evaluate the cause of dyspnea occurring with or without exercise.
- Evaluate lung compliance to determine changes in elasticity, as evidenced by changes in lung volumes (decreased in restrictive pulmonary disease, increased in COPD and in older adult patients).
- Evaluate pulmonary disability for legal or insurance claims.
- Evaluate pulmonary function after surgical pneumonectomy, lobectomy, or segmental lobectomy.
- Evaluate the respiratory system to determine the patient's ability to tolerate procedures such as surgery or diagnostic studies.
- Screen high-risk populations for early detection of pulmonary conditions (e.g., patients with exposure

P

to occupational or environmental hazards, smokers, patients with a hereditary predisposition).

POTENTIAL MEDICAL DIAGNOSIS

Normal adult lung volumes, capacities, and flow rates are as follows:

TV	500 mL at rest
RV	1,200 mL (approximate)
IRV	3,000 mL (approximate)
ERV	1,100 mL (approximate)
VC	4,600 mL (approximate)
TLC	5,800 mL (approximate)
IC	3,500 mL (approximate)
FRC	2,300 mL (approximate)
FVC	3,000–5,000 mL (approximate)
FEV_1/FVC	81%–83%
MMEF	25%–75%
FIF	25%–75%
MVV	25%–35% or 170 L/min
PIFR	300 L/min
PEFR	450 L/min
F-V loop	Normal curve
DCOL	25 mL/min per mm Hg (approximate)
CV	10%–20% of VC
V_{iso}	Based on age formula
Bronchial provocation	No change, or less than 20% reduction in FEV_1

Note: Normal values listed are estimated values for adults. Actual pediatric and adult values are based on age, height, and gender. These normal values are included on the patient's pulmonary function laboratory report.

CV = closing volume; DCOL = diffusing capacity of the lungs; ERV = expiratory reserve volume; FEV_1 = forced expiratory volume in 1 sec; FIF = forced inspiratory flow rate; FRC = functional residual capacity; FVC = forced vital capacity; F-V loop = flow-volume loop; IC = inspiratory capacity; IRV = inspiratory reserve volume; MMEF = maximal midexpiratory flow (also known as FEF_{25-75}); MVV = maximal voluntary ventilation; PEFR = peak expiratory flow rate; PIFR = peak inspiratory flow rate; RV = residual volume; TLC = total lung capacity; TV = tidal volume; VC = vital capacity; V_{iso} = isoflow volume. (See Figure 2.)

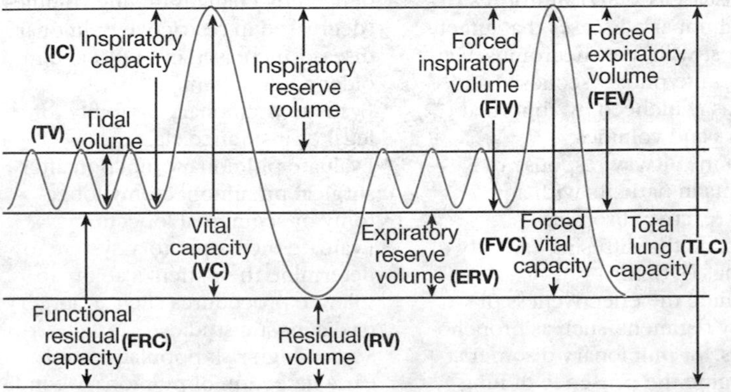

Figure 2 Showing lung volumes measured during PFT.

Normal findings

- Normal respiratory volume and capacities, gas diffusion, and distribution
- No evidence of COPD or restrictive pulmonary disease

Abnormal findings related to

- Allergy
- Asbestosis
- Asthma
- Bronchiectasis
- Chest trauma
- COPD
- Curvature of the spine
- Myasthenia gravis
- Obesity
- Pulmonary fibrosis
- Pulmonary tumors
- Respiratory infections
- Sarcoidosis

CRITICAL FINDINGS:

Hypoxia occurs at oxygen saturation levels less than 90%. Significant hypoxia, levels less than 85%, require immediate evaluation and treatment.

Note and immediately report to the requesting health-care provider (HCP) any critical findings and related symptoms. A listing of these findings varies among facilities. Timely notification of a critical finding for laboratory or diagnostic studies is a role expectation of the professional nurse. The notification processes vary among facilities. Upon receipt of the critical finding, the information should be read back to the caller to verify accuracy.

INTERFERING FACTORS

- The aging process can cause decreased values (FVC, DCOL) depending on the study done.
- Inability of the patient to put forth the necessary breathing effort affects the results.
- Medications such as bronchodilators can affect results.
- Improper placement of the nose clamp or mouthpiece that allows for leakage can affect volume results.
- Confusion or inability to understand instructions or cooperate during the study can cause inaccurate results.
- Exercise caution with patients who have upper respiratory infections, such as a cold or acute bronchitis.

NURSING IMPLICATIONS AND PROCEDURE

See Potential Nursing Problems on Fast Find at davispl.us/vanleeuwen7.

PRETEST:

- Positively identify the patient using at least two person-specific identifiers before services, treatments, or procedures are performed.
- ***Patient Teaching:*** Inform the patient this procedure can assist in assessing lung function.
- Obtain a history of the patient's health concerns, symptoms, surgical procedures, and results of previously performed laboratory and diagnostic studies. Include a list of known allergens, especially allergies or sensitivities to latex.
- Obtain a list of the patient's current medications, including over-the-counter medications and dietary supplements (see Effects of Natural Products on Laboratory Values online at Davis*Plus*).
- Review the procedure with the patient. Address concerns about pain related to the procedure and explain that no discomfort will be experienced during the test. Explain that the procedure is generally performed in a specially equipped room or in an office by a HCP specializing in this procedure and usually lasts 1 hr.
- ***Sensitivity to social and cultural issues,*** as well as concern for modesty, is important in providing psychological support before, during, and after the procedure.

- Record the patient's height and weight.
- Instruct the patient to avoid bronchodilators (oral or inhalant) for at least 4 hr before the study, as directed by the HCP.
- Instruct the patient to refrain from smoking tobacco or eating a heavy meal for 4 to 6 hr prior to the study. Protocols may vary among facilities.

INTRATEST:

Potential Complications: N/A

- Observe standard precautions, and follow the general guidelines in Patient Preparation and Specimen Collection online at Davis*Plus*. Positively identify the patient.
- Ensure the patient has complied with dietary and medication restrictions and pretesting preparations.
- Obtain an inhalant bronchodilator to treat any bronchospasms that may occur with testing.
- Avoid the use of equipment containing latex if the patient has a history of allergic reaction to latex.
- Instruct the patient to void and to loosen any restrictive clothing.
- Instruct the patient to cooperate fully and to follow directions.
- Place the patient in a sitting position on a chair near the spirometry equipment.
- Place a soft clip on the patient's nose to restrict nose breathing, and instruct the patient to breathe through the mouth.
- Place a mouthpiece in the mouth and instruct the patient to close his or her lips around it to form a seal.
- Tubing from the mouthpiece attaches to a cylinder that is connected to a computer that measures, records, and calculates the values for the tests done.
- Instruct the patient to inhale deeply and then to quickly exhale as much air as possible into the mouthpiece.
- Additional breathing maneuvers are performed on inspiration and expiration (normal, forced, and breath-holding).

POST-TEST:

- Inform the patient that a report of the results will be made available to the requesting HCP, who will discuss the results with the patient.
- Assess the patient for dizziness or weakness after the testing.
- Allow the patient to rest as long as needed to recover.
- Instruct the patient to resume usual diet and medications, as directed by the HCP. Inform the patient of smoking cessation programs as appropriate.
- Recognize anxiety related to test results, and be supportive of perceived loss of independent function. Discuss the implications of abnormal test results on the patient's lifestyle. Provide teaching and information regarding the clinical implications of the test results, as appropriate.
- Reinforce information given by the patient's HCP regarding further testing, treatment, or referral to another HCP. Answer any questions or address any concerns voiced by the patient or family.
- Depending on the results of this procedure, additional testing may be performed to evaluate or monitor progression of the disease process and determine the need for a change in therapy. Evaluate test results in relation to the patient's symptoms and other tests performed.

Patient Education:

- Teach the patient to report signs of bleeding (bleeding gums, black tarry stools, blood in urine, hematoma).
- Teach the patient the symptoms of pulmonary embolism and the importance of timely reporting.

Expected Patient Outcomes:

Understanding

- The patient and family state the importance of the patient remaining on bedrest to prevent movement of the embolus.
- The patient and family state the importance of keeping oxygen on at all times.

Ability

- The patient demonstrates effective coping mechanisms to decrease anxiety.
- The patient demonstrates how to use controlled breathing to improve breathing patterns.

Response

- The patient agrees to visit the HCP's office for follow-up coagulation studies.
- The patient agrees to take pain medication to decrease breathing discomfort and improve oxygenation.

RELATED STUDIES:

- Related tests include α_1-AT, anion gap, arterial/alveolar oxygen ratio, biopsy lung, blood gases, bronchoscopy, carboxyhemoglobin, chest x-ray, chloride sweat, CBC, CBC hemoglobin, CBC WBC count and differential, CT angiography, CT thoracic, culture and smear for mycobacteria, culture bacterial sputum, culture viral, cytology sputum, echocardiography, ECG, Gram stain, IgE, lactic acid, lung perfusion scan, lung ventilation scan, MR angiography, MRI chest, osmolality, phosphorus, plethysmography, pleural fluid analysis, potassium, PET chest, pulse oximetry, sodium, and TB skin test.
- Refer to the Cardiovascular and Respiratory systems tables online at Davis*Plus* for related tests by body system.

Pulse Oximetry

SYNONYM/ACRONYM: Oximetry, pulse ox.

COMMON USE: To assess arterial blood oxygenation toward evaluating respiratory status during ventilation, acute illness, activity, and sleep and to evaluate the effectiveness of therapeutic interventions.

AREA OF APPLICATION: Earlobe, fingertip; for infants, use the large toe, top or bottom of the foot, or sides of the ankle.

DESCRIPTION: Pulse oximetry is a noninvasive study that provides continuous readings of arterial blood oxygen saturation (SpO_2) using a sensor site (earlobe or fingertip). The SpO_2 equals the ratio of the amount of O_2 contained in the hemoglobin to the maximum amount of O_2 contained, with hemoglobin expressed as a percentage. The results obtained may compare favorably with O_2 saturation levels obtained by arterial blood gas analysis without the need to perform successive arterial punctures. The device used is a clip or probe that produces a light beam with two different wavelengths on one side. A sensor on the opposite side measures the absorption of each of the wavelengths of light to determine the O_2 saturation reading. The displayed result is a ratio, expressed as a percentage, between the actual O_2 content of the hemoglobin and the potential maximum O_2-carrying capacity of the hemoglobin.

This procedure is contraindicated for: N/A

INDICATIONS

- Determine the effectiveness of pulmonary gas exchange function.
- Evaluate suspected nocturnal hypoxemia in chronic obstructive pulmonary disease.
- Monitor oxygenation during testing for sleep apnea.
- Monitor oxygenation perioperatively and during acute illnesses.

P

- Monitor oxygenation status in patients on a ventilator, during surgery, and during bronchoscopy.
- Monitor O_2 saturation during activities such as pulmonary exercise stress testing or pulmonary rehabilitation exercises to determine optimal tolerance.
- Monitor response to pulmonary drug regimens, especially flow and O_2 content.

POTENTIAL MEDICAL DIAGNOSIS

Normal findings

- Greater than or equal to 95% (values may be at the lower end of the normal range in older adults)

Abnormal findings related to

- Abnormal gas exchange
- Hypoxemia with levels less than 95%
- Impaired cardiopulmonary function

CRITICAL FINDINGS:

Hypoxia occurs at oxygen saturation levels less than 90%. Significant hypoxia, levels less than 85%, require immediate evaluation and treatment.

Note and immediately report to the requesting health-care provider (HCP) any critical findings and related symptoms. A listing of these findings varies among facilities. Timely notification of a critical finding for laboratory or diagnostic studies is a role expectation of the professional nurse. The notification processes vary among facilities. Upon receipt of the critical finding, the information should be read back to the caller to verify accuracy.

P

INTERFERING FACTORS

- Patients who smoke or have experienced carbon monoxide inhalation, because O_2 levels may be falsely elevated.

Factors that may result in incorrect values

- Patients with anemic conditions reflecting a reduction in hemoglobin, the O_2-carrying component in the blood.
- Excessive light surrounding the patient, such as from surgical lights.
- Impaired cardiopulmonary function.
- Lipid emulsion therapy and presence of certain dyes.
- Movement of the finger or ear or improper placement of probe or clip.
- Nail polish, artificial fingernails, and skin pigmentation when a finger probe is used.
- Vasoconstriction from cool skin temperature, drugs, hypotension, or vessel obstruction causing a decrease in blood flow.

Other considerations

- Accuracy for most units is plus or minus 2% to 3%.

NURSING IMPLICATIONS AND PROCEDURE

See Potential Nursing Problems on Fast Find at davispl.us/vanleeuwen7.

PRETEST:

- Positively identify the patient using at least two person-specific identifiers before services, treatments, or procedures are performed.
- ***Patient Teaching:*** Inform the patient this procedure can assist in monitoring oxygen in the blood.
- Obtain a history of the patient's health concerns, symptoms, surgical procedures, and results of previously performed laboratory and diagnostic studies. Include a list of known allergens, especially allergies or sensitivities to latex.
- Obtain a list of the patient's current medications, including over-the-counter medications and dietary supplements (see Effects of Natural Products on Laboratory Values online at Davis*Plus*).
- Review the procedure with the patient. Address concerns about pain

related to the procedure and explain that no pain is associated with the procedure. Inform the patient that the procedure is generally performed at the bedside, in the operating room during a surgical procedure, or in the office of an HCP. Explain that the procedure lasts as long as the monitoring is needed and could be continuous.

- *Sensitivity to social and cultural issues,* as well as concern for modesty, is important in providing psychological support before, during, and after the procedure.
- If a finger probe is used, instruct the patient to remove artificial fingernails and nail polish.
- When used in the presence of flammable gases, the equipment must be approved for that specific use.
- Instruct the patient not to smoke for 24 hr before the procedure.
- Note that there are no food, fluid, or medication restrictions unless by medical direction.

INTRATEST:

Potential Complications: N/A

- Observe standard precautions, and follow the general guidelines in Patient Preparation and Specimen Collection online at Davis*Plus*. Positively identify the patient.
- Ensure that the patient has complied with pretesting preparations prior to the study, as instructed.
- Avoid the use of equipment containing latex if the patient has a history of allergic reaction to latex.
- If a finger probe is used, instruct the patient not to grip treadmill rail or bed rail tightly; doing so restricts blood flow.
- Instruct the patient to cooperate fully and to follow directions.
- Massage or apply a warm towel to the upper earlobe or finger to increase the blood flow.
- The index finger is normally used, but if the patient's finger is too large for the probe, a smaller finger can be used.
- If the earlobe is used, make sure good contact is achieved.
- The big toe, top or bottom of the foot, or sides of the heel may be used in infants.
- Place the photodetector probe over the finger in such a way that the light beams and sensors are opposite each other. Turn the power switch to the oximeter monitor, which will display information about heart rate and peripheral capillary saturation (SaO_2).
- Remove the clip used for monitoring when the procedure is complete.

POST-TEST:

- Inform the patient that a report of the results will be made available to the requesting HCP, who will discuss the results with the patient.
- Closely observe SpO_2, and report to the HCP if it decreases to 90%.
- Recognize anxiety related to test results, and be supportive of perceived loss of independent function. Discuss the implications of abnormal test results on the patient's lifestyle. Provide teaching and information regarding the clinical implications of the test results, as appropriate.
- Reinforce information given by the patient's HCP regarding further testing, treatment, or referral to another HCP. Answer any questions or address any concerns voiced by the patient or family.
- Depending on the results of this procedure, additional testing may be performed to evaluate or monitor progression of the disease process and determine the need for a change in therapy. Evaluate test results in relation to the patient's symptoms and other tests performed.

Patient Education:

- Teach the patient the pathophysiology behind diminished oxygenation and disease process.
- Teach the patient the reportable signs and symptoms of poor oxygenation.

Expected Patient Outcomes:

Understanding

- The patient and family state the importance of keeping oxygen on at all times.

P

- The patient and family recognize that a HCP specializing in respiratory conditions may be consulted to assist with the disease management.

Ability

- The patient demonstrates how to use controlled breathing to improve breathing patterns.
- The patient demonstrates how to pace and bundle activities to improve activity tolerance.

Response

- The patient agrees to make required lifestyle changes to support positive health.
- The patient and family agree to work with the health-care team to discuss treatment options and expected outcomes.

RELATED STUDIES:

- Related tests include α_1-AT, anion gap, arterial/alveolar oxygen ratio, biopsy lung, blood gases, bronchoscopy, carboxyhemoglobin, chest x-ray, chloride sweat, CBC, CBC hemoglobin, CBC WBC count and differential, CT angiography, culture and smear for mycobacteria, culture bacterial sputum, culture viral, cytology sputum, ECG, Gram stain, IgE, lactic acid, lung perfusion scan, lung ventilation scan, MR angiography, MR chest, osmolality, phosphorus, plethysmography, pleural fluid analysis, potassium, pulmonary function tests, sodium, and TB skin test.
- Refer to the Cardiovascular and Respiratory systems tables online at Davis*Plus* for related tests by body system.

Pyruvate Kinase

SYNONYM/ACRONYM: PK.

COMMON USE: To assess for an enzyme deficiency to assist in diagnosis of hemolytic anemia.

SPECIMEN: Whole blood collected in yellow-top (acid-citrate-dextrose [ACD]) tube. Specimens collected in a lavender-top (EDTA) or green-top (heparin) tube also may be acceptable in some laboratories.

NORMAL FINDINGS: (Method: Enzymatic) 4.6–11.2 units/g Hgb.

POTENTIAL MEDICAL DIAGNOSIS

Increased in:

Related to release of skeletal and cardiac specific isoenzymes of PK from damaged tissue cells.

- Carriers of Duchenne's muscular dystrophy
- Muscle disease
- Myocardial infarction

Decreased in:

- Hereditary pyruvate kinase deficiency (evidenced by autosomal recessive trait for PK enzyme deficiency):
  Congenital nonspherocytic hemolytic anemia
- Acquired pyruvate kinase deficiency (related to interaction of medications used for therapy; related to release of leukocyte specific isoenzymes from damaged leukocytes):
  Acute leukemia
  Aplasias
  Other anemias

CRITICAL FINDINGS: N/A

Find and print out the full study on Fast Find at davispl.us/vanleeuwen7.

Radioactive Iodine Uptake

SYNONYM/ACRONYM: RAIU, thyroid uptake.

COMMON USE: To assess thyroid function toward diagnosing disorders such as hyperthyroidism and goiter.

AREA OF APPLICATION: Thyroid.

POTENTIAL MEDICAL DIAGNOSIS

Normal findings

- Variations in normal ranges of iodine uptake can occur with differences in dietary intake, geographic location, and protocols among laboratories:

Iodine Uptake	Percentage of Radionuclide
2-hr absorption	1%–13%
6-hr absorption	2%–25%
24-hr absorption	15%–45%

Abnormal findings related to

- Decreased iodine intake or increased iodine excretion
- Graves' disease
- Iodine-deficient goiter
- Hashimoto's thyroiditis (early)
- Hyperthyroidism, increased uptake of radionuclide:
  - Rebound thyroid hormone withdrawal
  - Drugs and hormones such as barbiturates, diuretics, estrogens, lithium carbonate, phenothiazines, and thyroid-stimulating hormone
- Hypothyroidism, decreased uptake of 0% to 10% radionuclide over 24-hr period:
  - Chronic kidney disease
  - Hypoalbuminemia
  - Malabsorption
  - Subacute thyroiditis
  - Thyrotoxicosis as a result of ectopic thyroid metastasis

CRITICAL FINDINGS: N/A

Find and print out the full study on Fast Find at davispl.us/vanleeuwen7.

Radiofrequency Ablation, Liver

SYNONYM/ACRONYM: RFA, RF ablation.

COMMON USE: To assist in treating tumors of the liver that are too small for surgery or have poor response to chemotherapy.

AREA OF APPLICATION: Liver.

DESCRIPTION: One minimally invasive therapy to eliminate tumors in organs such as the liver is called radiofrequency ablation (RFA). This technique works by passing electrical current in the range of radiofrequency waves between the needle electrode and the grounding pads placed on the patient's skin. A special needle electrode is placed in the tumor under the guidance of an imaging method such as ultrasound (US), computed tomography (CT) scanning (with or without iodinated contrast), or magnetic resonance

R

imaging (MRI). A radiofrequency current is then passed through the electrode to heat the tumor tissue near the needle tip and to ablate, or eliminate, it. The current creates heat around the electrode inside the tumor, and this heat spreads out to destroy the entire tumor but little of the surrounding normal liver tissue. The heat from radiofrequency energy also closes up small blood vessels, thereby minimizing the risk of bleeding. Because healthy liver tissue withstands more heat than a tumor, RFA is able to destroy a tumor and a small rim of normal tissue about its edges without affecting most of the normal liver. The dead tumor cells are gradually replaced by scar tissue that shrinks over time. This approach is used in destroying liver tumors that may have failed to respond to chemotherapy or have recurred after initial surgery. If there are multiple tumor nodules, they may be treated in one or more sessions. In general, RFA causes only minimal discomfort and may be done as an outpatient procedure without general anesthesia. The procedure can be performed percutaneously, laproscopically, or by open surgery. RFA is most effective if the tumor is less than 4 cm in diameter; results are not as good when RFA is used to treat larger tumors. Similar therapy is being used to treat tumors in the kidney, pancreas, bone, thyroid, breast, adrenal gland, and lung.

R

This procedure is contraindicated for

- Patients who are pregnant or suspected of being pregnant, unless the potential benefits of a procedure using radiation (if CT is performed with or without contrast) far outweigh the risk of radiation exposure to the fetus.
- Patients with conditions associated with adverse reactions to contrast medium (e.g., asthma, food allergies, or allergy to contrast medium).

  Although patients are asked specifically if they have a known allergy to iodine or shellfish, it has been well established that the reaction is not to iodine; an actual iodine allergy would be problematic because iodine is required for the production of thyroid hormones. In the case of shellfish, the reaction is to a muscle protein called tropomyosin; in the case of iodinated contrast medium, the reaction is to the noniodinated part of the contrast molecule. Patients with a known hypersensitivity to the medium may benefit from premedication with corticosteroids and diphenhydramine; the use of nonionic contrast or an alternative noncontrast imaging study, if available, may be considered for patients who have severe asthma or who have experienced moderate to severe reactions to ionic contrast medium.
- Patients with conditions associated with preexisting renal insufficiency (e.g., chronic kidney disease, single kidney transplant, nephrectomy, diabetes, multiple myeloma, treatment with aminoglycosides and NSAIDs) ***because iodinated contrast is nephrotoxic.***
- Patients who are chronically dehydrated before the test, especially older adults and patients whose health is already compromised, ***because of their risk of contrast-induced acute kidney injury.***
- Patients with the presence of large or numerous tumors (studies show that RFA is most successful if fewer than three tumors are present and each lesion is not greater than

3 cm in size; ablation of tumors that occupy greater than 40% of the liver may not leave sufficient liver capacity to support normal function).

- Patients with metastasis to the bile duct or surrounding hepatic vessel.
- Patients with bile duct or major vessel invasion.
- Patients with significant extrahepatic disease.
- Patients with bleeding disorders who are receiving an arterial or venous puncture, because the site may not stop bleeding.

INDICATIONS

- Ablation of metastases to the liver.
- Ablation of primary liver tumors, with hepatocellular carcinoma.
- Therapy for multiple small liver tumors that are too spread out to remove surgically.
- Therapy for recurrent liver tumors.
- Therapy for tumors that are less than 2 in. in diameter.
- Therapy for tumors that have failed to respond to chemotherapy.
- Therapy for tumors that have recurred after initial surgery.

POTENTIAL MEDICAL DIAGNOSIS

Normal findings

- Decrease in tumor size
- Normal size, position, contour, and texture of the liver

Abnormal findings related to: N/A

CRITICAL FINDINGS: N/A

INTERFERING FACTORS

Factors that may alter the results of the study

- Metallic objects (e.g., jewelry, rings, surgery clips) within the examination field, which may inhibit organ visualization and cause unclear images.
- Inability of the patient to cooperate or remain still during the procedure because of age, significant pain, or mental status.

Other considerations

- This procedure may be terminated if chest pain or severe cardiac dysrhythmias occur.
- Failure to follow dietary restrictions and other pretesting preparations before the procedure may cause the procedure to be canceled or repeated.

NURSING IMPLICATIONS AND PROCEDURE

PRETEST:

- Positively identify the patient using at least two person-specific identifiers before services, treatments, or procedures are performed.
- *Patient Teaching:* Inform the patient this procedure can assist in assessing liver function.
- Obtain a history of the patient's health concerns, symptoms, surgical procedures, and results of previously performed laboratory and diagnostic studies. Include a list of known allergens, especially allergies or sensitivities to latex, anesthetics, sedatives, or contrast medium.
- Obtain a history of the patient's hepatobiliary system, symptoms, and results of previously performed laboratory tests and diagnostic and surgical procedures.
- Note any recent procedures that can interfere with test results, including barium examinations.
- Record the date of the last menstrual period and determine the possibility of pregnancy in perimenopausal women.
- Obtain a list of the patient's current medications, including over-the-counter medications, dietary supplements, anticoagulants, aspirin and other salicylates (see Effects of Natural Products on Laboratory Values online at Davis*Plus*). Such

R

products should be discontinued by medical direction for the appropriate number of days prior to a surgical procedure. Note the last time and dose of medication taken.

- If iodinated contrast medium is scheduled to be used in patients receiving metformin (Glucophage) for type 2 diabetes, the drug should be discontinued on the day of the test and continue to be withheld for 48 hr after the test. Iodinated contrast can temporarily impair kidney function, and failure to withhold metformin may indirectly result in drug-induced lactic acidosis, a dangerous and sometimes fatal adverse effect of metformin ***related to renal impairment that does not support sufficient excretion of metformin.***
- Review the procedure with the patient. Address concerns about pain related to the procedure and explain that a sedative and/or analgesia will be administered to promote relaxation and reduce discomfort prior to the needle electrode insertion. Explain that any discomfort with the needle electrode will be minimized with local anesthetics and systemic analgesics. Inform the patient that the procedure is performed in the radiology department by a health-care provider (HCP), with support staff, and takes approximately 30 to 90 min.
- Explain that an intravenous (IV) line may be inserted to allow infusion of fluids such as saline, anesthetics, sedatives, contrast medium, or emergency medications.
- *Sensitivity to social and cultural issues,* as well as concern for modesty, is important in providing psychological support before, during, and after the procedure.
- Instruct the patient to remove jewelry and other metallic objects from the area to be examined prior to the procedure.
- Instruct the patient to fast and restrict fluids for 8 hr prior to the procedure. Instruct the patient to avoid taking anticoagulant medication or to reduce dosage as ordered prior to the procedure. Protocols may vary among facilities.
- *Make sure a written and informed consent has been signed prior to the procedure and before administering any medications.*

INTRATEST:

Potential Complications:

Complications related to the ablation are rare but may include brief or long-lasting shoulder pain, inflammation of the gallbladder, damage to the bile ducts with resulting biliary obstruction, thermal damage to the bowel, thermal damage to surrounding tissue resulting in cellulitis, hemorrhage, or flu-like symptoms that appear 3 to 5 days after the procedure and last for approximately 5 days.

Establishing an IV site and injecting contrast medium by catheter are invasive procedures. Complications are rare but do include risk for allergic reaction ***related to contrast reaction***; bleeding from the puncture site ***related to a bleeding disorder or the effects of natural products and medications with known anticoagulant, antiplatelet, and thrombolytic properties;*** hematoma ***related to blood leakage into the tissue following needle insertion;*** or infection ***that might occur if bacteria from the skin surface is introduced at the puncture site.***

- Observe standard precautions, and follow the general guidelines in Patient Preparation and Specimen Collection online at Davis*Plus*. Positively identify the patient.
- Ensure that the patient has complied with dietary, fluid, and medication restrictions and pretesting preparations prior to the procedure, as instructed.
- Ensure that the patient has removed all external metallic objects from the area to be examined prior to the procedure.
- Avoid the use of equipment containing latex if the patient has a history of allergic reaction to latex.

R

- Have emergency equipment readily available.
- Administer ordered prophylactic steroids or antihistamines before the procedure if the patient has a history of allergic reactions to any substance or drug.
- Instruct the patient to void and change into the gown, robe, and foot coverings provided.
- Instruct the patient to cooperate fully and to follow directions. Instruct the patient to remain still throughout the procedure because movement produces unreliable results.
- Record baseline vital signs and assess neurological status. Protocols may vary among facilities.
- Establish an IV fluid line for the injection of saline, sedatives, contrast medium, or emergency medications.
- Administer an antianxiety drug, as ordered, if the patient has claustrophobia. Administer a sedative to a child or to an uncooperative adult, as ordered.
- Place electrocardiographic electrodes on the patient for cardiac monitoring. Establish baseline rhythm; determine if the patient has ventricular dysrhythmias.
- Place the patient in the supine position on an examination table. Cleanse the selected area, and cover with a sterile drape.
- A local anesthetic is injected at the site, and a needle electrode is inserted under US, CT, or MRI guidance.
- A radiofrequency current is passed through the needle electrode, and the tumor is ablated.
- Instruct the patient to take slow, deep breaths if nausea occurs during the procedure. Monitor and administer an antiemetic drug if ordered. Ready an emesis basin for use.
- The needle electrode is removed, and a pressure dressing is applied over the puncture site.
- Observe/assess the needle electrode insertion site for bleeding, inflammation, or hematoma formation.
- Monitor the patient for complications related to the procedure (e.g., allergic reaction, anaphylaxis, bronchospasm).

POST-TEST:

- Inform the patient that a report of the results will be made available to the requesting HCP, who will discuss the results with the patient.
- Instruct the patient to resume usual diet, fluids, medications, and activity, as directed by the HCP. Kidney function should be assessed before metformin is resumed if contrast was used.
- Monitor vital signs and neurological status every 15 min for 1 hr, then every 2 hr for 4 hr, and as ordered. Take temperature every 6 hr for 24 hr. Compare with baseline values. Notify the HCP if temperature is elevated. Protocols may vary among facilities.
- Observe for delayed allergic reactions, such as rash, urticaria, tachycardia, hyperpnea, hypertension, palpitations, nausea, or vomiting.
- Instruct the patient to immediately report symptoms such as fast heart rate, difficulty breathing, skin rash, itching, chest pain, persistent right shoulder pain, or abdominal pain. Immediately report symptoms to the appropriate HCP.
- Instruct the patient to immediately report bile leakage, inflammation, any pleuritic pain, persistent right shoulder pain, or abdominal pain.
- Observe/assess the needle electrode insertion site for bleeding, inflammation, or hematoma formation.
- Instruct the patient in the care and assessment of the site.
- Instruct the patient to apply cold compresses to the puncture site as needed to reduce discomfort or edema.
- Instruct the patient to maintain bed rest for 4 to 6 hr after the procedure or as ordered.
- Recognize anxiety related to test results, and be supportive of impaired activity related to physical activity. Discuss the implications of abnormal test results on the patient's lifestyle. Provide teaching

R

and information regarding the clinical implications of the test results, as appropriate.
- Reinforce information given by the patient's HCP regarding further testing, treatment, or referral to another HCP. Answer any questions or address any concerns voiced by the patient or family.
- Depending on the results of this procedure, additional testing may be performed to evaluate or monitor progression of the disease process and determine the need for a change in therapy. Evaluate test results in relation to the patient's symptoms and other tests performed.

RELATED STUDIES:
- Related tests include ALT, angiography abdomen, AST, bilirubin, biopsy liver, CT liver, MRI abdomen, and US liver and biliary system.
- Refer to the Hepatobiliary System table online at Davis*Plus* for related tests by body system.

Radiography, Bone

SYNONYM/ACRONYM: Arm x-rays, bone x-rays, leg x-rays, orthopedic x-rays, rib x-rays, spine x-rays.

COMMON USE: To assist in evaluating bone pain, trauma, and abnormalities related to disorders or events such as dislocation, fracture, abuse, and degenerative disease.

AREA OF APPLICATION: Skeleton.

DESCRIPTION: Skeletal x-rays are noninvasive studies used to evaluate extremity pain or discomfort due to trauma, bone and spine abnormalities, or fluid within a joint. Serial skeletal x-rays are used to evaluate growth pattern. Radiation emitted from the x-ray machine passes through the patient onto an image receptor. X-rays pass through air freely and are absorbed by the anatomical structures of the body in varying degrees based on density. Bones are very dense and therefore absorb or attenuate most of the x-rays passing into the body and appear white; organs and muscles are denser than air but not as dense as bone, so they appear in various shades of gray. Metals absorb x-rays and appear white and thus facilitate the search for foreign bodies in the patient.

This procedure is contraindicated for

Patients who are pregnant or suspected of being pregnant, unless the potential benefits of a procedure using radiation far outweigh the risk of radiation exposure to the fetus and mother.

INDICATIONS
- Assist in detecting bone fracture, dislocation, deformity, and degeneration.
- Evaluate for child or elder abuse.
- Evaluate growth pattern.
- Identify abnormalities of bones, joints, and surrounding tissues.
- Monitor fracture healing process.

R

POTENTIAL MEDICAL DIAGNOSIS

Normal findings

- *Infants and children:* Thin plate of cartilage, known as growth plate or epiphyseal plate, between the shaft and both ends
- *Adolescents and adults:* By age 17, calcification of cartilage plate; no evidence of fracture, congenital abnormalities, tumors, or infection

Abnormal findings related to

- Arthritis
- Bone degeneration
- Bone spurs
- Foreign bodies
- Fracture
- Genetic disturbance (achondroplasia, dysplasia, dyostosis)
- Hormonal disturbance
- Infection, including osteomyelitis
- Injury
- Joint dislocation or effusion
- Nutritional or metabolic disturbances
- Osteoporosis or osteopenia
- Soft tissue abnormalities
- Tumor or neoplastic disease (osteogenic sarcoma, Paget's disease, myeloma)

CRITICAL FINDINGS: N/A

INTERFERING FACTORS:

Factors that may alter the results of the study

- Retained barium from a previous radiological procedure.
- Metallic objects (e.g., jewelry, body rings) within the examination field, which may inhibit organ visualization and can produce unclear images.
- Inability of the patient to cooperate or remain still during the procedure because of age, significant pain, or mental status.

Other considerations: N/A

NURSING IMPLICATIONS AND PROCEDURE

See Potential Nursing Problems on Fast Find at davispl.us/vanleeuwen7.

PRETEST:

- Positively identify the patient using at least two person-specific identifiers before services, treatments, or procedures are performed.
- *Patient Teaching:* Inform the patient this procedure can assist in examining bone structure.
- Obtain a history of the patient's health concerns, symptoms, surgical procedures, and results of previously performed laboratory and diagnostic studies. Include a list of known allergens, especially allergies or sensitivities to latex, anesthetics, or sedatives.
- Record the date of the last menstrual period and determine the possibility of pregnancy in perimenopausal women.
- Obtain a list of the patient's current medications, including over-the-counter medications and dietary supplements (see Effects of Natural Products on Laboratory Values online at Davis*Plus*).
- Review the procedure with the patient. Explain that numerous x-rays may be taken depending on the bones or joint affected. Address concerns about pain and explain that some pain may be experienced during the test, or there may be moments of discomfort. Inform the patient that the procedure is performed in the radiology department by a health-care provider (HCP), with support staff, and takes approximately 10 to 30 min.

  Pediatric Considerations: Preparation of children for a bone radiography depends on the age of the child. Encourage parents to be truthful about what the child may experience during the procedure and to use words that they know their child will understand. Toddlers and preschool-age children have short attention

R

spans, so the best time to talk about the test is right before the procedure. The child should be assured that he or she will be allowed to bring a favorite comfort item into the examination room, and if appropriate, that a parent will be with the child during the procedure. Provide older children with information about the test and allow them to participate in as many decisions as possible (e.g., choice of clothes to wear to the appointment) in order to reduce anxiety and encourage cooperation. If the child will be asked to maintain a certain position for the test, encourage the child to practice the required position, provide a CD that demonstrates the procedure, and teach strategies to remain calm, such as deep breathing, humming, or counting to himself or herself.

- *Sensitivity to social and cultural issues,* as well as concern for modesty, is important in providing psychological support before, during, and after the procedure.
- Instruct the patient to inhale deeply and hold his or her breath while the image is taken. Warn the patient that the extremity's position during the procedure may be uncomfortable, but ask the patient to hold still during the procedure because movement will produce unclear images.
- Instruct the patient to remove jewelry and other metallic objects from the area to be examined prior to the procedure.
- Note that there are no food, fluid, or medication restrictions unless by medical direction.

R

INTRATEST:

Potential Complications: N/A

- Observe standard precautions, and follow the general guidelines in Patient Preparation and Specimen Collection online at Davis*Plus*. Positively identify the patient.
- Ensure that the patient has removed all external metallic objects from the area to be examined prior to the procedure.
- Avoid the use of equipment containing latex if the patient has a history of allergic reaction to latex.
- Have emergency equipment readily available.
- Instruct the patient to void prior to the procedure and to change into the gown, robe, and foot coverings provided.
- Place patient in a standing, sitting, or recumbent position in front of the image receptor.
- Ask the patient to inhale deeply and hold his or her breath while the x-ray images are taken.
- Instruct the patient to cooperate fully and to follow directions. Ask the patient to remain still throughout the procedure because movement produces unreliable results.

POST-TEST:

- Inform the patient that a report of the examination will be sent to the requesting HCP, who will discuss the results with the patient.
- Recognize anxiety related to test results, and be supportive of impaired activity related to the perceived loss of daily function. Discuss the implications of abnormal test results on the patient's lifestyle. Provide teaching and information regarding the clinical implications of the test results, as appropriate. Provide contact information, if desired, for the American College of Rheumatology (www.rheumatology.org) or the Arthritis Foundation (www.arthritis.org). 🍁
- Reinforce information given by the patient's HCP regarding further testing, treatment, or referral to another HCP. Explain the importance of adhering to the therapy regimen. Answer any questions or address any concerns voiced by the patient or family.
- Depending on the results of this procedure, additional testing may be performed to evaluate or monitor progression of the disease process and determine the need for a change in therapy. Evaluate test results in relation to the patient's symptoms and other tests performed.

Patient Education:

- Teach the patient how to decrease fall risk by adhering to fall risk protocols.
- Teach the patient the signs and symptoms of impinged circulation due to cast or appliance application.

Expected Patient Outcomes:

Understanding

- The patient acknowledges the importance of participating in activity to maintain functional levels.
- The patient acknowledges the importance of adequate pain management to facilitate activity.

Ability

- The patient successfully demonstrates the use of assistive devices to support mobility.
- The patient and family demonstrate how to care for a cast or other assistive device (application and removal as appropriate).

Response

- The patient agrees to participate in recommend physical therapy to improve mobility.
- The patient agrees to participate in fall risk programs.

RELATED STUDIES:

- Related tests include antibodies anti-cyclic citrullinated peptide, ANA, arthrogram, arthroscopy, biopsy bone, BMD, bone scan, calcium, CBC, CRP, collagen cross-linked telopeptides, CT spine, ESR, MRI musculoskeletal, osteocalcin, phosphorus, synovial fluid analysis, RF, vitamin D, and WBC scan.
- Refer to the Musculoskeletal System table online at Davis*Plus* for related tests by body system.

Red Blood Cell Cholinesterase

SYNONYM/ACRONYM: Acetylcholinesterase (AChE), erythrocyte cholinesterase, true cholinesterase.

COMMON USE: To assess for pesticide toxicity and screen for cholinesterase deficiency, which may contribute to unrecoverable apnea after surgical induction with succinylcholine.

SPECIMEN: Whole blood collected in a lavender-top (EDTA) tube.

NORMAL FINDINGS: (Method: Enzymatic)

Test	Conventional Units
RBC cholinesterase	9,500–15,000 units/L

POTENTIAL MEDICAL DIAGNOSIS

Increased in:

- Hemolytic anemias (e.g., sickle cell anemia, thalassemias, spherocytosis, and acquired hemolytic anemias) ***(increased in hemolytic anemias as AChE is released from the hemolyzed RBCs)***

Decreased in:

- Insecticide exposure ***(organic phosphate insecticides inhibit AChE activity)***
- Late pregnancy ***(related to anemia of pregnancy)***
- Paroxysmal nocturnal hemoglobinuria ***(related to lack***

of RBC production by bone marrow)

- Relapse of megaloblastic anemia ***(related to underproduction of normal RBCs containing AChE)***

CRITICAL FINDINGS: N/A

Find and print out the full study on Fast Find at davispl.us/vanleeuwen7.

Refraction

SYNONYM/ACRONYM: N/A

COMMON USE: To assess the visual acuity of the eyes in patients of all ages, to evaluate visual acuity as required by driver licensing laws, and to assist in evaluating the eyes prior to therapeutic interventions such as eyeglasses, contact lenses, low vision aids, cataract surgery, or laser-assisted in situ keratomileusis (LASIK) surgery.

AREA OF APPLICATION: Eyes.

DESCRIPTION: This noninvasive procedure tests the visual acuity (VA) of the eyes and determines abnormalities or refractive errors that need correction. Refractions are performed using a combination of different pieces of equipment. Refractive error can be quickly and accurately measured using computerized automatic refractors or manually with a viewing system consisting of an entire set of trial lenses mounted on a circular wheel (phoropter). A projector may also be used to display test letters and characters from Snellen eye charts for use in assessing VA. If the VA is worse than 20/20, the pinhole test may be used to quickly assess the best corrected vision. Refractive errors of the peripheral cornea and lens can be reduced or eliminated by having the patient look through a pinhole at the vision test. Patients with cataracts or visual field defects will not show improved results using the pinhole test. The retinoscope is probably the most valuable instrument that can be used to objectively assess VA. It is also the only objective means of assessing refractive error in pediatric patients and patients who are unable to cooperate with other techniques of assessing refractive error due to illiteracy, senility, or inability to speak the same language as the examiner. Visual defects identified through refraction, such as hyperopia (farsightedness), in which the point of focus lies behind the retina; myopia (nearsightedness), in which the point of focus lies in front of the retina; and astigmatism, in which the refraction is unequal in different curvatures of the eyeball, can be corrected by glasses, contact lenses, or refractive surgery.

This procedure is contraindicated for

- Patients with narrow-angle glaucoma if pupil dilation is performed; dilation can initiate a severe and sight-threatening open-angle attack.

Patients with allergies to mydriatics if pupil dilation using mydriatics is performed.

INDICATIONS

- Determine if an optical defect is present and if light rays entering the eye focus correctly on the retina.
- Determine the refractive error prior to refractive surgery such as radial keratotomy, photorefractive keratotomy, LASIK, intracorneal rings, limbal relaxing incisions, implantable contact lens (phakic intraocular lens), clear lens replacement.
- Determine the type of corrective lenses (e.g., biconvex or plus lenses for hyperopia, biconcave or minus lenses for myopia, compensatory lenses for astigmatism) needed for refractive errors.
- Diagnose refractive errors in vision.

POTENTIAL MEDICAL DIAGNOSIS

Visual Acuity Scale

Foot	Meter	Decimal
20/200	6/60	0.1
20/160	6/48	0.13
20/120	6/36	0.17
20/100	6/30	0.2
20/80	6/24	0.25
20/60	6/18	0.33
20/50	6/15	0.4
20/40	6/12	0.5
20/30	6/9	0.67
20/25	6/7.5	0.8
20/20	6/6	1
20/16	6/4.8	1.25
20/12	6/3.6	1.67
20/10	6/3	2

VA can be expressed fractionally in feet, fractionally in meters, or as a decimal where perfect vision of 20/20 feet or 6/6 meters is equal to 1. Comparing the fraction in feet or meters to the decimal helps demonstrate that acuity less than 20/20, or less than 1.0, is “worse” vision, and acuity greater than 20/20, or greater than 1.0, is “better.” A patient who cannot achieve best corrected VA of 20/200 or above (greater than 0.1) in his or her better eye is considered legally blind in the United States.

Uncorrected Visual Acuity	Foot	Meter	Decimal
Mild vision loss	20/30–20/70	6/9–6/21	0.67–0.29
Moderate vision loss	20/80–20/160	6/24–6/48	0.25–0.13
Severe vision loss	20/200–20/400	6/60–6/120	0.1–0.05
Profound vision loss	20/500–20/1,000	6/150–6/300	0.04–0.02

Normal findings

- Normal visual acuity; 20/20 (with corrective lenses if appropriate)

Abnormal findings related to

- Refractive errors such as anisometropia, astigmatism, hyperopia, myopia, and presbyopia

CRITICAL FINDINGS: N/A

INTERFERING FACTORS

Factors that may alter the results of the study

- Improper pupil dilation may prevent adequate examination for refractive error.
- Inability of the patient to cooperate and remain still during the procedure because of age, significant pain, or mental status may interfere with the test results.
- Failure to follow medication restrictions before the procedure may cause the procedure to be canceled or repeated.

NURSING IMPLICATIONS AND PROCEDURE

PRETEST:

- Positively identify the patient using at least two person-specific identifiers before services, treatments, or procedures are performed.
- *Patient Teaching:* Inform the patient this procedure can assist in assessing visual acuity.
- Obtain a history of the patient's health concerns (especially known or suspected vision loss; changes in visual acuity, including type and cause; use of glasses or contact lenses; eye conditions with treatment regimens; eye surgery; and other tests and procedures to assess and diagnose visual deficit), symptoms, surgical procedures, and results of previously performed laboratory and diagnostic studies.
Include a list of known allergens, especially allergies or sensitivities to latex and mydriatics (if dilation is to be performed).
- Obtain a list of the patient's current medications, including over-the-counter medications and dietary supplements (see Effects of Natural Products on Laboratory Values online at Davis*Plus*).
- Instruct the patient to remove contact lenses or glasses, as appropriate. Instruct the patient regarding the importance of keeping the eyes open for the test.
- Review the procedure with the patient. Address concerns about pain and explain that mydriatics, if used, may cause blurred vision and sensitivity to light. There may also be a brief stinging sensation when the drop is put in the eye. Inform the patient that a health-care provider (HCP) performs the test, in a quiet, darkened room, and that to evaluate both eyes, the test can take up 30 min (including time for the pupils to dilate before the test is actually performed).
- *Sensitivity to social and cultural issues,* as well as concern for modesty, is important in providing psychological support before, during, and after the procedure.
- Note that there are no food or fluid restrictions unless by medical direction.
- Instruct the patient to withhold eye medications (particularly miotic eye drops which may constrict the pupil preventing a clear view of the fundus and mydriatic eyedrops in order to avoid instigation of an acute open angle attack in patients with narrow angle glaucoma) for at least 1 day prior to the test.
- Ensure that the patient understands that he or she must refrain from driving until the pupils return to normal (about 4 hr) after the test and has made arrangements to have someone else be responsible for transportation after the test.

INTRATEST:

Potential Complications:

Dilation can initiate a severe and sight-threatening open-angle attack in patients with narrow-angle glaucoma.

- Observe standard precautions, and follow the general guidelines in Patient Preparation and Specimen Collection online at Davis*Plus*. Positively identify the patient.
- Ensure that the patient has complied with medication restrictions and pretesting preparations prior to the procedure, as instructed.
- Instruct the patient to cooperate fully and to follow directions. Ask the patient to remain still during the procedure because movement produces unreliable results.
- If dilation is to be performed, administer the ordered mydriatic to each eye and repeat in 5 to 15 min. Drops are placed in the eye with the patient looking up and the solution directed at the six o'clock position of the sclera (white of the eye) near the limbus (gray, semitransparent area of the eyeball where the cornea and sclera meet). The dropper bottle should not touch the eyelashes.
- Ask the patient to place the chin in the chin rest and gently press the forehead against the support bar. The examiner will sit about 2 ft away at eye level with the patient. The retinoscope light is held in front of the eyes and directed through the pupil. Each eye is also examined for the characteristics of the red reflex, the reflection of the light from the retinoscope, which normally moves in the same direction as the light.
- Request that the patient look straight ahead while the eyes are examined with the instrument and while different lenses are tried to provide the best corrective lenses to be prescribed. When optimal VA is obtained with the trial lenses in each eye, a prescription for corrective lenses is written.

POST-TEST:

- Inform the patient that a report of the results will be made available to the requesting HCP, who will discuss the results with the patient.
- Instruct the patient to resume usual medications, as directed by the HCP.
- Recognize anxiety related to test results, and be supportive of impaired activity related to vision loss, anticipated loss of driving privileges, or the possibility of requiring corrective lenses (self-image). Discuss the implications of abnormal test results on the patient's lifestyle. Provide teaching and information regarding the clinical implications of the test results, as appropriate. Provide contact information, if desired, for a general patient education Web site on the topic of eye care (e.g., www.allaboutvision.com). 🍁
- Reinforce information given by the patient's HCP regarding further testing, treatment, or referral to another HCP. Inform the patient that visual acuity and responses to light may change. Suggest that the patient wear dark glasses after the test until the pupils return to normal size. Answer any questions or address any concerns voiced by the patient or family.
- Depending on the results of this procedure, additional testing may be performed to evaluate or monitor progression of the disease process and determine the need for a change in therapy. Evaluate test results in relation to the patient's symptoms and other tests performed.

RELATED STUDIES:

- Related tests include color perception test, intraocular muscle function, intraocular pressure, Schirmer tear test, and slit-lamp biomicroscopy.
- Refer to the Ocular System table online at Davis*Plus* for related tests by body system.

R

Renin

SYNONYM/ACRONYM: Plasma renin activity (PRA), angiotensinogenase.

COMMON USE: To assist in evaluating for a possible cause of hypertension.

SPECIMEN: Plasma collected in a lavender-top (EDTA) or pink-top (K_2EDTA) tube.

NORMAL FINDINGS: (Method: Radioimmunoassay)

Age and Position	Conventional Units	SI Units (Conventional Units × 1)
Newborn–12 mo	2–35 ng/mL/hr	2–35 mcg/L/hr
Supine, normal sodium diet		
1–3 yr	1.7–11.2 ng/mL/hr	1.7–11.2 mcg/L/hr
4–5 yr	1–6.5 ng/mL/hr	1.0–6.5 mcg/L/hr
6–10 yr	0.5–5.9 ng/mL/hr	0.5–5.9 mcg/L/hr
11–15 yr	0.5–3.3 ng/mL/hr	0.5–3.3 mcg/L/hr
Adult	0.2–2.3 ng/mL/hr	0.2–2.3 mcg/L/hr
Upright, normal sodium diet		
Adult–older adult	1.3–4 ng/mL/hr	1.3–4 mcg/L/hr

Values vary according to the laboratory performing the test, as well as the patient's age, gender, dietary pattern, state of hydration, posture, and physical activity.

DESCRIPTION: Renin is an enzymatic peptide hormone secreted by the granular cells of the juxtaglomerular apparatus in the kidney in response to sodium depletion and hypovolemia. Renin activates the renin-angiotensin system through the conversion of angiotensinogen to angiotensin I. Angiotensin I is converted to the biologically active angiotensin II by angiotensin-converting enzyme primarily within the capillaries of the lungs. Angiotensin II is a powerful vasoconstrictor that ultimately maintains the appropriate perfusion pressure in the kidneys. Angiotensin II stimulates aldosterone production in the adrenal cortex, secretion of antidiuretic hormone from the pituitary, and stimulates the thirst reflex from the hypothalmus. The net effect is regulation of blood pressure by regulating arterial vasoconstriction and the movement of extracellular fluids such as plasma, lymphatic fluid, and interstitial fluid. Excessive amounts of angiotensin II cause renal hypertension. The random collection of specimens without prior dietary preparations does not provide clinically significant information. Values should also be evaluated along with simultaneously collected aldosterone levels (see studies titled "Aldosterone" and "Angiotensin-Converting Enzyme").

R

This procedure is contraindicated for: N/A

INDICATIONS

- Assist in the identification of primary hyperaldosteronism resulting from aldosterone-secreting adrenal adenoma.
- Assist in monitoring patients on mineralocorticoid therapy.
- Assist in the screening of the origin of essential, renal, or renovascular hypertension.

POTENTIAL MEDICAL DIAGNOSIS

Increased in:

- Addison's disease ***(related to hyponatremia, which stimulates production of renin)***
- Bartter's syndrome ***(related to hereditary defect in loop of Henle that affects sodium resorption; hyponatremia stimulates renin production)***
- Cirrhosis ***(related to fluid buildup, which dilutes sodium concentration; hyponatremia is a strong stimulus for production of renin)***
- Gastrointestinal disorders with electrolyte loss ***(related to hyponatremia, which stimulates production of renin)***
- Heart failure ***(related to fluid buildup, which dilutes sodium concentration; hyponatremia is a strong stimulus for production of renin)***
- Hepatitis ***(related to fluid buildup, which dilutes sodium concentration; hyponatremia is a strong stimulus for production of renin)***
- Hypokalemia ***(related to decreased potassium levels, which stimulate renin production)***
- Malignant hypertension ***(related to secondary hyperaldosteronism that constricts the blood vessels and results in hypertension)***
- Nephritis ***(the kidneys can produce renin in response to inflammation or disease)***
- Nephropathies with sodium or potassium wasting ***(related to hyponatremia, which stimulates production of renin)***
- Pheochromocytoma ***(related to renin production in response to hypertension)***
- Pregnancy ***(related to retention of fluid and hyponatremia that stimulates renin production; normal pregnancy is associated with changes in the balance between renin and angiotensin)***
- Renin-producing kidney tumors
- Renovascular hypertension ***(related to decreased renal blood flow, which stimulates release of renin)***

Decreased in:

- Cushing's syndrome ***(related to excessive production of glucocorticoids, which increase sodium levels and decrease potassium levels, inhibiting renin production)***
- Primary hyperaldosteronism ***(related to aldosterone-secreting adrenal tumor; aldosterone inhibits renin production)***

CRITICAL FINDINGS: N/A

INTERFERING FACTORS

- Drugs and other substances that may increase renin levels include albuterol, amiloride, azosemide, benazepril, bendroflumethiazide, captopril, chlorthalidone, cilazapril, desmopressin, diazoxide, dihydralazine, doxazosin, enalapril, endralazine, felodipine, fenoldopam, fosinopril, furosemide, hydralazine, hydrochlorothiazide, laxatives, lisinopril, lithium, methyclothiazide, metolazone, muzolimine, nicardipine, nifedipine, opiates, oral contraceptives, perindopril, ramipril, spironolactone, triamterene, and xipamide.

- Drugs and other substances that may decrease renin levels include acetylsalicylic acid, angiotensin, angiotensin II, atenolol, bopindolol, bucindolol, carbenoxolone, carvedilol, clonidine, cyclosporin A, glycyrrhiza, ibuprofen, indomethacin, levodopa, metoprolol, naproxen, nicardipine, NSAIDs, oral contraceptives, oxprenolol, propranolol, sulindac, and vasopressin.
- Upright body posture, stress, and strenuous exercise can increase renin levels.
- Recent radioactive scans or radiation can interfere with test results when radioimmunoassay is the test method.
- Diet can significantly affect results (e.g., low-sodium diets stimulate the release of renin).
- Hyperkalemia, acute increase in blood pressure, and increased blood volume may suppress renin secretion.
- Failure to follow dietary restrictions before the procedure may cause the procedure to be canceled or repeated.

NURSING IMPLICATIONS AND PROCEDURE

R

PRETEST:

- Positively identify the patient using at least two person-specific identifiers before services, treatments, or procedures are performed.
- *Patient Teaching:* Inform the patient this test can assist in evaluating for high blood pressure.
- Obtain a history of the patient's health concerns, symptoms, surgical procedures, and results of previously performed laboratory and diagnostic studies. Include a list of known allergens, especially allergies or sensitivities to latex.
- Note any recent procedures that can interfere with test results.
- Obtain a list of the patient's current medications, including over-the-counter medications and dietary supplements (see Effects of Natural Products on Laboratory Values online at Davis*Plus*).
- Review the procedure with the patient. Inform the patient or family member that the position required (supine or upright) must be maintained for 2 hr before specimen collection. Inform the patient that multiple specimens may be required. Inform the patient that specimen collection takes approximately 5 to 10 min. Address concerns about pain and explain that there may be some discomfort during the venipuncture.
- *Sensitivity to social and cultural issues,* as well as concern for modesty, is important in providing psychological support before, during, and after the procedure.
- The patient should be on a normal sodium diet (1 to 2 g sodium per day) for 2 to 4 wk before the test. Protocols may vary among facilities.
- By medical direction, the patient should avoid diuretics, antihypertensive drugs, herbals, cyclic progestogens, and estrogens for 2 to 4 wk before the test.
- Prepare an ice slurry in a cup or plastic bag to have ready for immediate transport of the specimen to the laboratory.

INTRATEST:

Potential Complications: N/A

- Ensure that the patient has complied with diet and medication restrictions prior to the study, as instructed.
- Avoid the use of equipment containing latex if the patient has a history of allergic reaction to latex.
- Instruct the patient to cooperate fully and to follow directions. Direct the patient to breathe normally and to avoid unnecessary movement.

- Observe standard precautions, and follow the general guidelines in Patient Preparation and Specimen Collection online at Davis*Plus*. Positively identify the patient, and label the appropriate tubes with the corresponding patient demographics, date, and time of collection. Specify patient position (upright or supine) and exact source of specimen (peripheral vs. arterial). Perform a venipuncture after the patient has been in the upright (sitting or standing) position for 2 hr. If a supine specimen is requested on an inpatient, the specimen should be collected early in the morning before the patient rises.
- Remove the needle and apply direct pressure with dry gauze to stop bleeding. Observe/assess venipuncture site for bleeding or hematoma formation and secure gauze with adhesive bandage.
- The sample should be placed in an ice slurry immediately after collection. Information on the specimen label should be protected from water in the ice slurry by first placing the specimen in a protective plastic bag. Promptly transport the specimen to the laboratory for processing and analysis.

POST-TEST:

- Inform the patient that a report of the results will be made available to the requesting health-care provider (HCP), who will discuss the results with the patient.
- Instruct the patient to resume usual medications, as directed by the HCP.
- ***Nutritional Considerations:*** Instruct the patient to notify the requesting HCP of any signs and symptoms of dehydration or fluid overload related to abnormal renin levels or compromised sodium regulatory mechanisms. Fluid loss or dehydration is signaled by the thirst response. Decreased skin turgor, dry mouth, and multiple longitudinal furrows in the tongue are symptoms of dehydration. Fluid overload may be signaled by a loss of appetite and nausea. Excessive fluid also causes pitting edema: When firm pressure is placed on the skin over a bone (e.g., the ankle), the indentation will remain after 5 sec.
- ***Nutritional Considerations:*** Educate patients of the importance of proper water balance. In buildings with hard water, untreated tap water contains minerals such as calcium, magnesium, and iron. Water-softening systems replace these minerals with sodium, and therefore patients on a low-sodium diet should avoid drinking treated tap water and drink bottled water instead.
- ***Nutritional Considerations:*** Renin levels affect the regulation of fluid balance and electrolytes. If appropriate, educate patients with low sodium levels that the major source of dietary sodium is found in table salt. Many foods, such as milk and other dairy products, are also good sources of dietary sodium. Most other dietary sodium is available through the consumption of processed foods. Patients on low-sodium diets should be advised to avoid beverages such as colas, ginger ale, sports drinks, lemon-lime sodas, and root beer. Many over-the-counter medications, including antacids, laxatives, analgesics, sedatives, and antitussives, contain significant amounts of sodium. The best advice is to emphasize the importance of reading all food, beverage, and medicine labels. The requesting HCP or nutritionist should be consulted before the patient on a low-sodium diet begins using salt substitutes. Potassium is present in all plant and animal cells, making dietary replacement fairly simple to achieve.
- Reinforce information given by the patient's HCP regarding further testing, treatment, or referral to another HCP. Answer any questions or address any concerns voiced by the patient or family.
- Depending on the results of this procedure, additional testing may be performed to evaluate or monitor progression of the disease process and determine the need for a change

R

in therapy. Evaluate test results in relation to the patient's symptoms and other tests performed.

RELATED STUDIES:

- Related tests include ACTH, ALT, aldosterone, ACE, AST, ANP, BNP, bilirubin, biopsy kidney, BUN, calcium, chloride, cortisol, creatinine, DHEAS, fecal fat, GGT, glucose, GTT, magnesium, metanephrines, potassium, protein total and fractions, renogram, sodium, UA, and VMA.
- Refer to the Endocrine and Genitourinary systems tables online at Davis*Plus* for related tests by body system.

Renogram

SYNONYM/ACRONYM: Radioactive renogram, renocystography, renocystogram, renal scintigraphy.

COMMON USE: To assist in diagnosing kidney disorders such as embolism, obstruction, infection, inflammation, trauma, stones, and bleeding.

AREA OF APPLICATION: Kidneys.

DESCRIPTION: A renogram is a nuclear medicine study performed to assist in diagnosing renal disorders, such as abnormal blood flow, collecting-system defects, and excretion dysfunction. Because renography uses no iodinated contrast medium, it is safe to use in patients who have iodine allergies or compromised renal function.

After intravenous (IV) administration of the radioisotope, information about the structures of the kidneys is obtained. The radioactive material is detected by a gamma camera, which can detect the gamma rays emitted by the radionuclide in the kidney. Renography simultaneously tracks the rate at which the radionuclide flows into *(vascular phase),* through *(tubular phase),* and out of *(excretory phase)* the kidneys. The times are plotted on a graph and compared to normal parameters of organ function. Differential estimates of left and right kidney contributions to glomerular filtration rate and effective renal plasma flow can be calculated. With the use of diuretic stimulation during the excretory phase, it is possible to differentiate between anatomic obstruction and nonobstructive residual dilation from previous hydronephrosis. All information obtained is stored in a computer to be used for further interpretation and computations. Kidney function can be monitored by serially repeating this test and comparing results.

This procedure is contraindicated for

Patients who are pregnant or suspected of being pregnant, unless the potential benefits of a procedure using radiation far outweigh the risk of radiation exposure to the fetus and mother.

INDICATIONS

- Aid in the diagnosis of renal artery embolism or renal infarction causing obstruction.
- Aid in the diagnosis of renal artery stenosis resulting from renal

R

dysplasia or atherosclerosis and causing arterial hypertension and reduced glomerular filtration rate.
- Aid in the diagnosis of renal vein thrombosis resulting from dehydration in infants or obstruction of blood flow in the presence of renal tumors in adults.
- Detect infectious or inflammatory diseases of the kidney, such as acute or chronic pyelonephritis, abscess, or nephritis.
- Determine the presence and effects of kidney trauma, such as arterial injury, renal contusion, hematoma, rupture, arteriovenous fistula, or urinary extravasation.
- Determine the presence, location, and cause of obstructive uropathy, such as calculi, neoplasm, congenital disorders, scarring, or inflammation.
- Evaluate acute kidney injury and chronic kidney disease.
- Evaluate chronic urinary tract infections, especially in children.
- Evaluate kidney transplant for acute or chronic rejection.
- Evaluate obstruction caused by stones or tumor.

POTENTIAL MEDICAL DIAGNOSIS

Normal findings

- Normal shape, size, position, symmetry, vasculature, perfusion, and function of the kidneys
- Radionuclide material circulates bilaterally, symmetrically, and without interruption through the renal parenchyma, ureters, and urinary bladder, with 50% of the radionuclide excreted within the first 10 min

Abnormal findings related to

- Acute tubular necrosis
- Chronic kidney disease, infarction, cyst, or abscess
- Congenital anomalies (e.g., absence of a kidney)
- Decreased kidney function
- Diminished blood supply
- Infection or inflammation (pyelonephritis, glomerulonephritis)
- Masses
- Obstructive uropathy
- Renal vascular disease, including renal artery stenosis or renal vein thrombosis
- Trauma

CRITICAL FINDINGS: N/A

INTERFERING FACTORS

Factors that may alter the results of the study

- Inability of the patient to cooperate or remain still during the procedure because of age, significant pain, or mental status.
- Serum creatinine levels greater than or equal to 3 mg/dL (depending on the radionuclide used), which can decrease renal perfusion.
- Other nuclear medicine studies done within the previous 24 to 48 hr.
- Medications such as antihypertensives, angiotensin-converting enzyme (ACE) inhibitors, and β-blockers taken within 24 hr of the test.
- Dehydration, which can accentuate abnormalities, or overhydration, which can mask abnormalities.
- Metallic objects (e.g., jewelry, body rings) within the examination field, which may inhibit organ visualization.

Other considerations

- Inaccurate timing of imaging after the radionuclide injection can affect the results.

NURSING IMPLICATIONS AND PROCEDURE

See Potential Nursing Problems on Fast Find at davispl.us/vanleeuwen7.

PRETEST:

- Positively identify the patient using at least two person-specific identifiers

before services, treatments, or procedures are performed.

- ***Patient Teaching:*** Inform the patient this procedure can assist in assessing the renal system.
- Obtain a history of the patient's health concerns, symptoms, surgical procedures, and results of previously performed laboratory and diagnostic studies. Include a list of known allergens, especially allergies or sensitivities to latex, anesthetics, sedatives, or radionuclides.
- Obtain a history of the patient's genitourinary system, symptoms, and results of previously performed laboratory tests and diagnostic and surgical procedures.
- Record the date of the last menstrual period and determine the possibility of pregnancy in perimenopausal women.
- Obtain a list of the patient's current medications, including over-the-counter medications and dietary supplements (see Effects of Natural Products on Laboratory Values online at Davis*Plus*).
- Review the procedure with the patient. Address concerns about pain related to the procedure and explain that some pain may be experienced during the test, and there may be moments of discomfort. Reassure the patient that radioactive material poses minimal radioactive hazard because of its short half-life and rarely produces adverse effects. Inform the patient that the procedure is performed in a nuclear medicine department by a health-care provider (HCP) and usually takes approximately 60 to 90 min, and that delayed images are needed 2 to 24 hr later. The patient may leave the department and return later to undergo delayed imaging.
- ***Sensitivity to social and cultural issues,*** as well as concern for modesty, is important in providing psychological support before, during, and after the procedure.
- Explain that an IV line may be inserted to allow infusion of fluids such as saline, anesthetics, sedatives, radionuclides, medications used in the procedure, or emergency medications.
- Instruct the patient to remove jewelry and other metallic objects from the area to be examined prior to the procedure.
- Inform the patient that he or she will be asked to drink several glasses of fluid before the study for hydration, unless the patient has a restricted fluid intake for other reasons.
- Note that there are no food or medication restrictions unless by medical direction.

INTRATEST:

Potential Complications:

Although it is rare, there is the possibility of allergic reaction to the radionuclide. Have emergency equipment and medications readily available. If the patient has a history of allergic reactions to any substance or drug, administer ordered prophylactic steroids or antihistamines before the procedure.

Establishing an IV site and injecting radionuclides is an invasive procedure. Complications are rare but do include bleeding from the puncture site ***related to a bleeding disorder or the effects of natural products and medications with known anticoagulant, antiplatelet, or thrombolytic properties;*** hematoma ***related to blood leakage into the tissue following needle insertion;*** infection ***that might occur if bacteria from the skin surface is introduced at the puncture site;*** or nerve injury ***that might occur if the needle strikes a nerve.***

- Observe standard precautions, and follow the general guidelines in Patient Preparation and Specimen Collection online at Davis*Plus*. Positively identify the patient.
- Ensure that the patient has removed external metallic objects from the area to be examined prior to the procedure.

R

- Instruct the patient to void and change into the gown, robe, and foot coverings provided.
- Avoid the use of equipment containing latex if the patient has a history of allergic reaction to latex.
- Have emergency equipment readily available.
- Record baseline vital signs and assess neurological status. Protocols may vary among facilities.
- Establish an IV fluid line for the injection of saline, anesthetics, sedatives, radionuclides, or emergency medications.
- Administer sedative to a child or to an uncooperative adult, as ordered.
- Place the patient in a supine position on a flat table with foam wedges to help maintain position and immobilization.
- The radionuclide is administered IV, and the kidney area is scanned immediately with images taken every minute for 30 min.
- During the flow and static imaging, the diuretic furosemide or ACE inhibitor (captopril) can be administered IV and images obtained.
- Urine and blood laboratory studies are done after the renogram to correlate findings before diagnosis.
- If a study for vesicoureteral reflux is done, the patient is asked to void, and a catheter is inserted into the bladder. The radionuclide is instilled into the bladder, and multiple images are obtained during bladder filling. The patient is then requested to void, with the catheter in place or after catheter removal, depending on department policy. Imaging is continued during and after voiding. Reflux is determined by calculating the urine volume and counts obtained by imaging.
- Gloves should be worn during the radionuclide administration and while handling the patient's urine.
- Remove the needle or catheter and apply a pressure dressing over the puncture site.
- Observe/assess the needle/catheter insertion site for bleeding, inflammation, or hematoma formation.

POST-TEST:

- Inform the patient that a report of the results will be made available to the requesting HCP, who will discuss the results with the patient.
- Unless contraindicated, advise patient to drink increased amounts of fluids for 24 hr to eliminate the radionuclide from the body. Inform the patient that radionuclide is eliminated from the body within 6 to 24 hr.
- Instruct the patient to immediately flush the toilet and to meticulously wash hands with soap and water after each voiding for 24 hr after the procedure.
- Instruct all caregivers to wear gloves when discarding urine for 24 hr after the procedure. Wash gloved hands with soap and water before removing gloves; then wash ungloved hands.
- Observe/assess the needle/catheter site for bleeding, hematoma formation, and inflammation.
- Instruct the patient in the care and assessment of the site.
- Instruct the patient to apply cold compresses to the puncture site as needed to reduce discomfort or edema.
- Recognize anxiety related to test results. Discuss the implications of abnormal test results on the patient's lifestyle. Provide teaching and information regarding the clinical importance of the test results, as appropriate.
- Reinforce information given by the patient's HCP regarding further testing, treatment, or referral to another HCP. Answer any questions or address any concerns voiced by the patient or family.
- Depending on the results of this procedure, additional testing may be needed to evaluate or monitor progression of the disease process and determine the need for a change in therapy. Evaluate test results in relation to the patient's symptoms and other tests performed.

Patient Education:

- Teach the patient to avoid foods that facilitate stone formation (tea, beer,

R

chocolate) when diagnosed with stones.
- Teach the patient foods that can discourage stone formation, such as milk and milk products.

Expected Patient Outcomes:

Understanding
- The patient and family acknowledge the importance of increased oral intake to renal health.
- The patient and family acknowledge the importance of completing the prescribed antibiotic regime.

Ability
- The patient successfully demonstrates the ability to strain the urine.
- The patient successfully demonstrates how to measure and record intake an output.

Response
- The patient agrees to diet changes that will facilitate renal health.
- The patient agrees to HCP recommended follow-up evaluations.

RELATED STUDIES:
- Related tests include angiography kidneys, antibodies antiglomerular basement membrane, biopsy kidney, bladder cancer markers, BUN, calculus kidney stone panel, C4, CT abdomen, CT kidneys, CT pelvis, creatinine, creatinine clearance, cystoscopy, IVP, KUB studies, MRA, MRI abdomen, retrograde ureteropyelography, strep group A, US abdomen, US kidney, and UA.
- Refer to the Genitourinary System table online at Davis*Plus* for related tests by body system.

Reticulocyte Count

SYNONYM/ACRONYM: Retic count.

COMMON USE: To assess reticulocyte count in relation to bone marrow activity toward diagnosing anemias such as pernicious iron deficiency, and hemolytic; to monitor response of therapeutic interventions.

SPECIMEN: Whole blood collected in a lavender-top (EDTA) tube.

NORMAL FINDINGS: (Method: Automated analyzer or microscopic examination of specially stained peripheral blood smear)

Age	Reticulocyte Count %
Newborn	3%–6%
Infant	0.4%–2.8%
Child	0.8%–2.1%
Adult–older adult	0.5%–1.5%
	Reticulocyte Count (Absolute Number)
Birth–older adult	0.02–0.10 (10^6 cells/microL)
	Immature Reticulocyte Fraction %
Birth	2.5%–6.5%
Newborn–older adult	2.5%–17%
	Reticulocyte Hemoglobin
Birth	22–32 pg/cell
Newborn–18 yr	23–34 pg/cell
Adult–older adult	30–35 pg/cell

DESCRIPTION: Normally, as it matures, the red blood cell (RBC) loses its nucleus. The remaining ribonucleic acid (RNA) produces a characteristic color when special stains are used, making these cells easy to identify and enumerate. Some automated cell counters have the ability to provide a reticulocyte panel, which includes the enumeration of circulating reticulocytes as an absolute count and as a percentage of total RBCs; the immature reticulocyte fraction, which reflects the number of reticulocytes released into the circulation within the past 24 to 48 hours; and the reticulocyte hemoglobin content, which reflects the amount of iron incorporated into the maturing RBCs. The presence of reticulocytes is an indication of the level of erythropoietic activity in the bone marrow. The information provided by the reticulocyte panel is useful in the evaluation of anemias, bone marrow response to therapy, degree of bone marrow engraftment following transplant, and the effectiveness of altitude training in high-performance athletes. In abnormal conditions, reticulocytes are prematurely released into circulation. (See studies titled "Complete Blood Count, RBC Count" and "Complete Blood Count, RBC Morphology and Inclusions.")

This procedure is contraindicated for: N/A

INDICATIONS

- Evaluate erythropoietic activity.
- Monitor response to therapy for anemias.

POTENTIAL MEDICAL DIAGNOSIS

The reticulocyte production index (RPI) is a good estimate of RBC production. The calculation corrects the count for anemia and for the premature release of reticulocytes into the peripheral blood during periods of hemolysis or significant bleeding. The RPI also takes into consideration the maturation time of large polychromatophilic cells or nucleated RBCs seen on the peripheral smear:

RPI = % reticulocytes × [patient hematocrit (Hct)/normal Hct] × (1/maturation time)

As the formula shows, the RPI is inversely proportional to Hct, as follows:

Hematocrit (%)	Maturation Time (d)
45	1
35	1.5
25	2
15	2.5

Increased in:

Conditions that result in excessive RBC loss or destruction stimulate a compensatory bone marrow response by increasing production of RBCs.

- Blood loss
- Hemolytic anemias
- Iron-deficiency anemia
- Malaria
- Megaloblastic anemia

Other

- Pregnancy
- Treatment for anemia

Decreased in:

- Alcoholism ***(decreased production related to nutritional deficit)***
- Anemia of chronic disease
- Aplastic anemia ***(related to overall lack of RBC)***
- Bone marrow replacement ***(new marrow fails to produce RBCs until it engrafts)***

R

- Endocrine disease ***(hypometabolism related to hypothyroidism is reflected by decreased bone marrow activity)***
- Kidney disease ***(diseased kidneys cannot produce erythropoietin, which stimulates the bone marrow to produce RBCs)***
- RBC aplasia ***(related to overall lack of RBCs)***
- Sideroblastic anemia ***(RBCs are produced but are abnormal in that they cannot incorporate iron into hemoglobin, resulting in anemia)***

CRITICAL FINDINGS: N/A

INTERFERING FACTORS

- Drugs and other substances that may increase reticulocyte counts include acetylsalicylic acid, amyl nitrate, antimalarials, antipyretics, antipyrine, arsenicals, corticotropin, dimercaprol, etretinate, furazolidone, levodopa, methyldopa, nitrofurans, penicillin, procainamide, and sulfones.
- Drugs and other substances that may decrease reticulocyte counts include azathioprine, dactinomycin, hydroxyurea, methotrexate, and zidovudine.
- Reticulocyte count may be falsely increased by the presence of RBC inclusions (Howell-Jolly bodies, Heinz bodies, and Pappenheimer bodies) that stain with methylene blue.
- Reticulocyte count may be falsely decreased as a result of the dilutional effect after a recent blood transfusion.
- Specimens that are clotted or hemolyzed should be rejected for analysis.

NURSING IMPLICATIONS AND PROCEDURE

PRETEST:

- Positively identify the patient using at least two person-specific identifiers before services, treatments, or procedures are performed.
- *Patient Teaching:* Inform the patient this test can assist in assessing for anemia.
- Obtain a history of the patient's health concerns, symptoms, surgical procedures, and results of previously performed laboratory and diagnostic studies. Include a list of known allergens, especially allergies or sensitivities to latex.
- Note any recent procedures that can interfere with test results.
- Obtain a list of the patient's current medications, including over-the-counter medications and dietary supplements (see Effects of Natural Products on Laboratory Values online at Davis*Plus*).
- Review the procedure with the patient. Inform the patient that specimen collection takes approximately 5 to 10 min. Address concerns about pain and explain that there may be some discomfort during the venipuncture.
- *Sensitivity to social and cultural issues,* as well as concern for modesty, is important in providing psychological support before, during, and after the procedure.
- Note that there are no food, fluid, or medication restrictions unless by medical direction.

INTRATEST:

Potential Complications: N/A

- Avoid the use of equipment containing latex if the patient has a history of allergic reaction to latex.
- Instruct the patient to cooperate fully and to follow directions. Direct the patient to breathe normally and to avoid unnecessary movement.

R

- Observe standard precautions, and follow the general guidelines in Patient Preparation and Specimen Collection online at Davis*Plus*. Positively identify the patient, and label the appropriate specimen container with the corresponding patient demographics, initials of the person collecting the specimen, date, and time of collection. Perform a venipuncture.
- Remove the needle and apply direct pressure with dry gauze to stop bleeding. Observe/asses venipuncture site for bleeding or hematoma formation and secure gauze with adhesive bandage.
- Promptly transport the specimen to the laboratory for processing and analysis.

POST-TEST:

- Inform the patient that a report of the results will be made available to the requesting health-care provider (HCP), who will discuss the results with the patient.
- Reinforce information given by the patient's HCP regarding further testing, treatment, or referral to another HCP. Answer any questions or address any concerns voiced by the patient or family.
- Depending on the results of this procedure, additional testing may be performed to evaluate or monitor progression of the disease process and determine the need for a change in therapy. Evaluate test results in relation to the patient's symptoms and other tests performed.

RELATED STUDIES:

- Related tests include biopsy bone marrow, complement, CBC, CBC hematocrit, CBC hemoglobin, CBC RBC count, CBC RBC indices, CBC RBC morphology, Coomb's antiglobulin direct and indirect, erythropoietin, iron/TIBC, ferritin, folate, G6PD, Ham's test, Hgb electrophoresis, lead, osmotic fragility, PK, sickle cell screen, and vitamin B_{12}.
- Refer to the Hematopoietic System table online at Davis*Plus* for related tests by body system.

Retrograde Ureteropyelography

SYNONYM/ACRONYM: Retrograde.

COMMON USE: To assess the urinary tract for trauma, obstruction, stones, infection, and abscess that can interfere with function.

AREA OF APPLICATION: Renal calyces, ureter.

DESCRIPTION: Retrograde ureteropyelography uses a contrast medium introduced through a ureteral catheter during cystography and radiographic visualization to view the renal collecting system (calyces, renal pelvis, and urethra). During a cystoscopic examination, a catheter is advanced through the ureters and into the kidney and contrast medium is injected through the catheter into the kidney. This procedure is primarily used in patients who are known to be hypersensitive to intravenous (IV) injected iodine-based contrast medium and when excretory ureterography does not adequately reveal the renal collecting system. The incidence of allergic reaction to the contrast medium is reduced because there is less systemic absorption of the contrast medium when injected into the kidney than when injected IV. Retrograde ureteropyelography sometimes provides more information about the anatomy of the different parts of the collecting system than can be obtained by excretory ureteropyelography. Computed tomography (CT) and ultrasound studies are replacing retrograde pyelography because they are less invasive and the quality of the technology has significantly improved.

This procedure is contraindicated for

Patients who are pregnant or suspected of being pregnant, unless the potential benefits of a procedure using radiation far outweigh the risk of radiation exposure to the fetus and mother.

Patients with conditions associated with adverse reactions to contrast medium (e.g., asthma, food allergies, or allergy to contrast medium).

Although patients are asked specifically if they have a known allergy to iodine or shellfish, it has been well established that the reaction is not to iodine; an actual iodine allergy would be problematic because iodine is required for the production of thyroid hormones. In the case of shellfish, the reaction is to a muscle protein called tropomyosin; in the case of iodinated contrast medium, the reaction is to the noniodinated part of the contrast molecule. Patients with a known hypersensitivity to the medium may benefit from premedication with corticosteroids and diphenhydramine; the use of nonionic contrast or an alternative noncontrast imaging study, if available, may be considered for patients who have severe asthma or who have experienced moderate to severe reactions to ionic contrast medium.

Patients with conditions associated with preexisting renal insufficiency (e.g., chronic kidney disease, single kidney transplant, nephrectomy, diabetes, multiple myeloma, treatment with aminoglycosides and NSAIDs) ***because iodinated contrast is nephrotoxic.***

Patients who are chronically dehydrated before the test, especially older adults and patients whose health is already compromised, ***because of their risk of contrast-induced acute kidney injury.***

Patients with bleeding disorders because the puncture site may not stop bleeding.

INDICATIONS

- Evaluate the effects of urinary system trauma.
- Evaluate known or suspected ureteral obstruction.
- Evaluate placement of a ureteral stent or catheter.
- Evaluate the presence of calculi in the kidneys, ureters, or bladder.
- Evaluate the renal collecting system when excretory urography is unsuccessful.
- Evaluate space-occupying lesions or congenital anomalies of the urinary system.
- Evaluate the structure and integrity of the renal collecting system.

POTENTIAL MEDICAL DIAGNOSIS

Normal findings

- Normal outline and opacification of renal pelvis and calyces
- Normal size and uniform filling of the ureters
- Symmetrical and bilateral outline of structures

Abnormal findings related to

- Congenital renal or urinary tract abnormalities
- Hydronephrosis
- Neoplasms

- Obstruction as a result of tumor, blood clot, stricture, or calculi
- Obstruction of ureteropelvic junction
- Perinephric abscess
- Perinephric inflammation or suppuration
- Polycystic kidney disease
- Prostatic enlargement
- Tumor of the kidneys or the collecting system

CRITICAL FINDINGS: N/A

INTERFERING FACTORS

Factors that may alter the results of the study

- Gas or feces in the gastrointestinal tract resulting from inadequate cleansing or failure to restrict food intake before the study.
- Retained barium from a previous radiological procedure.
- Metallic objects (e.g., jewelry, body rings) within the examination field, which may inhibit organ visualization and cause unclear images.
- Inability of the patient to cooperate or remain still during the procedure because of age, significant pain, or mental status.

Other considerations

- Failure to follow dietary restrictions and other pretesting preparations may cause the procedure to be canceled or repeated.
- This procedure may be terminated if chest pain, severe cardiac dysrhythmias, or signs of a cerebrovascular accident occur.

NURSING IMPLICATIONS AND PROCEDURE

See Potential Nursing Problems on Fast Find at davispl.us/vanleeuwen7.

PRETEST:

- Positively identify the patient using at least two person-specific identifiers before services, treatments, or procedures are performed.
- *Patient Teaching:* Inform the patient this procedure can assist in assessing the urinary tract.
- Obtain a history of the patient's health concerns, symptoms, surgical procedures, and results of previously performed laboratory and diagnostic studies. Include a list of known allergens, especially allergies or sensitivities to latex, anesthetics, sedatives, or contrast medium. Ensure results of coagulation testing are obtained and recorded prior to the procedure; a creatinine level is also needed before contrast medium is to be used.
- Note any recent procedures that can interfere with test results, including examinations using barium.
- Record the date of the last menstrual period and determine the possibility of pregnancy in perimenopausal women.
- Obtain a list of the patient's current medications, including over-the-counter medications and dietary supplements (see Effects of Natural Products on Laboratory Values online at Davis*Plus*).
- Note that if iodinated contrast medium is scheduled to be used in patients receiving metformin (Glucophage) for type 2 diabetes, the drug should be discontinued on the day of the test and continue to be withheld for 48 hr after the test. Iodinated contrast can temporarily impair kidney function, and failure to withhold metformin may indirectly result in drug-induced lactic acidosis, a dangerous and sometimes fatal adverse effect of metformin ***related to renal impairment that does not support sufficient excretion of metformin.***
- Review the procedure with the patient. Address concerns about pain related to the procedure and explain that some pain may be experienced during the test, or there may be moments of discomfort. Inform the patient that the procedure is performed in a special department, usually in a radiology or vascular suite, by a health-care provider (HCP), with

R

support staff, and takes approximately 30 to 60 min.

- *Sensitivity to social and cultural issues,* as well as concern for modesty, is important in providing psychological support before, during, and after the procedure.
- Inform the patient that he or she may receive a laxative the night before the test and an enema or a cathartic the morning of the test, as ordered.
- Explain that an IV line may be inserted to allow infusion of fluids such as saline, anesthetics, sedatives, or emergency medications. Explain that the contrast medium will be injected, by catheter, at a separate site from the IV line.
- Inform the patient that if a local anesthetic is used, the patient may feel (1) some pressure in the kidney area as the catheter is introduced and contrast medium injected and (2) the urgency to void.
- Instruct the patient to remove jewelry and other metallic objects from the area to be examined prior to the procedure.
- Instruct the patient to fast and restrict fluids for 8 hr prior to the procedure. Instruct the patient to avoid taking anticoagulant medication or to reduce dosage as ordered prior to the procedure. Protocols may vary among facilities.
- *Make sure a written and informed consent has been signed prior to the procedure and before administering any medications.*

INTRATEST:

Potential Complications:

Establishing an IV site and injecting contrast medium by catheter are invasive procedures. Complications are rare but do include risk for allergic reaction ***related to contrast reaction;*** bleeding from the puncture site ***related to a bleeding disorder, or the effects of natural products and medications with known anticoagulant, antiplatelet, and thrombolytic properties;*** hematoma ***related to blood leakage into the tissue following needle insertion;*** infection ***that might occur if bacteria from the skin surface is introduced at the puncture site;*** urinary tract infection ***related to insertion of cystoscope or catheter;*** hematuria ***related to insertion of cystoscope;*** and sepsis ***related to bacterial contamination from infected urine.***

- Observe standard precautions, and follow the general guidelines in Patient Preparation and Specimen Collection online at Davis*Plus*. Positively identify the patient.
- Ensure that the patient has complied with dietary, fluid, and medication restrictions prior to the procedure, as instructed.
- Ensure the patient has removed all external metallic objects from the area to be examined prior to the procedure.
- Administer ordered prophylactic steroids or antihistamines before the procedure if the patient has a history of allergic reactions to any substance or drug. Use nonionic contrast medium for the procedure.
- Avoid the use of equipment containing latex if the patient has a history of allergic reaction to latex.
- Have emergency equipment readily available.
- Instruct the patient to void prior to the procedure and to change into the gown, robe, and foot coverings provided.
- Instruct the patient to cooperate fully and to follow directions. Instruct the patient to remain still throughout the procedure because movement produces unreliable results.
- Record baseline vital signs and assess neurological status. Protocols may vary among facilities.
- Establish an IV fluid line for the injection of saline, sedatives, or emergency medications.
- Administer an antianxiety drug, as ordered, if the patient has claustrophobia. Administer a sedative to a child or to an uncooperative adult, as ordered.

R

- Place electrocardiographic electrodes on the patient for cardiac monitoring. Establish baseline rhythm; determine if the patient has ventricular dysrhythmias.
- Place patient supine on the table in the lithotomy position.
- A kidney, ureter, and bladder (KUB) or plain image is taken to ensure that no barium or stool will obscure visualization of the urinary system. The patient may be asked to hold his or her breath to facilitate visualization.
- The patient is given a local anesthetic, and a cystoscopic examination is performed and the bladder is inspected.
- A catheter is inserted, and the renal pelvis is emptied by gravity. Contrast medium is introduced into the catheter. Inform the patient that the contrast medium may cause a temporary flushing of the face, a feeling of warmth, or nausea.
- X-ray images are made and the results processed. Inform the patient that additional images may be necessary to visualize the area in question.
- Additional contrast medium is injected through the catheter to outline the ureters as the catheter is withdrawn.
- The catheter may be kept in place and attached to a gravity drainage unit until urinary flow has returned or is corrected.
- Additional x-ray images are taken 10 to 15 min after the catheter is removed to evaluate retention of the contrast medium, indicating urinary stasis.
- Remove the needle or catheter and apply a pressure dressing over the puncture site.
- Observe/assess the needle/catheter insertion site for bleeding, inflammation, or hematoma formation.

POST-TEST:

- Inform the patient that a report of the results will be made available to the requesting HCP, who will discuss the results with the patient.
- Instruct the patient to resume usual diet, fluids, medications, and activity, as directed by the HCP. Kidney function should be assessed before metformin is resumed, if contrast is used.
- Monitor vital signs and neurological status every 15 min for 1 hr, then every 2 hr for 4 hr, and then as ordered. Take temperature every 4 hr for 24 hr. Monitor intake and output at least every 8 hr. Compare with baseline values. Notify the HCP if temperature is elevated. Protocols may vary among facilities.
- Observe for delayed allergic reactions, such as rash, urticaria, tachycardia, hyperpnea, hypertension, palpitations, nausea, or vomiting.
- Instruct the patient to immediately report symptoms such as fast heart rate, difficulty breathing, skin rash, itching, chest pain, persistent right shoulder pain, or abdominal pain. Immediately report symptoms to the appropriate HCP.
- Observe/assess the needle/catheter insertion site for bleeding, inflammation, or hematoma formation.
- Instruct the patient in the care and assessment of the site.
- Instruct the patient to apply cold compresses to the puncture site as needed to reduce discomfort or edema.
- Monitor for signs of sepsis and severe pain in the kidney area.
- Maintain the patient on adequate hydration after the procedure. Encourage the patient to drink lots of fluids to prevent stasis and to prevent the buildup of bacteria.
- Recognize anxiety related to test results, and be supportive of perceived loss of independent function. Discuss the implications of abnormal test results on the patient's lifestyle. Provide teaching and information regarding the clinical implications of the test results, as appropriate.
- Reinforce information given by the patient's HCP regarding further testing, treatment, or referral to another HCP. Answer any questions or address any concerns voiced by the patient or family.

R

- Instruct the patient in the use of any ordered medications. Explain the importance of adhering to the therapy regimen. As appropriate, instruct the patient in significant adverse effects associated with the prescribed medication. Encourage him or her to review corresponding literature provided by a pharmacist.
- Depending on the results of this procedure, additional testing may be needed to evaluate or monitor progression of the disease process and determine the need for a change in therapy. Evaluate test results in relation to the patient's symptoms and other tests performed.

Patient Education:

- Teach the patient how to strain urine and to report any blood noted in the urine.
- Teach the patient the symptoms of infection that should be reported to the HCP.

Expected Patient Outcomes:

Understanding

- The patient states the importance of increasing oral fluid intake to facilitate stone removal.
- The patient states the importance of straining all urine to identify when a stone has passed.

Ability

- The patient successfully demonstrates the knees-to-chest position to decrease discomfort.
- The patient demonstrates relaxation techniques that successfully decrease pain.

Response

- The patient agrees to avoid high-calcium fluids (dairy, chocolate).
- The patient agrees to maintain in increased oral intake to mitigate stone reoccurrence.

RELATED STUDIES:

- Related tests include angiography kidneys, BUN, calculus kidney stone panel, CT abdomen, CT kidneys, creatinine, cystoscopy, IVP, KUB, MRI abdomen, PT/INR, PSA, renogram, US kidney, UA, and voiding cystourethrography.
- Refer to the Genitourinary System table online at Davis*Plus* for related tests by body system.

Rheumatoid Factor

SYNONYM/ACRONYM: RF, RA.

COMMON USE: To primarily assist in diagnosing rheumatoid arthritis.

SPECIMEN: Serum collected in a gold-, red-, or red/gray-top tube.

R

NORMAL FINDINGS: (Method: Immunoturbidimetric) Less than 14 international units/mL. Elevated values may be detected in healthy adults 60 yr and older. ✦

DESCRIPTION: Rheumatoid arthritis (RA) is a chronic, systemic autoimmune disease that damages the synovium or membrane surrounding the joints. Collagen, the main fibrous protein in tendons, bone, and other types of connective tissue, is gradually destroyed, narrowing the joint space. As the disease progresses, a pannus or growth of thickened synovial tissue forms and permeates the bone and cartilage, leading to permanent damage and joint deformity. Inflammation caused by autoimmune responses can affect other organs and body systems. The American College of Rheumatology and European League Against Rheumatism jointly developed the current criteria (2010) that focuses on earlier diagnosis of newly presenting patients who have at least one swollen joint unrelated to another condition. The criteria includes four determinants: joint involvement (number and size of joints involved), serological test results (rheumatoid factor [RF] and/or anticitrullinated protein antibody), indications of acute inflammation (C-reactive protein and/or erythrocyte sedimentation rate), and duration of symptoms. A score of 6 or greater defines the presence of RA. Patients with longstanding RA, whose condition is inactive, or whose prior history would have satisfied the previous classification criteria by having four of seven findings—morning stiffness, arthritis of three or more joint areas, arthritis of hand joints, symmetric arthritis, rheumatoid nodules, abnormal amounts of rheumatoid factor, and radiographic changes—should remain classified as having RA. 🍁 The study of RA is complex, and it is believed that multiple genes may be involved in the manifestation of RA. Individuals with RA harbor a macroglobulin-type antibody called *rheumatoid factor* in their blood. Patients with other diseases (e.g., systemic lupus erythematosus [SLE] and occasionally tuberculosis, chronic hepatitis, infectious mononucleosis, and subacute bacterial endocarditis) may also test positive for RF. RF antibodies are usually immunoglobulin M (IgM) but may also be IgG or IgA. Women are two to three times more likely than men to develop RA. Although RA is most likely to affect people aged 35 to 50, it can affect all ages.

This procedure is contraindicated for: N/A

INDICATIONS

Assist in the diagnosis of rheumatoid arthritis, especially when clinical diagnosis is difficult.

POTENTIAL MEDICAL DIAGNOSIS

Increased in:

Pathophysiology is unclear, but RF is present in numerous conditions, including rheumatoid arthritis.

- Chronic hepatitis
- Chronic viral infections
- Cirrhosis
- Dermatomyositis
- Infectious mononucleosis
- Leishmaniasis
- Leprosy
- Malaria
- Rheumatoid arthritis
- Sarcoidosis
- Scleroderma
- Sjögren's syndrome
- SLE
- Syphilis
- Tuberculosis
- Waldenström's macroglobulinemia

Decreased in: N/A

CRITICAL FINDINGS: N/A

INTERFERING FACTORS

- Older healthy patients may have higher values.
- Recent blood transfusion, multiple vaccinations or transfusions, or an inadequately activated complement may affect results.
- Serum with cryoglobulin or high lipid levels may cause a false-positive test and may require that the test be repeated after a fat-restriction diet.

R

NURSING IMPLICATIONS AND PROCEDURE

POTENTIAL NURSING PROBLEMS:

Problem	Signs & Symptoms	Interventions
Self-care ***(related to immune system dysfunction)***	Joint stiffness; joint swelling; joint pain; self-reports of difficulty in completing activities of daily living (ADLs); limited range of motion	Assess range of motion; administer prescribed anti-inflammatory drugs; teach exercises that will increase joint mobility and increase ability to participate in ADLs; teach the patient to take analgesics prior to activity to decrease pain and facilitate self-care
Mobility ***(related to deformed joints secondary to immune system dysfunction; fatigue; pain)***	Unsteady gait; lack of coordination; difficult purposeful movement; inadequate range of motion	Assess gait; assess muscle strength; assess weakness and coordination; assess physical endurance and level of fatigue; assess ability to perform independent ADLs; assess ability for safe independent movement; identify need for assistive device; encourage safe self-care; administer prescribed steroids
Body image ***(related to deformed joints secondary to immune system dysfunction)***	Negative self remarks; expressions of feelings or concerns over visual physical changes; fear of rejection by others due to appearance	Assess feelings related to body image changes (refusal to discuss changes, participate in care, withdraw from social situations); encourage participation in support groups; emphasize strengths; determine the patient's expectations regarding appearance; identify the influence of the patient's culture, religion, ethnicity, and gender on body image perceptions; monitor verbalization of self-criticism
Fatigue ***(related to chronic illness; discomfort; immobility; psychological stress; pain)***	Disturbed sleep pattern; chronic pain; verbal report of fatigue	Suggest bedtime routine that will promote rest (warm bath, warm milk); pace activities, balancing them with rest periods; assess the level of psychological stress and suggest assistive coping strategies; facilitate use of assistive devices

PRETEST:

- Positively identify the patient using at least two person-specific identifiers before services, treatments, or procedures are performed.
- *Patient Teaching:* Inform the patient this test can assist in diagnosing arthritic disorders.
- Obtain a history of the patient's health concerns, symptoms, surgical procedures, and results of previously performed laboratory and diagnostic studies. Include a list of known allergens, especially allergies or sensitivities to latex.
- Obtain a list of the patient's current medications, including over-the-counter medications and dietary supplements (see Effects of Natural Products on Laboratory Values online at Davis*Plus*).
- Review the procedure with the patient. Inform the patient that specimen collection takes approximately 5 to 10 min. Address concerns about pain and explain that there may be some discomfort during the venipuncture.
- *Sensitivity to social and cultural issues,* as well as concern for modesty, is important in providing psychological support before, during, and after the procedure.
- Note that there are no food, fluid, or medication restrictions unless by medical direction.

INTRATEST:

Potential Complications: N/A

- Avoid the use of equipment containing latex if the patient has a history of allergic reaction to latex.
- Instruct the patient to cooperate fully and to follow directions. Direct the patient to breathe normally and to avoid unnecessary movement.
- Observe standard precautions, and follow the general guidelines in Patient Preparation and Specimen Collection online at Davis*Plus*. Positively identify the patient, and label the appropriate specimen container with the corresponding patient demographics, initials of the person collecting the specimen, date, and time of collection. Perform a venipuncture.
- Remove the needle and apply direct pressure with dry gauze to stop bleeding. Observe venipuncture site for bleeding or hematoma formation and secure gauze with adhesive bandage.
- Promptly transport the specimen to the laboratory for processing and analysis.

POST-TEST:

- Inform the patient that a report of the results will be made available to the requesting health-care provider (HCP), who will discuss the results with the patient.
- Recognize anxiety related to test results, and be supportive of impaired activity related to anticipated chronic pain resulting from joint inflammation, impairment in mobility, musculoskeletal deformity, and loss of independence. Discuss the implications of abnormal test results on the patient's lifestyle. Provide teaching and information regarding the clinical implications of the test results, as appropriate. Educate the patient regarding access to counseling services, as appropriate. Provide contact information, if desired, for the American College of Rheumatology (www.rheumatology.org) or for the Arthritis Foundation (www.arthritis.org). 🍁
- Depending on the results of this procedure, additional testing may be performed to evaluate or monitor progression of the disease process and determine the need for a change in therapy. Anemia is a common complication of RA. Evaluate test results in relation to the patient's symptoms and other tests performed.

Patient Education:

- Reinforce information given by the patient's HCP regarding further testing, treatment, or referral to another HCP.

R

- Advise the patient, as appropriate, that additional studies may be undertaken to determine treatment regimen or to determine the possible causes of symptoms if the test is negative for RA.
- Answer any questions or address any concerns voiced by the patient or family.

Expected Patient Outcomes:

Understanding

- The patient and family state that taking anti-inflammatory medication prior to activity may improve mobility.
- The patient and family state the risks and benefits of steroid use.

Ability

- The patient demonstrates positive coping strategies and seeks support as appropriate.
- The patient demonstrates the proficient use of assistive devices to support mobility and decrease fatigue.

Response

- The patient complies with the request to attend a rheumatoid arthritis support group.
- The patient and family comply with the request to minimize exposure to sick individuals when immunocompromised.

RELATED STUDIES:

- Related laboratory tests include antibodies anticyclic citrullinated peptide, ANA, arthrogram, arthroscopy, biopsy bone, BMD, bone scan, calcium, collagen cross-linked telopeptides, CBC, CT spine, CRP, ESR, MRI musculoskeletal, osteocalcin, phosphorus, radiography bone, synovial fluid analysis, uric acid, vitamin D, and WBC scan.
- Refer to the Immune and Musculoskeletal systems tables online at Davis*Plus* for related tests by body system.

Rubella Antibodies, IgG and IgM

SYNONYM/ACRONYM: German measles serology.

COMMON USE: To assess for antibodies related to rubella immunity or for presence of rubella infection.

SPECIMEN: Serum collected in a gold-, red-, or red/gray-top tube. Place separated serum into a standard transport tube within 2 hr of collection.

NORMAL FINDINGS: (Method: Chemiluminescent immunoassay)

	IgM	Interpretation	IgG	Interpretation
Negative	0.9 index or less	No significant level of detectable antibody	Less than 8 units/mL	No significant level of detectable antibody; indicative of nonimmunity
Indeterminate	0.91–1.09 index	Equivocal results; retest in 10–14 d	8–12 units/mL	Equivocal results; retest in 10–14 d

	IgM	Interpretation	IgG	Interpretation
Positive	1.1 index or greater	Antibody detected; indicative of recent immunization, current or recent infection	Greater than 12 units/mL	Antibody detected; indicative of immunization, current or past infection

DESCRIPTION: Rubella, commonly known as German measles, is a communicable viral disease transmitted by contact with respiratory secretions and aerosolized droplets of the secretions. The incubation period is 14 to 21 days. This disease produces a pink, macular rash that disappears in 2 to 3 days. Rubella infection induces immunoglobulin (Ig) G and IgM antibody production. This test can determine current infection or immunity from past infection. Rubella serology is part of the TORCH (*to*xoplasmosis, other [congenital syphilis and viruses], *r*ubella, *c*ytomegalovirus, and *h*erpes simplex type 2) panel routinely performed on pregnant women. Fetal infection during the first trimester can affect all organs in the developing fetus and cause spontaneous abortion, fetal demise, or congenital defects. Up to 90% of infants born to mothers infected during the first trimester will develop a pattern of birth defects called congenital rubella syndrome (CRS). The rate of CRS decreases when infection occurs later in the gestational period. Ideally, the immune status of women of childbearing age should be ascertained before pregnancy, when vaccination can be administered to provide lifelong immunity. The presence of IgM antibodies indicates acute infection. The presence of IgG antibodies indicates current or past infection. Susceptibility to rubella is indicated by a negative reaction. Many laboratories use a qualitative assay that detects the presence of both IgM and IgG rubella antibodies. IgM- and IgG-specific enzyme immunoassays are also available to help distinguish acute infection from immune status. Either the rubella-combined or IgG-specific assay should be used in routine prenatal testing of maternal serum.

This procedure is contraindicated for: N/A

INDICATIONS

- Assist in the diagnosis of rubella infection.
- Determine presence of rubella antibodies.
- Determine susceptibility to rubella, particularly in pregnant women.
- Perform as part of routine prenatal serological testing.

POTENTIAL MEDICAL DIAGNOSIS

Positive findings in

- Rubella infection (past or present)

CRITICAL FINDINGS:

A nonimmune status in pregnant patients may present significant health consequences for the developing fetus if the mother is exposed to an infected individual.

Note and immediately report to the requesting health-care provider (HCP) any critical findings and related symptoms. A listing of these findings varies among facilities. Timely notification of a critical finding for laboratory or diagnostic studies is a role expectation of the professional nurse. The notification processes vary among facilities. Upon receipt of the critical finding, the information should be read back to the caller to verify accuracy.

INTERFERING FACTORS: N/A

NURSING IMPLICATIONS AND PROCEDURE

POTENTIAL NURSING PROBLEMS:

Problem	Signs & Symptoms	Interventions
Knowledge ***(related to new condition or diagnosis; lack of familiarity with or understanding of disease and treatment)***	Lack of interest or questions; multiple questions; anxiety in relation to disease process and management	Teach the patient or parents that this disease is accompanied by a rash and fever that lasts for 2 to 3 d; explain that the disease can be spread to others through coughing and sneezing of the infected person; explain that measles, mumps, rubella vaccination is recommended
Infection ***(related to exposure to viral organism from an infected individual)***	Fever and rash lasting 2 to 3 d; runny nose; headache; malaise	Explain that those infected can expose others to the virus from 1 wk before the rash is present up to 2 wk after the rash is gone; administer prescribed acetaminophen for headache and fever; discuss the fetal risk associated with infection during pregnancy (miscarriage, stillbirth); teach good hygiene
Grief ***(related to loss of potential child; loss secondary to rubella viral infection)***	Crying; report of grief; expression of emotional shock; psychological distress; disturbed sleep; loss of appetite; detachment; withdrawal; anger; blame; despair	Monitor for manifestation of grief (crying, loud grief vocalization); assess for the stage of grief; assess for the effectiveness of coping strategies; consider the cultural norm for grief expression; encourage sharing feelings; recommend grief support group; recommend psychosocial counseling as appropriate; administer prescribed medication to offset the emotional impact of grief (as appropriate); recognize the need to relive the loss

R

PRETEST:

- Positively identify the patient using at least two person-specific identifiers before services, treatments, or procedures are performed.
- ***Patient Teaching:*** Inform the patient this test can indicate rubella infection or immunity.
- Obtain a history of the patient's health concerns (especially exposure to rubella), symptoms, surgical procedures, and results of previously performed laboratory and diagnostic studies. Include a list of known allergens, especially allergies or sensitivities to latex.
- Obtain a list of the patient's current medications, including over-the-counter medications and dietary supplements (see Effects of Natural Products on Laboratory Values online at Davis*Plus*).
- Review the procedure with the patient. Inform the patient that several tests may be necessary to confirm diagnosis. Any individual positive result should be repeated in 7 to 14 days to monitor a change in detectable level of antibody. Inform the patient that specimen collection takes approximately 5 to 10 min. Address concerns about pain and explain that there may be some discomfort during the venipuncture.
- ***Sensitivity to social and cultural issues,*** as well as concern for modesty, is important in providing psychological support before, during, and after the procedure.
- Note that there are no food, fluid, or medication restrictions unless by medical direction.

INTRATEST:

Potential Complications: N/A

- Avoid the use of equipment containing latex if the patient has a history of allergic reaction to latex.
- Instruct the patient to cooperate fully and to follow directions. Direct the patient to breathe normally and to avoid unnecessary movement.
- Observe standard precautions, and follow the general guidelines in Patient Preparation and Specimen Collection online at Davis*Plus*. Positively identify the patient, and label the appropriate specimen container with the corresponding patient demographics, initials of the person collecting the specimen, date, and time of collection. Perform a venipuncture.
- Remove the needle and apply direct pressure with dry gauze to stop bleeding. Observe/assess venipuncture site for bleeding or hematoma formation and secure gauze with adhesive bandage.
- Promptly transport the specimen to the laboratory for processing and analysis.

POST-TEST:

- Inform the patient that a report of the results will be made available to the requesting HCP, who will discuss the results with the patient.
- ***Vaccination Considerations:*** Record the date of the last menstrual period and determine the possibility of pregnancy prior to administration of rubella vaccine to female rubella-nonimmune patients. Instruct patient not to become pregnant for 1 mo after being vaccinated with the rubella vaccine to protect any fetus from contracting the disease and having serious birth defects. Instruct the patient on birth control methods to prevent pregnancy, if appropriate. Delay rubella vaccination in pregnancy until after childbirth, and give immediately prior to discharge from the hospital.
- Recognize anxiety related to test results, and provide emotional support if results are positive and the patient is pregnant. Encourage the family to seek counseling if concerned with pregnancy termination. Provide teaching and information regarding the clinical implications of the test results, as appropriate. Decisions regarding elective abortion should take place in the presence of both parents. Provide a nonjudgmental, nonthreatening atmosphere for discussing the risks and difficulties of delivering and raising a developmentally challenged infant as well as for exploring other options (e.g., termination of

R

pregnancy or adoption). Educate the patient regarding access to counseling services, as appropriate.

- Depending on the results of this procedure, additional testing may be performed to evaluate or monitor progression of the disease process and determine the need for a change in therapy. Evaluate test results in relation to the patient's symptoms and other tests performed.

Patient Education:

- Reinforce information given by the patient's HCP regarding further testing, treatment, or referral to another HCP.
- Instruct the patient in isolation precautions during time of communicability or contagion.
- Emphasize the need to return to have a convalescent blood sample taken in 7 to 14 days.
- Provide information regarding vaccine-preventable diseases where indicated (e.g., rubella).
- Provide contact information, if desired, for the Centers for Disease Control and Prevention (www.cdc.gov/vaccines/vpd-vac) and (www.cdc.gov/DiseasesConditions). 🍁
- Answer any questions or address any concerns voiced by the patient or family.

Expected Patient Outcomes:

Understanding

- The patient and family state the stages of grief that may be experienced with a loss.
- The patient and family accurately describe the dose and frequency of acetaminophen to treat fever and headache.

Ability

- The patient and family demonstrate proficient hand washing.
- The patient and family accurately describe precautions that should be taken to prevent the exposure of others to the infecting pathogen.

Response

- The patient complies with the recommendation to provide a secondary blood sample up to 14 days after diagnosis.
- The patient and family agree to seek grief counseling to assist in coping with the loss of a potential child.

RELATED STUDIES:

- Related tests include culture viral, CMV, rubeola, *Toxoplasma,* and varicella antibody.
- Refer to the Immune and Reproductive systems tables online at Davis*Plus* for related tests by body system.

Rubeola Antibodies

SYNONYM/ACRONYM: Measles serology.

COMMON USE: To assess for a rubeola infection or immunity.

SPECIMEN: Serum collected in a gold-, red-, or red/gray-top tube. Place separated serum into a standard transport tube within 2 hr of collection.

NORMAL FINDINGS: (Method: Enzyme immunoassay)

	IgM	Interpretation	IgG	Interpretation
Negative	0.79 AU or less	No significant level of detectable antibody	0.89 index or less	No significant level of detectable antibody; indicative of nonimmunity

	IgM	Interpretation	IgG	Interpretation
Indeterminate	0.8–1.2 AU	Equivocal results; retest in 10–14 d	0.9–1 index	Equivocal results; retest in 10–14 d
Positive	1.3 AU or greater	Antibody detected; indicative of recent immunization, current or recent infection	1.1 index or greater	Antibody detected; indicative of immunization, current or past infection

DESCRIPTION: Measles is caused by a single-stranded ribonucleic acid (RNA) paramyxovirus that invades the respiratory tract and lymphoreticular tissues. It is transmitted by respiratory secretions and aerosolized droplets of the secretions. The incubation period is 10 to 11 days. Symptoms initially include conjunctivitis, cough, and fever. Koplik's spots develop 4 to 5 days later, followed by papular eruptions, body rash, and lymphadenopathy. The presence of immunoglobulin M (IgM) antibodies indicates acute infection. The presence of IgG antibodies indicates current or past infection. Susceptibility to measles is indicated by a negative reaction. Many laboratories use a qualitative assay that detects the presence of both IgM and IgG rubeola antibodies. IgM- and IgG-specific enzyme immunoassays are also available to help distinguish acute infection from immune status.

This procedure is contraindicated for: N/A

INDICATIONS

- Determine resistance to or protection against measles virus.
- Differential diagnosis of viral infection, especially in pregnant women with a history of exposure to measles.

POTENTIAL MEDICAL DIAGNOSIS

Positive findings in

- Measles infection

CRITICAL FINDINGS: N/A

INTERFERING FACTORS: N/A

NURSING IMPLICATIONS AND PROCEDURE

PRETEST:

- Positively identify the patient using at least two person-specific identifiers before services, treatments, or procedures are performed.
- *Patient Teaching:* Inform the patient this test is to assess for measles.
- Obtain a history of the patient's health concerns (especially exposure to measles), symptoms, surgical procedures, and results of previously performed laboratory and diagnostic studies. Include a list of known allergens, especially allergies or sensitivities to latex.
- Obtain a list of the patient's current medications, including over-the-counter medications and dietary supplements (see Effects of Natural Products on Laboratory Values online at Davis*Plus*).
- Review the procedure with the patient. Inform the patient that several tests may be necessary to confirm the diagnosis. Any individual

R

positive result should be repeated in 7 to 14 days to monitor a change in detectable levels of antibody. Inform the patient that specimen collection takes approximately 5 to 10 min. Address concerns about pain and explain that there may be some discomfort during the venipuncture.
- *Sensitivity to social and cultural issues,* as well as concern for modesty, is important in providing psychological support before, during, and after the procedure.
- Note that there are no food, fluid, or medication restrictions, unless by medical direction.

INTRATEST:

Potential Complications: N/A

- Avoid the use of equipment containing latex if the patient has a history of allergic reaction to latex.
- Instruct the patient to cooperate fully and to follow directions. Direct the patient to breathe normally and to avoid unnecessary movement.
- Observe standard precautions, and follow the general guidelines in Patient Preparation and Specimen Collection online at Davis*Plus.* Positively identify the patient, and label the appropriate specimen container with the corresponding patient demographics, initials of the person collecting the specimen, date, and time of collection. Perform a venipuncture.
- Remove the needle and apply direct pressure with dry gauze to stop bleeding. Observe/assess venipuncture site for bleeding or hematoma formation and secure gauze with adhesive bandage.
- Promptly transport the specimen to the laboratory for processing and analysis.

POST-TEST:

- Inform the patient that a report of the results will be made available to the requesting health-care provider (HCP), who will discuss the results with the patient.
- *Vaccination Considerations:* Record the date of the last menstrual period and determine the possibility of pregnancy prior to administration of rubeola vaccine to female rubeola-nonimmune patients. Instruct patient not to become pregnant for 1 mo after being vaccinated with the rubeola vaccine to protect any fetus from contracting the disease. The danger of contracting measles while pregnant include the possibilities of miscarriage, stillbirth, or preterm delivery. Instruct the patient on birth control methods to prevent pregnancy, if appropriate. Delay rubeola vaccination in pregnancy until after childbirth, and give immediately prior to discharge from the hospital.
- Reinforce information given by the patient's HCP regarding further testing, treatment, or referral to another HCP. Instruct the patient in isolation precautions during time of communicability or contagion. Emphasize the need to return to have a convalescent blood sample taken in 7 to 14 days. Provide information regarding vaccine-preventable diseases where indicated (e.g., measles) for the Centers for Disease Control and Prevention (www.cdc.gov/vaccines/vpd-vac) and (www.cdc.gov/DiseasesConditions). 🍁 Answer any questions or address any concerns voiced by the patient or family.
- Depending on the results of this procedure, additional testing may be performed to evaluate or monitor progression of the disease process and determine the need for a change in therapy. Evaluate test results in relation to the patient's symptoms and other tests performed.

RELATED STUDIES:

- Related tests include culture viral, rubella, and varicella.
- Refer to the Immune System table online at Davis*Plus* for related tests by body system.

R

Schirmer Tear Test

SYNONYM/ACRONYM: N/A

COMMON USE: To assess tear duct function.

AREA OF APPLICATION: Eyes.

DESCRIPTION: The tear film, secreted by the lacrimal, Krause, and Wolfring glands, covers the surface of the eye. Blinking spreads tears over the eye and moves them toward an opening in the lower eyelid known as the *punctum*. Tears drain through the punctum into the nasolacrimal duct and into the nose. The Schirmer tear test simultaneously tests both eyes to assess lacrimal gland function by determining the amount of moisture accumulated on standardized filter paper or strips held against the conjunctival sac of each eye. The Schirmer test measures both reflex and basic secretion of tears. The Schirmer II test measures basic tear secretion and is used to evaluate the accessory glands of Krause and Wolfring. The Schirmer test is performed by instilling a topical anesthetic before insertion of filter paper. The topical anesthetic inhibits reflex tearing of major lacrimal glands by the filter paper, allowing testing of the accessory glands. The Schirmer II test is performed by irritating the nostril with a cotton swab to stimulate tear production.

This procedure is contraindicated for: N/A

INDICATIONS
- Assess adequacy of tearing for contact lens comfort and for successful LASIK surgery.
- Assess suspected tearing deficiency.

POTENTIAL MEDICAL DIAGNOSIS

Normal findings
- 10 mm of moisture on test strip after 5 min. It may be slightly less than 10 mm in older adult patients.

Abnormal findings related to
- Tearing deficiency related to aging, dry eye syndrome, or Sjögren's syndrome
- Tearing deficiency secondary to leukemia, lupus erythemastosus, lymphoma, rheumatoid arthritis, or scleroderma

CRITICAL FINDINGS: N/A

INTERFERING FACTORS

Factors that may impair the results of the examination
- Inability of the patient to remain still and cooperative during the test may interfere with the test results.
- Rubbing or squeezing the eyes may affect results.
- Clinical conditions such as pregnancy may temporarily result in dry eye due to hormonal fluctuations.

NURSING IMPLICATIONS AND PROCEDURE

PRETEST:
- Positively identify the patient using at least two person-specific identifiers before services, treatments, or procedures are performed.
- *Patient Teaching:* Inform the patient this procedure can assist in evaluating tear duct function.
- Obtain a history of the patient's health concerns (especially known

S

or suspected vision loss; changes in visual acuity, including type and cause; use of glasses or contact lenses; eye conditions with treatment regimens; eye surgery; and other tests and procedures to assess and diagnose visual deficit), symptoms, surgical procedures, and results of previously performed laboratory and diagnostic studies. Include a list of known allergens, especially allergies or sensitivities to latex or topical anesthetic eyedrops.

- Obtain a list of the patient's current medications, including over-the-counter medications and dietary supplements (see Effects of Natural Products on Laboratory Values online at Davis*Plus*).
- Instruct the patient to remove contact lenses or glasses, as appropriate. Instruct the patient regarding the importance of keeping the eyes open for the test.
- Review the procedure with the patient. Address concerns about pain and explain that no pain will be experienced during the test, but there may be moments of discomfort. Explain to the patient that some discomfort may be experienced after the test when the numbness wears off from anesthetic drops administered prior to the test. Inform the patient that the test is performed by a health-care provider (HCP) and takes about 15 min to complete.
- ***Sensitivity to social and cultural issues,*** as well as concern for modesty, is important in providing psychological support before, during, and after the procedure.
- Note that there are no food, fluid, or medication restrictions unless by medical direction.

S

INTRATEST:

Potential Complications:

Corneal abrasion caused by patient rubbing the eye before topical anesthetic has worn off.

- Observe standard precautions, and follow the general guidelines in Patient Preparation and Specimen Collection online at Davis*Plus*. Positively identify the patient.
- Instruct the patient to cooperate fully and to follow directions. Ask the patient to remain still during the procedure because movement produces unreliable results.
- Seat the patient comfortably. Instruct the patient to look straight ahead, keeping the eyes open and unblinking.
- Instill topical anesthetic in each eye, as ordered, and provide time for it to work. Topical anesthetic drops are placed in the eye with the patient looking up and the solution directed at the six o'clock position of the sclera (white of the eye) near the limbus (gray, semitransparent area of the eyeball where the cornea and sclera meet). Neither the dropper nor the bottle should touch the eyelashes. Insert a test strip in each eye. The strip should be folded over the mid-portion of both lower eyelids. Instruct the patient to gently close both eyes for approximately 5 min then remove the strips and measure the amount of moisture on the strips.

POST-TEST:

- Inform the patient that a report of the results will be made available to the requesting HCP, who will discuss the results with the patient.
- Assess for corneal abrasion caused by patient rubbing the eye before topical anesthetic has worn off.
- Instruct the patient to avoid rubbing the eyes for 30 min after the procedure.
- If appropriate, instruct the patient not to reinsert contact lenses for 2 hr.
- Recognize anxiety related to test results, and be supportive of pain related to decreased lacrimation or inflammation. Discuss the implications of abnormal test results on the patient's lifestyle. Provide teaching and information regarding the clinical implications of the test results, as appropriate. Provide contact information, if desired, for a general patient education Web site

on the topic of eye care (e.g., www.allaboutvision.com). 🍁
- Reinforce information given by the patient's HCP regarding further testing, treatment, or referral to another HCP. Answer any questions or address any concerns voiced by the patient or family.
- Instruct the patient in the use of any ordered medications. Explain the importance of adhering to the therapy regimen. As appropriate, instruct the patient in significant adverse effects associated with the prescribed medication. Encourage him or her to review corresponding literature provided by a pharmacist.
- Depending on the results of this procedure, additional testing may be performed to evaluate or monitor progression of the disease process and determine the need for a change in therapy. Evaluate test results in relation to the patient's symptoms and other tests performed.

RELATED STUDIES:
- Related tests include antibodies ANA, refraction, rheumatoid factor, and slit-lamp biomicroscopy.
- Refer to the Ocular System table online at Davis*Plus* for related tests by body system.

Semen Analysis

SYNONYM/ACRONYM: N/A

COMMON USE: To assess for male infertility related to disorders such as obstruction, testicular failure, and atrophy.

SPECIMEN: Semen from ejaculate specimen collected in a clean, dry, glass container known to be free of detergent. The specimen container should be kept at body temperature (37°C) during transportation.

NORMAL FINDINGS: (Method: Macroscopic and microscopic examination)

Test	Normal Result
Volume	2–5 mL
Color	White or opaque
Appearance	Viscous (pours in droplets, not clumps or strings)
Clotting and liquefaction	Complete in 15–20 min, rarely over 60 min
pH	7.2–8
Sperm count	Greater than 15 million/mL
Total sperm count	Greater than 39 million/ejaculate
Motility	At least 40% at 60 min
Vitality (membrane intact)	At least 58%
Morphology	Greater than 25%–30% normal oval-headed forms

The number of normal sperm is calculated by multiplying the total sperm count by the percentage of normal forms.

DESCRIPTION: Semen analysis is a valid measure of overall male fertility. Semen contains a combination of elements produced by various parts of the male reproductive system. Spermatozoa are produced in the testes and account for only a small volume of seminal fluid. Fructose and other nutrients are provided by fluid produced in the seminal vesicles. The prostate gland provides acid phosphatase and other enzymes required for coagulation and liquefaction of semen. Sperm motility depends on the presence of a sufficient level of ionized calcium. If the specimen has an abnormal appearance (e.g., bloody, oddly colored, turbid), the patient may have an infection. Specimens can be tested with a leukocyte esterase strip to detect the presence of white blood cells.

This procedure is contraindicated for: N/A

INDICATIONS

- Assist in the diagnosis of azoospermia and oligospermia.
- Evaluate infertility.
- Evaluate effectiveness of vasectomy.
- Evaluate the effectiveness of vasectomy reversal.
- Support or disprove sterility in paternity suit.

POTENTIAL MEDICAL DIAGNOSIS

There is marked intraindividual variation in sperm count. Indications of suboptimal fertility should be investigated by serial analysis of two to three samples collected over several months. If abnormal results are obtained, additional testing may be requested.

Abnormality	Test Ordered	Normal Result
Decreased count	Fructose	Present (greater than 150 mg/dL)
Decreased motility with clumping	Male antisperm antibodies	Absent
Normal semen analysis with infertility	Female antisperm antibodies	Absent

Increased in: N/A

Decreased in:

- Hyperpyrexia ***(unusual and abnormal elevation in body temperature may result in insufficient sperm production)***
- Infertility ***(related to insufficient production of sperm)***
- Obstruction of ejaculatory system
- Orchitis ***(insufficient sperm production usually related to viral infection, rarely bacterial infection)***
- Postvasectomy period ***(related to obstruction of the vas deferens)***
- Primary and secondary testicular failure ***(congenital, as in Klinefelter's syndrome, or acquired via infection)***
- Testicular atrophy (e.g., recovery from mumps)
- Varicocele ***(abnormal enlargement of the blood vessels in the scrotal area eventually damages testicular tissue and affects sperm production)***

CRITICAL FINDINGS: N/A

INTERFERING FACTORS

- Drugs and other substances that may decrease sperm count include

S

arsenic, azathioprine, cannabis, cimetidine, cocaine, cyclophosphamide, estrogens, ketoconazole, lead, methotrexate, methyltestosterone, nitrofurantoin, nitrogen mustard, procarbazine, sulfasalazine, and vincristine.

- **Testicular radiation may decrease sperm counts.**
- **Cigarette smoking is associated with decreased production of semen.**
- **Caffeine consumption is associated with increased sperm density and number of abnormal forms.**
- **Delays in transporting the specimen and failure to keep the specimen warm during transportation are the most common reasons for specimen rejection.**

NURSING IMPLICATIONS AND PROCEDURE

PRETEST:

- Positively identify the patient using at least two person-specific identifiers before services, treatments, or procedures are performed.
- ***Patient Teaching:*** Inform the patient this test can assess for infertility.
- Obtain a history of the patient's health concerns, symptoms, surgical procedures, and results of previously performed laboratory and diagnostic studies. Include a list of known allergens, especially allergies or sensitivities to latex.
- Obtain a list of the patient's current medications, including over-the-counter medications and dietary supplements (see Effects of Natural Products on Laboratory Values online at Davis*Plus*).
- Note any recent procedures that can interfere with test results.
- Review the procedure with the patient. Instruct the patient to refrain from any sexual activity for 3 days before specimen collection. Instruct the patient to bring the specimen to the laboratory within 30 to 60 min of collection and to keep the specimen warm (close to body temperature) during transportation. The requesting health-care provider (HCP) usually provides the patient with instructions for specimen collection. Address concerns about pain and explain that there should be no discomfort during the procedure.
- ***Sensitivity to social and cultural issues,*** as well as concern for modesty, is important in providing psychological support before, during, and after the procedure.
- Note that there are no food, fluid, or medication restrictions unless by medical direction.

INTRATEST:

Potential Complications: N/A

- Instruct the patient to cooperate fully and to follow directions.
- Observe standard precautions, and follow the general guidelines in Patient Preparation and Specimen Collection online at Davis*Plus*. Positively identify the patient, and label the appropriate specimen container with the corresponding patient demographics, initials of the person collecting the specimen, date, and time of collection.

Ejaculated Specimen

- Ideally, the specimen is obtained by masturbation in a private location close to the laboratory. In cases in which the patient expresses psychological or religious concerns about masturbation, the specimen can be obtained during coitus interruptus, through the use of a condom, or through postcoital collection of samples from the cervical canal and vagina of the patient's sexual partner. The patient should be warned about the possible loss of the sperm-rich portion of the sample if coitus interruptus is the collection approach. If a condom is used, the patient must be instructed to carefully wash and dry the condom completely before use to prevent contamination of the specimen with spermicides.

S

Cervical Vaginal Specimen

- Assist the patient's partner to the lithotomy position on the examination table. A speculum is inserted, and the specimen is obtained by direct smear or aspiration of saline lavage.

Specimens Collected From Skin or Clothing

- Dried semen may be collected by sponging the skin with a gauze soaked in saline or by soaking the material in a saline solution.

General

- Promptly transport the specimen to the laboratory for processing and analysis.

POST-TEST:

- Inform the patient that a report of the results will be made available to the requesting HCP, who will discuss the results with the patient.
- Recognize anxiety related to test results. Provide a supportive, nonjudgmental environment when assisting a patient through the process of fertility testing. Discuss the implications of abnormal test results on the patient's lifestyle. Provide teaching and information regarding the clinical implications of the test results, as appropriate. Encourage the patient or family to seek counseling and other support services if concerned with infertility.
- Reinforce information given by the patient's HCP regarding further testing, treatment, or referral to another HCP. Answer any questions or address any concerns voiced by the patient or family.
- Depending on the results of this procedure, additional testing may be performed to evaluate or monitor progression of the disease process and determine the need for a change in therapy. Evaluate test results in relation to the patient's symptoms and other tests performed.

RELATED STUDIES:

- Related tests include antisperm antibodies, cancer antigens, *Chlamydia* group antibodies, estradiol, FSH, hysterosalpingography, laparoscopy gynecologic, LH, testosterone, and US scrotal.
- Refer to the Immune and Reproductive systems tables online at Davis*Plus* for related tests by body system.

Sialography

SYNONYM/ACRONYM: Salivary gland studies.

COMMON USE: To assess parotid, submaxillary, sublingual, and submandibular ducts for structure, tumors, and inflammation related to pain, swelling, and tenderness.

AREA OF APPLICATION: Base of the tongue, mandible, parotid gland, submandibular gland, sublingual gland.

S

POTENTIAL MEDICAL DIAGNOSIS

Normal findings

- Normal salivary ducts with no indication of gland abnormalities

Abnormal findings related to

- Calculi
- Fistulas
- Mixed parotid tumors
- Sialectasia (dilation of a duct)
- Strictures of the ducts

CRITICAL FINDINGS: N/A

Find and print out the full study on Fast Find at davispl.us/vanleeuwen7.

Sickle Cell Screen

SYNONYM/ACRONYM: Sickle cell test.

COMMON USE: To assess for hemoglobin S to assist in diagnosing sickle cell anemia.

SPECIMEN: Whole blood collected in a lavender-top (EDTA) tube.

NORMAL FINDINGS: (Method: Hemoglobin high-salt solubility) Negative.

DESCRIPTION: The sickle cell screen is one of several screening tests for a group of hereditary hemoglobinopathies. The test is positive in the presence of rare sickling hemoglobin (Hgb) variants such as Hgb S and Hgb C Harlem. Electrophoresis and high-performance liquid chromatography as well as molecular genetics testing for beta-globin mutations can also be used to identify Hgb S. Hgb S results from an amino acid substitution during Hgb synthesis whereby valine replaces glutamic acid. Hemoglobin C Harlem results from the substitution of lysine for glutamic acid. Individuals with sickle cell disease have chronic anemia because the abnormal Hgb is unable to carry oxygen. The red blood cells of affected individuals are also abnormal in shape, resembling a crescent or sickle rather than the normal disk shape. This abnormality, combined with cell-wall rigidity, prevents the cells from passing through smaller blood vessels. Blockages in blood vessels result in hypoxia, damage, and pain. Knowledge of genetics assists the nurse in identifying patients and family members who may benefit from additional education, risk assessment, and counseling. Genetics is the study and identification of genes, genetic mutations, and inheritance. For example, genetics provides some insight into the likelihood of inheriting a trait such as blue eyes or a medical condition such as a hemogloinopathy. Some conditions are the result of mutations involving a single gene, whereas other conditions may involve multiple genes and/or multiple chromosomes. Sickle cell disease is an example of an autosomal recessive disorder in which the offspring inherits a copy of the defective gene from each parent. Individuals with the sickle cell trait do not have the clinical manifestations of the disease but may pass the disease on to children if the other parent has the trait (or the disease) as well. Further information regarding inheritance of genes can be found in the study titled "Genetic Testing."

This procedure is contraindicated for: N/A

INDICATIONS

- Detect sickled red blood cells.
- Evaluate hemolytic anemias.

POTENTIAL MEDICAL DIAGNOSIS

Positive findings in

Deoxygenated Hgb S is insoluble in the presence of a high-salt solution

S

and will form a cloudy turbid suspension when present.

- Combination of Hgb S with other hemoglobinopathies
- Hgb C Harlem anemia
- Sickle cell anemia
- Sickle cell trait
- Thalassemias

Negative findings in: N/A

CRITICAL FINDINGS: N/A

INTERFERING FACTORS

- Drugs and other substances that may increase sickle cells in vitro include prostaglandins.
- A positive test does not distinguish between the sickle trait and sickle cell anemia; to make this determination, follow-up testing by Hgb electrophoresis should be performed.
- False-negative results may occur in children younger than 3 mo of age.
- False-negative results may occur in patients who have received a recent blood transfusion before specimen collection, as a result of the dilutional effect.
- False-positive results may occur in patients without the trait or disease who have received a blood transfusion from a sickle cell–positive donor; this effect can last for 4 mo after the transfusion.
- Test results are unreliable if the patient has pernicious anemia or polycythemia.

S

NURSING IMPLICATIONS AND PROCEDURE

PRETEST:

- Positively identify the patient using at least two person-specific identifiers before services, treatments, or procedures are performed.
- ***Patient Teaching:*** Inform the patient this test can assist in diagnosing anemia.
- Obtain a history of the patient's health concerns, symptoms, surgical procedures, and results of previously performed laboratory and diagnostic studies. Include a list of known allergens, especially allergies or sensitivities to latex.
- Note any recent procedures that can interfere with test results.
- Obtain a list of the patient's current medications, including over-the-counter medications and dietary supplements (see Effects of Natural Products on Laboratory Values online at Davis*Plus*).
- Review the procedure with the patient. Inform the patient that specimen collection takes approximately 5 to 10 min. Address concerns about pain and explain that there may be some discomfort during the venipuncture.
- ***Sensitivity to social and cultural issues,*** as well as concern for modesty, is important in providing psychological support before, during, and after the procedure.
- Note that there are no food, fluid, or medication restrictions unless by medical direction.

INTRATEST:

Potential Complications: N/A

- Avoid the use of equipment containing latex if the patient has a history of allergic reaction to latex.
- Instruct the patient to cooperate fully and to follow directions. Direct the patient to breathe normally and to avoid unnecessary movement.
- Observe standard precautions, and follow the general guidelines in Patient Preparation and Specimen Collection online at Davis*Plus*. Positively identify the patient, and label the appropriate specimen container with the corresponding patient demographics, initials of the person collecting the specimen, date, and time of collection. Perform a venipuncture.
- Remove the needle and apply direct pressure with dry gauze to stop bleeding. Observe/assess

venipuncture site for bleeding or hematoma formation and secure gauze with adhesive bandage.
- Promptly transport the specimen to the laboratory for processing and analysis.

POST-TEST:
- Inform the patient that a report of the results will be made available to the requesting health-care provider (HCP), who will discuss the results with the patient.
- Advise the patient with sickle cell disease to avoid situations in which hypoxia may occur, such as strenuous exercise, staying at high altitudes, or traveling in an unpressurized aircraft. Obstetric and surgical patients with sickle cell anemia are at risk for hypoxia and therefore require close observation: Obstetric patients are at risk for hypoxia during the stress of labor and delivery, and surgical patients may become hypoxic while under general anesthesia.
- Recognize anxiety related to test results, and offer support, as appropriate. Discuss the implications of abnormal test results on the patient's lifestyle. Provide teaching and information regarding the clinical implications of the test results, as appropriate. Educate the patient regarding access to counseling services. Provide contact information, if desired, for the Sickle Cell Disease Association of America (www.sicklecelldisease.org). 🍁
- Reinforce information given by the patient's HCP regarding further testing, treatment, or referral to another HCP. Inform the patient that further testing may be indicated if results are positive. Answer any questions or address any concerns voiced by the patient or family.
- Depending on the results of this procedure, additional testing may be performed to evaluate or monitor progression of the disease process and determine the need for a change in therapy. Evaluate test results in relation to the patient's symptoms and other tests performed.

RELATED STUDIES:
- Related tests include biopsy bone marrow, CBC, CBC RBC morphology, CBC RBC indices, ESR, genetic testing, Hgb electrophoresis, hemosiderin, LAP, MRI musculoskeletal, newborn screening, RBC cholinesterase, and US spleen.
- Refer to the Hematopoietic System table online at Davis*Plus* for related tests by body system.

Slit-Lamp Biomicroscopy

SYNONYM/ACRONYM: Slit-lamp examination.

COMMON USE: To detect abnormalities in the external and anterior eye structures to assist in diagnosing disorders such as corneal injury, hemorrhage, ulcers, and abrasion.

AREA OF APPLICATION: Eyes.

POTENTIAL MEDICAL DIAGNOSIS

Normal findings
- Normal anterior tissues and structures of the eyes

Abnormal findings related to
- Blepharitis
- Conjunctivitis
- Corneal abrasions

S

- Corneal foreign bodies
- Corneal ulcers
- Diabetes
- Ectropion
- Entropion
- Glaucoma
- Hordeolum
- Iritis
- Keratoconus (abnormal curvatures)
- Lens opacities
- Scleritis
- Trachoma

CRITICAL FINDINGS: N/A

Find and print out the full study on Fast Find at davispl.us/vanleeuwen7.

Sodium, Blood

SYNONYM/ACRONYM: Serum Na^+.

COMMON USE: To assess electrolyte balance related to hydration levels and disorders such as diarrhea and vomiting and to monitor the effect of diuretic use.

SPECIMEN: Serum collected in a gold-, red-, or red/gray-top tube. Plasma collected in a green-top (heparin) tube is also acceptable.

NORMAL FINDINGS: (Method: Ion-selective electrode)

Age	Conventional & SI Units
Cord	126–166 mEq/L or mmol/L
1–12 hr	124–156 mEq/L or mmol/L
12–24 hr	132–159 mEq/L or mmol/L
24–48 hr	134–160 mEq/L or mmol/L
48–72 hr	139–162 mEq/L or mmol/L
Newborn	135–145 mEq/L or mmol/L
7 d–1 mo	134–144 mEq/L or mmol/L
2 mo–5 mo	134–142 mEq/L or mmol/L
6 mo–1 yr	133–142 mEq/L or mmol/L
Child–Adult–older adult	135–145 mEq/L or mmol/L

Note: Older adults are at increased risk for both hypernatremia and hyponatremia. Diminished thirst, illness, and lack of mobility are common causes for hypernatremia in older adults. There are multiple causes of hyponatremia in older adults, but the most common factor may be related to the use of thiazide diuretics.

S

DESCRIPTION: Electrolytes dissociate into electrically charged ions when dissolved. Cations, including sodium, carry a positive charge. Body fluids contain approximately equal numbers of anions and cations, although the nature of the ions and their mobility differs between the intracellular and extracellular compartments. Both types of ions affect the electrical and osmolar functions of the body. Electrolyte quantities and the balance among them are controlled by oxygen and carbon dioxide exchange in the lungs; absorption, secretion, and excretion of many substances by the kidneys; and secretion of regulatory hormones by the endocrine glands. Sodium is the most abundant extracellular cation that together with chloride and bicarbonate participate in a number of essential functions to include maintaining the osmotic pressure of extracellular fluid, regulating renal retention and excretion of water, maintaining acid-base balance, regulating potassium levels, stimulating neuromuscular reactions, and maintaining systemic blood pressure. *Hypernatremia* (elevated sodium level) occurs when there is excessive water loss or abnormal retention of sodium. *Hyponatremia* (low sodium level) occurs when there is inadequate sodium retention or inadequate intake.

This procedure is contraindicated for: N/A

INDICATIONS

- Determine whole-body stores of sodium, because the ion is predominantly extracellular.
- Monitor the effectiveness of drug therapy, especially diuretics, on serum sodium levels.

POTENTIAL MEDICAL DIAGNOSIS

Increased in:

- Azotemia ***(related to increased renal retention)***
- Burns ***(hemoconcentration related to excessive loss of free water)***
- Cushing's disease
- Dehydration
- Diabetes ***(dehydration related to frequent urination)***
- Diarrhea ***(related to water loss in excess of salt loss)***
- Excessive intake
- Excessive saline therapy ***(related to administration of intravenous (IV) fluids)***
- Excessive sweating ***(related to loss of free water, which can cause hemoconcentration)***
- Fever ***(related to loss of free water through sweating)***
- Hyperaldosteronism ***(related to excessive production of aldosterone, which increases renal absorption of sodium and increases blood levels)***
- Lactic acidosis ***(related to diabetes)***
- Nasogastric feeding with inadequate fluid ***(related to dehydration and hemoconcentration)***
- Vomiting ***(related to dehydration)***

Decreased in:

- Central nervous system disease
- Cystic fibrosis ***(related to loss from chronic diarrhea; poor intestinal absorption)***
- Excessive antidiuretic hormone production ***(related to excessive loss through renal excretion)***
- Excessive use of diuretics ***(related to excessive loss through renal excretion, renal absorption is blocked)***
- Heart failure ***(diminished renal blood flow due to reduced cardiac capacity decreases urinary excretion and increases blood sodium levels)***
- Hepatic failure ***(hemodilution related to fluid retention)***
- Hypoproteinemia ***(related to fluid retention)***
- Insufficient intake
- IV glucose infusion ***(hypertonic glucose draws water into extracellular fluid and sodium is diluted)***
- Mineralocorticoid deficiency (Addison's disease) ***(related to inadequate production of aldosterone, which results in decreased absorption by the kidneys)***
- Nephrotic syndrome ***(related to decreased ability of renal tubules to reabsorb sodium)***

S

CRITICAL FINDINGS:

- *Hyponatremia:* Less than 120 mEq/L or mmol/L (SI: Less than 120 mmol/L)
- *Hypernatremia:* Greater than 160 mEq/L or mmol/L (SI: Greater than 160 mmol/L)

Note and immediately report to the requesting health-care provider (HCP) any critical findings and related symptoms. A listing of these findings varies among facilities. Timely notification of a critical finding for laboratory or diagnostic studies is a role expectation of the professional nurse. The notification processes vary among facilities. Upon receipt of the critical finding, the information should be read back to the caller to verify accuracy.

Consideration may be given to verification of critical findings before action is taken. Policies vary among facilities and may include requesting immediate recollection and retesting by the laboratory or retesting using a rapid point-of-care testing instrument at the bedside, if available.

Signs and symptoms of hyponatremia include confusion, irritability, convulsions, tachycardia, nausea, vomiting, and loss of consciousness. Possible interventions include maintenance of airway, monitoring for convulsions, fluid restriction, and performance of hourly neurological checks. Administration of saline for replacement requires close attention to serum and urine osmolality.

Signs and symptoms of hypernatremia include restlessness, intense thirst, weakness, swollen tongue, seizures, and coma. Possible interventions include treatment of the underlying cause of water loss or sodium excess, which includes sodium restriction and administration of diuretics combined with IV solutions of 5% dextrose in water (D_5W).

INTERFERING FACTORS

- Drugs and other substances that may increase serum sodium levels include anabolic steroids, angiotensin, bicarbonate, cisplatin, corticotropin, cortisone, gamma globulin, and mannitol.
- Drugs and other substances that may decrease serum sodium levels include amphotericin B, bicarbonate, cathartics (excessive use), chlorpropamide, chlorthalidone, diuretics, ethacrynic acid, fluoxetine, furosemide, laxatives (excessive use), methyclothiazide, metolazone, nicardipine, quinethazone, theophylline (IV infusion), thiazides, and triamterene.
- Specimens should never be collected above an IV line because of the potential for dilution when the specimen and the IV solution combine in the collection container, falsely decreasing the result. There is also the potential of contaminating the sample with the substance of interest, if it is present in the IV solution, falsely increasing the result.

NURSING IMPLICATIONS AND PROCEDURE

S

POTENTIAL NURSING PROBLEMS:

Problem	Signs & Symptoms	Interventions
Fluid volume ***(related to an excess or deficit of sodium***	**Deficient:** Decreased urinary output, fatigue, sunken eyes, dark	Record daily weight and monitor trends; record accurate intake and output; collaborate with HCP with

Problem	Signs & Symptoms	Interventions
associated with electrolyte disturbance and associated disease process)	urine, decreased blood pressure, increased heart rate, and altered mental status **Overload:** Edema, shortness of breath, increased weight, ascites, rales, rhonchi, and diluted laboratory values	administration of IV fluids to support hydration; monitor laboratory values that reflect alterations in fluid status (potassium, blood urea nitrogen, creatinine, calcium, hemoglobin, hematocrit, sodium); manage underlying cause of fluid alteration; monitor urine characteristics and respiratory status; establish baseline assessment data; collaborate with HCP to adjust oral and IV fluids to provide optimal hydration status; administer replacement electrolytes as ordered; adjust diuretics as appropriate
Electrolyte imbalance: **Excess *(related to excess fluid loss, watery diarrhea; inability to take oral fluids; excess perspiration; large area burns; excess sodium intake)* Deficit *(related to excess sodium loss through kidneys; diuretic use; adrenal insufficiency with altered cortisol and aldosterone production; vomiting and diarrhea; heart failure; renal failure; cirrhosis)***	**Excess:** Furrowed tongue; dry mouth; headache; dry skin; seizures; coma; tachycardia; hypotension; vascular collapse; restlessness; increased urine; output; weight gain; altered mental status **Deficit:** Muscle cramps; weakness; fatigue; confusion; anorexia; nausea; vomiting; abdominal cramps; diarrhea; headache; depression; personality changes; irritability; muscle twitching; coma; anxiety	Correlate sodium imbalance with disease process, nutritional intake, kidney function, medications; monitor electrocardiogram status; monitor for respiratory changes; minimize metabolic complications; provide a safe environment to prevent injury; collaborate with the pharmacist and HCP for appropriate pharmacologic interventions; adjust medication dosage to compensate for renal impairment; collaborate with dietitian for dietary modifications; use kidney dialysis as necessary; reduce or increase intake of high-sodium foods and salts; if deficit avoid thiazide diuretics; if excess use diuretics to increase sodium excretion; if excess use IV fluids to remedy dehydration; if excess use IV NaCl infusion as prescribed

(table continues on page 1414)

S

Problem	Signs & Symptoms	Interventions
Diarrhea ***(related to gastric irritation from diet or disease; stress; drug adverse effect; laxative misuse; malabsorption; alcohol abuse; chemotherapy; enteric infections)***	Abdominal pain; cramping; frequent stools that exceed three per d; watery stools; gastrointestinal (GI) urgency; hyperactive bowel sounds	Assess bowel sounds; send stool for culture as ordered; assess for food intolerances that can irritate the GI tract; review tolerance to dairy products; check for a history of GI disease or surgery; ask about foreign travel; administer prescribed antidiarrheal; evaluate and replace lost fluids; consider dietary bulk
Confusion ***(related to sodium excess or deficit secondary to metabolic alterations, disease process, or burns)***	Disorganized thinking; restlessness; irritability; altered concentration and attention span; changeable mental function over the d; hallucinations	Treat the medical condition; correlate confusion with the need to reverse altered electrolytes; evaluate medications; prevent falls and injury through appropriate use of postural support, bed alarm, or the restraints; consider pharmacological interventions; record accurate intake and output to assess fluid status

PRETEST:

- Positively identify the patient using at least two person-specific identifiers before services, treatments, or procedures are performed.
- *Patient Teaching:* Inform the patient this test can assist in evaluating electrolyte balance.
- Obtain a history of the patient's health concerns, symptoms, surgical procedures, and results of previously performed laboratory and diagnostic studies. Include a list of known allergens, especially allergies or sensitivities to latex.
- Obtain a list of the patient's current medications, including over-the-counter medications and dietary supplements (see Effects of Natural Products on Laboratory Values online at Davis*Plus*).
- Review the procedure with the patient. Inform the patient that specimen collection takes approximately 5 to 10 min. Address concerns about pain and explain that there may be some discomfort during the venipuncture.
- *Sensitivity to social and cultural issues,* as well as concern for modesty, is important in providing psychological support before, during, and after the procedure.
- Note that there are no food, fluid, or medication restrictions unless by medical direction.

INTRATEST:

Potential Complications: N/A

- Avoid the use of equipment containing latex if the patient has a history of allergic reaction to latex.
- Instruct the patient to cooperate fully and to follow directions. Direct the patient to breathe normally and to avoid unnecessary movement.

S

- Observe standard precautions, and follow the general guidelines in Patient Preparation and Specimen Collection online at Davis*Plus*. Positively identify the patient, and label the appropriate specimen container with the corresponding patient demographics, initials of the person collecting the specimen, date, and time of collection. Perform a venipuncture.
- Remove the needle and apply direct pressure with dry gauze to stop bleeding. Observe/assess venipuncture site for bleeding or hematoma formation and secure gauze with adhesive bandage.
- Promptly transport the specimen to the laboratory for processing and analysis.

POST-TEST:

- Inform the patient that a report of the results will be made available to the requesting HCP, who will discuss the results with the patient.
- *Nutritional Considerations:* Evaluate the patient for signs and symptoms of dehydration. Decreased skin turgor, dry mouth, and multiple longitudinal furrows in the tongue are symptoms of dehydration. Dehydration is a significant and common finding in older adults and other patients in whom kidney function has deteriorated.
- *Nutritional Considerations:* If appropriate, educate patients with low sodium levels that the major source of dietary sodium is found in table salt. Many foods, such as milk and other dairy products, are also good sources of dietary sodium. Most other dietary sodium is available through the consumption of processed foods; some examples are baking mixes (pancakes or muffins), sauces (barbecue), butter, canned soups and sauces, dry soup mixes, frozen or microwave meals, ketchup, pickles, and snack foods (potato chips, pretzels). Patients on low-sodium diets should be advised to avoid beverages such as colas, ginger ale, sports drinks, lemon-lime sodas, and root beer. Many over-the-counter medications, including antacids, laxatives, analgesics, sedatives, and antitussives, contain significant amounts of sodium. The best advice is to emphasize the importance of reading all food, beverage, and medicine labels.
- Depending on the results of this procedure, additional testing may be performed to evaluate or monitor progression of the disease process and determine the need for a change in therapy. Evaluate test results in relation to the patient's symptoms and other tests performed.

Patient Education:

- Reinforce information given by the patient's HCP regarding further testing, treatment, or referral to another HCP.
- Recognize anxiety related to test results and answer any questions or address any concerns voiced by the patient or family.
- Educate the patient regarding access to nutritional counseling services.
- Provide contact information, if desired, for the Institute of Medicine of the National Academies (www.iom.edu) or USDA's resource for nutrition (http://www.choosemyplate.gov). 🍁
- Teach the patient and family to recognize symptoms of both an excess and deficit of sodium.
- Teach the importance of fluid replacement with multiple diarrhea episodes.

Expected Patient Outcomes:

Understanding

- The patient and family acknowledge that an altered sodium level can have a significant impact on cognitive function.
- The patient and family acknowledge that excessive watery stools can result in an altered sodium level.

Ability

- The patient and family identify foods to select that will support a healthy sodium level.
- The patient and family select dietary supplements to what is required to support a healthy sodium level.

Response

- The patient complies with the recommendation to monitor diarrhea and report excessive stools to the HCP.
- The patient complies with the recommendation to increase oral fluid intake to replace lost fluids that can affect sodium levels.

RELATED STUDIES:

- Related tests include ACTH, aldosterone, anion gap, ANP, BNP, blood gases, BUN, calculus kidney stone panel, BUN, calcium, carbon dioxide, chloride, chloride sweat, cortisol, creatinine, DHEAS, echocardiography, glucose, insulin, ketones, lactic acid, lung perfusion scan, magnesium, osmolality, potassium, renin, US abdomen, urine sodium, and UA.
- Refer to the Cardiovascular, Endocrine, and Genitourinary systems tables online at Davis*Plus* for related tests by body system.

Sodium, Urine

SYNONYM/ACRONYM: Urine Na^+.

COMMON USE: To assist in evaluating for acute renal failure, acute oliguria, and to assist in the differential diagnosis of hyponatremia.

SPECIMEN: Urine from an unpreserved random or timed specimen collected in a clean plastic collection container.

NORMAL FINDINGS: (Method: Ion-selective electrode)

Age	Conventional Units	SI Units (Conventional Units × 1)
6–10 yr		
Male	41–115 mEq/24 hr or mmol/24 hr	41–115 mmol/24 hr
Female	20–69 mEq/24 hr or mmol/24 hr	20–69 mmol/24 hr
10–14 yr		
Male	63–177 mEq/24 hr or mmol/24 hr	63–177 mmol/24 hr
Female	48–168 mEq/24 hr or mmol/24 hr	48–168 mmol/24 hr
Adult–older adult	27–287 mEq/24 hr or mmol/24 hr	27–287 mmol/24 hr

Values vary markedly depending on dietary intake and hydration state.

DESCRIPTION: Sodium balance is dependent on a number of influences in addition to dietary intake, including aldosterone, renin, and atrial natriuretic hormone levels. Regulating electrolyte balance is a major function of the kidneys. In normally functioning kidneys, urine sodium levels increase when serum levels are high and decrease when serum levels are low to maintain homeostasis. Analyzing these urinary levels can provide important clues to the functioning of the kidneys and other major organs. There is diurnal variation in excretion of sodium, with values lower at night. Urine sodium tests usually involve timed urine collections over a 12- or 24-hr period. Measurement of random specimens may also be requested.

This procedure is contraindicated for: N/A

INDICATIONS

- Determine potential cause of renal calculi.
- Evaluate known or suspected endocrine disorder.
- Evaluate known or suspected kidney disease.
- Evaluate malabsorption disorders.

POTENTIAL MEDICAL DIAGNOSIS

Increased in:

- Adrenal failure ***(inadequate production of aldosterone results in decreased renal sodium absorption)***
- Dehydration ***(related to decreased water excretion, which results in higher concentration of the urine constituents)***
- Diabetes ***(increased glucose levels result in hypertonic extracellular fluid; dehydration from excessive urination can cause hemoconcentration)***
- Diuretic therapy ***(medication causes sodium to be lost by the kidneys)***
- Excessive intake
- Salt-losing nephritis ***(related to diminished capacity of the kidneys to reabsorb sodium)***
- Syndrome of inappropriate antidiuretic hormone secretion ***(related to increased reabsorption of water by the kidneys, which results in higher concentration of the urine constituents)***

Decreased in:

- Adrenal hyperfunction, such as Cushing's disease and hyperaldostronism ***(overproduction of aldosterone and other corticosteroids stimulate renal absorption of sodium decreasing urine sodium levels)***
- Heart failure ***(decreased renal blood flow related to diminished cardiac output)***
- Diarrhea ***(related to decreased intestinal absorption; a decrease in blood levels will cause sodium to be retained by the kidneys and will lower urine sodium levels)***
- Excessive sweating ***(excessive loss of sodium through sweat; sodium will be retained by the kidneys)***
- Extrarenal sodium loss with adequate hydration
- Insufficient intake
- Postoperative period (first 24 to 48 hr)
- Prerenal azotemia
- Sodium retention ***(premenstrual)***

CRITICAL FINDINGS: N/A

INTERFERING FACTORS

- Drugs and other substances that may increase urine sodium levels include acetazolamide, acetylsalicylic acid, amiloride, ammonium chloride, azosemide, benzthiazide, bumetanide, calcitonin, chlorothiazide, clopamide, cyclothiazide, diapamide, dopamine, ethacrynic acid, furosemide, hydrocortisone, isosorbide, levodopa, mercurial diuretics, methyclothiazide, metolazone, polythiazide, quinethazone, spironolactone, sulfates, tetracycline, thiazides, torasemide, triamterene, trichlormethiazide, triflocin, verapamil, and vincristine.
- Drugs and other substances that may decrease urine sodium levels include aldosterone, anesthetics, angiotensin, corticosteroids, cortisone, etodolac, indomethacin, levarterenol, lithium, and propranolol.
- Sodium levels are subject to diurnal variation (output being lowest at night), which is why 24-hr collections are recommended.

S

NURSING IMPLICATIONS AND PROCEDURE

PRETEST:

- Positively identify the patient using at least two person-specific identifiers before services, treatments, or procedures are performed.
- ***Patient Teaching:*** Inform the patient this test can assist in evaluating kidney function.
- Obtain a history of the patient's health concerns, symptoms, surgical procedures, and results of previously performed laboratory and diagnostic studies. Include a list of known allergens, especially allergies or sensitivities to latex.
- Obtain a list of the patient's current medications, including over-the-counter medications and dietary supplements (see Effects of Natural Products on Laboratory Values online at DavisPlus).
- Review the procedure with the patient. Provide a nonmetallic urinal, bedpan, or toilet-mounted collection device. Address concerns about pain and explain that there should be no discomfort during the procedure.
- ***Sensitivity to social and cultural issues,*** as well as concern for modesty, is important in providing psychological support before, during, and after the procedure.
- Usually a 24-hr time frame for urine collection is ordered. Inform the patient that all urine must be saved during that 24-hr period. Instruct the patient not to void directly into the laboratory collection container. Instruct the patient to avoid defecating in the collection device and to keep toilet tissue out of the collection device to prevent contamination of the specimen. Place a sign in the bathroom to remind the patient to save all urine.
- Instruct the patient to void all urine into the collection device and then to pour the urine into the laboratory collection container. Alternatively, the specimen can be left in the collection device for a health care staff member to add to the laboratory collection container.
- Note that there are no food, fluid, or medication restrictions unless by medical direction.

INTRATEST:

Potential Complications: N/A

- Avoid the use of equipment containing latex if the patient has a history of allergic reaction to latex.
- Instruct the patient to cooperate fully and to follow directions.
- Observe standard precautions, and follow the general guidelines in Patient Preparation and Specimen Collection online at Davis*Plus*. Positively identify the patient, and label the appropriate specimen container with the corresponding patient demographics, initials of the person collecting the specimen, date, and time of collection.

Random Specimen (Collect in Early Morning)

Clean-Catch Specimen

- Instruct the male patient to (1) thoroughly wash his hands, (2) cleanse the meatus, (3) void a small amount into the toilet, and (4) void directly into the specimen container.
- Instruct the female patient to (1) thoroughly wash her hands; (2) cleanse the labia from front to back; (3) while keeping the labia separated, void a small amount into the toilet; and (4) without interrupting the urine stream, void directly into the specimen container.

Indwelling Catheter

- Put on gloves. Empty drainage tube of urine. It may be necessary to clamp off the catheter for 15 to 30 min before specimen collection. Cleanse specimen port with antiseptic swab, and then aspirate 5 mL of urine with a 21- to 25-gauge needle and syringe. Transfer urine to a sterile container.

S

Timed Specimen

- Obtain a clean 3 L urine specimen container, toilet-mounted collection device, and plastic bag (for transport of the specimen container). The specimen must be refrigerated or kept on ice throughout the entire collection period. If an indwelling urinary catheter is in place, the drainage bag must be kept on ice.
- Begin the test between 0600 and 0800, if possible. Collect first voiding and discard. Record the time the specimen was discarded as the beginning of the timed collection period. The next morning, ask the patient to void at the same time the collection was started and add this last voiding to the container. Urinary output should be recorded throughout the collection time.
- If an indwelling catheter is in place, replace the tubing and container system at the start of the collection time. Keep the container system on ice during the collection period, or empty the urine into a larger container periodically during the collection period; monitor to ensure continued drainage, and conclude the test the next morning at the same hour the collection was begun.
- At the conclusion of the test, compare the quantity of urine with the urinary output record for the collection; if the specimen contains less than what was recorded as output, some urine may have been discarded, invalidating the test.
- Include on the collection container's label the amount of urine, test start and stop times, and any foods or medications that can affect test results.

General

- Promptly transport the specimen to the laboratory for processing and analysis.

POST-TEST:

- Inform the patient that a report of the results will be made available to the requesting health-care provider (HCP), who will discuss the results with the patient.
- Instruct the patient to resume usual diet, fluids, medications, and activity, as directed by the HCP.
- ***Nutritional Considerations:*** If appropriate, educate patients with low sodium levels that the major source of dietary sodium is found in table salt. Many foods, such as milk and other dairy products, are also good sources of dietary sodium. Most other dietary sodium is available through the consumption of processed foods. Patients on low-sodium diets should be advised to avoid beverages such as colas, ginger ale, sports drinks, lemon-lime sodas, and root beer. Many over-the-counter medications, including antacids, laxatives, analgesics, sedatives, and antitussives, contain significant amounts of sodium. The best advice is to emphasize the importance of reading all food, beverage, and medicine labels.
- Recognize anxiety related to test results. Discuss the implications of abnormal test results on the patient's lifestyle. Provide teaching and information regarding the clinical implications of the test results, as appropriate.
- Reinforce information given by the patient's HCP regarding further testing, treatment, or referral to another HCP. Answer any questions or address any concerns voiced by the patient or family.
- Depending on the results of this procedure, additional testing may be performed to evaluate or monitor progression of the disease process and determine the need for a change in therapy. Evaluate test results in relation to the patient's symptoms and other tests performed.

RELATED STUDIES:

- Related tests include ACTH, aldosterone, anion gap, ANP, BNP, blood gases, BUN, calcium, calculus kidney stone panel, carbon dioxide, chloride, chloride sweat, cortisol, creatinine,

S

DHEAS, echocardiography, glucose, insulin, ketones, lactic acid, lung perfusion scan, magnesium, osmolality, potassium, renin, sodium, and UA.

- Refer to the Endocrine and Genitourinary system tables online at Davis*Plus* for related tests by body system.

Spondee Speech Recognition Threshold

SYNONYM/ACRONYM: SRT, speech reception threshold, speech recognition threshold.

COMMON USE: To evaluate for hearing loss related to speech discrepancies.

AREA OF APPLICATION: Ears.

POTENTIAL MEDICAL DIAGNOSIS

Normal findings

- Normal spondee threshold of about 6 to 10 dB (decibels) of the normal pure tone threshold with 50% of the words presented being correctly repeated at the appropriate intensity (see study titled "Audiometry, Hearing Loss")
- Normal speech recognition with 90% to 100% of the words presented being correctly repeated at an appropriate intensity

Abnormal findings related to

- Conductive hearing loss
- Impacted cerumen
- Obstruction of external ear canal ***(related to presence of a foreign body)***
- Otitis externa ***(related to infection in ear canal)***
- Otitis media ***(related to poor eustachian tube function or infection)***
- Otitis media serus ***(related to fluid in middle ear due to allergies or a cold)***
- Otosclerosis
- High-frequency hearing loss ***(normal hearing range is 20 Hz to 20,000 Hz; high-frequency range begins at 4,000 Hz)***
- Presbycusis ***(related to gradual hearing loss experienced in advancing age, which occurs in the high-frequency range)***
- Noise induced ***(related to exposure over long periods of time)***
- Sensorineural hearing loss (acoustic nerve impairment)
- Congenital damage or malformations of the inner ear
- Ménière's disease
- Ototoxic drugs ***(aminoglycosides, e.g., gentamicin or tobramycin; salicylates, e.g., aspirin)***
- Presbycusis ***(related to gradual hearing loss experienced in advancing age)***
- Serious infections ***(meningitis, measles, mumps, other viral infections, syphilis)***
- Trauma to the inner ear ***(related to exposure to noise in excess of 90 dB or as a result of physical trauma)***
- Tumor ***(e.g., acoustic neuroma, cerebellopontine angle tumor, meningioma)***
- Vascular disorders

CRITICAL FINDINGS: N/A

Find and print out the full study on Fast Find at davispl.us/vanleeuwen7.

Stereotactic Biopsy, Breast

SYNONYM/ACRONYM: N/A

COMMON USE: To assess suspicious breast tissue for cancer.

SPECIMEN: Breast tissue or cells.

NORMAL FINDINGS: (Method: Macroscopic and microscopic examination of tissue) No abnormal cells or tissue.

POTENTIAL MEDICAL DIAGNOSIS

- Positive findings in carcinoma of the breast

CRITICAL FINDINGS: N/A

Find and print out the full study on Fast Find at davispl.us/vanleeuwen7.

Synovial Fluid Analysis

SYNONYM/ACRONYM: Arthrocentesis, joint fluid analysis, knee fluid analysis.

COMMON USE: To identify the presence and assist in the management of joint disease related to disorders such as arthritis and gout.

SPECIMEN: Synovial fluid collected in a red-top tube for antinuclear antibodies (ANAs), complement, crystal examination, protein, rheumatoid factor (RF), and uric acid; sterile (red-top) tube for microbiological testing; lavender-top (EDTA) tube for mucin clot/viscosity, complete blood count (CBC) and differential; gray-top (sodium fluoride [NaFl]) tube for glucose; green-top (heparin) tube for lactic acid and pH.

NORMAL FINDINGS: (Method: Macroscopic evaluation of appearance; spectrophotometry for glucose, lactic acid, protein, and uric acid; Gram stain, acid-fast stain, and culture for microbiology; microscopic examination of fluid for cell count and evaluation of crystals; ion-selective electrode for pH; nephelometry for RF and C3 complement; indirect fluorescence for ANAs)

Test	Normal Result
Color	Colorless to pale yellow
Clarity	Clear
Viscosity	High
ANA	Parallels serum level
C3	Parallels serum level
Glucose	Less than 10 mg/dL of blood level

(table continues on page 1422)

S

Test	Normal Result
Lactic acid	5–20 mg/dL
pH	7.2–7.4
Protein	Less than 3 g/dL
RF	Parallels serum level
Uric acid	Parallels serum level
Crystals	None present
RBC count	None
WBC count	Less than 200 cells/microL
Neutrophils	Less than 25%
WBC morphology	No abnormal cells or inclusions
Gram stain and culture	No organisms present
AFB smear and culture	No AFB present

AFB = acid-fast bacilli; ANA = antinuclear antibodies; C3 = complement; RBC = red blood cell; RF = rheumatoid factor; WBC = white blood cell.

DESCRIPTION: Synovial fluid analysis is performed via arthrocentesis, an invasive procedure involving insertion of a needle into the joint space. Synovial effusions are associated with disorders or injuries involving the joints. The most commonly aspirated joint is the knee, although samples also can be obtained from the shoulder, hip, elbow, wrist, and ankle if clinically indicated. Joint disorders can be classified into five categories: noninflammatory, inflammatory, septic, crystal-induced, and hemorrhagic. The mucin clot test is used to correlate the qualitative assessment of synovial fluid viscosity with the presence of hyaluronic acid. The test is performed by mixing equal amounts of synovial fluid and 5% acetic acid solution on a glass slide and grading the ropiness of the subsequent clot as good, fair, or poor. Long, ropy strands are seen in normal synovial fluid.

This procedure is contraindicated for: N/A

INDICATIONS

- Administration of anti-inflammatory medications by injection.
- Assist in the diagnosis of arthritis.
- Assist in the evaluation of joint effusions.
- Assist in the diagnosis of joint infection.
- Differentiate gout from pseudogout.

POTENTIAL MEDICAL DIAGNOSIS

Fluid values increased in

- *Acute bacterial infection:* Elevated WBC count with marked predominance of neutrophils (greater than 90% neutrophils), positive Gram stain, positive cultures, possible presence of rice bodies, increased lactic acid (produced by bacteria), and complement levels paralleling those found in serum (may be elevated or decreased)
- *Gout:* Elevated WBC count with a predominance of neutrophils (90% neutrophils), presence of monosodium urate crystals, increased uric acid, and complement levels paralleling those of serum (may be elevated or decreased)
- *Osteoarthritis, traumatic arthritis degenerative joint disease:* Elevated WBC count with less than

S

25% neutrophils and the presence of cartilage cells
- *Pseudogout:* Presence of calcium pyrophosphate crystals
- *Rheumatoid arthritis:* Elevated WBC count with a predominance of neutrophils (greater than 70% neutrophils), presence of ragocyte cells and possibly rice bodies, presence of cholesterol crystals if effusion is chronic, increased protein, increased lactic acid, and presence of rheumatoid factor
- *Systemic lupus erythematosus (SLE):* Elevated WBC count with a predominance of neutrophils, presence of SLE cells, and presence of antinuclear antibodies
- *Trauma, joint tumors, or hemophilic arthritis:* Elevated RBC count, increased protein level, and presence of fat droplets (if trauma involved)
- *Tuberculous arthritis:* Elevated WBC count with a predominance of neutrophils (up to 90% neutrophils), possible presence of rice bodies, presence of cholesterol crystals if effusion is chronic, in some cases a positive culture and smear for acid-fast bacilli (results frequently negative), and lactic acid

Fluid values decreased in (analytes in parentheses are decreased)
- Acute bacterial arthritis (glucose and pH)
- Gout (glucose)
- Rheumatoid arthritis (glucose, pH, and complement)
- SLE (glucose, pH, and complement)
- Tuberculous arthritis (glucose and pH)

CRITICAL FINDINGS:

Positive culture findings in any sterile body fluid.

Note and immediately report to the requesting health-care provider (HCP) any critical findings and related symptoms. A listing of these findings varies among facilities. Timely notification of a critical finding for laboratory or diagnostic studies is a role expectation of the professional nurse. The notification processes vary among facilities. Upon receipt of the critical finding, the information should be read back to the caller to verify accuracy.

INTERFERING FACTORS
- Blood in the sample from traumatic arthrocentesis may falsely elevate the RBC count.
- Undetected hypoglycemia or hyperglycemia may produce misleading glucose values.
- Refrigeration of the sample may result in an increase in monosodium urate crystals secondary to decreased solubility of uric acid; exposure of the sample to room air with a resultant loss of carbon dioxide and rise in pH encourages the formation of calcium pyrophosphate crystals.

NURSING IMPLICATIONS AND PROCEDURE

PRETEST:
- Positively identify the patient using at least two person-specific identifiers before services, treatments, or procedures are performed.
- *Patient Teaching:* Inform the patient this procedure can assist in assessing joint health.
- Obtain a history of the patient's health concerns, symptoms, surgical procedures, and results of previously performed laboratory and diagnostic studies. Include a list of known allergens, especially allergies or sensitivities to latex.
- Note any recent procedures that can interfere with test results.
- Record the date of the last menstrual period and determine the possibility of pregnancy in perimenopausal women.

S

- Obtain a list of the patient's current medications, including over-the-counter medications, dietary supplements, anticoagulants, aspirin and other salicylates (see Effects of Natural Products on Laboratory Values online at Davis*Plus*). Such products should be discontinued by medical direction for the appropriate number of days prior to a surgical procedure. Note the last time and dose of medication taken.
- Review the procedure with the patient. Inform the patient that it may be necessary to remove hair from the site before the procedure. Address concerns about pain and explain that a sedative and/or analgesia will be administered to promote relaxation and reduce discomfort prior to needle insertion through the joint space. Explain that any discomfort with the needle insertion will be minimized with local anesthetics and systemic analgesics. Explain that the anesthetic injection may cause an initial stinging sensation. Explain that, after the skin has been anesthetized, a large needle will be inserted through the joint space, and a "popping" sensation may be experienced as the needle penetrates the joint. Inform the patient that the procedure is performed by an HCP specializing in this procedure. The procedure usually takes approximately 20 min to complete.
- ***Sensitivity to social and cultural issues,*** as well as concern for modesty, is important in providing psychological support before, during, and after the procedure.
- Note that there are no fluid restrictions unless by medical direction. Fasting for at least 12 hr before the procedure is recommended if fluid glucose measurements are included in the analysis. Instruct the patient to avoid taking anticoagulant medication or to reduce dosage as ordered prior to the procedure. Protocols may vary among facilities.
- *Make sure a written and informed consent has been signed prior to the procedure and before administering any medications.*

INTRATEST:

Potential Complications: N/A

- Ensure that the patient has complied with dietary and medication restrictions and pretesting preparations prior to the procedure, as instructed. Notify the HCP if patient anticoagulant therapy has not been withheld.
- Assemble the necessary equipment, including an arthrocentesis tray with solution for skin preparation, local anesthetic, a 20-mL syringe, needles of various sizes, sterile drapes, and sterile gloves for the tests to be performed.
- Avoid the use of equipment containing latex if the patient has a history of allergic reaction to latex.
- Instruct the patient to cooperate fully and to follow directions. Direct the patient to breathe normally and to avoid unnecessary movement during the local anesthetic and the procedure.
- Observe standard precautions, and follow the general guidelines in Patient Preparation and Specimen Collection online at Davis*Plus*. Positively identify the patient, and label the appropriate specimen container with the corresponding patient demographics, initials of the person collecting the specimen, date and time of collection, and site location, especially, right or left knee, shoulder, hip, elbow, wrist, or ankle.
- Assist the patient into a comfortable sitting or supine position, as appropriate.
- Use clippers to remove hair from the site prior to the administration of general or local anesthesia, cleanse the site with an antiseptic solution, and drape the area with sterile towels.
- After the local anesthetic is administered, the needle is inserted at the collection site, and fluid is removed by syringe. Manual pressure may be applied to facilitate fluid removal.
- If medication is injected into the joint, the syringe containing the sample

S

is detached from the needle and replaced with the one containing the drug. The medication is injected with gentle pressure. The needle is withdrawn, and digital pressure is applied to the site for a few minutes. If there is no evidence of bleeding, a sterile dressing is applied to the site. An elastic bandage can be applied to the joint.

- Monitor the patient for complications related to the procedure (allergic reaction, anaphylaxis).
- Place samples in properly labelled specimen containers and promptly transport the specimens to the laboratory for processing and analysis. If bacterial culture and sensitivity tests are to be performed, record on the specimen containers any antibiotic therapy the patient is receiving.

POST-TEST:

- Inform the patient that a report of the results will be made available to the requesting HCP, who will discuss the results with the patient.
- Instruct the patient to resume usual diet and medications, as directed by the HCP.
- After local anesthesia, monitor vital signs and compare with baseline values. Notify the HCP if temperature is elevated. Protocols may vary among facilities.
- Observe/assess puncture site for bleeding, bruising, inflammation, and excessive drainage of synovial fluid approximately every 4 hr for 24 hr and daily thereafter for several days.
- Instruct the patient to report excessive pain, bleeding, or swelling to the requesting HCP immediately. Report to HCP if severe pain is present or the patient is unable to move the joint.
- Observe/assess for nausea and pain. Administer antiemetic and analgesic medications as needed and as directed by the HCP.
- Instruct the patient to apply an ice pack to the site for 24 to 48 hr.
- Administer antibiotics, as ordered, and instruct the patient in the importance of completing the entire course of antibiotic therapy even if no symptoms are present.
- Recognize anxiety related to test results, and be supportive of impaired activity related to anticipated chronic pain resulting from joint inflammation, impairment in mobility, musculoskeletal deformity, and loss of independence. Discuss the implications of abnormal test results on the patient's lifestyle. Provide teaching and information regarding the clinical implications of the test results, as appropriate. Educate the patient regarding access to counseling services, as appropriate. Provide contact information, if desired, for the American College of Rheumatology (www.rheumatology.org) or for the Arthritis Foundation (www.arthritis.org). 🍁
- Reinforce information given by the patient's HCP regarding further testing, treatment, or referral to another HCP. Instruct the patient or caregiver to handle linen and dispose of dressings cautiously, especially if septic arthritis is suspected. Instruct the patient to avoid excessive use of the joint for several days to prevent pain and swelling. Instruct the patient to return for a follow-up visit as scheduled. Answer any questions or address any concerns voiced by the patient or family.
- Depending on the results of this procedure, additional testing may be performed to evaluate or monitor progression of the disease process and determine the need for a change in therapy. Evaluate test results in relation to the patient's symptoms and other tests performed.

RELATED STUDIES:

- Related tests include antibodies anticyclic citrullinated, ANA, arthrogram, arthroscopy, BMD, bone scan, CRP, cholesterol, CBC, CBC WBC count and differential, ESR, MRI musculoskeletal, radiography bone, RF, synovial fluid analysis, and uric acid.
- Refer to the Immune and Musculoskeletal systems tables online at Davis*Plus* for related tests by body system.

Syphilis Serology

SYNONYM/ACRONYM: Automated reagin testing (ART), fluorescent treponemal antibody testing (FTA-ABS), microhemagglutination-***Treponema pallidum*** (MHA-TP), rapid plasma reagin (RPR), treponemal studies, Venereal Disease Research Laboratory (VDRL) testing.

COMMON USE: To indicate past or present syphilis infection.

SPECIMEN: Serum collected in a gold-, red-, or red/gray-top tube. Place separated serum into a standard transport tube within 2 hr of collection.

NORMAL FINDINGS: (Method: Dark-field microscopy, rapid plasma reagin, enzyme-linked immunosorbent assay [ELISA], microhemagglutination, fluorescence) Nonreactive or absence of treponemal organisms.

DESCRIPTION: Syphilis is a sexually transmitted infection (STI) with three stages. On average, symptoms start within 3 wk of infection but can appear as soon as 10 days or as late as 90 days after infection. The primary stage of syphilis is usually marked by the appearance of a single sore, called a chancre, at the site where the organism entered the body. The chancre is small and round in appearance, is firm, and is usually painless. The chancre lasts 3 to 6 wk and heals with or without treatment. If untreated, the infection progresses to the secondary stage as the chancre is healing or several weeks after the chancre has healed. The secondary stage is characterized by a skin rash and lesions of the mucous membranes. Other symptoms may include fever, swollen lymph glands, sore throat, patchy hair loss, headaches, weight loss, muscle aches, and fatigue. As with the primary stage, the signs and symptoms of secondary syphilis will resolve either with or without treatment. If untreated, the infection will progress to the latent or hidden stage in which the infection and ability to transmit infection is present even though the infected person is asymptomatic. The latent stage begins when the primary and secondary symptoms disappear, and it can last for years. About 15% of people in the latent stage, who have not been treated, will develop late-stage syphilis, which can appear 10 to 20 yr after infection. Untreated disease at this stage can result in significant damage to the brain, nerves, eyes, heart, blood vessels, liver, bones, and joints—damage serious enough to cause death. Signs and symptoms of the late stage of syphilis include difficulty coordinating muscle movements, numbness, paralysis, blindness, and dementia.

There are numerous methods for detecting *Treponema pallidum*, the gram-negative spirochete bacterium known to cause syphilis. Syphilis serology is routinely ordered as part of a prenatal work-up and is required for evaluating donated blood units before release for transfusion. Selection of the proper testing method is important. ART, RPR, and VDRL testing have

S

traditionally been used for screening purposes. These nontreponemal assays detect antibodies directed against lipoidal antigens from damaged host cells. Nontreponemal assays can produce false-positive results, which are associated with older age or conditions unrelated to syphilis, such as autoimmune disorders or injection drug use, and require confirmation by a treponemal test method. FTA-ABS, MHA-TP, and *T.* by particle agglutination (TP-PA) are confirmatory methods for samples that screen positive or reactive. Some laboratories have begun using a reverse-screening approach. Highly automated, rapid-testing treponemal enzyme immunoassays (EIA) and chemiluminescent assays (CIA) detect antibodies directed against T. pallidum proteins. These assays detect early primary infections as well as past treated infections. The problem with the EIAs and CIAs is that they are very sensitive but less specific; therefore, positive test results should be confirmed using a nontreponemal assay. If reverse screening is used, the Centers for Disease Control and Prevention (CDC) recommends (1) positive EIA/CIA be confirmed using the RPR and reactive RPR test results should be reported as the endpoint titer of reactivity; (2) a positive EIA/CIA followed by a nonreactive RPR should be tested by a direct treponemal assay such as the TP-PA or FTA-ABS to ensure a false-positive result is not reported and acted upon. Cerebrospinal fluid should be tested only by the FTA-ABS method. Cord blood should not be submitted for testing by any of the aforementioned methods; instead, the mother's serum should be tested to establish whether the infant should be treated.

This procedure is contraindicated for: N/A

INDICATIONS

- Monitor effectiveness of treatment for syphilis.
- Screen for and confirm the presence of syphilis.

POTENTIAL MEDICAL DIAGNOSIS

Positive findings in

- Syphilis

False-positive or false-reactive findings in screening (RPR, VDRL) tests

- Infectious:
  - Bacterial endocarditis
  - Chancroid
  - Chickenpox
  - HIV
  - Infectious mononucleosis
  - Leprosy
  - Leptospirosis
  - Lymphogranuloma venereum
  - Malaria
  - Measles
  - Mumps
  - Mycoplasma pneumoniae
  - Pneumococcal pneumonia
  - Psittacosis
  - Relapsing fever
  - Rickettsial disease
  - Scarlet fever
  - Trypanosomiasis
  - Tuberculosis
  - Vaccinia (live or attenuated)
  - Viral hepatitis
- Noninfectious:
  - Advanced cancer
  - Advancing age
  - Chronic liver disease
  - Connective tissue diseases
  - Intravenous drug use
  - Multiple blood transfusions
  - Multiple myeloma and other immunological disorders
  - Narcotic addiction
  - Pregnancy

S

False-positive or false-reactive findings in confirmatory (FTA-ABS, MHA-TP) tests

- Infectious:
  - Infectious mononucleosis
  - Leprosy
  - Leptospirosis
  - Lyme disease
  - Malaria
  - Relapsing fever
- Noninfectious:
  - Systemic lupus erythematosus

False-positive findings in confirmatory (TP-PA) tests

- Infectious:
  - Pinta
  - Yaws

Negative findings in: N/A

CRITICAL FINDINGS: N/A

INTERFERING FACTORS: N/A

NURSING IMPLICATIONS AND PROCEDURE

POTENTIAL NURSING PROBLEMS:

Problem	Signs & Symptoms	Interventions
Knowledge ***(related to new condition or diagnosis; lack of familiarity with or understanding of disease and treatment)***	Lack of interest or questions; multiple questions; anxiety in relation to disease process and management	Identify sexual orientation; teach the process of infection transmission, heterosexual or homosexual activity; teach the patient that infection risk increases with the number of sexual partners over time; identify the patient's sexual activity; discuss importance of notifying sexual partners of disease exposure; assess for cultural, literacy, or vision and hearing concerns that would interfere with learning; teach the importance of taking the entire course of prescribed medication to treat the disease; administer prescribed medication; explore with the patient the value of monogamous relationship to support positive health
Infection	Rash on body; rash on the palms of the hands; rash on the soles of the feet; small firm nodules on genitalia, anus, or mouth; lack	Assess for signs and symptoms of syphilis; ensure understanding that the infection is transmitted through direct contact with syphilis sores (located in genitalia, vagina, anus, inside

Problem	Signs & Symptoms	Interventions
	of coordinated movement; paralysis; gradual blindness; numbness; dementia; internal organ damage (brain, nerves, eyes, heart, liver, bones, joints); death at end stage	the rectum, in the mouth); ensure understanding that it is a sexually transmitted infection; identify sexual partners who are at risk, notify them; assess for mucocutaneous infections; administer prescribed antibiotic
Body image ***(related to the presence of lesions; rash)***	Focus on appearance (lesions, rash); states feelings of worthlessness due to physical changes; reports difficulty in coping with syphilis diagnosis; change in social interaction; withdrawal	Assess the patient's perception of physical changes; note the frequency of negative comments about changed physical state; assist in the identification of positive coping strategies to address changed physical appearance
Sexuality ***(related to alterations in sexual role secondary to syphilis infection)***	Hesitancy to discuss sexual relationship with significant other	Facilitate a discussion of realistic changes to sexual intimacy associated with syphilis infection; provide a relaxed atmosphere in which to discuss sexuality concerns; provide contact information for a support group

PRETEST:

- Positively identify the patient using at least two person-specific identifiers before services, treatments, or procedures are performed.
- *Patient Teaching:* Inform the patient this test can assist in diagnosing syphilis.
- Obtain a history of the patient's health concerns (especially exposure to syphilis), symptoms, surgical procedures, and results of previously performed laboratory and diagnostic studies. Include a list of known allergens, especially allergies or sensitivities to latex.
- Obtain a list of the patient's current medications, including over-the-counter medications and dietary supplements (see Effects of Natural Products on Laboratory Values online at Davis*Plus*).
- Review the procedure with the patient. Inform the patient that specimen collection takes approximately 5 to 10 min. Address concerns about pain and explain that there may be some discomfort during the venipuncture.
- ***Sensitivity to social and cultural issues,*** as well as concern for modesty, is important in providing psychological support before, during, and after the procedure.
- Note that there are no food, fluid, or medication restrictions unless by medical direction.

INTRATEST:

Potential Complications: N/A

- Avoid the use of equipment containing latex if the patient has a history of allergic reaction to latex.

S

- Instruct the patient to cooperate fully and to follow directions. Direct the patient to breathe normally and to avoid unnecessary movement.
- Observe standard precautions, and follow the general guidelines in Patient Preparation and Specimen Collection online at Davis*Plus*. Positively identify the patient, and label the appropriate specimen container with the corresponding patient demographics, initials of the person collecting the specimen, date, and time of collection. Perform a venipuncture.
- Remove the needle and apply direct pressure with dry gauze to stop bleeding. Observe/assess venipuncture site for bleeding or hematoma formation and secure gauze with adhesive bandage.
- Promptly transport the specimen to the laboratory for processing and analysis.

POST-TEST:

- Inform the patient that a report of the results will be made available to the requesting health-care provider (HCP), who will discuss the results with the patient.
- Recognize anxiety related to test results, and offer support. Counsel the patient, as appropriate, regarding the risk of transmission and proper prophylaxis, and reinforce the importance of strict adherence to the treatment regimen. Inform the patient that positive findings must be reported to local health department officials, who will question him or her regarding sexual partners. Provide teaching and information regarding the clinical implications of the test results, as appropriate. Educate the patient regarding access to counseling services.
- Offer support, as appropriate, to patients who may be the victim of sexual assault. Provide a nonjudgmental, nonthreatening atmosphere for a discussion during which risks of STIs are explained. It is also important to discuss problems the patient may experience (e.g., guilt, depression, anger).
- Depending on the results of this procedure, additional testing may be performed to evaluate or monitor progression of the disease process and determine the need for a change in therapy. Evaluate test results in relation to the patient's symptoms and other tests performed.

Patient Education:

- Reinforce information given by the patient's HCP regarding further testing, treatment, or referral to another HCP.
- Inform the patient that repeat testing may be needed at 3-mo intervals for 1 yr to monitor the effectiveness of treatment.
- Provide information regarding vaccine-preventable diseases where indicated (e.g., sexually transmitted infections such as hepatitis B and human papillomavirus). Provide contact information, if desired, for the CDC (www.cdc.gov/vaccines/vpd-vac). 🍁
- Answer any questions or address any concerns voiced by the patient or family.
- Educate the patient regarding access to counseling services.

Expected Patient Outcomes:

Understanding

- The patient states the importance of notifying sexual partners of disease exposure.
- The patient states that untreated syphilis can be passed to an unborn child, resulting in multiple health problems, including the possibility of death if untreated.

Ability

- The patient describes the importance of a yearly gynecological examination to assess for STI.
- The patient demonstrates proficiency in the self-administration of antibiotic to treat syphilis infection.

S

Response

- The patient complies with the request to notify exposed current sexual partners about diagnoses to decrease community risk.
- The patient complies with the request to attend a support group to address specific concerns of self and sexual partner.

RELATED STUDIES:

- Related tests include cerebrospinal fluid analysis, *Chlamydia* group antibody, culture bacterial anal, Gram stain, hepatitis B, hepatitis C, HIV, and β_2-microglobulin.
- Refer to the Immune and Reproductive systems tables online at Davis*Plus* for related tests by body system.

S

Testosterone, Total and Free

SYNONYM/ACRONYM: N/A

COMMON USE: To evaluate testosterone to assist in identification of disorders related to early puberty, late puberty, and infertility while assessing gonadal and adrenal function.

SPECIMEN: Serum collected in a red- or red/gray-top tube. Plasma collected in green-top (heparin) tube is also acceptable.

NORMAL FINDINGS: (Method: HPLC/tandem MS for total and immunochemiluminometric assay [ICMA] for free testosterone)

Free Testosterone

Age	Conventional Units	SI Units (Conventional Units × 3.47)
1–12 yr		
Male and female	Less than 2 pg/mL	Less than 6.94 pmol/L
12–14 yr		
Male	Less than 60 pg/mL	Less than 208 pmol/L
Female	Less than 2 pg/mL	Less than 6.94 pmol/L
14–18 yr		
Male	4–100 pg/mL	13.88–347 pmol/L
Female	Less than 4 pg/mL	Less than 13.88 pmol/L
Adult		
Male	50–224 pg/mL	173.5–777.28 pmol/L
Female	1–8.5 pg/mL	3.47–29.5 pmol/L
Older adult		
Male	5–75 pg/mL	17.35–260.25 pmol/L
Female	1–8.5 pg/mL	3.47–29.5 pmol/L

Total Testosterone

Age	Conventional Units	SI Units (Conventional Units × 0.0347)
Newborn		
Male	17–61 ng/dL	0.59–2.12 nmol/L
Female	16–44 ng/dL	0.56–1.53 nmol/L
1–5 mo		
Male	Less than 300 ng/dL	Less than 10.41 nmol/L
Female	Less than 20 ng/dL	Less than 0.69 nmol/L
6–11 mo		
Male	Less than 40 ng/dL	Less than 1.39 nmol/L
Female	Less than 9 ng/dL	Less than 0.31 nmol/L

Age	Conventional Units	SI Units (Conventional Units × 0.0347)
1–5 yr		
Male and female	Less than 10 ng/dL	Less than 0.35 nmol/L
6–7 yr		
Male	Less than 20 ng/dL	Less than 0.69 nmol/L
Female	Less than 10 ng/dL	Less than 0.35 nmol/L
8–10 yr		
Male	2–25 ng/dL	0.07–0.87 nmol/L
Female	1–30 ng/dL	0.04–1 nmol/L
11–12 yr		
Male	Less than 350 ng/dL	Less than 12.1 nmol/L
Female	Less than 50 ng/dL	Less than 1.74 nmol/L
13–15 yr		
Male	15–500 ng/dL	0.52–17.35 nmol/L
Female	Less than 50 ng/dL	Less than 1.74 nmol/L
Adult		
Male	241–827 ng/dL	8.36–28.7 nmol/L
Female	15–70 ng/dL	0.52–2.43 nmol/L
Older adult		
Male	300–720 ng/dL	10.41–24.98
Female	5–32 ng/dL	0.17–1.11

Post menopausal levels are about half the normal adult level for females; levels in women who are pregnant are 3 to 4 times the normal adult level for females who are not pregnant.

DESCRIPTION: Testosterone is the major androgen responsible for sexual differentiation. In males, testosterone is made by the Leydig cells in the testicles and is responsible for spermatogenesis and the development of secondary sex characteristics. In females, the ovary and adrenal gland secrete small amounts of this hormone; however, most of the testosterone in females comes from the metabolism of androstenedione. Testosterone levels have a slight diurnal variation with the highest levels occurring around 0800 and lowest levels around 2000. Measurements of total testosterone levels are used most often in evaluating suspected hormone imbalances. Free testosterone is the active form of the hormone. It is used in conjunction with total testosterone to evaluate hormone levels in conditions known to alter the effectiveness of testosterone-binding protein, also called *sex hormone-binding globulin*, or SHBG. Alterations in the affinity of SHBG to bind free testosterone are known to occur with obesity, liver disease, and hyperthyroidism. In males, a testicular, adrenal, or pituitary tumor can cause an overabundance of testosterone, triggering precocious puberty. In females, adrenal tumors, hyperplasia, and medications can cause an overabundance of this hormone, resulting in masculinization or hirsutism.

T

This procedure is contraindicated for: N/A

INDICATIONS

- Assist in the diagnosis of hypergonadism.
- Assist in the diagnosis of male sexual precocity before age 10.
- Distinguish between primary and secondary hypogonadism.
- Evaluate hirsutism.
- Evaluate male infertility.

POTENTIAL MEDICAL DIAGNOSIS

Increased in:

- Adrenal hyperplasia ***(oversecretion of the androgen precursor dehydroepiandrosterone [DHEA])***
- Adrenocortical tumors ***(oversecretion of the androgen precursor DHEA)***
- Hirsutism ***(any condition that results in increased production of testosterone or its precursors)***
- Hyperthyroidism ***(high thyroxine levels increase the production of sex hormone–binding protein, which increases measured levels of total testosterone)***
- Idiopathic sexual precocity ***(related to stimulation of testosterone production by elevated levels of luteinizing hormone)***
- Polycystic ovaries ***(high estrogen levels increase the production of sex hormone–binding protein, which increases measured levels of total testosterone)***
- Syndrome of androgen resistance
- Testicular or extragonadal tumors ***(related to excessive secretion of testosterone)***
- Trophoblastic tumors during pregnancy
- Virilizing ovarian tumors

Decreased in:

- Anovulation
- Cryptorchidism ***(related to dysfunctional testes)***
- Delayed puberty
- Down syndrome ***(related to diminished or dysfunctional testes)***
- Excessive alcohol intake ***(alcohol inhibits secretion of testosterone)***
- Hepatic insufficiency ***(related to decreased binding protein and reflects decreased measured levels of total testosterone)***
- Impotence ***(decreased testosterone levels can result in impotence)***
- Klinefelter's syndrome ***(chromosome abnormality XXY associated with testicular failure)***
- Malnutrition
- Myotonic dystrophy ***(related to testicular atrophy)***
- Orchiectomy ***(testosterone production occurs in the testes)***
- Primary and secondary hypogonadism
- Primary and secondary hypopituitarism
- Uremia

CRITICAL FINDINGS: N/A

INTERFERING FACTORS

- Drugs and other substances that may increase testosterone levels include barbiturates, bromocriptine, cimetidine, flutamide, gonadotropin, levonorgestrel, mifepristone, moclobemide, nafarelin (males), nilutamide, oral contraceptives, rifampin, and tamoxifen.
- Drugs and other substances that may decrease testosterone levels include cyclophosphamide, cyproterone, danazol, dexamethasone, diethylstilbestrol, digoxin,

T

D-Trp-6-LHRH, fenoldopam, goserelin, ketoconazole, leuprolide, magnesium sulfate, medroxyprogesterone, methylprednisone, oral contraceptives, pravastatin, prednisone, pyridoglutethimide, spironolactone, tetracycline, and thioridazine.

NURSING IMPLICATIONS AND PROCEDURE

POTENTIAL NURSING PROBLEMS:

Problem	Signs & Symptoms	Interventions
Sexuality ***(related to insufficient testosterone level)***	Delayed puberty; poor development of muscle mass; minimal body hair; insufficient penile and testicle growth; gynecomastia (breast development); arms and legs grow faster than the body trunk; erectile dysfunction; infertility; osteoporosis	Explain the importance of testosterone replacement therapy; administer prescribed testosterone replacement medication
Body image ***(related to altered male sexual development secondary to lack of testosterone)***	Negative verbalization of physical appearance and lack of male attributes; preoccupation with lack of physical body changes; distress and refusal to talk about appearance; negative verbalization about physical appearance	Assess the patient's perception of physical appearance; note the frequency of negative comments about lack of male attributes associated with physical appearance; assist in the identification of positive coping strategies to address inadequate male attribute physical appearance; provide reassurance that physical appearance may change with testosterone therapy; provide a referral to local support groups

(table continues on page 1436)

Problem	Signs & Symptoms	Interventions
Self-esteem ***(related to altered body image; functional impairment [erectile dysfunction])***	Negative self comments; comments regarding difficulty dealing with health situation; indecisive behavior	Assess feelings regarding patient's sense of control over health management; provide an environment that will encourage the expression of feelings; assess the patient's feeling of being accepted and loved by others; use active listening; provide guidance as necessary to decrease anxiety

PRETEST:

- Positively identify the patient using at least two person-specific identifiers before services, treatments, or procedures are performed.
- ***Patient Teaching:*** Inform the patient this test can assist with evaluating hormone levels.
- Obtain a history of the patient's health concerns, symptoms, surgical procedures, and results of previously performed laboratory and diagnostic studies. Include a list of known allergens, especially allergies or sensitivities to latex.
- Obtain a list of the patient's current medications, including over-the-counter medications and dietary supplements (see Effects of Natural Products on Laboratory Values online at Davis*Plus*).
- Review the procedure with the patient. Inform the patient that specimen collection takes approximately 5 to 10 min. Address concerns about pain and explain that there may be some discomfort during the venipuncture.
- ***Sensitivity to social and cultural issues,*** as well as concern for modesty, is important in providing psychological support before, during, and after the procedure.
- Note that there are no food, fluid, or medication restrictions unless by medical direction.

INTRATEST:

Potential Complications: N/A

- Avoid the use of equipment containing latex if the patient has a history of allergic reaction to latex.
- Instruct the patient to cooperate fully and to follow directions. Direct the patient to breathe normally and to avoid unnecessary movement.
- Observe standard precautions, and follow the general guidelines in Patient Preparation and Specimen Collection online at Davis*Plus*. Positively identify the patient, and label the appropriate specimen container with the corresponding patient demographics, initials of the person collecting the specimen, date, and time of collection. Perform a venipuncture.
- Remove the needle and apply direct pressure with dry gauze to stop bleeding. Observe/assess venipuncture site for bleeding or hematoma formation and secure gauze with adhesive bandage.
- Promptly transport the specimen to the laboratory for processing and analysis.

POST-TEST:

- Inform the patient that a report of the results will be made available to the requesting health-care provider (HCP), who will discuss the results with the patient.
- Recognize anxiety related to test results, and offer support, as

T

appropriate. Discuss the implications of abnormal test results on the patient's lifestyle. Provide teaching and information regarding the clinical implications of the test results, as appropriate. Educate the patient regarding access to counseling services.

- Depending on the results of this procedure, additional testing may be performed to evaluate or monitor progression of the disease process and determine the need for a change in therapy. Evaluate test results in relation to the patient's symptoms and other tests performed.

Patient Education:

- Reinforce information given by the patient's HCP regarding further testing, treatment, or referral to another HCP.
- Answer any questions or address any concerns voiced by the patient or family.

Expected Patient Outcomes:

Understanding

- The patient and family acknowledge that lack of development of male attributes is due to inadequate testosterone.
- The patient and family acknowledge the importance of testosterone replacement to supporting male characteristic development.

Ability

- The patient expresses the harmful effects of negative self-talk on self-esteem.
- The patient reads provided referral information and agrees to attend an introductory meeting.

Response

- The patient refrains from making negative self-comments associated with physical appearance.
- The patient agrees to counseling in relation to concerns related to erectile dysfunction and intimacy.

RELATED STUDIES:

- Related tests include angiography adrenal gland scan, ACE, antibodies antisperm, biopsy thyroid, chromosome analysis, CT kidneys, DHEAS, estradiol, FSH, LH, PTH, RAIU, semen analysis, thyroid scan, TSH, thyroxine, and US scrotal.
- Refer to the Endocrine and Reproductive systems tables online at Davis*Plus* for related test by body system.

Thyroglobulin

SYNONYM/ACRONYM: Tg.

COMMON USE: To evaluate thyroid gland function related to disorders such as tumor, inflammation, structural damage, and cancer.

SPECIMEN: Serum collected in a gold-, red-, or red/gray-top tube.

NORMAL FINDINGS: (Method: Chemiluminescent enzyme immunoassay)

Age	Conventional Units	SI Units (Conventional Units × 1)
6 mo–3 yr	7–50 ng/mL	7–50 mcg/L
4–7 yr	4–40 ng/mL	4–40 mcg/L
8–17 yr	0.8–27 ng/mL	0.8–27 mcg/L
Adult–older adult	0.5–40 ng/mL	0.5–40 mcg/L

Access Canadian content on Fast Find: Lab and Dx at davispl.us/vanleeuwen7

POTENTIAL MEDICAL DIAGNOSIS

Increased in:

Thyroglobulin is secreted by normal, abnormal, and cancerous thyroid tissue cells.

- Differentiated thyroid cancer
- Graves' disease (untreated) ***(autoimmune destruction of thyroid tissue cells)***
- Surgery or irradiation of the thyroid ***(elevated levels indicate residual or disseminated carcinoma)***
- T_4-binding globulin deficiency
- Thyroiditis ***(related to leakage from inflamed, damaged thyroid tissue cells)***
- Thyrotoxicosis

Decreased in:

- Administration of thyroid hormone ***(feedback loop suppresses production)***
- Congenital athyrosis (neonates) ***(related to insufficient synthesis)***
- Thyrotoxicosis factitia

CRITICAL FINDINGS: N/A

Find and print out the full study on Fast Find at davispl.us/vanleeuwen7.

Thyroid-Binding Inhibitory Immunoglobulins

SYNONYM/ACRONYM: Thyrotropin receptor antibodies, thyrotropin-binding inhibitory immunoglobulin, TBII, TRAb (TSH receptor antibodies).

COMMON USE: To assist in diagnosing Graves' disease related to thyroid function.

SPECIMEN: Serum collected in a red-top tube.

NORMAL FINDINGS: (Method: Radioreceptor assay) Less than 17% of basal activity.

POTENTIAL MEDICAL DIAGNOSIS

Increased in:

Evidenced by antibodies that block the action of TSH and result in hyperthyroid conditions.

- Graves' disease
- Hyperthyroidism (various forms)
- Maternal thyroid disease
- Neonatal thyroid disease
- Toxic goiter

Decreased in: N/A

CRITICAL FINDINGS: N/A

Find and print out the full study on Fast Find at davispl.us/vanleeuwen7.

Thyroid Scan

T

SYNONYM/ACRONYM: Iodine thyroid scan, technetium thyroid scan, thyroid scintiscan.

COMMON USE: To assess thyroid gland size, structure, function, and shape toward diagnosing disorders such as tumor, inflammation, cancer, and bleeding.

AREA OF APPLICATION: Thyroid.

DESCRIPTION: The thyroid scan is a nuclear medicine study performed to assess thyroid size, shape, position, and function. It is useful for evaluating thyroid nodules, multinodular goiter, and thyroiditis; assisting in the differential diagnosis of masses in the neck, base of the tongue, and mediastinum; and ruling out possible ectopic thyroid tissue in these areas. Thyroid scanning is performed after oral administration of radioactive iodine-123 (I-123) or I-131 or intravenous (IV) injection of technetium-99m (Tc-99m). Increased or decreased uptake by the thyroid gland and surrounding area and tissue is noted: Areas of increased radionuclide uptake ("hot spots") are caused by hyperfunctioning thyroid nodules, which are usually nonmalignant; areas of decreased uptake ("cold spots") are caused by hypofunctioning nodules, which are more likely to be malignant. Ultrasound imaging may be used to determine if the cold spot is a solid, semicystic lesion or a pure cyst (cysts are rarely cancerous). To determine whether the cold spot depicts a malignant neoplasm, however, a biopsy must be performed.

This procedure is contraindicated for

Patients who are pregnant or suspected of being pregnant, unless the potential benefits of a procedure using radiation far outweigh the risk of radiation exposure to the fetus and mother.

INDICATIONS

- Assess palpable nodules and differentiate between a benign tumor or cyst and a malignant tumor.
- Assess the presence of a thyroid nodule or enlarged thyroid gland.
- Detect benign or malignant thyroid tumors.
- Detect causes of neck or substernal masses.
- Detect forms of thyroiditis (e.g., acute, chronic, Hashimoto's).
- Detect thyroid dysfunction.
- Differentiate between Graves' disease and Plummer's disease, both of which cause hyperthyroidism.
- Evaluate thyroid function in hyperthyroidism and hypothyroidism (analysis combined with interpretation of laboratory tests, thyroid function panel including thyroxine and triiodothyronine, and thyroid uptake tests).

POTENTIAL MEDICAL DIAGNOSIS

Normal findings

- Normal size, contour, position, and function of the thyroid gland with homogeneous uptake of the radionuclide

Abnormal findings related to

- Adenoma
- Cysts
- Fibrosis
- Goiter
- Graves' disease (diffusely enlarged, hyperfunctioning gland)
- Hematoma
- Metastasis
- Plummer's disease (nodular hyperfunctioning gland)
- Thyroiditis (Hashimoto's)
- Thyrotoxicosis
- Tumors, benign or malignant

CRITICAL FINDINGS: N/A

INTERFERING FACTORS

Factors that may alter the results of the study

- Inability of the patient to cooperate or remain still during the procedure because of age, significant pain, or mental status.

T

- Other nuclear scans or iodinated contrast medium radiographic studies done within the previous 24 to 48 hr.
- Ingestion of foods containing iodine (iodized salt) or medications containing iodine (cough syrup, potassium iodide, vitamins, Lugol's solution, thyroid replacement medications), which can decrease the uptake of the radionuclide.
- Antihistamines, antithyroid medications (propylthiouracil), corticosteroids, isoniazid, nitrates, sulfonamides, thyroid hormones, and warfarin, which can decrease the uptake of the radionuclide.
- Increased uptake of iodine in persons with an iodine-deficient diet or who are on phenothiazine therapy.
- Vomiting and severe diarrhea, which can affect absorption of orally administered radionuclide.
- Gastroenteritis, which can interfere with absorption of orally administered radionuclide.
- Metallic objects (e.g., jewelry, body rings) within the examination field, which may inhibit organ visualization and cause unclear images.

Other considerations

- Improper injection of the radionuclide that allows the tracer to seep deep into the muscle tissue can produce erroneous hot spots.

NURSING IMPLICATIONS AND PROCEDURE

PRETEST:

- Positively identify the patient using at least two person-specific identifiers before services, treatments, or procedures are performed.
- ***Patient Teaching:*** Inform the patient this procedure can assist in evaluating the thyroid glands structure and function.
- Obtain a history of the patient's health concerns, symptoms, surgical procedures, and results of previously performed laboratory and diagnostic studies. Include a list of known allergens, especially allergies or sensitivities to latex, anesthetics, sedatives, or radionuclides.
- Ensure thyroid blood tests are completed prior to this procedure.
- Note any recent procedures that can interfere with test results, including examinations using iodinated contrast medium or radioactive nuclides.
- Ensure that this procedure is performed before all radiographic procedures using iodinated contrast medium.
- Record the date of the last menstrual period and determine the possibility of pregnancy in perimenopausal women.
- Obtain a list of the patient's current medications, including over-the-counter medications and dietary supplements (see Effects of Natural Products on Laboratory Values online at Davis*Plus*).
- Review the procedure with the patient. Address concerns about pain related to the procedure and explain that some pain may be experienced during the test. Inform the patient that the procedure is performed in a nuclear medicine department, usually by a health-care provider (HCP) specializing in this procedure, with support staff, and takes approximately 30 to 60 min.
- ***Sensitivity to social and cultural issues,*** as well as concern for modesty, is important in providing psychological support before, during, and after the procedure.
- Explain that an IV line may be inserted to allow infusion of fluids such as saline, anesthetics, sedatives, radionuclides, medications used in the procedure, or emergency medications.
- Instruct the patient to remove jewelry and other metallic objects from the area to be examined.
- Instruct the patient to fast for 8 to 12 hr prior to the procedure. Protocols may vary among facilities.

T

- *Make sure a written and informed consent has been signed prior to the procedure and before administering any medications.*

INTRATEST:

Potential Complications:

Although it is rare, there is the possibility of allergic reaction to the radionuclide. Have emergency equipment and medications readily available. If the patient has a history of allergic reactions to any substance or drug, administer ordered prophylactic steroids or antihistamines before the procedure.

Establishing an IV site and injecting radionuclides are invasive procedures. Complications are rare but do include bleeding from the puncture site ***related to a bleeding disorder or the effects of natural products and medications with known anticoagulant, antiplatelet, and thrombolytic properties;*** hematoma ***related to blood leakage into the tissue following needle insertion;*** infection ***that might occur if bacteria from the skin surface is introduced at the puncture site;*** or nerve injury ***that might occur if the needle strikes a nerve.***

- Observe standard precautions, and follow the general guidelines in Patient Preparation and Specimen Collection online at Davis*Plus*. Positively identify the patient.
- Ensure that the patient has complied with dietary restrictions prior to the procedure, as instructed.
- Ensure that the patient has removed all external metallic objects from the area to be examined prior to the procedure.
- Instruct the patient to void prior to the procedure and to change into the gown, robe, and foot coverings provided.
- Avoid the use of equipment containing latex if the patient has a history of allergic reaction to latex.
- Have emergency equipment readily available.
- Instruct the patient to cooperate fully and to follow directions. Ask the patient to lie still during the procedure because movement produces unclear images.
- Administer sedative to a child or to an uncooperative adult, as ordered.
- Tc-99m pertechnetate is injected IV 20 min before scanning.
- If oral radioactive nuclide is used instead, administer I-123 24 hr before scanning.
- Place the patient in a supine position on a flat table to obtain images of the neck area.
- Remove the needle or catheter and apply a pressure dressing over the puncture site.
- Observe/assess the needle/catheter insertion site for bleeding, inflammation, or hematoma formation.

POST-TEST:

- Inform the patient that a report of the results will be made available to the requesting HCP, who will discuss the results with the patient.
- Observe/assess the needle/catheter insertion site for bleeding, inflammation, or hematoma formation.
- Instruct the patient in the care and assessment of the injection site.
- Advise the patient to drink increased amounts of fluids for 24 to 48 hr to eliminate the radionuclide from the body, unless contraindicated. Tell the patient that radionuclide is eliminated from the body within 6 to 24 hr.
- If a woman who is breastfeeding must have a nuclear scan, she should not breastfeed the infant until the radionuclide has been eliminated. This could take as long as 3 days. She should be instructed to express the milk and discard it during the 3-day period to prevent cessation of milk production.
- Instruct the patient to flush the toilet immediately and to meticulously wash hands with soap and water after each voiding for 24 hr after the procedure.
- Instruct all caregivers to wear gloves when discarding urine for 24 hr after the procedure. Wash gloved hands with soap and water before removing gloves; then wash ungloved hands.
- Recognize anxiety related to test results, and be supportive of

T

perceived loss of independent function. Discuss the implications of abnormal test results on the patient's lifestyle. Provide teaching and information regarding the clinical implications of the test results, as appropriate.

- Reinforce information given by the patient's HCP regarding further testing, treatment, or referral to another HCP. Answer any questions or address any concerns voiced by the patient or family.
- Depending on the results of this procedure, additional testing may be needed to evaluate or monitor progression of the disease process and determine the need for a change in therapy. Evaluate test results in relation to the patient's symptoms and other tests performed.

RELATED STUDIES:

- Related tests include ACTH, angiography adrenal, biopsy thyroid, calcium, CT kidneys, cortisol, glucose, radioactive iodine uptake, sodium, thyroglobulin, thyroid antibodies, TBII, thyroid scan, TSH, TT_3, T_4, FT_4, and US thyroid.
- Refer to the Endocrine System table online at Davis*Plus* for related tests by body system.

Thyroid-Stimulating Hormone

SYNONYM/ACRONYM: Thyrotropin, TSH.

COMMON USE: To evaluate thyroid gland function related to the primary cause of hypothyroidism and assess for congenital disorders, tumor, and inflammation.

SPECIMEN: Serum collected in a gold-red- or tiger-top tube; for a neonate, use filter paper.

NORMAL FINDINGS: (Method: Immunoassay)

Age	Conventional Units	SI Units (Conventional Units × 1)
Neonates–3 d	Less than 40 micro-international units/mL	Less than 40 milli-international units/L
2 wk–5 mo	1.7–9.1 micro-international units/mL	1.7–9.1 milli-international units/L
6 mo–1 yr	0.7–6.4 micro-international units/mL	0.7–6.4 milli-international units/L
2 yr–19 yr	0.5–4.5 micro-international units/mL	0.5–4.5 milli-international units/L
Greater than 20 yr	0.4–4.2 micro-international units/mL	0.4–4.2 milli-international units/L
Pregnancy		
First trimester	0.3–2.7 micro-international units/mL	0.3–2.7 milli-international units/L
Second trimester	0.5–2.7 micro-international units/mL	0.5–2.7 milli-international units/L
Third trimester	0.4–2.9 micro-international units/mL	0.4–2.9 milli-international units/L

T

DESCRIPTION: Thyroid-stimulating hormone (TSH) is produced by the pituitary gland in response to stimulation by thyrotropin-releasing hormone (TRH), a hypothalamic-releasing factor. TRH regulates the release and circulating levels of thyroid hormones in response to variables such as cold, stress, and increased metabolic need. Thyroid and pituitary function can be evaluated by TSH measurement. TSH exhibits diurnal variation, peaking between midnight and 0400 and troughing between 1700 and 1800. TSH values are high at birth but reach adult levels in the first week of life. Elevated TSH levels combined with decreased thyroxine (T_4) levels indicate hypothyroidism and thyroid gland dysfunction. In general, decreased TSH and T_4 levels indicate secondary congenital hypothyroidism and pituitary hypothalamic dysfunction. A normal TSH level and a depressed T_4 level may indicate (1) hypothyroidism owing to a congenital defect in T_4-binding globulin or (2) transient congenital hypothyroidism owing to hypoxia or prematurity. Early diagnosis and treatment in the neonate are crucial for the prevention of congenital hypothyroidism (cretinism).

This procedure is contraindicated for: N/A

INDICATIONS
- Assist in the diagnosis of congenital hypothyroidism.
- Assist in the diagnosis of hypothyroidism or hyperthyroidism or suspected pituitary or hypothalamic dysfunction.
- Differentiate functional euthyroidism from true hypothyroidism in debilitated individuals.

POTENTIAL MEDICAL DIAGNOSIS

Increased in:

A decrease in thyroid hormone levels activates the feedback loop to increase production of TSH.

- Congenital hypothyroidism in the neonate (filter paper test)
- Ectopic TSH-producing tumors (lung, breast)
- Primary hypothyroidism ***(related to a dysfunctional thyroid gland)***
- Secondary hyperthyroidism owing to pituitary hyperactivity
- Thyroid hormone resistance
- Thyroiditis (Hashimoto's autoimmune disease)

Decreased in:

An increase in thyroid hormone levels activates the feedback loop to decrease production of TSH.

- Excessive thyroid hormone replacement
- Graves' disease
- Primary hyperthyroidism
- Secondary hypothyroidism ***(related to pituitary involvement that decreases production of TSH)***
- Tertiary hypothyroidism ***(related to hypothalamic involvement that decreases production of TRH)***

CRITICAL FINDINGS: N/A

INTERFERING FACTORS
- Drugs and other substances that may increase TSH levels include amiodarone, benserazide, erythrosine, flunarizine (males), iobenzamic acid, iodides, lithium, methimazole, metoclopramide, morphine, propranolol, radiographic medium, TRH, and valproic acid.

- Drugs and other substances that may decrease TSH levels include acetylsalicylic acid, amiodarone, anabolic steroids, carbamazepine, corticosteroids, glucocorticoids, hydrocortisone, interferon-alfa-2b, iodamide, levodopa (in hypothyroidism), levothyroxine, methergoline, nifedipine, T_4, and triiodothyronine (T_3).
- Failure to let the filter paper sample dry may affect test results.

NURSING IMPLICATIONS AND PROCEDURE

POTENTIAL NURSING PROBLEMS:

Problem	Signs & Symptoms	Interventions
Nutrition ***(related to slow metabolism)***	Decreased appetite with weight gain; selection of high-calorie, high-sodium foods; sedentary lifestyle; caloric intake greater than metabolic needs; constipation; decreased activity	Teach the patient to avoid foods with high sodium, saturated fat, and cholesterol content; teach the patient to eat a diet high in protein and low in calories to promote weight loss; encourage the patient to eat small, frequent meals to prevent overeating and enhance weight control; encourage the consumption of high-fiber foods such as fruits and vegetables with the skins and whole-grain breads to improve gastric motility; monitor daily weight; accurately assess appetite and measure caloric intake over a 24-hr period; arrange dietary consult
Decreased cardiac output ***(related to a deficit of thyroid hormone)***	Bradycardia; lethargy; hypotension; decreased thyroid hormone levels; fatigue; activity intolerance; poor peripheral perfusion; cool skin; shortness of breath	Assess and trend vital signs and blood pressure; monitor and trend thyroid laboratory studies (TSH, T3, T4, radioactive iodine uptake); assess cardiac status indicators (peripheral pulses, skin color, skin temperature, dry scaly skin); assess for periorbital edema; administer prescribed thyroid hormone replacement medication; facilitate measures to improve patient warmth (blankets, warm clothing and liquids, warmer environment); pace activity and schedule rest periods to manage fatigue; use pulse oximetry to monitor oxygen saturation; assess respiratory status checking for crackles and increased respiratory rate; monitor for fluid overload

T

Problem	Signs & Symptoms	Interventions
Altered thought processes ***(related to decreased cardiac output and impaired cerebral perfusion secondary to a deficit of thyroid hormone)***	Altered memory; mental impairment; decreased concentration; depression; inaccurate environmental perception; inappropriate thinking; memory deficits	Minimize apprehension and dread; collaborate with the health-care provider (HCP) to manage medical problem associated with decreased cerebral perfusion; promote comprehension and understanding of current events; provide a modified environment that promotes safety; monitor the ability to provide self-care (activities of daily living); monitor injury risk (violence, fall risk, self-harm risk); administer prescribed thyroid hormone replacement medication
Self-esteem ***(related to chronic illness; physiologic impairment associated with thyroid hormone deficiency)***	Negative self-evaluation; negative evaluation of personal abilities; expressions of shame or guilt; seeks excessive reassurance; exaggerates negative feedback; indecisive; passive; nonassertive; conforming	Facilitate a positive outlook based on real rather than exaggerated factors that influence health; facilitate acknowledgment of personal strengths and values; provide a safe environment for verbalization of concerns; collaborate with patient in designing an appropriate plan of care; collaborate with patient in promoting effective decision making; monitor frequency of negative self-comments; promote the concept of counseling to improve the concept of self-worth; use role-play and modeling to improve positive behavioral skills; provide information about community resources for continued counseling

PRETEST:

- Positively identify the patient using at least two person-specific identifiers before services, treatments, or procedures are performed.
- *Patient Teaching:* Inform the patient this test can assist in evaluating thyroid function.
- Obtain a history of the patient's health concerns, symptoms, surgical procedures, and results of previously performed laboratory and diagnostic studies. Include a list of known allergens, especially allergies or sensitivities to latex.
- Obtain a list of the patient's current medications, including over-the-counter medications and dietary supplements (see Effects of Natural Products on Laboratory Values online at Davis*Plus*).
- Review the procedure with the patient. Inform the patient that specimen collection takes approximately

5 to 10 min. Address concerns about pain and explain that there may be some discomfort during the venipuncture.

- ***Sensitivity to social and cultural issues,*** as well as concern for modesty, is important in providing psychological support before, during, and after the procedure.
- Note that there are no food, fluid, or medication restrictions unless by medical direction.

INTRATEST:

Potential Complications: N/A

- Avoid the use of equipment containing latex if the patient has a history of allergic reaction to latex.
- Instruct the patient to cooperate fully and to follow directions. Direct the patient to breathe normally and to avoid unnecessary movement.
- Observe standard precautions, and follow the general guidelines in Patient Preparation and Specimen Collection online at Davis*Plus*. Positively identify the patient, and label the appropriate specimen container with the corresponding patient demographics, initials of the person collecting the specimen, date, and time of collection. Perform a venipuncture.
- Remove the needle and apply direct pressure with dry gauze to stop bleeding. Observe/assess venipuncture site for bleeding or hematoma formation and secure gauze with adhesive bandage.
- Promptly transport the specimen to the laboratory for processing and analysis.

Filter Paper Test (Neonate)

- Obtain kit and cleanse heel with antiseptic. Observe standard precautions, and follow the general guidelines in Patient Preparation and Specimen Collection online at Davis*Plus*. Perform heel stick, gently squeeze infant's heel, and touch filter paper to the puncture site. Use gauze to dry the stick area completely. When collecting samples for newborn screening, it is important to apply each blood drop to the correct side of the filter paper card and fill each circle with a single application of blood. Overfilling or underfilling the circles will cause the specimen card to be rejected by the testing facility. Additional information is required on newborn screening cards and may vary by testing facility. Newborn screening cards should be allowed to air dry for several hours on a level, nonabsorbent, unenclosed area. If multiple patients are tested, do not stack cards. Testing facility regulations usually require the specimen cards to be submitted within 24 hr of collection.

POST-TEST:

- Inform the patient that a report of the results will be made available to the requesting HCP, who will discuss the results with the patient.
- Depending on the results of this procedure, additional testing may be performed to evaluate or monitor progression of the disease process and determine the need for a change in therapy. Evaluate test results in relation to the patient's symptoms and other tests performed.

Patient Education:

- Reinforce information given by the patient's HCP regarding further testing, treatment, or referral to another HCP.
- Recognize anxiety related to test results and answer any questions or address any concerns voiced by the patient or family.
- Educate the patient and family regarding the effects of hypothyroidism on the body over time.
- Educate the family regarding safety interventions that can be taken in the event that the patient becomes confused.

Expected Patient Outcomes:

Understanding

- The patient and family agree to report to the HCP when the patient experiences difficulty breathing, to facilitate timely interventions.

- The patient and family state the importance of taking thyroid replacement therapy to overall health.

Ability

- The patient and family demonstrate proficiency in designing a dietary strategy that encompasses the concept of six small meals a day to better manage caloric needs.
- The patient and family identify ways to conserve energy and prevent fatigue associated with compromised cardiac status.

Response

- The patient complies with the HCP's recommendation of a dietary consult to assist in managing caloric needs appropriately.
- The patient complies with taking thyroid replacement medication as prescribed.

RELATED STUDIES:

- Related tests include albumin, antibodies antithyroglobulin, biopsy thyroid, copper, newborn screening, PTH, protein, RAIU, thyroglobulin, TSI, TBII, thyroid scan, T_4, free T_4, T_3, free T_3, and US thyroid.
- Refer to the Endocrine System table online at Davis*Plus* for related tests by body system.

Thyroid-Stimulating Immunoglobulins

SYNONYM/ACRONYM: Thyrotropin receptor antibodies, thyroid-stimulating immunoglobulins, TRAb (TSH receptor antibodies).

COMMON USE: To differentiate between antibodies that stimulate or inhibit thyroid hormone production related to disorders such as Graves' disease.

SPECIMEN: Serum collected in a red-top tube.

NORMAL FINDINGS: (Method: Animal cell transfection with luciferase marker) Less than 130% of basal activity.

POTENTIAL MEDICAL DIAGNOSIS

Increased in:

- Graves' disease ***(this form of hyperthyroidism has an autoimmune component; the antibodies stimulate release of thyroid hormones outside the feedback loop that regulates TSH levels)***

Decreased in: N/A

CRITICAL FINDINGS: N/A

Find and print out the full study on Fast Find at davispl.us/vanleeuwen7.

Thyroxine-Binding Globulin

SYNONYM/ACRONYM: TBG.

COMMON USE: To evaluate thyroid hormone levels related to deficiency or excess to assist in diagnosing disorders such as hyperthyroidism and hypothyroidism.

SPECIMEN: Serum collected in a gold-, red-, or red/gray-top tube.

NORMAL FINDINGS: (Method: Immunochemiluminometric assay [ICMA])

Age	Conventional Units	SI Units (Conventional Units × 10)
0–1 wk	3–8 mg/dL	30–80 mg/L
1–12 mo	1.6–3.6 mg/dL	16–36 mg/L
14–19 yr	1.2–2.5 mg/dL	12–25 mg/L
Greater than 20 yr	1.3–3.3 mg/dL	13–33 mg/L
Pregnancy, third trimester	4.7–5.9 mg/dL	47–59 mg/L
Oral contraceptives	1.5–5.5 mg/dL	15–55 mg/L

POTENTIAL MEDICAL DIAGNOSIS

Increased in:

- Acute intermittent porphyria ***(pathophysiology is unclear)***
- Estrogen therapy ***(TBG is increased in the presence of exogenous or endogenous estrogens)***
- Genetically high TBG (rare)
- Hyperthyroidism ***(related to increased levels of total thyroxine available for binding)***
- Infectious hepatitis and other liver diseases ***(pathophysiology is unclear)***
- Neonates
- Pregnancy ***(TBG is increased in the presence of exogenous or endogenous estrogens)***

Decreased in:

- Acromegaly
- Chronic hepatic disease ***(related to general decrease in protein synthesis)***
- Genetically low TBG
- Major illness ***(related to general decrease in protein synthesis)***
- Marked hypoproteinemia, malnutrition ***(related to general decrease in protein synthesis)***
- Nephrotic syndrome ***(related to general increase in protein loss)***
- Ovarian hypofunction ***(TBG is decreased in the absence of estrogens)***
- Surgical stress ***(related to general decrease in protein synthesis)***
- Testosterone-producing tumors ***(TBG is decreased in the presence of testosterone)***

CRITICAL FINDINGS: N/A

Find and print out the full study on Fast Find at davispl.us/vanleeuwen7.

Thyroxine, Free

T

SYNONYM/ACRONYM: Free T_4, $Free_4$.

COMMON USE: A reflex test for thyroid function to assist in diagnosing hyperthyroidism and hypothyroidism in the presence of an abnormal TSH level.

SPECIMEN: Serum collected in a gold-, red-, or red/gray-top tube. Plasma collected in a green-top (heparin) tube is also acceptable.

NORMAL FINDINGS: (Method: Immunoassay)

Age	Conventional Units	SI Units (Conventional Units × 12.9)
Newborn	0.8–2.8 ng/dL	10–36 pmol/L
1–12 mo	0.8–2 ng/dL	10–26 pmol/L
1–18 yr	0.8–1.7 ng/dL	10–22 pmol/L
Adult–older adult	0.8–1.5 ng/dL	10–19 pmol/L
Pregnancy	0.7–1.4 ng/dL	9–18 pmol/L

DESCRIPTION: Thyroxine (T_4) is a hormone produced and secreted by the thyroid gland. Most T_4 in the serum (99.97%) is bound to thyroxine-binding globulin (TBG), prealbumin, and albumin. The remainder (0.03%) circulates as unbound or free T_4, which is the physiologically active form. Levels of free T_4 are proportional to levels of total T_4. The advantage of measuring free T_4 instead of total T_4 is that, unlike total T_4 measurements, free T_4 levels are not affected by fluctuations in TBG levels; as a result, free T_4 levels are considered the most accurate indicator of T_4 and its thyrometabolic activity. Free T_4 measurements are useful in evaluating thyroid disease when thyroid-stimulating hormone (TSH) levels alone provide insufficient information. Free T_4 and TSH levels are inversely proportional. Measurement of free T_4 is also recommended during treatment for hyperthyroidism until symptoms have abated and levels have decreased into the normal range.

This procedure is contraindicated for: N/A

INDICATIONS

- Evaluate signs of hypothyroidism or hyperthyroidism.
- Monitor response to therapy for hypothyroidism or hyperthyroidism.

POTENTIAL MEDICAL DIAGNOSIS

Increased in:

- Hyperthyroidism ***(thyroxine is produced independently of stimulation by TSH)***
- Hypothyroidism treated with T_4 ***(laboratory tests do not distinguish between endogenous and exogenous sources)***

Decreased in:

- Hypothyroidism ***(thyroid hormones are not produced in sufficient quantities regardless of TSH levels)***
- Pregnancy (late)

CRITICAL FINDINGS: N/A

INTERFERING FACTORS

- Drugs and other substances that may increase free T_4 levels include acetylsalicylic acid, amiodarone, halofenate, heparin, iopanoic acid, levothyroxine, methimazole, and radiographic medium.
- Drugs and other substances that may decrease free T_4 levels include amiodarone, anabolic steroids, asparaginase, methadone, methimazole, oral contraceptives, and phenylbutazone.

T

NURSING IMPLICATIONS AND PROCEDURE

POTENTIAL NURSING PROBLEMS:

Problem	Signs & Symptoms	Interventions
Decreased cardiac output ***(related to a deficit of thyroid hormone)***	Bradycardia; lethargy; hypotension; decreased thyroid hormone levels; fatigue; activity intolerance; poor peripheral perfusion; cool skin; shortness of breath	Assess and trend vital signs and blood pressure; monitor and trend thyroid laboratory studies (TSH, T3, T4, radioactive iodine uptake); assess cardiac status indicators (peripheral pulses, skin color, skin temperature, dry scaly skin); assess for periorbital edema; administer prescribed thyroid hormone replacement medication; facilitate measures to improve patient warmth (blankets, warm clothing and liquids, warmer environment); pace activity and schedule rest periods to manage fatigue; use pulse oximetry to monitor oxygen saturation; assess respiratory status checking for crackles and increased respiratory rate; monitor for fluid overload
Altered thought processes ***(related to decreased cardiac output and impaired cerebral perfusion secondary to a deficit of thyroid hormone)***	Altered memory; mental impairment; decreased concentration; depression; inaccurate environmental perception; inappropriate thinking; memory deficits	Minimize apprehension and dread; collaborate with the health-care provider (HCP) to manage medical problem associated with decreased cerebral perfusion; promote comprehension and understanding of current events; provide a modified environment that promotes safety; monitor the ability to provide self-care (activities of daily living); monitor injury risk (violence, fall risk, self-harm risk); administer prescribed thyroid hormone replacement medication

T

Problem	Signs & Symptoms	Interventions
Body image ***(related to the presence of goiter and exophthalmos)***	Eye bulging from exophthalmos; enlarged neck from goiter; distress and refusal to talk about changed appearance; negative verbalization about changes in appearance; uses clothing or other devices to hide changed appearance (scarves, high necks, sunglasses)	Assess the patient's perception of physical changes; note the frequency of negative comments about changed physical state; assist in the identification of positive coping strategies to address changed physical appearance
Elevated temperature ***(related to increased basal metabolic rate)***	Elevated temperature; flushed; warm skin; diaphoresis	Assess the patient's temperature frequently; monitor for emotionally labile events that could precipitate a thyroid storm or crisis and precipitate an elevation in temperature; ensure the patient's immediate environment remains cool; encourage the use of light bedding and lightweight clothing to prevent overheating; increase fluid intake to offset insensible fluid loss; encourage bathing with tepid water for comfort and promotion of cooling; administer prescribed antithyroid therapy

PRETEST:

- Positively identify the patient using at least two person-specific identifiers before services, treatments, or procedures are performed.
- *Patient Teaching:* Inform the patient this test can assist in assessing thyroid gland function.
- Obtain a history of the patient's health concerns, symptoms, surgical procedures, and results of previously performed laboratory and diagnostic studies. Include a list of known allergens, especially allergies or sensitivities to latex.
- Obtain a list of the patient's current medications, including over-the-counter medications and dietary supplements (see Effects of Natural Products on Laboratory Values online at Davis*Plus*).

- Review the procedure with the patient. Inform the patient that specimen collection takes approximately 5 to 10 min. Address concerns about pain and explain that there may be some discomfort during the venipuncture.
- ***Sensitivity to social and cultural issues,*** as well as concern for modesty, is important in providing psychological support before, during, and after the procedure.
- Note that there are no food, fluid, or medication restrictions unless by medical direction.

INTRATEST:

Potential Complications: N/A

- Avoid the use of equipment containing latex if the patient has a history of allergic reaction to latex.
- Instruct the patient to cooperate fully and to follow directions. Direct the patient to breathe normally and to avoid unnecessary movement.
- Observe standard precautions, and follow the general guidelines in Patient Preparation and Specimen Collection online at Davis*Plus*. Positively identify the patient, and label the appropriate specimen container with the corresponding patient demographics, initials of the person collecting the specimen, date, and time of collection. Perform a venipuncture.
- Remove the needle and apply direct pressure with dry gauze to stop bleeding. Observe/assess venipuncture site for bleeding or hematoma formation and secure gauze with adhesive bandage.
- Promptly transport the specimen to the laboratory for processing and analysis.

POST-TEST:

- Inform the patient that a report of the results will be made available to the requesting HCP, who will discuss the results with the patient.
- Depending on the results of this procedure, additional testing may be performed to evaluate or monitor progression of the disease process and determine the need for a change in therapy. Evaluate test results in relation to the patient's symptoms and other tests performed.

Patient Education:

- Reinforce information given by the patient's HCP regarding further testing, treatment, or referral to another HCP.
- Recognize anxiety related to test results, and answer any questions or address any concerns voiced by the patient or family.
- Teach the family and patient about the relationship between the development of goiter and exophthalmos and hyperthyroidism.

Expected Patient Outcomes:

Understanding

- The patient and family identify symptoms that may indicate a thyroid storm.
- The patient and family identify symptoms that would indicate hypothyroidism.

Ability

- The patient and family demonstrate proficiency in selecting clothing that will assist in remaining cool and prevent overheating.
- The patient demonstrates proficiency in the self-administration of thyroid or antithyroid medication correctly as prescribed.

Response

- The patient displays acceptance of changed appearance and refrains from negative self-comments.
- The patient complies with recommended medication regime.

RELATED STUDIES:

- Related tests include albumin, antibodies antithyroglobulin, biopsy thyroid, copper, PTH, prealbumin, protein, RAIU, thyroglobulin, TBII, thyroid scan, TSH, TSI, T_4, T_3, free T_3, and US thyroid.
- Refer to the Endocrine System table online at Davis*Plus* for related tests by body system.

T

Thyroxine, Total

SYNONYM/ACRONYM: T_4.

COMMON USE: A complementary laboratory test in evaluating thyroid hormone levels, a screening test for newborns to detect thyroid dysfunction, and a tool to evaluate the effectiveness of therapeutic thyroid therapy.

SPECIMEN: Serum collected in a gold-, red-, or red/gray-top tube. Plasma collected in a green-top (heparin) tube is also acceptable.

NORMAL FINDINGS: (Method: Immunoassay)

Age	Conventional Units	SI Units (Conventional Units × 12.9)
Cord blood	6.6–17.5 mcg/dL	85–226 nmol/L
1–30 d	5.4–22.6 mcg/dL	70–292 nmol/L
1 mo–23 mo	5.4–16.6 mcg/dL	70–214 nmol/L
2–6 yr	5.3–15 mcg/dL	68–194 nmol/L
7–11 yr	5.7–14.1 mcg/dL	74–182 nmol/L
12–19 yr	4.7–14.6 mcg/dL	61–188 nmol/L
Adult	4.6–12 mcg/dL	59–155 nmol/L
Pregnant female	5.5–16 mcg/dL	71–206 nmol/L
Over 60 yr	5–10.7 mcg/dL	64–138 nmol/L

DESCRIPTION: Thyroxine (T_4) is a hormone produced and secreted by the thyroid gland. Most T_4 in the serum (99.97%) is bound to thyroxine-binding globulin (TBG), prealbumin, and albumin. The remainder (0.03%) circulates as unbound or free T_4, which is the physiologically active form. Levels of free T_4 are proportional to levels of total T_4. The advantage of measuring free T_4 instead of total T_4 is that, unlike total T_4 measurements, free T_4 levels are not affected by fluctuations in TBG levels; as a result, free T_4 levels are considered the most accurate indicator of T_4 and its thyrometabolic activity (see study titled "Thyroxine, Free"). Untreated deficiency of T_4 in newborns can result in untreatable, severe intellectual deficits and growth impairment. Neonatal screening for hypothyroidism is mandatory in all 50 states. 🍁

This procedure is contraindicated for: N/A

INDICATIONS

- Evaluate signs of hypothyroidism or hyperthyroidism and neonatal screening for congenital hypothyroidism.
- Evaluate thyroid response to protein deficiency associated with severe illnesses.
- Monitor response to therapy for hypothyroidism or hyperthyroidism.

POTENTIAL MEDICAL DIAGNOSIS

Increased in:

- Acute mental health illnesses ***(pathophysiology is unknown, although there is a relationship between thyroid hormone levels and certain types of mental illness)***
- Excessive intake of iodine ***(iodine is rapidly taken up by the body to form thyroxine)***
- Hepatitis ***(related to decreased production of TBG by damaged liver cells)***
- Hyperthyroidism ***(thyroxine is produced independently of stimulation by TSH)***
- Obesity
- Thyrotoxicosis due to Graves' disease ***(thyroxine is produced independently of stimulation by TSH)***
- Thyrotoxicosis factitia ***(laboratory tests do not distinguish between endogenous and exogenous sources)***

Decreased in:

- Decreased TBG ***(nephrotic syndrome, liver disease, gastrointestinal protein loss, malnutrition)***
- Hypothyroidism ***(thyroid hormones are not produced in sufficient quantities regardless of TSH levels)***
- Panhypopituitarism ***(dysfunctional pituitary gland does not secrete enough thyrotropin to stimulate the thyroid to produce thyroxine)***
- Strenuous exercise

CRITICAL FINDINGS:

- *Hypothyroidism:* Less than 2 mcg/dL (SI: Less than 25.8 nmol/L)
- *Hyperthyroidism:* Greater than 20 mcg/dL (Greater than 258 nmol/L)

Note and immediately report to the requesting health-care provider (HCP) any critical findings and related symptoms. A listing of these findings varies among facilities. Timely notification of a critical finding for laboratory or diagnostic studies is a role expectation of the professional nurse. The notification processes vary among facilities. Upon receipt of the critical finding, the information should be read back to the caller to verify accuracy.

Consideration may be given to verification of critical findings before action is taken. Policies vary among facilities and may include requesting immediate recollection and retesting by the laboratory.

At levels less than 2 mcg/dL (SI: less than 25.8 nmol/L), the patient is at risk for myxedema coma. Signs and symptoms of severe hypothyroidism include hypothermia, hypotension, bradycardia, hypoventilation, lethargy, and coma. Possible interventions include airway support, hourly monitoring for neurological function and blood pressure, and administration of intravenous thyroid hormone.

At levels greater than 20 mcg/dL (greater than 258 nmol/L), the patient is at risk for thyroid storm. Signs and symptoms of severe hyperthyroidism include hyperthermia, diaphoresis, vomiting, dehydration, and shock. Possible interventions include supportive treatment for shock, fluid and electrolyte replacement for dehydration, and administration of antithyroid drugs (propylthiouracil and Lugol's solution).

INTERFERING FACTORS

- Drugs and other substances that may increase T_4 levels include amiodarone, amphetamines, corticosteroids, ether, fluorouracil, glucocorticoids, halofenate, insulin, iobenzamic acid, iopanoic acid, iopodate, levarterenol, levodopa, levothyroxine, opiates, oral contraceptives, phenothiazine, and prostaglandins.

T

- **Drugs and other substances that may decrease T_4 levels include acetylsalicylic acid, aminoglutethimide, aminosalicylic acid, amiodarone, anabolic steroids, anticonvulsants, asparaginase, barbiturates, carbimazole, chlorpromazine, chlorpropamide, cholestyramine, clofibrate, cobalt, colestipol, corticotropin, cortisone, cotrimoxazole, cytostatic therapy, danazol, dehydroepiandrosterone, dexamethasone, diazepam, diazo dyes (e.g., Evans blue), ethionamide, fenclofenac, halofenate, interferon alfa-2b, iron, isotretinoin, liothyronine, lithium, lovastatin, methimazole, methylthiouracil, mitotane, norethindrone, penicillamine, penicillin, phenylbutazone, potassium iodide, propylthiouracil, reserpine, salicylate, sodium nitroprusside, sulfonylureas, tolbutamide, and triiodothyronine (T_3).**

NURSING IMPLICATIONS AND PROCEDURE

PRETEST:

- Positively identify the patient using at least two person-specific identifiers before services, treatments, or procedures are performed.
- *Patient Teaching:* Inform the patient this test can assist in assessing thyroid gland function.
- Obtain a history of the patient's health concerns, symptoms, surgical procedures, and results of previously performed laboratory and diagnostic studies. Include a list of known allergens, especially allergies or sensitivities to latex.
- Obtain a history of the patient's endocrine system, symptoms, and results of previously performed laboratory tests and diagnostic and surgical procedures.
- Obtain a list of the patient's current medications, including over-the-counter medications and dietary supplements (see Effects of Natural Products on Laboratory Values online at Davis*Plus*).
- Review the procedure with the patient. Inform the patient that specimen collection takes approximately 5 to 10 min. Address concerns about pain and explain that there may be some discomfort during the venipuncture.
- *Sensitivity to social and cultural issues,* as well as concern for modesty, is important in providing psychological support before, during, and after the procedure.
- Note that there are no food, fluid, or medication restrictions unless by medical direction.

INTRATEST:

Potential Complications: N/A

- Avoid the use of equipment containing latex if the patient has a history of allergic reaction to latex.
- Instruct the patient to cooperate fully and to follow directions. Direct the patient to breathe normally and to avoid unnecessary movement.
- Observe standard precautions, and follow the general guidelines in Patient Preparation and Specimen Collection online at Davis*Plus*. Positively identify the patient, and label the appropriate specimen container with the corresponding patient demographics, initials of the person collecting the specimen, date, and time of collection. Perform a venipuncture.
- Remove the needle and apply direct pressure with dry gauze to stop bleeding. Observe/assess venipuncture site for bleeding or hematoma formation and secure gauze with adhesive bandage.
- Promptly transport the specimen to the laboratory for processing and analysis.

POST-TEST:

- Inform the patient that a report of the results will be made available to the requesting HCP, who will discuss the results with the patient.
- Reinforce information given by the patient's HCP regarding further testing, treatment, or referral to another

T

HCP. Answer any questions or address any concerns voiced by the patient or family.

- Depending on the results of this procedure, additional testing may be performed to evaluate or monitor progression of the disease process and determine the need for a change in therapy. Evaluate test results in relation to the patient's symptoms and other tests performed.

RELATED STUDIES:

- Related tests include albumin, antibodies antithyroglobulin, biopsy thyroid, copper, newborn screening, PTH, prealbumin, protein, RAIU, thyroglobulin, TBII, thyroid scan, TSH, TSI, free T_4, T_3, free T_3, and US thyroid.
- Refer to the Endocrine System table online at Davis*Plus* for related tests by body system.

Toxoplasma Antibody

SYNONYM/ACRONYM: Toxoplasmosis serology, toxoplasmosis titer.

COMMON USE: To assess for a past or present toxoplasmosis infection and to assess for the presence of antibodies.

SPECIMEN: Serum collected in a gold-, red-, or red/gray-top tube. Place separated serum into a standard transport tube within 2 hr of collection.

NORMAL FINDINGS: (Method: Chemiluminescent immunoassay)

	IgM and IgG	Interpretation
Negative	0.89 index or less	No significant level of detectable antibody
Indeterminate	0.9–1 index	Equivocal results; retest in 10–14 days
Positive	1.1 index or greater	Antibody detected; indicative of recent immunization, current or recent infection

DESCRIPTION: Toxoplasmosis is a severe, generalized granulomatous central nervous system disease caused by the protozoan *Toxoplasma gondii*. The disease is more common in warm, humid climates at lower altitudes. Domestic and related cats are the only known definitive hosts for oocysts of *Toxoplasma gondii*. Intermediate hosts become infected by ingesting the oocysts which then transform into the tachyzoite form. Tachyzoites migrate to neural and muscle tissue and develop into tissue cysts. Transmission to humans occurs by ingesting undercooked meat of infected animals, handling contaminated matter such as cat litter, drinking contaminated water, receiving a blood product transfusion or organ transplant from an infected donor, or across the placenta from mother to fetus. Immunoglobulin M (IgM) antibodies develop approximately 5 days after infection and can remain elevated for 3 wk to several months. Immunoglobulin G (IgG) antibodies develop 1 to 2 wk after

T

infection and can remain elevated for months or years. Healthy patients who become infected may not exhibit any symptoms or if symptoms are present they may be vague and common to other conditions. Some patients may develop lesions in the eye which can inflame the retina and form scars upon resolution. Successive reactivation of the inflammation can lead to progressive loss of vision. *T. gondii* serology is part of the TORCH (*t*oxoplasmosis, *o*ther [congenital syphilis and viruses], *r*ubella, *c*ytomegalovirus, and *h*erpes simplex type 2) panel routinely performed on pregnant women. Fetal infection during the first trimester can cause spontaneous abortion or congenital defects such as microcephaly, microphthalmia, hydranencephaly, and hydrocephalus. Immunocompromised individuals are also at high risk for serious complications if infected. While most healthy people recover without treatment, pregnant women, newborns, infants, and immunocompromised patients receive effective treatment until the worst symptoms have passed and the infection resolves. However, the location of the parasite makes it difficult to completely eradicate with medications. The presence of IgM antibodies indicates acute or congenital infection; the presence of IgG antibodies indicates current or past infection.

This procedure is contraindicated for: N/A

INDICATIONS

- Assist in establishing a diagnosis of toxoplasmosis.
- Document past exposure or immunity.
- Serological screening during pregnancy.

POTENTIAL MEDICAL DIAGNOSIS

Positive findings in

- *Toxoplasma* infection

CRITICAL FINDINGS: N/A

INTERFERING FACTORS: N/A

NURSING IMPLICATIONS AND PROCEDURE

POTENTIAL NURSING PROBLEMS:

Problem	Signs & Symptoms	Interventions
Knowledge ***(related to recent diagnosis; complexity of treatment; poor understating of provided information; cultural or language barriers; anxiety; emotional disturbance; unfamiliarity with medical management)***	Possibility that there will not be symptoms if the individual has a healthy immune system	Teach the patient and family that toxoplasmosis infection is caused by the *Toxoplasma gondii* parasite; teach the patient and family that parasite infection is caused from eating undercooked or contaminated pork, lamb, venison

(table continues on page 1458)

Problem	Signs & Symptoms	Interventions
Infection ***(related to inadequate meat preparation [pork, lamb, venison]; accidental ingestion after handling contaminated meat and not washing hands; drinking contaminated water; swallowing contaminated cat feces; accidentally ingesting contaminated soil; pregnancy [mother-child])***	Absence of symptoms; flu-like symptoms (muscular aches, pains, swollen glands); reduced or blurred vision; eye redness; tearing; eye lesion; infected newborns can have serious eye and brain damage at birth	Teach the patient that if the immune system is healthy and the patient is not pregnant, treatment may not be necessary; teach the patient that if eye lesions are present, an ophthalmologist may need to be consulted; administer prescribed medications to patients who are HIV positive or are immunosuppressed
Fear ***(related to fetal injury secondary to parasite infection during pregnancy)***	Verbalization of fear; restlessness; increased tension; continuous questioning; increased blood pressure, heart rate, respiratory rate	Evaluate verbal and nonverbal indicators of fear; assess for the cause of fear; acknowledge the patient's awareness of his or her fear; explain all procedures with simple, age-appropriate, and culturally appropriate language; administer prescribed mild tranquilizer; maintain a confident, assured professional manner in all patient interactions
Noncompliance ***(related to refusal to accept new diagnosis; financial instability; cultural norms; complexity of the medical management; lack of knowledge)***	Insufficient disease management; continued use of raw or contaminated food or water for diet and food preparation	Assess the patient's ability to understand and comply with health recommendations; assess for personal factors that may limit the patient's ability to understand, such as cognitive and hearing factors; assess the level of family support; ensure the patient knows the signs and symptoms related to the disease process; teach

T

Problem	Signs & Symptoms	Interventions
		correct food preparation and how to prevent at-risk activities related to contamination by soil or cat feces; refer to social services as appropriate

PRETEST:

- Positively identify the patient using at least two person-specific identifiers before services, treatments, or procedures are performed.
- ***Patient Teaching:*** Inform the patient this test can assist in assessing for toxoplasmosis infection.
- Obtain a history of the patient's health concerns (especially exposure to toxoplasma), symptoms, surgical procedures, and results of previously performed laboratory and diagnostic studies. Include a list of known allergens, especially allergies or sensitivities to latex.
- Obtain a list of the patient's current medications, including over-the-counter medications and dietary supplements (see Effects of Natural Products on Laboratory Values online at Davis*Plus*).
- Review the procedure with the patient. Inform the patient that several tests may be necessary to confirm the diagnosis. Any individual positive result should be repeated in 3 wk to monitor a change in detectable level of antibody. Inform the patient that specimen collection takes approximately 5 to 10 min. Address concerns about pain and explain that there may be some discomfort during the venipuncture.
- ***Sensitivity to social and cultural issues,*** as well as concern for modesty, is important in providing psychological support before, during, and after the procedure.
- Note that there are no food, fluid, or medication restrictions unless by medical direction.

INTRATEST:

Potential Complications: N/A

- Avoid the use of equipment containing latex if the patient has a history of allergic reaction to latex.
- Instruct the patient to cooperate fully and to follow directions. Direct the patient to breathe normally and to avoid unnecessary movement.
- Observe standard precautions, and follow the general guidelines in Patient Preparation and Specimen Collection online at Davis*Plus*. Positively identify the patient, and label the appropriate specimen container with the corresponding patient demographics, initials of the person collecting the specimen, date, and time of collection. Perform a venipuncture.
- Remove the needle and apply direct pressure with dry gauze to stop bleeding. Observe/assess venipuncture site for bleeding or hematoma formation and secure gauze with adhesive bandage.
- Promptly transport the specimen to the laboratory for processing and analysis.

POST-TEST:

- Inform the patient that a report of the results will be made available to the requesting health-care provider (HCP), who will discuss the results with the patient.
- Recognize anxiety related to test results, and provide emotional support if results are positive and the patient is pregnant and/or immunocompromised. Discuss the implications of abnormal test results on the patient's lifestyle. Provide teaching and information regarding the clinical implications

T

of the test results, as appropriate. Educate the patient regarding access to counseling services.

- Depending on the results of this procedure, additional testing may be performed to evaluate or monitor progression of the disease process and determine the need for a change in therapy. Evaluate test results in relation to the patient's symptoms and other tests performed.

Patient Education:

- Reinforce information given by the patient's HCP regarding further testing, treatment, or referral to another HCP.
- Instruct the patient in isolation precautions during time of communicability or contagion.
- Emphasize the need to return to have a convalescent blood sample taken in 3 wk.
- Answer any questions or address any concerns voiced by the patient or family.

Expected Patient Outcomes:

Understanding

- The patient and family state that raw or undercooked pork, lamb, or venison can cause a parasitic infection
- The patient and family state the importance of washing hands after emptying cat litter box to prevent parasitic infection.

Ability

- The patient and family describe food preparation activities that demonstrate understanding of correct meat preparation and cooking time.
- The patient and family demonstrate proficient hand-washing technique.

Response

- The patient and family recognize the importance of making lifestyle changes to support the health of themselves and family.
- The patient and family comply with the recommendation to take special precautions to avoid at-risk activities during pregnancy.

RELATED STUDIES:

- Related tests include CMV, fetal fibronectin, rubella, and viral culture.
- Refer to the Immune and Reproductive systems tables online at Davis*Plus* for related tests by body system.

Transferrin

SYNONYM/ACRONYM: Siderophilin, TRF.

COMMON USE: To assess circulating iron levels related to dietary intake to assist in diagnosing disorders such as iron deficiency anemia or hemochromatosis.

SPECIMEN: Serum collected in a gold-, red-, or red/gray-top tube.

NORMAL FINDINGS: (Method: Nephelometry)

Age	Conventional Units	SI Units (Conventional Units × 0.01)
Newborn	130–275 mg/dL	1.3–2.75 g/L
1–9 yr	180–330 mg/dL	1.8–3.3 g/L
10–19 yr	195–385 mg/dL	1.95–3.85 g/L
Adult		
Male	215–365 mg/dL	2.2–3.6 g/L
Female	250–380 mg/dL	2.5–3.8 g/L

T

DESCRIPTION: Transferrin is a glycoprotein formed in the liver. Its role is the transportation of iron, obtained from dietary intake or RBC breakdown; normally one-third of available transferrin is saturated. Inadequate transferrin levels can lead to impaired hemoglobin synthesis and anemia. Transferrin is subject to diurnal variation, and it is responsible for the variation in levels of serum iron throughout the day. (See study titled "Iron-Binding Capacity (Total), Transferrin, and Iron Saturation.")

This procedure is contraindicated for: N/A

INDICATIONS

- Determine the iron-binding capacity of the blood.
- Evaluate iron metabolism in iron-deficiency anemia.
- Evaluate nutritional status.
- Screen for hemochromatosis.

POTENTIAL MEDICAL DIAGNOSIS

Increased in:

- Estrogen therapy ***(estrogen stimulates the liver to produce transferrin)***
- Iron-deficiency anemia ***(the liver produces transferrin in response to decreased iron levels)***
- Pregnancy ***(the liver produces transferrin in response to anemia of pregnancy)***

Decreased in:

- Acute or chronic infection ***(a negative acute-phase reactant protein whose levels decrease in response to inflammation)***
- Cancer (especially of the gastrointestinal tract) ***(related to malnutrition)***
- Excessive protein loss from kidney disease ***(related to increased loss from damaged kidney)***
- Hepatic damage ***(related to decreased synthesis in the liver)***
- Hereditary atransferrinemia
- Malnutrition ***(related to a protein-deficient diet that does not provide the nutrients required for synthesis)***

CRITICAL FINDINGS: N/A

INTERFERING FACTORS

- Drugs and other substances that may increase transferrin levels include carbamazepine, danazol, mestranol, and oral contraceptives.
- Drugs and other substances that may decrease transferrin levels include cortisone and dextran. 🍁
- Transferrin levels are subject to diurnal variation and should be collected in the morning, when levels are highest.
- Failure to follow dietary restrictions before the procedure may cause the procedure to be canceled or repeated.

NURSING IMPLICATIONS AND PROCEDURE

PRETEST:

- Positively identify the patient using at least two person-specific identifiers before services, treatments, or procedures are performed.
- *Patient Teaching:* Inform the patient this test can assist in evaluating for anemia.
- Obtain a history of the patient's health concerns, symptoms, surgical procedures, and results of previously performed laboratory and diagnostic studies. Include a list of known allergens, especially allergies or sensitivities to latex.
- Obtain a list of the patient's current medications, including over-the-counter medications and dietary supplements (see Effects of Natural Products on Laboratory Values online at Davis*Plus*).

- Review the procedure with the patient. Inform the patient that specimen collection takes approximately 5 to 10 min. Address concerns about pain and explain that there may be some discomfort during the venipuncture.
- ***Sensitivity to social and cultural issues,*** as well as concern for modesty, is important in providing psychological support before, during, and after the procedure.
- Instruct the patient to fast for at least 12 hr before specimen collection.
- Note that there are no fluid or medication restrictions unless by medical direction.

INTRATEST:

Potential Complications: N/A

- Ensure that the patient has complied with dietary restrictions prior to the study, as instructed.
- Avoid the use of equipment containing latex if the patient has a history of allergic reaction to latex.
- Instruct the patient to cooperate fully and to follow directions. Direct the patient to breathe normally and to avoid unnecessary movement.
- Observe standard precautions, and follow the general guidelines in Patient Preparation and Specimen Collection online at Davis*Plus*. Positively identify the patient, and label the appropriate specimen container with the corresponding patient demographics, initials of the person collecting the specimen, date, and time of collection. Perform a venipuncture.
- Remove the needle and apply direct pressure with dry gauze to stop bleeding. Observe/assess venipuncture site for bleeding or hematoma formation and secure gauze with adhesive bandage.
- Promptly transport the specimen to the laboratory for processing and analysis.

POST-TEST:

- Inform the patient that a report of the results will be made available to the requesting health-care provider (HCP), who will discuss the results with the patient.
- Instruct the patient to resume usual diet, as directed by the HCP.
- ***Nutritional Considerations:*** Educate the patient with abnormal iron values that numerous factors affect the absorption of iron, enhancing or decreasing absorption regardless of the original content of the iron-containing dietary source. Patients must be educated to either increase or avoid intake of iron and iron-rich foods depending on their specific condition; for example, a patient with hemochromatosis or acute pernicious anemia should be educated to avoid foods rich in iron. Consumption of large amounts of alcohol damages the intestine and allows increased absorption of iron. A high intake of calcium and ascorbic acid also increases iron absorption. Iron absorption after a meal is also increased by factors in meat, fish, and poultry. Iron absorption is decreased by the absence (gastric resection) or diminished presence (use of antacids) of gastric acid. Phytic acids from cereals, tannins from tea and coffee, oxalic acid from vegetables, and minerals such as copper, zinc, and manganese interfere with iron absorption.
- Reinforce information given by the patient's HCP regarding further testing, treatment, or referral to another HCP. Answer any questions or address any concerns voiced by the patient or family. Educate the patient regarding access to nutritional counseling services. Provide contact information, if desired, for the Institute of Medicine of the National Academies (www.iom.edu) and USDA's resource for nutrition (www.choosemyplate.gov). 🍁
- Depending on the results of this procedure, additional testing may be performed to evaluate or monitor progression of the disease process and determine the need for a change in therapy. Evaluate test results in relation to the patient's symptoms and other tests performed.

RELATED STUDIES:

- Related tests include A/G, CBC, CBC RBC count, CBC RBC indices, CBC RBC morphology, ferritin, iron/TIBC, prealbumin, and total protein.
- Refer to the Hematopoietic System table online at Davis*Plus* for related tests by body system.

Triglycerides

SYNONYM/ACRONYM: Trigs, TG.

COMMON USE: To evaluate triglyceride (TG) levels to assess cardiovascular disease risk and evaluate the effectiveness of therapeutic interventions.

SPECIMEN: Serum collected in a gold-, red-, or red/gray-top tube. Plasma collected in a green-top (heparin) tube is also acceptable.

NORMAL FINDINGS: (Method: Spectrophotometry)

ATP III Classification	Conventional Units	SI Units (Conventional Units × 0.0113)
Normal	Less than 150 mg/dL	Less than 1.7 mmol/L
Borderline high	150–199 mg/dL	1.7–2.2 mmol/L
High	200–499 mg/dL	2.2–5.6 mmol/L
Very high	Greater than 500 mg/dL	Greater than 5.6 mmol/L

DESCRIPTION: Fat or adipose is an important source of energy. TGs are a combination of three fatty acids and one glycerol molecule. Much of the fatty acids used in various metabolic processes come from dietary sources. However, the body also generates fatty acids, from available glucose and amino acids, that are converted into glycogen or stored energy by the liver. Beyond TG, total cholesterol, high-density lipoprotein (HDL), and low-density lipoprotein (LDL) cholesterol values, other important risk factors must be considered. Guidelines for the prevention of cardiovascular disease (CVD) have been developed by the American College of Cardiology (ACC) and the American Heart Association (AHA) in conjunction with members of the National Heart, Lung, and Blood Institute's (NHLBI) ATP intravenous (IV) Expert Panel. The updated, evidence-based guidelines redefine the condition of concern as *atherosclerotic cardiovascular disease* (ASCVD) and expand ASCVD to include cardiovascular disease (CVD), stroke, and peripheral arterial disease. Some of the important highlights include the following:

- Movement away from the use of LDL cholesterol targets in determining treatment with statins. Recommendations that focus on selecting (1) the patients who fall into four groups most likely to benefit from statin therapy, and (2) the level of statin intensity

T

most likely to affect or reduce development of ASCVD.

- Development of a new 10-yr risk assessment tool based on findings from a large, diverse population. Evidence-based risk factors include age, sex, ethnicity, total cholesterol, HDL cholesterol, blood pressure, blood-pressure treatment status, diabetes, and current use of tobacco products.
- Recommendations for aspects of lifestyle that would encourage prevention of ASCVD, including adherence to a Mediterranean-style or DASH (Dietary Approaches to Stop Hypertension)-style diet; dietary restriction of saturated fats, trans fats, sugar, and sodium; and regular participation in aerobic exercise. The guidelines contain reductions in body mass index (BMI) cutoffs for men and women designed to promote discussions between health-care providers (HCPs) and their patients regarding the benefits of maintaining a healthy weight.
- Recognition that additional biological markers, such as family history, high-sensitivity C-reactive protein, ankle-brachial index, and coronary artery calcium score, may be selectively used with the assessment tool to assist in predicting and evaluating risk.
- Recognition that other biomarkers, such as apolipoprotein B, estimated glomerular filtration rate, creatinine, lipoprotein (a) or Lp(a), and microalbumin, warrant further study and may be considered for inclusion in future guidelines. 🍁

TG levels vary by age, gender, weight, and ethnicity:

Levels increase with age.
Levels are higher in men than in women (among women, those who take oral contraceptives have levels that are 20 to 40 mg/dL 🍁 higher than those who do not).
Levels are higher in overweight and obese people than in those with normal weight.
Levels in African Americans are approximately 10 to 20 mg/dL 🍁 lower than in people of European descent.

This procedure is contraindicated for: N/A

INDICATIONS

- Evaluate known or suspected disorders associated with altered TG levels.
- Identify hyperlipoproteinemia (hyperlipidemia) in patients with a family history of the disorder.
- Monitor the response to drugs known to alter TG levels.
- Screen adults who are either over 40 yr or obese to estimate the risk for atherosclerotic cardiovascular disease.

POTENTIAL MEDICAL DIAGNOSIS

Increased in:

- Acute myocardial infarction (AMI) ***(elevated TG is identified as an independent risk factor in the development of coronary artery disease [CAD])***
- Alcoholism ***(related to decreased breakdown of fats in the liver and increased blood levels)***
- Anorexia nervosa ***(compensatory increase secondary to starvation)***
- Chronic ischemic heart disease ***(elevated TG is identified as an independent risk factor in the development of CAD)***
- Cirrhosis ***(increased TG blood levels related to decreased breakdown of fats in the liver)***
- Glycogen storage disease ***(G6PD deficiency, e.g., von Gierke's disease, results in hepatic overproduction of very-low-density***

lipoprotein [VLDL] cholesterol, the TG-rich lipoprotein)
- Gout ***(TG is frequently elevated in patients with gout, possibly related to alterations in apolipoprotein E genotypes)***
- Hyperlipoproteinemia ***(related to increase in transport proteins)***
- Hypertension ***(associated with elevated TG, which is identified as an independent risk factor in the development of CAD)***
- Hypothyroidism ***(significant relationship between elevated TG and decreased metabolism)***
- Impaired glucose tolerance ***(increase in insulin stimulates production of TG by liver)***
- Metabolic syndrome ***(syndrome consisting of obesity, high blood pressure, and insulin resistance)***
- Nephrotic syndrome ***(related to absence or insufficient levels of lipoprotein lipase to remove circulating TG and to decreased catabolism of TG-rich VLDL lipoproteins)***
- Obesity ***(significant and complex relationship between obesity and elevated TG)***
- Pancreatitis ***(acute and chronic; related to effects on insulin production)***
- Pregnancy ***(increased demand for production of hormones related to pregnancy)***
- Kidney failure ***(related to diabetes; elevated insulin levels stimulate production of TG by liver)***
- Respiratory distress syndrome ***(related to artificial lung surfactant used for therapy)***
- Stress ***(related to poor diet; effect of hormones secreted under stressful situations that affect glucose levels)***
- Werner's syndrome ***(clinical features resemble metabolic syndrome)***

Decreased in:
- End-stage liver disease ***(related to cessation of liver function that results in decreased production of TG and TG transport proteins)***
- Hyperthyroidism ***(related to increased catabolism of VLDL transport proteins and general increase in metabolism)***
- Hypolipoproteinemia and abetalipoproteinemia ***(related to decrease in transport proteins)***
- Intestinal lymphangiectasia
- Malabsorption disorders ***(inadequate supply from dietary sources)***
- Malnutrition ***(inadequate supply from dietary sources)***

CRITICAL FINDINGS: N/A

INTERFERING FACTORS
- Drugs and other substances that may increase TG levels include acetylsalicylic acid, atenolol, bisoprolol, β blockers, bendroflumethiazide, cholestyramine, conjugated estrogens, cyclosporine, estrogen/progestin therapy, estropipate, ethynodiol, etretinate, furosemide, glucocorticoids, hydrochlorothiazide, isotretinoin, labetalol, levonorgestrel, medroxyprogesterone, mepindolol, methyclothiazide, metoprolol, miconazole, mirtazapine, nadolol, nafarelin, oral contraceptives, oxprenolol, pindolol, prazosin, propranolol, tamoxifen, thiazides, ticlopidine, timolol, and tretinoin.
- Drugs and other substances that may decrease TG levels include anabolic steroids, ascorbic acid, beclobrate, bezafibrate, captopril, carvedilol, celiprolol, chenodiol, cholestyramine, cilazapril, ciprofibrate, clofibrate, colestipol, danazol, doxazosin, enalapril, eptastatin (type IIb only), fenofibrate, flaxseed oil, fluvastatin,

T

gemfibrozil, halofenate, insulin, levonorgestrel, levothyroxine, lifibrol, lovastatin, medroxyprogesterone, metformin, niacin, niceritrol, Norplant, pentoxifylline, pindolol, pravastatin, prazosin, probucol, simvastatin, and verapamil.

- Failure to follow dietary restrictions before the procedure may cause the procedure to be canceled or repeated.

NURSING IMPLICATIONS AND PROCEDURE

POTENTIAL NURSING PROBLEMS:

Problem	Signs & Symptoms	Interventions
Nutrition ***(related to excess caloric intake with large amounts of dietary sodium and fat; cultural lifestyle; overeating associated with anxiety, depression, compulsive disorder; genetics; inadequate or unhealthy food resources)***	Observable obesity; high fat or sodium food selections; high BMI; high consumption of ethnic foods; sedentary lifestyle; dietary religious beliefs and food selections; binge eating; diet high in refined sugar; repetitive dieting and failure	Discuss ideal body weight and the purpose of and relationship between ideal weight and caloric intake to support cardiac health; review ways to decrease intake of saturated fats and increase intake of polyunsaturated fats; discuss limiting cholesterol intake to less than 300 mg per day; discuss limiting the intake of refined processed sugar; teach limiting sodium intake to the HCP's recommended restriction; encourage intake of fresh fruits and vegetables, unprocessed carbohydrates, poultry, and grains
Health management ***(related to failure to regulate diet; lack of exercise; alcohol use; smoking)***	Inability or failure to recognize or process information toward improving health and preventing illness with associated mental and physical effects	Encourage regular participation in weight-bearing exercise; assess diet, smoking, and alcohol use; teach the importance of adequate calcium intake with diet and supplements; refer to smoking cessation and alcohol treatment programs; collaborate with HCP for bone density evaluation
Tissue perfusion ***(related to hypovolemia; decreased hemoglobin; interrupted arterial flow;***	Hypotension; dizziness; cool extremities; pallor; capillary refill greater than 3 sec in fingers and toes; weak pedal pulses;	Monitor blood pressure; assess for dizziness; assess extremities for skin temperature, color, warmth; assess capillary refill; assess pedal pulses; monitor for numbness, tingling,

T

Problem	Signs & Symptoms	Interventions
interrupted venous flow)	altered level of consciousness; altered sensation	hyperesthesia, hypoesthesia; monitor for deep venous thrombosis; instruct in careful use of heat and cold on affected areas; use foot cradle to keep pressure off of affected body parts
Fear ***(related to loss of control; ineffective coping; change in life expectancy; unfamiliar surroundings; illness; disease; unknown)***	Expression of fear; preoccupation with fear; increased tension; increased blood pressure; increased heart rate; vomiting; diarrhea; nausea; fatigue; weakness; insomnia; shortness of breath; increased respiratory rate; withdrawal; panic attacks	Access social services; provide specific and culturally appropriate education; assist the patient and family to recognize effective coping strategies; assist the patient to acknowledge his or her fear; provide a safe environment to decrease fear; explore cultural influences that may enhance fear; utilize therapeutic touch as appropriate to decrease fear; collaborate with social services, respiratory services, physical therapy, and occupational therapy to address specific medical problems associated with fear

PRETEST:

- Positively identify the patient using at least two person-specific identifiers before services, treatments, or procedures are performed.
- *Patient Teaching:* Inform the patient this test can assist in monitoring and evaluating lipid levels.
- Obtain a history of the patient's health concerns, symptoms, surgical procedures, and results of previously performed laboratory and diagnostic studies. Include a list of known allergens, especially allergies or sensitivities to latex. The presence of other risk factors, such as family history of heart disease, smoking, obesity, diet, lack of physical activity, hypertension, diabetes, previous MI, and previous vascular disease, should be investigated. Knowledge of genetics assists the nurse in identifying patients and family members who may benefit from additional education, risk assessment, and counseling. Genetics is the study and identification of genes, genetic mutations, and inheritance. For example, genetics provides some insight into the likelihood of inheriting a trait such as blue eyes or a medical condition such as CAD. Genomic studies evaluate the interaction of groups of genes. The combined activity or combined expression of groups of genes allows assumptions or predictions to be made. As an example, genomic studies measure the levels of activity in multiple genes to predict how they, along with environmental and lifestyle decisions, influence the development of type 2 diabetes, CAD, MI, or ischemic stroke. Further information regarding inheritance of genes can be found in the study titled "Genetic Testing."

T

- Obtain a list of the patient's current medications, including over-the-counter medications and dietary supplements (see Effects of Natural Products on Laboratory Values online at Davis*Plus*).
- Review the procedure with the patient. Inform the patient that specimen collection takes approximately 5 to 10 min. Address concerns about pain and explain that there may be some discomfort during the venipuncture.
- ***Sensitivity to social and cultural issues,*** as well as concern for modesty, is important in providing psychological support before, during, and after the procedure.
- Instruct the patient to fast for 12 hr before specimen collection; fasting is required prior to measurement of TG levels. Ideally, the patient should be on a stable diet for 3 wk and avoid alcohol consumption for 3 days before specimen collection; alcohol increases TG levels. Protocols may vary among facilities.
- Note that there are no medication restrictions unless by medical direction.

INTRATEST:

Potential Complications: N/A

- Ensure that the patient has complied with dietary restrictions and other pretesting preparations prior to the study, as instructed.
- Avoid the use of equipment containing latex if the patient has a history of allergic reaction to latex.
- Instruct the patient to cooperate fully and to follow directions. Direct the patient to breathe normally and to avoid unnecessary movement.
- Observe standard precautions, and follow the general guidelines in Patient Preparation and Specimen Collection online at Davis*Plus*. Positively identify the patient, and label the appropriate specimen container with the corresponding patient demographics, initials of the person collecting the specimen, date, and time of collection. Perform a venipuncture.
- Remove the needle and apply direct pressure with dry gauze to stop bleeding. Observe/assess venipuncture site for bleeding or hematoma formation and secure gauze with adhesive bandage.
- Promptly transport the specimen to the laboratory for processing and analysis.

POST-TEST:

- Inform the patient that a report of the results will be made available to the requesting HCP, who will discuss the results with the patient.
- Instruct the patient to resume usual diet, as directed by the HCP.
- ***Nutritional Considerations:*** Increased TG levels may be associated with atherosclerosis and CAD. Nutritional therapy is recommended for the patient identified to be at risk for developing CAD or for individuals who have specific risk factors and/or existing medical conditions (e.g., elevated LDL cholesterol levels, other lipid disorders, type 1 diabetes, type 2 diabetes, insulin resistance, or metabolic syndrome). Other changeable risk factors warranting patient education include strategies to encourage patients, especially those who are overweight and with high blood pressure, to safely decrease sodium intake, achieve a normal weight, ensure regular participation in moderate aerobic physical activity three to four times per week, eliminate tobacco use, and adhere to a heart-healthy diet. If TGs also are elevated, the patient should be advised to eliminate or reduce alcohol. A variety of dietary patterns are beneficial for people with CAD, and there are many meal-planning approaches with nutritional goals endorsed by the American Diabetes Association (ADA). The Guideline on Lifestyle Management to Reduce Cardiovascular Risk published by the ACC and AHA in conjunction with the NHLBI recommends a Mediterranean-style diet rather than

T

a low-fat diet. The guideline emphasizes inclusion of vegetables, whole grains, fruits, low-fat dairy, nuts, legumes, and nontropical vegetable oils (e.g., olive, canola, peanut, sunflower, flaxseed) along with fish and lean poultry. 🍁 A similar dietary pattern, the DASH diet, makes additional recommendations for the reduction of dietary sodium. Both dietary styles emphasize a reduction in consumption of red meats, which are high in saturated fats and cholesterol, and other foods containing sugar, saturated fats, trans fats, and sodium. The ADA also includes a vegetarian diet as well as other potential weight loss diets such as Weight Watchers. 🍁 The nutritional needs of each patient need to be determined individually (especially during pregnancy) with the appropriate HCPs, particularly professionals educated in nutrition.

- *Sensitivity to social and cultural issues:* Numerous studies point to the prevalence of excess body weight in American children and adolescents. Experts estimate that obesity is present in 25% of the population aged 6 to 11 yr. The medical, social, and emotional consequences of excess body weight are significant. Special attention should be given to instructing the pediatric patient and caregiver regarding health risks and weight control education. 🍁
- Recognize anxiety related to test results, and be supportive of fear of shortened life expectancy.
- Depending on the results of this procedure, additional testing may be performed to evaluate or monitor progression of the disease process and determine the need for a change in therapy. Evaluate test results in relation to the patient's symptoms and other tests performed.

Patient Education:

- Discuss the implications of abnormal test results on the patient's lifestyle.
- Provide teaching and information regarding the clinical implications of the test results, as appropriate.
- Educate the patient regarding access to counseling services.
- Provide contact information, if desired, for the AHA (www.americanheart.org), NHLBI (www.nhlbi.nih.gov), Institute of Medicine of the National Academies (www.iom.edu), and USDA's resource for nutrition (www.choosemyplate.gov). 🍁
- Reinforce information given by the patient's HCP regarding further testing, treatment, or referral to another HCP.
- Answer any questions or address any concerns voiced by the patient or family.
- Teach the patient the negative effects that elevated TGs can have on cardiac health.
- Teach the patient to follow a diet of protein and complex carbohydrates.

Expected Patient Outcomes:

Understanding

- The patient and family state that increased TGs can increase the risk of heart attack.
- The patient and family compare traditionally ethnic foods to heart-healthy selections toward making dietary changes.

Ability

- The patient and family exhibit proficiency in making dietary selections that are heart healthy.
- The patient identifies strategies for effective coping that do not involve overeating.

Response

- The patient and family discuss the correlation between selected diet and increased TG levels.
- The patient and family complies with HCP's recommended lifestyle changes to improve TG levels.

RELATED STUDIES:

- Related tests include antidysrhythmic drugs, apolipoproteins A, B, and C, atrial natriuretic peptide, blood gases, BNP, calcium, cholesterol (total, HDL, and LDL), CT cardiac scoring, C-reactive protein, CK and isoenzymes, echocardiography, genetic testing, glucose, glycated hemoglobin, Holter monitor, homocysteine, ketones, LDH and isoenzymes, lipoprotein electrophoresis, magnesium, MRI chest, myocardial infarct scan, myocardial perfusion heart scan, myoglobin, PET heart, potassium, and troponin.

- Refer to the Cardiovascular System table online at Davis*Plus* for related tests by body system.

Triiodothyronine, Free

SYNONYM/ACRONYM: Free T_3, FT_3.

COMMON USE: A complementary adjunct to evaluate thyroid hormone levels primarily related to hyperthyroidism and to assess causes of hypothyroidism.

SPECIMEN: Serum collected in a gold-, red-, or red/gray-top tube.

NORMAL FINDINGS: (Method: Immunoassay)

Age	Conventional Units	SI Units (Conventional Units × 1.54)
0–3 d	2–7.9 pg/mL	3.1–12.2 pmol/L
4–30 d	2–5.2 pg/mL	3.1–8 pmol/L
1–23 mo	1.6–6.4 pg/mL	2.5–9.9 pmol/L
2–6 yr	2–6 pg/mL	3.1–9.2 pmol/L
7–17 yr	2.9–5.1 pg/mL	4.5–7.8 pmol/L
Adults and older adults	2.6–4.8 pg/mL	4–7.4 pmol/L
Pregnant women (4–9 mo gestation)	2–3.4 pg/mL	3–5.2 pmol/L

DESCRIPTION: Unlike the thyroid hormone thyroxine (T_4), most T_3 is converted enzymatically from T_4 in the tissues rather than being produced directly by the thyroid gland (see study titled "Thyroxine, Total"). Approximately one-third of T_4 is converted to T_3. Most T_3 in the serum (99.97%) is bound to thyroxine-binding globulin (TBG), prealbumin, and albumin. The remainder (0.03%) circulates as unbound or free T_3, which is the physiologically active form. Levels of free T_3 are proportional to levels of total T_3. The advantage of measuring free T_3 instead of total T_3 is that, unlike total T_3 measurements, free T_3 levels are not affected by fluctuations in TBG levels. T_3 is four to five times more biologically potent than T_4. This hormone, along with T_4, is responsible for maintaining a euthyroid state. Free T_3 measurements are rarely required, but they are indicated in the diagnosis of T_3 toxicosis and when certain drugs are being administered that interfere with the conversion of T_4 to T_3.

This procedure is contraindicated for: N/A

T

INDICATIONS

- Adjunctive aid to thyroid-stimulating hormone (TSH) and free T_4 assessment.
- Assist in the diagnosis of T_3 toxicosis.

POTENTIAL MEDICAL DIAGNOSIS

Increased in:

- High altitude
- Hyperthyroidism ***(triiodothyronine is produced independently of stimulation by TSH)***
- T_3 toxicosis

Decreased in:

- Hypothyroidism ***(thyroid hormones are not produced in sufficient quantities regardless of TSH levels)***
- Malnutrition ***(related to protein or iodine deficiency; iodine is needed for thyroid hormone synthesis and proteins are needed for transport)***
- Nonthyroidal chronic diseases
- Pregnancy (late)

CRITICAL FINDINGS: N/A

INTERFERING FACTORS

- Drugs and other substances that may increase free T_3 include acetylsalicylic acid, amiodarone, and levothyroxine.
- Drugs and other substances that may decrease free T_3 include amiodarone, methimazole, phenytoin, propranolol, and radiographic medium.

NURSING IMPLICATIONS AND PROCEDURE

PRETEST:

- Positively identify the patient using at least two person-specific identifiers before services, treatments, or procedures are performed.
- *Patient Teaching:* Inform the patient this test can assist in assessing thyroid gland function.
- Obtain a history of the patient's health concerns, symptoms, surgical procedures, and results of previously performed laboratory and diagnostic studies. Include a list of known allergens, especially allergies or sensitivities to latex.
- Obtain a list of the patient's current medications, including over-the-counter medications and dietary supplements (see Effects of Natural Products on Laboratory Values online at Davis*Plus*).
- Review the procedure with the patient. Inform the patient that specimen collection takes approximately 5 to 10 min. Address concerns about pain and explain that there may be some discomfort during the venipuncture.
- *Sensitivity to social and cultural issues,* as well as concern for modesty, is important in providing psychological support before, during, and after the procedure.
- Note that there are no food, fluid, or medication restrictions unless by medical direction.

INTRATEST:

Potential Complications: N/A

- Avoid the use of equipment containing latex if the patient has a history of allergic reaction to latex.
- Instruct the patient to cooperate fully and to follow directions. Direct the patient to breathe normally and to avoid unnecessary movement.
- Observe standard precautions, and follow the general guidelines in Patient Preparation and Specimen Collection online at Davis*Plus*. Positively identify the patient, and label the appropriate specimen container with the corresponding patient demographics, initials of the person collecting the specimen, date, and time of collection. Perform a venipuncture.
- Remove the needle and apply direct pressure with dry gauze to stop bleeding. Observe/assess

T

venipuncture site for bleeding or hematoma formation and secure gauze with adhesive bandage.
- Promptly transport the specimen to the laboratory for processing and analysis.

POST-TEST:
- Inform the patient that a report of the results will be made available to the requesting health-care provider (HCP), who will discuss the results with the patient.
- Reinforce information given by the patient's HCP regarding further testing, treatment, or referral to another HCP. Answer any questions or address any concerns voiced by the patient or family.
- Depending on the results of this procedure, additional testing may be performed to evaluate or monitor progression of the disease process and determine the need for a change in therapy. Evaluate test results in relation to the patient's symptoms and other tests performed.

RELATED STUDIES:
- Related tests include albumin, antibodies antithyroglobulin, biopsy thyroid, copper, PTH, prealbumin, protein, RAIU, thyroglobulin, TBII, thyroid scan, TSH, TSI, T_4, free T_4, T_3, and US thyroid.
- Refer to the Endocrine System table online at Davis*Plus* for related tests by body system.

Triiodothyronine, Total

SYNONYM/ACRONYM: T_3.

COMMON USE: To assist in evaluating thyroid function primarily related to diagnosing hyperthyroidism and monitoring the effectiveness of therapeutic interventions.

SPECIMEN: Serum collected in a gold-, red-, or red/gray-top tube. Plasma collected in a green-top (heparin) tube is also acceptable.

NORMAL FINDINGS: (Method: Immunoassay)

Age	Conventional Units	SI Units (Conventional Units × 0.0154)
Cord blood	14–86 ng/dL	0.22–1.32 nmol/L
1–3 d	100–292 ng/dL	1.54–4.5 nmol/L
4–30 d	62–243 ng/dL	0.96–3.74 nmol/L
1–12 mo	105–245 ng/dL	1.62–3.77 nmol/L
1–5 yr	105–269 ng/dL	1.62–4.14 nmol/L
6–10 yr	94–241 ng/dL	1.45–3.71 nmol/L
16–20 yr	80–210 ng/dL	1.23–3.23 nmol/L
Adult	70–204 ng/dL	1.08–3.14 nmol/L
Older adult	40–181 ng/dL	0.62–2.79 nmol/L
Pregnant woman (last 4 mo gestation)	116–247 ng/dL	1.79–3.8 nmol/L

T

DESCRIPTION: Unlike the thyroid hormone thyroxine (T_4), most T_3 is converted enzymatically from T_4 in the tissues rather than being produced directly by the thyroid gland (see study titled "Thyroxine, Total"). Approximately one-third of T_4 is converted to T_3. Most T_3 in the serum (99.97%) is bound to thyroxine-binding globulin (TBG), prealbumin, and albumin. The remainder (0.03%) circulates as unbound or free T_3, which is the physiologically active form. Levels of free T_3 are proportional to levels of total T_3. The advantage of measuring free T_3 instead of total T_3 is that, unlike total T_3 measurements, free T_3 levels are not affected by fluctuations in TBG levels. T_3 is four to five times more biologically potent than T_4. This hormone, along with T_4, is responsible for maintaining a euthyroid state.

This procedure is contraindicated for: N/A

INDICATIONS

Adjunctive aid to thyroid-stimulating hormone (TSH) and free T_4 assessment.

POTENTIAL MEDICAL DIAGNOSIS

Increased in:

- Conditions with increased TBG ***(e.g., pregnancy and estrogen therapy)***
- Early thyroid failure
- Hyperthyroidism ***(triiodothyronine is produced independently of stimulation by TSH)***
- Iodine-deficiency goiter
- T_3 toxicosis
- Thyrotoxicosis factitia ***(laboratory tests do not distinguish between endogenous and exogenous sources)***
- Treated hyperthyroidism

Decreased in:

- Acute and subacute nonthyroidal disease ***(pathophysiology is unclear)***
- Conditions with decreased TBG ***(TBG is the major transport protein)***
- Hypothyroidism ***(thyroid hormones are not produced in sufficient quantities regardless of TSH levels)***
- Malnutrition ***(related to insufficient protein sources to form albumin and TBG)***

CRITICAL FINDINGS: N/A

INTERFERING FACTORS

- Drugs and other substances that may increase total T_3 levels include amiodarone, amphetamine, clofibrate, fluorouracil, halofenate, insulin, levothyroxine, methadone, opiates, oral contraceptives, phenothiazine, phenytoin, prostaglandins, and T_3.
- Drugs and other substances that may decrease total T_3 levels include acetylsalicylic acid, amiodarone, anabolic steroids, asparaginase, carbamazepine, cholestyramine, clomiphene, colestipol, dexamethasone, fenclofenac, furosemide, glucocorticoids, hydrocortisone, interferon alfa-2b, iobenzamic acid, iopanoic acid, ipodate, isotretinoin, lithium, methimazole, netilmicin, oral contraceptives, penicillamine, phenylbutazone, phenytoin, potassium iodide, prednisone, propranolol, propylthiouracil, radiographic medium, sodium ipodate, salicylate, sulfonylureas, and tyropanoic acid.

T

NURSING IMPLICATIONS AND PROCEDURE

PRETEST:

- Positively identify the patient using at least two person-specific identifiers before services, treatments, or procedures are performed.
- *Patient Teaching:* Inform the patient this test can assist in assessing thyroid gland function.
- Obtain a history of the patient's health concerns, symptoms, surgical procedures, and results of previously performed laboratory and diagnostic studies. Include a list of known allergens, especially allergies or sensitivities to latex.
- Obtain a list of the patient's current medications, including over-the-counter medications and dietary supplements (see Effects of Natural Products on Laboratory Values online at Davis*Plus*).
- Review the procedure with the patient. Inform the patient that specimen collection takes approximately 5 to 10 min. Address concerns about pain and explain that there may be some discomfort during the venipuncture.
- ***Sensitivity to social and cultural issues,*** as well as concern for modesty, is important in providing psychological support before, during, and after the procedure.
- Note that there are no food, fluid, or medication restrictions unless by medical direction.

INTRATEST:

Potential Complications: N/A

- Avoid the use of equipment containing latex if the patient has a history of allergic reaction to latex.
- Instruct the patient to cooperate fully and to follow directions. Direct the patient to breathe normally and to avoid unnecessary movement.
- Observe standard precautions, and follow the general guidelines in Patient Preparation and Specimen Collection online at Davis*Plus*. Positively identify the patient, and label the appropriate specimen container with the corresponding patient demographics, initials of the person collecting the specimen, date, and time of collection. Perform a venipuncture.
- Remove the needle and apply direct pressure with dry gauze to stop bleeding. Observe/assess venipuncture site for bleeding or hematoma formation and secure gauze with adhesive bandage.
- Promptly transport the specimen to the laboratory for processing and analysis.

POST-TEST:

- Inform the patient that a report of the results will be made available to the requesting health-care provider (HCP), who will discuss the results with the patient.
- Reinforce information given by the patient's HCP regarding further testing, treatment, or referral to another HCP. Answer any questions or address any concerns voiced by the patient or family.
- Depending on the results of this procedure, additional testing may be performed to evaluate or monitor progression of the disease process and determine the need for a change in therapy. Evaluate test results in relation to the patient's symptoms and other tests performed.

RELATED STUDIES:

- Related tests include albumin, antibodies antithyroglobulin, biopsy thyroid, copper, PTH, prealbumin, protein, RAIU, thyroglobulin, TBII, thyroid scan, TSH, TSI, T_4, free T_4, free T_3, and US thyroid.
- Refer to the Endocrine System table online at Davis*Plus* for related tests by body system.

Troponins I and T

SYNONYM/ACRONYM: Cardiac troponin, cardiac troponin I (cTnI), cardiac troponin T (cTnT).

COMMON USE: To assist in evaluating myocardial muscle damage related to disorders such as myocardial infarction.

SPECIMEN: Serum collected in a gold-, red-, or red/gray-top tube. Plasma collected in a green-top (heparin) tube is also acceptable. Serial sampling is highly recommended. Care must be taken to use the same type of collection container if serial measurements are to be taken.

NORMAL FINDINGS: (Method: Enzyme immunoassay)

Troponin I	Conventional Units	SI Units (Conventional Units × 1)
0–30 d	Less than 4.8 ng/mL	Less than 4.8 mcg/L
1–3 mo	Less than 0.4 ng/mL	Less than 0.4 mcg/L
3–6 mo	Less than 0.3 ng/mL	Less than 0.3 mcg/L
7–12 mo	Less than 0.2 ng/mL	Less than 0.2 mcg/L
1–18 yr	Less than 0.1 ng/mL	Less than 0.1 mcg/L
Adult	Less than 0.05 ng/mL	Less than 0.05 mcg/L
Troponin T	Less than 0.2 ng/mL	Less than 0.2 mcg/L

Normal values can vary significantly due to differences in test kit reagents and instrumentation. The testing laboratory should be consulted for comparison of results to the corresponding reference range.

DESCRIPTION: Troponin is a complex of three contractile proteins that regulate the interaction of actin and myosin. Troponin C is the calcium-binding subunit; it does not have a cardiac muscle-specific subunit. Troponin I and troponin T, however, do have cardiac muscle–specific subunits. They are detectable a few hours to 7 days after the onset of symptoms of myocardial damage. Troponin I is thought to be a more specific marker of cardiac damage than troponin T. Cardiac troponin I begins to rise 2 to 6 hr after myocardial infarction (MI). It has a biphasic peak: It initially peaks at 15 to 24 hr after MI and then exhibits a lower peak after 60 to 80 hr. Cardiac troponin T levels rise 2 to 6 hr after MI and remain elevated. Both proteins return to the reference range 7 days after MI.

Timing for Appearance and Resolution of Serum/Plasma Cardiac Markers in Acute MI

Cardiac Marker	*Appearance (hr)*	*Peak (hr)*	*Resolution (d)*
CK (total)	4–6	24	2–3

(table continues on page 1476)

Timing for Appearance and Resolution of Serum/Plasma Cardiac Markers in Acute MI

Cardiac Marker	*Appearance (hr)*	*Peak (hr)*	*Resolution (d)*
CK-MB	4–6	15–20	2–3
LDH	12	24–48	10–14
Myoglobin	1–3	4–12	1
Troponin I	2–6	15–20	5–7

CK = creatine kinase; CK-MB = creatine kinase MB fraction; LDH = lactate dehydrogenase.

This procedure is contraindicated for: N/A

INDICATIONS

- Assist in establishing a diagnosis of MI.
- Evaluate myocardial cell damage.

POTENTIAL MEDICAL DIAGNOSIS

Increased in:

Conditions that result in cardiac tissue damage; troponin is released from damaged tissue into the circulation.

- Acute MI
- Minor myocardial damage
- Myocardial damage after coronary artery bypass graft surgery or percutaneous transluminal coronary angioplasty 🍁
- Unstable angina pectoris

Decreased in: N/A

CRITICAL FINDINGS: N/A

INTERFERING FACTORS: N/A

NURSING IMPLICATIONS AND PROCEDURE

POTENTIAL NURSING PROBLEMS:

Problem	Signs & Symptoms	Interventions
Cardiac output ***(prolonged myocardial ischemia; acute MI; reduced cardiac muscle contractility; rupture papillary muscle; mitral insufficiency)***	Weak peripheral pulses; slow capillary refill; decreased urinary output; cool, clammy skin; tachypnea; dyspnea; altered level of consciousness; abnormal heart sounds; fatigue; hypoxia; loud holosystolic murmur; electrocardiogram (ECG) changes; increased jugular venous distention	Assess peripheral pulses and capillary refill; monitor blood pressure and check for orthostatic changes; assess respiratory rate, breath sounds, and orthopnea; assess skin color and temperature; assess level of consciousness; monitor urinary output; use pulse oximetry to monitor oxygenation; monitor ECG; administer ordered inotropic and peripheral vasodilator medications, nitrates; provide oxygen administration

T

Problem	Signs & Symptoms	Interventions
Pain ***(related to myocardial ischemia; MI)***	Reports of chest pain; new onset of angina; shortness of breath; pallor; weakness; diaphoresis; palpitations; nausea; vomiting; epigastric pain or discomfort; increased blood pressure; increased heart rate	Assess pain characteristics, squeezing pressure, location in substernal back neck or jaw; assess pain duration and onset (minimal exertion, sleep, or rest); identify pain modalities that have relieved pain in the past; monitor cardiac biomarkers (CK-MB, troponin, myoglobin); collaborate with ancillary departments to complete ordered echocardiography, exercise stress testing, pharmacological stress testing; administer prescribed pain medication; monitor and trend vital signs; administer prescribed oxygen; administer prescribed anticoagulants, antiplatelets, beta blockers, calcium channel blockers, ACE inhibitors, ARBs, thrombolytic drugs
Health management ***(related to failure to regulate diet; lack of exercise; alcohol use; smoking)***	Inability or failure to recognize or process information toward improving health and preventing illness with associated mental and physical effects	Collaborate with health-care provider (HCP) to develop a plan of care that supports cardiac health; assist patient to adhere to recommended medication regime; ensure patient attends a smoking cessation program; encourage patient to comply with health-care follow-up appointments; assess diet and lifestyle choices
Fear ***(related to threat of MI, possible death; recurrent pain)***	Verbalization of fear; restlessness; increased tension; continuous questioning; increased blood pressure, heart rate, respiratory rate	Evaluate verbal and nonverbal indicators of fear; assess for the cause of fear; acknowledge the patient's awareness of his or her fear; explain all procedures with simple age-appropriate and culturally appropriate language; administer prescribed mild tranquilizer; maintain a confident, assured professional manner in all patient interactions

T

PRETEST:

- Positively identify the patient using at least two person-specific identifiers before services, treatments, or procedures are performed.
- ***Patient Teaching:*** Inform the patient this test can assist in evaluating heart damage.
- Obtain a history of the patient's health concerns, symptoms, surgical procedures, and results of previously performed laboratory and diagnostic studies. Include a list of known allergens, especially allergies or sensitivities to latex. The presence of other risk factors, such as family history of heart disease, smoking, obesity, diet, lack of physical activity, hypertension, diabetes, previous myocardial infarction, and previous vascular disease, should be investigated. Knowledge of genetics assists the nurse in identifying patients and family members who may benefit from additional education, risk assessment, and counseling. Genetics is the study and identification of genes, genetic mutations, and inheritance. For example, genetics provides some insight into the likelihood of inheriting a trait such as blue eyes or a medical condition such as coronary artery disease (CAD). Genomic studies evaluate the interaction of groups of genes. The combined activity or combined expression of groups of genes allows assumptions or predictions to be made. As an example, genomic studies measure the levels of activity in multiple genes to predict how they, along with environmental and life style decisions, influence the development of type 2 diabetes, CAD, MI, or ischemic stroke. Further information regarding inheritance of genes can be found in the study titled "Genetic Testing."
- Obtain a list of the patient's current medications, including over-the-counter medications and dietary supplements (see Effects of Natural Products on Laboratory Values online at Davis*Plus*).
- Review the procedure with the patient. Inform the patient that a number of samples will be collected. Collection at time of admission, 2 to 4 hr, 6 to 8 hr, and 12 hr after admission are the minimal recommendations. Additional samples may be requested. Inform the patient that specimen collection takes approximately 5 to 10 min. Address concerns about pain and explain that there may be some discomfort during the venipuncture.
- ***Sensitivity to social and cultural issues,*** as well as concern for modesty, is important in providing psychological support before, during, and after the procedure.
- Note that there are no food, fluid, or medication restrictions unless by medical direction.

INTRATEST:

Potential Complications: N/A

- Avoid the use of equipment containing latex if the patient has a history of allergic reaction to latex.
- Instruct the patient to cooperate fully and to follow directions. Direct the patient to breathe normally and to avoid unnecessary movement.
- Observe standard precautions, and follow the general guidelines in Patient Preparation and Specimen Collection online at Davis*Plus*. Positively identify the patient, and label the appropriate specimen container with the corresponding patient demographics, initials of the person collecting the specimen, date, and time of collection. Perform a venipuncture.
- Remove the needle and apply direct pressure with dry gauze to stop bleeding. Observe/assess venipuncture site for bleeding or hematoma formation and secure gauze with adhesive bandage.
- Promptly transport the specimen to the laboratory for processing and analysis.

POST-TEST:

- Inform the patient that a report of the results will be made available to the requesting HCP, who will discuss the results with the patient.

T

- *Nutritional Considerations:* Increased troponin levels are associated with CAD. Nutritional therapy is recommended for the patient identified to be at risk for developing CAD or for individuals who have specific risk factors and/or existing medical conditions (e.g., elevated LDL cholesterol levels, other lipid disorders, type 1 diabetes, type 2 diabetes, insulin resistance, or metabolic syndrome). Other changeable risk factors warranting patient education include strategies to encourage patients, especially those who are overweight and with high blood pressure, to safely decrease sodium intake, achieve a normal weight, ensure regular participation in moderate aerobic physical activity three to four times per week, eliminate tobacco use, and adhere to a heart-healthy diet. If triglycerides also are elevated, the patient should be advised to eliminate or reduce alcohol. A variety of dietary patterns are beneficial for people with CAD, and there are many meal-planning approaches with nutritional goals endorsed by the American Diabetes Association (ADA). The Guideline on Lifestyle Management to Reduce Cardiovascular Risk published by the American College of Cardiology (ACC) and the American Heart Association (AHA) in conjunction with the National Heart, Lung, and Blood Institute (NHLBI) recommends a Mediterranean-style diet rather than a low-fat diet. The guideline emphasizes inclusion of vegetables, whole grains, fruits, low-fat dairy, nuts, legumes, and nontropical vegetable oils (e.g., olive, canola, peanut, sunflower, flaxseed) along with fish and lean poultry. 🍁 A similar dietary pattern known as the Dietary Approaches to Stop Hypertension (DASH) diet makes additional recommendations for the reduction of dietary sodium. Both dietary styles emphasize a reduction in consumption of red meats, which are high in saturated fats and cholesterol, and other foods containing sugar, saturated fats, trans fats, and sodium. The ADA also includes a vegetarian diet as well as other potential weight loss diets such as Weight Watchers. 🍁 The nutritional needs of each patient need to be determined individually (especially during pregnancy) with the appropriate HCPs, particularly professionals educated in nutrition.
- Recognize anxiety related to test results, and be supportive of fear of shortened life expectancy.
- Depending on the results of this procedure, additional testing may be performed to evaluate or monitor progression of the disease process and determine the need for a change in therapy. Evaluate test results in relation to the patient's symptoms and other tests performed.

Patient Education:

- Discuss the implications of abnormal test results on the patient's lifestyle.
- Provide teaching and information regarding the clinical implications of the test results, as appropriate.
- Educate the patient regarding access to counseling services.
- Provide contact information, if desired, for the AHA (www.americanheart.org), NHLBI (www.nhlbi.nih.gov), Institute of Medicine of the National Academies (www.iom.edu), and USDA's resource for nutrition (www.choosemyplate.gov). 🍁
- Reinforce information given by the patient's HCP regarding further testing, treatment, or referral to another HCP.
- Answer any questions or address any concerns voiced by the patient or family.
- Teach the patient and family to report chest pain as soon as it starts.
- Teach the patient about the disease progression and pathophysiology.

Expected Patient Outcomes:

Understanding

- The patient and family state the signs and symptoms of heart attack.
- The patient and family state the purpose of prescribed medications to treat medical condition.

Ability

- The patient and family identify actions that can be taken to improve cardiac health (e.g., maintain a healthy diet, participate in regular physical activities, eliminate the use of tobacco products, and limit the use of alcohol), as appropriate.
- The patient and family identify positive coping strategies that can be used to reduce fear.

Response

- The patient complies with the recommendation to undergo smoking cessation.
- The patient and family comply with recommendations for lifestyle improvements to decrease the risk of future cardiac injury.

RELATED STUDIES:

- Related tests include antidysrhythmic drugs, apolipoproteins A, B, and C, ANP, blood gases, blood pool imaging, BNP, calcium, cholesterol (total, HDL, and LDL), CRP, CT cardiac scoring, CK and isoenzymes, culture viral, echocardiography, echocardiography transesophageal, ECG, exercise stress test, glucose, glycated hemoglobin, Holter monitor, homocysteine, ketones, LDH and isoenzymes, lipoprotein electrophoresis, magnesium, MRI chest, MI infarct scan, myocardial perfusion heart scan, myoglobin, pericardial fluid analysis, PET heart, potassium, and triglycerides.
- Refer to the Cardiovascular System table online at Davis*Plus* for related tests by body system.

Tuberculosis: Skin and Blood Tests

SYNONYM/ACRONYM: TST, TB tine test, PPD, Mantoux skin test, QuantiFERON-TB Gold blood test (QFT-G), QuantiFERON-TB Gold In-Tube test (QFT-GIT), T-SPOT.TB test (T-SPOT).

COMMON USE: To evaluate for current or past tuberculin infection or exposure.

SPECIMEN: Whole blood collected in a green-top (LiHep) tube (QuantiFERON-TB Gold and T-SPOT.TB blood tests), whole blood collected in each of three special (nil, antigen, and mitogen) specimen containers (QuantiFERON-TB Gold In-Tube test).

NORMAL FINDINGS: (Method: Intradermal skin test, enzyme-linked immunosorbent assay [ELISA] blood test for QuantiFERON assays, enzyme-linked ImmunoSpot [ELISPOT] for T-SPOT.TB test) Negative.

DESCRIPTION: Routine screening for tuberculosis (TB) has not been needed for some time because, until recently, the disease had largely been eradicated. Recommendations for the timing of initial and subsequent screening may vary according to state laws, practitioners' guidelines, and specific circumstances (foreign adoptions or immigration from areas where TB is endemic, or in high-risk environments such as health-care or congregated settings). Children and adults are screened on the basis of a risk assessment. For example, the American Academy of Pediatrics recommends identifying individuals at highest risk by means of a questionnaire before testing, and adults who either work or reside

T

in a high-risk environment are required to submit to annual Mantoux testing or chest x-ray (for individuals with a previously positive Mantoux test or individuals from other countries who have received the Bacillus Calmette-Guérin [BCG] vaccine). ✦ Tuberculin skin tests are done to determine past or present exposure to tuberculosis (TB). The multipuncture or tine test is no longer used as a screening technique and has been largely replaced by the more definitive Mantoux test using Aplisol or Tubersol, purified protein derivatives (PPDs) of the mycobacterial cell wall, administered by intradermal injection. The Mantoux test is the test of choice in symptomatic patients. It is also used in some settings as a screening test. A negative result is judged if there is no sign of redness or induration at the site of the injection or if the zone of redness and induration is less than 5 mm in diameter. TB skin tests are classified in three categories depending on the measured diameter (in millimeters) of the induration and the person's risk of being infected or of progressing to developing TB if infected.

1. A positive result evidenced by an area of erythema and induration at the injection site greater than 5 mm is considered to be positive in persons infected with HIV, persons who have been in recent contact with an individual who has TB, persons with chest x-ray findings consistent with a previous TB infection, persons who have received transplanted organs, or persons who are immunosuppressed from other causes.
2. A positive result evidenced by an area of erythema and induration at the injection site greater than 10 mm is considered to be positive in persons who have immigrated or are foreign adoptees from a country with a high prevalence of TB within the past 5 yr; persons who misuse drugs by injection; persons who work in mycobacteriology laboratories; persons who work or live in highly congregated settings; children less than 4 yr of age; any person with a clinical condition whose immune system is immature, suppressed, or otherwise compromised; and any younger person (infant through adolescent) who has been exposed to adults in a high-risk group.
3. A positive result evidenced by an area of erythema and induration at the injection site greater than 15 mm is considered to be positive in any person.

A positive result does not distinguish between active and dormant infection. A positive response to the Mantoux test is followed up with chest radiography and bacteriological sputum testing to confirm diagnosis.

The QuantiFERON-TB Gold (QFT-G), QuantiFERON-TB Gold In-Tube (QFT-GIT), and T-SPOT TB interferon-gamma release blood tests, also known as *interferon—gamma release assays* (IGRAs), are approved by the U.S. Food and Drug Administration for all applications in which the TB skin test is used. ✦ The blood tests are procedures in which T lymphocytes from the patient, either in whole blood or harvested from whole blood, are incubated with a reagent cocktail of peptides that simulate two or three proteins made only by *Mycobacterium tuberculosis*. These proteins are not found in the blood of previously vaccinated individuals or individuals who do not have TB. The blood test offers the advantage of eliminating many of the false reactions encountered with skin testing, only a single patient visit is required, and results can be available within 24 hr. Results obtained by the QFT-G test are not affected by BCG vaccination. The blood tests and skin tests are approved as indirect tests for *Mycobacterium tuberculosis*, and the Centers for Disease Control and Prevention (CDC) recommends their use in conjunction with risk assessment, chest x-ray, and other appropriate medical and diagnostic evaluations.

This procedure is contraindicated for: N/A

INDICATIONS

- Evaluate cough, weight loss, fatigue, hemoptysis, and abnormal x-rays to determine if the cause of symptoms is TB.
- Evaluate known or suspected exposure to TB, with or without symptoms, to determine if TB is present.
- Evaluate patients with medical conditions placing them at risk for TB (e.g., AIDS, lymphoma, diabetes).
- Screen populations at risk for developing TB (e.g., health-care workers, residents of long-term care facilities, correctional facility personnel, prison inmates, and residents of the inner city living in poor hygienic conditions).

POTENTIAL MEDICAL DIAGNOSIS

Positive findings in

- Pulmonary TB

CRITICAL FINDINGS:

- Positive results

Note and immediately report to the requesting health-care provider (HCP) any critical findings and related symptoms. A listing of these findings varies among facilities. Timely notification of a critical finding for laboratory or diagnostic studies is a role expectation of the professional nurse. The notification processes vary among facilities. Upon receipt of the critical finding, the information should be read back to the caller to verify accuracy.

INTERFERING FACTORS

General

- Each of the blood and skin tests evaluate different facets of the immune response and use different methodologies and reagents; interpretations may not be interchangeable.

Skin Test

- Drugs such as immunosuppressive drugs or steroids can alter results.
- Diseases such as hematological cancers or sarcoidosis can alter results.
- Recent or present bacterial, fungal, or viral infections may affect results. False-positive results may be caused by the presence of nontuberculous mycobacteria or by serial testing.
- False-negative results can occur if sensitized T cells are temporarily decreased. False-negative results also can occur in the presence of bacterial infections, immunological deficiencies, immunosuppressive agents, live-virus vaccinations (e.g., measles, mumps, varicella, rubella), malnutrition, old age, overwhelming TB, kidney disease, and active viral infections (e.g., chickenpox, measles, mumps).
- Improper storage of the tuberculin solution (e.g., with respect to

temperature, exposure to light, and stability on opening) may affect the results.

- Improper technique when performing the intradermal injection (e.g., injecting into subcutaneous tissue) may cause false-negative results.
- Incorrect amount or dilution of antigen injected or delayed injection after drawing the antigen up into the syringe may affect the results.
- Incorrect reading of the measurement of response or timing of the reading may interfere with results.
- It is not known whether the test has teratogenic effects or reproductive implications; the test should be administered to pregnant women only when clearly indicated.
- The test should not be administered to a patient with a previously positive tuberculin skin test because of the danger of severe reaction, including vesiculation, ulceration, and necrosis.
- The test does not distinguish between current and past infection.

Blood Test

- The performance of these blood tests has not been evaluated in large studies with patients who have impaired or altered immune function, have or are highly likely to develop TB, are younger than 17, are pregnant, or have diseases other than TB. These individuals are either immunosuppressed, immunocompromised, or have immature immune function and may not produce sufficient numbers of T lymphocytes for accurate results. The testing laboratory should be consulted for interpretation of results or limitations for use with patients in these categories.
- False-negative results are possible due to exposure or infection prior to development of detectable immune response.
- False-positive results are possible due to some cross-reactivity to some strains of environmental mycobacteria.
- False-negative results are possible due to exposure or infection prior to development of detectable immune response.

NURSING IMPLICATIONS AND PROCEDURE

POTENTIAL NURSING PROBLEMS:

Problem	Signs & Symptoms	Interventions
Breathing ***(related to productive cough; fatigue; inflammation)***	Tachypnea; dyspnea; orthopnea; change in the rate and depth of respirations; retractions; nasal flare; use of accessory muscles	Assess and trend respiratory rate and effort; monitor for retractions, nasal flare, and use of accessory muscles; evaluate cough effectiveness; auscultate lungs for adventitious breath sounds; monitor pulse oximetry and trend results; administer prescribed oxygen therapy; prepare for possible mechanical intubation; encourage oral fluids; encourage cough and deep breathing; pace activities

(table continues on page 1484)

T

Problem	Signs & Symptoms	Interventions
Infection ***(related to exposure to M. tuberculosis)***	Productive cough of bloody sputum; fever with temperature spikes; positive acid-fast bacilli (AFB) smear; fatigue; night sweats; weight loss; chills; lack of appetite	Send ordered sputum specimen for culture; monitor and trend temperature; monitor AFB smear results; induce sputum as ordered if patient is unable to provide one through cough; place in respiratory isolation (negative airflow); administer prescribed medications; instruct the patient to cover the mouth when coughing or sneezing; teach the patient to wash his or her hands after coming into contact with contaminated sputum; teach the patient and family the importance of wearing masks when visiting; report all confirmed TB cases to the department of health 🍁
Health maintenance ***(related to knowledge deficit; financial or cultural barriers; lack of social support; no motivation; complexity of health-care system)***	Inability or failure to recognize or process information toward improving health and preventing illness with associated mental and physical effects; self-report of difficulty managing health regime; resistance to treatment; increased symptoms; chest x-ray confirmation of disease reactivation	Assess for evidence of therapeutic regime noncompliance (increased productive cough, drug-resistant culture results); identify the cause of noncompliance; arrange social services consult; teach the patient about the disease process and treatment modality in understandable, culturally appropriate terms (transmission, symptoms, length of treatment, risk to others, follow-up appointments); consider referral of the continued noncompliant to a direct observation therapy program; explain the importance of taking prescribed medication; encourage smoking abstinence
Nutrition ***(related to poor appetite secondary to M. tuberculosis infection)***	Unintended weight loss; pale dry skin; dry mucous membranes; documented	Encourage a high-calorie, high-protein diet; encourage an increased intake of oral fluids; record accurate daily weight at the same time each day

Problem	Signs & Symptoms	Interventions
	inadequate caloric intake; subcutaneous tissue loss; hair pulls out easily; self-report of no appetite	with the same scale; obtain an accurate nutritional history; assess attitude toward eating; promote a dietary consult to evaluate current eating habits and best method of nutritional supplementation; monitor nutritional laboratory values such as albumin; assess swallowing ability; encourage cultural home foods; provide a pleasant environment for eating; alter food seasoning to enhance flavor; provide parenteral or enteral nutrition as prescribed

PRETEST:

Blood and Skin Tests

- Positively identify the patient using at least two person-specific identifiers before services, treatments, or procedures are performed.
- *Patient Teaching:* Inform the patient this test can assess for a tuberculin infection or exposure.
- Obtain a history of the patient's health concerns, symptoms, surgical procedures, and results of previously performed laboratory and diagnostic studies. Include a list of known allergens, especially allergies or sensitivities to latex.
- Obtain a history of the patient's immune and respiratory systems, symptoms, and results of previously performed laboratory tests and diagnostic and surgical procedures. Obtain a history of TB or TB exposure, signs and symptoms indicating possible TB, and other skin tests or vaccinations and sensitivities.
- Obtain a list of the patient's current medications, including over-the-counter medications and dietary supplements (see Effects of Natural Products on Laboratory Values online at Davis*Plus*).
- Review the procedure with the patient.

Skin Test

- Before beginning the test, ensure that the patient does not currently have TB and has not previously had a positive skin test. Do not administer the test if the patient has a skin rash or other eruptions at the test site. Inform the patient that the procedure takes approximately 5 min. Address concerns about pain and explain that a moderate amount of pain may be experienced when the intradermal injection is performed.
- Emphasize to the patient that the area should not be scratched or disturbed after the injection and before the reading.

Blood Test

- Inform the patient that specimen collection takes approximately 5 to 10 min. Address concerns about pain and explain that there may be some discomfort during the venipuncture.

Blood and Skin Tests

- ***Sensitivity to social and cultural issues,*** as well as concern for modesty, is important in providing psychological support before, during, and after the procedure.
- Note that there are no food, fluid, or medication restrictions unless by medical direction.

T

INTRATEST:

Potential Complications: N/A

- Observe standard precautions, and follow the general guidelines in Patient Preparation and Specimen Collection online at Davis*Plus*. Positively identify the patient.

Blood and Skin Tests

- Avoid the use of equipment containing latex if the patient has a history of allergic reaction to latex.
- Instruct the patient to cooperate fully and to follow directions. Direct the patient to breathe normally and to avoid unnecessary movement.

Skin Test

- Have epinephrine hydrochloride solution (1:1,000) available in the event of anaphylaxis.
- Cleanse the skin site on the lower anterior forearm with alcohol swabs and allow to air-dry.

Mantoux (Intradermal) Test

- Prepare PPD or old tuberculin in a tuberculin syringe with a short, 26-gauge needle attached. Prepare the appropriate dilution and amount for the most commonly used intermediate strength (5 tuberculin units in 0.1 mL) or a first strength usually used for children (1 tuberculin unit in 0.1 mL). Inject the preparation intradermally at the prepared site as soon as it is drawn up into the syringe. When properly injected, a bleb or wheal 6 to 10 mm in diameter is formed within the layers of the skin. Record the site, and remind the patient to return in 48 to 72 hr to have the test read. At the time of the reading, use a plastic ruler to measure the diameter of the largest indurated area, making sure the room is sufficiently lighted to perform the reading. Palpate for thickening of the tissue; a positive result is indicated by a reaction of 5 mm or more with erythema and edema.

Blood Test

- Observe standard precautions, and follow the general guidelines in Patient Preparation and Specimen Collection online at Davis*Plus*. Positively identify the patient, and label the appropriate specimen container with the corresponding patient demographics, initials of the person collecting the specimen, date, and time of collection. Perform a venipuncture.
- Remove the needle and apply direct pressure with dry gauze to stop bleeding. Observe/assess venipuncture site for bleeding or hematoma formation and secure gauze with adhesive bandage.
- Promptly transport the specimen to the laboratory for processing and analysis.

POST-TEST:

- Inform the patient that a report of the results will be made available to the requesting HCP, who will discuss the results with the patient.
- Recognize anxiety related to test results and be supportive of perceived loss of independence and fear of shortened life expectancy. Discuss the implications of abnormal test results on the patient's lifestyle. Provide teaching and information regarding the clinical implications of the test results, as appropriate. Counsel the patient, as appropriate, regarding the risk of transmission and proper prophylaxis, and reinforce the importance of strict adherence to the treatment regimen. Inform the patient that positive findings must be reported to local health department officials, who will question him or her regarding other persons who may have been exposed through contact. Educate the patient regarding access to counseling services.
- Depending on the results of this procedure, additional testing may be performed to evaluate or monitor progression of the disease process and determine the need for a change in therapy. Evaluate test results in relation to the patient's symptoms and other tests performed.

Patient Education:

- Reinforce information given by the patient's HCP regarding further testing, treatment, or referral to another HCP.

T

- Emphasize to the patient who receives skin testing the need to return and have the test results read within the specified time frame of 48 to 72 hr after injection.
- Inform the patient that the effects from a positive response at the site can remain for 1 wk.
- Educate the patient that a positive result may put him or her at risk for infection related to impaired primary defenses, impaired gas exchange related to decrease in effective lung surface, and intolerance to activity related to an imbalance between oxygen supply and demand.
- Answer any questions or address any concerns voiced by the patient or family.

Expected Patient Outcomes:

Understanding

- The patient and family acknowledge the importance of covering the mouth during coughing or sneezing to decrease possibility of droplet contamination.
- The patient and family acknowledge the importance of an adequate fluid intake to liquefy secretions.

Ability

- The patient demonstrates the correct technique for covering the mouth and nose when coughing or sneezing.
- The patient demonstrates proficient cough and deep breathing.

Response

- The patient and family compy with the request to refrain from smoking.
- The patient complies with the recommendation to take prescribed medication as ordered.

RELATED STUDIES:

- Related tests include alveolar/arterial gradient, angiography pulmonary, biopsy lung, blood gases, bronchoscopy, calcium, carbon dioxide, chest x-ray, CBC WBC count and differential, CT thoracic, culture and smear mycobacteria, culture blood, culture sputum, cytology sputum, eosinophil count, ESR, gallium scan, Gram stain, lung perfusion scan, lung ventilation scan, mediastinoscopy, pleural fluid analysis, PFT, and zinc.
- Refer to the Immune and Respiratory systems tables online at Davis*Plus* for related tests by body system.

Tuning Fork Tests

SYNONYM/ACRONYM: Bing test, Rinne test, Schwabach test, Weber test.

COMMON USE: To assess for and determine type of hearing loss.

AREA OF APPLICATION: Ears.

POTENTIAL MEDICAL DIAGNOSIS

Normal findings

- Normal air and bone conduction in both ears; no evidence of hearing loss
- Bing test: Pulsating sound that gets louder and softer when the opening to the ear canal is alternately opened and closed (*Note:* This result, observed in patients with normal hearing, is also observed in patients with sensorineural hearing loss.)
- Rinne test: Longer and louder tone heard by air conduction than by bone conduction (*Note:* This result, observed in patients with normal hearing, is also observed in patients with sensorineural hearing loss.)
- Schwabach test: Same tone loudness heard equally long by the examiner and the patient

T

- Weber test: Same tone loudness heard equally in both ears

Abnormal findings related to

- Conduction hearing loss related to or evidenced by:
  Impacted cerumen
  Obstruction of external ear canal ***(presence of a foreign body)***
  Otitis externa ***(infection in ear canal)***
  Otitis media ***(poor eustachian tube function or infection)***
  Otitis media serous ***(fluid in middle ear due to allergies or a cold)***
  Otosclerosis
  Bing test: No change in the loudness of the sound
  Rinne test: Tone louder or detected for a longer time than the air-conducted tone
  Schwabach test: Prolonged duration of tone when compared to that heard by the examiner
  Weber test: Lateralization of tone to one ear, indicating loss of hearing on that side (i.e., tone is heard in the poorer ear)
- Sensorineural hearing loss related to or evidenced by:
  Congenital damage or malformations of the inner ear
  Ménière's disease
  Ototoxic drugs ***(aminoglycosides, e.g., gentamicin or tobramycin; salicylates, e.g., aspirin)***
  Presbycusis ***(gradual hearing loss experienced in advancing age)***
  Serious infections ***(meningitis, measles, mumps, other viral, syphilis)***
  Trauma to the inner ear ***(related to exposure to noise in excess of 90 dB or as a result of physical trauma)***
  Tumor ***(e.g., acoustic neuroma, cerebellopontine angle tumor, meningioma)***
  Vascular disorders
  Bing test: Pulsating sound that gets louder and softer when the opening to the ear canal is alternately opened and closed
  Rinne test: Tone heard louder by air conduction
  Schwabach test: Shortened duration of tone when compared to that heard by the examiner
  Weber test: Lateralization of tone to one ear indicating loss of hearing on the other side (i.e., tone is heard in the better ear)

CRITICAL FINDINGS: N/A

Find and print out the full study on Fast Find at davispl.us/vanleeuwen7.

Ultrasound, Abdomen

SYNONYM/ACRONYM: Abdominal ultrasound, abdomen sonography.

COMMON USE: To visualize and assess the solid organs of the abdomen, including the aorta, bile ducts, gallbladder, kidneys, pancreas, spleen, and other large abdominal blood vessels. This study is used to perform biopsies and assist in diagnosing disorders such as aortic aneurysm, infections, fluid collections, masses, and obstructions. This procedure can also be used to evaluate therapeutic interventions such as organ transplants.

AREA OF APPLICATION: Abdomen from the xiphoid process to the umbilicus.

DESCRIPTION: Ultrasound (US) procedures are diagnostic, noninvasive, and relatively inexpensive. They take a short time to complete, do not use radiation, and cause no harm to the patient. High-frequency sound waves of various intensities are delivered by a transducer, a flashlight-shaped device, pressed against the skin. The waves are bounced back off internal anatomical structures and fluids, converted to electrical energy, amplified by the transducer, and displayed as images on a monitor. US is often used as a diagnostic and therapeutic tool for guiding minimally invasive procedures such as needle biopsies and fluid aspiration (paracentesis). The contraindications and complications for biopsy and fluid aspiration are discussed in detail in the individual related studies.

Different types of transducers and imaging systems are sometimes used in clinical settings. Conventional US systems assume that sound waves pass through tissue at a constant speed. Advances in technology have led to the development of "smart" transducers that can compensate for tissue aberrations in technically difficult patients. Other advancements in imaging systems include three-dimensional and Doppler US. Color Doppler US uses color to indicate the velocity and direction of blood flow. Power Doppler is a more sensitive Doppler variation, capable of providing detailed images of blood flow; a limitation of power Doppler is that it cannot provide information regarding the direction of blood flow. Spectral Doppler provides data from blood flow measurements in formats other than color—for example, it can convert the measurements into a graph representing distance of blood flow against time or as a unique sound heard with every heartbeat.

Abdominal US is valuable in determining aortic aneurysms, determining the internal components of organ masses (solid versus cystic), and evaluating other abdominal diseases, ascites, and abdominal obstruction. Abdominal US can be performed on the same day as a radionuclide scan or other radiological procedure and is especially valuable in patients who have hypersensitivity to contrast medium or are pregnant. US is also widely used for pediatric patients to help diagnose appendicitis and for infants to assign cause for recurrent vomiting.

This procedure is contraindicated for: N/A

U

INDICATIONS

- Determine the patency and function of abdominal blood vessels, including the abdominal aorta; vena cava; and portal, splenic, renal, and superior and inferior mesenteric veins.
- Detect and measure an abdominal aortic aneurysm.
- Monitor abdominal aortic aneurysm expansion to prevent rupture.
- Determine changes within small aortic aneurysms pre- and postsurgery.
- Evaluate abdominal ascites.
- Evaluate size, shape, and pathology of intra-abdominal organs.

POTENTIAL MEDICAL DIAGNOSIS

Normal findings

- Absence of ascites, aortic aneurysm, cysts, obstruction, or tumors
- Normal size, position, and shape of intra-abdominal organs and associated structures

Abnormal findings related to

Identification of abnormal findings is assisted by comparison of parameters such as size, shape, symmetry, and location; for example, areas of altered echo patterns in either an expected or unexpected location may indicate enlargement of an organ or the presence of blood or other fluids, tumors, or cysts. Comparison by type of abnormal findings may also assist in evaluating areas of altered patterns; for example, small round or oval areas with well-defined borders and clear central areas can differentiate a fluid-filled cyst from a solid tumor.

- Abdominal abscess, ascitic fluid, or hematoma
- Aortic aneurysm greater than 4 cm
- Congenital absence or malplacement of organs
- Gallbladder or renal calculi
- Tumor, liver, spleen, or retroperitoneal space

CRITICAL FINDINGS:

- Aortic aneurysm measuring 5 cm or more in diameter.

Note and immediately report to the requesting health-care provider (HCP) any critical findings and related symptoms. A listing of these findings varies among facilities. Timely notification of a critical finding for laboratory or diagnostic studies is a role expectation of the professional nurse. The notification processes vary among facilities. Upon receipt of the critical finding, the information should be read back to the caller to verify accuracy.

INTERFERING FACTORS

Factors that may alter the results of the study

- Attenuation of the sound waves by bony structures which can impair clear imaging of the upper abdominal structures.
- Incorrect placement of the transducer over the desired test site; quality of the US study is very dependent upon the skill of the ultrasonographer.
- Metallic objects (e.g., jewelry, body rings) within the examination field, which may inhibit organ visualization and cause unclear images.
- Inability of the patient to cooperate or remain still during the procedure because of age, significant pain, or mental status.
- Retained air, barium, or gas from a previous radiological procedure may block the transmission of sound waves.
- Gas or feces in the gastrointestinal (GI) tract resulting from inadequate cleansing or failure to restrict food intake before the study.
- Patients who are technically difficult and who present challenges in obtaining reliable results (e.g., who are obese; have reduced rib spaces; present with fatty liver;

U

have postoperative incisions, bandages, or dressings; have significant scarring in the area of interest). Aberrations in tissue composition may attenuate the sound waves and alter findings.

Other considerations

- Failure to follow dietary and fluid restrictions and other pretesting preparations may cause the procedure to be canceled or repeated.
- The procedure may be canceled if the patient's weight exceeds the safety limit for the equipment.

NURSING IMPLICATIONS AND PROCEDURE

See Potential Nursing Problems on Fast Find at davispl.us/vanleeuwen7.

PRETEST:

- Positively identify the patient using at least two person-specific identifiers before services, treatments, or procedures are performed.
- Inform the patient this procedure can assist in assessing abdominal abnormalities.
- Obtain a history of the patient's health concerns, symptoms, surgical procedures, and results of previously performed laboratory and diagnostic studies. Include a list of known allergens, especially allergies or sensitivities to latex.
- Note any recent procedures that can interfere with test results (e.g., surgery, biopsy, barium studies, colonoscopy, endoscopic retrograde cholangiopancreatography). Ensure that interfering studies were performed at least 24 hr before this test or can be rescheduled after this procedure.
- Obtain a list of the patient's current medications, including over-the-counter medications and dietary supplements (see Effects of Natural Products on Laboratory Values online at Davis*Plus*).
- Review the procedure with the patient. Address concerns about pain related to the procedure. Explain to the patient that there may be moments of discomfort experienced during the test. Inform the patient that the procedure is performed in a US department, by a HCP specializing in this procedure, with support staff, and takes approximately 30 to 60 min.

  Pediatric Considerations Preparing children for an abdominal US depends on the age of the child. Encourage parents to be truthful about what the child may experience during the procedure and to use words that they know their child will understand. Toddlers and preschool-age children have a short attention span, so the best time to talk about the test is right before the procedure. The child should be assured that he or she will be allowed to bring a favorite comfort item into the examination room and, if appropriate, that a parent will be with the child during the procedure. Provide older children with information about the test, and allow them to participate in as many decisions as possible (e.g., choice of clothes to wear to the appointment) in order to reduce anxiety and encourage cooperation. If the child will be asked to maintain a certain position for the test, encourage the child to practice the required position, provide a CD that demonstrates the procedure, and teach strategies to remain calm, such as deep breathing, humming, or counting to himself or herself.
- ***Sensitivity to social and cultural issues,*** as well as concern for modesty, is important in providing psychological support before, during, and after the procedure.
- Instruct the patient to remove jewelry and other metallic objects in the area to be examined.
- Instruct the patient to fast and restrict fluids for 8 hr prior to the procedure; instruct the caregiver of a pediatric patient to have the patient fast and restrict fluids for 8 hr prior to the procedure or as ordered.

Food restrictions help ensure reduction of bowel gas, which can interfere with the transmission of US waves. Protocols may vary among facilities.

INTRATEST:

Potential Complications: N/A

- Observe standard precautions, and follow the general guidelines in Patient Preparation and Specimen Collection online at Davis*Plus*. Positively identify the patient.
- Ensure that the patient has complied with dietary and fluid restrictions prior to the procedure, as instructed.
- Ensure that the patient has removed external metallic objects prior to the procedure.
- Instruct the patient to void prior to the procedure and to change into the gown, robe, and foot coverings provided.
- Instruct the patient to cooperate fully and to follow directions. Instruct the patient to remain still throughout the procedure because movement produces unreliable results.
- Place the patient in the supine position on an examination table. The right- or left-side-up positions may be used to allow gravity to reposition the liver, gas, and fluid to facilitate better organ visualization.
- Expose the abdominal area and drape the patient.
- Conductive gel is applied to the skin, and a Doppler transducer is moved over the skin to obtain images of the area of interest.
- Ask the patient to breathe normally during the examination. If necessary for better organ visualization, ask the patient to inhale deeply and hold his or her breath.

POST-TEST:

- Inform the patient that a report of the results will be sent to the requesting HCP, who will discuss the results with the patient.
- When the study is completed, remove the gel from the skin.
- Instruct the patient to resume usual diet and fluids, as directed by the HCP.
- Recognize anxiety related to test results. Discuss the implications of abnormal test results on the patient's lifestyle. Provide teaching and information regarding the clinical implications of the test results, as appropriate.
- Reinforce information given by the patient's HCP regarding further testing, treatment, or referral to another HCP. Answer any questions or address any concerns voiced by the patient or family.
- Depending on the results of this procedure, additional testing may be needed to evaluate or monitor progression of the disease process and determine the need for a change in therapy. Evaluate test results in relation to the patient's symptoms and other tests performed.

Patient Education:

- Teach the pathophysiology associated with the diagnosis.
- Teach the patient treatment options for diagnosis.

Expected Patient Outcomes:

Understanding

- The patient and family accurately describe treatment options in relation to diagnosis.
- The patient and family state the effects selected treatment options may have on current lifestyle.

Ability

- The patient demonstrates grief over personal concerns appropriately with the support of family and significant other.
- The patient demonstrates effective coping mechanisms to decrease anxiety.

Response

- The patient agrees to discuss concerns with identified support (family, friends, group, spiritual advisor).
- The patient agrees to lifestyle modifications to control disease process and symptoms.

U

RELATED STUDIES:

- Related tests include ACTH and challenge tests, albumin, ALKP, ALT, amylase, angiography abdomen, AST, biopsy intestinal, biopsy liver, bilirubin and fractions, BUN, calcium, calculus kidney stone panel, cancer antigens, carbon dioxide, CBC, CBC hematocrit, CBC hemoglobin, CBC WBC and differential, chloride, cortisol and challenge tests, creatinine, CT abdomen, GGT, HCG, hepatobiliary scan, infectious mononucleosis, IVP, KUB, LDH, lipase, magnesium, MRI abdomen, peritoneal fluid analysis, phosphorus, potassium, PT/INR, renogram, sodium, US kidney, US liver and biliary, US pancreas, US spleen, uric acid, urinalysis, and WBC scan.
- Refer to the Cardiovascular, Gastrointestinal, Genitourinary, and Hepatobiliary systems tables online at Davis*Plus* for related tests by body system.

Ultrasound, Arterial Doppler, Carotid Studies

SYNONYM/ACRONYM: Carotid Doppler, carotid ultrasound, arterial ultrasound, cerebrovascular ultrasound.

COMMON USE: To visualize and assess blood flow through the carotid arteries toward evaluating risk for stroke related to atherosclerosis.

AREA OF APPLICATION: Arteries.

DESCRIPTION: Ultrasound (US) procedures are diagnostic, noninvasive, and relatively inexpensive. They take a short time to complete, do not use radiation, and cause no harm to the patient. High-frequency sound waves of various intensities are delivered by a transducer, a flashlight-shaped device, pressed against the skin. The waves are bounced back off internal anatomical structures and fluids, converted to electrical energy, amplified by the transducer, and displayed as images on a monitor.

Different types of transducers and imaging systems are sometimes used in clinical settings. Conventional US systems assume that sound waves pass through tissue at a constant speed. Advances in technology have led to the development of "smart" transducers that can compensate for tissue aberrations in technically difficult patients. Other advancements in imaging systems include three-dimensional and Doppler US. Color Doppler US uses color to indicate the velocity and direction of blood flow. Power Doppler is a more sensitive Doppler variation, capable of providing detailed images of blood flow; a limitation of power Doppler is that it cannot provide information regarding the direction of blood flow. Spectral Doppler provides data from blood flow measurements in formats other than color—for example, it can convert the measurements into a graph representing distance of blood flow against time or as a unique sound heard with every heartbeat.

Using the duplex scanning method, carotid US records sound

waves to obtain information about the carotid arteries. The amplitude and waveform of the carotid pulse are measured, resulting in a two-dimensional image of the artery. Carotid arterial sites used for the studies include the common carotid, external carotid, and internal carotid. Blood flow direction, velocity, and the presence of flow disturbances can be readily assessed. The sound waves that hit the moving red blood cells and are reflected back to the transducer correspond to the velocity of the blood flow through the vessel. Color Doppler US can be used with the duplex method whereby red and blue are assigned to represent the direction of blood flow, and the intensity of the color is an indication of velocity. The result is the visualization of the artery to assist in the diagnosis (i.e., presence, amount, location) of plaque causing vessel stenosis or atherosclerotic occlusion affecting the flow of blood to the brain. Depending on the degree of stenosis causing a reduction in vessel diameter, additional testing can be performed to determine the effect of stenosis on the hemodynamic status of the artery.

The combined information obtained from carotid US and ankle-brachial index (ABI) provides significant support for predicting coronary artery disease. ABI is a noninvasive, simple comparison of blood pressure measurements in the arms and legs and can be used to detect peripheral arterial disease (PAD). A Doppler stethoscope is used to obtain the systolic pressure in either the dorsalis pedis or the posterior tibial artery. This ankle pressure is then divided by the highest brachial systolic pressure acquired after taking the blood pressure in both of the patient's arms. This index should be greater than 1 with a range of 0.85 to 1.4. When the index falls below 0.5, blood flow impairment is considered significant. Patients should be scheduled for a vascular consult for an abnormal ABI. Patients with diabetes or kidney disease, and some older adult patients, may have a falsely elevated ABI due to calcifications of the vessels in the ankle causing an increased systolic pressure. The ABI test approaches 95% accuracy in detecting PAD. However, a normal ABI value does not absolutely rule out the possibility of PAD for some individuals, and additional tests should be done to evaluate symptoms.

This procedure is contraindicated for: N/A

INDICATIONS

- Assist in the diagnosis of carotid artery occlusive disease, as evidenced by visualization of blood flow disruption.
- Detect irregularities in the structure of the carotid arteries.
- Detect plaque or stenosis of the carotid artery, as evidenced by turbulent blood flow or changes in Doppler signals indicating occlusion.

POTENTIAL MEDICAL DIAGNOSIS

Normal findings

- Normal blood flow through the carotid arteries with no evidence of occlusion or narrowing

Abnormal findings related to

- Arterial aneurysm
- Carotid artery occlusive disease (atherosclerosis)
- Plaque or stenosis of carotid artery

U

- Reduction in vessel diameter of more than 16%, indicating stenosis
- Tumor

CRITICAL FINDINGS: N/A

INTERFERING FACTORS

Factors that may alter the results of the study

- Attenuation of the sound waves by bony structures, which can impair clear imaging of the vessels.
- Incorrect placement of the transducer over the desired test site; quality of the US study is very dependent upon the skill of the ultrasonographer.
- Metallic objects (e.g., jewelry, body rings) within the examination field, which may inhibit organ visualization and cause unclear images.
- Inability of the patient to cooperate or remain still during the procedure because of age, significant pain, or mental status.
- Patients who are technically difficult and who present challenges in obtaining reliable results (e.g., who are obese; have reduced rib spaces; present with fatty liver; have postoperative incisions, bandages, or dressings; have significant scarring in the area of interest). Aberrations in tissue composition may attenuate the sound waves and alter findings.

Other considerations

- The procedure may be canceled if the patient's weight exceeds the safety limit for the equipment.

NURSING IMPLICATIONS AND PROCEDURE

See Potential Nursing Problems on Fast Find at davispl.us/vanleeuwen7.

PRETEST:

- Positively identify the patient using at least two person-specific identifiers before services, treatments, or procedures are performed.
- ***Patient Teaching:*** Inform the patient this procedure can assist in assessing the carotid arteries in the neck.
- Obtain a history of the patient's health concerns, symptoms, surgical procedures, and results of previously performed laboratory and diagnostic studies. Include a list of known allergens, especially allergies or sensitivities to latex. The presence of other risk factors, such as family history of heart disease, smoking, obesity, diet, lack of physical activity, hypertension, diabetes, previous myocardial infarction (MI), and previous vascular disease, should be investigated. Knowledge of genetics assists the nurse in identifying patients and family members who may benefit from additional education, risk assessment, and counseling. Genetics is the study and identification of genes, genetic mutations, and inheritance. For example, genetics provides some insight into the likelihood of inheriting a trait such as blue eyes or a medical condition such as coronary artery disease (CAD). Genomic studies evaluate the interaction of groups of genes. The combined activity or combined expression of groups of genes allows assumptions or predictions to be made. As an example, genomic studies measure the levels of activity in multiple genes to predict how they, along with environmental and lifestyle decisions, influence the development of type 2 diabetes, CAD, MI, or ischemic stroke. Further information regarding inheritance of genes can be found in the study titled "Genetic Testing."
- Obtain a list of the patient's current medications, including over-the-counter medications and dietary supplements (see Effects of Natural Products on Laboratory Values online at Davis*Plus*).
- Review the procedure with the patient. Address concerns about pain related to the procedure and explain that some pain may be experienced during the test, and

U

there may be moments of discomfort. Inform the patient that the procedure is performed in a US department by a health-care provider (HCP) who specializes in this procedure, with support staff, and takes approximately 30 to 60 min.

- ***Sensitivity to social and cultural issues,*** as well as concern for modesty, is important in providing psychological support before, during, and after the procedure.
- Instruct the patient to remove jewelry and other metallic objects from the area to be examined.
- Note that there are no food, fluid, or medication restrictions unless by medical direction. Some protocols may require the patient to restrict nicotine and caffeine for 1 to 2 hr before the procedure in order to avoid vasoconstriction or vasodilation.

INTRATEST:

Potential Complications: N/A

- Observe standard precautions, and follow the general guidelines in Patient Preparation and Specimen Collection online at Davis*Plus*. Positively identify the patient.
- Ensure that the patient has removed all external metallic objects from the area to be examined prior to the procedure.
- Instruct the patient to void and change into the gown, robe, and foot coverings provided.
- Avoid the use of equipment containing latex if the patient has a history of allergic reaction to latex.
- Instruct the patient to cooperate fully and to follow directions. Ask the patient to remain still throughout the procedure because movement produces unreliable results.
- Place the patient in the supine position on an examination table; other positions may be used during the examination.
- Expose the neck and drape the patient.
- Conductive gel is applied to the skin, and a Doppler transducer is moved over the skin to obtain images of the area of interest.
- Ask the patient to breathe normally during the examination. If necessary for better organ visualization, ask the patient to inhale deeply and hold his or her breath.

POST-TEST:

- Inform the patient that a report of the results will be made available to the requesting HCP, who will discuss the results with the patient.
- When the study is completed, remove the gel from the skin.
- Instruct the patient to continue with diet, fluids, and medications, as directed by the HCP.
- ***Nutritional Considerations:*** Abnormal findings may be associated with cardiovascular disease. Nutritional therapy is recommended for the patient identified to be at risk for developing CAD or for individuals who have specific risk factors and/or existing medical conditions (e.g., elevated low-density lipoprotein cholesterol levels, other lipid disorders, type 1 diabetes, type 2 diabetes, insulin resistance, or metabolic syndrome). Other changeable risk factors warranting patient education include strategies to encourage patients, especially those who are overweight and with high blood pressure, to safely decrease sodium intake, achieve a normal weight, ensure regular participation in moderate aerobic physical activity three to four times per week, eliminate tobacco use, and adhere to a heart-healthy diet. If triglycerides also are elevated, the patient should be advised to eliminate or reduce alcohol. A variety of dietary patterns are beneficial for people with CAD, and there are many meal-planning approaches with nutritional goals endorsed by the American Diabetes Association (ADA). The Guideline on Lifestyle Management to Reduce Cardiovascular Risk published by the American College of Cardiology and the American Heart Association (AHA) in conjunction with the

National Heart, Lung, and Blood Institute (NHLBI) recommends a Mediterranean-style diet rather than a low-fat diet. The guideline emphasizes inclusion of vegetables, whole grains, fruits, low-fat dairy, nuts, legumes, and nontropical vegetable oils (e.g., olive, canola, peanut, sunflower, flaxseed) along with fish and lean poultry. 🍁 A similar dietary pattern known as the Dietary Approaches to Stop Hypertension (DASH) diet makes additional recommendations for the reduction of dietary sodium. Both dietary styles emphasize a reduction in consumption of red meats, which are high in saturated fats and cholesterol, and other foods containing sugar, saturated fats, trans fats, and sodium. The ADA also includes a vegetarian diet as well as other potential weight loss diets such as Weight Watchers. 🍁 The nutritional needs of each patient need to be determined individually (especially during pregnancy) with the appropriate HCPs, particularly professionals educated in nutrition.

- *Sensitivity to social and cultural issues:* Numerous studies point to the prevalence of excess body weight in American children and adolescents. Experts estimate that obesity is present in 25% of the population aged 6 to 11 yr. The medical, social, and emotional consequences of excess body weight are significant. Special attention should be given to instructing the pediatric patient and caregiver regarding health risks and weight control education. 🍁
- Recognize anxiety related to test results, and be supportive of fear of shortened life expectancy and perceived loss of independent function. Discuss the implications of abnormal test results on the patient's lifestyle. Provide teaching and information regarding the clinical implications of the test results, as appropriate. Educate the patient regarding access to counseling services. Provide contact information, if desired, for the AHA (www.americanheart.org), NHLBI (www.nhlbi.nih.gov), Institute of Medicine of the National Academies (www.iom.edu), and USDA's resource for nutrition (http://www.choosemyplate.gov). 🍁
- Reinforce information given by the patient's HCP regarding further testing, treatment, or referral to another HCP. Answer any questions or address any concerns voiced by the patient or family.
- Instruct the patient in the use of any ordered medications. Explain the importance of adhering to the therapy regimen. As appropriate, instruct the patient in significant adverse effects associated with the prescribed medication. Encourage him or her to review corresponding literature provided by a pharmacist.
- Depending on the results of this procedure, additional testing may be performed to evaluate or monitor progression of the disease process and determine the need for a change in therapy. Evaluate test results in relation to the patient's symptoms and other tests performed.

Patient Education:

- Teach the patient, parent, or significant other reportable symptoms related to bleeding due to medication use.
- Teach the patient, parent, or significant other bleeding precautions that should be used with specific medications.

Expected Patient Outcomes:

Understanding

- The patient and family state the importance of refraining from risky activity that would result in trauma and bleeding.
- The patient and family state the importance of frequent positioning to decrease risk of pressure ulcer development.

Ability

- The patient successfully demonstrates range-of-motion technique.
- The patient successfully demonstrates the use of assistive devices.

Response

- The patient and family agree to follow-up laboratory studies to manage medications to prevent stroke.
- The patient agrees to call for assistance when getting out of bed to decrease fall risk.

RELATED STUDIES:

- Related tests include angiography carotid, angiography coronary, antidysrhythmic drugs, apolipoproteins A, B, and C, blood gases, calcium, cholesterol (total, HDL, LDL), CT angiography, CT cardiac scoring, echocardiography, CRP, CK and isoenzymes, genetic testing, glucose, glycated hemoglobin, Holter monitor, homocysteine, ketones, LDH and isoenzymes, lipoprotein electrophoresis, magnesium, MRI angiography, MRI chest, MRI venography, myocardial infarction scan, myocardial perfusion heart scan, myoglobin, PET heart, triglycerides, troponin, US arterial Doppler upper and lower extremities, and US venous Doppler extremity.
- Refer to the Cardiovascular System table online at Davis*Plus* for related tests by body system.

Ultrasound, Arterial Doppler, Lower and Upper Extremity Studies

SYNONYM/ACRONYM: Doppler, arterial ultrasound, duplex scan.

COMMON USE: To visualize and assess blood flow through the arteries of the upper and lower extremities toward diagnosing disorders such as occlusion and aneurysm and evaluate for the presence of plaque and stenosis. This procedure can also be used to assess the effectiveness of therapeutic interventions such as arterial graphs and blood flow to transplanted organs.

AREA OF APPLICATION: Arteries of the lower and upper extremities.

DESCRIPTION: Ultrasound (US) procedures are diagnostic, noninvasive, and relatively inexpensive. They take a short time to complete, do not use radiation, and cause no harm to the patient. High-frequency sound waves of various intensities are delivered by a transducer, a flashlight-shaped device, pressed against the skin. The waves are bounced back off internal anatomical structures and fluids, converted to electrical energy, amplified by the transducer, and displayed as images on a monitor. Color Doppler US can be used with the duplex method whereby red and blue are assigned to represent the direction of blood flow, and the intensity of the color is an indication of velocity. Using the duplex scanning method, arterial leg US records sound waves to obtain information about the arteries of the lower extremities from the common femoral arteries and their branches as they extend into the calf area. The amplitude and waveform of the pulses are measured, resulting in a two-dimensional image of the artery. Blood flow direction, velocity, and the presence of flow disturbances can be readily assessed, and for diagnostic studies, the technique is done bilaterally. The sound waves hit the moving red blood cells and are reflected back to the transducer corresponding to the velocity of the blood flow through the vessel. The result is the visualization of the artery to assist in the diagnosis (i.e., presence, amount, and location) of plaque causing vessel stenosis or occlusion and to help determine the cause of claudication. Arterial reconstruction and graft condition and patency can also be evaluated.

In arterial Doppler studies, arteriosclerotic disease of the peripheral vessels can be detected by slowly deflating blood pressure cuffs that are placed on an extremity such as the calf, ankle, or upper extremity. The systolic pressure of the various arteries of the extremities can be measured. The Doppler transducer can detect the first sign of blood flow through the cuffed artery, even the most minimal blood flow, as evidenced by a swishing noise. There is normally a reduction in systolic blood pressure from the arteries of the arms to the arteries of the legs; a reduction exceeding 20 mm Hg is indicative of occlusive disease (deep vein thrombosis) proximal to the area being tested. This procedure may also be used to monitor the patency of a graft, status of previous corrective surgery, vascular status of the blood flow to a transplanted organ, blood flow to a mass, or the extent of vascular trauma.

The ankle-brachial index (ABI) can also be assessed during this study. This noninvasive, simple comparison of blood pressure measurements in the arms and legs can be used to detect peripheral arterial disease (PAD). A Doppler stethoscope is used to obtain the systolic pressure in either the dorsalis pedis or the posterior tibial artery. This ankle pressure is then divided by the highest brachial systolic pressure acquired after taking the blood pressure in both of the patient's arms. This index should be greater than 1 with a range of 0.85 to 1.4. When the index falls below 0.5, blood flow impairment is considered significant. Patients should be scheduled for a vascular consult for an abnormal ABI. Patients with diabetes or kidney disease, and some older adult patients, may have a falsely elevated ABI due to calcifications of the vessels in the ankle causing an increased systolic pressure. The ABI test approaches 95% accuracy in detecting PAD. However, a normal ABI value does not absolutely rule out the possibility of PAD for some individuals, and additional tests should be done to evaluate symptoms.

This procedure is contraindicated for: N/A

INDICATIONS

- Aid in the diagnosis of small or large vessel PAD.
- Aid in the diagnosis of spastic arterial disease, such as Raynaud's phenomenon.
- Assist in the diagnosis of aneurysm, pseudoaneurysm, hematoma, arteriovenous malformation, or hemangioma.
- Assist in the diagnosis of ischemia, arterial calcification, or plaques, as evidenced by visualization of blood flow disruption.
- Detect irregularities in the structure of the arteries.
- Detect plaque or stenosis of the lower extremity artery, as evidenced by turbulent blood flow or changes in Doppler signals indicating occlusion.

U

- Determine the patency of a vascular graft, stent, or previous surgery.
- Evaluate possible arterial trauma.

POTENTIAL MEDICAL DIAGNOSIS

Normal findings

- Normal blood flow through the lower extremity arteries with no evidence of vessel occlusion or narrowing
- Normal arterial systolic and diastolic Doppler signals
- Normal reduction in systolic blood pressure (i.e., less than 20 mm Hg) when compared to a normal extremity
- Normal ABI (greater than 0.85)

Abnormal findings related to

- ABI less than 0.85, indicating significant arterial occlusive disease within the extremity
- Aneurysm
- Arterial calcification or plaques
- Embolic arterial occlusion
- Graft diameter reduction
- Hemangioma
- Hematoma
- Ischemia
- PAD
- Pseudoaneurysm
- Reduction in vessel diameter of more than 16%, indicating stenosis
- Spastic arterial occlusive disease, such as Raynaud's phenomenon

CRITICAL FINDINGS: N/A

INTERFERING FACTORS

Factors that may impair the results of the examination

- Attenuation of the sound waves by bony structures, which can impair clear imaging of the vessels.
- Incorrect placement of the transducer over the desired test site; quality of the US study is very dependent upon the skill of the ultrasonographer.
- Metallic objects (e.g., jewelry, body rings) within the examination field, which may inhibit organ visualization and cause unclear images.
- Inability of the patient to cooperate or remain still during the procedure because of age, significant pain, or mental status.
- Patients who are technically difficult and who present challenges in obtaining reliable results (e.g., who are obese; have reduced rib spaces; present with fatty liver; have postoperative incisions, bandages, or dressings; have significant scarring in the area of interest). Aberrations in tissue composition may attenuate the sound waves and alter findings.

Other considerations

- Cold extremities, resulting in vasoconstriction, which can cause inaccurate measurements.
- Occlusion proximal to the site being studied, which would affect blood flow to the area.
- Cigarette smoking, because nicotine can cause constriction of the peripheral vessels.
- An abnormally large leg, making direct examination difficult.
- The procedure may be canceled if the patient's weight exceeds the safety limit for the equipment.

NURSING IMPLICATIONS AND PROCEDURE

See Potential Nursing Problems on Fast Find at davispl.us/vanleeuwen7.

PRETEST:

- Positively identify the patient using at least two person-specific identifiers before services, treatments, or procedures are performed.
- ***Patient Teaching:*** Inform the patient this procedure can assist in assessing blood flow to the upper and lower extremities.

U

- Obtain a history of the patient's health concerns, symptoms, surgical procedures, and results of previously performed laboratory and diagnostic studies. Include a list of known allergens, especially allergies or sensitivities to latex.
- Report the presence of a lesion that is open or draining; maintain clean, dry dressing for the ulcer; protect the limb from trauma.
- Note any recent procedures that can interfere with test results (e.g., surgery, biopsy).
- Obtain a list of the patient's current medications, including over-the-counter medications and dietary supplements (see Effects of Natural Products on Laboratory Values online at Davis*Plus*).
- Review the procedure with the patient. Address concerns about pain related to the procedure and explain that some pain may be experienced during the test, and there may be moments of discomfort. Inform the patient that the procedure is performed in a US department by a health-care provider (HCP) specializing in this procedure, with support staff, and takes approximately 30 to 60 min.
- ***Sensitivity to social and cultural issues,*** as well as concern for modesty, is important in providing psychological support before, during, and after the procedure.
- Instruct the patient to remove jewelry and other metallic objects from the area to be examined.
- Note that there are no food, fluid, or medication restrictions unless by medical direction. Some protocols may require the patient to restrict nicotine and caffeine for 1 to 2 hr before the procedure in order to avoid vasoconstriction or vasodilation.

INTRATEST:

Potential Complications: N/A

- Observe standard precautions, and follow the general guidelines in Patient Preparation and Specimen Collection online at Davis*Plus*. Positively identify the patient.
- Ensure that the patient has removed all external metallic objects from the area to be examined prior to the procedure.
- Instruct the patient to void and change into the gown, robe, and foot coverings provided.
- Avoid the use of equipment containing latex if the patient has a history of allergic reaction to latex.
- Instruct the patient to cooperate fully and to follow directions. Ask the patient to remain still throughout the procedure because movement produces unreliable results.
- Place the patient in the supine position on an examination table; other positions may be used during the examination.
- Expose the area of interest and drape the patient.
- Place blood pressure cuffs on the thigh, calf, and ankle.
- Apply conductive gel to the skin over the area distal to each of the cuffs to promote the passage of sound waves as a Doppler transducer is moved over the skin to obtain images of the area of interest.
- Inflate the thigh cuff to a level above the patient's systolic pressure found in the normal extremity.
- Place the Doppler transducer in the gel, distal to the inflated cuff, and slowly release the pressure in the cuff.
- When the swishing sound of blood flow is heard, record it at the highest point along the artery at which it is audible. The test is repeated at the calf and then the ankle.

POST-TEST:

- Inform the patient that a report of the results will be made available to the requesting HCP, who will discuss the results with the patient.
- When the study is completed, remove the gel from the skin.
- Instruct the patient to continue diet, fluids, and medications, as directed by the HCP.
- ***Nutritional Considerations:*** Patients on low-sodium diets should be advised to avoid beverages such as colas,

U

ginger ale, sports drinks, lemon-lime sodas, and root beer. Many over-the-counter medications, including antacids, laxatives, analgesics, sedatives, and antitussives, contain significant amounts of sodium. The best advice is to emphasize the importance of reading all food, beverage, and medicine labels.
- Recognize anxiety related to test results, and be supportive of perceived loss of independent function. Discuss the implications of abnormal test results on the patient's lifestyle. Provide teaching and information regarding the clinical implications of the test results, as appropriate.
- Reinforce information given by the patient's HCP regarding further testing, treatment, or referral to another HCP. Answer any questions or address any concerns voiced by the patient or family.
- Depending on the results of this procedure, additional testing may be performed to evaluate or monitor progression of the disease process and determine the need for a change in therapy. Evaluate test results in relation to the patient's symptoms and other tests performed.

Patient Education:
- Teach the patient how to decrease fall risk by adhering to fall risk protocols.
- Encourage the patient to work with the health-care team to discuss treatment options and expected outcomes.

Expected Patient Outcomes:

Understanding
- The patient and family state the importance of follow-up diagnostic and laboratory studies associated with disease management.
- The patient and family state the importance of refraining from risky activity that would result in trauma and bleeding.

Ability
- The patient and family demonstrate positive coping strategies.
- The patient successfully demonstrates the use of assistive devices.

Response
- The patient agrees to HCP recommended follow-up evaluations.
- The patient agrees to make required lifestyle changes to support positive health.

RELATED STUDIES:
- Related tests include alveolar/arterial ratio, ANA, angiography pulmonary, aPTT, blood gases, CBC platelet count, CT angiography, D-Dimer, FDP, fibrinogen, lung perfusion scan, lung ventilation scan, MRI abdomen, MRI angiography, plethysmography, PT/INR, US venous Doppler lower extremities, and venography lower extremity.
- Refer to the Cardiovascular System table online at Davis*Plus* for related tests by body system.

Ultrasound, A-scan

SYNONYM/ACRONYM: Amplitude modulation scan, A-scan ultrasound biometry.

COMMON USE: To assess for ocular tissue abnormality and to determine the power of the intraocular lens required for replacement in cataract surgery.

AREA OF APPLICATION: Eyes.

U

DESCRIPTION: Diagnostic techniques such as A-scan ultrasonography can be used to identify abnormal tissue. The A-scan employs a single-beam, linear sound wave to detect abnormalities by returning an echo when interference disrupts its straight path. When the sound wave is directed at lens vitreous, the normal homogeneous tissue does not return an echo; an opaque lens with a cataract will produce an echo. The returning waves produced by abnormal tissue are received by a microfilm that converts the sound energy into electrical impulses that are amplified and displayed on an oscilloscope as an ultrasonogram or echogram. The A-scan echo can be used to indicate the position of the cornea and retina. The A-scan is most commonly used to measure the axial length of the eye. This measurement is used to determine the power requirement for an intraocular lens used to replace the abnormal, opaque lens of the eye removed in cataract surgery. There are two different methods currently in use. The applanation method involves placement of an ultrasound (US) probe directly on the cornea. The immersion technique is more popular because it does not require direct contact and compression of the cornea. The immersion technique protects the cornea by placement of a fluid layer between the eye and the US probe. The accuracy of the immersion technique is thought to be greater than applanation because no corneal compression is caused by the immersion method. Therefore, the measured axial length achieved by immersion is closer to the true axial length of the cornea.

This procedure is contraindicated for: N/A

INDICATIONS

- Determination of power requirement for replacement intraocular lens in cataract surgery.

POTENTIAL MEDICAL DIAGNOSIS

Normal findings

- Normal homogeneous ocular tissue

Abnormal findings related to

- Cataract

CRITICAL FINDINGS: N/A

INTERFERING FACTORS

Factors that may impair the results of the examination

- Inability of the patient to cooperate and remain still during the procedure may interfere with the test results.
- Rubbing or squeezing the eyes may affect results.
- Improper placement of the probe tip to the surface of the eye may produce inaccurate results.

NURSING IMPLICATIONS AND PROCEDURE

PRETEST:

- Positively identify the patient using at least two person-specific identifiers before services, treatments, or procedures are performed.
- *Patient Teaching:* Inform the patient this procedure determines the strength of the lens that will be replaced during cataract surgery.
- Obtain a history of the patient's health concerns (especially known or suspected vision loss; changes in visual acuity, including type and cause; use of glasses or contact lenses; eye conditions with treatment regimens; eye surgery; and other tests and procedures to assess and diagnose visual deficit), symptoms, surgical procedures, and results of previously performed laboratory and diagnostic studies. Include a list of known allergens, especially allergies or sensitivities to latex and topical anesthetic eyedrops.
- Obtain a list of the patient's current medications, including over-the-counter medications and dietary

U

supplements (see Effects of Natural Products on Laboratory Values online at Davis*Plus*).

- Instruct the patient to remove contact lenses or glasses, as appropriate. Instruct the patient regarding the importance of keeping the eyes open for the test.
- Review the procedure with the patient. Explain that the patient will be requested to fixate the eyes during the procedure. Address concerns about pain and explain that no discomfort will be experienced during the test but that some discomfort may be experienced after the test when the numbness wears off from the anesthetic drops administered prior to the test. Inform the patient that a health-care provider (HCP) performs the test in a quiet, darkened room and that evaluation of the eye upon which surgery is to be performed can take up 10 min.
- ***Sensitivity to social and cultural issues,*** as well as concern for modesty, is important in providing psychological support before, during, and after the procedure.
- Note that there are no food, fluid, or medication restrictions unless by medical direction.

INTRATEST:

Potential Complications: N/A

- Observe standard precautions, and follow the general guidelines in Patient Preparation and Specimen Collection online at Davis*Plus*. Positively identify the patient.
- Instruct the patient to cooperate fully and to follow directions. Ask the patient to remain still during the procedure because movement produces unreliable results.
- Seat the patient comfortably. Instruct the patient to look straight ahead, keeping the eyes open and unblinking.
- Avoid the use of equipment containing latex if the patient has a history of allergic reaction to latex.
- Instill topical anesthetic in each eye, as ordered, and provide time for it to work. Topical anesthetic drops are placed in the eye with the patient looking up and the solution directed at the six o'clock position of the sclera (white of the eye) near the limbus (gray, semitransparent area of the eyeball where the cornea and sclera meet). Neither the dropper nor the bottle should touch the eyelashes.
- Ask the patient to place the chin in the chin rest and gently press the forehead against the support bar. When the US probe is properly positioned on the patient's surgical eye, a reading is automatically taken.
- Multiple measurements may be taken in order to ensure that a consistent and accurate reading has been achieved. Variability between serial measurements is unavoidable using the applanation technique.

POST-TEST:

- Inform the patient that a report of the results will be made available to the requesting HCP, who will discuss the results with the patient.
- Recognize anxiety related to test results, and be supportive of impaired activity related to vision loss, anticipated loss of driving privileges, or the possibility of requiring corrective lenses (self-image). Discuss the implications of test results on the patient's lifestyle. Reassure the patient regarding concerns related to the impending cataract surgery. Provide teaching and information regarding the clinical implications of the test results, as appropriate.
- Reinforce information given by the patient's HCP regarding further testing, treatment, or referral to another HCP. Answer any questions or address any concerns voiced by the patient or family.
- Depending on the results of this procedure, additional testing may be performed to evaluate or monitor progression of the disease process and determine the need for a change in therapy. Evaluate test results in relation to the patient's symptoms and other tests performed.

U

RELATED STUDIES:
- Related tests include refraction and slit-lamp biomicroscopy.
- Refer to the Ocular System table online at Davis*Plus* for related tests by body system.

Ultrasound, Biophysical Profile, Obstetric

SYNONYM/ACRONYM: BPP ultrasound, fetal age sonogram, gestational age sonogram, OB sonography, pregnancy ultrasound, pregnancy echo, pregnant uterus ultrasonography.

COMMON USE: To visualize and assess the fetus in utero to monitor fetal health related to growth, congenital abnormalities, distress, and demise. Also used to identify gender and multiple pregnancy and to obtain amniotic fluid for analysis.

AREA OF APPLICATION: Pelvis and abdominal region.

DESCRIPTION: Ultrasound (US) procedures are diagnostic, noninvasive, and relatively inexpensive. They take a short time to complete, do not use radiation, and cause no harm to the patient. High-frequency sound waves of various intensities are delivered by a transducer, a flashlight-shaped device, pressed against the skin. The waves are bounced back off internal anatomical structures and fluids, converted to electrical energy, amplified by the transducer, and displayed as images on a monitor to visualize the fetus and placenta. US is often used as a diagnostic and therapeutic tool for guiding minimally invasive procedures such as needle biopsies and fluid aspiration (amniocentesis). The contraindications and complications for biopsy and fluid aspiration are discussed in detail in the individual studies. This procedure is done by a transabdominal or transvaginal approach, depending on when the procedure is performed (first trimester [transabdominal or transvaginal or combination] vs. second or third trimester [transabdominal]). It is the safest method of examination to evaluate the uterus and determine fetal size, growth, and position; fetal structural abnormalities; ectopic pregnancy; placenta position and amount of amniotic fluid; and multiple gestation.

Obstetric US is used to secure different types of information regarding the fetus and placenta, varying with the trimester during which the procedure is done. This procedure may also include a nonstress test (NST) in combination with Doppler monitoring of amniotic fluid volume, fetal heart, gross fetal movements, fetal muscle tone, and fetal respiratory movements to detect high-risk pregnancy. The procedure is indicated as a guide for amniocentesis, cordocentesis, fetoscopy, aspiration of multiple oocytes for in vitro fertilization, and other intrauterine interventional procedures.

The biophysical profile (BPP) considers five antepartum parameters measured to predict

U

fetal wellness. The BPP is indicated in women with high-risk pregnancies to identify a fetus in distress or in jeopardy of demise. It includes fetal heart rate (FHR) measurement, fetal breathing movements, fetal body movements, fetal muscle tone, and amniotic fluid volume. Each of the five parameters is assigned a score of either 0 or 2, allowing a maximum or perfect score of 10. The NST is an external US monitoring of FHR performed either as part of the BPP or when one or more of the US procedures have abnormal results. The NST is interpreted as either reactive or nonreactive.

BPP Parameter	Normal: Score = 2	Abnormal: Score = 0
Fetal heart rate reactivity	Two or more movement-associated FHR accelerations of 15 or more beats/min above baseline, lasting 15 sec, in a 20-min interval	One or no movement-associated FHR accelerations of 15 or more beats/min above baseline in a 20-min interval
Fetal breathing movements	One or more breathing movements lasting 20–60 sec in a 30-min interval	Absent or no breathing movements lasting longer than 19 sec in a 30-min interval
Fetal body movements	Two or more discrete body or limb movements in a 30-min interval	Less than two discrete body or limb movements in a 30-min interval
Fetal muscle tone	One or more episodes of active limb extension and return to flexion (to include opening and closing of hand)	Absent movement, slow extension with partial return to flexion, partial opening of hand
Amniotic fluid volume	One or more pockets of fluid that are 2 cm or more in the vertical axis	No pockets of fluid or no pocket measuring at least 2 cm in the vertical axis

A contraction stress test (CST, or oxytocin challenge test) may be requested in the event of an abnormal fetal heart rate in the BPP or NST. The CST is used to assess the fetus's ability to tolerate low oxygen levels as experienced during labor contractions. The CST includes external FHR monitoring by US and measurement of oxytocin (Pitocin)-induced uterine contractions. Pressure changes during contractions are monitored on an external tocodynamometer. Results of the two tests are interpreted as negative or positive. A negative or normal finding is no late decelerations of FHR during three induced contractions over a 10-min period. A positive or abnormal finding is identified when frequent contractions of 90 sec or more occur and FHR decelerates beyond the time of the contractions. The amniotic fluid index is another application of US used to estimate amniotic fluid volume. The abdomen is

U

divided into four quadrants using the umbilicus to delineate upper and lower halves and linea nigra to delineate the left and right halves. The numbered score is determined by adding the sum in centimeters of fluid in pockets seen in each of the four quadrants. The score is interpreted in relation to gestational age. The median index is considered normal between 8 and 12 cm. Oligohydramnios (too little amniotic fluid) is associated with an index between 5 and 6 cm, and polyhydramnios (too much amniotic fluid) with an index between 18 and 22 cm.

This procedure is contraindicated for: N/A

INDICATIONS

- Detect blighted ovum (missed abortion), as evidenced by empty gestational sac.
- Detect fetal death, as evidenced by absence of movement and fetal heart tones.
- Detect fetal position before birth, such as breech or transverse presentations.
- Detect tubal and other forms of ectopic pregnancy.
- Determine and confirm pregnancy or multiple gestation by determining the number of gestational sacs in the first trimester.
- Determine cause of bleeding, such as placenta previa or abruptio placentae.
- Determine fetal effects of Rh incompatibility due to maternal sensitization.
- Determine fetal gestational age by uterine size and measurements of crown-rump length, biparietal diameter, fetal extremities, head, and other parts of the anatomy at key phases of fetal development.
- Determine fetal heart and body movements and detect high-risk pregnancy by monitoring fetal heart and respiratory movements in combination with Doppler US or real-time grayscale scanning.
- Determine fetal structural anomalies, usually at the 20th week of gestation or later.
- Determine the placental size, location, and site of implantation.
- Differentiate a tumor (hydatidiform mole) from a normal pregnancy.
- Guide the needle during amniocentesis and fetal transfusion.
- Measure fetal gestational age and evaluate umbilical artery, uterine artery, and fetal aorta by Doppler examination to determine fetal intrauterine growth retardation.
- Monitor placental growth and amniotic fluid volume.

POTENTIAL MEDICAL DIAGNOSIS

Normal findings

- Normal age, size, viability, position, and functional capacities of the fetus.
- Normal placenta size, position, and structure; adequate volume of amniotic fluid.
- BPP score of 8 to 10 is considered normal. Each of the fetal movements evaluated in the BPP is related to oxygen-dependent activities that originate from the central nervous system. Their presence is assumed to indicate normal brain function and absence of systemic hypoxia.

Abnormal findings related to

- Abruptio placentae
- Cardiac abnormalities
- Ectopic pregnancy
- Fetal death
- Fetal deformities (organs or skeleton)

U

- Fetal hydrops (nonimmune)
- Fetal intestinal atresia
- Fetal malpresentation (breech, transverse)
- Hydrocephalus
- Myelomeningocele
- Multiple pregnancy
- Placenta previa
- Renal or skeletal defects
- BPP score between 4 and 6 is considered equivocal. Gestational age is important in determining intervals for retesting and/or a decision to deliver.

CRITICAL FINDINGS:

- Abruptio placentae
- BPP score between 0 and 2 is abnormal and indicates the need for assessment and decisions regarding early or immediate delivery.
- Ectopic pregnancy
- Fetal death
- Placenta previa

Note and immediately report to the requesting health-care provider (HCP) any critical findings and related symptoms. A listing of these findings varies among facilities.

INTERFERING FACTORS

- Patients with latex allergy; use of the vaginal probe requires the probe to be covered with a condom-like sac, usually made from latex. Latex-free covers are available.

Factors that may alter the results of the study

- Attenuation of the sound waves by bony structures, which can impair clear imaging in the area of interest.
- Incorrect placement of the transducer over the desired test site; quality of the US study is very dependent upon the skill of the ultrasonographer.
- Metallic objects (e.g., jewelry, body rings) within the examination field, which may inhibit organ visualization and cause unclear images.
- Inability of the patient to cooperate or remain still during the procedure because of age, significant pain, or mental status.
- Retained air, barium, or gas from a previous radiological procedure may block the transmission of sound waves.
- Dehydration, which can cause failure to demonstrate the boundaries between organs and tissue structures.
- Insufficiently full bladder, which fails to push the bowel from the pelvis and the uterus from the symphysis pubis, thereby prohibiting clear imaging of the pelvic organs in transabdominal imaging.
- Patients who are technically difficult and who present challenges in obtaining reliable results (e.g., who are obese; have reduced rib spaces; present with fatty liver; have postoperative incisions, bandages, or dressings; have significant scarring in the area of interest). Aberrations in tissue composition may attenuate the sound waves and alter findings.

Other considerations

- The procedure may be canceled if the patient's weight exceeds the safety limit for the equipment.
- Absence of activity in a particular parameter of the BPP may be related to fetal sleep pattern; gestational age less than 33 wk or greater than 42 wk; maternal ingestion of glucose, nicotine, or alcohol; maternal administration of magnesium or medications; artificial or premature rupture of membranes; and/or labor.

NURSING IMPLICATIONS AND PROCEDURE

PRETEST:

- Positively identify the patient using at least two person-specific identifiers before services, treatments, or procedures are performed.
- ***Patient Teaching:*** Inform the patient this procedure can assess abdomen and pelvic organ function.
- Obtain a history of the patient's health concerns, symptoms, surgical procedures, and results of previously performed laboratory and diagnostic studies. Include a list of known allergens, especially allergies or sensitivities to latex.
- Note any recent procedures that can interfere with test results (i.e., surgery, biopsy, barium studies, colonoscopy, endoscopic retrograde cholangiopancreatography). There should be 24 hr between administration of barium and this test.
- Record the date of the last menstrual period. Obtain a history of menstrual dates, previous pregnancy, and treatment received for high-risk pregnancy.
- Obtain a list of the patient's current medications, including over-the-counter medications and dietary supplements (see Effects of Natural Products on Laboratory Values online at Davis*Plus*).
- Review the procedure with the patient. Address concerns about pain related to the procedure and explain that some pain may be experienced during the test, and there may be moments of discomfort. Inform the patient the procedure is performed in a US department, usually by an HCP specializing in this procedure, and takes approximately 30 to 60 min.
- For the transvaginal approach, inform the patient that a sterile latex- or sheath-covered probe will be inserted into the vagina.
- ***Sensitivity to social and cultural issues,*** as well as concern for modesty, is important in providing psychological support before, during, and after the procedure.
- Instruct the patient receiving transabdominal US to drink three to four glasses of fluid 90 min before the procedure, and not to void, because the procedure requires a full bladder. Patients receiving transvaginal US only do not need to have a full bladder.
- Instruct the patient to remove jewelry and other metallic objects from the area to be examined prior to the procedure.
- Note that there are no food or medication restrictions unless by medical direction. The test may be scheduled in relation to mealtime because fetal activity is highest 1 to 3 hr after the mother ingests a meal.

INTRATEST:

Potential Complications: N/A

- Observe standard precautions, and follow the general guidelines in Patient Preparation and Specimen Collection online at Davis*Plus*. Positively identify the patient.
- Ensure that the patient has removed all external metallic objects from the area to be examined prior to the procedure.
- Ensure that the patient receiving transabdominal US drank three to four glasses of fluid and has not voided.
- Instruct the patient to change into the gown, robe, and foot coverings provided.
- Instruct the patient to cooperate fully and to follow directions. Ask the patient to remain still throughout the procedure because movement produces unreliable results.
- Avoid the use of equipment containing latex if the patient has a history of allergic reaction to latex.
- Place the patient in the supine position on an examination table. The right- or left-side-up position may be used to allow gravity to reposition the liver, gas, and fluid to facilitate better organ visualization.
- Expose the abdominal area and drape the patient.

U

- ***Transabdominal approach:*** Conductive gel is applied to the skin, and a transducer is moved over the skin while the bladder is distended to obtain images of the area of interest.
- ***Transvaginal approach:*** A lubricated, covered probe is inserted into the vagina and moved to different levels to obtain images.
- Ask the patient to breathe normally during the examination. If necessary for better organ visualization, ask the patient to inhale deeply and hold her breath.

POST-TEST:

- Inform the patient that a report of the results will be made available to the requesting HCP, who will discuss the results with the patient.
- Allow the patient to void, as needed.
- When the study is completed, remove the gel from the skin.
- Recognize anxiety related to test results. Discuss the implications of abnormal test results on the patient's lifestyle. Provide teaching and information regarding the clinical implications of the test results, as appropriate. Encourage the family to seek appropriate counseling if concerned with pregnancy termination and to seek genetic counseling if a chromosomal abnormality is determined. Decisions regarding elective abortion should take place in the presence of both parents. Provide a nonjudgmental, nonthreatening atmosphere for discussing the risks and difficulties of delivering and raising a developmentally challenged infant and for exploring other options (termination of pregnancy or adoption). It is also important to discuss problems the mother and father may experience (guilt, depression, anger) if fetal abnormalities are detected.
- Reinforce information given by the patient's HCP regarding further testing, treatment, or referral to another HCP. Answer any questions or address any concerns voiced by the patient or family.
- Depending on the results of this procedure, additional testing may be performed to evaluate or monitor progression of the disease process and determine the need for a change in therapy. There are numerous tests for fetal genetic testing associated with inherited diseases and congenital abnormalities. The tests can be performed from amniotic fluid by methods that include polymerase chain reaction, microarray, and cell culture with karyotyping comparison. Evaluate test results in relation to the patient's symptoms and other tests performed.

RELATED STUDIES:

- Related tests include amniotic fluid analysis and L/S ratio, biopsy chorionic villus, blood groups and antibodies, chromosome analysis, culture bacterial anal/genital, culture viral, fetal fibronectin, α_1-fetoprotein, genetic testing, hexosaminidase A and B, human chorionic gonadotropin, KUB, Kleihauer-Betke test, MRI abdomen, and prolactin.
- Refer to the Reproductive System table online at Davis*Plus* for related tests by body system.

Ultrasound, Bladder

SYNONYM/ACRONYM: Bladder sonography.

COMMON USE: To visualize and assess the bladder toward diagnosing disorders such as retention, obstruction, distention, cancer, infection, bleeding, and inflammation.

AREA OF APPLICATION: Bladder.

Access Canadian content on Fast Find: Lab and Dx at davispl.us/vanleeuwen7

DESCRIPTION: Ultrasound (US) procedures are diagnostic, noninvasive, and relatively inexpensive. They take a short time to complete, do not use radiation, and cause no harm to the patient. High-frequency sound waves of various intensities are delivered by a transducer, a flashlight-shaped device, pressed against the skin. The waves are bounced back off internal anatomical structures and fluids, converted to electrical energy, amplified by the transducer, and displayed as images on a monitor. US is often used as a diagnostic and therapeutic tool for guiding minimally invasive procedures such as needle biopsies and fluid aspiration. The contraindications and complications for biopsy and fluid aspiration are discussed in detail in the individual related studies.

Different types of transducers and imaging systems are sometimes used in clinical settings. Conventional US systems assume that sound waves pass through tissue at a constant speed. Advances in technology have lead to the development of "smart" transducers that can compensate for tissue aberrations in technically difficult patients. Other advancements in imaging systems include three-dimensional and Doppler US. Color Doppler US uses color to indicate the velocity and direction of blood flow. Power Doppler is a more sensitive Doppler variation, capable of providing detailed images of blood flow; a limitation of power Doppler is that it cannot provide information regarding the direction of blood flow. Spectral Doppler provides data from blood flow measurements in formats other than color—for example, it can convert the measurements into a graph representing distance of blood flow against time or as a unique sound heard with every heartbeat.

Bladder US evaluates the structure and position of the contents of the bladder and identifies disorders of the bladder, such as masses or lesions. The methods for imaging may include the transrectal, transurethral, and transvaginal approaches. The examination is helpful for monitoring a patient's response to therapy for bladder disease. Bladder images can be included in other US studies such as the kidneys, ureters, bladder, urethra, and gonads in diagnosing renal/neurological disorders.

The bladder scan is another noninvasive US study commonly used to assess post-void residual. Advantages of the bladder scan over other studies, such as cystometry, is that the study can be performed at the bedside and does not require the patient to be catheterized, thereby eliminating the possibility of the patient developing a catheter-related UTI. The patient's gynecological history should be obtained prior to using the scanner in order to select the proper setting. The scanners have settings for male, female, and child, but scanning a female patient who has had a hysterectomy and is without a uterus should be performed using the settings for a male patient. This test is not usually performed on pregnant women. Normal findings are less than 30 to 50 mL.

This procedure is contraindicated for: N/A

INDICATIONS

- Assess residual urine after voiding to diagnose urinary tract obstruction causing overdistention.
- Detect tumor of the bladder wall or pelvis, as evidenced by distorted position or changes in bladder contour.
- Determine end-stage malignancy of the bladder caused by extension of a primary tumor of the ovary or other pelvic organ.
- Evaluate the cause of urinary tract infection, urine retention, and flank pain.
- Evaluate hematuria, urinary frequency, dysuria, and suprapubic pain.
- Measure urinary bladder volume by transurethral or transvaginal approach.

POTENTIAL MEDICAL DIAGNOSIS

Normal findings

- Normal size, position, and contour of the bladder

Abnormal findings related to

Identification of abnormal findings is assisted by comparison of parameters such as size, shape, symmetry, and location; for example, areas of altered echo patterns in either an expected or unexpected location may indicate enlargement of an organ or the presence of blood or other fluids, tumors, or cysts. Comparison by type of abnormal findings may also assist in evaluating areas of altered patterns; for example, small round or oval areas with well-defined borders and clear central areas can differentiate a fluid-filled cyst from a solid tumor.

- Bladder diverticulum
- Cyst
- Cystitis
- Malignancy of the bladder
- Tumor
- Ureterocele
- Urinary tract obstruction

CRITICAL FINDINGS: N/A

INTERFERING FACTORS

Factors that may alter the results of the study

- Attenuation of the sound waves by bony structures, which can impair clear imaging of the area of interest.
- Incorrect placement of the transducer over the desired test site; quality of the US study is very dependent upon the skill of the ultrasonographer.
- Metallic objects (e.g., jewelry, body rings) within the examination field, which may inhibit organ visualization and cause unclear images.
- Inability of the patient to cooperate or remain still during the procedure because of age, significant pain, or mental status.
- Retained air, barium, or gas from a previous radiological procedure may block the transmission of sound waves.
- Gas or feces in the gastrointestinal (GI) tract resulting from inadequate cleansing or failure to restrict food intake before the study.
- Patients who are technically difficult and who present challenges in obtaining reliable results (e.g., who are obese; have reduced rib spaces; present with fatty liver; have postoperative incisions, bandages, or dressings; have significant scarring in the area of interest). Aberrations in tissue composition may attenuate the sound waves and alter findings.

Other considerations

- Failure to follow pretesting preparations may cause the procedure to be canceled or repeated.
- The procedure may be canceled if the patient's weight exceeds the safety limit for the equipment.

U

NURSING IMPLICATIONS AND PROCEDURE

See Potential Nursing Problems on Fast Find at davispl.us/vanleeuwen7.

PRETEST:

- Positively identify the patient using at least two person-specific identifiers before services, treatments, or procedures are performed.
- *Patient Teaching:* Inform the patient this procedure can assist in assessing the bladder and pelvic organs.
- Obtain a history of the patient's health concerns, symptoms, surgical procedures, and results of previously performed laboratory and diagnostic studies. Include a list of known allergens, especially allergies or sensitivities to latex.
- Note any recent procedures that can interfere with test results (e.g., surgery, biopsy, barium studies, colonoscopy, endoscopic retrograde cholangiopancreatography). Ensure that interfering studies were performed at least 24 hr before this test or can be rescheduled after this procedure.
- Record the date of the last menstrual period and determine the possibility of pregnancy in perimenopausal women.
- Obtain a list of the patient's current medications, including over-the-counter medications and dietary supplements (see Effects of Natural Products on Laboratory Values online at Davis*Plus*Patient Preparation and Specimen Collection online at Davis*Plus*).
- Review the procedure with the patient. Address concerns about pain related to the procedure. Explain to the patient that some pain may be experienced during the test, and there may be moments of discomfort. Inform the patient that the procedure is performed in a US department by a health-care provider (HCP) with support staff, and takes approximately 30 to 60 min.
- *Sensitivity to social and cultural issues,* as well as concern for modesty, is important in providing psychological support before, during, and after the procedure.
- Instruct the patient to remove jewelry and other metallic objects from the area to be examined prior to the procedure.
- If required, instruct the patient receiving transabdominal US to drink three to four glasses of fluid 90 min before the procedure, and not to void, because the procedure requires a full bladder.
- Note that there are no food, fluid, or medication restrictions unless by medical direction.

INTRATEST:

Potential Complications: N/A

- Observe standard precautions, and follow the general guidelines in Patient Preparation and Specimen Collection online at Davis*Plus*. Positively identify the patient.
- Ensure that the patient has removed all external metallic objects from the area to be examined prior to the procedure.
- Ensure that the patient receiving transabdominal US drank three to four glasses of fluid and has not voided.
- Avoid the use of equipment containing latex if the patient has a history of allergic reaction to latex.
- Instruct the patient to change into the gown, robe, and foot coverings provided.
- Instruct the patient to cooperate fully and to follow directions. Instruct the patient to remain still throughout the procedure because movement produces unreliable results.
- Place the patient in the supine position on an examination table. The right- or left-side-up positions may be used to allow gravity to reposition the liver, gas, and fluid to facilitate better organ visualization.
- Expose the abdominal area and drape the patient.

U

- Conductive gel is applied to the skin, and a transducer is moved over the skin while the bladder is distended to obtain images of the area of interest.
- Ask the patient to breathe normally during the examination. If necessary for better organ visualization, ask the patient to inhale deeply and hold his or her breath.
- Instruct the patient who is to be examined for residual urine volume to empty the bladder; repeat the procedure and calculate the volume.

POST-TEST:

- Inform the patient that a report of the results will be made available to the requesting HCP, who will discuss the results with the patient.
- Allow the patient to void, as needed.
- When the study is completed, remove the gel from the skin.
- Recognize anxiety related to test results. Discuss the implications of abnormal test results on the patient's lifestyle. Provide teaching and information regarding the clinical implications of the test results, as appropriate.
- Reinforce information given by the patient's HCP regarding further testing, treatment, or referral to another HCP. Answer any questions or address any concerns voiced by the patient or family.
- Depending on the results of this procedure, additional testing may be performed to evaluate or monitor progression of the disease process and determine the need for a change in therapy. Evaluate test results in relation to the patient's symptoms and other tests performed.

Patient Education:

- Teach the patient the pathophysiology associated with the disease process.
- Teach the patient the medical and surgical treatment options.

Expected Patient Outcomes:

Understanding

- The patient and family state the importance of completing an entire course of antibiotics to treat infection.
- The patient and family correctly state symptoms that would indicate bladder distention.

Ability

- The patient and family correctly describe treatment options related to disease process.
- The patient demonstrates the correct method of measuring and documenting intake and output.

Response

- The patient agrees to HCP recommended follow-up evaluations
- The patient agrees to avoid alcohol consumption to decrease urinary retention.

RELATED STUDIES:

- Related tests include bladder cancer markers urine, CT pelvis, cystoscopy, IVP, KUB study, and MRI pelvis.
- Refer to the Genitourinary System table online at Davis*Plus* for related tests by body system.

Ultrasound, Breast

SYNONYM/ACRONYM: Mammographic ultrasound.

COMMON USE: Used in place of or in conjunction with mammography to assist in diagnosing disorders such as tumor, cancer, and cysts.

U

AREA OF APPLICATION: Breast.

DESCRIPTION: Ultrasound (US) procedures are diagnostic, noninvasive, and relatively inexpensive. They take a short time to complete, do not use radiation, and cause no harm to the patient. High-frequency sound waves of various intensities are delivered by a transducer, a flashlight-shaped device, pressed against the skin. The waves are bounced back off internal anatomical structures and fluids, converted to electrical energy, amplified by the transducer, and displayed as images on a monitor. US is often used as a diagnostic and therapeutic tool for guiding minimally invasive procedures such as needle biopsies and fluid aspiration. The contraindications and complications for biopsy and fluid aspiration are discussed in detail in the individual studies.

Different types of transducers and imaging systems are sometimes used in clinical settings. Conventional US systems assume that sound waves pass through tissue at a constant speed. Advances in technology have led to the development of "smart" transducers that can compensate for tissue aberrations in patients who are technically difficult. Other advancements in imaging systems include three-dimensional and Doppler US. Color Doppler US uses color to indicate the velocity and direction of blood flow. Power Doppler is a more sensitive Doppler variation, capable of providing detailed images of blood flow; a limitation of power Doppler is that it cannot provide information regarding the direction of blood flow. Spectral Doppler provides data from blood flow measurements in formats other than color—for example, it can convert the measurements into a graph representing distance of blood flow against time or as a unique sound heard with every heartbeat.

When used in conjunction with mammography and clinical examination, breast US is indispensable in the diagnosis and management of benign and malignant processes. Both breasts are usually examined during this procedure. Images displayed on a monitor can determine the presence of palpable and nonpalpable masses; size and structure of the mass can also be evaluated. This procedure is useful in patients with an abnormal mass on a mammogram, because it can determine whether the abnormality is cystic or solid; that is, it can differentiate between a palpable, fluid-filled cyst and a palpable, solid breast lesion (benign or malignant). It is especially useful in patients with dense breast tissue and in those with silicone prostheses, because the US beam easily penetrates in these situations, allowing routine examination that cannot be performed with x-ray mammography. The procedure can be done as an adjunct to mammography, or it can be done in place of mammography in patients who refuse x-ray exposure or in whom it is contraindicated (e.g., pregnant women, women less than 25 yr ***related to increased breast tissue density that produces unclear images.***

Knowledge of genetics assists the nurse in identifying patients and family members who may benefit from additional education, risk assessment, and counseling. Genetics is the study and

U

identification of genes, genetic mutations, and inheritance. For example, genetics provides some insight into the likelihood of inheriting a trait such as blue eyes or a condition associated with a type of cancer such as breast cancer. Genomic studies evaluate the interaction of groups of genes. The combined activity or combined expression of groups of genes allows assumptions or predictions to be made. As an example, genomic studies measure the levels of activity in multiple genes to predict how they influence the development and growth of a tumor. Further information regarding inheritance of genes can be found in the study titled "Genetic Testing."

This procedure is contraindicated for: N/A

INDICATIONS

- Detect tiny tumors in combination with mammography for diagnostic validation.
- Determine the presence of nonpalpable abnormalities viewed on mammography of dense breast tissue and monitor changes in these abnormalities.
- Differentiate among types of breast masses (e.g., cyst, solid tumor, other lesions) in dense breast tissue.
- Evaluate palpable masses in young (less than age 25), pregnant, and lactating patients.
- Guide interventional procedures such as cyst aspiration, large-needle core biopsy, fine-needle aspiration biopsy, abscess drainage, presurgical localization, and galactography.
- Identify an abscess in a patient with mastitis.

POTENTIAL MEDICAL DIAGNOSIS

Normal findings

- Normal subcutaneous, mammary, and retromammary layers of tissue in both breasts; no evidence of pathological lesions (cyst or tumor) in either breast

Abnormal findings related to

Identification of abnormal findings is assisted by comparison of parameters such as size, shape, symmetry, and location; for example, areas of altered echo patterns in either an expected or unexpected location may indicate enlargement of an organ or the presence of blood or other fluids, tumors, or cysts. Comparison by type of abnormal findings may also assist in evaluating areas of altered patterns; for example, small round or oval areas with well-defined borders and clear central areas can differentiate a fluid-filled cyst from a solid tumor.

- Abscess
- Breast solid tumor, lesions
- Cancer (ductal carcinoma, infiltrating lobular carcinoma, medullary carcinoma, tubular carcinoma, and papillary carcinoma)
- Cystic breast disease
- Fibroadenoma
- Focal fibrosis
- Galactocele
- Hamartoma (fibroadenolipoma)
- Hematoma
- Papilloma
- Phyllodes tumor
- Radial scar

CRITICAL FINDINGS: N/A

INTERFERING FACTORS

Factors that may alter the results of the study

- Excessively large breasts.
- Incorrect placement of the transducer over the desired test site; quality of the US study is very

U

dependent upon the skill of the ultrasonographer.

- Metallic objects (e.g., jewelry, body rings) within the examination field, which may inhibit organ visualization and cause unclear images.
- Inability of the patient to cooperate or remain still during the procedure because of age, significant pain, or mental status.
- Patients who are technically difficult and who present challenges in obtaining reliable results (e.g., who are obese; have reduced rib spaces; present with fatty liver; have postoperative incisions, bandages, or dressings; have significant scarring in the area of interest). Aberrations in tissue composition may attenuate the sound waves and alter findings.

Other considerations

- The procedure may be canceled if the patient's weight exceeds the safety limit for the equipment.

NURSING IMPLICATIONS AND PROCEDURE

See Potential Nursing Problems on Fast Find at davispl.us/vanleeuwen7.

PRETEST:

- Positively identify the patient using at least two person-specific identifiers before services, treatments, or procedures are performed.
- ***Patient Teaching:*** Inform the patient this procedure can assist in assessing the breast.
- Obtain a history of the patient's health concerns, symptoms, surgical procedures, and results of previously performed laboratory and diagnostic studies. Include a list of known allergens, especially allergies or sensitivities to latex.
- Note any recent procedures that can interfere with test results (e.g., surgery or biopsy).
- Obtain a list of the patient's current medications, including over-the-counter medications and dietary supplements (see Effects of Natural Products on Laboratory Values online at Davis*Plus*).
- Review the procedure with the patient. Address concerns about pain related to the procedure and explain that some pain may be experienced during the test, and there may be moments of discomfort. Inform the patient that the procedure is performed in a US department by a health-care provider (HCP) who specializes in this procedure, with support staff, and takes approximately 30 to 60 min..
- ***Sensitivity to social and cultural issues,*** as well as concern for modesty, is important in providing psychological support before, during, and after the procedure.
- Instruct the patient not to apply lotions, deodorant, bath powder, or other substances to the chest and breast area before the examination.
- Instruct the patient to remove jewelry and other metallic objects from the area to be examined.
- Note that there are no food, fluid, or medication restrictions unless by medical direction.

INTRATEST:

Potential Complications: N/A

- Observe standard precautions, and follow the general guidelines in Patient Preparation and Specimen Collection online at Davis*Plus*. Positively identify the patient.
- Ensure that the patient has not applied lotions, deodorant, bath powder, or other substances to the chest and breast area before the examination.
- Ensure that the patient has removed all external metallic objects from the area to be examined prior to the procedure.
- Instruct the patient to change into the gown and robe provided.

- Avoid the use of equipment containing latex if the patient has a history of allergic reaction to latex.
- Instruct the patient to cooperate fully and to follow directions. Instruct the patient to remain still throughout the procedure because movement produces unreliable results.
- Place the patient in the supine position on an examination table. The right- and left-side-up positions are also used during the scan to facilitate better organ visualization.
- Expose the breast area and drape the patient.
- Conductive gel is applied to the skin and a transducer is moved over the skin to obtain images of the area of interest.
- Ask the patient to breathe normally during the examination. If necessary for better organ visualization, ask the patient to inhale deeply and hold her breath.

POST-TEST:

- Inform the patient that a report of the results will be made available to the requesting HCP, who will discuss the results with the patient.
- When the study is completed, remove the gel from the skin.
- Recognize anxiety related to test results. Discuss the implications of abnormal test results on the patient's lifestyle. Provide teaching and information regarding the clinical implications of the test results, as appropriate. Educate the patient regarding access to counseling services.
- Reinforce information given by the patient's HCP regarding further testing, treatment, or referral to another HCP. Decisions regarding the need for and frequency of breast self-examination, mammography, magnetic resonance imaging (MRI) of the breast, or other cancer screening procedures should be made after consultation between the patient and HCP. The most current guidelines for breast cancer screening of the general population as well as of individuals with increased risk are available from the American Cancer Society (ACS) (www.cancer.org), American College of Obstetricians and Gynecologists (ACOG) (www.acog.org), and American College of Radiology (www.acr.org). The ACS recommends breast examinations be performed every 3 yr for women between the ages of 20 and 39 yr and annually for women over 40 yr of age; annual mammograms should be performed on women 40 yr and older as long as they are in good health. The ACS also recommends annual MRI testing, in addition to an annual mammogram, for women at high risk of developing breast cancer. 🍁 Genetic testing for inherited mutations (BRCA1 and BRCA2) associated with increased risk of developing breast cancer may be ordered for women at risk. The test is performed on a blood specimen.
- Depending on the results of this procedure, additional testing may be performed to evaluate or monitor progression of the disease process and determine the need for a change in therapy. Evaluate test results in relation to the patient's symptoms and other tests performed.

Patient Education:

- Provide information on disease signs and symptoms and management.
- Provide information on possible diagnostic and laboratory studies associated with disease management.

Expected Patient Outcomes:

Understanding

- The patient and family acknowledge the medical and surgical options offered by the HCP.
- The patient and family correctly state disease pathophysiology and prognosis.

Ability

- The patient and family demonstrate positive coping strategies.
- The patient and family successfully demonstrate care of surgical site.

Response

- The patient agrees to attend cancer support group meetings.

- The patient agrees to seek psychological counseling to adjust to body changes and intimacy concerns.

RELATED STUDIES:

- Related tests include biopsy breast, cancer antigens, chest x-ray, CT thorax, ductograpy, genetic testing, mammogram, MRI breast, and stereotactic biopsy breast.
- Refer to the Reproductive System table online at Davis*Plus* for related tests by body system.

Ultrasound, Kidney

SYNONYM/ACRONYM: Renal ultrasound, renal sonography.

COMMON USE: To visualize and assess the kidneys, to perform biopsies, and assist in diagnosing disorders such as tumor, cancer, stones, and congenital anomalies. This procedure can also be used to evaluate therapeutic interventions such as transplants.

AREA OF APPLICATION: Kidney.

DESCRIPTION: Ultrasound (US) procedures are diagnostic, noninvasive, and relatively inexpensive. They take a short time to complete, do not use radiation, and cause no harm to the patient. High-frequency sound waves of various intensities are delivered by a transducer, a flashlight-shaped device, pressed against the skin. The waves are bounced back off internal anatomical structures and fluids, converted to electrical energy, amplified by the transducer, and displayed as images on a monitor. US is often used as a diagnostic and therapeutic tool for guiding minimally invasive procedures such as needle biopsies and fluid aspiration. The contraindications and complications for biopsy and fluid aspiration are discussed in detail in the individual studies.

Different types of transducers and imaging systems are sometimes used in clinical settings. Conventional US systems assume that sound waves pass through tissue at a constant speed. Advances in technology have led to the development of "smart" transducers that can compensate for tissue aberrations in technically difficult patients. Other advancements in imaging systems include three-dimensional and Doppler US. Color Doppler US uses color to indicate the velocity and direction of blood flow. Power Doppler is a more sensitive Doppler variation, capable of providing detailed images of blood flow; a limitation of power Doppler is that it cannot provide information regarding the direction of blood flow. Spectral Doppler provides data from blood flow measurements in formats other than color—for example, it can convert the measurements into a graph representing distance of blood flow against time or as a unique sound heard with every heartbeat.

Renal US is used to evaluate the structure, size, and position of the kidneys and to identify renal system disorders. It is valuable for determining the internal components of renal masses (solid versus cystic) and for evaluating other renal diseases, renal parenchyma, perirenal tissues, and obstruction. Renal US can be performed on the same day as a radionuclide scan or other radiological procedure and is especially valuable in patients who are in acute kidney injury, chronic kidney disease, or end-stage renal disease; have hypersensitivity to contrast medium; have a kidney that did not visualize on intravenous pyelography (IVP); or are pregnant. It does not rely on renal function or the injection of contrast medium to obtain a diagnosis. The procedure is indicated for evaluation after a kidney transplant and is used as a guide for biopsy and other interventional procedures, abscess drainage, and nephrostomy tube placement. Renal US may be the diagnostic examination of choice because no radiation is used and, in most cases, the accuracy is sufficient to make the diagnosis without further imaging procedures.

This procedure is contraindicated for: N/A

INDICATIONS

- Aid in the diagnosis of the effect (e.g., decrease in size) of chronic glomerulonephritis or chronic kidney disease on the kidneys.
- Detect an accumulation of fluid in the kidney caused by backflow of urine, hemorrhage, or perirenal fluid.
- Detect masses and differentiate between cysts or solid tumors, as evidenced by specific waveform patterns or absence of sound waves.
- Determine the presence and location of renal or ureteral calculi and obstruction.
- Determine the size, shape, and position of a nonfunctioning kidney to identify the cause.
- Evaluate or plan therapy for renal tumors.
- Evaluate renal transplantation for changes in kidney size.
- Locate the site of and guide percutaneous renal biopsy, aspiration needle insertion, or nephrostomy tube insertion.
- Monitor kidney development in children when renal disease has been diagnosed.
- Provide the location and size of renal masses in patients who are unable to undergo IVP because of poor renal function or an allergy to iodinated contrast medium.

POTENTIAL MEDICAL DIAGNOSIS

Normal findings

- Absence of calculi, cysts, hydronephrosis, obstruction, or tumor
- Normal size, position, and shape of the kidneys and associated structures

Abnormal findings related to

Identification of abnormal findings is assisted by comparison of parameters such as size, shape, symmetry, and location; for example, areas of altered echo patterns in either an expected or unexpected location may indicate enlargement of an organ or the presence of blood or other fluids, tumors, or cysts. Comparison by type of abnormal findings may also assist in evaluating areas of altered patterns; for example, small round or oval areas with well-defined borders and clear central areas can differentiate a fluid-filled cyst from a solid tumor.

- Acute glomerulonephritis
- Acute pyelonephritis

- Chronic kidney disease
- Congenital anomalies, such as absent, horseshoe, ectopic, or duplicated kidney
- Hydronephrosis
- Obstruction of ureters
- Perirenal abscess or hematoma
- Polycystic kidney
- Rejection of kidney transplant
- Renal calculi
- Renal cysts, hypertrophy, or tumors
- Ureteral obstruction

CRITICAL FINDINGS: N/A

INTERFERING FACTORS

Factors that may alter the results of the study

- Attenuation of the sound waves by bony structures, which can impair clear imaging of the area of interest.
- Incorrect placement of the transducer over the desired test site; quality of the US study is very dependent upon the skill of the ultrasonographer.
- Metallic objects (e.g., jewelry, body rings) within the examination field, which may inhibit organ visualization and cause unclear images.
- Inability of the patient to cooperate or remain still during the procedure because of age, significant pain, or mental status.
- Retained air, barium, or gas from a previous radiological procedure may block the transmission of sound waves.
- Patients who are technically difficult and who present challenges in obtaining reliable results (e.g., who are obese; have reduced rib spaces; present with fatty liver; have postoperative incisions, bandages, or dressings; have significant scarring in the area of interest). Aberrations in tissue composition may attenuate the sound waves and alter findings.

Other considerations

- The procedure may be canceled if the patient's weight exceeds the safety limit for the equipment.

NURSING IMPLICATIONS AND PROCEDURE

See Potential Nursing Problems on Fast Find at davispl.us/vanleeuwen7.

PRETEST:

- Positively identify the patient using at least two person-specific identifiers before services, treatments, or procedures are performed.
- ***Patient Teaching:*** Inform the patient this procedure can assist in assessing kidney function.
- Obtain a history of the patient's health concerns, symptoms, surgical procedures, and results of previously performed laboratory and diagnostic studies. Include a list of known allergens, especially allergies or sensitivities to latex.
- Note any recent procedures that can interfere with test results (e.g., surgery, biopsy, barium studies, colonoscopy, endoscopic retrograde cholangiopancreatography). Ensure that interfering studies were performed at least 24 hr before this test or can be rescheduled after this procedure.
- Record the date of the last menstrual period and determine the possibility of pregnancy in perimenopausal women.
- Obtain a list of the patient's current medications, including over-the-counter medications and dietary supplements (see Effects of Natural Products on Laboratory Values online at Davis*Plus*).
- Review the procedure with the patient. Address concerns about pain related to the procedure. Explain to the patient that some pain may be experienced during the test, and there may be moments of discomfort. Inform the patient that the procedure is performed in a US

U

department, usually by a health-care provider (HCP) who specializes in this procedure, with support staff, and takes approximately 30 to 60 min.

- ***Sensitivity to social and cultural issues,*** as well as concern for modesty, is important in providing psychological support before, during, and after the procedure.
- Instruct the patient to remove jewelry and other metallic objects from the area to be examined.
- Note that there are no food, fluid, or medication restrictions unless by medical direction.

INTRATEST:

Potential Complications: N/A

- Observe standard precautions, and follow the general guidelines in Patient Preparation and Specimen Collection online at Davis*Plus*. Positively identify the patient.
- Ensure that the patient has removed all external metallic objects from the area to be examined prior to the procedure.
- Instruct the patient to void and change into the gown, robe, and foot coverings provided.
- Avoid the use of equipment containing latex if the patient has a history of allergic reaction to latex.
- Instruct the patient to cooperate fully and to follow directions. Instruct the patient to remain still throughout the procedure because movement produces unreliable results.
- Place the patient in the supine position on an examination table. The right- or left-side-up positions may be used to allow gravity to reposition the liver, gas, and fluid to facilitate better organ visualization.
- Expose the abdominal and kidney area and drape the patient.
- Conductive gel is applied to the skin, and a transducer is moved over the skin to obtain images of the area of interest.
- Ask the patient to breathe normally during the examination. If necessary for better organ visualization, ask the patient to inhale deeply and hold his or her breath.

POST-TEST:

- Inform the patient that a report of the results will be made available to the requesting HCP, who will discuss the results with the patient.
- When the study is completed, remove the gel from the skin.
- Recognize anxiety related to test results. Discuss the implications of abnormal test results on the patient's lifestyle. Provide teaching and information regarding the clinical implications of the test results, as appropriate.
- Reinforce information given by the patient's HCP regarding further testing, treatment, or referral to another HCP. Answer any questions or address any concerns voiced by the patient or family.
- Depending on the results of this procedure, additional testing may be performed to evaluate or monitor progression of the disease process and determine the need for a change in therapy. Evaluate test results in relation to the patient's symptoms and other tests performed.

Patient Education:

- Teach the patient to avoid foods that facilitate stone formation (tea, beer, chocolate) when diagnosed with stones.
- Teach the patient foods that can discourage stone formation, such as milk and milk products.

Expected Patient Outcomes:

Understanding

- The patient and family acknowledge the importance of increased oral intake to kidney health (as appropriate).
- The patient and family acknowledge the importance of completing the prescribed antibiotic regime.

Ability

- The patient successfully demonstrates the ability to strain the urine.
- The patient and family successfully demonstrate how to measure and record intake and output.

U

Response

- The patient agrees to diet changes that will facilitate kidney health.
- The patient agrees to HCP-recommended follow-up evaluations.

RELATED STUDIES:

- Related tests include angiography kidneys, anti-glomerular basement membrane antibody, biopsy kidney, BUN, calculus kidney stone panel, CT abdomen, CT kidneys, creatinine, creatinine clearance, cytology urine, erythropoietin, group A streptococcal screen, IVP, KUB study, MRI abdomen, renogram, retrograde ureteropyelography, UA, and US abdomen.
- Refer to the Genitourinary System table online at Davis*Plus* for related tests by system.

Ultrasound, Liver and Biliary System

SYNONYM/ACRONYM: Gallbladder ultrasound, liver ultrasound, hepatobiliary sonography.

COMMON USE: To visualize and assess liver and gallbladder structure and function, assist in obtaining a biopsy, and diagnose disorders such as gallstones, cancer, tumors, cysts, and bleeding. Also used to evaluate the effectiveness of therapeutic interventions.

AREA OF APPLICATION: Liver, gallbladder, bile ducts.

DESCRIPTION: Ultrasound (US) procedures are diagnostic, noninvasive, and relatively inexpensive. They take a short time to complete, do not use radiation, and cause no harm to the patient. High-frequency sound waves of various intensities are delivered by a transducer, a flashlight-shaped device, pressed against the skin. The waves are bounced back off internal anatomical structures and fluids, converted to electrical energy, amplified by the transducer, and displayed as images on a monitor. US is often used as a diagnostic and therapeutic tool for guiding minimally invasive procedures such as needle biopsies, tube placement, and fluid aspiration. The contraindications and complications for biopsy and fluid aspiration are discussed in detail in the individual related studies.

Different types of transducers and imaging systems are sometimes used in clinical settings. Conventional US systems assume that sound waves pass through tissue at a constant speed. Advances in technology have led to the development of "smart" transducers that can compensate for tissue aberrations in technically difficult patients. Other advancements in imaging systems include three-dimensional and Doppler US. Color Doppler ultrasound uses color to indicate the velocity and direction of blood flow. Power Doppler is a more sensitive Doppler variation, capable of providing detailed images of blood flow; a limitation of power Doppler is that it cannot provide information regarding the direction of blood flow. Spectral Doppler provides data from blood flow measurements in formats other than color—for example, it can convert the measurements into a graph representing distance of blood flow against time or as a unique sound heard with every heartbeat.

Hepatobiliary US is used to evaluate the structure, size, and position of the liver and gallbladder in the right upper quadrant (RUQ) of the abdomen. The gallbladder and biliary system collect, store, concentrate, and transport bile to the intestines to aid in digestion. This procedure allows visualization of the gallbladder and bile ducts when the patient may have impaired liver function, and it is especially helpful when done on patients in whom gallstones cannot be visualized with oral or intravenous radiological studies. Liver US can be done in combination with a nuclear scan to obtain information about liver function and density differences in the liver.

This procedure is contraindicated for: N/A

INDICATIONS

- Detect cysts, polyps, hematoma, abscesses, hemangioma, adenoma, metastatic disease, hepatitis, or solid tumor of the liver or gallbladder, as evidenced by echoes specific to tissue density and sharply or poorly defined masses.
- Detect gallstones or inflammation when oral cholecystography is inconclusive.
- Detect hepatic lesions, as evidenced by density differences and echo-pattern changes.
- Determine the cause of unexplained hepatomegaly and abnormal liver function tests.
- Determine cause of unexplained RUQ pain.
- Determine patency and diameter of the hepatic duct for dilation or obstruction.
- Differentiate between obstructive and nonobstructive jaundice by determining the cause.
- Evaluate response to therapy for tumor, as evidenced by a decrease in size of the organ.
- Guide biopsy or tube placement.
- Guide catheter placement into the gallbladder for stone dissolution and gallbladder fragmentation.

POTENTIAL MEDICAL DIAGNOSIS

Normal findings

- Normal size, position, and shape of the liver and gallbladder as well as patency of the cystic and common bile ducts

Abnormal findings related to

Identification of abnormal findings is assisted by comparison of parameters such as size, shape, symmetry, and location. For example, areas of altered echo patterns in either an expected or unexpected location may indicate enlargement of an organ or the presence of blood or other fluids, tumors, or cysts. Comparison by type of abnormal findings may also assist in evaluating areas of altered patterns; for example, small round or oval areas with well-defined borders and clear central areas can differentiate a fluid-filled cyst from a solid tumor.

- Biliary or hepatic duct obstruction/dilation
- Cirrhosis
- Gallbladder inflammation, stones, carcinoma, polyps
- Hematoma or trauma
- Hepatic tumors, metastasis, cysts, hemangioma, hepatitis
- Hepatocellular disease, adenoma
- Hepatomegaly
- Intrahepatic abscess
- Subphrenic abscesses

CRITICAL FINDINGS: N/A

INTERFERING FACTORS

Factors that may alter the results of the study

- Attenuation of the sound waves by bony structures, which can impair clear imaging of the right lobe of the liver.
- Incorrect placement of the transducer over the desired test site; quality of the US study is dependent upon the skill of the ultrasonographer.
- Metallic objects (e.g., jewelry, body rings) within the examination field, which may inhibit organ visualization and cause unclear images.
- Inability of the patient to cooperate or remain still during the procedure because of age, significant pain, or mental status.
- Retained air, barium, or gas from a previous radiological procedure may block the transmission of sound waves.
- Gas or feces in the gastrointestinal tract resulting from inadequate cleansing or failure to restrict food intake before the study.
- Patients who are technically difficult and who present challenges in obtaining reliable results (e.g., who are obese; have reduced rib spaces; present with fatty liver; have postoperative incisions, bandages, or dressings; have significant scarring in the area of interest). Aberrations in tissue composition may attenuate the sound waves and alter findings.

Other considerations

- Failure to follow dietary restrictions may cause the procedure to be canceled or repeated.
- The procedure may be canceled if the patient's weight exceeds the safety limit for the equipment.

NURSING IMPLICATIONS AND PROCEDURE

See Potential Nursing Problems on Fast Find at davispl.us/vanleeuwen7.

PRETEST:

- Positively identify the patient using at least two person-specific identifiers before services, treatments, or procedures are performed.
- ***Patient Teaching:*** Inform the patient this procedure can assist in assessing liver and biliary function.
- Obtain a history of the patient's health concerns, symptoms, surgical procedures, and results of previously performed laboratory and diagnostic studies. Include a list of known allergens, especially allergies or sensitivities to latex.
- Note any recent procedures that can interfere with test results (e.g., surgery, biopsy, barium studies, colonoscopy, endoscopic retrograde cholangiopancreatography). Ensure that interfering studies were performed at least 24 hr before this test or can be rescheduled after this procedure.
- Obtain a list of the patient's current medications, including over-the-counter medications and dietary supplements (see Effects of Natural Products on Laboratory Values online at Davis*Plus*).
- Review the procedure with the patient. Address concerns about pain related to the procedure and explain that some pain may be experienced during the test, and there may be moments of discomfort. Inform the patient that the procedure is performed in a US department, usually by a health-care provider (HCP) who specializes in this procedure, with support staff, and takes approximately 30 to 60 min.
- ***Sensitivity to social and cultural issues,*** as well as concern for modesty, is important in providing psychological support before, during, and after the procedure.

U

- Instruct the patient to remove jewelry and other metallic objects from the area to be examined.
- Instruct the patient to fast and restrict fluids for 8 hr prior to the procedure. Patients may be asked to eat a low-or fat-free diet for the last meal before the procedure. Food restrictions help ensure reduction of bowel gas, which can interfere with the transmission of US wave. Protocols may vary among facilities.

INTRATEST:

Potential Complications: N/A

- Observe standard precautions, and follow the general guidelines in Patient Preparation and Specimen Collection online at Davis*Plus*. Positively identify the patient.
- Ensure that food and fluids have been restricted for at least 8 hr prior to the procedure.
- Ensure that the patient has removed all external metallic objects from the area to be examined prior to the procedure.
- Instruct the patient to void and change into the gown, robe, and foot coverings provided.
- Avoid the use of equipment containing latex if the patient has a history of allergic reaction to latex.
- Instruct the patient to cooperate fully and to follow directions. Instruct the patient to remain still throughout the procedure because movement produces unreliable results.
- Place the patient in the supine position on an examination table. The right- or left-side-up positions may be used to allow gravity to reposition the liver, gas, and fluid to facilitate better organ visualization.
- Expose the abdominal area and drape the patient.
- Conductive gel is applied to the skin, and a transducer is moved over the skin to obtain images of the area of interest.
- Ask the patient to breathe normally during the examination. If necessary for better organ visualization, ask the patient to inhale deeply and hold his or her breath.

POST-TEST:

- Inform the patient that a report of the results will be made available to the requesting HCP, who will discuss the results with the patient.
- When the study is completed, remove the gel from the skin.
- Instruct the patient to resume usual diet and fluids, as directed by the HCP.
- Recognize anxiety related to test results. Discuss the implications of abnormal test results on the patient's lifestyle. Provide teaching and information regarding the clinical implications of the test results, as appropriate.
- Reinforce information given by the patient's HCP regarding further testing, treatment, or referral to another HCP. Answer any questions or address any concerns voiced by the patient or family.
- Depending on the results of this procedure, additional testing may be performed to evaluate or monitor progression of the disease process and determine the need for a change in therapy. Evaluate test results in relation to the patient's symptoms and other tests performed.

Patient Education:

- Teach the patient to call for pain relief medication as soon as it is needed.
- Teach coping strategies that can be used to decrease anxiety and manage grief and fear.

Expected Patient Outcomes:

Understanding

- The patient describes pain management strategies that work and those that do not work.
- The patient and family state the pathophysiology related to the patient's specific disease process.

Ability

- The patient demonstrates effective coping mechanisms to decrease anxiety.
- The patient makes lifestyle changes that will support health and wellness.

U

Response

- The patient agrees to discuss concerns with identified support (family, friends, group, chaplain).
- The patient agrees to lifestyle modifications to control disease process and symptoms.

RELATED STUDIES:

- Related tests include ALP, ALT, AST, bilirubin, biopsy liver, cholangiography, colonoscopy, CT abdomen, endoscopy, ERCP, GGT, haptoglobin, hepatitis (A, B, C antigens and/or antibodies), hepatobiliary scan, laparoscopy abdominal, MRI abdomen, radiofrequency ablation liver, and US abdomen.
- Refer to the Hepatobiliary System table online at Davis*Plus* for related tests by body system.

Ultrasound, Pancreas

SYNONYM/ACRONYM: Pancreatic ultrasonography.

COMMON USE: To visualize and assess the pancreas toward diagnosing disorders such as tumor, cancer, obstruction, and cysts. Also used as a tool for biopsy and to evaluate the effectiveness of therapeutic interventions.

AREA OF APPLICATION: Pancreas and upper abdomen.

DESCRIPTION: Ultrasound (US) procedures are diagnostic, noninvasive, and relatively inexpensive. They take a short time to complete, do not use radiation, and cause no harm to the patient. High-frequency sound waves of various intensities are delivered by a transducer, a flashlight-shaped device, pressed against the skin. The waves are bounced back off internal anatomical structures and fluids, converted to electrical energy, amplified by the transducer, and displayed as images on a monitor. US is often used as a diagnostic and therapeutic tool for guiding minimally invasive procedures such as needle biopsies and fluid aspiration. The contraindications and complications for biopsy and fluid aspiration are discussed in detail in the individual studies.

Different types of transducers and imaging systems are sometimes used in clinical settings. Conventional US systems assume that sound waves pass through tissue at a constant speed. Advances in technology have led to the development of "smart" transducers that can compensate for tissue aberrations in technically difficult patients. Other advancements in imaging systems include three-dimensional and Doppler US. Color Doppler US uses color to indicate the velocity and direction of blood flow. Power Doppler is a more sensitive Doppler variation, capable of providing detailed images of blood flow; a limitation of power Doppler is that it cannot provide information regarding the direction of blood flow. Spectral Doppler provides data from blood flow measurements in formats

U

other than color—for example, it can convert the measurements into a graph representing distance of blood flow against time or as a unique sound heard with every heartbeat.

Pancreatic US is used to determine the size, shape, and position of the pancreas; determine the presence of masses or other abnormalities of the pancreas; and examine the surrounding viscera. Pancreatic US is usually done in combination with computed tomography (CT) or magnetic resonance imaging (MRI) of the pancreas.

This procedure is contraindicated for: N/A

INDICATIONS

- Detect anatomic abnormalities as a consequence of pancreatitis.
- Detect pancreatic cancer, as evidenced by a poorly defined mass or a mass in the head of the pancreas that obstructs the pancreatic duct.
- Detect pancreatitis, as evidenced by pancreatic enlargement with increased echoes.
- Detect pseudocysts, as evidenced by a well-defined mass with absence of echoes from the interior.
- Monitor therapeutic response to tumor treatment.
- Provide guidance for percutaneous aspiration and fine-needle biopsy of the pancreas.

POTENTIAL MEDICAL DIAGNOSIS

Normal findings

- Normal size, position, contour, and texture of the pancreas

Abnormal findings related to

Identification of abnormal findings is assisted by comparison of parameters such as size, shape, symmetry, and location; for example, areas of altered echo patterns in either an expected or unexpected location may indicate enlargement of an organ or the presence of blood or other fluids, tumors, or cysts. Comparison by type of abnormal findings may also assist in evaluating areas of altered patterns; for example, small round or oval areas with well-defined borders and clear central areas can differentiate a fluid-filled cyst from a solid tumor.

- Acute pancreatitis
- Calculi
- Pancreatic duct obstruction
- Pancreatic tumor
- Pseudocysts

CRITICAL FINDINGS: N/A

INTERFERING FACTORS

Factors that may alter the results of the study

- Attenuation of the sound waves bony structures, which can impair clear imaging of the area of interest.
- Incorrect placement of the transducer over the desired test site; quality of the US study is very dependent upon the skill of the ultrasonographer.
- Metallic objects (e.g., jewelry, body rings) within the examination field, which may inhibit organ visualization and cause unclear images.
- Inability of the patient to cooperate or remain still during the procedure because of age, significant pain, or mental status.
- Retained air, barium, or gas from a previous radiological procedure may block the transmission of sound waves.
- Gas or feces in the gastrointestinal (GI) tract resulting from inadequate cleansing or failure to restrict food intake before the study.

- Patients who are technically difficult and who present challenges in obtaining reliable results (e.g., who are obese; have reduced rib spaces; present with fatty liver; have postoperative incisions, bandages, or dressings; have significant scarring in the area of interest). Aberrations in tissue composition may attenuate the sound waves and alter findings.

Other considerations

- Failure to follow dietary and fluid restrictions and other pretesting preparations may cause the procedure to be canceled or repeated.
- The procedure may be canceled if the patient's weight exceeds the safety limit for the equipment.

NURSING IMPLICATIONS AND PROCEDURE

See Potential Nursing Problems on Fast Find at davispl.us/vanleeuwen7.

PRETEST:

- Positively identify the patient using at least two person-specific identifiers before services, treatments, or procedures are performed.
- *Patient Teaching:* Inform the patient this procedure can assist in assessing pancreatic function.
- Obtain a history of the patient's health concerns, symptoms, surgical procedures, and results of previously performed laboratory and diagnostic studies. Include a list of known allergens, especially allergies or sensitivities to latex.
- Note any recent procedures that can interfere with test results (e.g., surgery, biopsy, barium studies, colonoscopy, endoscopic retrograde cholangiopancreatography). Ensure that interfering studies were performed at least 24 hr before this test or can be rescheduled after this procedure.
- Record the date of the last menstrual period and determine the possibility of pregnancy in perimenopausal women.
- Obtain a list of the patient's current medications, including over-the-counter medications and dietary supplements (see Effects of Natural Products on Laboratory Values online at Davis*Plus*).
- Review the procedure with the patient. Address concerns about pain related to the procedure and explain that some pain may be experienced during the test, and there may be moments of discomfort. Inform the patient that the procedure is performed in a US department, usually by a health-care provider (HCP) specializing in this procedure, with support staff, and takes approximately 30 to 60 min.
- ***Sensitivity to social and cultural issues,*** as well as concern for modesty, is important in providing psychological support before, during, and after the procedure.
- Instruct the patient to remove jewelry and other metallic objects from the area to be examined.
- Instruct the patient to fast and restrict fluids for 8 hr prior to the procedure. Patients may be asked to eat a low- or fat-free diet the night before the procedure. Food restrictions help ensure reduction of bowel gas, which can interfere with the transmission of US waves. Protocols may vary among facilities.

INTRATEST:

Potential Complications: N/A

- Observe standard precautions, and follow the general guidelines in Patient Preparation and Specimen Collection online at Davis*Plus*. Positively identify the patient.
- Ensure that food and fluids have been restricted prior to the procedure, as instructed.
- Ensure that the patient has removed all external metallic objects from

the area to be examined prior to the procedure.

- Instruct the patient to void and change into the gown, robe, and foot coverings provided.
- Avoid the use of equipment containing latex if the patient has a history of allergic reaction to latex.
- Instruct the patient to cooperate fully and to follow directions. Ask the patient to remain still throughout the procedure because movement produces unreliable results.
- Place the patient in the supine position on an examination table. The right- or left-side-up position may be used to allow gravity to reposition the liver, gas, and fluid to facilitate better organ visualization.
- Expose the abdominal area and drape the patient.
- Conductive gel is applied to the skin, and a transducer is moved over the skin to obtain images of the area of interest.
- Ask the patient to breathe normally during the examination. If necessary for better organ visualization, ask the patient to inhale deeply and hold his or her breath.

POST-TEST:

- Inform the patient that a report of the results will be made available to the requesting HCP, who will discuss the results with the patient.
- When the study is completed, remove the gel from the skin.
- Instruct the patient to resume usual diet and fluids, as directed by the HCP.
- Recognize anxiety related to test results. Discuss the implications of abnormal test results on the patient's lifestyle. Provide teaching and information regarding the clinical implications of the test results, as appropriate.
- Reinforce information given by the patient's HCP regarding further testing, treatment, or referral to another HCP. Answer any questions or address any concerns voiced by the patient or family.
- Depending on the results of this procedure, additional testing may be needed to evaluate or monitor progression of the disease process and determine the need for a change in therapy. Evaluate test results in relation to the patient's symptoms and other tests performed.

Patient Education:

- Teach the patient that the consumption of alcohol can exacerbate the pain due to pancreatic stimulation.
- Facilitate a dietary consult to assist the patient in managing his or her nutritional status.

Expected Patient Outcomes:

Understanding

- The patient and family acknowledge the importance of progressing the diet slowly to evaluate food tolerance and make adjustments as needed.
- The patient and family acknowledge the importance of taking dietary supplements to support positive nutrition.

Ability

- The patient and family demonstrate the ability to select low-fat foods to include in the diet plan.
- The patient and family demonstrate the ability to accurately record intake and output.

Response

- The patient agrees to avoid drinking alcoholic and caffeinated beverages.
- The patient participates in a pain management plan that provides a level of relief acceptable to the patient.

RELATED STUDIES:

- Related tests include amylase, cancer antigens, CT abdomen, CT pancreas, C peptide, ERCP, KUB study, laparoscopy abdominal, lipase, MRI abdomen, MRI pancreas, peritoneal fluid analysis, and US abdomen.
- Refer to the Gastrointestinal System table online at Davis*Plus* for related tests by body system.

U

Ultrasound, Pelvis (Gynecologic, Nonobstetric)

SYNONYM/ACRONYM: Lower abdominal ultrasound, pelvic gynecologic (GYN) sonogram, pelvic sonography.

COMMON USE: To visualize and assess the pelvis for disorders such as uterine mass, tumor, cancer, cysts, and fibroids. This procedure can also be useful in evaluating ovulation and fallopian tube function related to fertility issues.

AREA OF APPLICATION: Pelvis and appendix region.

DESCRIPTION: Ultrasound (US) procedures are diagnostic, noninvasive, and relatively inexpensive. They take a short time to complete, do not use radiation, and cause no harm to the patient. High-frequency sound waves of various intensities are delivered by a transducer, a flashlight-shaped device, pressed against the skin. The waves are bounced back off internal anatomical structures and fluids, converted to electrical energy, amplified by the transducer, and displayed as images on a monitor. US is often used as a diagnostic and therapeutic tool for guiding minimally invasive procedures such as needle biopsies and fluid aspiration. The contraindications and complications for biopsy and fluid aspiration are discussed in detail in the individual related studies.

Different types of transducers and imaging systems are sometimes used in clinical settings. Conventional US systems assume that sound waves pass through tissue at a constant speed. Advances in technology have led to the development of "smart" transducers that can compensate for tissue aberrations in technically difficult patients. Other advancements in imaging systems include three-dimensional and Doppler US. Color Doppler US uses color to indicate the velocity and direction of blood flow. Power Doppler is a more sensitive Doppler variation, capable of providing detailed images of blood flow; a limitation of power Doppler is that it cannot provide information regarding the direction of blood flow. Spectral Doppler provides data from blood flow measurements in formats other than color—for example, it can convert the measurements into a graph representing distance of blood flow against time or as a unique sound heard with every heartbeat.

Gynecologic US is used to determine the presence, size, and structure of masses and cysts and determine the position of an intrauterine contraceptive device (IUD); evaluate postmenopausal bleeding; and examine other abnormalities of the uterus, ovaries, fallopian tubes, and vagina. This procedure is done by a transabdominal or transvaginal approach. The transabdominal approach provides a view of the pelvic organs posterior to the bladder. It requires a full bladder, thereby allowing a window for

U

transmission of the US waves, pushing the uterus away from the pubic symphysis, pushing the bowel out of the pelvis, and acting as a reference for comparison in the evaluation of the internal structures of a mass or cyst being examined. The transvaginal approach focuses on the female reproductive organs and is often used to monitor ovulation over a period of days in patients undergoing fertility assessment. This approach is also used in patients who are obese or in patients with retroversion of the uterus because the sound waves are better able to reach the organ from the vaginal site. Transvaginal images are significantly more accurate compared to anterior transabdominal images in identifying paracervical, endometrial, and ovarian pathology, and the transvaginal approach does not require a full bladder.

This procedure is contraindicated for: N/A

INDICATIONS

- Detect and monitor the treatment of pelvic inflammatory disease (PID) when done in combination with other laboratory tests.
- Detect bleeding into the pelvis resulting from trauma to the area or ascites associated with tumor metastasis.
- Detect masses in the pelvis and differentiate them from cysts or solid tumors, ***as evidenced by differences in sound-wave patterns.***
- Detect pelvic abscess or peritonitis caused by a ruptured appendix or diverticulitis.
- Detect the presence of ovarian cysts and malignancy and determine the type, if possible, as evidenced by size, outline, and change in position of other pelvic organs.
- Evaluate the effectiveness of tumor therapy, ***as evidenced by a reduction in mass size.***
- Evaluate suspected fibroid tumor or bladder tumor.
- Evaluate the thickness of the uterine wall.
- Monitor placement and location of an IUD.
- Monitor follicular size associated with fertility studies or to remove follicles for in vitro transplantation.

POTENTIAL MEDICAL DIAGNOSIS

Normal findings

- Normal size, position, location, and structure of pelvic organs (e.g., uterus, ovaries, fallopian tubes, vagina); IUD properly positioned within the uterine cavity

Abnormal findings related to

Identification of abnormal findings is assisted by comparison of parameters such as size, shape, symmetry, and location; for example, areas of altered echo patterns in either an expected or unexpected location may indicate enlargement of an organ or the presence of blood or other fluids, tumors, or cysts. Comparison by type of abnormal findings may also assist in evaluating areas of altered patterns; for example, small round or oval areas with well-defined borders and clear central areas can differentiate a fluid-filled cyst from a solid tumor.

- Abscess
- Adnexal torsion
- Appendicitis
- Endometrioma
- Fibroids (leiomyoma)
- Infection
- Nonovarian cyst
- Ovarian cysts
- Ovarian tumor

U

- Peritonitis
- PID
- Uterine tumor or adnexal tumor

CRITICAL FINDINGS:

- Abscess
- Adnexal torsion
- Appendicitis
- Infection
- Tumor with significant mass effect

Note and immediately report to the requesting health-care provider (HCP) any critical findings and related symptoms. A listing of these findings varies among facilities. Timely notification of a critical finding for laboratory or diagnostic studies is a role expectation of the professional nurse. The notification processes vary among facilities. Upon receipt of the critical finding, the information should be read back to the caller to verify accuracy.

INTERFERING FACTORS

Factors that may alter the results of the study

- Attenuation of the sound waves by bony structures, which can impair clear imaging in the area of interest.
- Incorrect placement of the transducer over the desired test site; quality of the US study is very dependent upon the skill of the ultrasonographer.
- Metallic objects (e.g., jewelry, body rings) within the examination field, which may inhibit organ visualization and cause unclear images.
- Inability of the patient to cooperate or remain still during the procedure because of age, significant pain, or mental status.
- Retained air, barium, or gas from a previous radiological procedure may block the transmission of sound waves.
- Dehydration, which can cause failure to demonstrate the boundaries between organs and tissue structures.
- Insufficiently full bladder, which fails to push the bowel from the pelvis and the uterus from the symphysis pubis, thereby prohibiting clear imaging of the pelvic organs in transabdominal imaging.
- Patients who are technically difficult and who present challenges in obtaining reliable results (e.g., who are obese; have reduced rib spaces; present with fatty liver; have postoperative incisions, bandages, or dressings; have significant scarring in the area of interest). Aberrations in tissue composition may attenuate the sound waves and alter findings.

Other considerations

- Failure to follow pretesting preparations may cause the procedure to be canceled or repeated.
- The procedure may be canceled if the patient's weight exceeds the safety limit for the equipment.
- Patients with latex allergy; use of the vaginal probe requires the probe to be covered with a condom-like sac, usually made from latex. Latex-free covers are available.

NURSING IMPLICATIONS AND PROCEDURE

See Potential Nursing Problems on Fast Find at davispl.us/vanleeuwen7.

PRETEST:

- Positively identify the patient using at least two person-specific identifiers before services, treatments, or procedures are performed.
- ***Patient Teaching:*** Inform the patient that this procedure can assist in assessing pelvic organ function.
- Obtain a history of the patient's health concerns, symptoms, surgical procedures, and results of previously

U

performed laboratory and diagnostic studies. Include a list of known allergens, especially allergies or sensitivities to latex.

- Note any recent procedures that can interfere with test results (e.g., surgery, biopsy, barium studies, colonoscopy, endoscopic retrograde cholangiopancreatography). Ensure that interfering studies were performed at least 24 hr before this test or can be rescheduled after this procedure.
- Record the date of the last menstrual period and determine the possibility of pregnancy in perimenopausal women.
- Obtain a list of the patient's current medications, including over-the-counter medications and dietary supplements (see Effects of Natural Products on Laboratory Values online at Davis*Plus*).
- Review the procedure with the patient. Address concerns about pain related to the procedure and explain that some pain may be experienced during the test, and there may be moments of discomfort. Inform the patient that the procedure is performed in a US department by an HCP who specializes in this procedure, with support staff, and takes approximately 30 to 60 min.
- ***Sensitivity to social and cultural issues,*** as well as concern for modesty, is important in providing psychological support before, during, and after the procedure.
- Instruct the patient to remove jewelry and other metallic objects from the area to be examined.
- Instruct the patient that a latex or sterile sheath-covered probe will be inserted into the vagina for the transvaginal approach.
- Note that there are no food, fluid, or medication restrictions unless by medical direction.
- Instruct the patient receiving transabdominal US to drink three to four glasses of fluid 90 min before the examination and not to void, because the procedure requires a full bladder. Patients receiving transvaginal US only do not need to have a full bladder.

INTRATEST:

Potential Complications: N/A

- Observe standard precautions, and follow the general guidelines in Patient Preparation and Specimen Collection online at Davis*Plus*. Positively identify the patient.
- Ensure that the patient receiving transabdominal US drank three to four glasses of fluid and has not voided.
- Ensure that the patient has removed all external metallic objects from the area to be examined prior to the procedure.
- Avoid the use of equipment containing latex if the patient has a history of allergic reaction to latex.
- Instruct the patient to change into the gown, robe, and foot coverings provided. Remind her not to void before the procedure. Patients receiving transvaginal US do not need to have a full bladder.
- Instruct the patient to cooperate fully and to follow directions. Ask the patient to remain still throughout the procedure because movement produces unreliable results.
- Place the patient in the supine position on an examination table. The right- or left-side-up positions may be used to allow gravity to reposition the liver, gas, and fluid to facilitate better organ visualization.
- Expose the abdominal and pelvic area and drape the patient.
- ***Transabdominal approach:*** Observe that conductive gel is applied to the skin, and a transducer is moved over the skin while the bladder is distended to obtain images of the area of interest.
- ***Transvaginal approach:*** Observe that a covered and lubricated probe is inserted into the vagina and moved to different levels. Images are obtained and recorded.
- Ask the patient to breathe normally during the examination. If necessary for better organ visualization, ask the

U

patient to inhale deeply and hold her breath.

POST-TEST:

- Inform the patient that a report of the results will be made available to the requesting HCP, who will discuss the results with the patient.
- Allow the patient to void, as needed.
- When the study is completed, remove the gel from the skin.
- Recognize anxiety related to test results. Discuss the implications of abnormal test results on the patient's lifestyle. Provide teaching and information regarding the clinical implications of the test results, as appropriate. Educate the patient regarding access to counseling services. Provide contact information, if desired, for the American Cancer Society (www.cancer.org). 🍁
- Reinforce information given by the patient's HCP regarding further testing, treatment, or referral to another HCP. Answer any questions or address any concerns voiced by the patient or family.
- Depending on the results of this procedure, additional testing may be needed to evaluate or monitor progression of the disease process and determine the need for a change in therapy. Evaluate test results in relation to the patient's symptoms and other tests performed.

Patient Education:

- Teach the pathophysiology of the disease process.
- Teach the patient the importance of calling for pain medication as soon as it is needed for effective pain management.

Expected Patient Outcomes:

Understanding

- The patient and family correctly describe treatment options related to disease process.
- The patient and family acknowledge the importance of family or group counseling related to end-of-life issues.

Ability

- The patient and family demonstrate the ability to maintain a quiet environment for emotional and physical rest.
- The patient and family demonstrate successful coping strategies.

Response

- The patient and family agree to family or individual support group counseling related to prognosis and end of life.
- The patient and family agrees to all follow-up diagnostic and laboratory studies needed to monitor health status and the effectiveness of treatment modalitics.

RELATED STUDIES:

- Related tests include cancer antigens, colposcopy, CT abdomen, hysterosalpingography, KUB study, laparoscopy gynecologic, MRI abdomen, Pap smear, and PET pelvis.
- Refer to the Reproductive System table online at Davis*Plus* for related tests by body system.

Ultrasound, Prostate (Transrectal)

SYNONYM/ACRONYM: Prostate sonography, TRUS.

COMMON USE: To visualize and assess the prostate gland as an adjunct of prostate-specific antigen (PSA) blood testing and examination to assist in diagnosing disorders such as tumor and cancer. Also used to assist in guiding biopsy of the prostate.

AREA OF APPLICATION: Prostate, seminal vesicles.

DESCRIPTION: Ultrasound (US) procedures are diagnostic, noninvasive, and relatively inexpensive. They take a short time to complete, do not use radiation, and cause no harm to the patient. High-frequency sound waves of various intensities are delivered by a transducer, a candle-shaped device, which is lubricated, sheathed with a condom, and inserted a few inches into the rectum. The waves are bounced back off internal anatomical structures and fluids, converted to electrical energy, amplified by the transducer, and displayed as images on a monitor. US is often used as a diagnostic and therapeutic tool for guiding minimally invasive procedures such as needle biopsies and fluid aspiration. The contraindications and complications for biopsy and fluid aspiration are discussed in detail in the individual related studies.

Different types of transducers and imaging systems are sometimes used in clinical settings. Conventional US systems assume that sound waves pass through tissue at a constant speed. Advances in technology have lead to the development of "smart" transducers that can compensate for tissue aberrations in technically difficult patients. Other advancements in imaging systems include three-dimensional and Doppler US. Color Doppler US uses color to indicate the velocity and direction of blood flow. Power Doppler is a more sensitive Doppler variation, capable of providing detailed images of blood flow; a limitation of Power Doppler is that it cannot provide information regarding the direction of blood flow. Spectral Doppler provides data from blood flow measurements in formats other than color—for example, it can convert the measurements into a graph representing distance of blood flow against time or as a unique sound heard with every heartbeat.

Prostate US is used to evaluate the structure, size, and position of the contents of the prostate (e.g., masses). This procedure can evaluate abnormal pathology in prostate tissue, the seminal vesicles, and surrounding perirectal tissue. Prostate US aids in the diagnosis of prostatic cancer by evaluating palpable nodules as a complement to a digital rectal examination (DRE) or in response to an elevated PSA level. The DRE is a simple procedure used to examine, by palpation, the lower rectum and prostate gland. It is performed by the health-care provider (HCP) who inserts a lubricated, gloved finger into the rectum while the patient is properly positioned. Prostate US can also be used to stage carcinoma and to assist in radiation seed placement. Micturition disorders can also be evaluated by this procedure. The examination is helpful in monitoring patient response to therapy for prostatic disease.

This procedure is contraindicated for

Patients with latex allergy; use of the rectal probe requires the probe to be covered with a condom, usually made from latex. Latex-free covers are available.

INDICATIONS

- Aid in the diagnosis of micturition disorders.
- Aid in prostate cancer diagnosis.

U

- Assess prostatic calcifications.
- Assist in guided needle biopsy of a suspected tumor.
- Assist in radiation seed placement.
- Determine prostatic cancer staging.
- Detect prostatitis.

POTENTIAL MEDICAL DIAGNOSIS

Normal findings

- Normal size, consistency, and contour of the prostate gland

Abnormal findings related to

Identification of abnormal findings is assisted by comparison of parameters such as size, shape, symmetry, and location; for example, areas of altered echo patterns in either an expected or unexpected location may indicate enlargement of an organ or the presence of blood or other fluids, tumors, or cysts. Comparison by type of abnormal findings may also assist in evaluating areas of altered patterns; for example, small round or oval areas with well-defined borders and clear central areas can differentiate a fluid-filled cyst from a solid tumor.

- Benign prostatic hyperplasia
- Micturition disorders
- Perirectal abscess
- Perirectal tumor
- Prostate abscess
- Prostate cancer
- Prostatitis
- Rectal tumor
- Seminal vesicle tumor

CRITICAL FINDINGS: N/A

INTERFERING FACTORS

Factors that may alter the results of the study

- Attenuation of the sound waves by pelvic bones, which can impair clear imaging of the prostate.
- Incorrect placement of the transducer over the desired test site; quality of the US study is very dependent upon the skill of the ultrasonographer.
- Metallic objects (e.g., jewelry, body rings) within the examination field, which may inhibit organ visualization and cause unclear images.
- Inability of the patient to cooperate or remain still during the procedure because of age, significant pain, or mental status.
- Retained air, barium, or gas from a previous radiological procedure may block the transmission of sound waves.
- Gas or feces in the gastrointestinal tract resulting from inadequate cleansing before the study.
- Patients who are technically difficult and who present challenges in obtaining reliable results (e.g., who are obese; have reduced rib spaces; present with fatty liver; have postoperative incisions, bandages, or dressings; have significant scarring in the area of interest). Aberrations in tissue composition may attenuate the sound waves and alter findings.

Other considerations

- Failure to follow pretesting preparations may cause the procedure to be canceled or repeated.
- The procedure may be canceled if the patient's weight exceeds the safety limit for the equipment.

NURSING IMPLICATIONS AND PROCEDURE

See Potential Nursing Problems on Fast Find at davispl.us/vanleeuwen7.

PRETEST:

- Positively identify the patient using at least two person-specific identifiers before services, treatments, or procedures are performed.

U

- ***Patient Teaching:*** Inform the patient this procedure can assist in evaluating the prostate gland.
- Obtain a history of the patient's health concerns, symptoms, surgical procedures, and results of previously performed laboratory and diagnostic studies. Include a list of known allergens, especially allergies or sensitivities to latex.
- Note any recent procedures that can interfere with test results (e.g., surgery, biopsy, barium studies, colonoscopy, endoscopic retrograde cholangiopancreatography). Ensure that interfering studies were performed at least 24 hr before this test or can be rescheduled after this procedure.
- Obtain a list of the patient's current medications, including over-the-counter medications, dietary supplements, anticoagulants, aspirin and other salicylates (see Effects of Natural Products on Laboratory Values online at Davis*Plus*). Such products should be discontinued by medical direction for the appropriate number of days prior to a surgical procedure. Note the last time and dose of medication taken.
- Review the procedure with the patient. Address concerns about pain related to the procedure and explain that some pain may be experienced during the test, and there may be moments of discomfort. Inform the patient that the procedure is performed in a US department by an HCP who specializes in this procedure, with support staff, and takes approximately 30 to 60 min.
- Inform the patient that a small volume enema will be administered prior to the procedure to help remove gas or feces that could interfere with the rectal probe; after the enema a sterile latex- or sheath-covered probe will be inserted into the rectum.
- ***Sensitivity to social and cultural issues,*** as well as concern for modesty, is important in providing psychological support before, during, and after the procedure.
- Note that there are no food or fluid restrictions unless by medical direction.

INTRATEST:

Potential Complications: N/A

- Observe standard precautions, and follow the general guidelines in Patient Preparation and Specimen Collection online at Davis*Plus*. Positively identify the patient.
- Instruct the patient to void and change into the gown, robe, and foot coverings provided.
- Avoid the use of equipment containing latex if the patient has a history of allergic reaction to latex.
- Instruct the patient to cooperate fully and to follow directions. Ask the patient to remain still throughout the procedure because movement produces unreliable results.
- Place the patient on the examination table on his left side with his knees bent toward the chest; other positions may be used during the examination.
- Expose the rectal area and drape the patient.
- Cover the rectal probe with a lubricated condom and insert it into the rectum. Inform the patient that he may feel slight pressure as the transducer is inserted. Water may be introduced through the sheath surrounding the transducer.
- Ask the patient to breathe normally during the examination. If necessary for better organ visualization, ask the patient to inhale deeply and hold his breath.

POST-TEST:

- Inform the patient that a report of the results will be made available to the requesting HCP, who will discuss the results with the patient.
- When the study is completed, remove the gel from the skin.
- ***Nutritional Considerations:*** There is growing evidence that inflammation and oxidation play key roles in the development of numerous

U

diseases, including prostate cancer. Research also indicates that diets containing dried beans, fresh fruits and vegetables, nuts, spices, whole grains, and smaller amounts of red meats can increase the amount of protective antioxidants. Regular exercise, especially in combination with a healthy diet, can bring about changes in the body's metabolism that decrease inflammation and oxidation.

- Recognize anxiety related to test results. Discuss the implications of abnormal test results on the patient's lifestyle. Provide teaching and information regarding the clinical implications of the test results, as appropriate. Administer antibiotics as ordered, after biopsy. Educate the patient regarding access to counseling services. Provide contact information, if desired, for the Prostate Cancer Foundation (www.prostatecancerfoundation.org).
- Reinforce information given by the patient's HCP regarding further testing, treatment, or referral to another HCP. Answer any questions or address any concerns voiced by the patient or family. Decisions regarding the need for and frequency of routine PSA testing or other cancer screening procedures should be made after consultation between the patient and HCP. Recommendations made by various medical associations and national health organizations regarding prostate cancer screening are moving away from routine PSA screening and toward informed decision making. The American Cancer Society (ACS) recommends that discussions about screening should begin at age 50 yr for men at average risk, 45 yr for men at high risk, and 40 yr for men at the highest risk of developing prostate cancer. The most current guidelines for prostate cancer screening of the general population as well as of individuals with increased risk are available from the ACS (www.cancer.org) and American Urological Association (www.aua.org).
- Depending on the results of this procedure, additional testing may be needed to evaluate or monitor progression of the disease process and determine the need for a change in therapy. Evaluate test results in relation to the patient's symptoms and other tests performed.

Patient Education:

- Reinforce information given by the HCP regarding further testing, treatment, or referral to another HCP.
- Consult the most current guidelines for prostate cancer screening and communicate that information to the patient.

Expected Patient Outcomes:

Understanding

- The patient acknowledges that postoperative urinary incontinence may take up to a year to resolve.
- The patient acknowledges that erectile dysfunction may occur as a postoperative complication.

Ability

- The patient successfully demonstrates the self-administration of a sitz bath.
- The patient correctly describes how to perform Kegel exercises to improve urinary control.

Response

- The patient complies with the request to perform sitz baths to facilitate postoperative healing.
- The patient agrees to meet with the HCP for scheduled follow-up appointments.

RELATED STUDIES:

- Related tests include biopsy prostate, CT pelvis, cystoscopy, cystourethrography voiding, IVP, KUB study, MRI pelvis, proctosigmoidoscopy, PSA, renogram, retrograde ureteropyelography, and semen analysis.
- Refer to the Genitourinary System table online at Davis*Plus* for related tests by body system.

U

Ultrasound, Scrotal

SYNONYM/ACRONYM: Scrotal sonography, ultrasound of the testes, testicular ultrasound.

COMMON USE: To visualize and assess scrotum structure and function toward diagnosing disorders such as tumor, cancer, undescended testes, and chronic inflammation.

AREA OF APPLICATION: Scrotum.

DESCRIPTION: Ultrasound (US) procedures are diagnostic, noninvasive, and relatively inexpensive. They take a short time to complete, do not use radiation, and cause no harm to the patient. High-frequency sound waves of various intensities are delivered by a transducer, a flashlight-shaped device, pressed against the skin. The waves are bounced back off internal anatomical structures and fluids, converted to electrical energy, amplified by the transducer, and displayed as images on a monitor. US is often used as a diagnostic and therapeutic tool for guiding minimally invasive procedures such as needle biopsies and fluid aspiration. The contraindications and complications for biopsy and fluid aspiration are discussed in detail in the individual studies.

Different types of transducers and imaging systems are sometimes used in clinical settings. Conventional US systems assume that sound waves pass through tissue at a constant speed. Advances in technology have led to the development of "smart" transducers that can compensate for tissue aberrations in technically difficult patients. Other advancements in imaging systems include three-dimensional and Doppler US. Color Doppler US uses color to indicate the velocity and direction of blood flow. Power Doppler is a more sensitive Doppler variation, capable of providing detailed images of blood flow; a limitation of power Doppler is that it cannot provide information regarding the direction of blood flow. Spectral Doppler provides data from blood flow measurements in formats other than color—for example, it can convert the measurements into a graph representing distance of blood flow against time or as a unique sound heard with every heartbeat.

Scrotal US is used to evaluate the structure, size, and position of the contents of the scrotum and for the evaluation of disorders of the scrotum. It is valuable in determining the internal components of masses (solid versus cystic) and for the evaluation of the testicle, extratesticular and intrascrotal tissues, benign and malignant tumors, and other scrotal pathology. Scrotal US can be performed before or after a radionuclide scan for further clarification of a testicular mass. Extratesticular lesions such as hydrocele, hematocele (blood in the scrotum), and pyocele (pus in the scrotum) can be identified, as can cryptorchidism (undescended testicles).

This procedure is contraindicated for: N/A

INDICATIONS

- Aid in the diagnosis of a chronic inflammatory condition such as epididymitis.
- Aid in the diagnosis of a mass and differentiate between a cyst and a solid tumor, as evidenced by specific waveform patterns or the absence of sound waves respectively.
- Aid in the diagnosis of scrotal or testicular size, abnormality, or pathology.
- Aid in the diagnosis of testicular torsion and associated testicular infarction.
- Assist guided needle biopsy of a suspected testicle tumor.
- Determine the cause of chronic scrotal swelling or pain.
- Determine the presence of a hydrocele, pyocele, spermatocele, or hernia before surgery.
- Evaluate the effectiveness of treatment for testicular infections.
- Locate an undescended testicle.

POTENTIAL MEDICAL DIAGNOSIS

Normal findings

- Normal size, position, and shape of the scrotum and structure of the testes

Abnormal findings related to

Identification of abnormal findings is assisted by comparison of parameters such as size, shape, symmetry, and location; for example, areas of altered echo patterns in either an expected or unexpected location may indicate enlargement of an organ or the presence of blood or other fluids, tumors, or cysts. Comparison by type of abnormal findings may also assist in evaluating areas of altered patterns; for example, small round or oval areas with well-defined borders and clear central areas can differentiate a fluid-filled cyst from a solid tumor.

- Abscess
- Epididymal cyst
- Epididymitis
- Hematoma
- Hydrocele
- Infarction
- Microlithiasis
- Orchitis
- Pyocele
- Scrotal hernia
- Spermatocele
- Testicular torsion
- Tumor, benign or malignant
- Tunica albuginea cyst
- Undescended testicle (cryptorchidism)
- Varicocele

CRITICAL FINDINGS:

- Testicular torsion

Note and immediately report to the requesting health-care provider (HCP) any critical findings and related symptoms. A listing of these findings varies among facilities. Timely notification of a critical finding for laboratory or diagnostic studies is a role expectation of the professional nurse. The notification processes vary among facilities. Upon receipt of the critical finding, the information should be read back to the caller to verify accuracy.

INTERFERING FACTORS

Factors that may alter the results of the study

- Incorrect placement of the transducer over the desired test site; quality of the US study is very dependent upon the skill of the ultrasonographer.
- Metallic objects (e.g., jewelry, body rings) within the examination field, which may inhibit organ visualization and cause unclear images.

- Inability of the patient to cooperate or remain still during the procedure because of age, significant pain, or mental status.
- Patients who are technically difficult and who present challenges in obtaining reliable results (e.g., who are obese; have reduced rib spaces; present with fatty liver; have postoperative incisions, bandages, or dressings; have significant scarring in the area of interest). Aberrations in tissue composition may attenuate the sound waves and alter findings.

Other considerations

- The procedure may be canceled if the patient's weight exceeds the safety limit for the equipment.

NURSING IMPLICATIONS AND PROCEDURE

See Potential Nursing Problems on Fast Find at davispl.us/vanleeuwen7.

PRETEST:

- Positively identify the patient using at least two person-specific identifiers before services, treatments, or procedures are performed.
- ***Patient Teaching:*** Inform the patient this procedure can assist in assessing the scrotum.
- Obtain a history of the patient's health concerns, symptoms, surgical procedures, and results of previously performed laboratory and diagnostic studies. Include a list of known allergens, especially allergies or sensitivities to latex.
- Note any recent procedures that can interfere with test results (e.g., surgery or biopsy).
- Obtain a list of the patient's current medications, including over-the-counter medications and dietary supplements (see Effects of Natural Products on Laboratory Values online at Davis*Plus*).
- Review the procedure with the patient. Address concerns about pain related to the procedure and explain that some pain may be experienced during the test, and there may be moments of discomfort. Inform the patient that the procedure is performed in a US department, by a health-care provider (HCP) who specializes in this procedure, with support staff, and takes approximately 30 to 60 min.
- ***Sensitivity to social and cultural issues,*** as well as concern for modesty, is important in providing psychological support before, during, and after the procedure.
- Instruct the patient to remove jewelry and other metallic objects from the area to be examined.
- Note that there are no food, fluid, or medication restrictions unless by medical direction.

INTRATEST:

Potential Complications: N/A

- Observe standard precautions, and follow the general guidelines in Patient Preparation and Specimen Collection online at Davis*Plus*. Positively identify the patient.
- Ensure that the patient has removed all external metallic objects from the area to be examined prior to the procedure.
- Instruct the patient to void and change into the gown, robe, and foot coverings provided.
- Avoid the use of equipment containing latex if the patient has a history of allergic reaction to latex.
- Instruct the patient to cooperate fully and to follow directions. Ask the patient to remain still throughout the procedure because movement produces unreliable results.
- Place the patient in the supine position on an examination table; other positions may be used during the examination.
- Expose the abdomen/pelvic area and drape the patient.
- Lift the penis upward and gently tape it to the lower part of the abdomen. Elevate the scrotum with a rolled towel or sponge for immobilization.

U

- Conductive gel is applied to the skin, and a transducer is moved over the skin to obtain images of the area of interest.
- Ask the patient to breathe normally during the examination. If necessary for better organ visualization, ask the patient to inhale deeply and hold his breath.

POST-TEST:

- Inform the patient that a report of the results will be made available to the requesting HCP, who will discuss the results with the patient.
- When the study is completed, remove the gel from the skin.
- Recognize anxiety related to test results. Discuss the implications of abnormal test results on the patient's lifestyle. Provide teaching and information regarding the clinical implications of the test results, as appropriate.
- Reinforce information given by the patient's HCP regarding further testing, treatment, or referral to another HCP. Answer any questions or address any concerns voiced by the patient or family.
- Depending on the results of this procedure, additional testing may be needed to evaluate or monitor progression of the disease process and determine the need for a change in therapy. Evaluate test results in relation to the patient's symptoms and other tests performed.

Patient Education:

- Provide information on disease signs and symptoms and management.
- Provide preoperative teaching as appropriate.

Expected Patient Outcomes:

Understanding

- The patient acknowledges and is able to discuss prognosis and treatment options.
- The patient states possible diagnostic and laboratory studies associated with disease management.

Ability

- The patient demonstrates positive coping strategies.
- The patient successfully demonstrates care of surgical site.

Response

- The patient agrees to attend cancer support group meetings.
- The patient agrees to seek psychological counseling to adjust to body changes and intimacy concerns.

RELATED STUDIES:

- Related tests include AFP, CT pelvis, KUB study, MRI pelvis, and semen analysis.
- Refer to the Reproductive System table online at Davis*Plus* for related tests by body system.

Ultrasound, Spleen

SYNONYM/ACRONYM: Spleen ultrasonography.

COMMON USE: To visualize and assess the spleen for abscess, trauma, rupture, cancer, and tumor. Also used to evaluate the effectiveness of therapeutic interventions and assist with guided biopsy.

AREA OF APPLICATION: Spleen/left upper quadrant.

DESCRIPTION: Ultrasound (US) procedures are diagnostic, noninvasive, and relatively inexpensive. They take a short time to complete, do not use radiation, and cause no harm to the patient.

High-frequency sound waves of various intensities are delivered by a transducer, a flashlight-shaped device, pressed against the skin. The waves are bounced back off internal anatomical structures and fluids, converted to electrical energy, amplified by the transducer, and displayed as images on a monitor. US is often used as a diagnostic and therapeutic tool for guiding minimally invasive procedures such as needle biopsies and fluid aspiration. The contraindications and complications for biopsy and fluid aspiration are discussed in detail in the individual studies.

Different types of transducers and imaging systems are sometimes used in clinical settings. Conventional US systems assume that sound waves pass through tissue at a constant speed. Advances in technology have led to the development of "smart" transducers that can compensate for tissue aberrations in technically difficult patients. Other advancements in imaging systems include three-dimensional and Doppler US. Color Doppler US uses color to indicate the velocity and direction of blood flow. Power Doppler is a more sensitive Doppler variation, capable of providing detailed images of blood flow; a limitation of power Doppler is that it cannot provide information regarding the direction of blood flow. Spectral Doppler provides data from blood flow measurements in formats other than color—for example, it can convert the measurements into a graph representing distance of blood flow against time or as a unique sound heard with every heartbeat.

Spleen US is used to evaluate the structure, size, and position of the spleen. This test is valuable for determining the internal components of splenic masses (solid versus cystic) and evaluating other splenic pathology, splenic trauma, and left upper quadrant perisplenic tissues. It can be performed to supplement a radionuclide scan or computed tomography (CT). It is especially valuable in patients who are in renal failure, are hypersensitive to contrast medium, or are pregnant, because it does not rely on adequate kidney function or the injection of contrast medium to obtain a diagnosis.

This procedure is contraindicated for: N/A

INDICATIONS

- Detect the presence of a subphrenic abscess after splenectomy.
- Detect splenic masses; differentiate between cysts or solid tumors (in combination with CT), as evidenced by specific waveform patterns or absence of sound waves respectively; and determine whether they are intrasplenic or extrasplenic.
- Determine late-stage sickle cell disease, as evidenced by decreased spleen size and presence of echoes.
- Determine the presence of splenomegaly and assess the size and volume of the spleen in these cases, as evidenced by increased echoes and visibility of the spleen.
- Differentiate spleen trauma from blood or fluid accumulation between the splenic capsule and parenchyma.
- Evaluate the effect of medical or surgical therapy on the progression or resolution of splenic disease.

- Evaluate the extent of abdominal trauma and spleen involvement, including enlargement or rupture, after a recent trauma.
- Evaluate the spleen before splenectomy performed for thrombocytopenic purpura.

POTENTIAL MEDICAL DIAGNOSIS

Normal findings

- Normal size, position, and contour of the spleen and associated structures

Abnormal findings related to

Identification of abnormal findings is assisted by comparison of parameters such as size, shape, symmetry, and location; for example, areas of altered echo patterns in either an expected or unexpected location may indicate enlargement of an organ or the presence of blood or other fluids, tumors, or cysts. Comparison by type of abnormal findings may also assist in evaluating areas of altered patterns; for example, small round or oval areas with well-defined borders and clear central areas can differentiate a fluid-filled cyst from a solid tumor.

- Abscess
- Accessory or ectopic spleen
- Infection
- Lymphatic disease; lymph node enlargement
- Splenic calcifications
- Splenic masses, tumors, cysts, or infarction
- Splenic trauma
- Splenomegaly

CRITICAL FINDINGS: N/A

INTERFERING FACTORS

Factors that may alter the results of the study

- Attenuation of the sound waves by bony structures, which can impair clear imaging in the area of interest.
- Incorrect placement of the transducer over the desired test site; quality of the US study is very dependent upon the skill of the ultrasonographer.
- Metallic objects (e.g., jewelry, body rings) within the examination field, which may inhibit organ visualization and cause unclear images.
- Inability of the patient to cooperate or remain still during the procedure because of age, significant pain, or mental status.
- Masses near the testing site, which can displace the spleen and cause inaccurate results if confused with splenomegaly.
- Retained air, barium, or gas from a previous radiological procedure may block the transmission of sound waves.
- Gas or feces in the gastrointestinal tract resulting from inadequate cleansing or failure to restrict food intake before the study.
- Patients who are technically difficult and who present challenges in obtaining reliable results (e.g., who are obese; have reduced rib spaces; present with fatty liver; have postoperative incisions, bandages, or dressings; have significant scarring in the area of interest). Aberrations in tissue composition may attenuate the sound waves and alter findings.

Other considerations

- Failure to follow dietary restrictions and other pretesting preparations may cause the procedure to be canceled or repeated.
- The procedure may be canceled if the patient's weight exceeds the safety limit for the equipment.

NURSING IMPLICATIONS AND PROCEDURE

PRETEST:

- Positively identify the patient using at least two person-specific identifiers before services, treatments, or procedures are performed.
- ***Patient Teaching:*** Inform the patient this procedure can assist in assessing the function of the spleen.
- Obtain a history of the patient's health concerns, symptoms, surgical procedures, and results of previously performed laboratory and diagnostic studies. Include a list of known allergens, especially allergies or sensitivities to latex.
- Note any recent procedures that can interfere with test results (e.g., surgery, biopsy, barium studies, colonoscopy, endoscopic retrograde cholangiopancreatography). Ensure that interfering studies were performed at least 24 hr before this test or can be rescheduled after this procedure.
- Obtain a list of the patient's current medications, including over-the-counter medications and dietary supplements (see Effects of Natural Products on Laboratory Values online at Davis*Plus*).
- Review the procedure with the patient. Address concerns about pain related to the procedure and explain that some pain may be experienced during the test, and there may be moments of discomfort. Inform the patient that the procedure is performed in a US department by a health-care provider (HCP) who specializes in this procedure, with support staff, and takes approximately 30 to 60 min.
- ***Sensitivity to social and cultural issues,*** as well as concern for modesty, is important in providing psychological support before, during, and after the procedure.
- Instruct the patient to remove jewelry and other metallic objects in the area to be examined.
- Instruct the patient to fast and restrict fluids for 8 hr prior to the procedure. Food restrictions help ensure reduction of bowel gas, which can interfere with the transmission of US waves. Protocols may vary among facilities.

INTRATEST:

Potential Complications: N/A

- Observe standard precautions, and follow the general guidelines in Patient Preparation and Specimen Collection online at Davis*Plus*. Positively identify the patient.
- Ensure that food and fluids have been restricted prior to the procedure, as instructed.
- Ensure that the patient has removed all external metallic objects in the area prior to the procedure.
- Instruct the patient to void and change into the gown, robe, and foot coverings provided.
- Avoid the use of equipment containing latex if the patient has a history of allergic reaction to latex.
- Instruct the patient to cooperate fully and to follow directions. Ask the patient to remain still throughout the procedure because movement produces unreliable results.
- Place the patient in the supine position on an examination table. The right- or left-side-up position may be used to allow gravity to reposition the liver, gas, and fluid to facilitate better organ visualization.
- Expose the abdominal area and drape the patient.
- Conductive gel is applied to the skin, and a transducer is moved over the skin to obtain images of the area of interest.
- Ask the patient to breathe normally during the examination. If necessary for better organ visualization, ask the patient to inhale deeply and hold his or her breath.

POST-TEST:

- Inform the patient that a report of the results will be made available to the requesting HCP, who will discuss the results with the patient.

- When the study is completed, remove the gel from the skin.
- Instruct the patient to resume usual diet and fluids, as directed by the HCP.
- Recognize anxiety related to test results. Discuss the implications of abnormal test results on the patient's lifestyle. Provide teaching and information regarding the clinical implications of the test results, as appropriate.
- Reinforce information given by the patient's HCP regarding further testing, treatment, or referral to another HCP. Answer any questions or address any concerns voiced by the patient or family.
- Depending on the results of this procedure, additional testing may be performed to evaluate or monitor progression of the disease process and determine the need for a change in therapy. Evaluate test results in relation to the patient's symptoms and other tests performed.

RELATED STUDIES:

- Related tests include angiography abdomen, biopsy bone marrow, CBC platelet count, CBC WBC and differential, CT abdomen, KUB study, liver and spleen scan, MRI abdomen, sickle cell screen, US abdomen, and WBC scan.
- Refer to the Hematopoietic System table online at Davis*Plus* for related tests by body system.

Ultrasound, Thyroid and Parathyroid

SYNONYM/ACRONYM: Parathyroid sonography, thyroid echo, thyroid sonography.

COMMON USE: To visualize and assess the thyroid and parathyroid glands for tumor, cancer, and cyst. Also used to stage cancer, guide biopsies, and monitor the effectiveness of therapeutic interventions.

AREA OF APPLICATION: Anterior neck region, parathyroid, thyroid.

DESCRIPTION: Ultrasound (US) procedures are diagnostic, noninvasive, and relatively inexpensive. They take a short time to complete, do not use radiation, and cause no harm to the patient. High-frequency sound waves of various intensities are delivered by a transducer, a flashlight-shaped device, pressed against the skin. The waves are bounced back off internal anatomical structures and fluids, converted to electrical energy, amplified by the transducer, and displayed as images on a monitor. US is often used as a diagnostic and therapeutic tool for guiding minimally invasive procedures such as needle biopsies and fluid aspiration. The contraindications and complications for biopsy and fluid aspiration are discussed in detail in the individual studies.

Different types of transducers and imaging systems are sometimes used in clinical settings. Conventional US systems assume that sound waves pass through tissue at a constant speed. Advances in technology have led to the development of "smart" transducers that can compensate for tissue aberrations in technically difficult patients. Other advancements in imaging systems include three-dimensional and Doppler US. Color Doppler US

U

uses color to indicate the velocity and direction of blood flow. Power Doppler is a more sensitive Doppler variation, capable of providing detailed images of blood flow; a limitation of power Doppler is that it cannot provide information regarding the direction of blood flow. Spectral Doppler provides data from blood flow measurements in formats other than color—for example, it can convert the measurements into a graph representing distance of blood flow against time or as a unique sound heard with every heartbeat.

Thyroid and parathyroid US is used to determine the position, size, shape, weight, and presence of masses of the thyroid gland; enlargement of the parathyroid glands; and other abnormalities of the thyroid and parathyroid glands and surrounding tissues. The primary purpose of this procedure is to determine whether a nodule is a fluid-filled cyst (usually benign) or a solid tumor (possibly malignant). This procedure is useful in evaluating the glands' response to medical treatment or assessing the remaining tissue after surgical resection. US is clearly the procedure of choice when examining the glands of pregnant patients. This procedure is usually done in combination with nuclear medicine imaging procedures and computed tomography (CT) of the neck. Despite the advantages of the procedure, in some cases it may not detect small nodules and lesions (less than 1 cm), leading to false-negative findings.

This procedure is contraindicated for: N/A

INDICATIONS

- Assist in determining the presence of a tumor, as evidenced by an irregular border and shadowing at the distal edge, peripheral echoes, or high- and low-amplitude echoes, depending on the density of the tumor mass; and diagnosing tumor type (e.g., benign, adenoma, carcinoma).
- Assist in diagnosing the presence of a cyst, as evidenced by a smoothly outlined, echo-free amplitude except at the far borders of the mass.
- Assist in diagnosis in the presence of a parathyroid enlargement indicating a tumor or hyperplasia, as evidenced by an echo pattern of lower amplitude than that for a thyroid tumor.
- Determine the need for surgical biopsy of a tumor or fine-needle biopsy of a cyst.
- Differentiate among a nodule, solid tumor, or fluid-filled cyst.
- Evaluate the effect of a therapeutic regimen for a thyroid mass or Graves' disease by determining the size and weight of the gland.
- Evaluate thyroid abnormalities during pregnancy (mother or baby).

POTENTIAL MEDICAL DIAGNOSIS

Normal findings

- Normal size, position, contour, and structure of the thyroid and parathyroid glands with uniform echo patterns throughout the glands; no evidence of tumor cysts or nodules in the glands

Abnormal findings related to

Identification of abnormal findings is assisted by comparison of parameters such as size, shape, symmetry, and location; for example, areas of altered echo patterns in either an expected or unexpected location may indicate enlargement of an organ or the presence of

U

blood or other fluids, tumors, or cysts. Comparison by type of abnormal findings may also assist in evaluating areas of altered patterns; for example, small round or oval areas with well-defined borders and clear central areas can differentiate a fluid-filled cyst from a solid tumor.

- Glandular enlargement
- Goiter
- Graves' disease
- Parathyroid tumor or hyperplasia
- Thyroid cysts
- Thyroid tumors (benign or malignant)

CRITICAL FINDINGS: N/A

INTERFERING FACTORS

Factors that may alter the results of the study

- Attenuation of the sound waves by bony structures, which can impair clear imaging in the area of interest.
- Incorrect placement of the transducer over the desired test site; quality of the US study is very dependent upon the skill of the ultrasonographer.
- Metallic objects (e.g., jewelry, body rings) within the examination field, which may inhibit organ visualization and cause unclear images.
- Inability of the patient to cooperate or remain still during the procedure because of age, significant pain, or mental status.
- Retained air, barium, or gas from a previous radiological procedure may block the transmission of sound waves.
- Patients who are technically difficult and who present challenges in obtaining reliable results (e.g., who are obese; have reduced rib spaces; present with fatty liver; have postoperative incisions, bandages, or dressings; have significant scarring in the area of interest).

Aberrations in tissue composition may attenuate the sound waves and alter findings.

Other considerations

- The procedure may be canceled if the patient's weight exceeds the safety limit for the equipment.
- Nodules less than 1 cm in diameter may not be detected.
- Nonthyroid cysts may appear the same as thyroid cysts.

NURSING IMPLICATIONS AND PROCEDURE

See Potential Nursing Problems on Fast Find at davispl.us/vanleeuwen7.

PRETEST:

- Positively identify the patient using at least two person-specific identifiers before services, treatments, or procedures are performed.
- ***Patient Teaching:*** Inform the patient this procedure can assist in assessing thyroid and parathyroid gland function.
- Obtain a history of the patient's health concerns, symptoms, surgical procedures, and results of previously performed laboratory and diagnostic studies. Include a list of known allergens, especially allergies or sensitivities to latex.
- Note any recent procedures that can interfere with test results (e.g., surgery, biopsy, barium studies, surgery, or biopsy). There should be 24 hr between administration of barium and this test.
- Obtain a list of the patient's current medications, including over-the-counter medications and dietary supplements (see Effects of Natural Products on Laboratory Values online at Davis*Plus*).
- Review the procedure with the patient. Address concerns about pain related to the procedure and explain that some pain may be experienced during the test, and there may be moments of discomfort. Inform the patient that

U

the procedure is performed in a US department by a health-care provider (HCP) who specializes in this procedure with support staff, and takes approximately 30 to 60 min.

- ***Sensitivity to social and cultural issues,*** as well as concern for modesty, is important in providing psychological support before, during, and after the procedure.
- Instruct the patient to remove jewelry and other metallic objects from the area to be examined.
- Note that there are no food, fluid, or medication restrictions unless by medical direction.

INTRATEST:

Potential Complications: N/A

- Observe standard precautions, and follow the general guidelines in Patient Preparation and Specimen Collection online at Davis*Plus*. Positively identify the patient.
- Ensure that the patient has removed all external metallic objects from the area to be examined prior to the procedure.
- Instruct the patient to void and change into the gown, robe, and foot coverings provided.
- Avoid the use of equipment containing latex if the patient has a history of allergic reaction to latex.
- Instruct the patient to cooperate fully and to follow directions. Ask the patient to remain still throughout the procedure because movement produces unreliable results.
- Place the patient in the supine position on an examination table; other positions may be used during the examination.
- Expose the neck and chest area and drape the patient.
- Hyperextend the neck, and place a pillow under the patient's shoulders to maintain a comfortable position. (An alternative method of imaging includes the use of a bag filled with water or gel placed over the neck area.)
- Conductive gel is applied to the skin, and a transducer is moved over the skin to obtain images of the area of interest.
- Ask the patient to breathe normally during the examination. If necessary for better organ visualization, ask the patient to inhale deeply and hold his or her breath.

POST-TEST:

- Inform the patient that a report of the results will be made available to the requesting HCP, who will discuss the results with the patient.
- When the study is completed, remove the gel from the skin.
- Recognize anxiety related to test results. Discuss the implications of abnormal test results on the patient's lifestyle. Provide teaching and information regarding the clinical implications of the test results, as appropriate.
- Reinforce information given by the patient's HCP regarding further testing, treatment, or referral to another HCP. Answer any questions or address any concerns voiced by the patient or family.
- Depending on the results of this procedure, additional testing may be performed to evaluate or monitor progression of the disease process and determine the need for a change in therapy. Evaluate test results in relation to the patient's symptoms and other tests performed.

Patient Education:

- Teach the patient the pathophysiology associated with cancer, disease, as well as ongoing treatment and screenings.
- Explain that an HCP specialist may need to be consulted to manage the disease.

Expected Patient Outcomes:

Understanding

- The patient and family discuss the medical versus surgical options for disease management.
- The patient and family acknowledge end-of-life treatment options as appropriate.

U

Ability

- The patient and family demonstrate positive coping strategies.
- The patient and family successfully demonstrate care of surgical site, biopsy site.

Response

- The patient and family agree to attend disease-specific support group meetings.
- The patient agrees to seek psychological counseling to adjust to lifestyle changes associated with positive therapeutic management strategies.

RELATED STUDIES:

- Related tests include antibodies antithyroglobulin, biopsy thyroid, chest x-ray, CT thorax, MRI chest, PTH, parathyroid scan, radioactive iodine uptake, thyroid-binding inhibitory immunoglobulin, thyroglobulin, thyroid scan, TSH, thyroxine free, thyroxine total, triiodothyronine free, and triiodothyronine total.
- Refer to the Endocrine System table online at Davis*Plus* for related tests by body system.

Ultrasound, Venous Doppler, Extremity Studies

SYNONYM/ACRONYM: Vascular ultrasound, venous duplex, venous sonogram, venous ultrasound.

COMMON USE: To assess venous blood flow in the upper and lower extremities toward diagnosing disorders such as deep vein thrombosis, venous insufficiency, causation of pulmonary embolism, varicose veins, and monitor the effects of therapeutic interventions

AREA OF APPLICATION: Veins of the upper and lower extremities.

DESCRIPTION: Ultrasound (US) procedures are diagnostic, noninvasive, and relatively inexpensive. They take a short time to complete, do not use radiation, and cause no harm to the patient. High-frequency sound waves of various intensities are delivered by a transducer, a flashlight-shaped device, pressed against the skin. The waves are bounced back off internal anatomical structures and fluids, converted to electrical energy, amplified by the transducer, and displayed as images on a monitor. US is often used as a diagnostic and therapeutic tool for guiding minimally invasive procedures such as needle biopsies and fluid aspiration. The contraindications and complications for biopsy and fluid aspiration are discussed in detail in the individual studies.

Ultrasound (US) procedures are used to obtain information about the patency of the venous vasculature in the upper and lower extremities to identify narrowing or occlusions of the veins or arteries. In venous Doppler studies, the Doppler identifies moving red blood cells (RBCs) within the vein. The US beam is directed at the vein and through the Doppler transducer while the RBCs reflect the beam back to the transducer. The reflected sound waves or echoes are transformed by a computer into scans, graphs, or audible sounds. Blood flow direction, velocity, and the presence of flow disturbances can be readily assessed. The velocity of the blood flow is transformed as a "swishing" noise, audible through the audio speaker. If the vein is occluded, no swishing sound is heard. For diagnostic studies, the procedure is done bilaterally. The sound emitted by the equipment corresponds to the velocity of the blood flow through the vessel occurring with spontaneous respirations. Changes in these sounds during respirations indicate the possibility of abnormal venous flow secondary to occlusive disease; the absence of sound indicates complete obstruction. Compression with a transducer augments a vessel for evaluation of thrombosis. Noncompressibility of the vessel indicates a thrombosis. Plethysmography may be performed to determine the filling time of calf veins to diagnose thrombotic disorder of a major vein and to identify incompetent valves in the venous system. An additional method used to evaluate incompetent valves is the Valsalva technique combined with venous duplex imaging.

The ankle-brachial index (ABI) can also be assessed during this study. This noninvasive, simple comparison of blood pressure measurements in the arms and legs can be used to detect peripheral arterial disease (PAD). A Doppler stethoscope is used to obtain the systolic pressure in either the dorsalis pedis or the posterior tibial artery. This ankle pressure is then divided by the highest brachial systolic pressure acquired after taking the blood pressure in both of the patient's arms. This index should be greater than 1 with a range of 0.85 to 1.4. When the index falls below 0.5, blood flow impairment is considered significant. Patients should be scheduled for a vascular consult for an abnormal ABI. Patients with diabetes or kidney disease, and some older adult patients, may have a falsely elevated ABI due to calcifications of the vessels in the ankle causing an increased systolic pressure. The ABI test approaches 95% accuracy in detecting PAD. However, a normal ABI value does not absolutely rule out the possibility of PAD for some individuals, and additional tests should be done to evaluate symptoms.

This procedure is contraindicated for: N/A

INDICATIONS

- Aid in the diagnosis of venous occlusion secondary to thrombosis or thrombophlebitis.
- Aid in the diagnosis of superficial thrombosis or deep vein thrombosis (DVT) leading to venous occlusion or obstruction, as evidenced by absence of venous flow, especially upon augmentation of the extremity; variations in flow during respirations; or failure of the veins to compress completely when the extremity is compressed.
- Detect chronic venous insufficiency, as evidenced by reverse blood flow indicating incompetent valves.
- Determine if further diagnostic procedures are needed to make or confirm a diagnosis.
- Determine the source of emboli when pulmonary embolism is suspected or diagnosed.

U

- Determine venous damage after trauma to the site.
- Differentiate between primary and secondary varicose veins.
- Evaluate the patency of the venous system in patients with a swollen, painful leg.
- Evaluate peripheral vascular disease (PVD).
- Monitor the effectiveness of therapeutic interventions.

POTENTIAL MEDICAL DIAGNOSIS

Normal findings

- Normal Doppler venous signal that occurs spontaneously with the patient's respiration
- Normal blood flow through the veins of the extremities with no evidence of vessel occlusion

Abnormal findings related to

- Chronic venous insufficiency
- Primary varicose veins
- PVD
- Recannulization in the area of an old thrombus
- Secondary varicose veins
- Superficial thrombosis or DVT
- Venous narrowing or occlusion secondary to thrombosis or thrombophlebitis
- Venous trauma

CRITICAL FINDINGS:

- DVT

Note and immediately report to the requesting health-care provider (HCP) any critical findings and related symptoms. A listing of these findings varies among facilities. Timely notification of a critical finding for laboratory or diagnostic studies is a role expectation of the professional nurse. The notification processes vary among facilities. Upon receipt of the critical finding, the information should be read back to the caller to verify accuracy.

INTERFERING FACTORS

- Patients with an open or draining lesion.

Factors that may alter the results of the study

- Attenuation of the sound waves by bony structures, which can impair clear imaging of the vessels.
- Incorrect placement of the transducer over the desired test site; quality of the US study is very dependent upon the skill of the ultrasonographer.
- Metallic objects (e.g., jewelry, body rings) within the examination field, which may inhibit organ visualization and cause unclear images.
- Inability of the patient to cooperate or remain still during the procedure because of age, significant pain, or mental status.
- Patients who are technically difficult and who present challenges in obtaining reliable results (e.g., who are obese; have reduced rib spaces; present with fatty liver; have postoperative incisions, bandages, or dressings; have significant scarring in the area of interest). Aberrations in tissue composition may attenuate the sound waves and alter findings.

Other considerations

- Cigarette smoking, because nicotine can cause constriction of the peripheral vessels.
- Cold extremities, resulting in vasoconstriction that can cause inaccurate measurements.
- Occlusion proximal to the site being studied, which would affect blood flow to the area.
- An abnormally large or swollen leg, making sonic penetration difficult.
- The procedure may be canceled if the patient's weight exceeds the safety limit for the equipment.

U

NURSING IMPLICATIONS AND PROCEDURE

See Potential Nursing Problems on Fast Find at davispl.us/vanleeuwen7.

PRETEST:

- Positively identify the patient using at least two person-specific identifiers before services, treatments, or procedures are performed.
- ***Patient Teaching:*** Inform the patient this procedure can assist in assessing the veins.
- Obtain a history of the patient's health concerns, symptoms, surgical procedures, and results of previously performed laboratory and diagnostic studies. Include a list of known allergens, especially allergies or sensitivities to latex.
- Report the presence of a lesion that is open or draining; maintain clean, dry dressing for the ulcer; protect the limb from trauma.
- Note any recent procedures that can interfere with test results (e.g., surgery, biopsy, barium studies, colonoscopy, endoscopic retrograde cholangiopancreatography). Ensure that interfering studies were performed at least 24 hr before this test or can be rescheduled after this procedure.
- Obtain a list of the patient's current medications, including over-the-counter medications and dietary supplements (see Effects of Natural Products on Laboratory Values online at Davis).
- Review the procedure with the patient. Address concerns about pain related to the procedure and explain that some pain may be experienced during the test, and there may be moments of discomfort. Inform the patient that the procedure is performed in a US department by a health-care provider (HCP) who specializes in this procedure, with support staff, and takes approximately 30 to 60 min.
- ***Sensitivity to social and cultural issues,*** as well as concern for modesty, is important in providing psychological support before, during, and after the procedure.
- Instruct the patient to remove jewelry and other metallic objects from the area to be examined.
- Note that there are no food, fluid, or medication restrictions unless by medical direction. Some protocols may require the patient to restrict nicotine and caffeine for 1 to 2 hr before the procedure in order to avoid vasoconstriction or vasodilation.

INTRATEST:

Potential Complications: N/A

- Observe standard precautions, and follow the general guidelines in *Plus*Patient Preparation and Specimen Collection online at Davis*Plus*. Positively identify the patient.
- Ensure that the patient has removed all external metallic objects from the area to be examined prior to the procedure.
- Avoid the use of equipment containing latex if the patient has a history of allergic reaction to latex.
- Instruct the patient to void and change into the gown, robe, and foot coverings provided.
- Instruct the patient to cooperate fully and to follow directions. Ask the patient to remain still throughout the procedure because movement produces unreliable results.
- Place the patient in the supine position on an examination table; other positions may be used during the examination.
- Expose the area of interest and drape the patient.
- Conductive gel is applied to the skin, and a transducer is moved over the area to obtain images of the area of interest. Waveforms are visualized and recorded with variations in respirations. Images with and without compression are performed proximally or distally to an obstruction to obtain information about a venous occlusion or obstruction. The procedure can be performed for both arms and

U

legs to obtain bilateral blood flow determination.

- Do not place the transducer on an ulcer site when there is evidence of venous stasis or ulcer.
- Ask the patient to breathe normally during the examination. If necessary for better organ visualization, ask the patient to inhale deeply and hold his or her breath.

POST-TEST:

- Inform the patient that a report of the results will be made available to the requesting HCP, who will discuss the results with the patient.
- When the study is completed, remove the gel from the skin.
- Instruct the patient to continue diet, fluids, and medications, as directed by the HCP.
- Recognize anxiety related to test results, and be supportive of fear of shortened life expectancy. Discuss the implications of abnormal test results on the patient's lifestyle. Provide teaching and information regarding the clinical implications of the test results, as appropriate. Educate the patient regarding access to counseling services.
- Reinforce information given by the patient's HCP regarding further testing, treatment, or referral to another HCP. Answer any questions or address any concerns voiced by the patient or family.
- Depending on the results of this procedure, additional testing may be needed to evaluate or monitor progression of the disease process and determine the need for a change in therapy. Evaluate test results in relation to the patient's symptoms and other tests performed.

Patient Education:

- Teach the patient to refrain from sitting with the knees crossed.

Expected Patient Outcomes:

Understanding

- The patient acknowledges the importance of refraining from standing for a long time.
- The patient acknowledges the importance of frequently changing position.

Ability

- The patient makes diet choices that will result in weight reduction.
- The patient correctly self-administers diuretics.

Response

- The patient agrees to call for assistance when getting out of bed to decrease fall risk.
- The patient agrees to consider an appropriate exercise program.

RELATED STUDIES:

- Related tests include alveolar/arterial ratio, angiography pulmonary, blood gases, CBC platelet count, CT angiography, D-dimer, FDP, fibrinogen, lung perfusion scan, lung ventilation scan, MRI abdomen, MRI angiography, MRI venography, aPTT, plethysmography, PT/INR, US arterial Doppler lower and upper extremity studies, and venography lower extremities.
- Refer to the Cardiovascular System table online at Davis*Plus* for related tests by body system.

Upper Gastrointestinal and Small Bowel Series

SYNONYM/ACRONYM: Gastric radiography, stomach series, small bowel study, upper GI series, UGI.

COMMON USE: To assess the esophagus, stomach, and small bowel for disorders related to obstruction, perforation, weight loss, swallowing, pain, cancer, reflux disease, ulcers, and structural anomalies.

U

AREA OF APPLICATION: Esophagus, stomach, and small intestine.

DESCRIPTION: The upper gastrointestinal (GI) series is a radiological examination of the esophagus, stomach, and small intestine after ingestion of barium sulfate, which is a milkshake-like, radiopaque substance. A combination of x-ray and fluoroscopy techniques are used to record the study. Air or gas may be instilled to provide double contrast and better visualization of the lumen of the esophagus, stomach, and duodenum. If perforation or obstruction is suspected, a water-soluble iodinated contrast medium is used. This test is especially useful in the evaluation of patients experiencing dysphagia, regurgitation, gastroesophageal reflux (GER), epigastric pain, hematemesis, melena, and unexplained weight loss. This test is also used to evaluate the results of gastric surgery, especially when an anastomotic leak is suspected. When a small bowel series is included, the test detects disorders of the jejunum and ileum. The patient's position is changed during the examination to allow visualization of the various structures and their function. Images of the swallowed contrast medium as it moves through the digestive system are visualized on a fluoroscopic screen, recorded, and stored electronically for review. Drugs such as glucagon may be given during an upper GI series to relax the GI tract; drugs such as metoclopramide (Reglan) may be given to accelerate the passage of the barium through the stomach and small intestine.

When the small bowel series is performed separately, the patient may be asked to drink several glasses of barium, or enteroclysis may be used to instill the barium. With enteroclysis, a catheter is passed through the nose or mouth and advanced past the pylorus and into the duodenum. Barium, followed by methylcellulose solution, is instilled via the catheter directly into the small bowel.

Pediatrics: An upper GI series is usually done in the pediatric population to diagnose the cause of recurrent GI signs (bleeding) and symptoms. The etiology is often related to age. In infants, recurrent symptoms such as vomiting after feeding, poor feeding, poor weight gain, and abdominal pain (evidenced by frequent crying during or after a feeding) may trigger an investigation. The most common causes of upper or lower GI bleeding in infants up to 1 mo include allergies to milk proteins, anorectal fissures, bacterial enteritis, coagulopathy, esophagitis, Hirschsprung's disease, intussusception, peptic ulcer, stenosis, varices, or Meckel's diverticulum. Children between 2 to 23 mo are most commonly diagnosed with allergies to milk proteins, anorectal fissures, esophagitis caused by gastroesophageal reflux (GER), gastritis, intussusception, Meckel's diverticulum, NSAID-induced ulcer, and ingested foreign body. Pediatric patients 24 mo and older are most commonly diagnosed with esophageal varices, Mallory Weiss tears, peptic ulcer, related to *Helicobacter pylori* infection or peptic ulcer secondary to some other type of systemic disease (e.g., Crohn's disease or inflammatory bowel disease [IBD]). Other abnormal findings in this age group include IBD, polyps, malignancy, sepsis, and Meckel's diverticulum.

This procedure is contraindicated for

- Patients who are pregnant or suspected of being pregnant, unless the potential benefits of a procedure using radiation far outweigh the risk of radiation exposure to the fetus and mother.
- Patients suspected of having upper GI perforation, unless water-soluble iodinated contrast medium, such as Gastrografin, is used.
- Patients with conditions associated with adverse reactions to contrast medium (e.g., asthma, food allergies, or allergy to contrast medium).

Although patients are asked specifically if they have a known allergy to iodine or shellfish (shellfish contain high levels of iodine), it has been well established that the reaction is not to iodine; an actual iodine allergy would be problematic because iodine is required for the production of thyroid hormones. In the case of shellfish, the reaction is to a muscle protein called tropomyosin; in the case of iodinated contrast medium, the reaction is to the noniodinated part of the contrast molecule. Patients with a known hypersensitivity to the medium may benefit from premedication with corticosteroids and diphenhydramine; the use of nonionic contrast or an alternative noncontrast imaging study, if available, may be considered for patients who have severe asthma or who have experienced moderate to severe reactions to ionic contrast medium.

- Conditions associated with preexisting renal insufficiency (e.g., chronic kidney disease, single kidney transplant, nephrectomy, diabetes, multiple myeloma, treatment with aminoglycosides and NSAIDs) ***because iodinated contrast is nephrotoxic.***
- Patients who are chronically dehydrated before the test, especially older adults and patients whose health is already compromised, ***because of their risk of contrast-induced acute kidney injury.***
- Patients with an intestinal obstruction ***because the barium or water from the enema may make the condition worse.***

INDICATIONS

- Determine the cause of regurgitation or epigastric pain
- Determine the presence of neoplasms, ulcers, diverticula, obstruction, foreign body, and hiatal hernia
- Evaluate suspected GER, inflammatory process, congenital anomaly, motility disorder, or structural change
- Evaluate unexplained weight loss or anemia
- Identify and locate the origin of hematemesis

POTENTIAL MEDICAL DIAGNOSIS

Normal findings

- Normal size, shape, position, and functioning of the esophagus, stomach, and small bowel

Abnormal findings related to

- Achalasia
- Cancer of the esophagus
- Chalasis
- Congenital abnormalities
- Duodenal cancer, and ulcers
- Esophageal diverticula, motility disorders, ulcers, varices, and inflammation
- Foreign body
- Gastric cancer or tumors, and ulcers
- Gastritis
- Hiatal hernia
- Perforation of the esophagus, stomach, or small bowel
- Polyps

U

- Small bowel tumors
- Strictures

CRITICAL FINDINGS:

- Foreign body
- Perforated bowel
- Tumor with significant mass effect

Note and immediately report to the requesting health-care provider (HCP) any critical findings and related symptoms. A listing of these findings varies among facilities. Timely notification of a critical finding for laboratory or diagnostic studies is a role expectation of the professional nurse. The notification processes vary among facilities. Upon receipt of the critical finding, the information should be read back to the caller to verify accuracy.

INTERFERING FACTORS

Factors that may alter the results of the study

- Inability of the patient to cooperate or remain still during the procedure because of age, significant pain, or mental status.
- Metallic objects (e.g., jewelry, body rings) within the examination field, which may inhibit organ visualization and cause unclear images.

Other considerations

- Failure to follow dietary restrictions before the procedure may cause the procedure to be canceled or repeated.
- Patients with swallowing problems may aspirate the barium, which could interfere with the procedure and cause patient complications.
- Possible constipation or partial bowel obstruction caused by retained barium in the small bowel or colon may affect test results.
- This procedure should be done after a kidney x-ray (intravenous pyelography) or computed tomography of the abdomen or pelvis.

NURSING IMPLICATIONS AND PROCEDURE

See Potential Nursing Problems on Fast Find at davispl.us/vanleeuwen7.

PRETEST:

- Positively identify the patient using at least two person-specific identifiers before services, treatments, or procedures are performed.
- ***Patient Teaching:*** Inform the patient this procedure can assist in assessing the esophagus, stomach, and small intestine.
- Obtain a history of the patient's health concerns, symptoms, surgical procedures, and results of previously performed laboratory and diagnostic studies. Include a list of known allergens, especially allergies or sensitivities to latex, anesthetics, sedatives, or contrast medium. Ensure results of coagulation testing are obtained and recorded prior to the procedure; a creatinine level is also needed before contrast medium is to be used.
- Ensure that this procedure is performed before a barium swallow.
- Record the date of the last menstrual period and determine the possibility of pregnancy in perimenopausal women.
- Obtain a list of the patient's current medications, including over-the-counter medications, dietary supplements, anticoagulants, aspirin and other salicylates (see Effects of Natural Products on Laboratory Values online at Davis*Plus*). Such products should be discontinued by medical direction for the appropriate number of days prior to a surgical procedure. Note the last time and dose of medication taken.
- If iodinated contrast medium (e.g., Gastrografin) is scheduled to be used in patients receiving metformin (Glucophage) for type 2 diabetes, the drug should be discontinued on the day of the test and continue to be withheld for 48 hr after the test. Iodinated contrast can temporarily impair kidney function, and failure

U

to withhold metformin may indirectly result in drug-induced lactic acidosis, a dangerous and sometimes fatal adverse effect of metformin ***related to kidney impairment that does not support sufficient excretion of metformin.***

- Review the procedure with the patient. Address concerns about pain and explain that there may be moments of discomfort and some pain experienced during the procedure. Inform the patient that the procedure is usually performed in a radiology department by an HCP, with support staff, and takes approximately 30 to 60 min. **Pediatric Considerations:** Preparing children for an upper GI examination depends on the age of the child. Encourage parents to be truthful about unpleasant sensations the child may experience during the procedure and to use words that they know their child will understand. Toddlers and preschool-age children have a short attention span, so the best time to talk about the test is right before the procedure. The child should be assured that he or she will be allowed to bring a favorite comfort item into the examination room, and if appropriate, that a parent will be with the child during the procedure.
- ***Sensitivity to social and cultural issues,*** as well as concern for modesty, is important in providing psychological support before, during, and after the procedure.
- Explain to the patient that he or she will be asked to drink a milkshake-like solution that has an unpleasant chalky taste.
- Instruct the patient to remove jewelry and other metallic objects from the area to be examined prior to the procedure.
- Instruct the patient to fast and restrict fluids for 8 hr prior to the procedure. Protocols may vary among facilities. **Pediatric Considerations:** The fasting period prior to the time of the examination depends on the child's age. General guidelines are that the patient should not eat for the period of time between normal meals: newborn 2 to 3 hr; infants to 4 yr: 3 to 4 hr; 5 yr through adolescence: 6 to 8 hr.

INTRATEST:

Potential Complications:

Complications include allergic reaction to the contrast medium, aspiration of the barium, significant diarrhea ***related to use of Gastrografin,*** and partial bowel obstruction caused by thickened or congealed barium.

- Observe standard precautions, and follow the general guidelines in Patient Preparation and Specimen Collection online at Davis*Plus*. Positively identify the patient.
- Ensure that the patient has complied with dietary and fluid restrictions prior to the procedure, as instructed.
- Ensure that the patient has removed all external metallic objects from the area to be examined prior to the procedure.
- Avoid the use of equipment containing latex if the patient has a history of allergic reaction to latex.
- Have emergency equipment readily available.
- Instruct the patient to void prior to the procedure and to change into the gown, robe, and foot coverings provided.
- Instruct the patient to cooperate fully and to follow directions. Ask the patient to remain still throughout the procedure because movement produces unreliable results.

Upper GI Series

- Place the patient on the x-ray table in a supine position, or ask the patient to stand in front of a fluoroscopy screen.
- Instruct the patient to take several swallows of the barium mixture through a straw while images are taken of the pharyngeal motion. An effervescent contrast medium may also be administered to introduce air into the stomach. **Pediatric Considerations:** For infants, barium contrast may be mixed with a small amount of the infant's feeding to take in a bottle. If the patient is unable to drink the

U

barium, a thin, flexible tube may be placed through his or her nose to get the barium into the esophagus.

Small Bowel Series

- If the small bowel is to be examined after the upper GI series, instruct the patient to drink an additional glass of barium while the small intestine is observed for passage of barium. Images are taken at 30- to 60-min intervals until the barium reaches the ileocecal valve. This process can last up to 5 hr, with follow-up images taken at 24 hr.

POST-TEST:

- Inform the patient that a report of the results will be made available to the requesting HCP, who will discuss the results with the patient.
- Instruct the patient to resume usual diet and fluids, as directed by the HCP.
- Monitor for reaction to iodinated contrast medium, including rash, urticaria, tachycardia, hyperpnea, hypertension, palpitations, nausea, or vomiting, if iodine is used.
- Instruct the patient to immediately report symptoms such as fast heart rate, difficulty breathing, skin rash, itching, chest pain, persistent right shoulder pain, or abdominal pain. Immediately report symptoms to the appropriate HCP.
- Instruct the patient to take a mild laxative and increase fluid intake (4 glasses) to aid in the elimination of barium unless contraindicated. **Pediatric Considerations:** Instruct the parents of pediatric patients to hydrate the child with electrolyte fluid post barium enema. **Older Adult Considerations:** Chronic dehydration can also result in frequent bouts of constipation. Therefore, after the procedure, older adult patients should be encouraged to hydrate with fluids containing electrolytes (e.g., Gatorade, Gatorade low calorie for patients with diabetes, or Pedialyte) and to use a mild laxative daily until the stool is back to normal color.
- Inform the patient that his or her stool will be white or light in color for 2 to 3 days. If the patient is unable to eliminate the barium, or if the stool does not return to normal color, the patient should notify the HCP.
- Recognize anxiety related to test results, and be supportive of perceived loss of independence and fear of shortened life expectancy. Discuss the implications of abnormal test results on the patient's lifestyle. Provide teaching and information regarding the clinical implications of the test results, as appropriate. Educate the patient regarding access to counseling services.
- Reinforce information given by the patient's HCP regarding further testing, treatment, or referral to another HCP. Answer any questions or address any concerns voiced by the patient or family.
- Depending on the results of this procedure, additional testing may be needed to evaluate or monitor progression of the disease process and determine the need for a change in therapy. Evaluate test results in relation to the patient's symptoms and other tests performed.

Patient Education:

- Teach the patient about the medical and surgical options associated with the disease process.
- Teach the patient the pathophysiology associated with the disease process.

Expected Patient Outcomes:

Understanding

- The patient and family acknowledge the importance of remaining NPO to rest the bowel and treat the disease.
- The patient and family acknowledge the importance of adequate pain control as a facet of treating the disease.

Ability

- The patient and family demonstrate the ability to accurately record intake and output.
- The patient and family demonstrate the ability to position the patient comfortably to decrease pain.

U

Response

- The patient and family agree to consider a surgical alternative to disease management.
- The patient and family agree that the patient will refrain from eating or drinking restricted food or fluids, as appropriate to disease management.

RELATED STUDIES:

- Related tests include barium enema, barium swallow, capsule endoscopy, CT abdomen, endoscopic retrograde cholangiopancreatography, esophageal manometry, fecal analysis, gastric acid stimulation test, gastric emptying scan, gastrin stimulation test, gastroesophageal reflux scan, *H. pylori* antibody, KUB study, Meckel's diverticulum scan, MRI abdomen, and US pelvis.
- Refer to the Gastrointestinal System table online at Davis*Plus* for related tests by body system.

Urea Breath Test

SYNONYM/ACRONYM: PY test, C-14 urea breath test, breath test, pylori breath test, UBT.

COMMON USE: To assist in diagnosing a gastrointestinal infection and ulceration of the stomach or duodenum related to a *Helicobacter pylori* infection.

AREA OF APPLICATION: Stomach.

DESCRIPTION: The C-14 urea breath test (UBT) is used to assist in the diagnosis of *Helicobacter pylori* infection. *H. pylori* is a bacterium that can infect the stomach lining. It has been implicated as the cause of many gastrointestinal conditions, including the development of duodenal and gastric ulcers. The UBT is a simple, noninvasive diagnostic nuclear medicine procedure that requires the patient to swallow a small amount of radiopharmaceutical C-14–labelled urea in a capsule with lukewarm water. In the presence of urease, an enzyme secreted by *H. pylori* in the gut, the urea in the capsule is broken down into nitrogen and C-14–labelled carbon dioxide (CO_2). The labelled CO_2 is absorbed through the stomach lining into the blood and excreted by the lungs. Breath samples are collected and trapped in a Mylar balloon. The C-14 urea is counted and quantitated with a liquid scintillation counter. The UBT can also be used to indicate the elimination of *H. pylori* infection after treatment with antibiotics. Other tests used to detect the presence of *H. pylori* include a blood *H. pylori* antibody test, a stool antigen test, and stomach biopsy.

This procedure is contraindicated for

- Patients who are pregnant or suspected of being pregnant, unless the potential benefits of a procedure using radiation far outweigh the risk of radiation exposure to the fetus and mother.
- Patients who have taken antibiotics, Pepto-Bismol, or bismuth in the past 30 days.
- Patients who have taken sucralfate in the past 14 days.

U

Patients who have used a proton pump inhibitor within the past 14 days.

INDICATIONS

- Aid in detection of *H. pylori* infection in the stomach.
- Monitor eradication of *H. pylori* infection following treatment regimen.
- Evaluate new-onset dyspepsia.

POTENTIAL MEDICAL DIAGNOSIS

Normal findings

- Negative for *H. pylori:* Less than 50 dpm (disintegrations per minute)

Abnormal findings related to

- Indeterminate for *H. pylori:* 50 to 199 dpm
- Positive for *H. pylori:* Greater than 200 dpm

CRITICAL FINDINGS: N/A

INTERFERING FACTORS

Other considerations

- Failure to follow dietary restrictions and other pretesting preparations may cause the procedure to be canceled or repeated.
- Patients who have had resective gastric surgery have the potential for resultant bacterial overgrowth (non-*H. pylori* urease), which can cause a false-positive result.
- Achlorhydria can cause a false-positive result.

NURSING IMPLICATIONS AND PROCEDURE

PRETEST:

- Positively identify the patient using at least two person-specific identifiers before services, treatments, or procedures are performed.
- *Patient Teaching:* Inform the patient this procedure can assist in diagnosing an infection of the stomach or intestine.
- Obtain a history of the patient's health concerns, symptoms, surgical procedures, and results of previously performed laboratory and diagnostic studies. Include a list of known allergens, especially allergies or sensitivities to latex.
- Record the date of the last menstrual period and determine the possibility of pregnancy in premenopausal women.
- Obtain a list of the patient's current medications, including over-the-counter medications and dietary supplements (see Effects of Natural Products on Laboratory Values online at Davis*Plus*).
- Review the procedure with the patient. Reassure the patient that the radionuclide poses no radioactive hazard and rarely produces adverse effects. Address concerns about pain and explain that there should be no discomfort during the procedure. Inform the patient that the procedure is done in the nuclear medicine department by technologists and support staff and usually takes approximately 30 to 60 min.
- *Sensitivity to social and cultural issues,* as well as concern for modesty, is important in providing psychological support before, during, and after the procedure.
- Instruct the patient to fast, restrict fluids, and, by medical direction, withhold medication for 6 hr prior to the procedure. Protocols may vary among facilities.

INTRATEST:

Potential Complications: N/A

- Observe standard precautions, and follow the general guidelines in Patient Preparation and Specimen Collection online at Davis*Plus*. Positively identify the patient.
- Ensure the patient has complied with dietary and medication restrictions and pretesting preparations prior to the procedure, as instructed.
- Instruct the patient to blow into a balloon prior to the start of the procedure to collect a sample of breath.

U

- Instruct the patient to swallow the C-14 capsule directly from a cup, followed by 20 mL of lukewarm water. Provide an additional 20 mL of lukewarm water for the patient to drink at 3 min after the dose.
- Take breath samples at different periods of time by instructing the patient to take in a deep breath and hold it for approximately 5 to 10 sec before exhaling through a straw into a Mylar balloon.
- Note that samples are counted on a liquid scintillation counter (LSC) and recorded in disintegrations per minute.

POST-TEST:

- Inform the patient that a report of the results will be made available to the requesting health-care provider (HCP), who will discuss the results with the patient.
- Instruct the patient to resume usual diet and medication, as directed by the HCP.
- Unless contraindicated, advise patient to drink increased amounts of fluids for 12 to 24 hr to eliminate the radionuclide from the body.
- If a woman who is breastfeeding must have a breath test, she should not breastfeed the infant until the radionuclide has been eliminated. This could take as long as 3 days. Instruct her to express the milk and discard it during the 3-day period to prevent cessation of milk production.
- Instruct the patient to immediately flush the toilet and to meticulously wash hands with soap and water after each voiding for 48 hr after the procedure.
- Instruct all caregivers to wear gloves when discarding urine for 48 hr after the procedure. Wash gloved hands with soap and water before removing gloves; then wash ungloved hands.
- Recognize anxiety related to test results. Discuss the implications of abnormal test results on the patient's lifestyle. Provide teaching and information regarding the clinical implications of the test results, as appropriate.
- Reinforce information given by the patient's HCP regarding further testing, treatment, or referral to another HCP. Answer any questions or address any concerns voiced by the patient or family.
- Depending on the results of the procedure, additional testing may be performed to evaluate or monitor progression of the disease process and determine the need for change in therapy. Evaluate test results in relation to the patient's symptoms and other tests performed.

RELATED STUDIES:

- Related tests include EGD, gastric emptying scan, *H. pylori* antibody, KUB study, and UGI.
- See the Gastrointestinal System table online at Davis*Plus* for related tests by body system.

Urea Nitrogen, Blood

SYNONYM/ACRONYM: BUN.

COMMON USE: To assist in assessing for kidney function toward diagnosing disorders such as kidney disease and dehydration. Also used in monitoring the effectiveness of therapeutic interventions such as hemodialysis.

SPECIMEN: Serum collected in a gold-, red-, or red/gray-top tube. Plasma collected in a green-top (heparin) tube is also acceptable.

NORMAL FINDINGS: (Method: Spectrophotometry)

Age	Conventional Units	SI Units (Conventional Units × 0.357)
Newborn–3 yr	5–17 mg/dL	1.8–6.1 mmol/L
4–13 yr	7–17 mg/dL	2.5–6.1 mmol/L
14 yr–adult	8–21 mg/dL	2.9–7.5 mmol/L
Adult older than 90 yr	10–31 mg/dL	3.6–11.1 mmol/L

DESCRIPTION: Unlike fats and carbohydrates, protein cannot be stored by the body. The amino acids and nitrogen used to make proteins are either obtained from dietary sources or from the normal turnover of aging cells in the body. Urea is a nonprotein nitrogen (NPN) compound formed in the liver from ammonia and excreted by the kidneys as an end product of protein metabolism. Other NPN compounds excreted by the kidneys include uric acid and creatinine. Blood urea nitrogen (BUN) levels reflect the balance between the amount of nitrogen ingested and excreted which is a representation of overall protein metabolism. BUN and creatinine values are commonly evaluated together. The normal BUN/creatinine ratio is 15:1 to 24:1 (e.g., if a patient has a BUN of 15 mg/dL, ✱ the creatinine should be approximately 0.6 to 1 mg/dL). ✱ BUN is used in the following calculation to estimate serum osmolality: (2 × Na^+) + (glucose/18) + (BUN/2.8).

This procedure is contraindicated for: N/A

INDICATIONS
- Assess nutritional support.
- Evaluate hemodialysis therapy.
- Evaluate hydration.
- Evaluate liver function.
- Evaluate patients with lymphoma after chemotherapy (tumor lysis).
- Evaluate renal function.
- Monitor the effects of drugs known to be nephrotoxic or hepatotoxic.

POTENTIAL MEDICAL DIAGNOSIS

Increased in:
- Acute kidney injury ***(related to decreased renal excretion)***
- Chronic glomerulonephritis ***(related to decreased renal excretion)***
- Decreased renal perfusion ***(reflects decreased renal excretion and increased blood levels)***
- Diabetes ***(related to decreased renal excretion)***
- Excessive protein ingestion ***(related to increased protein metabolism)***
- Gastrointestinal (GI) bleeding ***(excessive blood protein in the GI tract and increased protein metabolism)***
- Heart failure ***(related to decreased blood flow to the kidneys, decreased renal excretion, and accumulation in circulating blood)***
- Hyperalimentation ***(related to increased protein metabolism)***
- Hypovolemia ***(related to decreased blood flow to the kidneys, decreased renal excretion, and accumulation in circulating blood)***
- Ketoacidosis ***(dehydration from ketoacidosis correlates with***

U

decreased renal excretion of urea nitrogen)

- Muscle wasting from starvation ***(related to increased protein metabolism)***
- Neoplasms ***(related to increased protein metabolism or to decreased renal excretion)***
- Nephrotoxic drugs ***(related to decreased renal excretion and accumulation in circulating blood)***
- Pyelonephritis ***(related to decreased renal excretion)***
- Shock ***(related to decreased blood flow to the kidneys, decreased renal excretion, and accumulation in circulating blood)***
- Urinary tract obstruction ***(related to decreased renal excretion and accumulation in circulating blood)***

Decreased in:

- Inadequate dietary protein ***(urea nitrogen is a by-product of protein metabolism; less available protein is reflected in decreased BUN levels)***
- Low-protein/high-carbohydrate diet ***(urea nitrogen is a by-product of protein metabolism; less available protein is reflected in decreased BUN levels)***
- Malabsorption syndromes ***(urea nitrogen is a by-product of protein metabolism; less available protein is reflected in decreased BUN levels)***
- Pregnancy
- Severe liver disease ***(BUN is synthesized in the liver, so liver damage results in decreased levels)***

CRITICAL FINDINGS:

Adults

- Greater than 100 mg/dL (SI: Greater than 35.7 mmol/L) (nondialysis patients)

Children

- Greater than 55 mg/dL (SI: Greater than 19.6 mmol/L) (nondialysis patients)

Note and immediately report to the requesting health-care provider (HCP) any critical findings and related symptoms. A listing of these findings varies among facilities. Timely notification of a critical finding for laboratory or diagnostic studies is a role expectation of the professional nurse. The notification processes vary among facilities. Upon receipt of the critical finding, the information should be read back to the caller to verify accuracy.

Consideration may be given to verification of critical findings before action is taken. Policies vary among facilities and may include requesting immediate recollection and retesting by the laboratory or retesting using a rapid point-of-care testing instrument at the bedside, if available.

A patient with a grossly elevated BUN may have signs and symptoms including acidemia, agitation, confusion, fatigue, nausea, vomiting, and coma. Possible interventions include treatment of the cause, administration of intravenous (IV) bicarbonate, a low-protein diet, hemodialysis, and caution with respect to prescribing and continuing nephrotoxic medications.

INTERFERING FACTORS

- Drugs and other substances that may increase BUN levels include acetaminophen, alanine, alkaline antacids, amphotericin B, antimony compounds, arsenicals, bacitracin, bismuth subsalicylate, capreomycin, cephalosporins, chloral hydrate, chloramphenicol, chlorthalidone, colistimethate, colistin, cotrimoxazole, dexamethasone, dextran, diclofenac, doxycycline, ethylene glycol, gentamicin, guanethidine, guanoxan, ibuprofen, ifosfamide,

U

ipodate, kanamycin, mephenesin, metolazone, mitomycin, neomycin, phosphorus, plicamycin, tertatolol, tetracycline, triamterene, triethylenemelamine, viomycin, and vitamin D.

- Drugs and other substances that may decrease BUN levels include chloramphenicol, fluorides, and streptomycin.

NURSING IMPLICATIONS AND PROCEDURE

POTENTIAL NURSING PROBLEMS:

Problem	Signs & Symptoms	Interventions
Infection ***(related to uremia and decreased immune response; venous catheters; Foley catheters; endotracheal tubes)***	Temperature; elevated white cell count; cloudy urine; sediment in urine; blood in urine	Monitor urinary output; assess urine color, odor, presence of blood; monitor and trend temperature and white cell count; obtain urine for culture and sensitivity as required; administer prescribed antibiotics; avoid long-term indwelling catheters; encourage frequent personal and oral hygiene; encourage use of gentle soaps; assist in preventing skin breakdown; use meticulous care and sterile technique in provision of care for peripheral or venous catheters
Kidney function ***(related to renal ischemia associated with shock, sepsis, hypovolemia; postoperative injury; trauma; nephrotoxic drugs [aminoglycoside, heavy metals, radiographic contrast]; renal vascular occlusion; hemolytic transfusion reaction; decreased***	Increased BUN; increased creatinine; decreased creatinine clearance; increased urine specific gravity (greater than 1.029); hematuria; proteinuria; decreased urine output less than 400 mL/day (with	Monitor, record, and trend intake and output; monitor urine specific gravity; monitor and trend renal specific urine and blood studies, BUN, creatinine, sodium, potassium, magnesium, pH, urinalysis, Hgb, Hct; monitor and trend weight daily; assess and monitor for edema, jugular vein distention (JVD), hypertension,

Problem	Signs & Symptoms	Interventions
cardiac output; tubular necrosis; obstruction; tumor; medications [NSAID, ACE inhibitors, immunosuppressants, antineoplastics, antifungals])	adequate intake and no fluid loss); weight gain; elevated potassium; elevated phosphate; decreased calcium; decreased sodium; increased magnesium; metabolic acidosis; decreased hemoglobin (Hgb) and hematocrit (Hct)	adventitious breath sounds, impaired gas exchange; use pulse oximetry; administer prescribed oxygen; administer prescribed hemodialysis; administer prescribed medications (diuretics); administer prescribed fluids; consider renal function with antibiotic administration
Cardiac output ***(related to excess fluid volume; pericarditis; electrolyte imbalance; toxin accumulation; dysrhythmias; altered cardiac muscle contractility secondary to heart failure)***	Weak peripheral pulses; slow capillary refill; decreased urinary output; cool, clammy skin; tachypnea; dyspnea; altered level of consciousness; abnormal heart sounds; fatigue; hypoxia; loud holosystolic murmur; electrocardiogram (ECG) changes; increased JVD	Assess peripheral pulses and capillary refill; monitor blood pressure and check for orthostatic changes; assess respiratory rate, breath sounds, and orthopnea; assess skin color and temperature; assess level of consciousness; monitor urinary output; use pulse oximetry to monitor oxygenation; monitor ECG; assess for third heart sound (indicative of heart failure or pericarditis); administer ordered inotropic and peripheral vasodilator medications, nitrates; provide oxygen administration; administer as prescribed (sodium bicarbonate, glucose, insulin drip, potassium excretion resin, calcium salt)

(table continues on page 1568)

Problem	Signs & Symptoms	Interventions
Fluid volume (water) ***(related to excess fluid and sodium intake; compromised kidney function)***	**Excess:** Edema, shortness of breath, increased weight, ascites, rales, rhonchi, and diluted laboratory values; distended neck veins; tachycardia; restlessness; presence of S3 heart sound	Record daily weight and monitor trends; record accurate intake and output; monitor laboratory values that reflect alterations in fluid status (potassium, BUN, creatinine, calcium, Hgb, Hct, sodium); manage underlying cause of fluid alteration; monitor urine characteristics and respiratory status; establish baseline assessment data; assess and trend heart rate and blood pressure; assess for symptoms of fluid overload such as JVD, shortness of breath, dyspnea, crackles; provide low-sodium diet; administer prescribed diuretic; administer prescribed antihypertensive; elevate feet when sitting; monitor oxygenation with pulse oximetry; administer oxygen as appropriate; elevate the head of the bed; administer prescribed antihypertensives; administer IV medications with the least amount of fluid; prepare for hemodialysis as appropriate

PRETEST:

- Positively identify the patient using at least two person-specific identifiers before services, treatments, or procedures are performed.
- ***Patient Teaching:*** Inform the patient this test can assist in assessing kidney function.
- Obtain a history of the patient's health concerns, symptoms, surgical procedures, and results of previously performed laboratory and diagnostic studies. Include a list of known allergens, especially allergies or sensitivities to latex.

U

- Obtain a list of the patient's current medications, including over-the-counter medications and dietary supplements (see Effects of Natural Products on Laboratory Values online at Davis*Plus*).
- Review the procedure with the patient. Inform the patient that specimen collection takes approximately 5 to 10 min. Address concerns about pain and explain that there may be some discomfort during the venipuncture.
- ***Sensitivity to social and cultural issues,*** as well as concern for modesty, is important in providing psychological support before, during, and after the procedure.
- Note that there are no food, fluid, or medication restrictions unless by medical direction.

INTRATEST:

Potential Complications: N/A

- Avoid the use of equipment containing latex if the patient has a history of allergic reaction to latex.
- Instruct the patient to cooperate fully and to follow directions. Direct the patient to breathe normally and to avoid unnecessary movement.
- Observe standard precautions, and follow the general guidelines in Patient Preparation and Specimen Collection online at Davis*Plus*. Positively identify the patient, and label the appropriate specimen container with the corresponding patient demographics, initials of the person collecting the specimen, date, and time of collection. Perform a venipuncture.
- Remove the needle and apply direct pressure with dry gauze to stop bleeding. Observe/assess venipuncture site for bleeding or hematoma formation and secure gauze with adhesive bandage.
- Promptly transport the specimen to the laboratory for processing and analysis.

POST-TEST:

- Inform the patient that a report of the results will be made available to the requesting HCP, who will discuss the results with the patient.
- Monitor intake and output for fluid imbalance in renal dysfunction and dehydration.
- ***Nutritional Considerations:*** Greater than 100 nitrogen balance is commonly used as a nutritional assessment tool to indicate protein change. In healthy individuals, protein anabolism and catabolism are in equilibrium. During various disease states, nutritional intake decreases, resulting in a negative balance. During recovery from illness and with proper nutritional support, the nitrogen balance becomes positive. BUN is an important analyte to measure during administration of total parenteral nutrition (TPN). Educate the patient, as appropriate, in dietary adjustments required to maintain proper nitrogen balance. Inform the patient that the requesting HCP may prescribe TPN as part of the treatment plan.
- ***Nutritional Considerations:*** An elevated BUN can be caused by a high-protein diet or dehydration. Unless medically restricted, a healthy diet should be consumed daily. Provide contact information, if desired, for the Institute of Medicine of the National Academies (www.iom.edu) and USDA's resource for nutrition (www.choosemyplate.gov). 🍁 Fluid consumption should include six to eight 8-oz 🍁 glasses of water or water containing fluid per day.
- Recognize anxiety related to test results.
- Depending on the results of this procedure, additional testing may be performed to evaluate or monitor progression of the disease process and determine the need for a change in therapy. Evaluate test results in relation to the patient's symptoms and other tests performed.

Patient Education:

- Discuss the implications of abnormal test results on the patient's lifestyle.
- Provide teaching and information regarding the clinical implications of the test results, as appropriate.

U

- Reinforce information given by the patient's HCP regarding further testing, treatment, or referral to another HCP.
- Answer any questions or address any concerns voiced by the patient or family.
- Teach the patient how to accurately measure and record urine output.

Expected Patient Outcomes:

Understanding

- The patient and family acknowledges that hemodialysis may be necessary if kidney function fails to improve.
- The patient and family state the importance of adhering to the specified fluid limit.

Ability

- The patient and family demonstrate proficiency in tracking and documenting intake and output.
- The patient and family demonstrate proficiency in taking and documenting temperature.

Response

- The patient complies with the request for frequent personal and oral hygiene to decrease infection risk.
- The patient complies with the request to take prescribed medication as ordered.

RELATED STUDIES:

- Related tests include anion gap, antimicrobial drugs, biopsy kidney, calcium, calculus kidney stone panel, CT spleen, creatinine, creatinine clearance, cytology urine, cystoscopy, electrolytes, gallium scan, glucose, glycated hemoglobin, 5–HIAA, IVP, ketones, magnesium, MRI venography, microalbumin, osmolality, oxalate, phosphorus, protein total and fractions, renogram, US abdomen, US kidney, UA, urea nitrogen urine, and uric acid.
- Refer to the Genitourinary and Hepatobiliary systems tables online at Davis*Plus* for related tests by body system.

Urea Nitrogen, Urine

SYNONYM/ACRONYM: N/A

COMMON USE: To assess kidney function related to the progression of disorders such as diabetes, liver disease, and kidney disease.

SPECIMEN: Urine from an unpreserved random or timed specimen collected in a clean plastic collection container.

NORMAL FINDINGS: (Method: Spectrophotometry)

Conventional Units	SI Units (Conventional Units × 35.7)
12–20 g/24 hr	428–714 mmol/24 hr

POTENTIAL MEDICAL DIAGNOSIS

Increased in:

- Diabetes ***(related to increased protein metabolism)***
- Hyperthyroidism
- Increased dietary protein ***(related to increased protein metabolism)***
- Postoperative period

Decreased in:

- Kidney disease ***(related to decreased renal excretion)***
- Liver disease ***(BUN is synthesized in the liver, so liver damage results in decreased levels)***
- Low-protein/high-carbohydrate diet ***(urea nitrogen is a by-product of protein metabolism; less available protein is reflected in decreased BUN levels)***
- Normal-growing pediatric patients ***(increased demand for protein; less available protein is reflected in decreased BUN levels)***
- Pregnancy ***(increased demand for protein; less available protein is reflected in decreased BUN levels)***
- Toxemia ***(related to hypertension and decreased renal excretion)***

CRITICAL FINDINGS: N/A

Find and print out the full study on Fast Find at davispl.us/vanleeuwen7.

Urethrography, Retrograde

SYNONYM/ACRONYM: Pyelography, retrograde.

COMMON USE: To assess urethral patency in order to evaluate the success of surgical interventions on patients who have urethral structures or other anomalies that interfere with urination.

AREA OF APPLICATION: Urethra.

DESCRIPTION: Retrograde urethrography uses contrast medium, either injected or instilled via a catheter into the urethra, to visualize the membranous, bulbar, and penile portions, particularly after surgical repair of the urethra to assess the success of the surgery in male patients. The posterior portion of the urethra is visualized better when the procedure is performed with voiding cystourethrography. In women, it may be performed after surgical repair of the urethra to assess the success of the surgery and to assess structural abnormalities in conjunction with an evaluation for voiding dysfunction.

This procedure is contraindicated for

Patients who are pregnant or suspected of being pregnant, unless the potential benefits of a procedure using radiation far outweigh the risk of radiation exposure to the fetus and mother.

Patients with conditions associated with adverse reactions to contrast medium (e.g., asthma, food allergies, or allergy to contrast medium).

Although patients are asked specifically if they have a known allergy to iodine or shellfish, it has been well established that the reaction is not to iodine; an actual iodine allergy would be problematic because iodine is required for the production of thyroid hormones. In the case of shellfish, the reaction is to a muscle protein called tropomyosin; in the case of iodinated contrast medium, the reaction is to the noniodinated part of the contrast molecule. Patients with a known hypersensitivity to the medium may benefit from premedication with corticosteroids and diphenhydramine; the use of nonionic contrast or an alternative noncontrast imaging study, if available, may be considered for patients who have severe asthma or who have experienced moderate to severe reactions to ionic contrast medium.

Patients with conditions associated with preexisting renal insufficiency (e.g., chronic kidney disease, single kidney transplant, nephrectomy, diabetes, multiple myeloma, treatment with aminoglycosides and NSAIDs) ***because iodinated contrast is nephrotoxic.***

Patients who are chronically dehydrated before the test, especially older adults and patients whose health is already compromised, ***because of their risk of contrast-induced acute kidney injury.***

Patients with bleeding disorders ***because the puncture site may not stop bleeding.***

INDICATIONS

- Aid in the diagnosis of urethral strictures, lacerations, diverticula, and congenital anomalies.

POTENTIAL MEDICAL DIAGNOSIS

Normal findings

- Normal size, shape, and course of the membranous, bulbar, and penile portions of the urethra in male patients
- If the prostatic portion can be visualized, it also should appear normal

Abnormal findings related to

- Congenital anomalies, such as urethral valves and perineal hypospadias
- False passages in the urethra
- Prostatic enlargement
- Tumors of the urethra
- Urethral calculi
- Urethral diverticula
- Urethral fistulas
- Urethral strictures indicated by a narrowing and lacerations

CRITICAL FINDINGS: N/A

INTERFERING FACTORS:

Factors that may alter the results of the study

- Inability of the patient to cooperate or remain still during the procedure because of age, significant pain, or mental status.
- Metallic objects (e.g., jewelry, body rings) within the examination field, which may inhibit organ visualization and cause unclear images.

Other considerations: N/A

NURSING IMPLICATIONS AND PROCEDURE

PRETEST:

- Positively identify the patient using at least two person-specific identifiers before services, treatments, or procedures are performed.
- *Patient Teaching:* Inform the patient this procedure can assist in assessing the urethral patency.
- Obtain a history of the patient's health concerns, symptoms, surgical procedures, and results of previously performed laboratory and diagnostic studies. Include a list of known allergens, especially allergies or sensitivities to latex, anesthetics, sedatives, or contrast medium. Ensure results of coagulation testing are obtained and recorded prior to the procedure; a creatinine level is also needed before contrast medium is to be used.
- Obtain a history of the patient's genitourinary system, symptoms, and results of previously performed laboratory tests and diagnostic and surgical procedures.

U

- Ensure that this procedure is performed before an upper gastrointestinal study or barium swallow.
- Record the date of the last menstrual period and determine the possibility of pregnancy in perimenopausal women.
- Obtain a list of the patient's current medications, including over-the-counter medications and dietary supplements (see Effects of Natural Products on Laboratory Values online at Davis*Plus*).
- If iodinated contrast medium is scheduled to be used in patients receiving metformin (Glucophage) for type 2 diabetes, the drug should be discontinued on the day of the test and continue to be withheld for 48 hr after the test. Iodinated contrast can temporarily impair kidney function, and failure to withhold metformin may indirectly result in drug-induced lactic acidosis, a dangerous and sometimes fatal adverse effect of metformin ***related to renal impairment that does not support sufficient excretion of metformin.***
- Review the procedure with the patient. Address concerns about pain and explain that there may be moments of discomfort and some pain experienced during the procedure. Inform the patient that the procedure is performed in a cystoscopy room by a health-care provider (HCP), with support staff, and takes approximately 30 min.
- ***Sensitivity to social and cultural issues,*** as well as concern for modesty, is important in providing psychological support before, during, and after the procedure.
- Inform the patient that some pressure may be experienced when the catheter is inserted and contrast medium is instilled.
- Instruct the patient to remove jewelry and other metallic objects from the area to be examined prior to the procedure.
- Note that there are no food or fluid restrictions unless by medical direction.
- *Make sure a written and informed consent has been signed prior to the procedure and before administering any medications.*

INTRATEST:

Potential Complications:

Complications include allergic reaction to the contrast medium and bleeding.

- Observe standard precautions, and follow the general guidelines in Patient Preparation and Specimen Collection online at Davis*Plus*. Positively identify the patient.
- Ensure the patient has removed all external metallic objects from the area to be examined prior to the procedure.
- Instruct the patient to void prior to the procedure and to change into the gown, robe, and foot coverings provided.
- Avoid the use of equipment containing latex if the patient has a history of allergic reaction to latex.
- Instruct the patient to cooperate fully and to follow directions. Ask the patient to lie still during the procedure because movement produces unclear images.
- Obtain and record the patient's baseline vital signs.
- Place the patient on the table in a supine position.
- A single plain film is taken of the bladder and urethra.
- A catheter is filled with contrast medium to eliminate air pockets and is inserted until the balloon reaches the meatus. Inform the patient that the contrast medium may cause a temporary flushing of the face, a feeling of warmth, urticaria, headache, vomiting, or nausea.
- After three-fourths of the contrast medium is injected, another image is taken while the remainder of the contrast medium is injected.
- The procedure may be done on female patients using a double balloon to occlude the bladder neck from above and below the external meatus.

U

POST-TEST:

- Inform the patient that a report of the results will be made available to the requesting HCP, who will discuss the results with the patient.
- Instruct the patient to resume usual activities, as directed by the HCP. Kidney function should be assessed before metformin is resumed if contrast was used.
- Monitor vital and neurological signs every 15 min until they return to preprocedure levels.
- Monitor fluid intake and urinary output for 24 hr after the procedure. Decreased urine output may indicate impending kidney injury.
- Monitor for signs and symptoms of sepsis, including fever, chills, and severe pain in the kidney area.
- Instruct the patient to drink plenty of fluids to prevent stasis and to prevent the buildup of bacteria.
- Reinforce information given by the patient's HCP regarding further testing, treatment, or referral to another HCP. Answer any questions or address any concerns voiced by the patient or family.
- Depending on the results of this procedure, additional testing may be needed to evaluate or monitor progression of the disease process and determine the need for a change in therapy. Evaluate test results in relation to the patient's symptoms and other tests performed.

RELATED STUDIES:

- Related tests include CT abdomen, CT kidneys, CT pelvis, cystometry, cystoscopy, IVP, MRI abdomen, PSA, renogram, retrograde ureteropyelography, urinalysis, and voiding cystourethrography.
- Refer to the Genitourinary System table online at Davis*Plus* for related tests by body system.

Uric Acid, Blood

SYNONYM/ACRONYM: Urate.

COMMON USE: To monitor uric acid levels during treatment for gout and evaluation of tissue destruction, liver damage, renal function, and monitor the effectiveness of therapeutic interventions.

SPECIMEN: Serum collected in a gold-, red-, or red/gray-top tube. Plasma collected in a green-top (heparin) tube is also acceptable. Note: Rasburicase will rapidly decrease uric acid in specimens left at room temperature. If patients are receiving this medication, collect the blood sample in a prechilled green-top (heparin) tube and transport in an ice slurry.

NORMAL FINDINGS: (Method: Spectrophotometry)

Age	Conventional Units	SI Units (Conventional Units × 0.059)
1–30 d		
Male	1.3–4.9 mg/dL	0.08–0.29 mmol/L
Female	1.4–6.2 mg/dL	0.08–0.37 mmol/L

U

Age	Conventional Units	SI Units (Conventional Units × 0.059)
1–3 mo		
Male	1.4–5.3 mg/dL	0.08–0.31 mmol/L
Female	1.4–5.8 mg/dL	0.08–0.34 mmol/L
4–12 mo		
Male	1.5–6.4 mg/dL	0.09–0.38 mmol/L
Female	1.4–6.2 mg/dL	0.08–0.37 mmol/L
1–3 yr		
Male & female	1.8–5 mg/dL	0.11–0.3 mmol/L
4–6 yr		
Male & female	2.2–4.7 mg/dL	0.13–0.28 mmol/L
7–9 yr		
Male & female	2–5 mg/dL	0.12–0.3 mmol/L
10–12 yr		
Male & female	2.3–5.9 mg/dL	0.14–0.35 mmol/L
13–15 yr		
Male	3.1–7 mg/dL	0.18–0.41 mmol/L
Female	2.3–6.4 mg/dL	0.14–0.38 mmol/L
16–18 yr		
Male	2.1–7.6 mg/dL	0.12–0.45 mmol/L
Female	2.4–6.6 mg/dL	0.14–0.39 mmol/L
19 yr–Adult		
Male	4–8 mg/dL	0.24—0.47 mmol/L
Female	2.5–7 mg/dL	0.15–0.41 mmol/L
Adult older than 60 yr		
Male	4.2–8.2 mg/dL	0.25–0.48 mmol/L
Female	3.5–7.3 mg/dL	0.21–0.43 mmol/L

Therapeutic target for patients with gout: Less than 6 mg/dL (SI: Less than 0.4 mmol/L).

DESCRIPTION: Uric acid is the end product of purine metabolism. Purines are important constituents of nucleic acids; purine turnover occurs continuously in the body, producing substantial amounts of uric acid even in the absence of purine intake from dietary sources such as organ meats (e.g., liver, thymus gland and/or pancreas [sweetbreads], kidney), legumes, and yeasts. Uric acid is filtered, absorbed, and secreted by the kidneys and is a common constituent of urine. Serum urate levels are affected by the amount of uric acid produced and by the efficiency of renal excretion. Values can vary based on diet, gender, body size, level of exercise, level of stress, and regularity in consumption of alcohol. Elevated uric acid levels can indicate conditions of critical cellular injury or destruction; hyperuricemia has an association with hypertension, hypertriglyceridemia, obesity, myocardial infarct, renal disease, and diabetes. Rasburicase is a medication used in the treatment and prevention of acute hyperuricemia related to tumor lysis syndrome in children and for leukemias and lymphomas related

U

to the toxic effects of chemotherapy. Rasburicase is a recombinant form of uricase oxidase, an enzyme that converts uric acid to allantoin, a much more soluble and effectively excreted substance than uric acid.

This procedure is contraindicated for: N/A

INDICATIONS

- Assist in the diagnosis of gout when there is a family history (autosomal dominant genetic disorder) or signs and symptoms of gout, indicated by elevated uric acid levels.
- Determine the cause of known or suspected renal calculi.
- Evaluate the extent of tissue destruction in infection, starvation, excessive exercise, malignancies, chemotherapy, or radiation therapy.
- Evaluate possible liver damage in eclampsia, indicated by elevated uric acid levels.
- Monitor the effects of drugs known to alter uric acid levels, either as a adverse effect or as a therapeutic effect.

POTENTIAL MEDICAL DIAGNOSIS

Increased in:

Conditions that result in high cellular turnover release nucleic acids into circulation, which are converted to uric acid by the liver.

- Acute tissue destruction as a result of starvation or excessive exercise ***(related to cellular destruction)***
- Alcoholism
- Chemotherapy and radiation therapy ***(related to high cellular turnover)***
- Chronic lead toxicity ***(cellular destruction related to hemolysis)***
- Diabetes ***(decreased renal excretion results in increased blood levels)***
- Down syndrome
- Eclampsia
- Excessive dietary purines ***(purines are nucleic acid bases converted to uric acid by the liver)***
- Glucose-6-phosphate dehydrogenase deficiency ***(cellular destruction related to hemolysis)***
- Gout ***(usually related to excess dietary intake)***
- Heart failure ***(related to cellular destruction)***
- Hyperparathyroidism
- Hypertension ***(related to effects on renal excretion)***
- Hypoparathyroidism ***(related to disturbances in calcium and phosphorus homeostasis)***
- Lactic acidosis ***(cellular destruction related to shock)***
- Lead poisoning ***(cellular destruction related to hemolysis)***
- Lesch-Nyhan syndrome ***(related to disorder of uric acid metabolism)***
- Multiple myeloma ***(related to high cell turnover)***
- Pernicious anemia ***(cellular destruction related to hemolysis)***
- Polycystic kidney disease ***(related to decreased renal excretion, which results in increased blood levels)***
- Polycythemia ***(related to increased cellular destruction)***
- Psoriasis
- Sickle cell anemia ***(cellular destruction related to hemolysis)***
- Tumors ***(related to high cell turnover)***
- Type III hyperlipidemia

Decreased in:

- Fanconi's syndrome ***(related to increased renal excretion)***
- Low-purine diet ***(related to insufficient nutrients for liver to synthesize uric acid)***
- Severe liver disease ***(uric acid synthesis occurs in the liver)***

- Wilson's disease ***(affects normal liver function and is related to impaired tubular absorption)***

CRITICAL FINDINGS:

Adults

- Greater than 13 mg/dL (SI: Greater than 0.8 mmol/L)

Children

- Greater than 12 mg/dL (SI: Greater than 0.7 mmol/L)

Note and immediately report to the requesting health-care provider (HCP) any critical findings and related symptoms. A listing of these findings varies among facilities. Timely notification of a critical finding for laboratory or diagnostic studies is a role expectation of the professional nurse. The notification processes vary among facilities. Upon receipt of the critical finding, the information should be read back to the caller to verify accuracy.

Symptoms of acute renal dysfunction and/or chronic kidney disease associated with hyperuricemia include altered mental status, nausea and vomiting, fluid overload, pericarditis, and seizures. Prophylactic measures against the development of hyperuricemia should be undertaken before initiation of chemotherapy. Possible interventions include discontinuing medications that increase serum urate levels or produce acidic urine (e.g., thiazides and salicylates); administration of fluids with sodium bicarbonate as an additive to intravenous (IV) solutions to promote hydration and alkalinization of the urine to a pH greater than 7; administration of allopurinol 1 to 2 days before chemotherapy; monitoring of serum electrolyte, uric acid, phosphorus, calcium, and creatinine levels; and monitoring for ureteral obstruction by urate calculi using computed tomography or ultrasound studies. Possible interventions for advanced renal insufficiency and subsequent chronic kidney disease may include peritoneal dialysis or hemodialysis.

INTERFERING FACTORS

- Drugs and other substances that may increase uric acid levels include acetylsalicylic acid (low doses), aminothiadiazole, anabolic steroids, antineoplastic drugs, atenolol, azathioprine, chlorambucil, chlorthalidone, cisplatin, corn oil, cyclosporine, cyclothiazide, cytarabine, diapamide, diuretics, ethacrynic acid, ethambutol, ethoxzolamide, flumethiazide, hydrochlorothiazide, hydroflumethiazide, ibufenac, ibuprofen, levarterenol, mefruside, mercaptopurine, methicillin, methotrexate, methyclothiazide, mitomycin, morinamide, polythiazide, prednisone, pyrazinamide, quinethazone, salicylate, spironolactone, tacrolimus, theophylline, thiazide diuretics, thioguanine, thiotepa, triamterene, trichlormethiazide, vincristine, and warfarin.
- Drugs and other substances that may decrease uric acid levels include allopurinol, aspirin (high doses), azathioprine, benzbromaron, canola oil, chlorothiazide (given IV), chlorpromazine, chlorprothixene, clofibrate, corticosteroids, corticotropin, coumarin, dicumarol, enalapril, fenofibrate, guaifenesin, iodipamide, iodopyracet, iopanoic acid, ipodate, lisinopril, mefenamic acid, methotrexate, oxyphenbutazone, phenolsulfonphthalein, probenecid, radiographic medium, rasburicase, seclazone, sulfinpyrazone, and verapamil.
- Rasburicase will rapidly decrease uric acid in specimens left at room temperature. Specimens must be collected in prechilled tubes, transported in an ice slurry, and tested within 4 hr of collection.

U

NURSING IMPLICATIONS AND PROCEDURE

POTENTIAL NURSING PROBLEMS:

Problem	Signs & Symptoms	Interventions
Fluid volume (water) ***(related to decreased glomerular filtration or the presence of the diuretic stage of kidney disease)***	**Overload:** Edema, shortness of breath, increased weight, ascites, rales, rhonchi, and diluted laboratory values **Deficit:** Decreased urinary output, fatigue, sunken eyes, dark urine, decreased blood pressure, increased heart rate, and altered mental status	Manage underlying cause of fluid alteration; record accurate intake and output; monitor urine characteristics and respiratory status; establish baseline assessment data; collaborate to adjust oral and IV fluids to provide optimal hydration status
Confusion ***(related to an alteration in fluid and electrolytes, hepatic disease, kidney disease)***	Disorganized thinking, restlessness, irritability, altered concentration and attention span, changeable mental function over the day, hallucinations	Treat the medical condition; correlate confusion with the need to reverse altered electrolytes; evaluate medications; prevent falls and injury through appropriate use of postural support, bed alarm, or restraints; consider pharmacological interventions; record accurate intake and output to assess fluid status
Electrolytes ***(related to compromised excretion; kidney function)***	Increased blood urea nitrogen, increased creatinine; decreased sodium, increased urine specific gravity; increased potassium; decreased sodium; decreased calcium; increased magnesium; increased phosphorus; altered uric acid	Monitor laboratory values; administer appropriate IV infusions and medications to correct altered electrolytes as ordered; collaborate with HCP in consideration of dialysis as appropriate to maintain homeostasis; monitor uric acid levels

Problem	Signs & Symptoms	Interventions
Nutrition ***(related to altered taste, decreased food intake, nausea, vomiting)***	Poor nutrition with inadequate caloric intake; progressive weight loss; decreasing muscle mass; thin, weak, and apathetic; poor skin turgor with breakdown; difficulty healing; anemic; decreased respiratory and cardiac status	Assess nutritional requirements; seek a consultation with a registered dietitian; use a calorie count; correlate baseline nutritional intake with medical status; consider individual and cultural food preferences; collaborate with HCP, pharmacist, and clinical dietitian in consideration of enteral and parenteral nutrition

PRETEST:

- Positively identify the patient using at least two person-specific identifiers before services, treatments, or procedures are performed.
- ***Patient Teaching:*** Inform the patient this test can assist in diagnosing gout and assessing kidney function.
- Obtain a history of the patient's health concerns, including a list of known allergens, especially allergies or sensitivities to latex. Especially note.
- Obtain a history of the patient's health concerns (especially pain and edema in joints and great toe (caused by precipitation of sodium urates), headache, fatigue, decreased urinary output, and hypertension), symptoms, surgical procedures, and results of previously performed laboratory and diagnostic studies. Include a list of known allergens, especially allergies or sensitivities to latex.
- Obtain a list of the patient's current medications, including over-the-counter medications and dietary supplements (see Effects of Natural Products on Laboratory Values online at Davis*Plus*).
- Review the procedure with the patient. Inform the patient that specimen collection takes approximately 5 to 10 min. Address concerns about pain and explain that there may be some discomfort during the venipuncture.
- ***Sensitivity to social and cultural issues,*** as well as concern for modesty, is important in providing psychological support before, during, and after the procedure.
- Note that there are no food, fluid, or medication restrictions unless by medical direction.

INTRATEST:

Potential Complications: N/A

- Avoid the use of equipment containing latex if the patient has a history of allergic reaction to latex.
- Instruct the patient to cooperate fully and to follow directions. Direct the patient to breathe normally and to avoid unnecessary movement.
- Observe standard precautions, and follow the general guidelines in Patient Preparation and Specimen Collection online at Davis*Plus*. Positively identify the patient, and label the appropriate specimen container with the corresponding patient demographics, initials of the person collecting the specimen, date, and time of collection. Perform a venipuncture.
- Remove the needle and apply direct pressure with dry gauze to stop

bleeding. Observe/assess venipuncture site for bleeding or hematoma formation and secure gauze with adhesive bandage.

- Promptly transport the specimen to the laboratory for processing and analysis.

POST-TEST:

- Inform the patient that a report of the results will be made available to the requesting HCP, who will discuss the results with the patient.
- *Nutritional Considerations:* Increased uric acid levels may be associated with the formation of kidney stones. Educate the patient, if appropriate, on the importance of drinking a sufficient amount of water when kidney stones are suspected.
- *Nutritional Considerations:* Increased uric acid levels may be associated with gout. Nutritional therapy may be appropriate for some patients identified as having gout. Educate the patient that foods high in oxalic acid include caffeinated beverages, raw blackberries, gooseberries and plums, whole-wheat bread, beets, carrots, beans, rhubarb, spinach, dry cocoa, and Ovaltine. Foods high in purines include organ meats, which should be restricted. In other cases, the requesting HCP may not prescribe a low-purine or purine-restricted diet for treatment of gout because medications can control the condition easily and effectively.
- Recognize anxiety related to test results. Discuss the implications of abnormal test results on the patient's lifestyle. Provide teaching and information regarding the clinical implications of the test results, as appropriate.
- Reinforce information given by the patient's HCP regarding further testing, treatment, or referral to another HCP. Answer any questions or address any concerns voiced by the patient or family.
- Depending on the results of this procedure, additional testing may be performed to evaluate or monitor progression of the disease process and determine the need for a change in therapy. Evaluate test results in relation to the patient's symptoms and other tests performed.

Patient Education:

- Discuss lifestyle alterations that may improve health.
- Provide written and verbal information on the anatomy and physiology of the disease process.

Expected Patient Outcomes:

Understanding

- The patient and family acknowledge the importance of recognizing and reporting disease signs and symptoms to HCP.
- The patient and family verbalize food selections that are appropriate to health maintenance.

Ability

- The patient demonstrates proficiency in performing and recording daily weight.
- The patient demonstrates proficiency in self-administration of medication for gout after meals as appropriate.

Response

- The patient expresses willingness to make necessary lifestyle changes to improve health management.
- The patient complies with the recommended therapeutic plan of care.

RELATED STUDIES:

- Related tests include arthroscopy, biopsy bone marrow, calcium, calculus kidney stone panel, cholesterol, collagen cross-linked telopeptide, CBC, CBC RBC count, CBC RBC indices, CBC RBC morphology, creatinine, creatinine clearance, gastrin stimulation, G6PD, lactic acid, lead, PTH, parathyroid scan, phosphorus, sickle cell screen, synovial fluid analysis, UA, US abdomen, and uric acid urine.
- Refer to the Genitourinary, Hepatobiliary, and Musculoskeletal systems tables online at Davis*Plus* for related tests by body system.

U

Uric Acid, Urine

SYNONYM/ACRONYM: Urine urate.

COMMON USE: To assist in confirming a diagnosis of gout, assess renal function, evaluate for genetic defects related to uric acid levels, and monitor the effectiveness of therapeutic interventions.

SPECIMEN: Urine from a random or timed specimen collected in a clean plastic, unrefrigerated collection container. Sodium hydroxide preservative may be recommended to prevent precipitation of urates.

NORMAL FINDINGS: (Method: Spectrophotometry)

Gender	Conventional Units	SI Units (Conventional Units × 0.0059)
Male	250–800 mg/24 hr	1.48–4.72 mmol/24 hr
Female	250–750 mg/24 hr	1.48–4.43 mmol/24 hr

Values reflect average purine diet.

POTENTIAL MEDICAL DIAGNOSIS

Increased in:

- Disorders associated with impaired renal tubular absorption, such as Fanconi's syndrome and Wilson's disease
- Disorders of purine metabolism
- Excessive dietary intake of purines
- Gout
- Neoplastic disorders, such as leukemia, lymphosarcoma, and multiple myeloma ***(related to increased cell turnover)***
- Pernicious anemia ***(related to increased cell turnover)***
- Polycythemia vera ***(related to increased cell turnover)***
- Renal calculus formation ***(related to increased urinary excretion)***
- Sickle cell anemia ***(related to increased cell turnover)***

Decreased in:

- Chronic alcohol ingestion ***(related to decreased excretion)***
- Hypertension ***(related to decreased excretion)***
- Severe kidney damage ***(possibly resulting from chronic glomerulonephritis, collagen disorders, diabetic glomerulosclerosis, lactic acidosis, ketoacidosis, or alcohol misuse)***

CRITICAL FINDINGS: N/A

Find and print out the full study on Fast Find at davispl.us/vanleeuwen7.

Urinalysis

SYNONYM/ACRONYM: UA.

COMMON USE: To screen urine for multiple substances such as infection, blood, sugar, bilirubin, urobilinogen, nitrates, and protein to assist in diagnosing disorders such as kidney and liver disease as well as assess hydration status.

Access Canadian content on Fast Find: Lab and Dx at davispl.us/vanleeuwen7

SPECIMEN: Urine from an unpreserved, random specimen collected in a clean plastic collection container.

NORMAL FINDINGS: (Method: Macroscopic evaluation by dipstick and microscopic examination) Urinalysis comprises a battery of tests including a description of the color and appearance of urine; measurement of specific gravity and pH; and semiquantitative measurement of protein, glucose, ketones, urobilinogen, bilirubin, hemoglobin, nitrites, and leukocyte esterase. Urine sediment may also be examined for the presence of crystals, casts, renal epithelial cells, transitional epithelial cells, squamous epithelial cells, white blood cells (WBCs), red blood cells (RBCs), bacteria, yeast, sperm, and any other substances excreted in the urine that may have clinical significance. Examination of urine sediment is performed microscopically under high power, and results are reported as the number seen per high-power field (hpf). The color of normal urine ranges from light yellow to deep amber. The color depends on the patient's state of hydration (more concentrated samples are darker in color), diet, medication regimen, and exposure to other substances that may contribute to unusual color or odor. The appearance of normal urine is clear. Cloudiness is sometimes attributable to the presence of amorphous phosphates or urates as well as blood, WBCs, fat, or bacteria.

Dipstick

pH	4.5–8
Protein	Less than 20 mg/dL
Glucose	Negative
Ketones	Negative
Hemoglobin	Negative
Bilirubin	Negative
Urobilinogen	Up to 1 mg/dL
Nitrite	Negative
Leukocyte esterase	Negative
Specific gravity	1.005–1.03

Microscopic Examination

RBCs	Less than 5/hpf
WBCs	Less than 5/hpf
Renal cells	None seen
Transitional cells	None seen
Squamous cells	Rare; usually no clinical significance
Casts	Rare hyaline; otherwise, none seen
Crystals in acid urine	Uric acid, calcium oxalate, amorphous urates
Crystals in alkaline urine	Triple phosphate, calcium phosphate, ammonium biurate, calcium carbonate, amorphous phosphates
Bacteria, yeast, parasites	None seen

DESCRIPTION: Routine urinalysis, one of the most widely ordered laboratory procedures, is used for basic screening purposes. It is a group of tests that evaluate the kidneys' ability to selectively excrete and reabsorb substances while maintaining proper water balance. The results can provide valuable information regarding the overall health of the patient and the patient's response to disease and treatment. The urine dipstick has a number of pads on it to indicate various biochemical markers. Urine pH is an indication of the kidneys' ability to help maintain balanced hydrogen ion concentration in the blood. Specific gravity is a reflection of the concentration ability of the kidneys. Urine protein is the most common indicator of kidney disease, although there are conditions that can cause benign proteinuria. Glucose is used as an indicator of diabetes. The presence of ketones indicates impaired carbohydrate metabolism. Hemoglobin indicates the presence of blood, which is associated with kidney disease. Bilirubin is used to assist in the detection of liver disorders. Urobilinogen indicates hepatic or hematopoietic conditions. Nitrites and leukocytes are used to test for bacteriuria and other sources of urinary tract infections (UTIs). Most laboratories have established criteria for the microscopic examination of urine based on patient population (e.g., pediatric, oncology, urology), unusual appearance, and biochemical reactions.

This procedure is contraindicated for: N/A

INDICATIONS

- Determine the presence of a genitourinary infection or abnormality.
- Monitor the effects of physical or emotional stress.
- Monitor fluid imbalances or treatment for fluid imbalances.
- Monitor the response to drug therapy and evaluate undesired reactions to drugs that may impair renal function.
- Provide screening as part of a general physical examination, especially on admission to a health-care facility or before surgery.

POTENTIAL MEDICAL DIAGNOSIS

Unusual Color

Color	Presence of
Deep yellow	Riboflavin
Orange	Bilirubin, chrysophanic acid (e.g., rhubarb), phenazopyridine, santonin
Pink	Beet pigment, hemoglobin, myoglobin, porphyrin, rhubarb
Red	Beet pigment, hemoglobin, myoglobin, porphyrin, uroerythrin
Green	Oxidized bilirubin, Clorets (breath mint)
Blue	Diagnex, indican, methylene blue
Brown	Bilirubin, hematin, methemoglobin, metronidazole, nitrofurantoin, metabolites of rhubarb, senna
Black	Homogentisic acid, melanin
Smoky	RBCs

U

Test	Increased in	Decreased in
pH	Ingestion of citrus fruits Vegetarian diets Metabolic and respiratory alkalosis	Ingestion of cranberries High-protein diets Metabolic or respiratory acidosis
Protein	Benign proteinuria owing to stress, physical exercise, exposure to cold, or standing Diabetic nephropathy Glomerulonephritis Nephrosis Toxemia of pregnancy	N/A
Glucose	Diabetes	N/A
Ketones	Diabetes Fasting Fever High-protein diets Isopropanol intoxication Postanesthesia period Starvation Vomiting	N/A
Hemoglobin	Diseases of the bladder Exercise (march hemoglobinuria) Glomerulonephritis Hemolytic anemia or other causes of hemolysis (e.g., drugs, parasites, transfusion reaction) Malignancy Menstruation Paroxysmal cold hemoglobinuria Paroxysmal nocturnal hemoglobinuria Pyelonephritis Snake or spider bites Trauma Tuberculosis Urinary tract infections Urolithiasis	N/A
Urobilinogen	Cirrhosis Heart failure Hemolytic anemia Hepatitis Infectious mononucleosis	Antibiotic therapy (suppresses normal intestinal flora) Obstruction of the bile duct

Test	Increased in	Decreased in
	Malaria Pernicious anemia	
Bilirubin	Cirrhosis Hepatic tumor Hepatitis	N/A
Nitrites	Presence of nitrite-forming bacteria (e.g., *Citrobacter*, *Enterobacter*, *Escherichia coli*, *Klebsiella*, *Proteus*, *Pseudomonas*, *Salmonella*, and some species of *Staphylococcus*)	N/A
Leukocyte esterase	Bacterial infection Calculus formation Fungal or parasitic infection Glomerulonephritis Interstitial nephritis Tumor	N/A
Specific gravity	Adrenal insufficiency Dehydration Diabetes Diarrhea Fever Diuresis Excess IV fluids Excess hydration	Hypothermia Impaired renal concentrating ability Heart failure Proteinuria Sweating Vomiting Water restriction X-ray dyes

Formed Elements in Urine Sediment

Cellular Elements

- Clue cells (cell wall of the bacteria causes adhesion to epithelial cells) are present in nonspecific vaginitis caused by *Gardnerella vaginitis, Mobiluncus curtisii,* and *M. mulieris*.
- RBCs are present in glomerulonephritis, lupus nephritis, focal glomerulonephritis, calculus, malignancy, infection, tuberculosis, infarction, renal vein thrombosis, trauma, hydronephrosis, polycystic kidney, urinary tract disease, prostatitis, pyelonephritis, appendicitis, salpingitis, diverticulitis, gout, scurvy, subacute bacterial endocarditis, infectious mononucleosis, hemoglobinopathies, coagulation disorders, heart failure, and malaria.
- Renal cells that have absorbed cholesterol and triglycerides are also known as oval fat bodies.
- Renal cells come from the lining of the collecting ducts, and increased numbers indicate acute tubular damage as seen in acute tubular necrosis, pyelonephritis, malignant nephrosclerosis, acute glomerulonephritis, acute drug or substance (salicylate, lead, or

ethylene glycol) intoxication, or chemotherapy, resulting in desquamation, urolithiasis, and kidney transplant rejection.
- Squamous cells line the vagina and distal portion of the urethra. The presence of normal squamous epithelial cells in female urine is generally of no clinical significance. Abnormal cells with enlarged nuclei indicate the need for cytological studies to rule out malignancy.
- Transitional cells line the renal pelvis, ureter, bladder, and proximal portion of the urethra. Increased numbers are seen with infection, trauma, and malignancy.
- WBCs are present in acute UTI, tubulointerstitial nephritis, lupus nephritis, pyelonephritis, kidney transplant rejection, fever, and strenuous exercise.

Casts
- Granular casts are formed from protein or by the decomposition of cellular elements. They may be seen in kidney disease, viral infections, or lead intoxication.
- Large numbers of hyaline casts may be seen in kidney diseases, hypertension, heart failure, or nephrotic syndrome and in more benign conditions such as fever, exposure to cold temperatures, exercise, or diuretic use.
- RBC casts may be found in acute glomerulonephritis, lupus nephritis, and subacute bacterial endocarditis.
- Waxy casts are seen in chronic kidney disease or conditions such as kidney transplant rejection, in which there is renal stasis.
- WBC casts may be seen in lupus nephritis, acute glomerulonephritis, interstitial nephritis, and acute pyelonephritis.

Crystals
- Crystals found in freshly voided urine have more clinical significance than crystals seen in a urine sample that has been standing for more than 2 to 4 hr.
- Calcium oxalate crystals are found in ethylene glycol poisoning, urolithiasis, high dietary intake of oxalates, and Crohn's disease.
- Cystine crystals are seen in patients with cystinosis or cystinuria.
- Leucine or tyrosine crystals may be seen in patients with severe liver disease.
- Large numbers of uric acid crystals are seen in patients with urolithiasis, gout, high dietary intake of foods rich in purines, or who are receiving chemotherapy (see study titled "Uric Acid, Urine").

Yeast
- Yeast cells, usually *Candida albicans* may be seen in diabetes and vaginal moniliasis.

CRITICAL FINDINGS:

Possible critical findings are the presence of uric acid, cystine, leucine, or tyrosine crystals.

The combination of grossly elevated urine glucose and ketones is also considered significant.

Note and immediately report to the requesting health-care provider (HCP) any critical findings and related symptoms. A listing of these findings varies among facilities. Timely notification of a critical finding for laboratory or diagnostic studies is a role expectation of the professional nurse. The notification processes vary among facilities. Upon receipt of the critical finding, the information should be read back to the caller to verify accuracy.

INTERFERING FACTORS

- Certain foods, such as onion, garlic, and asparagus, contain substances that may give urine an unusual odor. An ammonia-like odor may be produced by the presence of bacteria. Urine with a maple syrup-like odor may indicate a congenital metabolic defect (maple syrup urine disease).

- The various biochemical strips are subject to interference that may produce false-positive or false-negative results. Consult the laboratory for specific information regarding limitations of the method in use and a listing of interfering drugs.
- The dipstick method for protein detection is mostly sensitive to the presence of albumin; light-chain or Bence Jones proteins may not be detected by this method. Alkaline pH may produce false-positive protein results.
- Large amounts of ketones or ascorbic acid may produce false-negative or decreased color development on the glucose pad. Contamination of the collection container or specimen with chlorine, sodium hypochlorite, or peroxide may cause false-positive glucose results.
- False-positive ketone results may be produced in the presence of ascorbic acid, levodopa metabolites, valproic acid, phenazopyridine, phenylketones, or phthaleins.
- The hemoglobin pad may detect myoglobin, intact RBCs, and free hemoglobin. Contamination of the collection container or specimen with sodium hypochlorite or iodine may cause false-positive hemoglobin results. Negative or decreased hemoglobin results may occur in the presence of formalin, elevated protein, nitrite, ascorbic acid, or high specific gravity.
- False-negative nitrite results are common. Negative or decreased results may be seen in the presence of ascorbic acid and high specific gravity. Other causes of false-negative values relate to the amount of time the urine was in the bladder before voiding or the presence of pathogenic organisms that do not reduce nitrates to nitrites.
- False-positive leukocyte esterase reactions result from specimens contaminated by vaginal secretions. The presence of high glucose, protein, or ascorbic acid concentrations may cause false-negative results. Specimens with high specific gravity may also produce false-negative results. Patients with neutropenia (e.g., oncology patients) may also have false-negative results because they do not produce enough WBCs to exceed the sensitivity of the biochemical reaction.
- Specimens that cannot be delivered to the laboratory or tested within 1 hr should be refrigerated or should have a preservative added that is recommended by the laboratory. Specimens collected more than 2 hr before submission may be rejected for analysis.
- Because changes in the urine specimen occur over time, prompt and proper specimen processing, storage, and analysis are important to achieve accurate results. Changes that may occur over time include:

Production of a stronger odor and an increase in pH (bacteria in the urine break urea down to ammonia)
A decrease in clarity (as bacterial growth proceeds or precipitates form)
A decrease in bilirubin and urobilinogen (oxidation to biliverdin and urobilin)
A decrease in ketones (lost through volatilization)
Decreased glucose (consumed by bacteria)
An increase in bacteria (growth over time)
Disintegration of casts, WBCs, and RBCs
An increase in nitrite (overgrowth of bacteria)

NURSING IMPLICATIONS AND PROCEDURE

POTENTIAL NURSING PROBLEMS:

Problem	Signs & Symptoms	Interventions
Fluid volume (water) ***(related to hypovolemia associated with body fluid shifts to third space, body fluid loss, reduced oral intake; increased perspiration; diaphoresis; gastrointestinal [GI] tract loss from vomiting, diarrhea; overly aggressive diuresis)***	**Deficient:** Decreased urinary output, fatigue, sunken eyes, dark urine, decreased blood pressure, increased heart rate, and altered mental status	Record daily weight and monitor trends; record accurate intake and output; collaborate with HCP on administration of intravenous (IV) fluids to support hydration; monitor laboratory values that reflect alterations in fluid status (potassium, blood urea nitrogen [BUN], creatinine [Cr], calcium, hemoglobin [Hbg], and hematocrit [Hct]); manage underlying cause of fluid alteration; monitor urine characteristics and respiratory status; establish baseline assessment data; collaborate with HCP to adjust oral and IV fluids to provide optimal hydration status; administer replacement electrolytes as ordered
Confusion ***(related to an alteration in fluid and electrolytes secondary to hepatic disease and encephalopathy; acute alcohol consumption; hepatic metabolic insufficiency)***	Disorganized thinking, restlessness, irritability, altered concentration and attention span, changeable mental function over the day, hallucinations; altered attention span; inability to follow directions; disoriented to person, place, time, and purpose; inappropriate affect	Treat the medical condition; correlate confusion with the need to reverse altered electrolytes; evaluate medications; prevent falls and injury through appropriate use of postural support, bed alarm, or restraints; consider pharmacological interventions; record accurate intake and output to assess fluid status; monitor blood

Access Canadian content on Fast Find: Lab and Dx at davispl.us/vanleeuwen7

Problem	Signs & Symptoms	Interventions
		ammonia level; determine last alcohol use; assess for symptoms of hepatic encephalopathy such as confusion, sleep disturbances, incoherence; protect the patient from physical harm; administer lactulose as prescribed
Self-care ***(related to altered mental status; fatigue; weakness; secondary to renal insufficiency, hepatic disease, hypovolemia, dehydration)***	Difficulty fastening clothing; difficulty performing personal hygiene; unable to maintain appropriate appearance; difficulty with independent mobility	Reinforce self-care techniques as taught by occupational therapy; ensure the patient has adequate time to perform self-care; encourage use of assistive devices to maintain independence
Kidney function ***(related to renal ischemia associated with shock, sepsis, hypovolemia; postoperative injury; trauma; nephrotoxic drugs [aminoglycoside, heavy metals, radiographic contrast]; renal vascular occlusion; hemolytic transfusion reaction; decreased cardiac output; tubular necrosis; obstruction; tumor; medications [NSAID, angiotensin-converting enzyme, immunosuppressants, antineoplastics, antifungals])***	Increased BUN; increased Cr; decreased Cr clearance; increased urine specific gravity (greater than 1.029); hematuria; proteinuria; decreased urine output less than 400 mL/day (with adequate intake and no fluid loss); weight gain; elevated potassium; elevated phosphate; decreased calcium; decreased sodium; increased magnesium; metabolic acidosis; decreased Hgb/Hct	Monitor, record, and trend intake and output; monitor urine specific gravity; monitor and trend renal specific urine and blood studies, BUN, Cr, sodium, potassium, magnesium, pH, urinalysis, Hgb/Hct; monitor and trend weight daily; assess and monitor for edema, jugular vein distention, hypertension, adventitious breath sounds, impaired gas exchange; use pulse oximetry; administer prescribed oxygen; administer prescribed hemodialysis; administer prescribed medications (diuretics); administer prescribed fluids; consider renal function with antibiotic administration

PRETEST:

- Positively identify the patient using at least two person-specific identifiers before services, treatments, or procedures are performed.
- *Patient Teaching:* Inform the patient this test can assist in assessing for disease, infection, and inflammation and evaluate for dehydration.
- Obtain a history of the patient's health concerns, symptoms, surgical procedures, and results of previously performed laboratory and diagnostic studies. Include a list of known allergens, especially allergies or sensitivities to latex.
- Obtain a list of the patient's current medications, including over-the-counter medications and dietary supplements (see Effects of Natural Products on Laboratory Values online at Davis*Plus*).
- Review the procedure with the patient. If a catheterized specimen is to be collected, explain this procedure to the patient, and obtain a catheterization tray. Address concerns about pain and explain that there should be no discomfort during the procedure. Inform the patient that specimen collection takes approximately 5 to 10 min.
- *Sensitivity to social and cultural issues,* as well as concern for modesty, is important in providing psychological support before, during, and after the procedure.
- Note that there are no food, fluid, or medication restrictions unless by medical direction.

INTRATEST:

Potential Complications: N/A

- Avoid the use of equipment containing latex if the patient has a history of allergic reaction to latex.
- Instruct the patient to cooperate fully and to follow directions. Direct the patient to breathe normally and to avoid unnecessary movement.
- Observe standard precautions, and follow the general guidelines in Patient Preparation and Specimen Collection online at Davis*Plus*. Positively identify the patient, and label the appropriate specimen container with the corresponding patient demographics, initials of the person collecting the specimen, date, and time of collection.

Random Specimen (Collect in Early Morning)

Clean-Catch Specimen

- Instruct the male patient to (1) thoroughly wash his hands, (2) cleanse the meatus, (3) void a small amount into the toilet, and (4) void directly into the specimen container.
- Instruct the female patient to (1) thoroughly wash her hands; (2) cleanse the labia from front to back; (3) while keeping the labia separated, void a small amount into the toilet; and (4) without interrupting the urine stream, void directly into the specimen container.

Pediatric Urine Collector

- Put on gloves. Appropriately cleanse the genital area, and allow the area to dry. Remove the covering over the adhesive strips on the collector bag, and apply the bag over the genital area. Diaper the child. When specimen is obtained, place the entire collection bag in a sterile urine container.

Indwelling Catheter

- Put on gloves. Empty drainage tube of urine. It may be necessary to clamp off the catheter for 15 to 30 min before specimen collection. Cleanse specimen port with antiseptic swab, and then aspirate 5 mL of urine with a 21- to 25-gauge needle and syringe. Transfer urine to a sterile container.

Urinary Catheterization

- Place female patient in lithotomy position or male patient in supine position. Using sterile technique, open the straight urinary catheterization kit and perform urinary catheterization. Place the retained urine in a sterile specimen container.

Suprapubic Aspiration

- Place the patient in a supine position. Cleanse the area with antiseptic and drape with sterile drapes. A needle is inserted through the skin into the bladder. A syringe attached to the needle is used to aspirate the urine sample. The needle is then removed and a sterile dressing is applied to the site. Place the sterile sample in a sterile specimen container.

- Perform catheterization through the stoma. Do not collect urine from the pouch from the patient with a urinary diversion (e.g., ileal conduit).

General

- Include on the collection container's label whether the specimen is clean catch or catheter and any medications that may interfere with test results.
- Promptly transport the specimen to the laboratory for processing and analysis.

POST-TEST:

- Inform the patient that a report of the results will be made available to the requesting HCP, who will discuss the results with the patient.
- Instruct the patient to report symptoms such as pain related to tissue inflammation, pain or irritation during void, bladder spasms, or alterations in urinary elimination.
- Observe/assess for signs of inflammation if the specimen is obtained by suprapubic aspiration.
- Recognize anxiety related to test results. Discuss the implications of abnormal test results on the patient's lifestyle. Provide teaching and information regarding the clinical implications of the test results, as appropriate. Instruct the patient with a UTI, as appropriate, on the proper technique for wiping the perineal area (front to back) after a bowel movement. UTIs are more common in women who use diaphragm/spermicide contraception. These patients can be educated, as appropriate, in the proper insertion and removal of the contraceptive device to avoid recurrent UTIs.
- Depending on the results of this procedure, additional testing may be performed to evaluate or monitor progression of the disease process and determine the need for a change in therapy. Evaluate test results in relation to the patient's symptoms and other tests performed.

Patient Education:

- Reinforce information given by the patient's HCP regarding further testing, treatment, or referral to another HCP.
- Instruct the patient to begin antibiotic therapy, as prescribed, and instruct the patient in the importance of completing the entire course of antibiotic therapy even if symptoms are no longer present.
- Answer any questions or address any concerns voiced by the patient or family.
- Teach the patient to save urine for accurate measurement and evaluation of characteristics.

Expected Patient Outcomes:

Understanding

- The patient and family state symptoms of fluid overload, headache, tachycardia, shortness of breath, and understands to report symptoms to HCP.
- The patient states fluid preferences and identifies selections for fluid replacement.

Ability

- The patient proficiently describes normal urine characteristics and identifies concerns that should be reported to HCP.
- The patient demonstrates proficiency in recording intake and measuring and recording urine output.

Response

- The patient complies with recommended medication regime.
- The patient complies with follow-up appointment schedule to monitor kidney and urinary function.

RELATED STUDIES:

- Related tests include amino acids, angiography kidneys, antibodies, antiglomerular basement membrane, biopsy bladder, biopsy

U

kidney, bladder cancer marker, BUN, calcium, calculus kidney stone panel, CBC, CT kidneys, creatinine, culture urine, cystometry, cystoscopy, cystourethrography voiding, cytology urine, electrolytes, glucose, glycated hemoglobin, IFE, IVP, ketones, KUB study, microalbumin, osmolality, oxalate, protein total, phosphorus, renogram, retrograde ureteropyelography, urea nitrogen urine, uric acid (blood and urine), and US abdomen.

- Refer to the Endocrine, Genitourinary, Immune, Hematopoietic, and Hepatobiliary systems tables online at Davis*Plus* for related tests by body system.

Uterine Fibroid Embolization

SYNONYM/ACRONYM: UFE; uterine artery embolization.

COMMON USE: A less invasive modality used to assist in treating fibroid tumors found in the uterine lining, heavy menstrual bleeding, and pelvic pain.

AREA OF APPLICATION: Uterus.

DESCRIPTION: Uterine fibroid embolization (UFE) is a way of treating fibroid tumors of the uterus. Fibroid tumors, also known as myomas, are masses of fibrous and muscle tissue in the uterine wall that are benign but that may cause heavy menstrual bleeding, pain in the pelvic region, or pressure on the bladder or bowel. Using angiographic methods, a catheter is placed in each of the two uterine arteries, and small particles are injected to block the arterial branches that supply blood to the fibroids. The fibroid tissue dies, the mass shrinks, and the symptoms are relieved. This procedure, which is done under local anesthesia, is less invasive than open surgery done to remove uterine fibroids. Because the effects of uterine fibroid embolization on fertility are not yet known, the ideal candidate is a premenopausal woman with symptoms from fibroid tumors who no longer wishes to become pregnant. This technique is an alternative for women who do not want to receive blood transfusions or do not wish to receive general anesthesia. This procedure may be used to halt severe bleeding following childbirth or caused by gynecological tumors.

This procedure is contraindicated for

Patients who are pregnant or suspected of being pregnant, unless the potential benefits of a procedure using radiation far outweigh the risk of radiation exposure to the fetus and mother.

Patients with conditions associated with adverse reactions to contrast medium (e.g., asthma, food allergies, or allergy to contrast medium).

Although patients are asked specifically if they have a known allergy to iodine or shellfish, it has been well established that the reaction is not to iodine, in fact an actual iodine allergy would be problematic because iodine is required for the production of thyroid hormones. In the case of shellfish, the reaction is to a muscle protein

U

called tropomyosin; in the case of iodinated contrast medium, the reaction is to the noniodinated part of the contrast molecule. Patients with a known hypersensitivity to the medium may benefit from premedication with corticosteroids and diphenhydramine; the use of nonionic contrast or an alternative noncontrast imaging study, if available, may be considered for patients who have severe asthma or who have experienced moderate to severe reactions to ionic contrast medium.

- Patients with conditions associated with preexisting renal insufficiency (e.g., chronic kidney disease, single kidney transplant, nephrectomy, diabetes, multiple myeloma, treatment with aminoglycosides and NSAIDs) ***because iodinated contrast is nephrotoxic.***
- Patients who are chronically dehydrated before the test, especially older adults and patients whose health is already compromised, ***because of their risk of contrast-induced acute kidney injury.***
- Patients with bleeding disorders ***because the puncture site may not stop bleeding.***
- Patients in whom cancer is a possibility or who have inflammation or infection in the pelvis.

INDICATIONS

- Treatment for anemia from chronic blood loss.
- Treatment of fibroid tumors and tumor vascularity, for both single and multiple tumors.
- Treatment of tumors in lieu of surgical resection.

POTENTIAL MEDICAL DIAGNOSIS

Normal findings

- Decrease in uterine bleeding
- Decrease of pelvic pain or fullness

Abnormal findings related to

- No reduction in size of fibroid

CRITICAL FINDINGS: N/A

INTERFERING FACTORS

Factors that may alter the results of the study

- Gas or feces in the gastrointestinal tract resulting from inadequate cleansing or failure to restrict food intake before the study.
- Retained barium from a previous radiological procedure.
- Metallic objects (e.g., jewelry, body rings) within the examination field, which may inhibit organ visualization and cause unclear images.

Other considerations

- The procedure may be terminated if chest pain or severe cardiac dysrhythmias occur.
- Inability of the patient to cooperate or remain still during the procedure because of age, significant pain, or mental status, may interfere with the test results.
- Failure to follow dietary restrictions before the procedure may cause the procedure to be canceled or repeated.
- A small percentage of women may pass a small piece of fibroid tissue after the procedure. Women with this problem may require a procedure called a D & C (dilatation and curettage).
- Some women may experience menopause shortly after the procedure.

NURSING IMPLICATIONS AND PROCEDURE

PRETEST:

- Positively identify the patient using at least two person-specific identifiers before services, treatments, or procedures are performed.
- ***Patient Teaching:*** Inform the patient this procedure can assist in assessing and treating the uterus.

- Obtain a history of the patient's health concerns, symptoms, surgical procedures, and results of previously performed laboratory and diagnostic studies. Include a list of known allergens, especially allergies or sensitivities to latex, anesthetics, sedatives, or contrast medium. Ensure results of coagulation testing are obtained and recorded prior to the procedure; a creatinine level is also needed before contrast medium is to be used.
- Note any recent procedures that can interfere with test results; include examinations utilizing barium- or iodine-based contrast medium.
- Record the date of the last menstrual period and determine the possibility of pregnancy in perimenopausal women.
- Obtain a list of the patient's current medications, including over-the-counter medications, dietary supplements, anticoagulants, aspirin and other salicylates (see Effects of Natural Products on Laboratory Values online at Davis*Plus*). Such products should be discontinued by medical direction for the appropriate number of days prior to a surgical procedure. Note the last time and dose of medication taken.
- If iodinated contrast medium is scheduled to be used in patients receiving metformin (Glucophage) for type 2 diabetes, the drug should be discontinued on the day of the test and continue to be withheld for 48 hr after the test. Iodinated contrast can temporarily impair kidney function, and failure to withhold metformin may indirectly result in drug-induced lactic acidosis, a dangerous and sometimes fatal adverse effect of metformin ***related to renal impairment that does not support sufficient excretion of metformin.***
- Review the procedure with the patient. Address concerns about pain and explain that there may be moments of discomfort and some pain experienced during the test. Explain that a sedative and/or anesthetic may be administered before the procedure to promote relaxation. Inform the patient that the procedure is performed in a radiology or vascular department by a health-care provider (HCP), with support staff, and takes approximately 30 to 120 min.
- ***Sensitivity to social and cultural issues,*** as well as concern for modesty, is important in providing psychological support before, during, and after the procedure.
- Explain that an intravenous (IV) line may be inserted to allow infusion of fluids such as saline, anesthetics, sedatives, or emergency medications. Explain that the contrast medium will be injected, by catheter, at a separate site from the IV line.
- Inform the patient that a burning and flushing sensation may be felt throughout the body during injection of the contrast medium. After injection of the contrast medium, the patient may experience an urge to cough, flushing, nausea, or a salty or metallic taste.
- Instruct the patient to remove jewelry and other metallic objects from the area to be examined prior to the procedure.
- Instruct the patient to fast and restrict fluids for 8 hr prior to the procedure. Instruct the patient to avoid taking anticoagulant medication or to reduce dosage as ordered prior to the procedure. Protocols may vary among facilities.
- *Make sure a written and informed consent has been signed prior to the procedure and before administering any medications.*

INTRATEST:

Potential Complications:

Establishing an IV site and injecting contrast medium by catheter are invasive procedures. Complications are rare but do include risk for allergic reaction ***(related to contrast reaction)***; bleeding ***(related to a bleeding disorder or the effects of natural products and medications with known anticoagulant, antiplatelet, or thrombolytic properties;***

U

postprocedural bleeding from the site is rare because at the conclusion of the procedure a resorbable device, composed of non-latex-containing arterial anchor, collagen plug, and suture, is deployed to seal the puncture site); blood clot formation ***(related to thrombus formation on the tip of the catheter sheath surface or in the lumen of the catheter; the use of a heparinized saline flush during the procedure decreases the risk of emboli);*** cardiac dysrhythmias; hematoma ***(related to blood leakage into the tissue following insertion of the catheter);*** infection ***(which might occur if bacteria from the skin surface is introduced during catheter insertion);*** tissue damage ***(related to extravasation of the contrast during injection);*** nerve injury or damage to a nearby organ ***(which might occur if the catheter strikes a nerve or perforates an organ);*** detachment of small pieces of fibroid tissue during UFE, which will pass, but a D & C may be required to verify that all material is removed to prevent further bleeding or infection; and the occurrence of menopause following UFE, which is generally experienced in women older than 45 yr of age.

- Observe standard precautions, and follow the general guidelines in Patient Preparation and Specimen Collection online at Davis*Plus*. Positively identify the patient.
- Ensure the patient has complied with dietary, fluid, and medication restrictions prior to the procedure, as instructed.
- Ensure the patient has removed all external metallic objects from the area to be examined prior to the procedure.
- Administer ordered prophylactic steroids or antihistamines before the procedure if the patient has a history of allergic reactions to any substance or drug.
- Avoid the use of equipment containing latex if the patient has a history of allergic reaction to latex.
- Have emergency equipment readily available.
- Instruct the patient to void prior to the procedure and to change into the gown, robe, and foot coverings provided.
- Instruct the patient to cooperate fully and to follow directions. Instruct the patient to remain still throughout the procedure because movement produces unreliable results.
- Record baseline vital signs and assess neurological status. Protocols may vary among facilities.
- Establish an IV fluid line for the injection of saline, sedatives, or emergency medications.
- Administer an antianxiety drug, as ordered, if the patient has claustrophobia. Administer a sedative to an adult who is uncooperative, as ordered.
- Place electrocardiographic electrodes on the patient for cardiac monitoring. Establish baseline rhythm; determine if the patient has ventricular dysrhythmias.
- Using a pen, mark the site of the patient's peripheral pulses before angiography; this allows for quicker and more consistent assessment of the pulses after the procedure.
- Place the patient in the supine position on an examination table. Cleanse the selected area, and cover with a sterile drape.
- The contrast medium is injected, and a rapid series of images is taken during and after the filling of the vessels to be examined. Delayed images may be taken to examine the vessels after a time and to monitor the venous phase of the procedure.
- Ask the patient to inhale deeply and hold her breath while the x-ray images are taken, and then to exhale after the images are taken.
- Instruct the patient to take slow, deep breaths if nausea occurs during the procedure. Monitor and administer an antiemetic drug if ordered. Ready an emesis basin for use.
- Particles are injected through the catheter to block the blood flow to the fibroids. The particles include polyvinyl alcohol, gelatin sponge (Gelfoam), and micospheres.

- The needle or catheter is removed, and a pressure dressing is applied over the puncture site.
- Monitor the patient for complications related to the procedure (e.g., allergic reaction, anaphylaxis, bronchospasm).
- Observe/assess the needle/catheter insertion site for bleeding, inflammation, or hematoma formation.

POST-TEST:

- Inform the patient that a report of the results will be made available to the requesting HCP, who will discuss the results with the patient.
- Instruct the patient to resume usual diet, fluids, medications, or activity, as directed by the HCP. Kidney function should be assessed before metformin is resumed, if contrast was used.
- Monitor vital signs and neurological status every 15 min for 1 hr, then every 2 hr for 4 hr, and then as ordered by the HCP. Take temperature every 4 hr for 24 hr. Monitor intake and output at least every 8 hr. Compare with baseline values. Notify the HCP if temperature is elevated. Protocols may vary among facilities.
- Observe for delayed allergic reactions, such as rash, urticaria, tachycardia, hyperpnea, hypertension, palpitations, nausea, or vomiting.
- Instruct the patient to immediately report symptoms such as fast heart rate, difficulty breathing, skin rash, itching, chest pain, persistent right shoulder pain, or abdominal pain. Immediately report symptoms to the appropriate HCP.
- Inform the patient that she may experience pelvic cramps for several days after the procedure and possible mild nausea and fever.
- Assess extremities for signs of ischemia or absence of distal pulse caused by a catheter-induced thrombus.
- Instruct the patient in the care and assessment of the injection site.
- Instruct the patient to apply cold compresses to the puncture site as needed, to reduce discomfort or edema.
- Recognize anxiety related to test results, and be supportive of impaired activity related to genitourinary system. Discuss the implications of abnormal test results on the patient's lifestyle. Provide teaching and information regarding the clinical implications of the test results, as appropriate. Educate the patient regarding access to counseling services.
- Reinforce information given by the patient's HCP regarding further testing, treatment, or referral to another HCP. Answer any questions or address any concerns voiced by the patient or family.
- Instruct the patient in the use of any ordered medications. Explain the importance of adhering to the therapy regimen. As appropriate, instruct the patient in significant adverse effects associated with the prescribed medication. Encourage her to review corresponding literature provided by a pharmacist.
- Depending on the results of this procedure, additional testing may be performed to evaluate or monitor progression of the disease process and determine the need for a change in therapy. Evaluate test results in relation to the patient's symptoms and other tests performed.

RELATED STUDIES:

- Related tests include CBC, CT angiography, CT pelvis, hysterosalpingography, laparoscopy, MRA, MRI pelvis, PT/INR, and US pelvis.
- Refer to the Reproductive System table online at Davis*Plus* for related tests by body system.

U

Vanillylmandelic Acid, Urine

SYNONYM/ACRONYM: VMA.

COMMON USE: To assist in the diagnosis and follow up treatment of pheochromocytoma, neuroblastoma, and ganglioblastoma. This test can also be useful in evaluation and follow-up of hypertension.

SPECIMEN: Urine from a timed specimen collected in a clean plastic collection container with 6N hydrochloric acid as a preservative.

NORMAL FINDINGS: (Method: High-pressure liquid chromatography)

Age	Conventional Units	SI Units (Conventional Units × 5.05)
3–6 yr	1–2.6 mg/24 hr	5–13 micromol/24 hr
7–10 yr	2–3.2 mg/24 hr	10–16 micromol/24 hr
11–16 yr	2.3–5.2 mg/24 hr	12–26 micromol/24 hr
17–83 yr	1.4–6.5 mg/24 hr	7–33 micromol/24 hr

DESCRIPTION: Vanillylmandelic acid (VMA) is a major metabolite of epinephrine and norepinephrine. It is elevated in conditions that also are marked by over production of catecholamines. Creatinine is usually measured simultaneously to ensure adequate collection and to calculate an excretion ratio of metabolite to creatinine.

This procedure is contraindicated for: N/A

INDICATIONS

- Assist in the diagnosis of neuroblastoma, ganglioneuroma, or pheochromocytoma.
- Evaluate hypertension of unknown cause.

POTENTIAL MEDICAL DIAGNOSIS

Increased in:

Catecholamine-secreting tumors will cause an increase in VMA.

- Ganglioneuroma
- Hypertension secondary to pheochromocytoma
- Neuroblastoma
- Pheochromocytoma

Decreased in: N/A

CRITICAL FINDINGS: N/A

INTERFERING FACTORS

- Drugs and other substances that may increase VMA levels include ajmaline, chlorpromazine, glucagon, guaifenesin, guanethidine, isoproterenol, methyldopa, nitroglycerin, oxytetracycline, phenazopyridine, phenolsulfonphthalein, prochlorperazine, rauwolfia, reserpine, and sulfobromophthalein.
- Drugs and other substances that may decrease VMA levels include brofaromine, guanethidine, guanfacine, imipramine, isocarboxazid, methyldopa, monoamine oxidase inhibitors, morphine, nialamide (in patients with schizophrenia), and reserpine.
- Stress, hypoglycemia, hyperthyroidism, strenuous exercise, smoking, and drugs can produce elevated catecholamines.
- Recent radioactive scans within 1 wk of the test can interfere with test results.

V

- **Failure to collect all urine and store 24-hr specimen properly will result in a falsely low result.**
- **Failure to follow dietary restrictions before the procedure may cause the procedure to be canceled or repeated.**

NURSING IMPLICATIONS AND PROCEDURE

PRETEST:

- Positively identify the patient using at least two person-specific identifiers before services, treatments, or procedures are performed.
- *Patient Teaching:* Inform the patient this test can assist in evaluating or the presence of tumors.
- Obtain a history of the patient's health concerns, symptoms, surgical procedures, and results of previously performed laboratory and diagnostic studies. Include a list of known allergens, especially allergies or sensitivities to latex.
- Obtain a list of the patient's current medications, including over-the-counter medications and dietary supplements (see Effects of Natural Products on Laboratory Values online at Davis*Plus*).
- Review the procedure with the patient. Provide a nonmetallic urinal, bedpan, or toilet-mounted collection device. Address concerns about pain and explain that there should be no discomfort during the procedure.
- *Sensitivity to social and cultural issues,* as well as concern for modesty, is important in providing psychological support before, during, and after the procedure.
- Usually a 24-hr time frame for urine collection is ordered. Inform the patient that all urine must be saved during that 24-hr period. Instruct the patient not to void directly into the laboratory collection container. Instruct the patient to avoid defecating in the collection device and to keep toilet tissue out of the collection device to prevent contamination of the specimen. Place a sign in the bathroom to remind the patient to save all urine.
- Instruct the patient to void all urine into the collection device and then to pour the urine into the laboratory collection container. Alternatively, the specimen can be left in the collection device for a health-care staff member to add to the laboratory collection container.
- Note that there are no fluid restrictions unless by medical direction.
- Instruct the patient to abstain from smoking tobacco for 24 hr before testing.
- Inform the patient of the following dietary, medication, and activity restrictions in preparation for the test (protocols may vary among facilities):
- The patient should not consume foods high in amines (bananas, avocados, beer, aged cheese, chocolate, cocoa, coffee, fava beans, grains, tea, vanilla, walnuts, and red wine) for 48 hr before testing.
- The patient should not consume foods or fluids high in caffeine (coffee, tea, cocoa, and chocolate) for 48 hr before testing.
- The patient should not consume any foods or fluids containing vanilla or licorice.
- The patient should avoid self-prescribed medications (especially aspirin) and prescribed medications (especially pyridoxine, levodopa, amoxicillin, carbidopa, reserpine, and disulfiram) for 2 wk before testing and as directed.
- The patient should avoid excessive exercise and stress during the 24-hr collection of urine.

INTRATEST:

Potential Complications: N/A

- Ensure that the patient has complied with dietary, medication, and activity restrictions and pretesting preparations prior to the procedure, as instructed.
- Avoid the use of equipment containing latex if the patient has a history of allergic reaction to latex.

- Instruct the patient to cooperate fully and to follow directions.
- Observe standard precautions, and follow the general guidelines in Patient Preparation and Specimen Collection online at Davis*Plus*. Positively identify the patient, and label the appropriate specimen container with the corresponding patient demographics, initials of the person collecting the specimen, date, and time of collection.

Timed Specimen

- Obtain a clean 3-L urine specimen container, toilet-mounted collection device, and plastic bag (for transport of the specimen container). The specimen must be refrigerated or kept on ice throughout the entire collection period. If an indwelling urinary catheter is in place, the drainage bag must be kept on ice.
- Begin the test between 0600 and 0800 if possible. Collect first voiding and discard. Record the time the specimen was discarded as the beginning of the timed collection period. The next morning, ask the patient to void at the same time the collection was started and add this last voiding to the container. Urinary output should be recorded throughout the collection time.
- If an indwelling catheter is in place, replace the tubing and container system at the start of the collection time. Keep the container system on ice during the collection period, or empty the urine into a larger container periodically during the collection period; monitor to ensure continued drainage, and conclude the test the next morning at the same hour the collection was begun.
- At the conclusion of the test, compare the quantity of urine with the urinary output record for the collection; if the specimen contains less than what was recorded as output, some urine may have been discarded, invalidating the test.
- Include on the collection container's label the amount of urine, test start and stop times, and ingestion of any foods or medications that can affect test results.
- Promptly transport the specimen to the laboratory for processing and analysis.

POST-TEST:

- Inform the patient that a report of the results will be made available to the requesting health-care provider (HCP), who will discuss the results with the patient.
- Instruct the patient to resume usual diet, fluids, medications, and activity, as directed by the HCP.
- ***Nutritional Considerations:*** Instruct the patient to avoid foods or drinks containing caffeine. Over-the-counter medications should be taken only under the advice of the patient's HCP.
- Recognize anxiety related to test results, and be supportive of fear of shortened life expectancy. Discuss the implications of abnormal test results on the patient's lifestyle. Provide teaching and information regarding the clinical implications of the test results, as appropriate. Educate the patient regarding access to counseling services.
- Reinforce information given by the patient's HCP regarding further testing, treatment, or referral to another HCP. Answer any questions or address any concerns voiced by the patient or family.
- Depending on the results of this procedure, additional testing may be performed to evaluate or monitor progression of the disease process and determine the need for a change in therapy. Evaluate test results in relation to the patient's symptoms and other tests performed.

RELATED STUDIES:

- Related tests include angiography adrenal, calcium, catecholamines, CT kidneys, homovanillic acid, metanephrines, and renin.
- Related to Endocrine System table online at Davis*Plus* for related tests by body system.

Varicella Antibodies

V

SYNONYM/ACRONYM: Varicella-zoster antibodies, chickenpox, VZ.

COMMON USE: To assist in diagnosing chickenpox or shingles related to a varicella-zoster infection and to assess for immunity.

SPECIMEN: Serum collected in a gold-, red-, or red/gray-top tube. Place separated serum into a standard transport tube within 2 hr of collection.

NORMAL FINDINGS: (Method: Enzyme immunoassay)

	IgM and IgG	Interpretation
Negative	0.89 index or less	No significant level of detectable antibody
Indeterminate	0.9–1 index	Equivocal results; retest in 10–14 d
Positive	1.1 index or greater	Antibody detected; indicative of recent immunization, current or recent infection

DESCRIPTION: Varicella-zoster is a double-stranded DNA herpes virus that is responsible for two clinical syndromes: chickenpox and shingles. The incubation period for varicella infection is 2 to 3 wk, and it is highly contagious for about 2 wk beginning 2 days before a rash develops. It is transmitted via respiratory secretions and by direct contact with the secretions inside. Painful eruptions appear on the skin and mucus membranes. The primary exposure to the highly contagious virus usually occurs in susceptible school-age children. Adults without prior exposure and who become infected may have severe complications, including pneumonia. Neonatal infection from the mother is possible if exposure occurs during the last 3 wk of gestation. The second syndrome, shingles, results when the presumably latent virus is reactivated and produces painful skin eruptions along nerve tracks. In both syndromes, the presence of immunoglobulin (Ig) M antibodies indicates acute infection and the presence of IgG antibodies indicates current or past infection. A reactive varicella antibody result indicates immunity but does not protect an individual from shingles. There are also polymerase chain reaction methods that can detect varicella-zoster DNA in various specimen types.

This procedure is contraindicated for: N/A

INDICATIONS

- Determine susceptibility or immunity to chickenpox.

POTENTIAL MEDICAL DIAGNOSIS

Positive findings in

- Varicella infection

Negative findings in: N/A

CRITICAL FINDINGS: N/A

INTERFERING FACTORS: N/A

V

NURSING IMPLICATIONS AND PROCEDURE

POTENTIAL NURSING PROBLEMS:

Problem	Signs & Symptoms	Interventions
Pain ***(related to altered nerve root function secondary to viral infection)***	Pain that is burning, stabbing, tearing	Keep clothing or bedding from touching the affected area; use a foot cradle as appropriate; assess and monitor the location, duration, and characteristics of pain; explain the importance of pain medication and administer as prescribed; teach how to apply antipruritic lotion (e.g., calamine); discuss the application of wet compresses to decrease itching; consider the use of distraction and relaxation techniques as a pain management modality
Infection ***(related to exposure to** Varicella **zoster)***	Headache; fever; malaise; blister rash; chills; nausea; pain and tingling at area of rash before appearance; itching; open sores; loss of appetite	Encourage vaccination of all at-risk family members or friends; administer prescribed antiviral medication; monitor and trend white blood cell count; monitor and trend temperature; decrease exposure to noninfected individuals by limiting visitors; prevent exposure to others from cough or touching infected fluids; practice vigilant hand washing; keep infected individuals home
Skin ***(related to itching secondary to varicella infection)***	Scratching with open sores; drainage from open sores	Teach how to decrease the itch-scratch cycle (use warm water and pat dry rather than rub); administer prescribed antipruritic creams or lotion
Fluid volume (water) ***(related to inadequate fluid intake secondary to nausea and altered appetite associated***	Hypotension; decreased cardiac output; decreased urinary output; dry skin/mucous membranes; poor skin turgor; sunken eyeballs;	Monitor intake and output; assess for symptoms of dehydration (dry skin, dry mucous membranes, poor skin turgor, sunken eyeballs); monitor and trend vital signs; monitor for symptoms of poor cardiac output (rapid, weak,

(table continues on page 1602)

Problem	Signs & Symptoms	Interventions
with varicella infection)	increased urine specific gravity; hemoconcentration	thready pulse); record daily weight with monitoring of trends; collaborate with health-care provider (HCP) on administration of intravenous (IV) fluids to support hydration; monitor laboratory values that reflect alterations in fluid status (potassium, blood urea nitrogen, creatinine, calcium, hemoglobin, hematocrit, sodium); manage underlying cause of fluid alteration; monitor urine characteristics and respiratory status; establish baseline assessment data; collaborate with HCP to adjust oral and IV fluids to provide optimal hydration status; administer replacement electrolytes as ordered

PRETEST:

- Positively identify the patient using at least two person-specific identifiers before services, treatments, or procedures are performed.
- ***Patient Teaching:*** Inform the patient this test can assist in assessing for a viral infection or immunity.
- Obtain a history of the patient's health concerns (especially exposure to varicella), symptoms, surgical procedures, and results of previously performed laboratory and diagnostic studies. Include a list of known allergens, especially allergies or sensitivities to latex.
- Obtain a list of the patient's current medications, including over-the-counter medications and dietary supplements (see Effects of Natural Products on Laboratory Values online at Davis*Plus*).
- Review the procedure with the patient. Inform the patient that several tests may be necessary to confirm diagnosis. Any individual positive result should be repeated in 7 to 14 days to monitor a change in detectable level of antibody. Inform the patient that specimen collection takes approximately 5 to 10 min. Address concerns about pain and explain that there may be some discomfort during the venipuncture.
- ***Sensitivity to social and cultural issues,*** as well as concern for modesty, is important in providing psychological support before, during, and after the procedure.
- Note that there are no food, fluid, or medication restrictions unless by medical direction.

INTRATEST:

Potential Complications: N/A

- Avoid the use of equipment containing latex if the patient has a history of allergic reaction to latex.
- Instruct the patient to cooperate fully and to follow directions. Direct the patient to breathe normally and to avoid unnecessary movement.
- Observe standard precautions, and follow the general guidelines in

Patient Preparation and Specimen Collection online at Davis*Plus*. Positively identify the patient, and label the appropriate specimen container with the corresponding patient demographics, initials of the person collecting the specimen, date, and time of collection. Perform a venipuncture.

- Remove the needle and apply direct pressure with dry gauze to stop bleeding. Observe/assess venipuncture site for bleeding or hematoma formation and secure gauze with adhesive bandage.
- Promptly transport the specimen to the laboratory for processing and analysis.

POST-TEST:

- Inform the patient that a report of the results will be made available to the requesting HCP, who will discuss the results with the patient.
- ***Vaccination Considerations:*** Record the date of last menstrual period and determine the possibility of pregnancy prior to administration of varicella vaccine to female varicella-nonimmune patients. Instruct patient not to become pregnant for 1 mo after being vaccinated with the varicella vaccine to protect any fetus from contracting the disease and having serious birth defects. Instruct on birth control methods to prevent pregnancy, if appropriate.
- Recognize anxiety related to test results, and provide emotional support if results are positive and the patient is pregnant. Inform the patient with shingles about access to pain management. Discuss the implications of abnormal test results on the patient's lifestyle. Provide teaching and information regarding the clinical implications of the test results, as appropriate. Educate the patient regarding access to counseling services.
- Depending on the results of this procedure, additional testing may be performed to evaluate or monitor progression of the disease process and determine the need for a change in therapy. Evaluate test results in relation to the patient's symptoms and other tests performed.

Patient Education:

- Reinforce information given by the patient's HCP regarding further testing, treatment, or referral to another HCP.
- Instruct the patient in isolation precautions during the time of communicability or contagion.
- Emphasize the need to return to have a convalescent blood sample taken in 7 to 14 days. Provide information regarding vaccine-preventable diseases where indicated (e.g., varicella).
- Provide contact information, if desired, for the Centers for Disease Control and Prevention (www.cdc.gov/vaccines/vpd-vac) and (www.cdc.gov/DiseasesConditions). 🍁
- Answer any questions or address any concerns voiced by the patient or family.

Expected Patient Outcomes:

Understanding

- The patient and family state importance of taking prescribed antiviral in its entirety to treat infection.
- The patient and family state the importance of good hand washing to prevent disease transmission to others.

Ability

- The patient and family demonstrate proficiency in the application of antipruritic lotion.
- The patient and family demonstrate proficiency in taking and recording temperature.

Response

- The patient complies with the request to remain home to prevent spread of the varicella virus until no longer contagious.
- The patient complies with the request to increase oral fluid intake to decrease dehydration risk.

RELATED STUDIES:

- Refer to the Immune and Reproductive systems tables online at Davis*Plus* for related tests by body system.

Venography, Lower Extremity Studies

SYNONYM/ACRONYM: Lower limb venography, phlebography, venogram.

COMMON USE: To visualize and assess the venous vasculature in the lower extremities related to diagnosis of deep vein thrombosis and congenital anomalies.

AREA OF APPLICATION: Veins of the lower extremities.

DESCRIPTION: Venography allows x-ray visualization of the venous vasculature system of the extremities after injection of an iodinated contrast medium. Lower extremity studies identify and locate thrombi within the venous system of the lower limbs. After injection of the contrast medium, x-ray images are taken at timed intervals. Usually both extremities are studied, and the unaffected side is used for comparison with the side suspected of having deep vein thrombosis (DVT) or other venous abnormalities, such as congenital malformations or incompetent valves. Thrombus formation usually occurs in the deep calf veins and at the venous junction and its valves. If DVT is not treated, it can lead to femoral and iliac venous occlusion, or the thrombus can become an embolus, causing a pulmonary embolism. Venography is accurate for identifying thrombi in veins below the knee.

This procedure is contraindicated for

- Patients who are pregnant or suspected of being pregnant, unless the potential benefits of a procedure using radiation far outweigh the risk of radiation exposure to the fetus and mother.
- Patients with conditions associated with adverse reactions to contrast medium (e.g., asthma, food allergies, or allergy to contrast medium).

  Although patients are asked specifically if they have a known allergy to iodine or shellfish, it has been well established that the reaction is not to iodine; an actual iodine allergy would be problematic because iodine is required for the production of thyroid hormones. In the case of shellfish, the reaction is to a muscle protein called tropomyosin; in the case of iodinated contrast medium, the reaction is to the noniodinated part of the contrast molecule. Patients with a known hypersensitivity to the medium may benefit from premedication with corticosteroids and diphenhydramine; the use of nonionic contrast or an alternative noncontrast imaging study, if available, may be considered for patients who have severe asthma or who have experienced moderate to severe reactions to ionic contrast medium.
- Patients with conditions associated with preexisting renal insufficiency (e.g., chronic kidney disease, single kidney transplant, nephrectomy, diabetes, multiple myeloma, treatment with aminoglycosides and NSAIDs) ***because iodinated contrast is nephrotoxic.***
- Patients who are chronically dehydrated before the test, especially older adults and patients whose health is already compromised, ***because of their risk of contrast-induced acute kidney injury.***

Patients with bleeding disorders because the puncture site may not stop bleeding.

Patients with severe edema of the legs in whom venous access is not possible.

INDICATIONS

- Assess deep vein valvular competence.
- Confirm a diagnosis of DVT.
- Determine the cause of extremity swelling or pain.
- Determine the source of emboli when pulmonary embolism is suspected or diagnosed.
- Distinguish clot formation from venous obstruction.
- Evaluate congenital venous malformations.
- Locate a vein for arterial bypass graft surgery.

POTENTIAL MEDICAL DIAGNOSIS

Normal findings

No obstruction to flow and no filling defects after injection of radiopaque contrast medium; steady opacification of superficial and deep vasculature with no filling defects.

Abnormal findings related to

- Deep vein valvular incompetence
- DVT
- Pulmonary embolism
- Venous obstruction

CRITICAL FINDINGS:

- DVT
- Pulmonary embolism

Note and immediately report to the requesting health-care provider (HCP) any critical findings and related symptoms. A listing of these findings varies among facilities. Timely notification of a critical finding for laboratory or diagnostic studies is a role expectation of the professional nurse. The notification processes vary among facilities. Upon receipt of the critical finding, the information should be read back to the caller to verify accuracy.

INTERFERING FACTORS

Factors that may alter the results of the study

- Metallic objects (e.g., jewelry, body rings) within the examination field, which may inhibit organ visualization and cause unclear images.
- Movement of the leg being tested, excessive tourniquet constriction, insufficient injection of contrast medium, and delay between injection and the x-ray.
- Severe edema of the legs, making venous access impossible.

Other considerations

- Improper injection of the contrast medium that allows it to seep deep into the muscle tissue.
- Inability of the patient to cooperate or remain still during the procedure because of age, significant pain, or mental status, may interfere with the test results.

NURSING IMPLICATIONS AND PROCEDURE

PRETEST:

- Positively identify the patient using at least two person-specific identifiers before services, treatments, or procedures are performed.
- *Patient Teaching:* Inform the patient this procedure can assist in assessing the veins in the lower extremities.
- Obtain a history of the patient's health concerns, symptoms, surgical procedures, and results of previously performed laboratory and diagnostic studies. Include a list of known allergens, especially allergies or sensitivities to latex, anesthetics, sedatives, or contrast medium. Ensure results of coagulation testing are obtained and

V

recorded prior to the procedure; a creatinine level is also needed before contrast medium is to be used.

- Note any recent procedures that can interfere with test results, including examinations using barium- or iodine-based contrast medium.
- Record the date of the last menstrual period and determine the possibility of pregnancy in perimenopausal women.
- Obtain a list of the patient's current medications, including over-the-counter medications, dietary supplements, anticoagulants, aspirin and other salicylates (see Effects of Natural Products on Laboratory Values online at Davis*Plus*). Such products should be discontinued by medical direction for the appropriate number of days prior to a surgical procedure. Note the last time and dose of medication taken.
- If iodinated contrast medium is scheduled to be used in patients receiving metformin (Glucophage) for type 2 diabetes, the drug should be discontinued on the day of the test and continue to be withheld for 48 hr after the test. Iodinated contrast can temporarily impair kidney function, and failure to withhold metformin may indirectly result in drug-induced lactic acidosis, a dangerous and sometimes fatal adverse effect of metformin ***related to renal impairment that does not support sufficient excretion of metformin.***
- Review the procedure with the patient. Address concerns about pain and explain to the patient that there may be moments of discomfort and some pain experienced during the procedure. Inform the patient that the procedure is usually performed in a radiology or vascular suite by an HCP, with support staff, and takes approximately 30 to 60 min.
- ***Sensitivity to social and cultural issues,*** as well as concern for modesty, is important in providing psychological support before, during, and after the procedure.
- Explain that an intravenous (IV) line may be inserted to allow infusion of fluids such as saline, anesthetics, sedatives, or emergency medications. Explain that the contrast medium will be injected, by catheter, at a separate site from the IV line.
- Inform the patient that a burning and flushing sensation may be felt throughout the body during injection of the contrast medium. After injection of the contrast medium, the patient may experience an urge to cough, flushing, nausea, or a salty or metallic taste.
- Instruct the patient to remove jewelry and other metallic objects from the area to be examined prior to the procedure.
- Instruct the patient to fast and restrict fluids for 8 hr prior to the procedure. Protocols may vary among facilities.
- *Make sure a written and informed consent has been signed prior to the procedure and before administering any medications.*
- This procedure may be terminated if chest pain, severe cardiac dysrhythmias, or signs of a cerebrovascular accident occur.

INTRATEST:

Potential Complications:

Complications include allergic reaction to the contrast medium, venous thrombophlebitis ***that is caused by contrast,*** venous embolism ***related to dislodgement of a deep-vein clot,*** and cellulitis or pain ***related to infiltration at the injection site.***

- Observe standard precautions, and follow the general guidelines in Patient Preparation and Specimen Collection online at Davis*Plus*. Positively identify the patient.
- Ensure the patient has complied with dietary, fluid, and medication restrictions prior to the procedure, as instructed.
- Ensure the patient has removed all external metallic objects from the area to be examined prior to the procedure.
- Administer ordered prophylactic steroids or antihistamines before the procedure if the patient has a history

of allergic reactions to any substance or drug.

- Avoid the use of equipment containing latex if the patient has a history of allergic reaction to latex.
- Have emergency equipment readily available.
- Instruct the patient to void prior to the procedure and to change into the gown, robe, and foot coverings provided.
- Instruct the patient to cooperate fully and to follow directions. Ask the patient to remain still throughout the procedure because movement produces unreliable results.
- Record baseline vital signs, and continue to monitor throughout the procedure. Protocols may vary among facilities.
- Establish an IV fluid line for the injection of saline, sedatives, or emergency medications.
- Administer an antianxiety drug, as ordered, if the patient has claustrophobia. Administer a sedative to a child or to an uncooperative adult, as ordered.
- Place electrocardiographic electrodes on the patient for cardiac monitoring. Establish baseline rhythm; determine if the patient has ventricular dysrhythmias.
- Using a pen, mark the site of the patient's peripheral pulses before venography; this allows for quicker and more consistent assessment of the pulses after the procedure.
- Place the patient in the supine position on an examination table. Cleanse the selected area, and cover with a sterile drape.
- A local anesthetic is injected at the site, and a small incision is made or a needle inserted.
- The contrast medium is injected, and a rapid series of images is taken during and after the filling of the vessels to be examined.
- Instruct the patient to inhale deeply and hold his or her breath while the x-ray images are taken, and then to exhale.
- Instruct the patient to take slow, deep breaths if nausea occurs during the procedure.
- Monitor the patient for complications related to the procedure (e.g., allergic reaction, anaphylaxis, bronchospasm).
- The needle or catheter is removed, and a pressure dressing is applied over the puncture site.
- Observe/assess the needle/catheter insertion site for bleeding, inflammation, or hematoma formation.

POST-TEST:

- Inform the patient that a report of the results will be made available to the requesting HCP, who will discuss the results with the patient.
- Instruct the patient to resume diet, fluids, and medications, as directed by the HCP. Kidney function should be assessed before metformin is resumed, if contrast was used.
- Monitor vital signs and neurological status every 15 min for 1 hr, then every 2 hr for 4 hr, and then as ordered by the HCP. Take temperature every 4 hr for 24 hr. Monitor intake and output at least every 8 hr. Compare with baseline values. Notify the HCP if temperature is elevated. Protocols may vary among facilities.
- Observe for delayed allergic reactions, such as rash, urticaria, tachycardia, hyperpnea, hypertension, palpitations, nausea, or vomiting.
- Instruct the patient to immediately report symptoms such as fast heart rate, difficulty breathing, skin rash, itching, chest pain, persistent right shoulder pain, or abdominal pain. Immediately report symptoms to the appropriate HCP.
- Assess extremities for signs of ischemia or absence of distal pulse caused by a catheter-induced thrombus.
- Instruct the patient in the care and assessment of the site.
- Instruct the patient to apply cold compresses to the puncture site as needed to reduce discomfort or edema.
- Instruct the patient to maintain bed rest for 4 to 6 hr after the procedure or as ordered.

V

- Recognize anxiety related to test results, and be supportive of perceived loss of independent function. Discuss the implications of abnormal test results on the patient's lifestyle. Provide teaching and information regarding the clinical implications of the test results, as appropriate.
- Reinforce information given by the patient's HCP regarding further testing, treatment, or referral to another HCP. Answer any questions or address any concerns voiced by the patient or family.
- Depending on the results of this procedure, additional testing may be needed to evaluate or monitor progression of the disease process and determine the need for a change in therapy. Evaluate test results in relation to the patient's symptoms and other tests performed.

RELATED STUDIES:

- Related tests include alveolar/arterial gradient, angiography pulmonary, antibodies anticardiolipin, antithrombin III, blood gases, CT angiography, D-dimer, FDP, lactic acid, lung perfusion scan, lung ventilation scan, MRA, MRI abdomen, MRI venography, plethysmography, PT/INR, renogram, US peripheral Doppler, and US venous Doppler extremity studies.
- Refer to the Cardiovascular and Respiratory systems tables online at Davis*Plus* for related tests by body system.

Vertebroplasty

SYNONYM/ACRONYM: None.

COMMON USE: A minimally invasive procedure to treat the spine for disorders such as tumor, lesions, osteoporosis, and vertebral compression.

AREA OF APPLICATION: Spine.

POTENTIAL MEDICAL DIAGNOSIS

Normal findings

- Improvement in the ability to ambulate without pain
- Relief of back pain

Abnormal findings related to

- Failure to reduce the patient's pain
- Failure to improve the patient's mobility

CRITICAL FINDINGS: N/A

Find and print out the full study on Fast Find at davispl.us/vanleeuwen7.

Visual Fields Test

SYNONYM/ACRONYM: Perimetry, VF.

COMMON USE: To assess visual field function related to the retina, optic nerve, and optic pathways to assist in diagnosing visual loss disorders such as brain tumors, macular degeneration, and diabetes.

AREA OF APPLICATION: Eyes.

DESCRIPTION: The visual field (VF) is the area within which objects can be seen by the eye as it fixes on a central point. The central field is an area extending 25° surrounding the fixation point. The peripheral field is the remainder of the area within which objects can be viewed. This test evaluates the central VF, except within the physiological blind spot, through systematic movement of the test object across a tangent screen. It tests the function of the retina, optic nerve, and optic pathways. VF testing may be performed manually by the examiner (confrontation VF examination) or by using partially or fully automated equipment (tangent screen, Goldman, Humphrey VF examination). In the manual VF test, the patient is asked to cover one eye and fix his or her gaze on the examiner. The examiner moves his or her hand out of the patient's VF and then gradually brings it back into the patient's VF. The patient signals the examiner when the hand comes back into view. The test is repeated on the other eye. The manual test is frequently used for screening because it is quick and simple. Tangent screen or Goldman testing is an automated method commonly used to create a map of the patient's VF.

This procedure is contraindicated for: N/A

INDICATIONS

- Detect field vision loss and evaluate its progression or regression.

POTENTIAL MEDICAL DIAGNOSIS

Normal findings

- Normal central vision field extends in a circle approximately 25° to 30° on all sides of central fixation and out 60° superiorly (upward), 60° nasally (medially), 75° inferiorly (downward), and 90° temporally (laterally). There is a normal physiological blind spot, 12° to 15° temporal to the central fixation point and approximately 1.5° below the horizontal meridian which is approximately 7.5° high and 5.5° wide. The patient should be able to see the test object throughout the entire central vision field except within the physiological blind spot.

Abnormal findings related to

- Amblyopia
- Blepharochalasis
- Blurred vision
- Brain injury
- Brain tumors
- Cerebrovascular accidents
- Choroidal nevus
- Diabetes with ophthalmic manifestations
- Glaucoma
- Headache
- Macular degeneration
- Macular drusen
- Nystagmus
- Optic neuritis or neuropathy
- Ptosis of eyelid
- Retinal detachment, hole, or tear
- Retinal exudates or hemorrhage
- Retinal occlusion of the artery or vein
- Retinitis pigmentosa
- Rheumatoid arthritis
- Stroke
- Subjective visual disturbance
- Use of high-risk medications
- VF defect
- Vitreous traction syndrome

CRITICAL FINDINGS: N/A

INTERFERING FACTORS

Factors that may alter the results of the study

- A patient who is uncooperative or a patient with severe vision loss

V

who has difficulty seeing even a large vision screen may have test results that are invalid.

- Assess and make note of the patient's cooperation and reliability as good, fair, or poor, because it is difficult to evaluate factors such as general health, fatigue, or reaction time that affect test performance.

NURSING IMPLICATIONS AND PROCEDURE

PRETEST:

- Positively identify the patient using at least two person-specific identifiers before services, treatments, or procedures are performed.
- ***Patient Teaching:*** Inform the patient this procedure assesses visual field function and vision loss.
- Obtain a history of the patient's health concerns (especially known or suspected vision loss; changes in visual acuity, including type and cause; use of glasses or contact lenses; eye conditions with treatment regimens; eye surgery; and other tests and procedures to assess and diagnose visual deficit), symptoms, surgical procedures, and results of previously performed laboratory and diagnostic studies. Include a list of known allergens, especially allergies or sensitivities to latex.
- Obtain a list of the patient's current medications, including over-the-counter medications and dietary supplements (see Effects of Natural Products on Laboratory Values online at Davis*Plus*).
- Measure visual acuity with and without corrective lenses prior to testing. Instruct the patient to wear corrective lenses if appropriate and if worn to correct for distance vision. Instruct the patient regarding the importance of keeping the eyes open for the test.
- Review the procedure with the patient. Address concerns about pain and explain that no discomfort will be experienced during the test. Inform the patient that a health-care provider (HCP) performs the test in a quiet, darkened room and that to evaluate both eyes, the test can take up 30 min.
- ***Sensitivity to social and cultural issues,*** as well as concern for modesty, is important in providing psychological support before, during, and after the procedure.
- Note that there are no food, fluid, or medication restrictions unless by medical direction.

INTRATEST:

Potential Complications: N/A

- Observe standard precautions, and follow the general guidelines in Patient Preparation and Specimen Collection online at Davis*Plus*. Positively identify the patient.
- Instruct the patient to cooperate fully and to follow directions. Ask the patient to remain still during the procedure because movement produces unreliable results.
- Seat the patient 3 ft 🍁 away from the tangent screen with the eye being tested directly in line with the central fixation tangent, usually a white disk, on the screen. Cover the eye that is not being tested. Ask the patient to place the chin in the chin rest and gently press the forehead against the support bar. Reposition the patient as appropriate to ensure the eye(s) to be tested are properly aligned in front of the VF testing equipment. While the patient stares at the disk on the screen, the examiner moves an object toward the patient's visual field. The patient signals the examiner when the object enters his or her visual field. The patient's responses are recorded, and a map of the patient's VF, including areas of visual defect, can be drawn on paper manually or by a computer.

POST-TEST:

- Inform the patient that a report of the results will be made available to the requesting HCP, who will discuss the results with the patient.

- *Nutritional Considerations:* Increased glucose levels may be associated with diabetes. There is no "diabetic diet"; however, many meal-planning approaches with nutritional goals are endorsed by the American Diabetes Association (ADA). 🍁 Patients who adhere to dietary recommendations report a better general feeling of health, better weight management, greater control of glucose and lipid values, and improved use of insulin. Instruct the patient, as appropriate, in nutritional management of diabetes. A variety of dietary patterns are beneficial for people with diabetes. The Mediterranean-style diet emphasizes inclusion of vegetables, whole grains, fruits, low-fat dairy, nuts, legumes, and nontropical vegetable oils (e.g., olive, canola, peanut, sunflower, flaxseed) along with fish and lean poultry. A similar dietary pattern known as the Dietary Approaches to Stop Hypertension (DASH) diet makes additional recommendations for the reduction of dietary sodium. Both dietary styles emphasize a reduction in consumption of red meats, which are high in saturated fats and cholesterol, and other foods containing sugar, saturated fats, trans fats, and sodium. A vegetarian diet as well as other potential weight loss diets such as Weight Watchers are also supported by the ADA. 🍁 If triglycerides also are elevated, the patient should be advised to eliminate or reduce alcohol. The nutritional needs of each patient with diabetes need to be determined individually (especially during pregnancy) with the appropriate HCPs, particularly professionals educated in nutrition.
- *Social and Cultural Considerations:* Studies comparing risk for developing diabetes demonstrate that certain populations are disproportionately affected by type 2 diabetes and complications of type 2 diabetes as compared to the general population. Nonmodifiable risk factors include age, ethnicity, and family history of diabetes or metabolic syndrome. The risk of developing type 2 diabetes increases with age. In the United States, affected populations include African Americans, Asian Americans, Hispanics, native Hawaiians and Pacific Islanders, American Indians, and Alaska natives. 🍁 Modifiable risk factors include lifestyle choices related to making healthy dietary choices, maintaining a healthy body weight, and meeting recommended levels of physical activity. The financial and emotional burdens of diabetes and related complications continue to grow at an alarming rate. A system for the prevention, management, and support of patients with type 2 diabetes should be provided through the coordinated efforts of multidisciplinary partners using strategies that are culturally appropriate.
- Recognize anxiety related to test results, and be supportive of impaired activity related to vision loss, perceived loss of driving privileges, or the possibility of requiring corrective lenses (self-image). Discuss the implications of the test results on the patient's lifestyle. Provide teaching and information regarding the clinical implications of the test results, as appropriate. The American Optometric Association's recommendations for the frequency of eye examinations can be accessed at (www.aoa.org). 🍁 Emphasize, as appropriate, that good glycemic control delays the onset of and slows the progression of diabetic retinopathy, nephropathy, and neuropathy. Provide education regarding smoking cessation, as appropriate. Provide contact information, if desired, for a general patient education Web site on the topic of eye care (e.g., www.allaboutvision.com). Provide contact information regarding vision aids, if desired, for ABLEDATA (sponsored by the National Institute on Disability and Rehabilitation Research) (www.abledata.com), the American Macular Degeneration Foundation (www.macular.org), American Heart Association (www.americanheart.org), ADA (www.diabetes.org),

National Heart, Lung, and Blood Institute (www.nhlbi.nih.gov), Institute of Medicine of the National Academies (www.iom.edu), and the USDA's resource for nutrition (www.choosemyplate.gov).

- Reinforce information given by the patient's HCP regarding further testing, treatment, or referral to another HCP. Answer any questions or address any concerns voiced by the patient or family.
- Instruct the patient in the use of any ordered medications. Explain the importance of adhering to the therapy regimen. As appropriate, instruct the patient in significant adverse effects associated with the prescribed medication. Encourage him or her to review corresponding literature provided by a pharmacist.
- Depending on the results of this procedure, additional testing may be performed to evaluate or monitor progression of the disease process and determine the need for a change in therapy. Evaluate test results in relation to the patient's symptoms and other tests performed.

RELATED STUDIES:

- Related tests include CT brain, EEG, evoked brain potentials, fluorescein angiography, fructosamine, fundoscopy, glucagon, glucose, glycated hemoglobin, gonioscopy, insulin, intraocular pressure, microalbumin, plethysmography, PET brain, and slit-lamp biomicroscopy.
- Refer to the Ocular System table online at Davis*Plus* for related tests by body system.

Vitamin B_{12}

SYNONYM/ACRONYM: Cyanocobalamin.

COMMON USE: To assess vitamin B_{12} levels to assist in diagnosing disorders such as pernicious anemia and malabsorption syndromes.

SPECIMEN: Serum collected in a gold-, red-, or red/gray-top tube.

NORMAL FINDINGS: (Method: Immunochemiluminescent assay)

Age	Conventional Units	SI Units (Conventional Units × 0.738)
Newborn–10 yr	160–1,300 pg/mL	118–959 pmol/L
11–17 yr	260–900 pg/mL	192–664 pmol/L
Adult	200–1,100 pg/mL	148–812 pmol/L

Values tend to decrease in older adults.

DESCRIPTION: Vitamin B_{12} has a ringed crystalline structure that surrounds an atom of cobalt. It is essential in DNA synthesis, hematopoiesis, and central nervous system (CNS) integrity. It is derived solely from dietary intake. Animal products are the richest source of vitamin B_{12}. Its absorption depends on the presence of intrinsic factor. Circumstances that may result in a deficiency of this vitamin include the presence of stomach or intestinal disease as well as insufficient dietary intake of foods containing vitamin B_{12}. A significant increase in red blood cells (RBCs) mean corpuscular volume may be an important indicator of vitamin B_{12} deficiency.

This procedure is contraindicated for: N/A

INDICATIONS

- Assist in the diagnosis of CNS disorders.
- Assist in the diagnosis of megaloblastic anemia.
- Evaluate alcoholism.
- Evaluate malabsorption syndromes.

POTENTIAL MEDICAL DIAGNOSIS

Increased in:

Increases are noted in a number of conditions; pathophysiology is unclear.

- Chronic granulocytic leukemia
- Chronic kidney disease
- Chronic obstructive pulmonary disease
- Diabetes
- Leukocytosis
- Liver cell damage (hepatitis, cirrhosis) ***(stores in damaged hepatocytes are released into circulation; synthesis of transport proteins is diminished by liver damage)***
- Obesity
- Polycythemia vera
- Protein malnutrition ***(lack of transport proteins increases circulating levels)***
- Severe heart failure
- Some carcinomas

Decreased in:

- Abnormalities of cobalamin transport or metabolism
- Bacterial overgrowth ***(vitamin is consumed and utilized by the bacteria)***
- Crohn's disease ***(related to poor absorption)***
- Dietary deficiency ***(related to insufficient intake, e.g., in vegetarians)***
- *Diphyllobothrium* (fish tapeworm) infestation ***(vitamin is consumed and utilized by the parasite)***
- Gastric or small intestine surgery ***(related to dietary deficiency or poor absorption)***
- Hypochlorhydria ***(related to ineffective digestion resulting in poor absorption)***
- Inflammatory bowel disease ***(related to dietary deficiency or poor absorption)***
- Intestinal malabsorption
- Intrinsic factor deficiency ***(required for proper vitamin B_{12} absorption)***
- Late pregnancy ***(related to dietary deficiency or poor absorption)***
- Pernicious anemia ***(related to dietary deficiency or poor absorption)***

CRITICAL FINDINGS: N/A

INTERFERING FACTORS

- Drugs that may increase vitamin B_{12} levels include chloral hydrate.
- Drugs that may decrease vitamin B_{12} levels include alcohol, aminosalicylic acid, anticonvulsants, ascorbic acid, cholestyramine, cimetidine, colchicine, metformin, neomycin, oral contraceptives, ranitidine, and triamterene.
- Hemolysis or exposure of the specimen to light invalidates results.
- Specimen collection soon after blood transfusion can falsely increase vitamin B_{12} levels.
- Failure to follow dietary restrictions before the procedure may cause the procedure to be canceled or repeated.

V

NURSING IMPLICATIONS AND PROCEDURE

PRETEST:

- Positively identify the patient using at least two person-specific identifiers before services, treatments, or procedures are performed.
- ***Patient Teaching:*** Inform the patient this test can assist in diagnosing a vitamin toxicity or deficiency.
- Obtain a history of the patient's health concerns, symptoms, surgical procedures, and results of previously performed laboratory and diagnostic studies. Include a list of known allergens, especially allergies or sensitivities to latex.
- Obtain a list of the patient's current medications, including over-the-counter medications and dietary supplements (see Effects of Natural Products on Laboratory Values online at Davis*Plus*).
- Review the procedure with the patient. Inform the patient that specimen collection takes approximately 5 to 10 min. Address concerns about pain and explain that there may be some discomfort during the venipuncture.
- ***Sensitivity to social and cultural issues,*** as well as concern for modesty, is important in providing psychological support before, during, and after the procedure.
- Instruct the patient to fast for at least 12 hr before specimen collection. Protocols may vary among facilities.
- Note that there are no fluid or medication restrictions unless by medical direction.

INTRATEST:

Potential Complications: N/A

- Ensure that the patient has complied with dietary restrictions prior to the procedure, as instructed.
- Avoid the use of equipment containing latex if the patient has a history of allergic reaction to latex.
- Instruct the patient to cooperate fully and to follow directions. Direct the patient to breathe normally and to avoid unnecessary movement.
- Observe standard precautions, and follow the general guidelines in Patient Preparation and Specimen Collection online at Davis*Plus*. Positively identify the patient, and label the appropriate specimen container with the corresponding patient demographics, initials of the person collecting the specimen, date, and time of collection. Perform a venipuncture. Protect the specimen from light.
- Remove the needle and apply direct pressure with dry gauze to stop bleeding. Observe/assess venipuncture site for bleeding or hematoma formation and secure gauze with adhesive bandage.
- Promptly transport the specimen to the laboratory for processing and analysis.

POST-TEST:

- Inform the patient that a report of the results will be made available to the requesting health-care provider (HCP), who will discuss the results with the patient.
- Instruct the patient to resume usual diet, as directed by the HCP.
- ***Nutritional Considerations:*** Instruct the patient with vitamin B_{12} deficiency, as appropriate, in the use of vitamin supplements. Inform the patient, as appropriate, that the best dietary sources of vitamin B_{12} are meats, fish, poultry, eggs, and milk.
- Reinforce information given by the patient's HCP regarding further testing, treatment, or referral to another HCP. Answer any questions or address any concerns voiced by the patient or family. Educate the patient regarding access to nutritional counseling services. Provide contact information, if desired, for the Institute of Medicine of the National Academies (www.iom.edu) and USDA's resource for nutrition (www.choosemyplate.gov). 🍁
- Depending on the results of this procedure, additional testing may be performed to evaluate or monitor

progression of the disease process and determine the need for a change in therapy. Evaluate test results in relation to the patient's symptoms and other tests performed.

RELATED STUDIES:

- Related tests include CBC, CBC RBC count, CBC RBC indices, CBC RBC morphology, CBC WBC count and differential, folate, gastric acid stimulation, gastrin stimulation, homocysteine, and intrinsic factor antibodies.
- Refer to the Gastrointestinal and Hematopoietic systems tables online at Davis*Plus* for related tests by body system.

Vitamin D

SYNONYM/ACRONYM: Cholecalciferol, vitamin D 1,25-dihydroxy.

COMMON USE: To assess vitamin D levels toward diagnosing disorders such as vitamin toxicity, malabsorption, and vitamin deficiency.

SPECIMEN: Serum collected in a red-top tube. Plasma collected in a green-top (heparin) tube is also acceptable.

NORMAL FINDINGS: (Method: High-performance liquid chromatography)

Form	Conventional Units	SI Units (Conventional Units × 2.496)
Vitamin D 25-hydroxy		
Deficient	Less than 20 ng/mL	Less than 49.9 nmol/L
Insufficient	20–30 ng/mL	49.9–74.9 nmol/L
Optimal	30–100 ng/mL	74.9–249.6 nmol/L
Possible Toxicity	Greater than 150 ng/mL	Greater than 374.4 nmol/L
	Conventional Units	**SI Units (Conventional Units × 2.6)**
Vitamin D 1,25-dihydroxy	18–72 pg/mL	47–187 pmol/L

DESCRIPTION: Vitamin D is a group of interrelated sterols that have hormonal activity in multiple organs and tissues of the body, including the kidneys, liver, skin, and bones. There are two metabolically active forms of vitamin D: vitamin D 25-hydroxy and vitamin D 1,25-dihydroxy. Ergocalciferol (vitamin D_2) is formed when ergosterol in plants is exposed to sunlight. Ergocalciferol is absorbed by the stomach and intestine when orally ingested. Cholecalciferol (vitamin D_3) is formed when the skin is exposed to sunlight or ultraviolet light. Vitamins D_2 and D_3 enter the bloodstream after absorption. Vitamin D_3 is converted to vitamin D

V

25-hydroxy by the liver and is the major circulating form of the vitamin. Vitamin D_2 is converted to vitamin D 1,25-dihydroxy (calcitriol) by the kidneys and is the more biologically active form. Vitamin D acts with parathyroid hormone and calcitonin to regulate calcium metabolism and osteoblast function. The effects of vitamin D deficiency have been studied for many years, and continued research indicates a link between vitamin D deficiency and the development of diseases such as heart failure, stroke, hypertension, cancer, autism, multiple sclerosis, type 2 diabetes, systemic lupus erythematosus, depression, and immune function. The amount of vitamin D_3 produced by exposure of the skin to ultraviolet radiation depends on the intensity of the radiation as well as the duration of exposure. The use of lotions containing sun block significantly decreases production of vitamin D_3.

This procedure is contraindicated for: N/A

INDICATIONS

- Differential diagnosis of disorders of calcium and phosphorus metabolism.
- Evaluate deficiency or suspected toxicity.
- Investigate bone diseases.
- Investigate malabsorption.

POTENTIAL MEDICAL DIAGNOSIS

Increased in:

- Endogenous vitamin D intoxication ***(in conditions such as sarcoidosis, cat scratch disease, and some lymphomas, extrarenal conversion of 25-hydroxy to 1,25-dihydroxy vitamin D occurs with a corresponding abnormal elevation of calcium)***
- Exogenous vitamin D intoxication

Decreased in:

- Bowel resection ***(related to lack of absorption)***
- Celiac disease ***(related to lack of absorption)***
- Inflammatory bowel disease ***(related to lack of absorption)***
- Malabsorption ***(related to lack of absorption)***
- Osteomalacia ***(related to dietary insufficiency)***
- Pancreatic insufficiency ***(lack of digestive enzymes to metabolize fat-soluble vitamin D; malabsorption)***
- Rickets ***(related to dietary insufficiency)***
- Thyrotoxicosis ***(possibly related to increased calcium loss through sweat, urine, or feces with corresponding decrease in vitamin D levels)***

CRITICAL FINDINGS:

Note and immediately report to the requesting health-care provider (HCP) any critical findings and related symptoms. A listing of these findings varies among facilities. Timely notification of a critical finding for laboratory or diagnostic studies is a role expectation of the professional nurse. The notification processes vary among facilities. Upon receipt of the critical finding, the information should be read back to the caller to verify accuracy.

Vitamin toxicity can be as significant as problems brought about by vitamin deficiencies. The potential for toxicity is especially important to consider with respect to fat-soluble vitamins, which are not eliminated from the body as quickly as water-soluble vitamins and can accumulate in the body. Most cases of toxicity are brought about by oversupplementing and can be avoided by consulting a qualified nutritionist for recommended daily dietary and supplemental allowances. Signs and symptoms of vitamin D toxicity include nausea, loss of appetite, vomiting, polyuria, muscle weakness, and constipation.

INTERFERING FACTORS

- Drugs and other substances that may increase vitamin D levels include cholestyramine, orlistat (a medication for weight loss), and phenytoin.

V

NURSING IMPLICATIONS AND PROCEDURE

POTENTIAL NURSING PROBLEMS:

Problem	Signs & Symptoms	Interventions
Health maintenance ***(related to failure to regulate diet and dietary supplements; inadequate exposure to sunlight to support optimal vitamin D intake; inability to obtain or understand health-related information)***	Inability or failure to recognize or process information toward improving health and preventing illness with associated mental and physical effects	Assess health habits to obtain an interventional baseline; obtain a current health history; identify the patient's and family's learning style; refrain from using medical jargon; observe for altered literacy cues; provide most important information first and reinforce with additional education; ensure the patient understands the ramifications of a lack of vitamin D on the health of the patient's bones
Nutrition ***(related to lack of vitamin D–rich foods in the diet)***	Failure to select vitamin D–rich foods such as fish, fortified milk, breads, cereals, orange juice, eggs and mushrooms; difficulty in opening food containers and feeding self	Determine the patient's ability to select vitamin D–rich foods; discuss the efficacy of increasing exposure to sunlight; collaborate with the HCP in determining the need for vitamin D supplements
Body image ***(related to deformities associated with bone loss from osteoporosis and vitamin D insufficiency)***	Visible physical deformity; presence of kyphosis or lordosis; verbalized negative feelings about appearance; altered social interactions with others due to embarrassment about appearance	Acknowledge the patient's emotional distress; encourage a positive attitude; coordinate meetings with a support group within the community

(table continues on page 1618)

V

Problem	Signs & Symptoms	Interventions
Self-care ***(related to loss of bone mass and physical deformity; pain; and limited range of motion)***	Difficulty fastening clothing; difficulty performing personal hygiene; unable to maintain appropriate appearance; difficulty with independent mobility	Reinforce self-care techniques as taught by occupational therapy; ensure the patient has adequate time to perform self-care; encourage use of assistive devices to maintain independence

PRETEST:

- Positively identify the patient using at least two person-specific identifiers before services, treatments, or procedures are performed.
- ***Patient Teaching:*** Inform the patient this test can assist in diagnosing vitamin toxicity or deficiency.
- Obtain a history of the patient's health concerns, symptoms, surgical procedures, and results of previously performed laboratory and diagnostic studies. Include a list of known allergens, especially allergies or sensitivities to latex.
- Obtain a list of the patient's current medications, including over-the-counter medications and dietary supplements (see Effects of Natural Products on Laboratory Values online at Davis*Plus*).
- Review the procedure with the patient. Inform the patient that specimen collection takes approximately 5 to 10 min. Address concerns about pain and explain that there may be some discomfort during the venipuncture.
- ***Sensitivity to social and cultural issues,*** as well as concern for modesty, is important in providing psychological support before, during, and after the procedure.
- Note that there are no food, fluid, or medication restrictions unless by medical direction.

INTRATEST:

Potential Complications: N/A

- Avoid the use of equipment containing latex if the patient has a history of allergic reaction to latex.
- Instruct the patient to cooperate fully and to follow directions. Direct the patient to breathe normally and to avoid unnecessary movement.
- Observe standard precautions, and follow the general guidelines in Patient Preparation and Specimen Collection online at Davis*Plus*. Positively identify the patient, and label the appropriate specimen container with the corresponding patient demographics, initials of the person collecting the specimen, date, and time of collection. Perform a venipuncture.
- Remove the needle and apply direct pressure with dry gauze to stop bleeding. Observe/assess venipuncture site for bleeding or hematoma formation and secure gauze with adhesive bandage.
- Promptly transport the specimen to the laboratory for processing and analysis.

POST-TEST:

- Inform the patient that a report of the results will be made available to the requesting health-care provider (HCP), who will discuss the results with the patient.
- ***Nutritional Considerations:*** Educate the patient with vitamin D deficiency, as appropriate, that foods high in calcium and vitamin D should be included in the diet. Explain that vitamin D is also synthesized by the body, in the skin, and is activated by sunlight. Examples of foods rich in calcium and vitamin D are yogurt, cheese, cottage cheese, canned sardines with bones, flounder, salmon, dried figs, and dark green leafy vegetables such as spinach and

V

broccoli. Processed foods with added calcium, such as breads and cereals, can also be included. Avoiding red meat and high-fat foods that bind calcium in the intestine can reduce loss. The excess use of alcohol, salt, or caffeine can also decrease absorption. Explain to the patient that vitamin D is also synthesized by the body, in the skin, and is activated by sunlight. Daily recommendations for calcium and vitamin D intake are based on age. Calcium and vitamin D supplements may be used if dietary intake is insufficient. Provide contact information, if desired, for the Institute of Medicine of the National Academies (www.iom.edu) and USDA's resource for nutrition (www.choosemyplate.gov) 🍁

- Depending on the results of this procedure, additional testing may be performed to evaluate or monitor progression of the disease process and determine the need for a change in therapy. Evaluate test results in relation to the patient's symptoms and other tests performed.

Patient Education:

- Reinforce information given by the patient's HCP regarding further testing, treatment, or referral to another HCP.
- Recognize anxiety related to test results and answer any questions or address any concerns voiced by the patient or family.
- Educate the patient regarding access to nutritional counseling services.
- Provide contact information, if desired, for the National Osteoporosis Foundation (www.nof.org), National Institutes of Health (www.nih.org), and Centers for Disease Control and Prevention (www.cdc.gov). 🍁
- Use plain, culturally appropriate and age-appropriate language in providing education to the patient and family.
- Provide written material that is appropriate to the patient's language and literacy level.

Expected Patient Outcomes:

Understanding

- The patient and family discuss the importance of altering the diet to contain vitamin D–rich foods.
- The patient and family state that adherence to a recommended vitamin D intake can preserve bone integrity.

Ability

- The patient and family design a strategy to ensure the daily minimal sun exposure for vitamin D.
- The patient demonstrates proficiency in taking vitamin D supplements as recommended.

Response

- The patient follows the recommendation to take positive measures to improve health.
- The patient responds to the need to protect independent function related to lost bone mass by adhering to recommended vitamin D intake.

RELATED STUDIES:

- Related tests include amylase, ANCA, biopsy intestinal, calcium, capsule endoscopy, colonoscopy, fecal analysis, fecal fat, antibodies gliadin antibodies, kidney stone panel, laparoscopy abdominal, lipase, osteocalcin, oxalate, phosphorus, and proctosigmoidoscopy.
- Refer to the Gastrointestinal and Musculoskeletal systems tables online at Davis*Plus* for related tests by body system.

Vitamin E

SYNONYM/ACRONYM: Alpha-tocopherol.

COMMON USE: To assess vitamin E levels to assist in diagnosing vitamin toxicity, malabsorption, neuromuscular disorders, and vitamin deficiency.

V

SPECIMEN: Serum collected in a gold-, red-, or red/gray-top tube.

NORMAL FINDINGS: (Method: High-performance liquid chromatography)

Age	Conventional Units	SI Units (Conventional Units × 2.322)
Newborn	1–3.5 mg/L	2.3–8.1 micromol/L
Neonate	2.5–3.7 mg/L	5.8–8.6 micromol/L
2–5 mo	2–6 mg/L	4.6–13.9 micromol/L
6–12 mo	3.5–8 mg/L	8.1–18.6 micromol/L
1–6 yr	3–9 mg/L	7–20.9 micromol/L
7–12 yr	4–9 mg/L	9.3–20.9 micromol/L
13–19 yr	6–10 mg/L	13.9–23.2 micromol/L
Adult	5–18 mg/L	11.6–41.8 micromol/L

Values tend to decrease in older adults.

POTENTIAL MEDICAL DIAGNOSIS

Increased in:

- Obstructive liver disease ***(related to malabsorption associated with obstructive liver disease)***
- Vitamin E intoxication ***(related to excessive intake)***

Decreased in:

- Abetalipoproteinemia ***(rare inherited disorder of fat metabolism evidenced by poor absorption of fat and fat-soluble vitamin E)***
- Hemolytic anemia ***(related to deficiency of vitamin E, an important antioxidant that protects RBC membranes from weakening)***
- Malabsorption disorders, such as biliary atresia, cirrhosis, cystic fibrosis, chronic pancreatitis, pancreatic carcinoma, and chronic cholestasis

CRITICAL FINDINGS:

Note and immediately report to the requesting health-care provider (HCP) any critical findings and related symptoms. A listing of these findings varies among facilities. Timely notification of a critical finding for laboratory or diagnostic studies is a role expectation of the professional nurse. The notification processes vary among facilities. Upon receipt of the critical finding, the information should be read back to the caller to verify accuracy.

Vitamin toxicity can be as significant as problems brought about by vitamin deficiencies. The potential for toxicity is especially important to consider with respect to fat-soluble vitamins, which are not eliminated from the body as quickly as water-soluble vitamins and can accumulate in the body. Most cases of toxicity are brought about by oversupplementing and can be avoided by consulting a qualified nutritionist for recommended daily dietary and supplemental allowances. *Note:* Excessive supplementation of vitamin E (greater than 60 times the recommended dietary allowance over a period of 1 yr or longer) can result in excessive bleeding, delayed healing of wounds, and depression.

Find and print out the full study on Fast Find at davispl.us/vanleeuwen7.

Vitamin K

SYNONYM/ACRONYM: Phylloquinone, phytonadione.

COMMON USE: Assessment of vitamin K levels to assist in diagnosing bleeding disorders where etiology is unknown, identify vitamin toxicity, and evaluate symptoms related to chronic antibiotic use.

SPECIMEN: Serum collected in a red-top tube.

NORMAL FINDINGS: (Method: High-performance liquid chromatography)

Conventional Units	SI Units (Conventional Units × 2.22)
0.13–1.19 ng/mL	0.29–2.64 nmol/L

POTENTIAL MEDICAL DIAGNOSIS

Increased in:

- Excessive administration of vitamin K

Decreased in:

- Antibiotic therapy ***(related to decreased intestinal flora)***
- Chronic fat malabsorption ***(related to lack of digestive enzymes and poor absorption)***
- Cystic fibrosis ***(related to lack of digestive enzymes and poor absorption)***
- Diarrhea (in infants) ***(related to increased loss in feces)***
- Gastrointestinal disease ***(related to malabsorption)***
- Hemorrhagic disease of the newborn ***(newborns normally have low levels of vitamin K; neonates at risk are those who are not given a prophylactic vitamin K shot at birth or those receiving nutrition strictly from breast milk, which has less vitamin K than cow's milk)***
- Hypoprothrombinemia ***(related to insufficient levels of prothrombin, a vitamin K–dependent protein)***
- Liver disease ***(interferes with storage of vitamin K)***
- Obstructive jaundice ***(related to insufficient levels of bile salts required for absorption of vitamin K)***
- Pancreatic disease ***(related to insufficient levels of enzymes to metabolize vitamin K)***

CRITICAL FINDINGS:

Note and immediately report to the requesting health-care provider (HCP) any critical findings and related symptoms. A listing of these findings varies among facilities. Timely notification of a critical finding for laboratory or diagnostic studies is a role expectation of the professional nurse. The notification processes vary among facilities. Upon receipt of the critical finding, the information should be read back to the caller to verify accuracy.

Vitamin toxicity can be as significant as problems brought about by vitamin deficiencies. The potential for toxicity is especially important to consider with respect to fat-soluble vitamins, which are not eliminated from the body as quickly as water-soluble vitamins and can accumulate in the body. The naturally occurring forms, vitamins K_1 and K_2, do not cause toxicity. Signs and symptoms of vitamin K_3 toxicity include bleeding and jaundice. Possible interventions include withholding the source.

Find and print out the full study on Fast Find at davispl.us/vanleeuwen7.

Vitamins A, B_1, B_6, and C

SYNONYM/ACRONYM: Vitamin A: retinol, carotene; vitamin B_1: thiamine; vitamin B_6: pyroxidine, P-5′-P, pyridoxyl-5-phosphate; vitamin C: ascorbic acid.

COMMON USE: To assess vitamin deficiency or toxicity to assist in diagnosing nutritional disorders such as malabsorption; disorders that affect vision, skin, and bones; and other diseases.

SPECIMEN: Serum collected in a red-top tube each for vitamins A and C; plasma collected in a lavender-top (EDTA) tube each for vitamins B_1 and B_6.

NORMAL FINDINGS: (Method: High-performance liquid chromatography)

Vitamin	Age	Conventional Units	SI Units
Vitamin A			***(Conventional Units × 0.0349)***
	Birth–1 yr	14–52 mcg/dL	0.49–1.81 micromol/L
	1–6 yr	20–43 mcg/dL	0.7–1.5 micromol/L
	7–12 yr	26–49 mcg/dL	0.91–1.71 micromol/L
	13–19 yr	26–72 mcg/dL	0.91–2.51 micromol/L
	Adult	30–120 mcg/dL	1.05–4.19 micromol/L
Vitamin B_1			***(Conventional Units × 29.6)***
Serum or plasma		0.21–1 mcg/dL	6.2–30 nmol/L
Whole blood		2.5–7.5 mcg/dL	74–222 nmol/L
Vitamin B_6			***(Conversion Factor × 4.046)***
		5–30 ng/mL	20–121 nmol/L
Vitamin C			***(Conventional Units × 56.78)***
		0.6–1.9 mg/dL	34.1–107.9 micromol/L

Vitamin B_1, vitamin B_6, and vitamin C levels tend to decrease in older adults.

POTENTIAL MEDICAL DIAGNOSIS

Increased in:

- Vitamin A:
  Chronic kidney disease
  Idiopathic hypercalcemia in infants
  Vitamin A toxicity

Decreased in:

- Vitamin A:
  Abetalipoproteinemia ***(related to poor absorption)***
  Carcinoid syndrome ***(related to poor absorption)***

Chronic infections ***(vitamin A deficiency decreases ability to fight infection)***
Cystic fibrosis ***(related to poor absorption)***
Disseminated tuberculosis ***(related to poor absorption)***
Hypothyroidism ***(condition decreases ability of beta carotene to convert to vitamin A)***
Infantile blindness ***(related to dietary deficiency)***
Liver, gastrointestinal, or pancreatic disease ***(related to malabsorption or poor absorption)***
Night blindness ***(related to chronic dietary deficiency or lack of absorption)***
Protein malnutrition ***(related to dietary deficiency)***
Sterility and teratogenesis ***(related to dietary deficiency)***
Zinc deficiency ***(zinc is required for generation of vitamin A transport proteins)***

- Vitamin B_1:

Alcoholism ***(related to dietary deficiency)***
Carcinoid syndrome ***(related to dietary deficiency or lack of absorption)***
Hartnup's disease ***(related to dietary deficiency)***
Pellagra ***(related to dietary deficiency)***

- Vitamin B_6 ***(this vitamin is involved in many essential functions, such as nucleic acid synthesis, enzyme activation, antibody production, electrolyte balance, and RBC formation; deficiencies result in a variety of conditions):***

Alcoholism ***(related to dietary deficiency)***
Asthma
Carpal tunnel syndrome
Gestational diabetes
Kidney dialysis
Lactation ***(related to dietary deficiency and/or increased demand)***
Malabsorption
Malnutrition
Neonatal seizures
Normal pregnancies ***(related to dietary deficiency and/or increased demand)***
Occupational exposure to hydrazine compounds ***(enzymatic pathways are altered by hydralazines in a manner that increases excretion of vitamin B_6)***
Pellagra ***(related to dietary deficiency)***
Pre-eclamptic edema
Uremia

- Vitamin C:

Alcoholism ***(related to dietary deficiency)***
Anemia ***(related to dietary deficiency)***
Cancer ***(related to dietary deficiency or lack of absorption)***
Hemodialysis ***(vitamin C is lost during the treatment)***
Hyperthyroidism ***(related to dietary deficiency and/or increased demand)***
Kidney dialysis ***(vitamin C is lost during the treatment)***
Malabsorption
Pregnancy ***(related to dietary deficiency and/or increased demand)***
Rheumatoid disease
Scurvy ***(related to dietary deficiency or lack of absorption)***

CRITICAL FINDINGS:

Note and immediately report to the requesting health-care provider (HCP) any critical findings and related symptoms. A listing of these findings varies among facilities. Timely notification of a critical finding for laboratory or diagnostic studies is a role expectation of the professional nurse. The notification processes vary among facilities. Upon receipt of the critical finding, the information should be read back to the caller to verify accuracy.

Vitamin toxicity can be as significant as problems brought about by vitamin deficiencies. The potential for toxicity is especially important to consider with respect to fat-soluble vitamins (A, D, E, and K), which are not eliminated from the body as quickly as water-soluble vitamins and can accumulate in the body. Most cases of toxicity are brought about by oversupplementing and can be avoided by consulting a qualified nutritionist for recommended daily dietary and supplemental allowances. Signs and symptoms of vitamin A toxicity may include headache, blurred vision, bone pain, joint pain, dry skin, and loss of appetite.

West Nile Virus Testing

W

SYNONYM/ACRONYM: N/A

COMMON USE: To assist in the diagnosis of West Nile virus (WNV) infection.

SPECIMEN: Serum collected in a red-top tube or CSF collected in a sterile plastic container.

NORMAL FINDINGS: (Method: Enzyme immunoassay [EIA] is generally used for clinical specimens, and nucleic acid testing [NAT] is generally used for testing specimens from potential donors of blood products, cellular therapy, or solid organ transplants.) Normal findings for EIA/ELISA (IgG & IgM): no antibody detected; for NAT viral RNA: nonreactive.

DESCRIPTION: The WNV, a single-stranded RNA virus, is classified as a flavivirus. Prior to 1999, the virus was primarily found in Africa; since then, it is found worldwide throughout Australia, North America, Europe, the Middle East, South America, and West Asia. WNV is one of three types of arbovirus capable of transmitting encephalitis and other febrile type diseases in North America via an arthropod vector: *Togaviridae, Flaviviridae,* and *Bunyaviridae*. The primary mode of this arboviral transmission to humans is mosquito bite. Many mosquito species (notably Culex) can serve as the disease vector; birds serve as the reservoir hosts (mainly crows, sparrows, and blue jays). WNV is not transmitted directly from human to human, by handling infected birds (dead or alive), from exposure to an infected equine, or by eating meat from infected birds or animals. Horses and humans are classified as "dead" hosts because, when infected, they do not produce a sufficient viral load to transmit virus when bitten by an uninfected mosquito vector. WNV can cause severe illness or death in horses; a vaccine has been developed for horses. There are rare reports of transmission by an infected person via blood product, tissue, or solid organ transplant; for that reason, all human products are tested for WNV prior to transfusion or transplantation. Although the majority of babies born to infected mothers do not contract the disease or suffer any associated congenital abnormalities, there are rare cases of known transmission from mother to baby during pregnancy and breast feeding.

The incubation period for WNV disease is from 2 to 14 days but can extend beyond that range in immunocompromised patients. About 80% of WNV infections are subclinical or asymptomatic, but of those who develop symptoms, the onset is described as an acute systemic febrile illness that can rapidly escalate into life-threatening sequelae that could include viral meningitis, an acute flaccid paralysis that is indistinguishable from poliovirus-associated poliomyelitis, or a severe encephalitis. Conditions that present like radiculopathy and Guillain-Barré syndrome have also been associated with WNV infection and can be distinguished from WNV acute flaccid paralysis by clinical signs and symptoms and electrophysiologic studies. However, in most cases, the symptoms are non–life threatening and nonspecific: headache, lethargy, weakness, aching muscles and bones, gastrointestinal discomfort, and/or skin rash. Symptoms may last for a period of days or persist for weeks or months. Therapy is supportive, and there is no commercially available human vaccine at this time. WNV infection is a significant infectious disease, and the first human clinical trial for a vaccine, sponsored by the National Institutes of Health, was initiated in 2015 at Duke University.

Assays for immunoglobulin G [IgG] and immunoglobulin M [IgM] antibodies to WNV assist in differentiating recent infection from prior exposure in the general population. Cerebrospinal fluid (CSF) specimens are used to document central nervous system (CNS) infection by WNV. WNV IgM antibodies appear the earliest and are soon followed by development of IgG antibodies. Presence of antibodies is detectable within 3 to 10 days after reported onset of symptoms and remain in circulation for approximately 30 to 90 days. If results from the IgM-specific or from both assays are positive, recent infection is suspected. Absence of detectable antibody within 10 days of onset does not rule out infection, and testing should be repeated within a short period of time. If the IgM-specific test results are negative and the IgG-specific antibody test results are positive, past infection is indicated. WNV testing is not widely available in routine clinical laboratories. Testing may be sent to a referral laboratory for enzyme immunoassay (EIA) and enzyme-linked immunosorbent assay (ELISA) or to a public health testing facility for a more specific and quantitative confirmatory analysis known as *plaque reduction neutralization testing* (PRNT), depending on the situation. Aliquots of all specimens should be sequestered for a specified period of time after collection; protocols vary by facility. Positive results obtained by EIA/ELISA testing should be confirmed by neutralizing antibody testing on both acute and convalescent serum specimens that have been collected 2 to 3 weeks apart. PRNTs can also confirm acute infection by demonstrating a fourfold or greater increase in PRNT antibody titer between acute and convalescent serum samples. Other testing methods for WNV disease include viral cultures on blood or body fluid (to detect viral RNA [ribonucleic acid]), immunohistochemistry using formalin-fixed tissue (to detect viral antigen), and reverse transcriptase polymerase chain reaction on serum, CSF, and tissue specimens (to detect viral RNA).

This procedure is contraindicated for: N/A

INDICATIONS

- Assist in the diagnosis of WNV.
- Assist in the differential diagnosis of other arboviral causes of encephalitis (e.g., Eastern equine, La Crosse, Powassan, St. Louis encephalitis, and Western equine).

POTENTIAL MEDICAL DIAGNOSIS

Positive findings in

- WNV infection

W

CRITICAL FINDINGS: N/A

INTERFERING FACTORS

False-positive results may be obtained in the presence of cross-reacting antibodies produced by other members of the Flaviviridae family, such as the St. Louis encephalitis virus.

NURSING IMPLICATIONS AND PROCEDURE

PRETEST:

- Positively identify the patient using at least two person-specific identifiers before services, treatments, or procedures are performed.
- ***Patient Teaching:*** Inform the patient this test can indicate the presence of WNV infection.
- Obtain a history of the patient's health concerns, symptoms, surgical procedures, and results of previously performed laboratory and diagnostic studies. Include a list of known allergens, especially allergies or sensitivities to latex.
- Obtain a list of the patient's current medications, including over-the-counter medications and dietary supplements (see Effects of Natural Products on Laboratory Values online at Davis*Plus*).
- Review the procedure with the patient. Inform the patient that several tests may be necessary to confirm diagnosis. Any individual positive result should be repeated in 10 to 14 days. Inform the patient that specimen collection by venipuncture takes approximately 5 to 10 min. CSF specimens are collected by lumbar puncture, as described in the cerebrospinal fluid analysis study. Address concerns about pain, and explain that there may be some discomfort during specimen collection.
- ***Sensitivity to social and cultural issues,*** as well as concern for modesty, is important in providing psychological support before, during, and after the procedure.
- Note that there are no food, fluid, or medication restrictions unless by medical direction.

INTRATEST:

Potential Complications: N/A

- Avoid the use of equipment containing latex if the patient has a history of allergic reaction to latex.
- Instruct the patient to cooperate fully and to follow directions. Direct the patient to breathe normally and to avoid unnecessary movement.
- Observe standard precautions, and follow the general guidelines in Patient Preparation and Specimen Collection online at Davis*Plus*. Positively identify the patient, and label the appropriate specimen container with the corresponding patient demographics, initials of the person collecting the specimen, date, and time of collection. Perform a venipuncture.
- Remove the needle, and apply direct pressure with dry gauze to stop bleeding. Observe/assess puncture site for bleeding or hematoma formation, and secure gauze with adhesive bandage.
- Promptly transport the specimen to the laboratory for processing and analysis. Include specimen type and site, as appropriate. Include information pertaining to onset of symptoms.

POST-TEST:

- Inform the patient that a report of the results will be made available to the requesting health-care provider (HCP), who will discuss the results with the patient.
- Inform the patient that positive findings must be reported to local health department officials. 🍁
- Recognize anxiety related to test results, and provide emotional support if results are positive. If the patient is pregnant, explain that risk of transmission from mother to fetus is believed to be very low. However, it is believed that transmission may be passed to the baby through breast milk. All patients and breastfeeding mothers should be advised to take

precautions against exposure to mosquito bites by wearing protective clothing and insect repellent, especially during peak times of insect activity (at dawn and dusk, July through October). 🍁 Effective repellents include those containing diethyltoluamide (DEET), picaridin, and lemon eucalyptus oil. 🍁 Prevention strategies also include the elimination of mosquito breeding grounds, as can be found in sources of standing water (drinking stations for pets, flower pots, bird baths, water barrels, children's wading pools or gym sets, etc.). Provide teaching and information regarding the clinical implications of the test results, as appropriate.

- Reinforce information given by the patient's HCP regarding further testing, treatment, or referral to another HCP. Emphasize the need to return to have a convalescent blood sample taken in 7 to 14 days. Provide contact information, if desired, for the Centers for Disease Control and Prevention (www.cdc.gov/westnile/resources/pdfs/wnvFactsheet_508.pdf and www.cdc.gov/DiseasesConditions/az/w.html). 🍁 Answer any questions or address any concerns voiced by the patient or family.
- Depending on the results of this procedure, additional testing may be performed to evaluate or monitor progression of the disease process and determine the need for a change in therapy. Evaluate test results in relation to the patient's symptoms and other tests performed.

RELATED STUDIES:

- Related tests include cerebrospinal fluid analysis, culture viral, Gram stain, electromyography, electroneurography, and evoked brain potentials.
- Refer to the immune system tables online at Davis*Plus* for related tests by body system.

White Blood Cell Scan

SYNONYM/ACRONYM: Infection scintigraphy, inflammatory scan, labelled autologous leukocytes, labelled leukocyte scan, WBC imaging.

COMMON USE: To assist in identification of abscess, infection, and inflammation of the bone, bowel, wound, and skin.

AREA OF APPLICATION: Whole body.

DESCRIPTION: Because white blood cells (WBCs) naturally accumulate in areas of inflammation, the WBC scan uses radiolabelled WBCs to help determine the site of an acute infection or confirm the presence or absence of infection or inflammation at a suspected site. A gamma camera detects the radiation emitted from the injected radionuclide, and a representative image of the radionuclide distribution is obtained and recorded or stored electronically. Because of its better image resolution and greater specificity for acute infections, the WBC scan has replaced scanning with gallium-67 citrate (Ga-67). Some chronic infections associated with pulmonary disease, however, may be better imaged with Ga-67. The WBC scan is especially helpful in detecting postoperative infection sites and in documenting lack of residual infection after a course of therapy.

W

This procedure is contraindicated for

Patients who are pregnant or suspected of being pregnant, unless the potential benefits of a procedure using radiation far outweigh the risk of radiation exposure to the fetus and mother.

INDICATIONS

- Aid in the diagnosis of infectious or inflammatory diseases.
- Differentiate infectious from noninfectious process.
- Evaluate the effects of treatment.
- Evaluate inflammatory bowel disease (IBD).
- Evaluate patients with fever of unknown origin.
- Evaluate postsurgical sites and wound infections.
- Evaluate suspected infection of an orthopedic prosthesis.
- Evaluate suspected osteomyelitis.

POTENTIAL MEDICAL DIAGNOSIS

Normal findings

- No focal localization of the radionuclide, along with some slight localization of the radionuclide within the reticuloendothelial system (liver, spleen, and bone marrow)

Abnormal findings related to

- Abscess
- Arthritis
- Infection
- Inflammation
- IBD
- Osteomyelitis

CRITICAL FINDINGS: N/A

INTERFERING FACTORS

Factors that may alter the results of the study

- Inability of the patient to cooperate or remain still during the procedure because of age, significant pain, or mental status.
- Retained barium from a previous radiological procedure, which may inhibit visualization of an abdominal lesion.
- Metallic objects (e.g., jewelry, body rings) within the examination field, which may inhibit organ visualization and cause unclear images.
- Other nuclear scans done within 48 hr and Ga-67 scans within 4 wk before the procedure.
- Lesions smaller than 1 to 2 cm, which may not be detectable.
- A distended bladder, which may obscure pelvic detail.

Other considerations

- Improper injection of the radionuclide that allows the tracer to seep deep into the muscle tissue produces erroneous hot spots.
- Patients with a low WBC count may need donor WBCs to complete the radionuclide labelling process; otherwise, Ga-67 scanning should be performed instead.
- False-negative images may be a result of hemodialysis, hyperglycemia, hyperalimentation, steroid therapy, and antibiotic therapy.
- The presence of multiple myeloma or thyroid cancer can result in a false-negative scan for bone abnormalities.

NURSING IMPLICATIONS AND PROCEDURE

PRETEST:

- Positively identify the patient using at least two person-specific identifiers before services, treatments, or procedures are performed.
- *Patient Teaching:* Inform the patient this test can assist in assessing for the presence of infection or inflammation.
- Obtain a history of the patient's health concerns, symptoms, surgical procedures, and results of previously performed laboratory and diagnostic

studies. Include a list of known allergens, especially allergies or sensitivities to latex, anesthetics, sedatives, or radionuclides.

- Note any recent procedures that can interfere with test results, including barium examinations.
- Record the date of the last menstrual period and determine the possibility of pregnancy in perimenopausal women.
- Obtain a list of the patient's current medications, including over-the-counter medications, dietary supplements, anticoagulants, aspirin and other salicylates (see Effects of Natural Products on Laboratory Values online at Davis*Plus*). Such products should be discontinued by medical direction for the appropriate number of days prior to a surgical procedure. Note the last time and dose of medication taken.
- Review the procedure with the patient. Address concerns about pain related to the procedure and explain that some pain may be experienced during the test, and there may be moments of discomfort. Reassure the patient that the radionuclide poses no radioactive hazard and rarely produces adverse effects. Inform the patient that the procedure is performed in a nuclear medicine department by a health-care provider. It usually takes approximately 1 to 6 hr, and delayed images are needed 24 hr later. The patient may leave the department and return later to undergo delayed imaging.
- ***Sensitivity to social and cultural issues,*** as well as concern for modesty, is important in providing psychological support before, during, and after the procedure.
- Explain that an intravenous (IV) line may be inserted to allow infusion of fluids such as saline, anesthetics, sedatives, radionuclides, medications used in the procedure, or emergency medications.
- Instruct the patient to remove jewelry and other metallic objects from the area to be examined.
- Note that there are no dietary or medication restrictions prior to the procedure, unless by medical direction.
- *Make sure a written and informed consent has been signed prior to the procedure and before administering any medications.*

INTRATEST:

Potential Complications:

Although it is rare, there is the possibility of allergic reaction to the radionuclide. Have emergency equipment and medications readily available. If the patient has a history of allergic reactions to any substance or drug, administer ordered prophylactic steroids or antihistamines before the procedure.

Establishing an IV site and injecting radionuclides are invasive procedures. Complications are rare but do include bleeding from the puncture site ***related to a bleeding disorder or the effects of natural products and medications with known anticoagulant, antiplatelet, or thrombolytic properties;*** hematoma ***related to blood leakage into the tissue following needle insertion;*** infection ***that might occur if bacteria from the skin surface is introduced at the puncture site;*** or nerve injury ***that might occur if the needle strikes a nerve.***

- Observe standard precautions, and follow the general guidelines in Patient Preparation and Specimen Collection online at Davis*Plus*. Positively identify the patient.
- Ensure the patient has removed all external metallic objects prior to the procedure.
- Administer ordered prophylactic steroids or antihistamines before the procedure if the patient has a history of allergic reactions to any substance or drug to be used in the procedure.
- Avoid the use of equipment containing latex if the patient has a history of allergic reaction to latex.
- Have emergency equipment readily available.
- Instruct the patient to void prior to the procedure and to change into the

gown, robe, and foot coverings provided.

- Record baseline vital signs, and assess neurological status. Protocols may vary among facilities.
- Establish an IV fluid line for the injection of saline, anesthetics, sedatives, radionuclides, or emergency medications.
- Administer sedative to a child or to an uncooperative adult, as ordered.
- Draw a 50- to 80-mL sample of blood on the day of the test for separating the WBCs from the blood and an in vitro process of labelling with radionuclide.
- IV radionuclide-labelled autologous WBCs are administered.
- Images are recorded 1 to 6 hr postinjection depending on the radionuclide used. Delayed images may be required at 24 hr after the injection.
- Remove the needle or catheter and apply a pressure dressing over the puncture site.
- Observe/assess the needle/catheter insertion site for bleeding, inflammation, or hematoma formation.
- If abdominal abscess or infection is suspected, laxatives or enemas may be ordered before delayed imaging.

POST-TEST:

- Inform the patient that a report of the results will be made available to the requesting HCP, who will discuss the results with the patient.
- Unless contraindicated, advise patient to drink increased amounts of fluids for 24 to 48 hr to eliminate the radionuclide from the body. Inform the patient that radionuclide is eliminated from the body within 6 to 24 hr.
- No other radionuclide tests should be scheduled for 24 to 48 hr after this procedure.
- Observe/assess the needle/catheter insertion site for bleeding, inflammation, or hematoma formation.
- Instruct the patient in the care and assessment of the injection site.
- If a woman who is breastfeeding must have a nuclear scan, she should not breastfeed the infant until the radionuclide has been eliminated. This could take as long as 3 days. She should be instructed to express the milk and discard it during the 3-day period to prevent cessation of milk production.
- Instruct the patient to immediately flush the toilet and to meticulously wash hands with soap and water after each voiding for 24 hr after the procedure.
- Instruct all caregivers to wear gloves when discarding urine for 24 hr after the procedure. Wash gloved hands with soap and water before removing gloves; then wash ungloved hands.
- Recognize anxiety related to test results, and be supportive of perceived loss of independent function. Discuss the implications of abnormal test results on the patient's lifestyle. Provide teaching and information regarding the clinical implications of the test results, as appropriate.
- Reinforce information given by the patient's HCP regarding further testing, treatment, or referral to another HCP. Answer any questions or address any concerns voiced by the patient or family.
- Depending on the results of this procedure, additional testing may be needed to evaluate or monitor progression of the disease process and determine the need for a change in therapy. Evaluate test results in relation to the patient's symptoms and other tests performed.

RELATED STUDIES:

- Related tests include angiography pulmonary, bone scan, colonoscopy, CBC, CBC WBC count and differential, CT abdomen, CT pelvis, CT spine, culture (blood, skin, wound), ESR, fecal analysis, gallium scan, GI blood loss scan, KUB, MRI musculoskeletal, MRI pelvis, MRI spine, proctosigmoidoscopy, radiography bone, US abdomen, US pelvis, and vitamin D.
- Refer to the Immune System table online at Davis*Plus* for related tests by body system.

Zinc

SYNONYM/ACRONYM: Zn.

COMMON USE: To assist in assessing for vitamin deficiency or toxicity, monitor therapeutic interventions, and assist in diagnosing disorders such as acrodermatitis enteropathica.

SPECIMEN: Serum collected in a trace element-free, royal blue-top tube.

NORMAL FINDINGS: (Method: Atomic absorption spectrophotometry)

Age	Conventional Units	SI Units (Conventional Units × 0.153)
Newborn–6 mo	26–141 mcg/dL	4–21.6 micromol/L
6–11 mo	29–131 mcg/dL	4.4–20 micromol/L
1–4 yr	31–115 mcg/dL	4.7–17.6 micromol/L
4–5 yr	48–119 mcg/dL	7.3–18.2 micromol/L
6–9 yr	48–129 mcg/dL	7.3–19.7 micromol/L
10–13 yr	25–148 mcg/dL	3.8–22.6 micromol/L
14–17 yr	46–130 mcg/dL	7–19.9 micromol/L
Adult	70–120 mcg/dL	10.7–18.4 micromol/L

POTENTIAL MEDICAL DIAGNOSIS

Increased in:

Zinc is contained in and secreted by numerous types of cells in the body. Damaged cells release zinc into circulation and increase blood levels.

- Anemia ***(related to competitive relationship with copper; copper deficiency is associated with decreased production of red blood cells)***

Decreased in:

This trace metal is an essential component of enzymes that participate in protein and carbohydrate metabolism. It is involved in DNA replication, insulin storage, carbon dioxide gas exchange, cellular immunity and healing, promotion of body growth, and sexual maturity. Deficiencies result in a variety of conditions.

- Acrodermatitis enteropathica ***(congenital abnormality that affects zinc uptake and results in zinc deficiency)***
- AIDS
- Acute infections
- Acute stress
- Burns
- Cirrhosis
- Conditions that decrease albumin ***(related to lack of available transport proteins)***
- Diabetes
- Long-term total parenteral nutrition
- Malabsorption
- Myocardial infarction
- Nephrotic syndrome
- Nutritional deficiency
- Pregnancy ***(related to increased uptake by fetus; related to excessive levels of iron and folic acid prescribed during pregnancy and which interfere with absorption)***
- Pulmonary tuberculosis

CRITICAL FINDINGS: N/A

Find and print out the full study on Fast Find at davispl.us/vanleeuwen7.

Index

IND

IND

IND

B

IND

IND

IND

E

F

IND

I

IND

J

K

M

IND

IND

O

IND

IND

IND

IND

S

T

IND

U

V

X

IND

Y

Z

BD Vacutainer® Venous Blood Collection
Tube Guide

Tubes with BD Hemogard™ Closure	Tubes with Conventional Stopper	Additive	Inversions at Blood Collection*	Laboratory Use
Gold 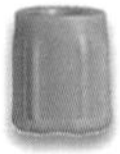	Red/Gray 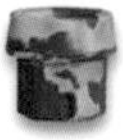	• Clot activator and gel for serum separation	5	For serum determinations in chemistry. May be used for routine blood donor screening and diagnostic testing of serum for infectious disease.** Tube inversions ensure mixing of clot activator with blood. Blood clotting time: 30 minutes.
Light Green 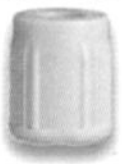	Green/Gray 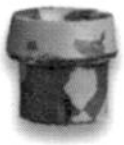	• Lithium heparin and gel for plasma separation	8	For plasma determinations in chemistry. Tube inversions ensure mixing of lot activator with blood. Blood clotting time: 60 minutes.
Red 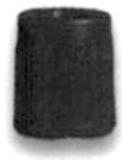	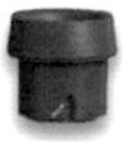	• None (glass) • Clot activator (plastic)	0 5	For serum determinations in chemistry. May be used for routine blood donor screening and diagnostic testing of serum for infectious disease.** Tube inversions ensure mixing of clot activator with blood. Blood clotting time: 60 minutes.
Orange 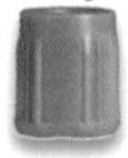		• Thrombin-based clot activator with gel for serum separation	5-6	For stat serum determinations in chemistry. Tube inversions ensure mixing of clot activator with blood. Blood clotting time: 5 minutes.
Orange 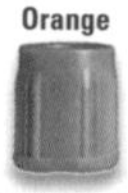		• Thrombin-based clot activator	8	For stat serum determinations in chemistry. Tube inversions ensure mixing of clot activator with blood. Blood clotting time: 5 minutes.
Royal Blue 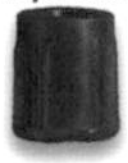		• Clot activator (plastic serum) • K_2EDTA (plastic)	8 8	For trace-element, toxicology, and nutritional chemistry determinations. Special stopper formulation provides low levels of trace elements (see package insert). Tube inversions ensure mixing of either clot activator or anticoagulant (EDTA) with blood.
Green 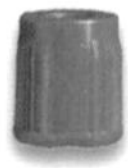	Green 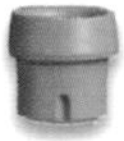	• Sodium heparin • Lithium heparin	8 8	For plasma determinations in chemistry. Tube inversions ensure mixing of anticoagulant (heparin) with blood to prevent clotting.
Gray 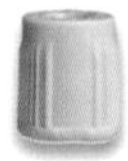	Gray 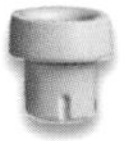	• Potassium oxalate/ sodium fluoride • Sodium fluoride/ Na_2 EDTA • Sodium fluoride (serum tube)	8 8 8	For glucose determinations. Oxalate and EDTA anticoagulants will give plasma samples. Sodium fluoride is the antiglycolytic agent. Tube inversions ensure proper mixing of additive and blood.
Tan 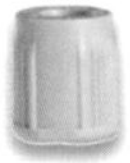		• K_2EDTA (plastic)	8	For lead determinations. This tube is certified to contain less than .01 µg/mL (ppm) lead. Tube inversions prevent clotting.